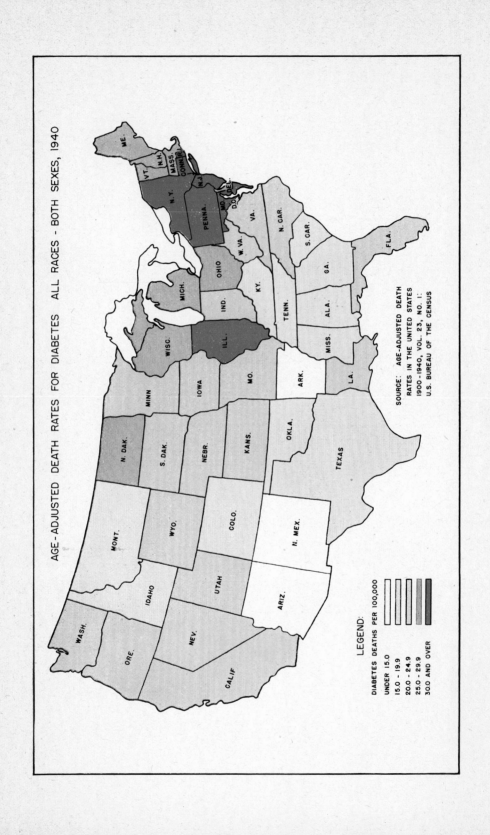

AGE-ADJUSTED DEATH RATES FOR DIABETES ALL RACES - BOTH SEXES, 1940

SOURCE: AGE-ADJUSTED DEATH
RATES IN THE UNITED STATES
1900-1940, VOL. 23, NO. 1:
U.S. BUREAU OF THE CENSUS

LEGEND:

DIABETES DEATHS PER 100,000

UNDER 15.0

15.0 - 19.9

20.0 - 24.9

25.0 - 29.9

30.0 AND OVER

ME.

VT.
N.H.
MASS.
CONN.
R.I.

N.Y.
N.J.
PENNA.
MD.
DEL.
D.C.
VA.
W.VA.
N. CAR.
S. CAR.
FLA.

OHIO
KY.
TENN.
GA.
ALA.
MISS.
MICH.
IND.
WISC.
ILL.
MO.
ARK.
LA.

MINN
IOWA
NEBR.
KANS.
OKLA.
TEXAS

N. DAK.
S. DAK.

MONT.
WYO.
COLO.
N. MEX.

IDAHO
UTAH
ARIZ.

WASH.
ORE.
NEV.
CALIF

THE TREATMENT OF DIABETES MELLITUS

BY

ELLIOTT P. JOSLIN, A.M., M.D., Sc.D.

*Medical Director, George F. Baker Clinic, New England Deaconess Hospital;
Clinical Professor of Medicine Emeritus, Harvard Medical School; Consulting
Physician, Boston City Hospital*

HOWARD F. ROOT, M.D.

*Physician-in-Chief, New England Deaconess Hospital; Consultant in Medicine,
Eastern Maine General Hospital; Massachusetts State Infirmary, Tewksbury, Mid-
dlesex County Sanatorium; Associate in Medicine, Harvard Medical School*

PRISCILLA WHITE, M.D.

*Physician, New England Deaconess Hospital; Instructor in Pediatrics, Tufts Col-
lege Medical School*

ALEXANDER MARBLE, A.M., M.D.

*Physician, New England Deaconess Hospital; Instructor in Medicine, Harvard
Medical School; Colonel, Medical Reserve Corps, U. S. Army; Chief, Section of
General Medicine, Branch No. 1 (New England), Veterans Administration*

C. CABELL BAILEY, M.D.

*Physician, New England Deaconess Hospital; Research Fellow in Medicine, Harvard
Medical School*

EIGHTH EDITION, THOROUGHLY REVISED, ILLUSTRATED

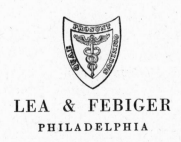

LEA & FEBIGER

PHILADELPHIA

To

BANTING AND BEST

DISCOVERERS OF INSULIN

ON THE

TWENTY-FIFTH ANNIVERSARY

OF THEIR

GIFT TO THE WORLD

PREFACE TO THE EIGHTH EDITION.

THIS book records the facts which have helped my associates and me treat 29,000 diabetics and glycosurics over a period of forty-eight years. It includes (1) the simple methods employed with office cases suitable for adoption by the general practitioner, (2) the plan used for the treatment of the growing number of ambulatory cases living in a nursing diabetic home which any doctor could create, and (3) the experience gained from patients, usually with complications and often with emergencies, intrusted to us by their physicians for investigation and care in a hospital.

From the very beginning of work with diabetic patients in 1898, the underlying purpose has been to be broad-minded. This was difficult in the days of undernutrition, but since the advent of insulin the field has steadily widened. Insulin has allowed surgery on a large scale and in all the specialties, and this has been augmented by the sulfonamides and penicillin. Insulin is keeping alive 1774 of the 2191 diabetic children we have seen, making the treatment of children and adolescents a compelling feature in the hospital and home and for many boys and girls in diabetic camps and boarding schools. Of course they fall in love and marry, and for the last decade obstetrics has thrust itself upon us so that 272 pregnant diabetics have been treated by Dr. Priscilla White and delivered by Dr. Raymond S. Titus. The aging of the patients from an average of forty-four to sixty-four years at death has brought of itself a multitude of complications in the cardiovascular-renal and nervous systems. All of these varied activities have entailed close coöperation with consultants in all specialties whose skill and advice become articulate in these pages.

It is easily seen that this expansion has necessitated too much detailed knowledge for one doctor, and the senior author is fortunate to have had join him in his work and in the publication of this volume, associates who have stamped their identity upon diabetic progress in this country, Dr. Howard F. Root, Dr. Priscilla White, Dr. Alexander Marble and Dr. C. Cabell Bailey. For a decade, except for his absence as a Major in the Army, my son, Dr. Allen P. Joslin, has borne much of the burden and heat of the day's work in office and hospital. I cannot overestimate the stimulus we have all received from the group of graduate physicians who have held Fellowships in our Clinic or have come to the Clinic for instruction and who have helped us in compiling material for a former or the present edition.

Statistics, physiology and pathology claim detailed attention.

One million diabetics in this country make diabetes a social problem which the laity, the medical profession and the government should face. Proof of the value of private statistics is afforded this year by the entrance of insurance companies into the field of the insurance of diabetics. In the compilation of our statistics we have received the help of the Metropolitan Life Insurance Company through its Vice-President and Statistician, Dr. Louis I. Dublin, and especially Mr. Herbert H. Marks, the Massachusetts State Department of Health through Dr. Herbert L. Lombard, and the aid of officials of the U. S. Bureau of the Census, Dr. Halbert L. Dunn and Mr. Frank S. Morrison, and others with a "passion for anonymity."

Progress in diabetes has always started in the laboratory. Who ever thought a chemical could cause the disease? Lasting credit should be given to the late Professor John Shaw Dunn of Glasgow and his associates for their discovery of the effect of alloxan. The prosecution of research along this line by Dr. C. Cabell Bailey and Mrs. Rachel Leech of our staff has been watched by us with intense interest.

The follow-up of our 8385 fatal cases is fundamental, because this discloses what the enemy is and where the fight is fiercest. This is the reason for Tables 26, 39, 40 and 41. We consider that they portray the justification of therapeutic methods which we consider are orthodox.

The periods during which we have treated diabetics have been named successively by us the Naunyn, Allen, Banting and Hagedorn Eras. The present is preëminently the era of investigation. It includes the twenty-fifth anniversary of the discovery of insulin. Therefore, we judge it appropriate to assign to this period the name of the co-discoverer of insulin, Charles H. Best, because he has exemplified for twenty-five years as medical student and professor the value of research.

Josiah Royce believed in the "fecundity of the aggregation" and I know this volume illustrates his concept. It represents the efforts and contributions of patients and doctors, of many, many clinicians throughout the world, of collaborators whose names unfortunately may not always appear in the text, and the painstaking efforts of our cheerful and untiring secretary, Frances Tilton, and her associates. More than ever do we wish to express our gratitude to our publishers, Messrs. Lea & Febiger, for their forbearance, counsel and aid.

E. P. J.

Boston, Massachusetts.

CONTENTS.

CHAPTER I.

CHAPTER VII.

THE EXAMINATION OF THE URINE AND THE BLOOD IN DIABETES.
Revised by ALEXANDER MARBLE, M.D.

CHAPTER VIII.

THE DIET IN HEALTH AND DIABETES.

CHAPTER IX.

THE DEFINITION, DIAGNOSIS, CLASSIFICATION, SYMPTOMATOLOGY AND PROGNOSIS OF DIABETES.

CHAPTER X.

THE TREATMENT OF DIABETES.

CHAPTER XI.

HYPOGLYCEMIA DUE TO INSULIN.
Revised by ALEXANDER MARBLE, M.D., and PRISCILLA WHITE, M.D.

CHAPTER XII.

HYPERINSULINISM.
By ALEXANDER MARBLE, M.D.

CHAPTER XIII.

DIABETIC COMA.

Revised by HOWARD F. ROOT, M.D., and ALEXANDER MARBLE, M.D.

CHAPTER XIV.

ALLERGY AND DIABETES.

Revised by C. CABELL BAILEY, M.D.

CHAPTER XV.

CARDIO-RENAL-VASCULAR DISEASE.

Revised by HOWARD F. ROOT, M.D.

CHAPTER XVI.

INFECTIONS IN DIABETES.

Revised by ALEXANDER MARBLE, M.D.

CHAPTER XVII.

THE DIGESTIVE SYSTEM IN DIABETES.

Revised by C. CABELL BAILEY, M.D.

CHAPTER XVIII.

The Nervous System and Diabetes.

Revised by C. Cabell Bailey, M.D., and Jean Murray, M.D.

CHAPTER XIX.

The Genito-urinary System in Diabetes.

Revised by Charles W. Styron, M.D.

CHAPTER XX.

Disorders of the Skin in Diabetes.

Revised by Priscilla White, M.D.

CHAPTER XXI.

Blood Complications in Diabetes.

Revised by Howard F. Root, M.D., and Eleanor A. Waskow, M.D.

CHAPTER XXII.

The Special Senses in Diabetes.

Revised by Howard F. Root, M.D.

CHAPTER XXIII.

TUBERCULOSIS.

Revised by HOWARD F. ROOT, M.D.

CHAPTER XXIV.

CANCER COMPLICATING DIABETES.

By ALEXANDER MARBLE, M.D.

CHAPTER XXV.

SYPHILIS AND DIABETES.

Revised by C. CABELL BAILEY, M.D.

CHAPTER XXVI.

SURGERY AND DIABETES.

Revised by HOWARD F. ROOT, M.D.

CHAPTER XXVII.

Clinical Disorders of the Glands of Internal Secretion Complicating Diabetes.

Revised by Howard F. Root, M.D., and Priscilla White, M.D.

CHAPTER XXVIII.

Diabetes in Childhood.

By Priscilla White, M.D.

CHAPTER XXIX.

Pregnancy Complicating Diabetes.

By Priscilla White, M.D.

CHAPTER XXX.

Non-diabetic Glycosuria.

By Alexander Marble, M.D.

CHAPTER XXXI.

Foods and Their Composition

Treatment of Diabetes Mellitus.

CHAPTER I.

PRESENT CONCEPTIONS OF DIABETES.

THE magnitude of the diabetic problem becomes more and more apparent. In my opinion, there are 1,000,000 diabetics in the United States today. The increase has been at the rate of about 50,000 new cases yearly since the last edition of this monograph. The number continues to grow, first, because more and more of the population are living into the sixth decade in which the onset of diabetes is most common; second, the duration of the life of a diabetic is three to four times as long as heretofore; third, doctors are more alert in discovering cases; fourth, people generally are more conscious medically and report their symptoms; and, fifth, the census continues to show more inhabitants, in 1940, 131,669,275 and in 1945 reported to be 139,682,000, a rise of more than 8,000,000 in the last five years or twice the increase in the preceding ten years.

Consider the repercussions from this growing army of diabetics upon physicians, patients and government! The medical profession will have many more patients to treat and each case for a longer period. Measles and mumps are soon over and there is only one appendix, but diabetes on the average will soon last for twenty years, while the life expectancy of a carefully treated diabetic child at ten years of age approaches forty years. Expansion of facilities for treatment, both in the doctors' offices, in nursing homes, and in hospitals, must follow. Since single tests of sugar in the blood and urine are relatively expensive and a knowledge of them is essential both for treatment and diagnosis, simpler methods already are being devised and coöperative laboratories must spring up in order to reap the economy of wholesale tests, and because for many a patient reports from the laboratory are life-saving.

Recognition of the changed status and growing importance of diabetes is attested by the entrance of insurance companies into the diabetic field, first in Canada and now in the United States. This is the answer to critics of our methods of treatment and emphasizes that what we have been doing has been productive. To the patients themselves the possibility of obtaining insurance will be an enormous stimulus to adherence to treatment. Moreover, it will encourage insurance companies to increase their own educational programs for the early detection and better treatment of diabetes, which already have been of such great value. Diabetes publicity is peculiarly their function. They can do what the medical profession could not do without inviting criticism. This year over a hundred insurance companies have combined to expend half a million dollars yearly for research in preventing arteriosclerosis and heart disease, the complications which carry off half of the diabetics and prematurely at that.

Diabetes is not a disease for specialists alone, not a disease solely for out-patient clinics with their medical personnel, not a disease for panel practice, but is *par excellence* a disease for interested family physicians to treat from its onset to its end throughout all the social, as well as physical, vicissitudes of patients' lives.

The diabetic child, onset under fifteen years, after a twenty year duration of his diabetes, is the patient who will blaze the pathway for the treatment of all diabetics in the next few years. He it is who, by his physical condition and ability to support himself, will furnish a standard of the efficacy of the type of treatment he has followed. At present his status leaves much to be desired, partly because he antedates the insulin era or began life when the use of insulin was largely experimental and handicapped by the low carbo-hydrate and undernutrition diets of the preceding epoch. At one time in visiting other clinics I always asked to see a six-year dura-tion diabetic; now I am eager to examine the eyes of a twenty-year diabetic child and to learn the condition of his arteries, his kidneys and heart.

For the younger diabetic patients, as I envisage it, the crux of the problem will be not how to secure treatment or how to get a job, but rather how to live so as to avoid complications fifteen or more years after the onset of the disease. And it is to present the facts about the disease and to portray the methods adopted by those diabetics who have lived most successfully and the pitfalls which the others have encountered that this monograph has been rewritten. Physical examinations, it is true, bar the way to certain occupations, but with the result that to a large degree the diabetic is forced to create his own job and to be individualistic and re-sourceful. Brains can or ought always to be utilized, and wherever there are jobs requiring brains there is a job for the diabetic. What kind of job? Experience has shown that the diabetic who uses his muscles does best and thus occupations requiring physical labor or those allowing time for exercise, going back and forth to work, are just the ones the diabetic needs. This is particularly true if the journey permits exposure to fresh air and sunshine and thus builds up resistance to infections and avoids contacts with tuberculosis, which remains still a real diabetic enemy. Diabetics need not worry unduly about the occupations from which they are or will be dis-barred. That problem will solve itself if each diabetic, particularly each child diabetic because he is destined to live the longest, is taught how to care for himself and to feel and take responsibility.

Naunyn believed that the diabetic who was treated aggressively was the one who in the long run did the best; conversely, and our own observations confirm it, he believed that the diabetic child or adult whose disease is uncontrolled is the one most susceptible to complications. In the child these include those serious conditions which may develop in after years in the kidneys and eyes.

For the government the extent of the diabetic situation is serious. It soon will be faced with the adaptation to the ways of healthy individuals of a million souls ranging from youth to old age, somewhat handicapped, who are living and not dying at the rapid rates common for those with cancer and tuberculosis. Strive the best we can to avert arteriosclerosis in the diabetic, one cannot blind one's eyes to the fact that the number of people above the age of three score years with one leg or none will increase and the ranks of the blind will include a disproportionately large number of diabetics. Already in the state sanatoria for tuberculosis in Massachusetts the diabetics number 2.6 per cent. At a Jewish home for the aged in Boston there are 275 inmates, of whom 15 are known to have diabetes mellitus, and in the tuberculosis section of the Montefiore Hospital in New York City Dr. E. M. Bluestone, Director, writes me that among 232 tuberculous patients the number of diabetics was 33 or 14.2 per cent for the year 1944. Despite the long duration of life of diabetics and their early entrance into the arteriosclerotic zone of life, it would appear that arteriosclerosis in diabetes has not yet reached its peak, because of the growing incidence of this complication in the later years of young diabetics. For older diabetics, however, death should occur as a result of the ills common to the rest of humanity. But there is this bright side to the picture—the diabetic, owing to his close contact with his family doctor, has an advantage over the non-diabetic. My non-diabetic patient in late middle life was most carefully examined in June, but in January returned with a cancer of the rectum. If he had been a diabetic this complication undoubtedly would have been observed during his quarterly routine examination in September when his earliest symptom appeared.

The cost of all this medical care may bring the remedy. The government will insist that the diabetes be prevented. It may not demand that the average individual above forty pay a tax for a pound overweight, as the girls do in some colleges for an extra inch around the waist, but something will be done by the government or insurance companies to make the foolish fat man or woman realize he is a candidate for diabetes. Of all the inciting causes of diabetes, obesity stands foremost. It is like the laws of the Medes and Persians—inexorable, and it holds for the Arizona Indian just as truly as for the Jew and Gentile.

Heredity is Naunyn's red thread which is intertwined in diabetes from youth to old age. It completely overshadows obesity in the first two decades but is ever to be found.   One-fourth of the inhabitants of this country have diabetic relatives and the percentage is so high that it makes one wonder if heredity would not be demonstrable in every case if we knew the facts.   Upon the family physician rest the responsibility and opportunity to attack diabetes from the hereditary angle and to prevent it.   My personal experience is that diabetics are extraordinarily cautious not to marry each other and try to avoid marriage into a heavily predisposed diabetic family.   However, it must be said that even in the most extreme case, of 100 children theoretically born of the marriage of diabetics to each other, only 44 will develop the disease, because the others will die too soon of other causes; and of the 44 there will be only 14 who will develop it under the age of forty years.   For the remaining, on account of improvement in the management of the disease, there will be less and less danger of invalidism and premature death. Shall we forbid marriage to diabetics?   If so, who will be left to halt the falling birth rate if all unsound individuals in the country are forbidden to have children?   There are many individuals one meets on the street who are far less desirable to choose for fathers and mothers than diabetics.

The improvement in control of the disease which protamine zinc insulin allows is extraordinary.   With protamine zinc insulin we know there are less coma, less tuberculosis, fewer insulin reactions, smaller livers, fewer injections, and there is a feeling of confidence on the part of the patient which allows him to live with comfort.   But I think perhaps the greatest benefit, after all, of the Hagedorn Era is that by doubling the duration of effect of regular insulin, which later Scott's addition of zinc quadrupled, protamine zinc insulin enticed thousands of mild diabetics, previously .appalled at the thought of multiple injections, to take one once a day.   By this means perhaps one or two hundred thousand individuals may avoid progression into diabetes of extreme or even moderate severity. Protamine zinc insulin, therefore, not only gives confidence and comfort, but it preserves the capacity for health and work throughout a lifetime.   It certainly was justifiable to name the epoch of its discovery for Hagedorn.

Experiments with other insulins are worth while, but these should be conducted not haphazardly but in clinics where the effect can be studied and compared under controlled conditions with protamine zinc insulin and standard regular or crystalline insulin.   Eventually, all physicians and patients hope for an insulin which will combine more of the good effects of both crystalline and protamine zinc insulin, but one must never expect that any insulin will have brains. Advances in the treatment of diabetes in the future must depend on new discoveries rather than on 5 or 10 per cent improvements in the insulins at present available.   Insulins are so efficacious that they are covering up a multitude of sins—diabetic complications.

By the grace of insulin a diabetic may escape disaster for a limited period of years.

The dietetic treatment of diabetes was not simplified by the discovery of insulin. When our patients were allowed 30 grams of carbohydrate they and we knew whether this was utilized. Now with the increase of carbohydrate to a minimum of 150 grams and in certain cases even to 200 or more grams daily, particularly in children, it makes inferences based upon the intake of carbohydrate less easily drawn, because insulin and exercise enter into the picture. It is easy to teach a patient a diet containing 150 to 200 grams of carbohydrate and to allow him protein and fat consistent with his age, weight and activity, but always today these must be balanced against the effect of insulin and exercise. The development of our knowledge of vitamins and minerals and their places in normal as well as in diabetic diets introduces new elements into the dietetic education of the patient. Whether vitamins are of direct benefit to a diabetic any more than to a non-diabetic, is open to some question, but there is little doubt that they are indirectly of value in the prevention and treatment of complications which may arise in the course of diabetes, especially if the disease is uncontrolled. The exact rôle of vitamins in carbohydrate metabolism still awaits clarification.

Spectacular changes in the causes of death of diabetics, such as have occurred in the last half century, will not continue. There is no cause of death today which, like tuberculosis and diabetic coma, can be lowered from over 50 per cent to 5 and 3 per cent. The predominant cause today is arteriosclerosis and that, of course, is linked with old age. We feared a short time ago that tuberculosis would rob the later lives of our diabetic children, because the relative incidence in them was high, but to our amazement in the last six years we have discovered but three instances of the fresh development of this complication in our patients under the age of twenty years. Of older diabetics with tuberculosis, we know of 58 who were alive in 1944. The incidence of tuberculosis in the total mortality of our own cases has not fallen for years, but this is readily explainable because the period of exposure, *i. e.*, the duration of life with diabetes, has trebled. On the other hand, deaths from cancer comprised 8.9 per cent of all deaths in the most recent era as contrasted with 1.5 in the Naunyn era when diabetics died twenty years younger and lived only one-third as long.

A pregnant diabetic woman was never seen by Bouchardat. Naunyn records but one instance. Later when pregnancy began to occur, the maternal mortality was terrific, but Priscilla White has demonstrated the safety with which diabetics can go through pregnancy, because there has been but 1 maternal death among two hundred and seventy-two of her cases treated since January 1, 1936. The fetal viability up to 1936 in our group in the last five months

2

of pregnancy was 50 per cent, but now has risen to 90 per cent and among those cases controlled for the greater period of pregnancy it has reached 95 per cent.

Infections of the genito-urinary tract are all too frequent in diabetic patients and exemplify the susceptibility of the diabetic to infection, particularly to blood-borne infections of the pyogenic type. We are indebted to Dr. C. W. Styron, our former associate, for a recent analysis of our material. It is evident from his studies that one should pay more attention to the presence of leukocytes in the urinary sediment, particularly in the urine of women, and that each case of this type should be investigated. It is still true that there is serious danger of infection following catheterization in coma or after operations in elderly patients, but fortunately today we have measures available to combat these infections if they occur and should use them.

Since the last edition of this monograph a third type of experimental diabetes, alloxan diabetes, has been added to those produced by pancreatectomy and injections of anterior pituitary extract. At first sight alloxan diabetes appeared quite different from the others, but as more and more studies have been carried out, its pathology and symptomatology approach rather than diverge from the others. The demonstration that diabetes could be caused by pancreatectomy was the impetus to modern research. Its production by injections of anterior pituitary extract was momentous, because so much of the pancreas was left intact and now its final causation by the injection of a chemical, alloxan, with its almost unbelievable specificity for attack upon the Beta cells of the islands of Langerhans is even more striking, because alloxan is so closely akin to uric acid and other substances which are known to exist in the body. We know that the effect of alloxan can be neutralized outside of the body and by the injection of various substances into the body prior to its administration. We know that diabetes can be produced with alloxan suddenly in five minutes or slowly in the course of five weeks. What will be the next step in our knowledge of alloxan? The subject is so new and so important we have set aside a special chapter for its consideration.

Neither von Noorden nor Benedict and I, in our studies at the Nutrition Laboratory, found a 100 per cent diabetic. Shields Warren, who has studied the diabetic pancreas as intensively as anyone, reports that only 74 per cent of glands obtained at autopsy had demonstrable lesions of the islands of Langerhans. It is true that it is often difficult to diagnose diabetes by the examination of the pancreas alone. We must ask pathologists to clarify for us clinicians their views upon the presence of diabetic lesions in the pancreas as compared with evidence of diabetes in the kidney and liver. To restore the functional activity of the remaining intact

β cells of the pancreas, which exist in all diabetics, should be the purpose of therapeutic endeavor.

The education of the diabetic is fundamental. It is so important that it is revolutionizing our approach to the treatment of diabetes. It holds both for the ambulatory and the seriously ill diabetic with complications. The latter group now constitutes the larger portion of hospital admissions due to the shortage of hospital beds, but it is increasingly evident that we must provide a certain section or unit in hospitals for the ambulatory or convalescent type of diabetic who requires less nursing and medical care, a shorter hospital stay but concentrated education. Education may protect this ambulatory type of diabetic from entering the stage of the seriously ill hospital diabetic and a dollar spent on the former group will save many dollars for the other. When I see a diabetic in a hospital with a sore toe occupying a bed for two months, I know that that patient has deprived at least eight other milder diabetics, whose expectancy of life may be many times as long, of an opportunity to learn how to care for themselves. · I know that beds now occupied by patients with these slowly healing surgical lesions could be transferred to less expensive quarters and thus allow more diabetic patients with early cataracts or cancer and younger patients with remediable surgical complications to be treated. Our group knows positively that our children learn more of diabetic treatment and learn it less expensively when at a diabetic camp than they do when in the hospital and, furthermore, that their treatment is better, because they not only have closer supervision but gain morale from association with other diabetic children.

In the future just as education helps in the management of these two groups, the hospital and the ambulatory, education should be made available to the greatest diabetic group of all, namely those whom the family doctor treats. This is the place where the government can step in and make available to the practicing physician opportunities for control of the disease which now are only available to a few physicians on hospital staffs.

Hypoglycemia in its various aspects now occupies as much time in the diabetic curriculum as does care of the skin and feet, but by no means is it routine for all diabetics to suffer from the symptoms of hypoglycemia. Insulin reactions are of vital importance to the diabetic; his education is not complete until he understands thoroughly the reasons for their origin, the mechanism by which they are brought about and the manifold symptoms and signs which accompany them, as well as their prevention and treatment. If a diabetic cannot avoid insulin reactions, his standing in the community and his self-respect are impaired. Diabetic coma may end the life of a patient, but frequent insulin reactions ruin it. Each is spectacular, but reactions are more common. Therefore, in this

monograph, as much emphasis will be laid upon hypoglycemia as
upon coma.

The detection of diabetes is claiming increasing attention because
of the advantages of early and energetic treatment, but this should
be accompanied by increasing vigilance in diagnosis. Errors in
diagnosis should be reported fully. The group of potential diabetics should receive regular periodic supervision. A number of these
may later turn out to be non-diabetic, but the diagnosis of diabetes, once made by any of the standard methods, will seldom
prove to be wrong. Quite as important and far more soul-satisfying
both to doctor and patient is the discovery of a renal glycosuric or
a pentosuric. To be able to tell a parent of a four-year-old child,
treated during two years with insulin, that diabetes is non-existent
and the reduction of copper in the Benedict test is due to pentose,
is a joy which technicians and doctors will never forget. A few
capillary blood sugars, not available at home, in the course of ten
days let out of a diabetic prison a six year old little girl who had
been in diabetic confinement for two years.

A diabetic who dies without investigation of the ultimate cause
has failed to render that service to his fellow men to which they
are entitled. Diabetics should lead the world in the percentage
submitting to autopsies, because diabetics are intelligent and their
disease and its treatment have led them along scientific paths from
which glimpses of modern medical progress are constantly afforded.
They have experienced in their own bodies the wonders and the
benefits of the outstanding triumph of the insulins over their own
disease. Even if they cannot endow a diabetic clinic, a laboratory
or a cell in it, or contribute to the care of a diabetic child in a camp,
at least they can allow an operation upon their bodies when they
no longer need them. And I repeat what I have said so often—an
operation during life is attended with pain and for the benefit of
the individual, but an operation after death is free from pain and
for the benefit of humanity.

I am proud of my diabetics. They were asked to contribute a
quota for the expansion of our hospital and not only were they the
first to go over the top, but they and their friends have given nearly
half again as much. The country and its million diabetics are just
beginning to appreciate the need for better facilities for the diagnosis
and care of diabetics and for research in the prevention and treatment of the disease. For tuberculosis and poliomyelitis millions of
dollars are given, but for diabetics, who greatly outnumber those
suffering from the two diseases mentioned, far too little has been
done. In seeking money for our diabetic clinic we have stressed the
point that one dollar from 1000 diabetics will accomplish more
good than $1000 from one, because if a diabetic gives a dollar, then
he shows his interest not only in the disease and its better treatment, but in his desire for further experimental work to produce

something even better than insulin upon which his present life depends. The demonstration that we have had 4787 separate contributions from diabetic patients to our Building Fund at the New England Deaconess Hospital and the Diabetic Funds, primarily for research, at the Boston Safe Deposit and Trust Company proves that not only are they tremendously interested in diabetes but in general are willing and anxious to take care of themselves. I am sure they will continue to do so if the opportunity is only brought to their attention.

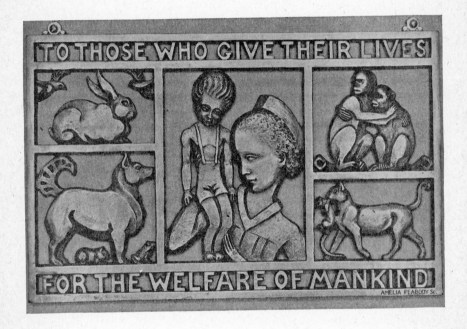

We doctors enjoy our medical practice, and our diabetic patients their lives, because of the victories over disease won by men and animals. There would be sorrow in our hearts if we were compelled to face a diabetic child without knowledge acquired by the scientific labors of physicians in many lands. But our minds linger as well on the animals who gave up their lives, not for their masters whom they loved but for diabetics whom they did not even know. And in recognition of what these lowly creatures have done we welcome the opportunity to insert again in this monograph a reproduction of the plaque created for us by Amelia Peabody and dedicated appropriately

"TO THOSE WHO GIVE THEIR LIVES FOR THE WELFARE OF MANKIND"

CHAPTER II.

THE INCIDENCE OF DIABETES.[1]

A. THE CENSUS AND DIABETIC MORTALITY.

THE United States Census reports 36,314 individuals as having died from diabetes in 1943 and 34,948 in 1944, representing rates respectively of 27.1 and 26.4 per 100,000. The ratio of diabetic deaths to total deaths was 2.48 per cent for 1943 and 2.47 per cent for 1944, or approximately 1 death from diabetes among 40 deaths from all causes in contrast to 1 death from diabetes among 181 deaths in 1900. The number living with the disease is problematical but in our opinion is about 1,000,000 (see page 40). The death rate from diabetes in the registration area of the continental United States more than trebled in the twenty years 1880–1900, but for the whole country forty years passed before this occurred again, namely, from 9.7 per 100,000 in 1900 to 27.1 in 1943. Pennsylvania is the only state in which the disease is legally reportable and the effect of this law upon the statistical incidence of diabetes in that state will be watched with interest. It ranked sixth among all the states, 30.6 per 100,000 in 1938 and third, 38.6 in 1943.

TABLE 1.—NUMBER OF DEATHS FROM ALL CAUSES, DEATHS AND RATES FROM DIABETES AND RATIO OF DEATHS FROM DIABETES TO DEATHS FROM ALL CAUSES: REGISTRATION AREA, 1900, 1910, 1920, 1930 AND 1940–1944.*

		Diabetes.		
Year.	Total deaths.	Number.	Rate per 100,000 population.	Ratio of diabetes deaths to total deaths (per cent).
1944 . . .	1,411,338	34,948	26.4	2.47
1943 . . .	1,459,544	36,314	27.1	2.48
1942 . . .	1,385,187	33,971	25.4	2.45
1941 . . .	1,397,642	33,879	25.5	2.42
1940 . . .	1,417,269	35,015	26.6	2.47
1930 . . .	1,343,356	22,528	19.0	1.67
1920 . . .	1,142,558	14,062	16.0	1.23
1910 . . .	805,412	8,040	14.9	1.00
1900 . . .	539,939	2,996	9.7	0.55

* Tables 1, 2, 13, 14 became available through the courtesy of Dr. Halbert L. Dunn and Mr. Frank S. Morrison of the U. S. Bureau of the Census.

[1] In this chapter as well as in Chapter III the authors have drawn freely upon five articles, published jointly with Dr. Louis I. Dublin, Second Vice-President and Statistician, and Mr. Herbert H. Marks, of the Metropolitan Life Insurance Company, in the Am. Jour. Med. Sci. (A, **186**, 753, 1933; B, **187**, 433, 1934; C, **189**, 163, 1935; D, **191**, 759, **192**, 9, 1936; E, **193**, 8, 1937). Many of the tables were originally prepared by the Statistical Bureau of the Metropolitan Life Insurance Company. The authors are deeply indebted to this organization, and to Dr. Dublin and Mr. Marks for the privilege of using this material, but it is only fair to state that the authors assume full responsibility for the manner in which they have utilized the data. In this chapter, Tables 3, 4, 5, 6, 7, 8, 11 and 12 and Figures 1 and 2 were prepared with the coöperation of the Statistical Bureau of the Metropolitan Life Insurance Company. To save space except in a few instances the references cited in these original articles are not repeated here.

(22)

The diabetic deaths recorded by the Census do not represent the total number of persons with diabetes who die, and for two main reasons. The first is the priority accorded by established rules of classification of deaths to a group of diseases of which tuberculosis, cancer, accidents, most puerperal conditions and most acute surgical conditions are examples. A second factor in the non-recognition of diabetic deaths is the omission of any reference to diabetes by the doctor when reporting the death. How frequently this takes place has been variously estimated. It occurs: (1) because a doctor new to the patient may sign the certificate without a knowledge of the existence of the diabetes; (2) the actual cause of death may seemingly and in fact bear little relation to diabetes and so the word diabetes is deliberately omitted; and (3) the diabetes may have so burned out in the old man or old woman that it is not recognized at the time of death or because of its mildness may never have been diagnosed. Lombard and Joslin[1] investigated the death certificates of 744 diabetic patients previously treated by me and found that only 62.9 per cent were so classified on the death records. This year we have repeated the study with the death certificates of 1000 patients and found that 64.9 per cent only were classified as diabetics. A detailed report of this investigation by Lombard and Joslin will be published. Even if all had had the word diabetes on the death certificate only 82.5 per cent of the total number would have been thus classified by the joint causes of death procedure. Thus the mortality from diabetes as recorded in the death records of Massachusetts represents about two-thirds of the mortality of individuals with the disease.[2]

Assuming that what has occurred in Massachusetts, namely, that only two-thirds of the individuals dying with diabetes are statistically reported as having the disease, then one must increase mortality figures from diabetes by approximately one-half, 50 per cent. This would increase the 36,314 deaths due to diabetes in the United States during 1943 to 54,471 persons and the 34,948 in 1944 to 52,422, or considerably more than 50,000 yearly *of persons dying with, even if not of, diabetes*. These computations are of great importance in any estimation of the incidence of diabetes or its prevalence in our midst. They suggest that more and more one must depend upon privately compiled statistics rather than upon officially reported death certificates. Similar compilations to those of Lombard and Joslin, comparing private and public data, should be repeated in other areas from time to time. One can venture the prediction that with the increasing duration of life of diabetics

---

[1] Joslin and Lombard: New Eng. Jour. Med., **214**, 7, 1936.

[2] One fears that the revision of the standard certificate of death, together with the instructions to physicians, contained in the latest (1939) Physicians' Handbook on Birth and Death Registration issued by the U. S. Bureau of the Census, will more than ever lead physicians to omit diabetes in recording the death of a patient unless this disease played a prominent part in the final illness.

and with the better control of the disease, less and less the word "diabetes" will take precedence on the death certificate.

TABLE 2.—CRUDE AND AGE-ADJUSTED DEATH RATES PER 100,000 FROM DIABETES IN THE UNITED STATES AND EVERY STATE IN 1940. BY RACE AND SEX.*

(Rates Adjusted on Basis of Age Distribution of Total Population in the United States in 1940.)

	Total persons.		White persons.					
			Total.		Males		Females.	
	Ad-justed.	Crude.	Ad-justed.	Crude.	Ad-justed.	Crude.	Ad-justed.	Crude.
United States . . .	26.6	26.6	26.7	27.6	20.6	20.9	32.9	34.3
Alabama	15.9	12.2	16.0	12.4	14.6	11.3	17.5	13.6
Arizona	14.3	11.0	14.1	11.0	13.6	11.4	14.8	10.6
Arkansas	12.4	10.5	12.9	11.1	11.5	10.3	14.5	11.9
California . . .	21.2	24.7	21.1	25.0	17.5	19.8	24.6	30.4
Colorado	16.4	17.8	16.5	17.9	13.7	15.0	19.6	20.9
Connecticut . . .	32.8	35.8	32.6	35.9	25.2	26.5	39.4	45.1
Delaware . . .	27.6	30.0	26.2	29.5	22.2	24.2	30.2	34.9
District of Clumbia	34.9	33.5	33.5	35.2	31.2	28.5	35.5	41.4
Florida	20.1	19.6	19.6	21.2	18.1	19.7	21.2	22.7
Georgia	15.5	12.2	16.8	13.8	17.4	14.0	16.3	13.6
Idaho	19.0	17.5	19.3	17.7	16.7	16.5	22.9	19.1
Illinois	32.0	34.1	31.5	34.1	24.2	25.6	39.0	42.6
Indiana	24.2	28.1	23.8	27.9	19.5	22.7	28.2	33.2
Iowa	23.1	28.4	22.9	28.3	18.9	23.2	27.1	33.5
Kansas	21.7	26.0	21.5	25.9	18.0	22.0	25.2	29.8
Kentucky . . .	16.9	15.7	16.5	15.2	14.6	13.4	18.6	17.1
Louisiana . . .	22.4	17.5	24.2	19.2	16.6	12.7	31.6	25.7
Maine	25.3	32.1	25.3	32.1	21.3	26.9	29.4	37.4
Maryland . . .	31.5	31.2	32.3	33.5	21.3	20.7	42.1	46.4
Massachusetts . .	29.8	35.7	29.8	35.8	22.7	25.5	35.9	45.6
Michigan	27.9	26.7	27.7	26.8	20.5	19.7	35.4	34.3
Minnesota . . .	24.5	26.8	24.4	26.8	18.3	20.5	31.2	33.3
Mississippi . . .	16.9	13.4	17.8	14.9	16.8	14.2	19.0	15.6
Missouri	21.6	25.3	21.4	25.5	18.2	21.6	24.5	29.4
Montana	19.3	19.3	19.7	19.8	11.4	12.1	31.2	28.6
Nebraska	24.7	28.1	24.8	28.2	21.0	24.4	28.7	32.1
Nevada	21.0	20.9	20.7	20.2	19.8	20.7	†	†
New Hampshire . .	28.1	37.0	28.1	37.1	25.0	31.9	31.0	42.2
New Jersey . . .	35.6	36.4	34.9	36.2	24.4	24.3	44.4	48.0
New Mexico . . .	12.1	8.3	12.7	8.7	10.9	8.3	15.1	9.1
New York . . .	39.0	40.6	38.8	41.2	29.0	29.6	48.0	52.7
North Carolina . .	20.0	14.2	20.2	14.8	20.3	14.5	20.3	15.0
North Dakota . .	28.7	26.6	28.6	26.6	22.9	22.7	36.3	30.9
Ohio	28.1	31.3	27.6	31.2	19.5	21.7	35.5	40.8
Oklahoma . . .	16.0	14.4	15.7	14.3	14.3	13.5	17.2	15.1
Oregon	21.6	25.9	21.6	25.9	18.7	22.7	24.9	29.4
Pennsylvania . .	35.9	36.3	35.4	36.3	22.4	22.3	48.1	50.3
Rhode Island . .	35.4	38.8	35.0	38.5	26.1	26.8	42.7	49.7
South Carolina . .	18.7	12.6	20.8	14.4	18.8	12.4	22.8	16.4
South Dakota . .	23.0	23.2	22.8	23.3	19.3	20.6	27.4	26.1
Tennessee . . .	16.4	14.2	14.9	13.0	15.2	13.3	14.8	12.8
Texas	17.2	14.4	16.9	14.3	15.3	12.9	18.8	15.7
Utah	23.4	19.4	23.7	19.7	16.4	13.1	31.1	26.5
Vermont	27.0	33.7	27.0	33.7	21.4	26.4	32.6	41.3
Virginia	23.5	20.1	22.5	19.9	19.1	16.5	25.9	23.5
Washington . . .	21.9	26.1	21.8	26.1	18.5	22.9	25.7	29.7
West Virginia . .	21.6	17.4	21.0	17.0	17.9	15.0	24.3	19.2
Wisconsin . . .	26.0	28.4	25.9	28.4	20.3	22.4	31.7	34.6
Wyoming	20.1	16.4	19.6	15.8	18.7	16.6	21.1	14.9

* Age-Adjusted Death Rates in the United States, 1900-1940, Bureau of the Census, **23**, No. 1, 27, 1945. Vital Statistics Rates in the United States, 1900-1940, Bureau of the Census, 434, 1943.

† Small population groups in which less than ten deaths from diabetes were reported.

In a similar analysis of known diabetic deaths in the State of Washington, Dr. Lester J. Palmer tells me that only 69.4 per cent, 168 of 242, fatal diabetics were classified as diabetes.

Wide variations occur in diabetic mortality data among the states. Thus the average mortality in 1940 in the ten states with the highest mortalities, including the District of Columbia as a state, was 35.3 crude, 32.9 adjusted, per 100,000, in contrast to 13 crude, 15.3 adjusted, for the ten states with the lowest mortalities. To only a trivial degree can the difference be explained by race, sex and age, though below the importance of all these factors will be discussed in connection with the evidence gained by the writer from his survey of living diabetics in Arizona.[1] The conclusions reached in that investigation regarding Arizona on the whole appear valid for the ten states with the lowest mortalities.

The Universality of Diabetes.—In the early months of 1940, studies were undertaken by the physicians of Arizona and the senior author to explain the low incidence of diabetes in that state as compared with Rhode Island, 10 in contrast to 42 per 100,000 for the year 1937, and for five recent years, 1934–1938, 9.8 versus 36.9. Age and sex adjustments alone accounted for a portion of the disparity in the death rates; thus for the single year 1937 the figures were changed to 13 versus 37 and for the average of nine years, 1930–1938, to 10.1 versus 22.4.

Factors other than age and sex also undoubtedly played a part in the reputedly low mortality of Arizona and the high mortality from diabetes in Rhode Island. The area of Arizona is 113,810 square miles and of Rhode Island 1067 square miles. The density of population of Arizona is 3.8 per square mile, while that of Rhode Island is 644, as compared with 41 for the United States as a whole. Although the number of physicians per residents of the two states does not greatly differ, their accessibility does, since two-thirds of the population of Arizona are in communities with population less than 2500. In Arizona Indians comprise 10 per cent and Mexicans 26 per cent of the population and the Jewish race about 0.5 per cent.

The results of the survey of diabetes in Arizona showed: (1) whereas Jews made up 0.5 per cent of the inhabitants they comprised 2 per cent of the total diabetics (755) reported by the doctors who replied to a questionnaire; (2) deaths of Indians from diabetes averaged 2 per year for the six years 1934 to 1939, but in the survey 73 Indians with diabetes were discovered or approximately the same percentage of all diabetics as of Indians in the whole population; (3) in the prison and in the mental hospital in Arizona more diabetics were found proportionately than in similar institutions in the East and more than would be expected from the National Health Survey; (4) diabetes was acknowledged by 1 in 42 doctors of 334 reporting

[1] Joslin: Jour. Am. Med. Assn., **115**, 2033, 1940.

in Arizona and by 1 in 36 of 393 reporting in Rhode Island. The returns from the clergy were similar; (5) in the state as a whole there were 755 diabetics reported by the 290 doctors who stated they had or had not diabetics in their care, or 2.8 per doctor.

In fact, normal ratios held for males, females, whites and Indians. Only for Mexicans was there a notable discrepancy, and during the survey it was considered that less of this nationality was surveyed than any other and, furthermore, doubt still exists as to the actual number of Mexicans in the state. Finally, it is significant that in Arizona death certificates marked cause of death "unknown" were three and one-half times as numerous as those certificates which ascribed the cause of death to diabetes.

At the Sage Memorial Hospital situated in Ganado, Arizona, in the heart of the Navajo section, Dr. C. G. Salsbury tells me there have been 22,790 admissions between 1930 and 1946. Among these there have been 7 patients with diabetes. Although those admitted are predominantly Navajos, only 4 of the diabetics were Navajos. I suspect this is explained by the nomadic life of this tribe and its scarcity of food in contrast to the frequency of diabetes among the Pimas in the southern part of the state, who are reputed to be more opulent. The hospital population is largely made up of children and young adults.

In the opinion of the authors this diabetic survey in Arizona supports the thesis that diabetes is universal. We believe the incidence of diabetes is highest where (1) the average age is the oldest, (2) women predominate, (3) obesity is most frequent, (4) the proportion of Jews is greatest, (5) medical supervision is closest and (6) deaths are most accurately reported.

B. THE INCREASE IN DIABETES IN NATION, STATE AND CITY.

Diabetes has advanced in importance as a cause of death in the United States from twenty-seventh place in 1900 to eighth place in 1943. If we exclude deaths from violence, it ranks seventh. In 1943 diabetes caused a greater number of deaths than did tuberculosis in 13 states. In 1943 in Massachusetts the number of deaths credited to diabetes was 1627 and to tuberculosis 1819. Among white women over forty-five years of age in 1943 in the United States diabetes caused three times as many deaths as tuberculosis and was fifth in rank among the causes of death. One can anticipate that within another decade diabetes may displace tuberculosis and pneumonia and thus reach fifth place for the entire population as a cause of death, and if we group all deaths from arteriosclerosis under one heading instead of three, cardiac, cerebral and renal, arteriosclerosis and cancer alone would exceed it.

A false impression regarding the increase in diabetes is created unless one compares crude with adjusted statistics. Crude statistics show the increase in total deaths, but when statistics are adjusted for changes in sex and age of the population, the information obtained is far different. A hint of this has already been mentioned in the discussion of diabetes in Arizona (See page 25.) It is strikingly evident if applied to nationwide[9] data. Thus the increase in the diabetic death rate without sex-age adjustments was 140 per cent between 1900 and 1940 but when adjusted was just a trifle over 100 per cent. Unadjusted between 1921 and 1940 the increase was 2.5 per cent yearly but if adjusted was only 1.4 per cent yearly. However, for the United States as a whole for 1940 the crude and adjusted death rates were identical, namely, 26.6 per 100,000.

TABLE 3.—DEATHS PER 100,000 OF POPULATION FROM THE CHIEF CAUSES OF DEATH IN THE REGISTRATION AREA OF THE UNITED STATES, 1943.

1. Heart disease (132.1—IV)* 318.3
2. Cancer (63—VIII) 124.5
3. Cerebral hemorrhage (71.5—VII) 95.0
4. Violence (accidents, suicides and homicides) (96—VI) . . . 89.3
5. Nephritis, acute, chronic, unspecified (89—V) 74.1
6. Pneumonia (180.5—II) 54.4
7. Tuberculosis, all forms (201.9—I) 42.6
8. Diabetes (9.7—XXVII) 27.1

* The first figure in the parenthesis represents the death rate and the Roman numeral the position occupied by the given disease in 1900.

Still more striking are the statistics of the Metropolitan Life Insurance Company for the periods 1931–1933 and 1941–1943 when the death rate from diabetes at all ages when adjusted to allow for changes in the age and sex composition of the insured population showed a moderate decline among white males, a very slight increase among colored males and a slight decrease among females both white and colored. For the years 1941–1943 it was 13.6 for white males and 25.9 for white females.

The crude death rate from diabetes among industrial policyholders of the Metropolitan Life Insurance Company in 1945 was 25.3 or almost 10 per cent less than in 1944. In fact, last year's figures were the lowest since 1938. However, comparison on the basis of standardized rates is even more favorable. The standardized rate in 1945 at ages one to seventy-four years was 16.1 as compared with 18.6 in 1944. Last year's standardized rate is the lowest since 1920. Nevertheless, when all is said and done, the doctor deals with the crude rates rather than with standardized rates and upon him will fall increasingly a greater number of diabetics to treat even though they may be at older ages. (See Figure 1.)

At times there are hints from statistical tables that the upper value for the diabetic death rate has been reached. In some years there has been a regression of death rates for the larger cities, but in contrast is the unexpected fact that the increase of the incidence of mortality from diabetes has gone up more rapidly in the states with the highest mortalities than in the states with the lowest mortalities, and this circumstance is so important that we record below the data upon which the statement is based. Thus a comparison for a ten-year period, 1930–1932 versus 1940–1942 shows that the percentage increase in diabetic mortality was actually 32.1 per cent for the ten states with the highest diabetic mortalities as compared with 19.8 per cent for the ten states with the lowest mortalities.[1] To the authors these figures indicate the end of the increase in diabetes is not in sight, because eventually we can expect the states with low mortalities to approach more closely those with high mortalities.

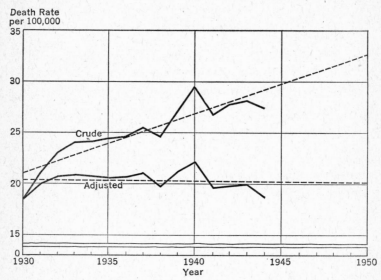

FIG. 1.—Diabetes. Crude and adjusted death rates 1930 to 1944, with trends projected to 1950. (Metropolitan Life Insurance Company, Industrial Department).

Space precludes detailed figures, but Table 4 shows the diabetic mortality in Massachusetts and New York and Table 5 in Boston and New York City.

TABLE 4.—DIABETIC MORTALITY IN MASSACHUSETTS AND NEW YORK STATE.*

	Massachusetts.			New York State.		
Year.	No.	Rate per 100,000 population.	Diabetic deaths to total deaths, per cent.	No.	Rate per 100,000 population.	Diabetic deaths to total deaths, per cent.
1900 . . .	358	12.8	0.70	827	11.4	0.62
1910 . . .	651	19.3	1.20	1694	18.6	1.15
1920 . . .	810	20.9	1.52	2439	23.2	1.69
1930 . . .	1018	23.9	2.06	3447	27.3	2.34
1940 . . .	1542	35.8	3.02	5471	40.6	3.64
1943 . . .	1627	38.2	2.99	5653	44.0	3.50

* Federal figures.

[1] See Diabetes Abstracts, **4**, 4, 1945.

TABLE 5.—DIABETIC MORTALITY IN BOSTON AND NEW YORK CITY.*

	Boston.			New York City.		
Year.	No.	Rate per 100,000 population.	Diabetic deaths to total deaths, per cent.	No.	Rate per 100,000 population.	Diabetic deaths to total deaths, per cent.
1900 . . .	85	15.2	0.74	392	11.4	0.55
1910 . . .	140	20.9	1.21	895	18.8	1.17
1920 . . .	182	24.3	1.57	1328	23.4	1.81
1930 . . .	240	30.7	2.18	1861	26.7	2.49
1935 . . .	288	35.0	2.51	2255	30.9	3.00
1940 . . .	264	34.2	2.70	3096	41.5	4.07
1943 . . .	289	37.6	2.74	3281	42.7	3.94
1944 . . .	265	34.6	2.59	3129	40.8	3.97
1945 . . .	269	35.1	2.69	3109	40.2	3.90

* Federal figures.

Writing from a most conservative point of view, Spiegelman and Marks[1] conclude that "during the next few decades, the number of diabetics in the United States will increase at a much greater rate than the total population. From 1940 to 1950, an increase of 18 per cent may be expected in the number of diabetics, while the total population is expected to grow only by 9 per cent.

"At least 50,000 persons in the United States became diabetic during 1940; about two-fifths were males and three-fifths females. Not quite half were under fifty-five at the onset of their diabetes; somewhat more than one-quarter became diabetic between ages fifty-five and sixty-four; and one-quarter were at ages sixty-five and over when they developed the disease.

"Of our population under age fifty, over 4 per cent of the females and more than 2 per cent of the males will eventually become diabetic."

Vermont, a state with the highest average age among all the states, has a crude diabetic mortality rate of only 33.7 (adjusted, 27.0) for 1940. I believe a personal survey of the state would show a far higher incidence.

C. AGE AND CHANGING INCIDENCE OF DIABETES AND DIABETIC MORTALITY.

The changing incidence of diabetic mortality is most apparent in the older decades of life, and, in fact, the increase in diabetic mortality depends upon individuals in the older age groups. Since the introduction of insulin, deaths from diabetes in individuals under fifty years of age have shown a marked decline, and this has been most prominent in the diabetic mortality of children. These facts are well brought out in Table 6. Thus, diabetic deaths, both in Massachusetts and among the insured of the Metropolitan Life Insurance Company, have declined in early life and risen in later life during five-year periods between 1900 and 1945.

[1] Spiegelman and Marks: Am. Journ. Public Health, **36**, 26, 1946.

Three factors have been instrumental in accomplishing this change: (1) the aging of the population in general and (2) the increasing duration of life of the modern diabetic—both of which bring those in the lower decades into the age zone of greatest diabetic incidence; (3) the greater attention to diagnosis of disease in aged people. However, thus far we have recognized among 28,000 patients consulting our group for glycosuria, 25,148 with diabetes, only 62 who have developed the disease above the age of eighty years, and of these but 7 over eighty-five years and only 1 with reasonably definite onset above the age of ninety years. The number of congenital diabetics reported in the world literature, concerning whom the data are not wholly satisfactory, is about the same as the number of cases we have seen with onset above the age of eighty-five years. We have recognized no congenital cases of diabetes.

TABLE 6.—AVERAGE DEATH-RATES FOR DIABETES IN MASSACHUSETTS AND AMONG INSURED OF THE METROPOLITAN LIFE INSURANCE COMPANY BY AGE.[1]

Years.	Massachusetts. Death-rate in age group.			Metropolitan. Death-rate in age group.		
	Under 20.	20–49.	50 and over.	Under 25.	25–44.	45–74.
1901 to 1905	3.4	6.8	54	?	?	?
1906 to 1910	3.6	7.3	63	?	?	?
1911 to 1915	4.3	8.3	73	3.0	7.2	63.7
1916 to 1920	4.1	8.7	77	3.2	7.3	66.3
1921 to 1925	2.9	7.0	86	2.8	7.1	73.2
1926 to 1930	1.6	5.2	97	2.2	5.9	83.3
1931 to 1935	1.1	5.6	120	1.8	5.8	95.5
1936 to 1940	1.2	5.3	136.6	1.5*	4.5*	100.8*
1941 to 1945†	1.0	5.0	136.7	1.5	4.4	89.0

* Age adjusted rates.
† Figures for Massachusetts are for 1941–44.

Between 1900–1914 and 1944–1946 the duration of life of the diabetic has increased from 4.9 years to 14.1 years. Those with onset in childhood have almost ceased to die of diabetes until the duration of the disease has passed twenty years. In 1900, 17.8 per cent of the population of the United States was forty-five years of age and over and 4.1 per cent sixty-five years and over. In 1940 these figures were respectively 26.5 and 6.8, but it is calculated that by 1960 they will rise to 32.6 for forty-five years and above, and 9.8 for sixty-five years and over.[1] In Boston for the year 1845, 80 per cent of the population died under the age of forty years in contrast to 1935 for the state of Massachusetts when 80 per cent died above the age of forty years. On the other hand, the total number of cases of diabetes in children may not increase because of a declining birth-rate. However, this is changing more slowly than is often indicated, and to offset it is the far greater decline in infant mortality.

[1] Thompson and Whelpton: Population Trends in the United States, New York, McGraw-Hill Company, 1933.

Recognizing the importance of the age of the population in the frequency of diabetes, the author has assembled data in Table 7 which show how greatly in the United States basic data have altered in the last three-quarters of a century. Between 1860 and 1945 the population increased from 31,443,000 to 139,621,000. The birth-rate on the whole has dropped, which partly accounts for the older average and median ages of the living as well as the average age at death. However, the birth-rate rose above 17.9 per 1000 for 1940, to 21.5 per 1000 for 1943, 20.2 for 1944 and 19.8 for 1945. Expectation of life at birth, particularly for women, has notably advanced; in 1943 for men to 63.16 years and for women to 68.27 years.

Evidently this country is far from having reached its maximum of the percentage of individuals over sixty years of age, despite the rapid strides it has made. Among the larger nations France is said to have the highest proportion of inhabitants more than sixty years old, 140 per 1000, compared with 115 in England, 110 in Germany, 108 in Italy, 85 in the United States, 74 in Japan and 66 in Russia.[1]

TABLE 7.—POPULATION, BIRTH-RATE, AVERAGE AGE, MEDIAN AGE, AVERAGE AGE
at DEATH, EXPECTATION OF LIFE IN THE UNITED STATES
BY DECADES, 1860 TO 1937.

Year.	Population (thousands).	Birth-rate (B.R.A.) per 1000.	Average age living.	Median age living.	Average age at death.	Expectation of life at birth, original registration states.	
						Male.	Female.
1860	31,443	..	23.3	19.4	22.7		
1870	38,588	..	24.2	20.1	25.2		
1880	50,156	..	24.8	20.9	26.9		
1890	62,948	..	25.8	21.4	31.1		
1900	75,995	..	26.3	22.9	35.2	48.2*	51.1*
1910	91,972	25.1†	27.2	24.0	38.7	50.2	53.6
1920	105,711	23.7	28.0	25.2	41.9	54.1	56.4
1930	122,775	18.9	29.5	26.4	48.7	59.1	62.6
1940	131,669	17.9	31.6	29.0	55.9	62.94	67.31
1943	136,497	21.5	31.8	29 5	56.6‡	63.16	68.27
1944	138,083	20.2	31.9	29 6	§	§	§
1945	139,621	19.8	32.0	29.7	§	§	§

* 1901. † 1915.
‡ Affected by absence of considerable number of young men overseas.
§ Figures not available.

The increasing duration of life of the diabetic and the part it plays in lowering diabetic mortality in the early decades and raising it in the later is shown in various ways. (Tables 6, 39, 40, 41.) The average age at death for 325 patients dying in the Naunyn era (1898–1914) was 44.5 years and in the Hagedorn era (January 1, 1937–December 31, 1943) for 2583 fatal cases was 64.9 years and for 651 fatal cases in the Charles H. Best era (January 1, 1944–May 15, 1946) was 64.5 years. For the 140 deaths of diabetics on our service at the George F. Baker Clinic at the New England Deaconess Hospital for 1933–1936 the average age at death was

[1] New York Times, January 22, 1939. Statistics reported to the Department of Commerce by the office of the United States Commercial Attaché in Paris.

58.3 years. For the 138 deaths in 1937, 1938 and 1939 it was 60.8 years and for 203 deaths betwen 1940 and 1945, inclusive, it was 62.0 years.

This increasing age at death is shown well by the diabetic mortality in Toronto. Dr. Gordon P. Jackson, Medical Officer, tells the authors that in 1914 the approximate average age of diabetics at death was 45.3 years, but in 1945 was 66.5 years. So, too, in the Metropolitan Life Insurance Company it has advanced from 51.5 years in 1911 to 61.5 years in 1945.

Direct proof of the lengthening duration of diabetes, as an illustration of its effect upon diabetic statistics, is also afforded by the authors' own series. The data have been gathered with extreme care and the date of onset of the disease has been determined by detailed questioning of the patient, often checked by two and even three of us, and has erred in placing the date too late rather than too early. The facts thus obtained are portrayed along with the average ages at death, discussed above, in Table 41 (page 319).

Thus in the Naunyn era, 1898–1914 the average duration of the diabetes was 4.9 years, in the Allen era, 1914–1922, 6.1 years, in the early Banting era, 1922–1925, 7.5 years, in the late Banting era, 1935–1936, 12.1 years, in the Hagedorn era, 1937–1943, 12.9 years, and in the Charles H. Best era, 1944–May 15, 1946, 14.1 years. Under Prognosis (page 316) and Diabetes in Childhood (page 741) the influences which children have exerted upon the lengthening duration of diabetes will be further considered.

Diabetes Not an Old Age Disease.—Hitherto in a sense, discussions and statistics upon the incidence of diabetes were all wrong, because they were based on dead diabetics instead of upon living diabetics. They have placed the cart before the horse. In Table 8 the authors submit the age at onset of diabetes for 9853 diabetics seen by them between the years 1898 and 1933, inclusive, and 2887 seen between 1936 and 1938, inclusive.

TABLE 8.—THE AGE OF ONSET OF DIABETES MELLITUS.
(Experience of E. P. Joslin, 1898–1933 and 1936–1938.)[1]

Decade.	Per cent appearing in each decade, 1898–1933.		Per cent appearing in each decade, 1936–1938.	
	Males.	Females.	Males.	Females.
1	5.0	4.4	6.7	4.6
2	7.2	6.4	9.0	6.2
3	9.6	6.1	8.6	6.2
4	13.8	10.8	13.1	11.0
5	23.3	22.9	19.8	21.0
6	24.2	30.3	22.1	28.1
7	13.6	15.8	16.2	18.1
8	3.2	3.1	4.3	4.4
9	0.1	0.2	0.2	0.4
	100.0	100.0	100.0	100.0
Number of cases	4639	5214	1265	1622

[1] Prepared by the Statistical Bureau of the Metropolitan Life Insurance Company

For comparison with Table 8 is a similar tabulation of the mortalities recorded as due to diabetes in the state of Massachusetts (Table 9), for the years 1901 to 1932 and 1933 to 1938. The onset rates are an attempt to represent the susceptibility to the development of diabetes in certain decades and the mortality rates represent the susceptibility to dying from diabetes in these same decades.

TABLE 9.—DIABETES AS A CAUSE OF DEATH.

(Massachusetts, 1901–1932 and 1933–1938.)

Decade.	Per cent appearing in each decade, 1901–1932.		Per cent appearing in each decade, 1933–1938.		Per cent appearing in each decade, 1941–1944.	
	Males.	Females.	Males.	Females.	Males.	Females.
1 . . .	2.7	1.9	0.5	0.3	0.4	0.2
2 . . .	4.7	2.9	1.3	0.6	0.8	0.5
3 . . .	4.7	3.2	1.6	0.9	1.1	0.6
4 . . .	6.2	4.0	2.3	1.2	1.9	0.8
5 . . .	9.7	8.0	5.6	4.7	6.2	3.2
6 . . .	20.0	21.7	18.4	16.8	16.7	16.5
7 . . .	28.8	32.8	32.6	37.3	32.0	34.5
8 . . .	18.5	20.3	30.3	30.4	30.5	32.8
9 . . .	4.7	5.2	7.4	7.8	9.9	10.3
10 . . .	..	..	..	..	0.5	0.6
	100.0	100.0	100.0	100.0	100.0	100.0
No. of cases	8744	13,492	2809	5392	2099	4212

An adaptation of the distribution of diabetes by age and sex, based upon the National Health Survey of 2,500,000 persons,[1] is shown in Table 10. One would not claim extraordinary accuracy for the table, but, on the other hand, it is extraordinarily valuable, because it shows in concrete form the rarity of diabetes in young people and its frequency in old age. Sex plays no rôle until the age of twenty-five years, but thereafter is of increasing importance, and at the age of sixty-five and over, 1 of 45 women has diabetes and 1 of 70 men.

In 1940 the total deaths in the United States from diabetes were 35,015. Of these 30 occurred in the first year of life and 19,101 over sixty-five years.

TABLE 10.—RATIO OF DIABETES IN THE POPULATION.

Age.	Males.	Females.	Age.	Total.	Males.	Females.
			Figures at left based on diabetics per 1000 Population from National Health Survey as follows:			
0–14	1:2500	1:2500	0–14	0.38	0.35	0.41
15–24	1:1700	1:1700	15–24	0.59	0.62	0.57
25–34	1:1100	1: 900	25–34	1.00	0.90	1.08
35–44	1: 500	1: 300	35–44	2.61	2.01	3.16
45–54	1: 225	1: 125	45–54	6.56	4.49	8.64
55–64	1: 100	1: 50	55–64	14.25	9.96	18.20
65 and over	1: 70	1: 45	65 and over	18.39	14.58	21.47
			All ages	3.67	2.73	4.53

The above data are based upon 9182 diabetics in a surveyed (urban) population of 2,502,391 persons.

[1] National Institute of Health, 1935-1936. The Magnitude of the Chronic Disease Problem in the United States. Division of Public Health Methods, National Institute of Health, U. S. Public Health Service, Washington, 1938.

3

Considering the onset-rates alone the figures demonstrate that for both males and females the maximum susceptibility to the development of diabetes occurs in the sixth decade, and our more detailed figures show that the ages of maximum susceptibility are 51 among males and 55 among females. The susceptibility of males to the development of diabetes rises steadily to this maximum and thereafter declines. The proportions of females, however, are on the whole somewhat less in the first 4 decades, about the same in the fifth, but decidedly more in the sixth, seventh, eighth and ninth.

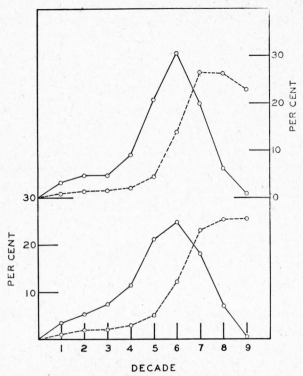

Fig. 2.—Relative onset and mortality-rates of diabetes mellitus in the various decades of life. Full lines, onset-rates; dashed lines, mortality-rates. The upper curves represent the data for females, the lower curves those for males. Abscissa, the decades of life; ordinates, relative mortality in per cent.

If it is assumed that the diabetes prevalence rates according to sex and age, as observed in the National Health Survey, prevailed in the general population of the United States during 1940, then over one-quarter of the total diabetics were under the age of fifty years, one-quarter between fifty and sixty years and a little under one-half at ages sixty and over. The average age of male diabetics was 55.6 years and of females 56.7 years.[1]

—————
[1] Loc. cit., page 33.

To our minds the most significant aspect of these onset-rates is the declining susceptibility in the later decades. This indicates that diabetes is not an old-age disease. It cannot be taken as a manifestation of senility. Its onset depends upon a complex of events (presumably of endocrine origin) which attain their maximum manifestation between the ages of forty and sixty years. Diabetics developing the disease after the age of sixty exhibit it generally in mild form; the exact time of onset of diabetes in older patients is not as easily ascertainable as in younger diabetics, because the condition develops more insidiously. These considerations favor the date of onset of the disease being placed late in the old.

If we take the mortality rates of diabetes as the basis of an incidence study, this situation would not be at all clear, for the mortality rates rise steadily until the eighth decade. The mortality rates imply that the older one grows up to the age of seventy, the greater are the chances of dying from diabetes, whereas the onset-rates indicate that certainly after the age of sixty is reached, the chances of developing diabetes decrease.

If we could only estimate accurately the exact date of onset of diabetes in a given individual, new data regarding the incidence of diabetes and its duration would be afforded. Unfortunately, the determination of onset is seldom definite. Thus, taking the new diabetics seen by us in 1945, of whom 1548 were available for the survey, the onset was definitely regarded as acute (in the course of twenty-four hours) in 0.5 per cent; rapid (in the course of six days) in 3.2 per cent; gradual (in the course of two months) in 10.2 per cent; and quite indefinite in 86.1 per cent.

From these statistical tables emerge two cardinal ideas: (1) That today emphasis should be put upon the prevention of the onset of diabetes in middle life; and (2) that the chief concern in the treatment of the disease should be with its late complications, because at present few die when young or of diabetes *per se*.

D. SEX AND DIABETES MELLITUS.

Sex likewise plays a more and more prominent part in diabetic incidence and mortality and this is also attributable to two causes. The first of these is the growing respect in which females are held throughout the world and the resulting greater investigation of their health.

Among the Arizona Indians a survey disclosed males 42, females 29 (2 unspecified), but in the entire State, females exceeded males. (See page 25.) However, it is true that years ago in Japan 80 per cent of the cases reported by Iwai were males, in Germany 70 per cent, whereas at that time in England and the United States only about 60 per cent were males.

The second is the increase in females in the upper ages. In the authors' practice the proportion of females with diabetes has risen from 41 per cent in their first 1000 patients consulting them for glycosuria in the years 1898–1916, to as high as 64 per cent in the tenth, 57.4 per cent in the eighteenth thousand and 53.0 per cent in the twenty-seventh thousand. Among the 1841 diabetic admissions to the George F. Baker Clinic at the New England Deaconess Hospital in 1941, females constituted 76 per cent. In Massachusetts for 1933–1938 the number of deaths among diabetic males was 2809, or 34.3 per cent, and for females 5392, or 65.7 per cent. In the National Health Survey,[1] which comprised a study of 2,502,391 individuals and among whom 9182 diabetics were found, males numbered 3285 and females numbered 5897, or 64.2 per cent (see Table 10). In the United States the definite increase of deaths of females over males from diabetes began in 1910, so that by 1940, when the total rate was 26.6 per 100,000 it was 20.0 for males and 34.3 for females; the females decidedly predominated from thirty-five years and over, nearly doubling the males between forty-five to seventy-four years.

This excess mortality from diabetes of women, as compared with men, is characteristic of the diabetes situation today. It is found in other countries besides the United States, although the actual excess differs appreciably from country to country. Thus, in England and Wales the diabetes death-rate of females at all ages is 25 per cent higher than the male rate. Up to age thirty-five years, female rates are about the same as those for males, and it is only after age forty-five years that there is any appreciable excess in the female rates. The maximum difference in the rates of the two sexes is as high as 50 per cent and occurs between ages fifty-five and sixty-four years.

In New Zealand the diabetes death rate of females is more than 75 per cent higher than that of males. In that country, also, the rate for women exceeds that for men beginning at age forty-five. The differences in the mortality of the two sexes are even larger than in the United States, reaching a maximum between ages fifty-five and seventy-four years. In Denmark the female death rate from diabetes is about one-third higher than the rate for males. In the Netherlands the difference in mortality between the two sexes is most marked; present rates for females are nearly double those for males. In Australia, too, the female rate is greatly in excess of that for males, and in the five-year period ending in 1930 the female rate averaged about two-thirds in excess of the male rate.

The diabetes death rates in Canada, Belgium, Switzerland, Norway and Germany are also higher among females than males. This is true to a lesser degree for Finland.[2] In all countries marked differences in diabetes mortality between the two sexes are limited to

---

[1] Loc. cit., page 33.
[2] Vartiainen and Vartiainen: Acta Med. Scandinav., 119, 364, 1944.

middle and old age. Of the countries for which these detailed data are available, Italy and Japan are exceptions to the rule. In those two countries the rates for males are slightly but not significantly higher than for females.

In Massachusetts between 1901 and 1932 and between 1933 and 1938 one notes a preponderance of males in the first five decades, of females in the sixth and seventh, but unimportant differences in the eighth and ninth.

Wilder *et al.* call attention to the preponderance of males at the Mayo Clinic, situated in Rochester, Minnesota, but this is evidently a localized, clinical experience, because for the entire state of Minnesota for 1943 the deaths from diabetes numbered 291 for males and 485 for females. Both in the urban and rural areas females preponderated. They likewise raise the possibility that the cause for the excess of females in our group and other groups on the eastern area of the United States might be due to the preponderance of Jews. It is true that up to the end of 1928 there was a preponderance of Jewish females of 46.3 per cent over Jewish males, whereas among non-Jewish patients the males preponderated. However, that was a temporary phenomenon, because in a subsequent series of 1000 of our diabetic patients the preponderance of females, both non-Jewish and Jews, is evident, Jewish males 46, females 58; non-Jewish males 372, females 524. And we might add that in New York City in 1931[2] there were 182 male Jewish deaths, female 420; non-Jewish males 192, females 478.

E. MARITAL CONDITION IN RELATION TO DIABETES.

The incidence of diabetes is higher in married women than in single women. This difference is not found in men. Indeed, only among the married is there a large difference between the sexes in regard to the frequency of diabetes. This was shown by Mosenthal and Bolduan,[3] from New York City mortality data, and is confirmed by similar Canadian data in the period from 1928 to 1932.[4]

TABLE 11.—DEATH RATES FOR DIABETES PER 100,000, IN UNITED STATES, 1940 BY SEX AND MARITAL STATUS, CRUDE AND SEX ADJUSTED.

Marital status.	Crude mortality.		Sex adjusted.	
	Male.	Female.	Male.	Female.
Single	12.7	13.7	24.3	23.0
Married	23.7	33.1	22.5	42.2
Widowed	89.5	135.2	30.5	50.4
Divorced	38.4	30.3	34.5	44.4

Table 11 shows for single persons, when adjustments are made for sex, that females are no more prone to diabetes than males, thus

[1] Wilder, Browne and Butt: Arch. Int. Med., **65**, 390, 1940.
[2] Bolduan and Weiner: New England Jour. Med., **208**, 407, 1933.
[3] Mosenthal and Bolduan: Am. Jour. Med. Sci., **186**, 605, 1933.
[4] Joslin, Dublin and Marks: Am. Jour. Med. Sci., **192**, 9, 1936.

conforming to the incidence of diabetes among both sexes up to the age of twenty-five years and almost to thirty-five years. (See Tables 8, 9, 10.) As so many of the single persons come in the younger age groups adjustments also should be made for age. The figures for married, widowed and divorced persons are about what we would expect for older age groups as suggested in Table 2, which records crude and adjusted rates for sex for whites.

In order to adjust for differences in age composition, estimated populations have been computed as no actual populations for 1936 and 1937 are available by marital status and age and sex. Such checks as could be made on this work lead us to believe that our tables are reasonably good and that the rates derived from them are equally good. However, it is possible that slight variations would occur due to faulty estimation. It would be impossible for the error to be sufficiently great to upset the general findings of this table which clearly indicates that there is very little difference between the four classifications in males and the single and divorced in females, but enormous differences in the married and widowed in the females.

Partial confirmation of the findings regarding the higher frequency of diabetes in married women is afforded also by analysis of the facts on the marital condition of the authors' group of patients. These have been tabulated as of the date of examination and compared with the marital distribution of the population of New England in 1920, that year being taken as an approximate mean. On this basis, there was a sizeable deficiency from ages 45 on in the proportion of single persons in this diabetic group, as compared with the general population, both among men and women, but more especially among women. At ages under 45, this relationship did not exist, for the proportion of single persons was higher among the diabetics at ages 20 to 24, and among women not greatly different at ages 25 to 44. This is not altogether surprising. To some extent, this is explained partly by the hesitation of young diabetics to marry, but to a far greater extent by the relatively large number of persons in this diabetic group from families in comfortable circumstances, where marriage tends to be delayed.

Mosenthal and Bolduan[1] suggest that the effect of pregnancy on the carbohydrate tolerance is a factor in the higher incidence of diabetes in married women. This accounts, however, for only part of the difference because diabetes even in married women usually has its onset many years after childbearing has ceased. More important than pregnancy itself would seem to be the effect of overfeeding and underexercise during and after pregnancy. Women usually gain weight during this period, some a considerable amount, and all or a large part of the added weight is often retained. Some

[1] Mosenthal and Bolduan: Loc. cit., p. 37.

indication of this is found in comparing the weights of single and married diabetic women. Among 1326 married women in this group[1] with onset of diabetes after 45, the average weight was 181 pounds, compared to only 161 pounds for 111 single women. No difference, however, was found in the average weights of childless and fertile married women. Another factor in the difference between the single and married women is the generally better economic status of the married. That means more frequent overnutrition and a greater probability of acquiring diabetes as indicated by the weight figures just quoted. It also means more medical care and a greater probability of correct diagnosis of the disease when it occurs.

As for the difference in the frequency of diabetes between married men and women, the extremely rapid increase in the frequency of onset among women in the late forties or fifties reflects the strain on the endocrine system during menopause. According to Rony[2] women maintain an almost even rate of gaining—0.6 to 0.7 pounds a year—between twenty-five and fifty years; there is no significant change in this rate during the menopausal period.

F.   TOTAL NUMBER OF DIABETICS IN THE UNITED STATES.

For the total number of diabetics in the United States no accurate figures are available. Although in 1943 one death out of each 40 deaths in the country was assigned to diabetes, one should not assume that 2.5 per cent of the population of 140,000,000, or 3,500,000, have or will have the disease before they die. Based on other reasoning, however, Spiegelman and Marks[3] of the Statistical Department of the Metropolitan Life Insurance Company estimate that 3,873,000 individuals now living eventually will have diabetes. According to these statisticians, the outlook for the next few decades is that the number of diabetics will increase at a much greater rate than the population, and that the problem of diabetes will gain in importance. If it is assumed that the course of the diabetes prevalence rates according to sex and age, as observed in the National Health Survey remain unchanged, then it is expected that the number of diabetics will increase 18 per cent in the decade from 1940 to 1950, while the total population may grow only by 9 per cent. Present indications are that our total population will be at a maximum about 1985, when it will be 22 per cent greater than it was in 1940;[4] however, over the same time the diabetic population may increase by 74 per cent.

The author is not unmindful of the various surveys conducted to

---

[1] Joslin: Bull. New York Acad. Med., **9**, 532, 1933.

[2] Rony: Obesity and Leanness, Philadelphia, Lea & Febiger, page 109, 1940.

[3] Spiegelman and Marks: Loc. cit., p. 29.

[4] These estimates are based upon the "medium" forecast of population published by Thompson and Whelpton in Estimates of the Future Population of the United States, 1940–2000, National Resources Planning Board, Washington, D. C., Table 7, page 68.

determine the incidence of diabetes in the country or of the opinions of outstanding statisticians. These will be presented in detail below, but first of all he will give his own estimate and his reasons therefor.

I believe there are 1,000,000 diabetics in the United States in 1946. Whenever in the past I have made an estimate of diabetes in the population, it has later proved to be too low. My friends, the statisticians, depending upon various sources of information have reached lower figures. Thus data obtained in the Massachusetts Survey of 1929–1931 by Bigelow and Lombard[1] applied to today would yield 560,000; the National Health Survey[2] of 1935-1936 projected to 1943 would be 725,000 and the careful estimate of Herbert H. Marks[3] of the Statistical Department of the Metropolitan Life Insurance Company is 675,000.

The crux of any estimates depends upon four variable factors. First, how closely the statistical death rates represent those who die with diabetes but not of it. Obviously, a diabetic dying of cancer escapes statistical enumeration. Second, for each diabetic death how many shall one conclude alive or what shall be taken as the average duration of the disease? I assume fifteen years. Third, crude and adjusted (for age and sex) death rates differ widely in the same state and in different sections of the country. Vermont, a state with older people, has a crude rate of 33.7 and an adjusted rate of 27 diabetic deaths per 100,000 in 1940. Arizona, a state with a younger population, has a crude rate of 11, an adjusted rate of 14.3. Fourth, statistical reports in certain states are more accurate than in others. Arizona had a death rate of one-fourth that of Rhode Island by crude computation, one-third by adjusted computation. For morbidity calculations for a single state I would choose the crude rates for that state, but when depending upon calculations for the entire country, based upon death rates for the ten states with the highest mortalities, the age adjusted average rate would be more conservative. I went to Arizona and I found the true incidence of living diabetics was practically the same as on the eastern seaboard.

Therefore, in computing the number of diabetics in the country, I base my estimate on (*a*) the average death rate for 1940 in those 10 states with the highest mortalities rather than in those 10 states where it is lowest, assuming that the more correctly reported and compiled figures are those of the 10 states with the highest mortalities; (*b*) the use of adjusted instead of crude ratios; (*c*) a duration of the disease of fifteen years and (*d*) a correction of death rates by the Lombard and Joslin factors of 1936[4] and 1946 in which of 754 of my diabetic patients dying in Massachusetts, only 62.9 per cent

[1] Bigelow and Lombard: Cancer and Other Chronic Diseases in Massachusetts, Boston, Houghton Mifflin Company, 1933.
[2] Loc. cit., p. 33.
[3] Marks: New Eng. Jour. Med., **235**, 289, 1946.
[4] Joslin and Lombard: Loc. cit., p. 23.

were reported statistically as having died of diabetes in the first series and 64.9 per cent of 1000 successive deaths in the second series, or approximately two-thirds of the total number who died with the disease. Thus one can assume for computation purposes the Lombard and Joslin correction adds 50 per cent. The average correction for the two series would be 63.9 per cent. The computation is as follows:

The average death rate of the 10 states with highest diabetic mortalities in the United States for 1940 was 32.9 adjusted and 35.3 crude per 100,000, and for the 10 states with lowest mortalities 15.3 adjusted and 13.0 crude per 100,000. Applying to this 32.9 adjusted rate the Lombard and Joslin correction of 50 per cent we have a rate of 52.6 diabetic deaths per 100,000, or for the present population of 140,000,000, the deaths would be 73,600. If diabetics are living fifteen years there would be 1,100,000 diabetics. Moreover, there would also be a considerable number of diabetics besides who were never diagnosed as such. Indeed, in one series of 500 cases, the disease had existed 5.4 months on the average before it was first recognized. In a forthcoming diabetic number of the Medical Clinics of North America, R. D. Lawrence will contribute a paper on Symptomless Glycosuria. These calculations lead me to conclude the number of diabetics in the country today is at least 1,000,000.

Sickness surveys in various parts of the country allow an estimate of the incidence of diabetes. Of these, the first extensive one was that of Bigelow and Lombard of the Massachusetts Department of Public Health.[1] From their investigation it was concluded that in 1931 there were 15,000 diabetics in Massachusetts or nearly 4 cases of the disease per 1000 inhabitants. If the incidence of 4 per 1000 registered in Massachusetts prevailed throughout the country the number of diabetics in the 140,000,000 population of the United States in 1946 would be 560,000. In 1931 the crude diabetic death rate for Massachusetts was 20.4, but in 1940 it had reached 35.7 per 100,000, the adjusted figure being 29.8 for 1940.

According to the National Health Survey[2] conducted during the winter of 1935–1936 under the auspices of the United States Public Health Service in which approximately 2,502,391 persons were interviewed, 9182 cases of diabetes were discovered, or about 3½ per thousand. Applying the rates by sex and age to the country as a whole, the resulting estimate for the total diabetics in the country was about 450,000 as of 1937 and with certain further adjustments which the authors made, their estimate was 660,000, or for the 1946 population of 140,000,000 is raised to 725,000.

A third estimate by Herbert H. Marks[3] of the Statistical Department of the Metropolitan Life Insurance Company places the number at 675,000. He arrives at this figure by citing that in 1940

[1] Bigelow and Lombard: Loc. cit., p. 40.
[2] Loc. cit., p. 33.
[3] Marks: Loc. cit., p. 40.

there were 35,015 persons dying in the United States in which diabetes was the primary cause of death. There were an additional 3991 deaths, or 11 per cent, more in which diabetes was the secondary cause, making in all 39,006 individuals who died with diabetes. Recognizing that even these deaths are an understatement because of the findings of Lombard and Joslin, he considers it conservative to add a correction of 25 per cent, thus raising the total mortality of persons dying with diabetes up to 45,000 annually. Multiplying the total deaths by 15 as representing the duration of life of the average diabetic today, he concludes that the total number of living diabetics in the country is 675,000. The same writer estimates that there are about 50,000 new cases of diabetes developing or discovered yearly and that this number may rise as high as 75,000 and, therefore, concludes that there is a net increase of at least 10,000 diabetics a year, although it may reach as high as 30,000.

An argument for the increasing number of diabetics in the country was formerly based on the diabetic admissions to hospitals. These grew rapidly but recently have fallen because of the scarcity of hospital beds. As a matter of fact, in a little frame house opposite the Deaconess Hospital, with crowded capacity for 14 patients, about one-fourth as many diabetics were treated in a year as in the Deaconess Hospital, because in the hospital the cases remain far longer because of serious complications.

Another type of estimate of living diabetics in our midst has been made. Diabetes and transient glycosuria in 45,650 consecutive selectees and volunteers aged eighteen to forty-five years in the Boston Armed Forces Induction Station were studied by Blotner and Hyde.[1] They found the incidence of diabetes was approximately three to four times that of the National Health Survey canvass. In contrast to the Health Survey, which was a house-to-house interrogative canvass, Blotner and Hyde's estimates were based on examinations of the urine one or more times and often on tests of the blood. The cases of diabetes found numbered 208, those of transient glycosuria 126 and of renal glycosuria, as interpreted by the authors, 33.

The average age of the diabetic patients was 34.4 years, the control group averaging 27.5 years. Incidentally, the diabetic selectees weighed on the average 158 pounds, about 18 pounds above the weights of 1000 consecutive selectees, and were of normal average height. A diabetic heredity was about six times as frequent in the diabetic patients. There were twice as many Jews and half again as many Irish in the diabetic group as in the control group.

To these studies I attach great importance, but before they are accepted as typical of the country as a whole, one should compare them with data similarly collected in other sections. Furthermore, it is a question whether the increased incidence, namely, three to four times that of the same age group, eighteen to forty-five years,

---

[1] Blotner and Hyde: New England Jour. Med., **229**, 885, 1943. For a critical review of this article see Editorial, Jour. Am. Med. Assn., **124**, 1062, 1944.

obtained by the National Health Survey, will apply to individuals under eighteen or over forty-five years. At any rate, studies of this nature may alter our entire conception of the incidence of diabetes in the country.

A survey of a similar nature in the New Orleans area by Spellberg and Leff[1] did not confirm the high incidence obtained in the district around Boston, but a subsequent survey of 69,088 selectees between the ages of eighteen and thirty-seven years in the Boston area by Blotner[2] has revealed a confirmation of the original findings. Blotner explains the difference between their results and those obtained in Louisiana in part on the ground that local boards screened out the diabetics in the latter State before they underwent final selective service examinations.

In this second study, the number of selectees with glycosuria was 2 per cent (1383 cases) and the number with diabetes 1.1 per cent, the latter figure being even greater than that found in the first survey.

The relatively high incidence of diabetes in the Canadian French and the Irish, about twice that of the controls, was striking. The rate for Jewish selectees in this second series was low, presumably due to their previous knowledge of the existence of glycosuria or diabetes. Of the 251 diabetics found in 479 tolerance tests, all except 39 had normal fasting blood sugar levels and in nearly all the fasting urines were sugar free. In this group of 1383 selectees with glycosuria a family history of diabetes was obtained in 24.3 per cent as compared with 5.2 per cent of a group of non-diabetic selectees.

Blotner's figures for the incidence of glycosuria in selectees find confirmation compiled in a study of the National Youth Administration.[3] Among 147,813 youths, ages fifteen to twenty-four, glycosuria was present in 2.6 per cent. There were 178 known diabetics. Negro youths had glycosuria more frequently than white youths, the incidence being 3.5 per cent in the negroes as compared with 2.4 per cent of the white youths. The glycosuria was recorded as slight in 3164 or 2.2 per cent of the cases, of medium degree in 335 or 0.2 per cent and marked in 235 or 0.2 per cent.

G. URBAN AND RURAL MORTALITY FROM DIABETES IN THE UNITED STATES.

Diabetes mortality in the cities and towns is usually much higher than in the country-side. In the United States, in 1940, the crude death-rate in the urban part of the registration states was 32.2 per 100,000, but only 19.3 in the rural areas. Thus, for the country as a whole, the excess of the urban rate in recent years has been approximately 67 per cent. This situation is a very general one. In only four states did the death rate in the rural areas exceed

[1] Spellberg and Leff: Jour. Am. Med. Assn., **129**, 246, 1945.
[2] Blotner: Jour. Am. Med. Assn., **131**, 1109, 1946.
[3] The Health Status of NYA Youth, Washington, U. S. Government Printing Office, 1942.

that in the cities during the two-year period, 1928 to 1929.   In these cases an exceptionally high proportion of old persons in the rural population or of young persons in the urban population is a prime reason for the excess of the rural rates.   The higher incidence of diabetes in urban areas, indicated by the mortality figures, was confirmed by the Massachusetts survey of chronic illness.   The trend of diabetes mortality in the cities of this country has been sharply upward; in the rural part it has been much steadier, and the authors believe it will continue to increase in the country rather rapidly as the upward tendency in the cities begins to slow down.

In the year 1943 the 10 states with the highest mortalities were in general the states with the highest urban population, namely, those in the New England and Middle Atlantic areas, in contrast to the 10 states with the lowest mortalities, for the most part the Southern states or those states most sparsely settled.   The low mortality recorded in the Southern states cannot be explained by the large negro population.

Particularly in cities over 100,000 inhabitants is the urban rate larger than the rural, yet regardless of the size of the city, the rates are higher than in the rural areas.   In 1940 the adjusted urban rate was over one and one-half times as high as the rural rate.

H.   RACE AND DIABETES MELLITUS.

The high incidence of diabetes in Jews is proverbial, but it is not so well known that a high mortality exists among the Irish. Mills,[1] who resided in China for two years, observed that among the Chinese diabetes was relatively infrequent and mild in character. He also quotes others on the rarity and mildness of the disease in Japan, the Philippines, India, the Sudan, West Africa and Venezuela. In the East it is reported with frequency only among the wealthy and leisured classes.   Bose,[2] who has described his experience with diabetes in India, does not believe the adoption of western diets a factor.   He points out the frequency of the disease in Bengal, especially among the large well-educated classes, among 2000 cases treated by him in India.   Hindus constituted 68.2 per cent, Mohammedans 14.6 per cent, other castes 2.1 per cent and Europeans (including Anglo-Indians) 15.1 per cent.   He also records a table for Calcutta in which the rate per 100,000 rose from 5.2 in 1929 to 10.4 in 1933 and to 20.7 in 1934.

Incidence of Diabetes Among Negroes.—Negroes appeared at one time to be almost immune to diabetes.   Today the mortality is only a little higher among the whites than among the colored.

[1] Mills: Arch. Int. Med., **46**, 569, 1930.
[2] Bose: A Handbook on Diabetes Mellitus and Its Modern Treatment, 2d ed., Calcutta, Thacker, Spink & Co., 1939.

In 1940, if adjustments are made for sex and age, the white diabetic death rate was but 15 per cent above the colored. Under fifty-five years at most ages the colored rates were actually higher, but after fifty-five years the white rates went ahead, and among older people the white rates are double those of the colored. Among females as a whole, irrespective of age, the white rates are 3 per cent higher than the colored and among males the white rates are nearly 40 per cent higher.

In 1940 the rate for all races in the United States was 26.6, for the whites 27.6, for the negroes 18. The percentage of deaths from diabetes to all causes was 2.6 for the whites but 1.3 for the negroes. In 1941–1943 for the Metropolitan Life Insurance Company Industrial Department, the rates per 100,000 were for all ages (one to seventy-four years) for males, white 12.9, negroes 12.9; for females, white 26.1, negroes 26.6.

In the period 1936–1938, according to the Metropolitan Life Insurance Company's experience, the rate of colored men at ages twenty-five to thirty-four years exceeded that of whites by 48 per cent; at ages thirty-five to forty-four years by 39 per cent; and at ages forty-five to fifty-four years by 22.4 per cent. Among females the differences were even greater. At ages twenty-five to thirty-four years, negro rates exceeded the white by 100 per cent; at ages thirty-five to forty-four years by 197.1 per cent; and at ages forty-five to fifty-four years by 80.7 per cent. In old age, rates of colored persons of both sexes were much below those for whites.

In 1940 more negroes were reported to have died of diabetes in New York (158) and Pennsylvania (172) than in any other states. In 1940 deaths from diabetes among negroes in the United States numbered 2310, males 716, females 1594. The peak age for mortality was fifty-five to sixty-four years. For white individuals the peak age for males and females was sixty-five to seventy-four years, or ten years older.

The negroes again contradict the assumption of a racial element in the origin of diabetes. Information concerning the incidence of diabetes in Africa is scanty. In the Southern states the rate is moderately low but relatively high.

Leopold[1] summarized the literature prior to 1931 of diabetes in the negro race. He says that in 1930 the death-rate of diabetes in Baltimore for negroes was 30.01 per 100,000, and for whites 28.02. On the other hand, white deaths from diabetes were 2.36 of all deaths, and negro deaths were 0.96. He noted that 86 per cent of the older negro females were obese. Syphilis did not play an etiological part in the cause or progress of the disease. Gangrene was seen only four times in 100 cases. Cataracts occurred in 15 per cent of the cases. He clearly foresaw that diabetes in negroes is not different in any way from the disease as found among white people.

[1] Leopold: Ann. Int. Med., 5, 285, 1931.

However, for the six years 1939–1944 the death rate per 100,000 for white people averaged 37.9 per 100,000 and for negroes 21.9.

In Baltimore for the six years 1939–1944 inclusive the average total death rate has been 34.9 per 100,000, but of whites 37.9 and of negroes only 22.

Incidence of Diabetes Among Jews.—According to Ernst Lyon[1] the Jewish race is not a pure race but has had many, many mixtures throughout the years and, therefore, it is hardly correct to attribute the increase in diabetes in Jews to a racial origin. He emphasizes the necessity for the standardization of statistics because the Jewish population is older due to a smaller number of children. The possibilities of obesity and in-breeding must be considered. Furthermore, the social status and occupations are factors. Lyon cites German statistics in which the mortality in Jews as compared with non-Jews in Germany was lower than had generally been considered. Of the 393,000 Jews in Germany in 1936, as estimated by E. Kahn,[2] 87,000 were over sixty years of age and one-half under forty-four years of age—an old group as compared to the Jews in Palestine that same year. There among 395,000 there were 17,000 over sixty years and one-half of the total under twenty years of age. Lyon also discussed the percentage of Jews among diabetic children. In our own group of 2191 diabetic children the percentage of Jews is 8, whereas the percentage of Jews in a recent 5000 cases of true diabetes (all ages) is 16.2.

The number of Jews in the United States has increased rapidly since the beginning of the century. In 1900 it is estimated their number was somewhat more than 1,000,000. Current estimates range from $4\frac{1}{4}$ to over 5,000,000. Today they constitute about 3.5 per cent of the population as compared with 1.3 per cent in 1900. The number of Jews in New York City is now estimated to exceed 2,000,000. The immigrant Jew was young, and only in the past decade or so have there been significant numbers in the older age groups in which diabetes is most frequent. In 1931 Bolduan and Weiner[3] found the proportion of diabetic deaths at all ages was nearly 80 per cent higher among Jews than among non-Jews. Under the age of forty-five years there was only a slight excess in the proportion of diabetes deaths among Jews. The proportion of diabetes deaths to total deaths among Jewish women between the ages fifty-five and sixty-four years reached the amazing figure of 11.5 per cent. From a study of diabetes deaths in Boston, between 1895 and 1913, Morrison[4] demonstrated that diabetes was nearly twice and a half as common among Jews.

The proportion of Jewish to total patients among one group of

[1] Lyon: Diabetes Mellitus and the Jewish Race, Jerusalem, Ludwig Mayer, 1940.
[2] Kahn: Jüd. Rundschau, vol. **41**, 1936.
[3] Bolduan and Weiner: Loc. cit., p. 37.
[4] Morrison: Boston Med. and Surg. Jour., **175**, 54, 1916.

6357 cases of the authors' series varied widely by sex and age. For all ages Jewish males constituted 11.6 per cent of all male patients, but females 16.3 of all female patients. Among males, the proportion of Jewish patients to total patients was relatively small at the younger ages of onset, but increased to the maximum of 18.9 per cent in the late thirties. Among females the proportion of Jewish patients is larger at every age than among the males. Even at the younger ages at onset, the proportion of Jewish females was well over 10 per cent and increased to a maximum of 24.2 per cent in the late thirties. Among 5000 of our new cases of diabetes in the immediate past, Jews constituted 810, or 16.2 per. cent. Of these, 429 were males, 53 per cent, and 381 were females, 47 per cent. In adults the greater number of Jews in the diabetic population appears to the authors understandable, first, because among them obesity is more frequent (see page 71), and second, because among the Jewish patients, both young and old, the incidence of heredity is higher than in the non-Jewish portion of our clientèle. See footnote, 1. E., page 22.

The age at onset of the authors' own Jewish cases compiled a few years ago both for males and females was somewhat different from that of other patients. The Jewish patients developed diabetes relatively early. The maximum numerical frequency of onset of diabetes in Jewish males was between forty and forty-four, compared with fifty and fifty-four years for all male patients. See Table 7 in Article D, Footnote page 22. In Jewish female patients, equal numbers of onsets were recorded in age periods forty-five to forty-nine and fifty to fifty-four years; whereas among all female patients the onset peak was definitely at ages fifty to fifty-four. The median age at onset of the Jewish patients was slightly over two years less than that of all patients.

In Koranyi's Clinic in Budapest, according to Benedict and St. Kemény,[1] the percentage of Jews is 23, which is also that of the Jews in Budapest, but of the diabetics 45 per cent are Jewish. Diabetic heredity was observed in 10.3 per cent among the non-Jewish portion of the clinic but reached 33.8 per cent among the Jews.

Irish.—A surprising feature is the high mortality found among the Irish. Recent data are not available. It has been generally assumed that the diabetes rate among the Irish was low. The basis for this assumption is probably the low diabetes rate prevailing in Ireland and the high mortality which the Irish suffer from tuberculosis. That high tuberculosis rates are associated with low diabetes rates and *vice versa* is an impression very general but not altogether well founded. The reason for the high diabetes mortality of the Irish here is not far to seek. The level of well-being and prosperity among the Irish in this country is far higher than in Ireland itself. Another item—not a negligible one—is that at the time covered in these

[1] Benedict and St. Kemény: Wiener Arch. f. inn. Med., **28**, 87, **1935**.

studies, a disproportionate number of the Irish engaged in the liquor business, an occupation in which diabetes mortality is exceptionally heavy.[1]

In contrast to data for Pennsylvania and New York are those for northern Ireland for 1941, where the death rate was 10.9 and the Irish Free State, 7.9

North American Indians.—(See page 25.) In 1945 there were 44 deaths from diabetes among the estimated 236,639 Indians (1.9 per 100,000).

I. INCIDENCE OF DIABETES IN OTHER COUNTRIES.

World conditions have prevented the compilation of detailed statistics in the last five years. Therefore, I consider myself fortunate to present data in Tables 13 and 14 assembled by Dr. Halbert L. Dunn and Mr. Frank S. Morrison of the United States Bureau of the Census in Washington. From other sources, and especially through the kindness of Mr. Herbert H. Marks, I have been able to gather fragmentary data to supplement the above.

Throughout the world the increase in diabetic mortality is obvious no matter whether countries or cities are compared. The United States leads in the frequency of the disease attributable in large measure, the authors trust, to a closer study of the inhabitants and our system of reporting disease. However, the change in the death-rates for diabetes at fifty-five years and over is even greater in England and Wales, Scotland and Denmark than in this country. It is notable that in Japan the disease doubled between 1910 and 1930, 1.8 to 3.5 per 100,000, in contrast to the United States, in which it increased only 36 per cent, and in New Zealand 27 per cent. In these same twenty years in the Netherlands it rose 77.7 per cent, and in Italy[2] 74.4 per cent, but in northern Ireland it decreased 10 per cent, a circumstance which makes that country almost unique; the rate has also fallen in Norway and the Netherlands, a circumstance it was hoped the 1940 census might explain.

In Germany, likewise, great interest was shown in the incidence of diabetes prior to the last war. A survey by Gottschalk of the whole population of Stettin, a city of 268,000 inhabitants, disclosed 640 diabetics (2.37 per 1000). On the basis of this study, the number of diabetics in Germany has been estimated to be 150,000. In 1938, during a vist to Germany by the senior author, as a result of con-

---

[1] Joslin, Dublin and Marks: Loc. cit., p. 22, 1 B.

[2] Coluzzi (Difesa Sociale, **18**, 577, 1939) states that in Italy the mortality-rate for diabetes increased from 1.8 per 100,000 in 1887–79 to 10 in 1935–37. All 18 provinces showed an increased rate from the year 1930 onward. The period 1935–37 compared with 1900–02 showed an increase in diabetic mortality for females of 333 per cent and for males 123 per cent. The increase was greatest in the age period over sixty-five years where the percentage increase was 297. Although the general death-rate in Italy has fallen from 30.5 per 1000 inhabitants for the period 1872–75 to 13.7 in 1936, due chiefly to the decline of deaths in childhood, a great increase in mortality ates for diseases of later life and especially diabetes has occurred.

versations with various reliable clinicians, he estimated the number of diabetics to be 300,000.

As for the diabetics in the United Kingdom, instead of an earlier figure of 70,000, R. D. Lawrence, in a personal note in 1939 writes, ". . . if asked to guess dogmatically would say somewhere in the nature of 150,000 to 200,000."

In Vienna the increase in fatal cases of diabetes from 1926 to 1935 was nearly 85 per cent, but wholly confined to the older ages.[1]

Canada shows an increase in diabetic mortality akin to that in the United States, but the population is younger. Furthermore, in certain provinces it labors under the same handicaps as were seen operative in Arizona, being sparsely settled and less favorably situated for the collection of accurate statistics. However, the rise in diabetic mortality per 100,000 has been, exclusive of the province of Quebec, from 9.5 in 1921 and 11.2 in 1926 to 19.5 in 1944; for the province of Quebec[2] for similar years provisional figures are 10.9 to 20 (1944). In 1942[3] the rate (provisional) for the whole of Canada without the Yukon and the Northwest Territories was 19.3 per 100,000. Even more striking have been the increases in Montreal, Toronto and Quebec. These are given in Table 12 and along with them for comparison death rates for certain cities in the United States and elsewhere.

TABLE 12.—DEATH RATES PER 100,000 FROM DIABETES
IN VARIOUS CITIES OF THE WORLD.

City.	1920.	Latest year available.
New York City	23.4	40.2 (1945)*
Philadelphia	18.2	37.0 (1945)*
Chicago	20.4	35.9 (1943)*
Boston	24.3	35.1 (1945)*
Montreal	12.0	29.0 (1945)*
Toronto	10.5	29.5 (1944)*
Quebec	8.8	17.7 (1942)*
Tokyo	2.2	2.5 (1937)
Greater Melbourne	16.4 (1932)	21.0 (1942)
Aukland†	13.0 (1926)	28.2 (1941)
Wellington†	10.7 (1926)	16.2 (1941)
London	8.0	11.0 (1941), civilians only
Berlin	10.9	19.8 (1937)
Copenhagen	15.7	28.3 (1940)
Paris	9.6	10.4 (1937)
Rome	18.3 (1930)	19.7 (1938)
Havana	8.4	14.2 (1941)
Buenos Aires	10.5	15.0 (1943)
Rio de Janeiro	7.8 (1922)	8.9 (1937)

* Provisional or estimated.
† Excluding Maioris.

[1] Fürth, E.: Münch. med. Wchnschr., II, 1259, 1936.
[2] Quebec not in Canadian Health Regulation Area until 1926.
[3] In 1944, 19.7 (Provisional).

4

The divergencies of death rates in countries where one would expect similarities deserve explanation. Why should Norway have a rate of 14.3 per 100,000 (1940), and Sweden 6.8 (1042), Denmark 19.1 (1942), Belgium 19.1 (1941) and the Netherlands 14 (1939 provisional)? The rate for civilians for nothern Ireland in 1941

TABLE 13.—POPULATION, DEATHS FROM ALL CAUSES AND FROM DIABETES, AND DEATH RATES FOR DIABETES: SPECIFIED COUNTRIES, LATEST AVAILABLE YEAR.

(Exclusive of still-births. By place of occurence. Rates are the number of deaths from diabetes per 100,000 population.)

Country.	Year.	Population.	Deaths from all causes.	Deaths from diabetes. No.	Deaths from diabetes. Rate.
United States[1]	1943	133,966,319	1,459,544	36,314	27.1
Australia[2]	1943	7,229,864*[3]	74,486[4]	1,504[4]	20.8*
Austria	1937	6,755,337	89,868	816	12.1
Belgium[5]	1941	8,257,392	121,134[6,7]	1,578	19.1
Canada[8]	1942	11,637,000	112,978	2,242	19.3
Cuba	1936	4,046,706	44,892[6]	190	4.7
Czechoslovakia	1937	15,239,000	202,359	1,867	12.3
Denmark[9]	1942	3,903,000	37,527	747	19.1
England and Wales	1944	42,449,000*[10]	492,188*[11]	4,063*[11]	9.6*
France	1936	41,907,056	642,318[6]	4,291	10.2
Irish Free State	1943	2,949,713*	43,494	232	7.9*
Italy	1942	45,400,000*	641,988*[12]	4,526*	10.0*
Japan (proper)	1938	72,222,700	1,259,805	3,043	4.2
Netherlands	1939	8,778,989	75,863*[6]	1,226*	14.0*
New Zealand [13,14]	1942	1,545,112	16,385	352	22.8
Northern Ireland[15]	1941	1,288,000	19,640	141	10.9
Norway	1940	2,953,028	32,045	423	14.3
Prussia	..	....	....	...	...
Russia	..	....	....	...	...
Scotland	1944	5,006,700*[16]	64,603*[7]	543*	10.8*
Spain[17]	1942	26,244,164*	384,749*[6]	1,718*	6.5*
Sweden	1942	6,432,337	63,741	437	6.8
Switzerland	1939	4,205,600	49,484	586	13.9
Union of South Africa[18]	1939	2,116,500	19,901	266	12.6

* Provisional. (....) data not available.
[1] Excludes data for armed forces overseas.
[2] Exclusive of full-blood aboriginals.
[3] Includes defense personnel, irrespective of location.
[4] Excludes deaths of defense personnel.
[5] Excludes data for 41 communes of Eupen, Malmedy, and Moresnet districts, not under Belgian administration.
[6] Excludes deaths of infants born alive but dying before registration of birth.
[7] Includes war losses, i. e., military and civilian deaths due to war.
[8] Exclusive of data for Yukon and the Northwest Territories.
[9] Exclusive of Faroe Islands.
[10] Includes armed forces and merchant seamen at home and abroad.
[11] Includes armed forces in home country and deaths of civilians due to war.
[12] Excludes war losses, i. e., military and civilian deaths due to war.
[13] Exclusive of Maoris.
[14] Excludes data for armed forces overseas and visiting servicemen and prisoners of war in New Zealand.
[15] Civilians only.
[16] 1939 midyear population.
[17] Includes Balearic and Canary Islands.
[18] European population only.

Source: Data taken from official vital statistics reports and year-books for each country. Rates computed in the Bureau of the Census.

was 10.9 and the provisional rate for the Irish Free State in 1943, 7.9, yet the Irish in this country rank high in diabetic morbidity. I cannot understand the reasons for the low provisional rates in Scotland, 10.8 (1944) and England and Wales, 9.6 (1944) per 100,000. Local surveys in many of these lands similar to that conducted by the Public Health Service here in 1936–1937 or by the senior author in Arizona would certainly help to calrify the situation. I wonder if polls of diabetic heredity in an audience outside of the United States would show as here that one in four of those present had a diabetic relative. As I recall, this is what I found to be true on a small scale in Norway and Sweden.

The Vartiainens[1] have estimated the number of diabetics in Finland and at the same time noted the variations in distribution according to age and sex. They reached the conclusion that in 1942 the number of diabetics was 5800, or 1.6 per 1000 of the total population, which is reported as 3,637,354. These figures are really estimates based largely upon the number of individuals receiving additional rations on account of diabetes, but are incomplete to this extent, that a certain percentage of the inquiries remained unanswered by the local Supply Committees and, secondly, because persons belonging to households with their own food supplies, chiefly in the country, did not receive any ration cards. According to the statistical data collected by the Ministry of Supply there were 2773 diabetics in Finland. By adding to these the estimated number of diabetics living in the area in which the inquiries remained unanswered, they obtained the figure 2834. Further, by adding to this figure those whose occupations were on farms, as compared with the total population, they increased the number of diabetics to their final estimate of 5800.

The total diabetic mortality in Finland from 1927 to 1941 showed a steady increase. The deaths among males have remained nearly stationary, but those among females have nearly doubled, the deaths being confined chiefly to those fifty years of age or above. The recent mortality figures show that the diabetic mortality has again decreased to the level of the years 1933–1935 and that the decrease chiefly concerns women, fifty years old and older. This decrease is attributed to the decrease in foodstuffs. People lost considerably in weight, particularly in the year 1942; for instance, in Helsinki often from 10 to 15 kilos.

Statistics in the nations of Central and South America are meager in the first place, in the second are again handicapped by a sparsely settled and scattered population, predominantly rural, deficient in medical supervision and of a distinctly younger character. With these factors in mind, and with appreciation of the courtesy of the Department of Commerce, Bureau of the Census, Mr. Herbert H. Marks and others attention is called to Table 14.

[1] Vartiainen and Vartiainen: Loc. cit., p. 36.

TABLE 14.—POPULATION, DEATHS FROM ALL CAUSES AND FROM DIABETES, AND
DEATH RATES FOR DIABETES: LATIN AMERICAN
REPUBLICS, LATEST AVAILABLE YEAR.

(Exclusive of still-births. By place of occurrence. Rates are the number of deaths
from diabetes per 100,000 population.)

Country.	Year.	Population.	Deaths from all causes.	Deaths from diabetes. No.	Deaths from diabetes. Rate.
Argentina	1936	12,562,262	150,149	885	7.0
Argentina (territories) . .	1941	702,234	11,982	46	6.6
Argentina (Buenos Aires) .	1943	2,457,494	28,670	368	15.0
Bolivia[1]	1940	3,457,000	13,177	9	0.3
Brazil (21 capital cities) .	1943	5,734,810*[2]	113,528*	562*	9.8*
Chile	1940	5,023,539	107,771	216	4.3
Colombia	1940	9,206,283	137,786	209	2.3
Costa Rica	1940	656,129	11,211	27	4.1
Cuba	1936	4,046,706	44,892	190	4.7
Dominican Republic[1] . .	1942	1,854,526	15,670	39	2.1
Ecuador	..	....	....	...	...
El Salvador	1943	1,896,168	38,366	42	2.2
Guatemala[3]	1943	3,450,732	77,837	23	0.7
Haiti[1]	1943	3,000,000	15,233	15	0.5
Honduras[4]	1943	1,173,032	23,391	9	0.8
Mexico	1941	20,520,810*	428,250*	793*	3.9*
Nicaragua	1942	1,030,700	17,186	22	2.1
Panama[5]	1943	601,200	8,248	31	5.2
Paraguay (25 biodemographic districts)[6]	1942	418,444	4,611	14	3.3
Peru	..	....	....	...	...
Uruguay	1942	2,202,936	20,646	123	5.6
Venezuela[7]	1943	4,003,707	64,131	98	2.4

* Provisional. (. . . .) data not available.

[1] Reported rates are not to be considered a measure of the true level of mortality because of the extreme incompleteness of death registration.

[2] 1941 population.

[3] Data are for period December 1 to November 30.

[4] Data are for year ending June 30.

[5] Excludes data for tribal Indians.

[6] Includes those districts in which there are established hospitals, health centers, dispensaries, or health units which are under the supervision of the *Ministerio de salud publica*, and which report to that agency.

[7] Excludes data for Indian tribes and Federal Dependencies.

Source: Data taken from official vital statistics reports and year-books for each country. Rates computed in the Bureau of the Census.

Argentina illustrates various factors just cited. As a whole in 1936 the rate was 7 per 100,000 and in the territories in 1941 it was essentially the same, 6.6, but in Buenos Aires, a city of 2,457,494, in 1943, the mortality was 15. This figure is the highest in the entire table.

Among the nations illustrative of a low mortality is Guatemala, where the rate for 1943 was 0.7 per 100,000. From information otherwise obtained, I learn that there are 300 physicians in Guatemala with a population somewhat over 3,000,000. Two hundred and twenty of these physicians practice in Guatemala City, which has a population of about 220,000. This leaves 80 physicians for the remaining 2,800,000 inhabitants. Moreover, this rural part of the population consists of about 70 to 75 per cent Indians. A visit to the General Hospital in Guatemala City revealed no case of diabetes, although its capacity was 1200 beds. However, I am assured by my friend, Dr. José Fajardo, who was in our clinic for a year, and also by patients that diabetes is not uncommon in the upper economic group.

In Costa Rica, likewise, the diagnosis of diabetes was extremely rare in the 1300 bed General Hospital. The physicians explained that the patients were from the low economic group and subsisted on an extremely low calorie diet—even below 1000 calories, and that their emotional level was extremely low.

Mexico is a huge country and factors already cited as fundamental in influencing the diabetic death rate hold here as well. The rate per 100,000 for 1941 was 3.9. Here again in the population of the General Hospital diabetes was rare, although a physician on service may see many patients in private practice. However, even among the latter the disease is apt to be mild. Although a scarcity of physicians existed and laboratory facilities were less than desired, it was evident that a phenomenal expansion along medical lines was in progress.

The figures for Cuba show a considerable increase in diabetic mortality. For the years 1933–1934 the average rate was 4.3 and for 1943–1944 it rose to 5.3 per 100,000, an increase of 23 per cent.

In 1942 the death rate from diabetes in the Dominican Republic is given as 2.1 per 100,000.

Data for Belgium during the recent war, when undernutrition was the rule, are lacking but certain facts stand out. Thus acidosis disappeared and coma was *tout à fait* exceptional. Likewise, cases of diabetes of the obesity type practically disappeared in the presence of emaciation due to famine. Contrariwise, with the return of food the former patients could not resist eating and "as a result I have seen acidosis reappear and my cured fat diabetics retrogress rapidly and their glycosuria reappear."[1]

From the administrative reports of the Surgeon General to the Government of Bombay it appears that 17 of the total 7334 deaths in 1927 were due to diabetes and 36 of 8377 in 1935, or 1 death in 233. For Bombay City for the three years 1934–1936 inclusive there were 92 deaths yearly or 1 death in 314, and this ratio was more than double that in 1925–1927. However, the number of diabetics admitted to the K.E.M. Hospital in Bombay in 1933 and 1934 was 129 or 1 in 159 of the total admissions.

[1] Mahaux: Personal communication.

CHAPTER III.

THE ETIOLOGY AND PREVENTION OF DIABETES.[1]

Preamble.—It is self-evident that the fields of etiology and prevention of diabetes are contiguous and that the inferences to be drawn from a survey of one make almost unnecessary a survey of the other. While cultivating one pasture the authors have found it difficult not to encroach upon the other, but they doubt if it greatly matters, because after all what we are after is to find out why diabetes begins and how to prevent it.

Heredity is the basis of diabetes. Heredity was noted in the seventh century A.D. in India in thin persons with severe diabetes, according to Ponteva,[2] and Rathery[3] states that Rondelet, a doctor of Montpellier, at the beginning of the sixteenth century suggested its etiological bearing. Morton[4] described it in 1696, and it was considered paramount by Naunyn, although the short duration of the diabetic life in his day and the somewhat less general examination of the urine allowed him to recognize heredity in only 18 per cent of his patients. For years the authors have taken a lively interest in securing information upon heredity from their clientèle and for years have requestioned their patients at their subsequent visits. The term heredity is divided into hereditary and familial. Under hereditary are included grandparents, parents, uncles, aunts and children; under the term familial, brothers, sisters and cousins. The total incidence of diabetes in families of 6357 of my patients seen between 1897 and 1928 studied by the Metropolitan Life Insurance Company was 24.5 per cent. (Table 15.) In 15.9 per cent it was hereditary, 8.6 per cent familial and 3.3 per cent both. The incidence of heredity among our 1619 cases treated at the New England Deaconess Hospital during 1941 was 41 per cent and for those with onset under fifteen years was 49 per cent. In the oldest age group, seventy-five years of age or over, it was 29 per cent. In fact, that is the lowest percentage of diabetic heredity of any age group in the 1941 series. Among our 249 children with a duration of diabetes of twenty or more years, the total heredity is 55 per cent. Of our 2191 children, the heredity is 35 per cent, hereditary

[1] In this chapter as well as in Chapter II the authors have drawn freely upon five articles, published jointly with Dr. Louis I. Dublin, Second Vice-President and Statistician, and Mr. Herbert H. Marks, of the Metropolitan Life Insurance Company, in the *American Journal of Medical Sciences* (A. **186**, 753, 1933; B. **187**, 433, 1934; C. **189**, 163, 1935; D. **191**, 759, **192**, 9, 1936; E. **193**, 8, 1937). Many of the tables were originally prepared by the Statistical Bureau of the Metropolitan Life Insurance Company. The authors are deeply indebted to this organization, and Dr. Dublin and Mr. Marks for the privilege of using this material, but it is only fair to state that the authors assume full responsibility for the manner in which they have utilized the data. In this chapter, Tables 15, 18 and 19 were prepared by the Statistical Bureau of the Metropolitan Life Insurance Company.

[2] Ponteva: Acta Med. Scandinav., Suppl. 88, 1, 1938.

[3] Rathery: Le Diabète Sucré, Leçons Cliniques, J. B. Baillière et Fils, p. 7, 1938.

[4] Cited by Allen, Stillman and Fitz: Total Dietary Regulation in the Treatment of Diabetes, New York, Rockefeller Inst. for Med. Res., p. 9, 1919.

33, familial 9 per cent. For the children of Jewish parentage the heredity is 49 per cent.

Blotner and Hyde[1] studied the family history of 126 cases of diabetes and 77 of glycosuria discovered in their survey of 45,650 selectees at the Boston Induction Station and found it to be 32 per cent for the diabetics and 9 per cent for the glycosurics in contrast to 5.2 per cent among a control group of 2293 non-diabetic selectees. In a subsequent survey of 1383 cases with glycosuria among 69,088 selectees by Blotner,[2] there was a family history of diabetes in 24.7 per cent and 43.7 per cent, respectively, for the 329 cases who knew they had diabetes or glycosuria. The incidence of diabetes in the families of diabetics in the clinical experience of others is shown in Table 16. Rathery[3] significantly reports that 16.9 per cent of his hospital diabetics disclosed a diabetic heredity in contrast to 49 per cent of those in his private practice. See also Chapter XXVIII, page 742, for data upon heredity in children.

At medical meetings we have often distributed ballots and asked for reports of heredity among the audiences largely composed of doctors and medical students with a lesser number of nurses and dietitians. The average incidence for all groups was 22.3 per cent.

TABLE 15.—INCIDENCE OF DIABETES IN THE FAMILIES OF DIABETICS. PERCENTAGE OF CASES REPORTING HEREDITARY AND FAMILIAL TYPES OF FAMILY HISTORY. EXPERIENCE OF E. P. JOSLIN, 1897–1928.[4]

Year of examination.	No. of cases.	Per cent with family history of diabetes.			
		Total hereditary and or familial.	Total hereditary.*	Familial only.	Hereditary and familial.
Total, 1897–1928 . . .	6,357	24.5	15.9	8.6	3.3
1925–1928	2,669	26.3	17.8	8.5	3.7
1920–1924	2,162	24.7	15.7	9.0	3.0
1915–1919	799	24.0	14.5	9.5	3.6
1897–1914	727	18.0	11.0	7.0	2.5

* Includes total hereditary cases with or without associated familial type of heredity.

Wilder[5] comments upon the evidence of Pincus and White, as published in a former edition and which follows with a few additions, as follows: "I am not sufficiently trained, either in statistics or eugenics, to be able to pass final judgment on this evidence, but it impresses me as being of more importance than anything else that we know about diabetes. If it is not adequate, the subject cries aloud for further study, because if the conclusions of Pincus and White are correct, it means that the biologic inferiority upon which diabetes depends is transmissible, not only by diabetics, but also by the siblings of diabetics." Would that experts in the genetic field would become interested in this problem.

[1] Blotner and Hyde: Loc. cit, p. 42.
[2] Blotner: Loc. cit., p. 43.
[3] Rathery, p. 6: Loc. cit., p. 54.
[4] Prepared by the Statistical Bureau of the Metropolitan Life Insurance Company.
[5] Wilder: Clinical Diabetes Mellitus and Hyperinsulinism, Philadelphia, W. B. Saunders Co., p. 53, 1940.

TABLE 16.—INCIDENCE OF DIABETES IN THE FAMILIES OF DIABETICS. PERCENTAGE
OF CASES REPORTING HEREDITARY AND/OR FAMILIAL TYPES OF FAMILY
HISTORY. RECENT CLINICAL EXPERIENCES.

	No. of cases.	Per cent with family history of diabetes.
Joslin, total children, 1946	2191	35.0
Joslin, 1946. Children of 20 or more years' duration	249	55.0
Joslin, 1941. Hospital cases	1619	41.0
Joslin, 1920–1928	4831	25.6
Barach, Pittsburgh, 1938	1030	44.5
John, Cleveland, 1938–1939	630	35.7*
Lawrence, London, to January 1939	5462	32.3
U. S. Veterans' Bureau, to August 1939	704	7.0†

* Includes 7 cases with combined hereditary and familial history.
† Includes 35 cases with combined hereditary and familial history.

A. HEREDITY IN DIABETES.

BY PRISCILLA WHITE, M.D., AND GREGORY PINCUS, D.SC.

So exact a science has the study of diabetes become that today certain predictions are possible. Thus we can predict where diabetes will develop, though not why. It was the diabetic child who revolutionized our conception of the underlying cause of the disease for, prior to two decades ago, we sought chiefly among the obese portion of the population for the potentially diabetic individual, since 80 out of 100 persons contracting the disease were not only overweight, but markedly overweight. Following the introduction of insulin therapy in 1922, the number of diabetic children coming for treatment became sufficiently large to give us reliable statistics, and it was found that only 2 per cent of our child diabetics were overweight prior to onset. Infections could not be blamed for their diabetes, because among the children in the year prior to onset 60 per cent had no acute infection. There was only one common denominator which could be found throughout all ages, namely, the potentiality for inheritance of the disease.

The conception of the hereditary nature of diabetes is not new. It has been emphasized by many students[1] of the disease, but

[1] Naunyn: Der Diabetes Melitus, Wien, Alfred Hölder, p. 37, 1906. Joslin: Treatment of Diabetes Melitus, 4th ed., Philadelphia, Lea & Febiger, 1928. Sherrill: Jour. Am. Med. Assn., 77, 1779, 1921. Allen and Mitchell: Arch. Int. Med., 25, 648, 1920. John: Ann. Int. Med., 8, 198, 1934. Rabinowitch: Proc. Assoc. Life Insurance Med. Directors of America, 20, 9, 1933. Umber: Klin. Wchnschr., 10, 5, 1931. Finke: Ztschr. f. klin. Med., 114, 713, 1930. Cammidge: Brit. Med. Jour., 2, 738, 1928. Priesel and Wagner: Die Zuckerkrankheit und ihre Behandlung im Kindesalter, Leipzig, George Thieme, p. 12, 1932. Fischer: Personal Communication. Labbé: Bull. Acad. de méd. de Paris, 105, 956, 1931. Ladd: Am. Jour. Dis. Child., 32, 812, 1926. Collens and Grayzel: Am. Jour. Dis. Child., 38, 275, 1929. Lion and Moreau: Arch. d. méd. d. enfants, 12, 21, 1909. Toverud: Brit. Jour. Child. Dis., 24, 185, 1927. Holt and Howland: Diseases of Infants and Children, 9th ed., New York, D. Appleton and Co., p. 966, 1926. Kennedy: Jour. Am. Med. Assn., 96, 241, 1931. Allan: Ann Int. Med., 6, 1272, 1933. Wright: Am. Jour. Med. Sci., 182, 484, 1931. Tyner: Am. Jour. Med. Sci., 185, 704, 1933. Lawrence: Diabetic Life: Its Control by Diet and Insulin, 10th ed., J. and A. Churchill, 1937. Barach: Am. Jour. Med. Sci., 172, 243, 1926. Bortz: Med. Clin. North America, 18, 269, 1934. Grote: Gazz. d. osp., 55, 1329, 1934. Kern: Tr. Assn. Am. Phys., 49, 23, 1934. Maddox and Scott: Med. Jour. Australia, 1, 7, 1934. Steiner: Deut. Arch. f. klin. Med., 178, 497, 1936.

inconsistencies were bound to arise (1) because prior to insulin therapy the duration of diabetes was so short that family histories were incomplete and the mode of transmission could not be demonstrated; and (2) because some schools believed in the unity and others in the manifold origin and character of this disease. Those who believed in the unity of diabetes would select for genetic analysis consecutive case histories, whereas those who believed in its manifold origin and character would analyze only cases with a positive family history of diabetes. The authors believe in the unity of the disease, unity of its symptoms, manifestations and underlying cause, and upon this conception of the unity of diabetes their analyses have been made.

Evidence in Favor of the Theory That Diabetes Is Inherited.—The evidence in favor of the theory that the potentiality for developing diabetes is inherited rests primarily upon four facts: (1) The almost simultaneous occurrence of diabetes in both members of pairs of similar twins; (2) the greater incidence of diabetes in the blood relatives of diabetics than in those of a control population; (3) the demonstration that Mendelian ratios of the recessive type are found in a large series of cases selected at random; and (4) the demonstration of expected ratios in presumably latent cases.

1. Diabetes in Twins.—The occurrence of diabetes in twins has been mentioned many times in the literature.[1] This has suggested inheritance, because 80 per cent of twin cases reported were similar in type. Much more can be learned, however, from a comparative analysis of the incidence of diabetes in similar and dissimilar twins, for, if diabetes is inherited, the incidence of the disease in both members of pairs of similar twins should far exceed the incidence in dissimilar twins. The expected incidence of diabetes among pairs of similar twins would be 100 per cent. The expected incidence of diabetes in both members of pairs of dissimilar twins, all other things being equal, would be no more than that of ordinary brothers and sisters of diabetics. In the authors' series of patients, 96 pairs of twins suitable for analysis were found. Of these twins, 33 were similar in type, 63 dissimilar. Many other pairs of twins were found in the total group of diabetics, but were excluded because of death of one of the pair in infancy or very early childhood.

Among at least 16 of the 33 sets of similar twins, both were diabetic (48.5 per cent) whereas in only 2 (3.2 per cent) of the 63 pairs of dissimilar twins did each twin have the disease. Theoretically it might be claimed that the excess of diabetics among our similar twins could be explained on the basis of age incidence or the genetic type of parents. The groups, however, are comparable, the chances

---

[1] Curtis: Jour. Am. Med. Assn., **92**, 952, 1929. White: Diabetes in Childhood and Adolescence, Philadelphia, Lea & Febiger, 1932. Umber: Jour. Am. Med. Assn., **102**, 1242, 1934. Peck: Jour. Mich. Med. Soc., **32**, 359, 1933. Watson: Canad. Med. Assn. Jour., **31**, 61, 1934. Bauer, Fischer and Lenz: Human Heredity, New York, The Macmillan Company, 1931.

for excess of diabetes in the dissimilar twin group being perhaps slightly greater, because 10 per cent of their parents were diabetic, compared with 5 per cent in the similar twin group, 9 per cent in the diabetic population and 2 per cent in the control population, as shown in a former compilation.

Similar results have been reported in a study of twins by Hildegard Then Berg.[1] One hundred thirty-three pairs of twins were studied at the Kaiser Wilhelm Institute of Geneology and Demography, Munich. Of these, 46 were similar and 87 pairs were dissimilar. Whenever possible a glucose tolerance test was performed on the twin mate who had no positive clinical evidence of diabetes. Among similar twins Berg found 17 pairs absolutely concordant, 13 others concordant according to tolerance test and 16 were probably discordant, or in a total of 65 per cent both twin mates had contracted diabetes. Of the dissimilar twins 9 pairs were concordant with clinical manifestations of the disease, 9 twin mates had lowered sugar tolerance and 62 pairs were probably discordant, or in 22 per cent both dissimilar twin mates had contracted diabetes. After the age of forty-three all similar twins studied by Berg were concordant. This was not true of our patients, but the non-diabetic partner had not been tested for sugar tolerance in all instances.

Umber[2] reports 15 instances of diabetes among 19 pairs of homologous twins, each of whom showed the disease. He notes that the severity of the diabetes is likewise hereditary, because its character in the twins was identical, namely, mild, moderate or severe. Avoidance of all those influences favoring diabetes may suppress the diabetic heredity.

2. Statistically Significant Excess of Diabetes in Blood Relatives of Our Patients.—The incidence of diabetes in the parents and siblings of diabetics was found to differ significantly from the incidence of diabetes in the parents and siblings of non-diabetics. This statement is based upon the analysis of a total of 4434 parents and siblings of diabetics and 1290 parents and siblings of non-diabetics. The total incidence of diabetics in the diabetic population was 300, or 6.7 per cent, compared with 16, or 1.23 per cent, in the control non-diabetic population. This difference between the incidence of diabetes in blood relatives of diabetics and of the control population is statistically significant.

Umber[3] found heredity in 26 per cent of 3500 of his cases, in contrast to 2.8 per cent in a control population numbering 1000. Cammidge[4] found 3.4 per cent of 500 non-diabetics with a family history of diabetes, and Kern[5] 6.2 per cent in 500 non-diabetics.

[1] Then Berg: Jour. Am. Med. Assn., 112, 1091, 1939.
[2] Umber: Klin. Wchnschr., 19, 45, 1940.
[3] Umber: Med. Welt, 9, 889, 1935.
[4] Cammidge: Lancet, 1, 393, 1934.
[5] Kern: Trans. Assn. Am. Phys., 49, 23, 1934.

Their data are not limited to parents and siblings, as was the case with the authors' analyses.

Actual and Expected Incidence in Direct Ancestry of Diabetic Children.—The actual and expected incidence of diabetes in the parents and grandparents has been studied for child diabetics by Joslin, Dublin and Marks.[1] They computed the expected number of diabetics among the parents and grandparents, derived from analysis of life tables by causes of death according to population mortality statistics. The estimate of the expected number is the sum of the products of the number of children times the separate probabilities of dying from diabetes for (1) the father, (2) the mother, (3) both grandfathers and (4) both grandmothers.

Of the 841 diabetic children (aged fifteen years or under at onset) seen between 1920 and 1934 and whose heredity record includes diabetic relatives reported up to May, 1935, 152 had diabetic parents or grandparents. In the great majority of these cases, only 1 of these relatives was diabetic, but in 13 cases there were 2 diabetics and in 5 cases 3 diabetics in the direct ancestry. There were 175 diabetic parents and grandparents distributed as follows: father 28, mother 21, grandfather 53, grandmother 73. The proportions were as follows: diabetic fathers 3.3 per cent, diabetic mothers 2.5 per cent, diabetic grandfathers 2.3 per cent, and diabetic grandmothers 4.3 per cent.

In comparison with the 175 cases actually recorded, only 99 were expected to be diabetic on the basis of the 1930 mortality statistics and 72 where the basis for grandparents was the 1910 mortality statistics. These figures indicate an incidence of diabetes among parents and grandparents at least twice that expected in a random sample.

3. Demonstration of Mendelian Ratios of the Recessive Type.—Although the excess of diabetes in the blood relatives of diabetics suggests inheritance, it does not prove it. Infections, dietary habits, etc., theoretically might be characteristic of these families and account for the manifestation of diabetes. To prove inheritance one must demonstrate a pattern of inheritance. It is not enough to say that obviously a trait is inherited, because one-third of such persons have relatives with the disease. If one is to believe it, one must see the mode of inheritance. Here we find a wide variety of results, because some investigators can discover no pattern,[2] others demonstrate double dominance[3] alternating dominance[4] and recessiveness or simple recessiveness.[5]

[1] Joslin, Dublin and Marks: Loc. cit., p. 22, 1 E.
[2] Allan: Ann. Int. Med., **6**, 1272, 1933. Buchanan: Am. Jour. Med. Sci., **155**, 675, 1923.
[3] Lawrence: Personal communication.
[4] Cammidge: Loc. cit., p. 58. Priesel and Wagner: Klin. Wchnschr., **8**, 1398, 1929. Rabinowitch: Loc. cit., p. 56.
[5] Danforth: Am. Jour. Phys. and Anthrop., **7**, 291, 1924. Pincus and White: Am. Jour. Med. Sci., **186**, 1, 1933.

Non-Mendelian type of inheritance the authors exclude, because it is rare and not generally conceded to occur in man; for example, maternal inheritance of plastid characteristics in plants. Simple dominance the authors could not demonstrate and think it improbable: (1) Because of the tendency of diabetes to skip one or more generations; (2) because of the low incidence of diabetes among the parents of their patients. The geneologies in the literature reported by Bauer, Fischer and Lenz,[1] as well as our own, support the notion that diabetes often skips a generation. If diabetes were transmitted as a dominant trait, eventually one parent in each family of our patients would be diabetic. According to the age behavior of diabetes (see page 61), about 50 per cent of the parents at the median age of the authors' group, namely, sixty-five years, should be identified as diabetic. Actually only 9 per cent were diabetic. This point the authors wish to emphasize, because to the average lay mind and to many medically trained minds, the low incidence of diabetes in the parents indicates that the disease is not inherited. Apparently one thinks more readily in terms of dominant than in terms of recessive types of transmission.

Tracing the transmission of the disease is difficult because recessive genes have no visible effects when carried by only one parent. Thus if we are dealing with a normal dominant state, designated "M," and a recessive anomaly, designated "m," three types of individuals are possible, according to the pairing of these genes, MM, normal, and mm, abnormal, Mm, no visible anomaly but a carrier of the anomaly. Such genes may thus pass undetected through an unlimited number of generations. Only if these heterozygenous Mm individuals (carriers) mate, then the corresponding character may, but even then not necessarily, come to light. Many persons adhere to the entirely erroneous conception that only those anomalies are hereditary which manifest themselves both in parents and offspring and do not realize that a strictly hereditary anomaly may be transmitted through outwardly normal individuals.

If the predisposition to develop diabetes is inherited as a recessive and we indicate those persons inheriting the potentiality as mm, those not capable of developing it but capable of transmitting it as Mm, and those neither potentially diabetic nor capable of transmitting it as MM, only three types of mating can produce (mm) diabetic individuals and in the following ratios: Mm $\times$ Mm = MM: 2Mm: 1mm or 25 per cent diabetics; in a cross between Mm $\times$ mm = 2 mm: 2Mm or 50 per cent diabetics; in a cross between mm $\times$ mm = mm or 100 per cent diabetics.

The expected ratios are altered by the manner of selection of cases, age at onset of diabetes, chances of dying before age at which diabetes would develop, the changing status of the population and

[1] Bauer, Fischer and Lenz: Loc. cit., p. 57.

inaccuracy of diagnosis and consequent incorrect genetic classification of parents.

(*a*) **Effect of Selection.**—The entire prediction could not be fulfilled, because each of these families in this study was chosen because at least one member was diabetic and thus the parents identified as carriers. We can calculate the expectation among siblings on the average number of children per family by the formula $\dfrac{p}{1-(q)_n}$, where p is the probability of diabetic individuals appearing, q the probability of diabetics not appearing, and n the number of children. When this is done, the expected number of diabetics among siblings in our diabetic (mm $\times$ mm) cross remains 100 per cent, in the diabetic-carrier cross (Mm $\times$ mm), becomes 40 per cent, and in the carrier-carrier (Mm $\times$ Mm) cross, 16 per cent in the assemblage of families in our series.

(*b*) **Effect of Age Behavior.**—Unlike many traits subject to genetic analysis, such as albinism, blood groups, color blindness, etc., which are present at birth or soon thereafter, diabetes appears at all ages, from birth to ninety years, and not until ninety years of age will all potential diabetics be identified. Not one of the authors' families satisfied this condition. On this basis of age at onset of diabetes the expected ratios would be only partially fulfilled, and 4 per cent were found where 16 per cent were expected, 10 per cent where 40 per cent were expected and 24 per cent where 100 per cent were expected, or, in other words, throughout one-quarter of the expectation, because 98 diabetics occurred in 2309 siblings of the carrier $\times$ carrier cross, 48 in the 475 siblings of the diabetic $\times$ carrier cross, and 8 in the 33 children of the diabetic $\times$ diabetic cross. The ratios were almost identical: 1:2.5 : 6.1 expected and 1:2.4:5.7 observed. Furthermore, the median age of these groups lies in the fifth decade, at the end of which time 25 per cent of all potential diabetics should be identified.

(*c*) **Effect of Chances of Death Before Onset of Diabetes.**—Our third problem concerns the chances of death before the opportunity for the onset of diabetes appears. Here we make one assumption, that the predestined diabetic, before the development of the disease, lives and dies at the same rate as those persons not predestined to diabetes. From ordinary life tables and tables giving diabetes age incidence for each decade we have, therefore, calculated the proportion of potential to identifiable diabetics. Glover's life tables for 1910 for the population of the United States and diabetic incidence data from three sources were used, namely, the first 6000 diabetic cases of the Joslin series, data of Adams from the Mayo Clinic, and the actual incidence among the patients of this study. It was demonstrated[1] that from these three sets of onset data essentially similar

[1] For details see Pincus and White: Loc. cit., p. 59.

life tables for potential diabetics are derived.   The expected number
of mm individuals actually identifiable as diabetics was calculated
by multiplying the Mendelian expectation by the expectation of
identification.   In any cross the true probability, p, is equal to the
Mendelian probability (P′) multiplied by the probability of identification (P″) and q, therefore equals 1 − (P′ × P″).   When this is
done, the expectation in a group of 523 cases so analyzed is closely
fulfilled.

Thus in the group where neither parent had diabetes, 64 of 1495
siblings of the patients were diabetic, as compared with 64.68 identifiable on the data of Joslin, 68.35 on the data of Adams, and 64.68
on the population studied.   Among the siblings of patients with
one parent diabetic, 32 diabetics were observed in 299 siblings,
32.85 identifiable by data of Joslin, 34.24 by Adams, and 32.43
identifiable by population studied.

(d) **Effect of Genetically Unidentified Diabetic Parents.**—All of this
analysis assumes correct genetic classification of parents which governs
the probability of diabetes among siblings and patients.   To such an
analysis an objection may be raised, because, while it is true that
once diabetic, always diabetic, it is not true that once non-diabetic,
always non-diabetic.   Although we found that on the basis of
Joslin's onset data the number of missing diabetic parents was
too small to alter the situation significantly, nonetheless we subsequently made this calculation, using a slightly different set of
standards, namely, life tables for potential diabetics prepared from
the age incidence of 9853 diabetics seen between 1898 and 1933,
and 1920 mortality-rates.[1]   Still another set of standards was prepared based upon Massachusetts data on deaths from diabetes,
corrected by Joslin's data on duration of diabetes.[1]   The table
prepared from Massachusetts mortalities we have recently discovered is about 38 per cent incorrect, because we know that among
our own diabetic patients, dying either under or outside of our
immediate care, the diagnosis of diabetes does not appear in mortality statistics because of omission on the death certificate in
24 per cent of the cases and precedence of other diseases in 13.5 per
cent.   Estimates of the incidence of diabetes taking into account
differential sex frequency and our two sets of data on age incidence
at onset showed that only 12 unidentified diabetics among the
parents are derived from Joslin's incidence data, whereas 175
are derived from the Massachusetts data.   Undoubtedly the true
age incidence of diabetes lies between the two.   We believe
Joslin's data contain an excess of very young patients, whereas the
Massachusetts data contain an excess probably of aged cases.   When,
to demonstrate the method of study, we distributed the 175 unidentified genetically diabetic parents derived from the Massachusetts

---

[1] Joslin: Treatment of Diabetes Mellitus, 6th ed., Philadelphia, Lea & Febiger,
1937. See also Am. Jour. Med. Sci., **188**, 159, 1934.

Life Table,[1] it was found that the expected and observed number of diabetic siblings agreed fairly well even when we used two definitely different estimates of diabetes onset incidences.

TABLE 17.—EXPECTED NUMBER OF DIABETIC SIBLINGS WHEN 175 UNIDENTIFIED GENETICALLY DIABETIC PARENTS ARE REDISTRIBUTED IN THE CALCULATIONS INVOLVING THE MASSACHUSETTS INCIDENCE DATA.

Type of cross.	Expected diabetic siblings based upon Joslin's incidence.	Expected diabetic siblings based upon Massachusetts incidence.	Diabetic siblings observed.
Mm × Mm	121	90	98
Mm × mm	63	39	48
mm × mm	13	8	8

(*e*) **Degree of Accuracy of Diagnosis and Consideration of Potential Diabetics.**—Still another theoretical source of error exists and another objection must be answered, because this analysis is based upon the accuracy of case histories and clinically revealed diabetes. Perhaps some people said they had diabetes when in reality they did not, or the reverse, and still others had latent diabetes. For this reason a series of controls and a series of relatives of diabetics have been studied in detail. In part it was hoped from this search to reveal potential diabetics. From the outset, however, we did not expect to identify all potential diabetics, because we know a normal tolerance curve does not preclude the future development of diabetes.

One hundred and sixty-nine close relatives of diabetics and 125 control individuals were studied by random blood sugars or tolerance tests. In many instances the tests confirmed case histories, but relative hyperglycemia was characteristic of the families of diabetic individuals no matter whether the examination was by routine or by tolerance test. Among the blood relatives of diabetics, 14 per cent by routine, 25 per cent by tolerance test had supernormal values, compared with 2 per cent in the control population. These supernormal values may not be clinically abnormal values, but are statistically supernormal in this series. The value of 0.14 per cent for the routine blood sugar two or more hours after a meal and the values for tolerance tests, using venous and capillary bloods, proved[2] to be statistically supernormal.

4. Demonstration of Mendelian Recessive Ratios in Presumably Latent Diabetics.—Not only did we find a significant excess of supernormal blood sugars in relatives of our diabetics, but the proportion of hyperglycemic individuals in the three types of mating was found to approximate closely simple Mendelian recessive probabilities, 1 : 2 : 4. The percentages were 7, 18 and 25 in the carrier × carrier, diabetic × carrier, and diabetic × diabetic cross, respectively, and these percentages are in the ratio, 1 : 2.6 : 3.7. The ratios

---

[1] Pincus and White: Am. Jour. Med. Sci., **188**, 159, 1934.
[2] Pincus and White: Am. Jour. Med. Sci., **188**, 782, 1934.

of presumed diabetics on the basis of Joslin's onset data are
1 : 2.2 : 3.9, and on the basis of Massachusetts tables, 1 : 2.1 : 4.7.

If we assume that these hyperglycemic individuals do represent
future diabetics, the actual and estimated number of cases added to
clinical diabetics give us the number of diabetics identifiable at
approximately fifty years of age, whereas the median age of this
group is thirty-five years. Will our blood-sugar examinations enable
us to foretell by many years the future diabetics?

The blood sugar of siblings of young diabetics was studied by
Mackler and Fischer and gave negative evidence.[1] Since these
examinations were made in a pediatric service, the youth of the
individuals tested must be taken into consideration. Tyner[2] found
that pre-diabetics were more frequent among those with a family
history of parental diabetes. Sherrill[3] reported 21 abnormal curves
in 40 supposedly normal relatives of diabetics. Pannhorst[4] studied
26 descendants of diabetics and found 11 showed anomalies of carbohydrate metabolism. Steiner,[5] Pannhorst,[4] Rudy and Keeler[6]
have reported the incidence of diabetes in the offspring of certain
crosses. Lemser[7] has investigated relatives of diabetics with carbohydrate tests, noted abnormal but not distinctively diabetic curves
and regretfully points out the inadequacy of present methods, but
emphasizes the necessity of following up such individuals. We cannot, however, compare their reports with our own since no correc-
tions could be made for manner of selection, number of children,
age behavior or chances of identity by survival.

Colwell,[8] Woodyatt[9], Penrose and Watson,[10] approaching the
problem differently, present data favoring the theory that the
tendency to develop diabetes is inherited. Thus, Colwell states that
if one employs the amount of insulin required daily for uniform control as a gauge of the severity of diabetes in groups of patients of
different ages and different stages of the disease, several interpretations appear justified, including the one that diabetes is inherent
and begins at birth. In this same article Colwell discusses the course
of diabetes in a novel way. He recalls that Woodyatt and Spetz[9]
reëmphasize, as did Bence-Jones in 1865,[11] Naunyn[12] and Von Noorden
and Isaac[13] later, the anticipation of diabetes. When diabetes occurs

[1] Mackler and Fischer: Jour. Am. Med. Assn., **103**, 240, 1934.
[2] Tyner: Loc. cit., p. 56.   [3] Sherrill: Loc. cit., p. 56.
[4] Pannhorst: Verhandl. d. deutsch. Gesellsch f. inn. Med. XLVIII Kongress,
Wiesbaden, p. 411, 1936.
[5] Steiner: Deutsch. Arch. f. klin. Med., **182**, 231, 1938.
[6] Rudy and Keeler: New England Jour. Med., **221**, 239, 1939.
[7] Lemser: Münch. med. Wchnschr., **85**, 1657, 1938.
[8] Colwell: Arch. Int. Med., **70**, 523, 1942.
[9] Woodyatt and Spetz: Jour. Am. Med. Assn., **120**, 602, 1942.
[10] Penrose and Watson: Proc. Amer. Diabetes Assn., **5**, 163, 1945.
[11] Bence-Jones: Medical Times and Gazette, **1**, 58, 1865.
[12] Naunyn: P. 96, loc. cit., p. 56.
[13] Von Noorden and Isaac: Die Zuckerkrankheit, 8th ed., Berlin, Julius Springer,
1927.

in three generations of a single family it may appear earlier in the second than in the first and earlier in the third than in the second, the same trend continuing through three generations; also it can be exhibited to some extent between older and younger members of a single generation.

When an inheritable character makes its appearance in one generation of a single family at a given age, in the following generation at an earlier age, and so on, the phenomenon is known as anticipation.

Evidence of the trend was definite beyond limits of probable error in determining actual ages of onset in 79, positive but less certain in 85, and suggestive in 90 of 100 families in which the disease occurred in two or more generations.

These observations have a bearing on our conception of the course of diabetes and on our understanding of the differences in the character of the disease in older and younger subjects. In those families in which the trend appeared, the differences between the ages of onset in two successive generations (or in two with a skipped generation between divided by 2) varied widely in different individual cases, but the general average was twenty years. So in a given typical or composite case (essentially similar to some actual cases) the disease might appear in a first generation in the forties, fifties, or later, in the second generation in the twenties, thirties, or forties, in a third generation in the first or second decade. Thus a parent could be affected at the age of fifty years, a child of the parent (or nephew or niece) at the age of thirty, a grandchild (or sibling) at the age of ten. Or the parent could be affected at the age of fifty and a grandchild at ten with no diabetes in the second generation. Then a continuance of the trend at the same average rate would bring the age of onset in a fourth generation to minus ten years or to whatever period this may imply in prenatal time. One might think perhaps of non-conception or of the development of the disease in intrauterine life with resultant death of the fetus. In any event, when last seen the trend is pointing in the direction of extinction of the strain (on one side of the family, if not on both).

The discussion of anticipation raises the question as to the chances run by a juvenile diabetic patient of producing a living child that would develop diabetes after birth. If the partner is also a juvenile diabetic patient it might seem that the probability would be most remote. If the partner is a diabetic (or potentially diabetic) but of a first or second generation of his or her family, the situation might differ, as a child conceivably could represent a later generation of the partner's family. The question can be settled only with the accumulation of data on the incidence of the disease in progeny of persons who have had diabetes in childhood.

Penrose and Watson[1] have presented data indicating the greater incidence of diabetes in like sex siblings.

[1] Penrose and Watson: Loc. cit., p. 64.

Linkage of Genes.—No positive evidence of sex linkage has been demonstrated. That one or more factor pairs may be involved in diabetic heredity is suggested by the high incidence of obesity, of congenital defects especially of mesenchymatous tissue (first reported by Priesel and Wagner), possibly such degenerative lesions as cataracts and arteriosclerosis in diabetic patients and the appearance of congenital anomalies, especially of the mesenchymatous tissues in the offspring of diabetic mothers. The high fetal mortality among infants of diabetic mothers, as well as the congenital anomalies, suggests a possible lethal effect in the gene now somewhat remediable by hormone therapy. (See pages 770 and 774.)

Race and Heredity.—Of adult Jewish patients,[1] 29.6 per cent reported 1 or more cases of diabetes in the family, as compared to 24.5 per cent for all patients. The percentage of positive family histories was 30.3 per cent for Jewish males, compared to 23 per cent for all males, whereas among females the incidence in Jewish cases was 29.1 per cent, compared to 26.5 per cent for all females. The higher incidence of family histories of diabetes among Jewish patients has been consistent throughout the experience. The incidence of hereditary type histories at younger ages is definitely higher among Jewish than non-Jewish patients, whereas at older ages the reverse is true.

Among Jewish children the percentage of positive family histories is higher than among adults. Of 80 Jewish children, 34 (42.5 per cent) reported cases of diabetes in their families. Hereditary type histories predominated, being reported by 35 per cent.

Müller,[2] Finke,[3] and Priesel and Wagner[4] report 33 per cent, 25.4 per cent, and 48 per cent respectively of Jewish diabetic patients as having diabetic relatives. Rudy and Keeler[5] report that 6.3 per cent of 1000 non-diabetic Jewish patients had diabetic heredity in contrast to 1.23 per cent in our unselected control group. However, 29.1 per cent of 1037 Jewish diabetic patients had one or more relatives with the disease as compared with 6.7 per cent in our unselected series. A study of blood groups (O, A, B and AB) and blood types (M, N and MN) was made. The distribution showed no significant difference from the distribution in non-diabetic Jews. In general the distribution of blood groups in all Jews in Boston most closely corresponds to that reported for groups of Jews in Russia.

Eugenic Considerations.—The chances of a diabetic and true non-diabetic reproducing a diabetic are nil. A broader scope of the problem, however, includes a consideration of out-breeding carriers of diabetics. This can be done only if diabetics and their descendants

[1] See page 54, Footnote, 1, E.
[2] Müller: Med. Klin., 31, 277, 1935.
[3] Finke: Loc. cit., p. 56.
[4] Priesel and Wagner: P. 121, loc. cit., p. 56. Their figures apply to children only.
[5] Rudy and Keeler: Loc. cit., p. 64.

consistently marry into non-diabetic families. In the first generation the offspring of a diabetic and non-diabetic are all carriers. In the next, providing a true non-diabetic partner is selected, the offspring stand 1 chance in 2 of being carriers, in the next generation 1 in 4, the next 1 in 8, etc., until the carrier tendency tends to disappear.

The children, grandchildren, nieces and nephews, brothers and sisters of diabetics want to know what their chances of developing the disease are, provided they live long enough. (1) If both parents have diabetes, the child will almost certainly have it. (2) If one parent has it and the other has not, but if in the family of the non-diabetic parent his father or mother has it, there is an even chance, for the non-diabetic parent is a carrier. If a child of this union has diabetes, that establishes the fact also that the non-diabetic parent is a carrier and that all of the other children stand a 50 per cent chance of developing diabetes.

If the brother or sister of the non-diabetic parent has diabetes, he may or may not be a carrier, so the chances of the child developing it are less than even. If a remote relative of the normal parent has it, the chances are possible but not probable.

(3) If neither parent has diabetes but if the disease has occurred in one of their parents, both are carriers and the chances are 1 in 4. If the brother or sister of the parents has it, the parents are probably carriers and the chances are probably 1 in 4.

If a child develops diabetes the parents are carriers and the chances of the other children of the family developing it are 1 in 4.

5. **Consideration of the Secondary Factors.**—Our problem in search for the fundamental etiology of diabetes remains only half solved—given the proper genic background, what determines that it shall be expressed as diabetes?

The age incidence of diabetes, we believe, rules out two possible etiological factors, namely, senility and infections. If diabetes were due to the process of aging, obviously the greater the age, the more the incidence of diabetes, and this is clearly not the case.[1] Second, it indicates that infections are not the likely precipitating factors, because they could not explain the rhythmic age appearance, pubescence and senescence, which occurs in each consecutive thousand of our cases and in our cases as compared with those in other American and European clinics. The onset of diabetes depends, we believe, upon a complex of events, presumably endocrinal, which obtain maximum manifestations between forty-five and fifty-five years of age. Endocrine functions are known to be controlled by recessive Mendelian genes; for example, dwarfism in mice is believed in this manner to be due to deficient secretion of the pituitary gland, and perhaps this is also true of the human cretin.[2] The gene here

[1] Pincus, Joslin and White: Am. Jour. Med. Sci., **188**, 116, 1934.
[2] Castle: Genetics and Eugenics, 4th ed., Cambridge, Harvard Univ. Press, p. 801, 1930.

may induce pituitary hyperactivity just as the gene for dwarfism induces hypoactivity. Evidence in favor of hyperpituitary activity in diabetes is the fact that the onset of the disease occurs (1) in childhood often at eleven years in the overgrown child, (2) in women especially at the menopause when anterior pituitary hormone content of the blood is high and changes in the anterior pituitary lobe take place, and (3) in the obese; (4) diabetes is altered by removal of the pituitary,[1] and (5) injections of anterior pituitary extracts produce permanent diabetes in the dog.[2] We believe, therefore, that the most probable mechanism is an action of the gene through the pituitary on the pancreas, liver and other tissues. (See p. 120.)

B. OBESITY AND DIABETES.[3]

1. An Intimate Illustration of the Relation of Obesity and Diabetes.
—Heredity determines the susceptible individuals, but since the disease is rarely, if ever, present at birth, search must be made for precipitating factors which will help to bring out the inherited disposition. Of all these factors obesity is by far the most important. For this we should be grateful, because obesity is preventable.

My attention was definitely focussed upon the etiological importance of obesity in diabetes by two sources of evidence. I was brought up in a country town in New England, and in it I found the first lead. On its peaceful, elm-lined, wide, Main street there once stood three houses side by side, as commodious and attractive as any in the village. In these three houses lived in succession 4 women and 3 men—heads of families—and of this number all but 1 subsequently succumbed to diabetes. This remaining member of the group never was fat, always was active, and at the age of seventy-seven years died of cancer of the stomach.

Although 6 of the 7 persons dwelling in these adjoining houses died from a single cause, no one spoke of an epidemic. Contrast the activities of the local and state boards of health if these deaths had occurred from scarlet fever, typhoid fever or tuberculosis. Consider the measures which would have been adopted to discover the source of the outbreak and to prevent a recurrence. Because the disease was diabetes, and because the deaths occurred over a considerable interval of time, the fatalities passed unnoticed. Even the insurance companies failed to grasp their significance, and yet probably no group of individuals in the community carried *per capita* a higher amount of insurance than did these 6 diabetics. At the time these individuals lived, ideas of exercise for pleasure and the benefit of the body had not penetrated this rural region. Consequently, in this, as in many other New England villages, fortunately to a less extent now, the well-to-do were unusually fat.

[1] Houssay and Biasotti: Jour. Am. Med. Assn., **94**, 2010, 1930.
[2] Young: Lancet, **2**, 372, 1937.
[3] The heights of adult diabetics are normal. For data about children see page 743.

2. **Statistical Relations Between Obesity and Diabetes, an Analysis of 1000 Diabetics.**—While compiling the data for age, height and weight of a series of 118 diabetics whose respiratory metabolism had been studied at the Nutrition Laboratory of the Carnegie Institution, it was found that persons above the age of fifty years rarely acquired diabetes if their weight remained a little below normal. These statistics, although striking, were too few for generalities. Therefore, data from 1000 successive cases of diabetes for whom the age, date of onset of the disease, weight and height were known, were compiled and such are recorded in Table 18.

From this table the statement is justified that among 1000 successive diabetics the maximum weights of only 8 per cent were below the standard weight zone, whereas 15 per cent were in that zone, and 77 per cent were above it. Between the years fifty-one and sixty there were but 2 diabetics in 252 whose maximum weights were below the normal zone prior to the onset of the disease. Among 2000 of my own cases of diabetes not one occurred who was more than 30 per cent under weight, and in Adams' series of 1000 cases at the Mayo Clinic no patient developed the disease who was more than 20 per cent under weight. From 31 years onwards 89 to 79 per cent of my cases were overweight.

TABLE 18.—VARIATION FROM NORMAL OF MAXIMUM WEIGHTS AT OR PRIOR TO ONSET OF 1000 CASES OF TRUE DIABETES, CALCULATED FOR HEIGHT, AGE AND SEX.

Age, years.	Number of cases.	Percentage in normal average zone. (+5 to −5 per cent.)	Percentage of each decade.	
			Below standard weight.	Above standard weight.
0 to 10	43	37	44	19
11 to 20	84	39	29	32
21 to 30	112	19	10	71
31 to 40	172	6	5	89
41 to 50	244	12	3	85
51 to 60	252	12	1	87
61 to 70	79	10	6	84
71 to 80	14	14	7	79

3. **Analysis by the Statistical Bureau of the Metropolitan Life Insurance Company of 4596 of the Authors' Diabetics.**—For a period of thirty years, 1898–1928, our clinical records have been analyzed with the help of Dr. Dublin and Mr. Marks, of the Metropolitan Life Insurance Company,[1] from two points of view: (1) The maximum weight prior to onset of the disease, and (2) weight at onset. Among 4596 patients (ages, twenty years and over) for whom facts were available, 78.5 per cent of the males and 83.3 per cent of the females were overweight (5 per cent or more above average for age) at the time of their maximum weight. The weight at onset gave somewhat lower figures. Of the 3094 cases for whom these facts were noted, 62.7 per cent of the males and 67.4 per cent

[1] See reference 1, p. 54.

of the females were overweight. Moreover, one-half of the men and close to 60 per cent of the women were at least 20 per cent overweight at their maximum weight. Large numbers were extremely fat. No less than 16.5 per cent of the men and 25.8 per cent of the women were 40 per cent or more overweight at their maximum. Data reported by John, by Adams, and by Palmer[1] are confirmatory. In all groups there is a greater frequency of overweight among diabetic women than among men. In contrast to these high figures, only 7.9 per cent of the diabetic men and 6.3 per cent of the diabetic women had always been underweight (5 per cent or more less than average for age) and less than 1 per cent of the whole group had always been 20 per cent or more underweight.

TABLE 19.—MAXIMUM WEIGHT PRIOR TO ONSET OF DIABETES AND WEIGHT AT ONSET OF ADULT DIABETIC PATIENTS (AGES, TWENTY YEARS AND OVER).*

Percentage in Groups Classified by Deviation from Average Weight for Height and Age. By Sex. Experience of Elliott P. Joslin, M.D., 1898–1928.

Weight group.	Per cent.			
	Previous maximum weight.		At onset.	
	Males.	Females.	Males.	Females
All cases	100.0	100.0	100.0	100.0
Overweight, total: (5% or more above average) .	78.5	83.3	62.7	67.4
20% or more	51.0	59.3	33.8	41.1
40% or more	16.5	25.8	8.6	15.4
30% to 39%	13.9	14.2	9.5	11.2
20% to 29%	20.6	19.3	15.7	14.5
5% to 19% . , ...	27.5	24.0	28.9	26.3
Normal weight (less than 5% above or below average)	13.6	10.4	17.9	13.6
Underweight, total: (5% or more below average) .	7.9	6.3	19.4	19.0
5% to 19%	7.1	5.5	16.3	14.9
20% or more	0.8	0.8	3.1	4.1
Number of cases	2251	2345	1613	1481

* Prepared by the Statistical Bureau of the Metropolitan Life Insurance Company.

In Jewish adult patients, the tendency to obesity is even more marked than among other patients. The proportion of diabetic

[1] See reference, Footnote 1, D., p. 54, which includes literature.

Jewish men who were overweight at their maximum prior to diagnosis was 86.8 per cent, compared with 78.5 per cent for all adult males in this experience. Among Jewish women, no less than 94.3 per cent were overweight at their maximum, compared with 83.3 per cent for all female diabetics. More of the Jewish patients were very stout, particularly the women. Of the diabetic Jewish men, 58.4 per cent were at least 20 per cent overweight as against 51 per cent for total males, and of the Jewish women, 77 per cent, compared with 59.3 per cent for total females. The proportion of the actually obese (40 per cent or more overweight) was about the same for the Jewish men (16.2 per cent) as for all males in this experience (16.5 per cent). Among Jewish women, however, 33.5 per cent were obese, compared with only 25.8 per cent for all of the diabetic women. The majority of the remaining Jewish patients were of average weight. Only 2 of the Jewish adult patients had always been thin, 1 male and 1 female, both of whom were under age thirty-five years at onset.

Diabetic children, in contrast to adults, are not overweight. This was noted by my colleagues Drs. Root and White and myself in 1925 and has been repeatedly confirmed by others. In the child overgrowth is vertical, in the adult it is lateral. Is not each type of endocrinal origin?

4. **Development of Diabetes Among Persons Accepted for Insurance.**—The importance of obesity in diabetes is also confirmed by insurance records, which show that its subsequent development among persons accepted for insurance after medical examination and known not to be diabetic is far more frequent among overweights than among persons of average weight or less. Thus, in the Medico-Actuarial investigation, covering the combined mortality experience of 43 insurance companies, between 1885 and 1909, on men insured at standard premium rates, three broad weight groups were distinguished, namely, 50 pounds or more overweight, 25 pounds or more underweight and "standard" weight, falling between these two extremes. Among those insured at ages under thirty years, the subsequent diabetes death-rate of overweights was 15 per 100,000, compared to 6 among "standard" weights and 2 among underweights. Among those between thirty and forty-five years when insured, the diabetes mortality was 59 per 100,000 for the overweights, 12 for "standard" weights and 5 for underweights. For those forty-five years or over when insured, the diabetes death-rate among overweights was 136, compared with 28 for the "standard" group and 6 for the underweights. In this study, therefore, a large disparity existed between the diabetes death-rates of overweights and persons of average weight or less, and this disparity increased with advancing age. In another Medical Impairment Study, an investigation of the same type as the earlier one, but

covering the experience of 39 companies, between 1909 and 1927, similar results were obtained.

5. Liability to Diabetes Increases With Degree of Overweight.— Furthermore, the toll of diabetes increases with the degree of overweight. A study of the experience of the Union Central Life Insurance Company[1] showed that men who were 5 to 14 per cent above average weight had a diabetes mortality only one and a half times that of normal weights, compared with three and a fifth times for those 15 to 24 per cent overweight, and eight and a third times for those 25 per cent or more overweight. These differences were even larger at the ages of forty-five years and over; those 5 to 14 per cent overweight suffered a mortality nearly twice that of normal weights, and those 15 to 24 per cent overweight, nearly four times, while those 26 per cent or more overweight had a mortality over ten times that of average men.

Similar studies on women show the same characteristics.[2]

6. Obesity and Heredity Closely Linked.— All fat people do not, of course, get diabetes. For example, in the Medico-Actuarial Investigation, only 5 per cent of the deaths of men 50 pounds or more overweight when insured were recorded as due to diabetes. I do not accept this figure as portraying the whole truth. It may be explained by the fact that the diabetes of the obese is apt to be mild and that the Lombard and Joslin correction would prevail here even more than among all diabetics. A detailed study of 1000 such cases would be a field for investigation. Other factors must be involved in the causation of the disease. Indeed, the factors of obesity and heredity are probably closely linked. Obese persons who become diabetic appear to be those with an inherited susceptibility to the disease, the obesity acting as the exciting factor to produce the disease. The hereditary predisposition to the disease is brought out by many careful analyses of family histories of diabetic patients, as shown in the earlier part of this chapter. It is also indicated by Tyner's study[3] of the weights of 500 patients with normal carbohydrate tolerance and 500 with impaired tolerance, but not frankly diabetic. Tyner found that "pre-diabetes" was more common in obese persons than in those of normal weight only where there was a family history of diabetes.

Rony[4] carried out glucose tolerance tests in 20 obese individuals at intervals over a period of from one to nine years. None of them developed diabetes despite the fact that 3 of the 20 patients gave a family history of diabetes. He found no direct evidence that low sugar tolerance in obesity is a precursor to diabetes. The number of individuals studied was so small and the period of observation

---

[1] Dublin and Marks: Human Biology, **2**, 159, 1930.
[2] Dublin and Marks: Proc. Assn. Life Ins. Med. Directors of America, **24**, 47, 1937; **25**, 203, 1938.
[3] Tyner: Loc. cit., p. 56.
[4] Rony: Endocrinology, **21**, 195, 1937.

so short that one should await further data before drawing conclusions. Embleton[1] noted high glucose tolerance curves were much more common in obese men above the age of thirty-five years than among women.

The authors recognize that the relationship between obesity and diabetes is as yet not clearly defined. Diabetes has not been produced by overfeeding alone, experimentally or otherwise. The nearest approach to this has been the work of Allen,[2] who produced symptoms of the disease by fattening partially depancreatized dogs. It is possible, or even likely, that the connection between obesity and diabetes is not entirely a causal one and that both reflect some underlying imbalance in the functioning of the body, probably of endocrine origin. Despite this, however, the association of diabetes with a preceding obesity is so close that conditions favoring obesity are undoubtedly related to concomitant variations in the incidence of diabetes.

Diabetes appears to be largely a penalty of obesity, and the greater the obesity, the more likely is Nature to enforce it. The sooner this is realized by physicians and the laity, the sooner will perhaps the advancing frequency of diabetes be checked. The penalty of taking too much alcohol is well-known, and a drunkard is looked on with pity or contempt. Rarely, persons who become fat deserve pity because of a real tendency to put on weight despite moderate eating, but usually most should be placed in somewhat the same category as the alcoholic. In the next generation one may be almost ashamed to have diabetes.

I feel quite justified in waging war against obesity in the adult in season and out of season, because even if the fat man or woman does not acquire diabetes, the obesity exposes him or her to premature breakdown of the circulatory system, renders them an easy prey to diseases of the biliary tract and adds an unfavorable factor to surgery. So dangerous is obesity that acquiring diabetes, losing weight and coming under medical supervision actually may prolong the fat man's life.

Rapid loss of weight by a fat individual, strange to say, may be followed by diabetes. How frequently this occurs, I cannot say, but it may be of considerable importance, because I recall several instances, among them Cases 406, 6338, 12570. The fat society woman in her zeal for fashion's lines takes black coffee for breakfast, bouillon and a few green vegetables at noon, in order to indulge in a liberal dinner. The total food calories for the day, it is true, are lowered but are replaced by the consumption of body calories to such an extent that the individual is actually living on a high-fat, low-carbohydrate diet. It is true he loses weight but at the expense of lowering his tolerance for carbohydrate. Moreover, by this dietetic plan a heavy load of carbohydrate is cast upon pancreas and liver, when the former's insulin-producing capacity has not

[1] Embleton: Brit. Med. Jour., 2, 739, 1938.
[2] Allen, Stillman and Fitz: Loc. cit., p. 54.

been trained by previous means to convert it into harmless glycogen, and when the latter's store of glycogen is so low that it functions with difficulty. Himsworth's conception of a diet relatively high in fat predisposing to diabetes is in line with these considerations. Moreover, the temporary loss of carbohydrate tolerance by living on a low-carbohydrate high-fat diet has been clearly and importantly demonstrated formerly by Sweeney and others and more recently by Himsworth.[1] (See page 162.) Indeed, it may also be true that the scant European breakfast after the long night's fast is safer than our heavier American breakfast. At any rate, after abstinence from food one should begin with small quantities of food in which carbohydrate finds a moderate place, and in losing weight, while one may omit all fat because the body has enough in store, one should never omit all carbohydrate from a meal.

7. **Obesity Explains Peculiarities in Distribution of Incidence of Diabetes.**—The preponderant influence of obesity in the development of diabetes explains many peculiarities in the distribution of the incidence of the disease. Thus, in conjugal diabetes I found in a study of 24 couples concerned that there was but 1 of the 27 partners seen by me who was thin. Husband and wife alike were fat, and the implication was strong that they contracted the disease from exposure to good food rather than to one another. The frequency of diabetes in the Jewish race has much to do with the obvious obesity which there exists, as stated above. See page 70. The increasing affluence of the Jewish race in this country and their readiness to acquire medical knowledge has notably decreased the frequency of obesity among the higher classes. One sees much less frequently today a Jewish doctor who is above normal weight.

The greater frequency of diabetes in the city in contradistinction to country workers can be explained by obesity, but here the activity of the muscles is undoubtedly an additional factor. So, too, the reputed greater incidence among locomotive engineers who tend to be fat, in contrast to all railroad employees. Old statistics showed 1 in 2000 of all trainmen had diabetes, but 1 engineer in 93. One would like to see new data, but I suspect it would be difficult to obtain such, because the existence of diabetes might be concealed. Likewise, figures about weights of train workers should be sought. Only a small part of this difference can be attributed to the higher average age of the engineers.

The apparent development of diabetes as a sequel to infectious diseases, rare as it is, may be explained by the rapid development of obesity, rather than due to the infections *per se*. Convalescents have big appetites, and unfortunately are almost fanatically overfed during a period of forced inactivity and at the very time when the pancreas must necessarily, like the rest of the body, be in a vulnerable state.

[1] Himsworth: Proc. Roy. Soc. Med., 29, 731, 1935-6.

Kisch[1] directed attention to the frequency of the development of diabetes in the later lives of fat children, and I never see a fat child without thinking of this possibility, because a fat child, as a result of early dietary habits, is likely to be a fat adult, and prone to develop diabetes. Particularly serious must it be for a child or adult of slight stature to put on weight which would be excessive even for a man of large frame. Case 1142 first consulted me at the age of forty-one years, and I can just remember his little spindling legs and delicate frame when he was a boy in the country village before he entered the primary school; many years later he entered a grocery store, "worked like the dickens and ate the same way," until at the age of forty years he was 60 pounds above the average weight, and sugar was found at a life insurance examination.

Chronic dietary excesses precede obesity and figure quite prominently in my records as precursors of diabetes. Allen's dogs, artificially predisposed to diabetes by removal of a considerable portion of the pancreas, became diabetic when overfed. It is, however, the excess of food rather than of available carbohydrate which does the harm. Indeed, a high percentage of carbohydrate in the diet does not appear to predispose to diabetes. Thus, the Japanese live upon a diet consisting largely of rice and barley, yet so far as statistics show, the disease is not only less frequent but milder in that country than in this. With the adoption of Occidental tastes both the frequency and severity of the disease have increased, according to my Japanese visitors.

8. Incidence of Diabetes in Very Tall Men.—With evidence pointing more and more strongly each year to the part played by the pituitary in diabetes, the incidence of the disease in very tall men, 6 feet, 2 inches or more, is important. This was investigated by the Metropolitan Life Insurance Company.[2] They found, first of all, that practically there was a normal mortality and a normal pattern of causes of death in this group. "The mortality from degenerative diseases was high only among the overweights, a condition which is also common in overweight men of lesser heights." Timme,[3] in his discussion of the paper, pointed out that the pituitary in the very tall usually reflects underactivity rather than overactivity.

9. Incidence of Diabetes and Consumption of Sugar.—An attempt has been made to correlate the increasing incidence of diabetes in this and other countries with the increasing consumption of sugar. Statistics, however, do not bear this out, particularly in the United States, where the consumption of sugar has been stationary in recent years, whereas diabetes has increased, and in certain other countries, where the consumption of sugar is high,

[1] Kisch: Jour. Am. Med. Assn., 64, 1038, 1915.
[2] Dublin and Marks: Proc. Assn. Life Ins. Med. Directors, 23, 153, 1936.
[3] Timme: Proc. Assn. Life Ins. Med. Directors, 23, 186, 1936.

the incidence of diabetes is relatively low. The consumption of sugar in the United States, as compared with diabetic mortality, is shown in Table 20. However, one must be cautious in the interpretation of the data, because the death-rates are not adjusted for sex, age and other factors. Nevertheless it is notable that in the period 1930–1937 the diabetic mortality continued to rise, although the yearly pounds of sugar per capita fell. In Australia where in 1937 the per capita consumption of sugar was 121 pounds (55 kilograms) per annum, diabetic death-rate 16.8 per 100,000, definite efforts were made to discourage its use, not that it was harmful per se, but that it destroyed appetite for more wholesome food. Recent data are invalidated by the exigencies of the war.

TABLE 20.—THE CONSUMPTION OF SUGAR IN THE UNITED STATES.

Years.	Population average for decade.	Pounds per capita, yearly average.	Diabetic death-rate per 100,000.
1880–1890	55,912,152	44	2.8– 5.5
1890–1900	68,818,801	56	5.5– 9.7
1900–1910	83,275,548	65	9.7–14.9
1910–1920	98,796,383	82	14.9–16.0
1920–1930	114,034,730	100	16.0–19.0
1930–1937	126,222,625	95	19.0–23.7

Acute dietary excesses are rarely, if ever, associated with the advent of diabetes. The incidence of diabetes in the employees of candy factories and candy shops would be of interest in this connection. Even yet this question has not been thoroughly investigated. The development of diabetes after glucose-tolerance tests has never been reported, or at least brought to my attention, but Dr. F. G. Brigham tells me Mrs. K. with multiple sclerosis developed diabetes after starting in to eat candy to gain weight.

Indeed, Himsworth[1] considers it is the high proportion of fat in the diet rather than carbohydrate which favors the development of diabetes. Data were painstakingly accumulated on a qualitative as well as a quantitative basis for 143 diabetics as a control group for the qualitative method and 137 subjects for the quantitative. By both methods the majority of diabetics prior to the onset of their disease reported diets containing an excessive proportion of fat. Both groups consumed the same proportion of protein. From the above Himsworth argues that since such diets with an increase of fat would impair sugar tolerance and insulin sensitivity in non-diabetic subjects the ingestion of such a diet by a potential diabetic would favor the occurrence of the disease. I must point out it is extremely difficult for diabetic patients even with the best intentions to divorce themselves from their present diabetic diets and to remember and record their previous, non-diabetic diets.

[1] Himsworth: Clinical Science, 2, 67, 95, 117, 1935; Lancet, 1, 127, 1936.

10. **Climate.**—Climate is closely related with the consumption of carbohydrate, although not with the use of sugar. The idea of climate being at all responsible for the high incidence of diabetes in northern regions and its low incidence in southern regions does not appeal to me. Those interested in another point of view should consult Mills,[1] Peterson[2] and Wilder.[3] I believe that the statistical incidence of diabetes is highest (1) where the urine of the inhabitants is most frequently examined, (2) where the inhabitants live the longest, and (3) where they weigh the most. The influence of heredity should be the same in all climates.[4] This paragraph was written prior to the Arizona survey which has only strengthened my belief in its trustworthiness. See p. 25.

11. **Seasonal Manifestations of Diabetes.**—Pannhorst and Rieger[5] reached the conclusion that diabetes cannot be regarded as a seasonal disorder. In Massachusetts Lombard[6] found during 1936 and 1937 there were decidedly more deaths in the winter months, December to May, than in June to November, 1779 as contrasted with 1459. The most significant increase was in respiratory diseases, including influenza, 219 versus 94. Mortality almost steadily decreased from January to August and then as steadily rose. New data should be gathered in which the incidence of onset rather than of death could be tabulated.

12. **Example of Multiple Etiology.**—Many diabetic patients appear to present multiple causes for their diabetes.

This is well exemplified by the history of a gentleman, aged forty-nine years, Case 954, who consulted me on December 12, 1915. One of his children died in 1901 at the age of two years and another in 1913 at the age of twelve years, both of diabetes. As a child he had measles, scarlet fever and whooping cough, and at twenty-four years was ill for eighteen months with inflammatory rheumatism, and the pericardium was tapped twice. At the age of thirty-four years his weight was 200 pounds, and for his height, 5 feet 11 inches, was 17 per cent above normal. Prior to this time he had indulged in considerable alcohol three evenings a week, and his use of tobacco was more than moderate. He was fond of sweets and occasionally ate ½ pound of candy in an evening. During the last two years he took little exercise, and recently led a strenuous life on account of his active business. An attack of gall stones, which was accompanied by an infection of the biliary tract, led to an operation on November 15, 1915. Prior to the operation the urine was examined and found normal. The anesthetic was ether. Convalescence from the operation was satisfactory, but while at the hospital his friends, knowing his fondness for sweets, sent him much candy, which he ate. On December 11, 1915, he

[1] Mills: Medical Climatology, Climatic and Weather Influences in Health and Disease, Springfield, Charles C Thomas, 1939.

[2] Peterson: The Patient and the Weather, Ann Arbor, Edwards Brothers, Inc., 4, Pt. 3, 269–300, 1938.

[3] Wilder, Browne and Butt: Loc. cit., p. 37. See also Wilder: Clinical Diabetes and Hyperinsulinism, Philadelphia, W. B. Saunders Company, p. 47, 1940.

[4] Mills: Arch. Int. Med., **46**, 569, 1930.

[5] Pannhorst and Rieger: Ztschr. f. klin. Med., **134**, 154, 1938.

[6] Personal communication from Herbert L. Lombard, Director, Division of Adult Hygiene, Department of Public Health, State of Massachusetts.

observed polyuria, and later he recalled that when nervous and working hard these symptoms had occurred off and on for a day's duration during several years. On December 11, 1915, sugar was demonstrated in the urine, and on the following day when he came for treatment the specific gravity was 1.045 and the percentage of sugar 7.2. The weight of the patient was approximately 185 pounds shortly after the operation, and on December 13 was 177 pounds naked. The patient began fasting by omitting his supper on December 12, and the twenty-four-hour quantity of urine, ending December 14, contained only a trace of sugar, and even this was absent the following day. Improvement was uninterrupted but (Moral!) he dropped from observation and I learned of his death from pneumonia in 1920, two years before the discovery of insulin.

The important etiological factors were all present in this case, namely, the optimum age, an hereditary tendency to diabetes, and obesity. Furthermore, he had led a strenuous life, had indulged in dietary excesses, and had taken little exercise.

13. **Incidence of Diabetes Varies With Chances of Becoming Overweight.**—Whatever increases the chances of becoming overweight in those hereditarily predisposed to the disease will tend to bring about a real increase in the incidence of diabetes. Consequently, whenever and wherever conditions of life are easy, food abundant and relatively cheap over long periods, and when large numbers of individuals become accustomed to partake of food in excess of their requirements for the expenditure of energy, the frequent development of obesity and of diabetes is favored.

Thus, in rural communities it is less frequent than in urban communities, and in rural communities hard manual work is usual among farm laborers, as it is among coal miners. An analysis of English occupational mortality, largely confirmed by recent American data, showed that the incidence of diabetes among workers of this type was among the lowest recorded. Farmers and their families, however, who, on the average, do less work and are generally better fed and circumstanced, had a diabetes rate more than twice that of their laborers. The high diabetes rates in cities, therefore, may be ascribed, in part, to the lighter work done by relatively large numbers of the urban population. But I wonder if closer medical supervision may be the explanation.

Of 2304 of my own patients, studied by the Metropolitan Life Insurance Company (see Footnote 1 B, page 54), whose occupation was definitely known, the proportion engaged in professional and semi-professional pursuits was 21.8 per cent.

(a) **Occupation and Income per Capita.**—In general, in those countries and cities where the level of *per capita* income is high it is reasonable to assume that the level of nutrition corresponds with *per capita* income. This has been studied carefully by the International Labor Office of the League of Nations and the data are analyzed by Joslin, Dublin and Marks. This holds also for regional variations in diabetes death-rates in the United States. Jordan, taking the percentage of those filing income tax reports in the various states as an index of economic well-being, found that those states where the percentage was high usually had above average rates from diabetes. Similar regional relationships exist between the incomes of wage workers and diabetes-rates.

The differences in the level of diabetes incidence in the various parts of the world, as well as within individual countries, also reflect the extent to which the inhabitants depend upon purely industrial, mercantile and professional pursuits, as opposed to farming and other activities requiring much physical labor. This phase of the problem is closely connected with the extent of urbanization. These tendencies are indicated both for nations and for the different sections of the regions of the United States and have been shown by various tabulations. From entirely different points of view one can note the effect of occupation on the incidence of diabetes. In the United States there have been great occupational shifts between 1870 and 1930. Thus, in the interval of sixty years the number of persons engaged in agriculture and allied occupations dropped from 52.8 to 21.3 per cent. Similar data are available for other countries. Contrariwise, manufacturing in this same period rose from 22 to 28.6 per cent, trade and transportation from 9.1 to 20.7 per cent, clerical service from 1.7 to 8.2 per cent, and professional service 2.7 to 6.5 per cent.

(*b*) **Increased Use of Power and Machines.**—The increased use of power to offset the need of human labor favors the development of obesity. The extent of this change in the United States is shown by comparing the changes in the number of wage earners engaged in manufacturing and the rated horsepower capacity of plant equipment. In the thirty-year period, 1899 to 1929, the number of wage earners increased only 88 per cent, compared with an increase of 331 per cent in power equipment capacity. In the decade between 1919 and 1929, despite a slight decrease in the number of wage earners, the power capacity increased nearly 50 per cent. The horsepower per worker rose from 2.1 in 1889 to 3.3 in 1919 and 4.9 in 1929. Industrial and mercantile nations, which tend to be those having a large percentage of their populations in urban areas, usually show high *per capita* incomes and high diabetes rates. The factors of industrialization and high earnings really reinforce each other. Despite their lower *per capita* food requirements, workers in industrial and mercantile countries are able to buy as much food as those in countries where the greater number of inhabitants depend upon more arduous occupations for their livelihood. Consequently, one should expect a great frequency of overweight and, therefore, of diabetes, in industrialized and urbanized communities. "The latest available occupational statistics are not exactly comparable with those of earlier years but they indicate a further decline in the proportion of persons engaged in agricultural and allied occupations, and further expansion of persons in clerical and selling jobs and in professional service." (H. H. M.)

(*c*) **Increase of Leisure.**—Another by-product of our mechanized civilization is the increased amount of leisure. Not only do men work less hard during their occupied hours, but they have more free hours. Fifty years ago the sixty-hour week was general in the United States, Germany, France and Belgium, a fifty-two-hour week in England, seventy-two hours in Italy, Russia and other countries. Even longer hours of work were not uncommon. Just before the first World War in many countries the eight-hour day already had obtained a strong foothold, and it became even more general after the war. Today a week of forty hours or less is not unusual.

The trend toward the cities has resulted in cutting down the expenditure of energy of large numbers of individuals. For women, especially, the removal to the city brings about a change to easier work inherent in the differences between the city and country households. Again, transportation facilities and their use are much greater among urban residents. Moreover, the greater availability of concentrated food rich in calories encourages overnutrition among urban residents, so that urbanization is a factor in the increase in diabetes. In 1900, 60 per cent of the people in the United States lived in the country, but in 1930 only 44 per cent were in rural areas. In one generation the population of our cities has increased 125 per cent, but our rural population has grown less than 20 per cent, and the actual farm population in the country decreased in the decade 1920 to 1930. In other countries this urbanization has gone on almost without exception. In England the change has been small because the rural population had diminished to about one-fifth of the total population three decades ago and yet the diabetic death rate is low in England.

(d) **The Changed Position of Women.**—Already this has been discussed under the heading, Sex (see page 35). Not only, however, has the recognition of women been greater, but the women have far less work to do. This comes about not because of the lower birthrate which is a characteristic development all over the world, but because families now live in small apartments, and many of the functions of the housewife, such as cooking, laundering and making of clothing, are now carried on in industry. Labor-saving devices have reduced the number of domestic servants, and they have sought lighter work in industry.

C. THE INCIDENCE OF DIABETES AS INFLUENCED BY VARIOUS FACTORS, ETIOLOGICAL AND OTHERWISE.

1. Incidence Varies With Degree of Interest and Skill Expended in Its Recognition.—Facilities for diagnosis are far greater today and in general in those countries where the medical services are better developed the chances for correct diagnosis of diabetes are as a rule better, and particularly for the more prosperous classes. Diabetes rates are usually high in areas which have the greater number of physicians and hospital beds. This holds for different sections of the United States and for other countries. To a certain extent this fits in with the incidence of diabetes in urban and rural regions. (See discussion of diabetes in Arizona, page 25.)

The quality of medical service has increased, although the number of physicians in the United States has dropped from 17.3 per 10,000 in 1900 to 12.2 in 1933, but risen to 13.0 in 1938. The return of physicians from military to civilian practice may be followed by an increase in the humber of cases of diabetes detected. Throughout the country the standards for admission to the practice of medicine have advanced. In foreign countries the number of physicians has increased, but today is far less than with us. Thus, in Germany in 1900 there were 4.6 doctors per 10,000, and in 1932, 6.4. In France, Belgium, Netherlands, Sweden, Norway and Switzerland, a similar though smaller increase took place. In England and Wales the number fell from 7 to 6.7 per 10,000. In Canada the proportion has stayed about constant, 10.2 *versus* 10.3. On the other hand in China in the occupied area in 1942 there was 1 doctor to 25,000; in India 1 to 10,000. The number of general hospitals and hospital beds has increased greatly in the United States, and in 1938 was 32.7 per 10,000. Out-patient departments doubled in fifteen years, and the number of visits to clinics reported in 24 of the 25 largest cities of the country increased from 7,000,000 in 1921 to 30,186,164 in 1944. Patients admitted to all hospitals in 1931 were 7,155,976 and in 1945, 16,257,402. In other countries there has been a similar increase. Industrial medical service favors the more frequent diagnosis of diabetes. In 1930–1931 it is known that 4,200,000 employees were furnished some form of medical service. One cannot go to college or to jail without an examination of the urine. Examinations for life insurance have increased greatly and the greater details in these examinations, which now frequently include blood-sugar tests, help to detect diabetes. Between 3,000,000 and 4,000,000 individuals yearly apply for life insurance, requiring medical examination. Between 1920 and 1928, 18 per cent of my own male patients of insurable age discovered their diabetes in this way. During the first thirty years of this century female applicants in the Metropolitan Life Insurance Company increased over eighty times, as compared with male applicants, who increased about twenty times. Life insurance companies have also contributed to the detection of diabetes by popularizing periodic health examinations. In one company alone more than 125,000 policy holders took advantage of this in 1938.

Among my own patients between 1897 and 1928, 426 were discovered by insurance examinations. For the insurable ages, twenty to sixty-four years, the percentages discovered by insurance are 15.9 per cent for males and 1.3 per cent for females. Among 1000 new diabetics seen since January 1, 1945, 85 were first diagnosed by insurance examinations. Of one group of these cases referred for diagnosis, but found not to be diabetic, insurance cases formed 25.3 per cent of the men. The insurance companies, represented by the Association of Life Insurance Medical Directors, spend $21,000,000 annually in death claims for diabetics, and the Metropolitan Life Insurance Company attributes to glycosuria the cause of 9.3 per cent of all rejections on medical grounds.

6

The routine examination of the urine for sugar is relatively recent. Bolduan[1] showed that in a large New York Hospital this did not become the practice until the decade 1880 to 1890. Estimations of the blood sugar began only about thirty years ago and did not become common until 1930. Unfortunately expense still prevents their general adoption and hampers treatment. I worked as a house pupil under a physician, the senior on the staff, at the Massachusetts General Hospital in 1895 who recorded, when he in his turn was house pupil, that the urine of the patient "tasted sweet." We need many more small laboratories and many more technicians in the smaller communities.

2. **Effect of Aging of the Population Upon the Incidence of Diabetes.**—The aging of the population accounts for a considerable part of the increase in diabetes. The favorite zone of onset of diabetes is between forty-five and fifty-five years. Among 2181 of my own cases, first seen in 1929 to 1938, inclusive, the acme of onset is between fifty and fifty-nine years. Since 1900 the total increase in population is approximately 70 per cent, but the increase in persons over forty-five years is twice as great, namely, 144 per cent. For females over forty-five years the increase is 150 per cent. By 1950 it is estimated that 28.8 per cent of our population will be forty-five years or over, compared to only 17.8 per cent at the beginning of the century. It is estimated that aging of the population alone will increase the number of diabetics in the country 20 per cent in the next ten years. The improved longevity of diabetics will raise the number even more.

3. **Racial Susceptibility.**—Racial susceptibility has been discussed in Chapter II.

4. **Is There a Nervous Element?**—A strenuous life or a worrying life was once considered as of importance in the etiology of diabetes, but I am not impressed with it as a factor. See discussion under Trauma, below.

5. **Influence of Infections.**—(See Chapter XVI, page 523.)

6. **Arteriosclerosis.**—Arteriosclerosis is a bad enough foe of the diabetic without blaming it for the causation of his disease. Diabetes is not an old-age disease as proved by the statistics of onset of 9853 of my patients. (See page 32.) Pathological evidence is against arteriosclerosis as a cause. (See page 219.) The duration of the diabetes itself is an argument against it, because, as a rule, the older the diabetic grows, the less severe the diabetes, and yet the greater the degree of arteriosclerosis.

7. **Trauma.**—Legal proceedings based upon trauma as a cause of or aggravating diabetes either should be avoided or entered upon after unusual deliberation by diabetics. A diabetic may go to court and win his suit, but this discourages employers from hiring or even keeping in their employ other diabetics. There are about

[1] Bolduan: New York Acad. Med., **9**, 523, 1933.

1,000,000 diabetics now living in the United States and in a peculiar sense each one is his "brother's keeper."

Concepts Concerning Trauma and Diabetes.[1]—1. The thesis that trauma *de novo* can cause diabetes has steadily lost support with the expanding knowledge of the nature of the disease.

2. Evidence has accumulated to show that trauma indirectly can activate, or accelerate, the appearance of a latent diabetes in the hereditarily predisposed, particularly if accompanied by infection, reduced muscular exercise, gain in weight or overeating.

3. Trauma in the course of diabetes has grown in importance, because the average duration of the disease has nearly trebled, thus lengthening the period of exposure. Moreover, the danger of exposure to trauma is intensified each successive year a diabetic lives, because time is provided for the disabling complications of the disease to appear and the physical infirmities of the normally aging process to advance.

The tissues of a diabetic are more vulnerable than those of a non-diabetic.

4. Trauma may make the diabetes more severe, but this effect is not necessarily permanent.

5. Emotional, nervous, so-called neurogenic diabetes, as von Noorden well said, was put "into the grave" by World War I, and there it is likely to remain, no data yet appearing to show that it was exhumed during the recent conflict.[2]

6. To prove that trauma is the cause of diabetes in any individual case evidence must be at hand to show: (*a*) that the disease did not exist before the trauma; (*b*) that the trauma was severe, injuring the pancreas; (*c*) that the symptoms and signs of the disease developed within a reasonable period following the trauma, the etiologic importance of the trauma waning with the prolongation of the interval; and (*d*) that the symptoms and signs of diabetes were not transitory but permanent.

7. This question of trauma as the cause of diabetes should be kept absolutely distinct from the question of compensation of an individual who is found to have diabetes following an accident. Too often, especially in foreign publications (Lommel, Troëll) the two are confused, and for social and governmental insurance reasons the court sitting in judgment on a case may vote to give the insured the benefit of a doubt which has no factual basis. Many European countries are saturated with social accident insurance, and if a citizen is not actually in the employ of the government, at least he expects a liberal interpretation of social or insurance benefits. If trauma were much of a factor in the causation of diabetes the World War of 1914–1918 would have shown it. That this was not

[1] This originally appeared in an article by Joslin: Ann. Surg., **117**, 607, 1943.
[2] See confirmatory view for World War II. Gendel and Benjamin: New Eng. Jour. Med., **234**, 556, 1946.

the case is evident from statistics upon the incidence of the disease in the United States, England, France and Germany. In not one of 600 diabetic soldiers in France did Labbé consider trauma an etiological factor. Joslin saw as Medical Consultant at Mesves, through which center passed 38,765 soldiers, of whom 12,498 were classified as battle casualties, 2 cases of diabetes and but 1 other was reported. In Germany diabetes in the army was less frequent than in the civil population in which it is universally recognized that diabetes decreased. Yet the World War I presented an ideal opportunity for the physical and psychic, traumatic origin of diabetes both in combatants and non-combatants and that the disease did not materialize is most significant. The fear of an operation or of the pain incident to child-bearing and the extraction of teeth do not bring on diabetes, nor do we know nor have we read in the literature of a surgeon who postponed an operation for fear that the trauma incident to it would cause diabetes.

Statistics of the incidence of diabetes among the armies of the world in the recent conflict are not yet available. So far as the incidence of diabetes in the United States armed forces is concerned, exact information is not known, but preliminary data indicate the incidence is insignificant although perhaps somewhat higher than for World War I, in which the rate per 1000 strength was 0.17. Undoubtedly the total deaths from diabetes in World War II will be much less, despite the larger number of troops and the longer duration of the war, due to the use of insulin. In World War I diabetic admissions were 718 and deaths 104.[1]

So far as my colleagues and I can remember, no definite instance in which we considered trauma a cause of diabetes has occurred among the 29,000 patients who have consulted us with diabetes mellitus and glycosuria. We know of no instance in which diabetes has been considered caused by cerebral shock, embolism or thrombosis. We know of no instance in which diabetes has been caused by accidents in the course of college athletics, particularly football, and to fortify our opinion in 1940 we consulted Dr. Arlie Bock of the Department of Hygiene of Harvard University. He wrote: "as far as I can determine, no case of diabetes following trauma has occurred among athletes at Harvard. We have had many types of injury but no known injury of the pancreas, and whether such trauma might result in diabetes, I do not know. You know there has been close medical supervision of athletes at Harvard for at least twenty-five years." We know of no instance in which Dr. Harvey Cushing reported diabetes following the development of a tumor in the brain save those instances in which diabetes occurred in connection with acromegaly and basophilism, and 2 patients (out of over 200) with chromophobe adenoma. "What is very

[1] The Medical Department of the United States Army in the World War. Vol. XV. Statistics Part 2. Medical and Casualty Statistics. War Department. Washington: U. S. Printing Office, 1925.
[2] Personal communication.

significant," according to Dr. Louise Eisenhardt,[2] "is that in Dr. Cushing's own long experience in operating for tumors of the hypophysis or third ventricle he found that such operations did not result in even a transient glycosuria." Dr. Gilbert Horrax writes: "I can certainly confirm what Dr. Eisenhardt has told you regarding pituitary cases, both from my experience with Dr. Cushing's patients and from my own. Furthermore, I have been unable to find in my own records any instance of glycosuria in tumors of the fourth ventricle or fourth ventricle region."[1]

Cushing[2] held that the glycosuria of diabetes in acromegaly is due actually to the type of secretion produced by the tumor, and not by pressure of the tumor upon neighboring structures.

We have on record in this office the signed statement of a medical observer of pugilistic contests as follows: "In my twenty-five years of experience in examining boys and men for both amateur and professional boxing throughout the United States, I have never come across one person who has ever had any symptoms or any knowledge on their part submitted to me by them that they had diabetes or had been suffering from diabetes. In all the injuries due to trauma I have never known one injury resulting from trauma that would in any way cause diabetes in any form or any symptoms which would pertain to that disease. During my years of experience, 90 per cent of the people who have participated in boxing exhibitions either in the amateur or professional ranks have had repeated examinations and none have ever showed any signs or symptoms of diabetes in any of its forms."

Dr. Donald Munro[3] writes: "I can cite the fact that in over 3000 craniocerebral injuries, I know of no case in which the trauma had produced either diabetes mellitus or glycosuria, by the time the patients had left the hospital after treatment for their injuries."

The demonstration of a neurogenic origin of diabetes has not yet been given (Falta,[4] Umber[5]) and, in general, has lost support, with the growing accuracy of knowledge of the central nervous system. Grafe subscribed to this in 1933,[6] but in 1938 changed his opinion.[7] The neurogenic conception of diabetes must not be dismissed in too cavalier a fashion; nor should one blind one's self to the fact of no

---

[1] Personal communication. Dr. Horrax writes further: "However, this much must be said regarding our present cases, that it would be perhaps impossible to tell definitely about a traumatic glycosuria from operations in this region since we now start all these patients with intravenous glucose at the beginning of the operation and then if necessary they can have a transfusion without any interruption of the flow of fluid. However, before this operative technic I know of no instance in our series." Dr. Horrax confirmed this statement in 1946.

[2] Cushing: Lancet, 119, 117, 1930.

[3] Munro: New England Jour. Med., **224**, 766, 1941.

[4] Falta: Die Zuckerkrankheit, Berlin und Wien, Urban & Schwarzenberg, p. 194, 1936.

[5] Umber: Handbuch der gesamten unfallheilkunde, Stuttgart, Ferdinand Enke, vol. **1**, 1932.

[6] Grafe: Metabolic Diseases and Their Treatment, Philadelphia, Lea & Febiger, 1933.

[7] Grafe: Med. Klin., **34**, 403, 1938; **34**, 430, 1938.

evident pathological change in the pancreas in 24 per cent of the
cases of diabetes, or to the existence of pathological anatomical
findings in the central nervous system, when such are disclosed by
experiment or postmortem examination.

Naturally, Young's experiments aroused new interest in the
pituitary gland, but, save for the rather frequent association of
diabetes with acromegaly (a follow-up by Coggeshall and Root[1] of
Cushing's 155 cases of proved acromegaly revealed 18 per cent
diabetic instead of the original 12 per cent), no proof is available
pathologically of its involvement in diabetes. Indeed, Eisenhardt
and Warren examined with extraordinary care the pituitaries of 55
of my diabetic patients without finding distinctive lesions.

Localized experimental destruction in areas of the hypothalamic
region of the brain, with the appearance of diabetes, was observed
in 1 of 50 monkeys, but in none of over 300 cats by Ranson.[2] Strieck[3]
observed glycosuria and hyperglycemia by producing lesions in the
hypothalamic area in dogs, and in 1 dog he believed that he definitely produced diabetes. The pancreas presented no abnormalities.

Is it surprising that with some 1,000,000 diabetics now alive in
this country, and approximately 4,000,000 other individuals whom
we can confidently expect to come down with it before they die,
one may discover glycosuria and even diabetes following the million, more or less, injuries annually which these people undergo?

The older literature upon trauma in relation to diabetes should be
discarded, because diagnoses were often inaccurate, due to lack of
tests for sugar in the blood and of differentiation of the various
kinds of urinary sugar or of renal glycosuria. It is notable in the
last nine years since the publication of the article on Trauma and
Diabetes Mellitus in the first edition of Trauma and Disease[4] how
few articles have appeared on the subject and how few cases apparently have come to trial in the courts. The spell of Claude Bernard[5]
hung over the disease and confusion regarding its etiology reigned
until in 1889 von Mering and Minkowski[6] demonstrated its dependence upon the pancreas and later Opie and Ssobolew its connection with the islands of Langerhans.

The recent experimental production of diabetes by two methods:
(a) the injection of an extract of the anterior pituitary into animals
and (b) the administration of alloxan are both linked with destruction of the islands of Langerhans.

In any consideration of trauma and diabetes one should bear in
mind that diabetes is universal, that 1 in 40 of the deaths in the

[1] Coggeshall and Root: Endocrinology, 26, 1, 1940.
[2] Ranson, Fisher and Ingram: Endocrinology, 23, 175, 1938.
[3] Strieck: Ztschr. f. d. ges. exper. Med., 104, 232, 1938.
[4] Joslin: Trauma and Diabetes, in Trauma and Disease, Brahdy and Kahn Eds.,
Philadelphia, Lea & Febiger, 1937; 2nd Ed., 1941.
[5] Bernard: Compt. rend. Soc. de Biol. 1849 (Paris), 1, 60, 1850.
[6] von Mering and Minkowski: Arch. f. exp. Path. u. Pharm., 26, 371, 1889–1890.

country in 1943 was reported due to it, and that 1 individual in 4 is a carrier of the disease. These facts are all important when the question of trauma arises, because they indicate how widespread the disease is and, therefore, the necessity of knowing whether the individual in question already had the disease before the accident. In Arizona in 1940 1 doctor in 42 of 339 responding, and in Rhode Island 1 in 36 of 392 who replied, reported he had diabetes.

The diagnosis of the diabetes must rest upon a sure foundation. The sugar in the urine must be glucose, not levulose or pentose, and be disclosed by a reliable test. The glycosuria must not be the result of dietetic or other tricks. Hyperglycemia is likewise essential and the methods employed to determine it should be investigated. Whereas a report of the presence of glycosuria usually can be accepted at its face value, the absence of glycosuria or hyperglycemia is by no means distinctive, because it is well known that even in diabetes, especially since the use of insulin, such conditions often prevail.

The investigation of any case of trauma as a possible factor in the causation of diabetes leads to a study of the family history of the patient for heredity, past or present overweight of the patient, and in children overheight, the presence of an infection, circumstances which might have prevented use of the muscles, because these states are favoring influences leading to the development of the disease. Bertram, in his second edition,[1] supplements the description in his first edition of a patient with no known heredity who, four weeks subsequent to a fall on the handlebars of a bicycle and followed by a long period of unconsciousness and marked abdominal pains, was found to have diabetes, by adding that subsequently the son developed true diabetes. He therefore now concludes that one must exclude a traumatic origin of diabetes in this case.

Trauma is practically never the primary cause of diabetes. Like von Noorden,[2] Umber[3] and Labbé,[4] I believe that it is only under extraordinary conditions that it can directly cause the disease.

With this view Viggo Thomsen agrees,[5] basing his opinion upon studies of blood and urine of 144 patients at the time of and subsequent to accidents, upon the absence of any essential difference in the frequency of diabetes in injured and non-injured persons in the Aarhus Hospital in Denmark between 1921 and 1935, upon a critical review of 81 cases reported in the literature as examples of traumatic diabetes, upon the lack of evidence that trauma can other than temporarily change the degree or course of the disease and, finally, upon his own experimental investigations.

[1] Bertram: Die Zuckerkrankheit, 2nd ed., Leipzig, Georg Thieme, p. 32, 1939.
[2] Von Noorden and Isaac: Loc. cit., p. 64.
[3] Umber: Loc. cit., p. 85.
[4] Labbé: Ann. de Med. leg., **7**, 541, 1927.
[5] Thomsen: Studies of Trauma and Carbohydrate Metabolism with Special Reference to the Existence of Traumatic Diabetes, Acta med. Scandin., Suppl. 91, 1938. See also Editorial, Jour. Am. Med. Assn., **112**, 1592, 1939.

An injury to the pancreas sufficient to produce diabetes would be so destructive that it is almost inconceivable that it could be compatible with life.   Among the more than 27,000 cases of diabetes seen by von Noorden, the 7,000 treated by Umber since 1923, and the 29,000 patients who have consulted me for sugar in the urine, there has been no patient whose diabetes they or I believe was directly caused by trauma.   It is true that various authors, but with less experience, particularly in years gone by, thought and do still believe otherwise.   Von Noorden in his early life, and I, too, suspected that trauma was a feature, but the more he and I saw of diabetes the less likely did either of us believe and certainly the less do I believe it to be a cause of diabetes directly or indirectly. On the other hand, it is recognized that frequently immediately following trauma an existing diabetes becomes apparent and exceptionally that the trauma indirectly may activate a tendency to diabetes hitherto dormant, latent, or, with Grote,[1] "potential," and thus allow the actual disease to break forth, but to subside to its quiescent state with the cessation of the effect of the trauma. Likewise, a severe trauma may, but not necessarily, make a diabetes more severe.   R. Herbst[2] also expresses views in line with those of the author.

It is conceivable that trauma might advance the date of onset of diabetes in an hereditarily predisposed individual who was predestined to become diabetic at a given age.   I believe such an individual would develop the disease earlier in life if he were fat, subjected to an infection, particularly in the region of the biliary tract, was incapacitated to such an extent that he could not use his muscles normally, or acquired a permanent lesion of the pituitary, thyroid, adrenal glands, or liver, but not as a result of mental or emotional strain.   Suppose a man is born with a diabetic tendency, escapes the disease in childhood, but when he comes of age realizes the tendency exists and in consequence tries to avert the development of diabetes by guarding against obesity, does the best he can to prevent the onset of infections, and, if they appear, seeks quick alleviation of the same, utilizes his muscles, and fortunately is free from evidence of disease of the endocrine glands or the liver.   If this man has an accident which interferes with the further carrying out of a life's program and diabetes develops, who could say that the accident did not hasten the appearance of the diabetes?   Furthermore, would not the same answer hold if by chance or environment, rather than by design, all these precautionary measures against the onset of diabetes had been fulfilled?

If one should grant that diabetes developed prematurely in a predisposed individual, what effect would it have upon him?   Above all else it would mean health *versus* chronic illness and his expectancy

---

[1] Grote: Deutsche med. Wchnschr., **57**, 984, 1931.
[2] Herbst: Münch. med. Wchnschr., **II**, 1262, 1936.

for life would be shortened. How much this would be is not certain, but it has been calculated by the Statistical Department of the Metropolitan Life Insurance Company, based upon death-rates of my patients, subsequent to first observation, regardless of duration of diabetes. Thus a diabetic child of ten years has an expectancy of forty years compared with fifty-seven years for the ordinary child and a diabetic at sixty-five years an expectancy of eight years instead of the ordinary expectancy of twelve years. See Table 42, page 321. These calculations were based on the death-rates of my patients in 1929–1938.

The situation alters materially, however, when one compares the effect of an injury upon a diabetic and a non-diabetic. Here the effect of the injury must be calculated upon the diabetic's life expectancy and not from that of the total population.

The rarity of trauma as an etiological factor in diabetes, direct or indirect, is in striking contrast to its frequency during the course of the disease. Perhaps one-sixth, recently one-fourth to one-third due to the shortage of beds and the acceptance of those requiring emergency care, of my patients treated in the New England Deaconess Hospital have lesions of the legs and here trauma plays a large factor. Trauma in the course of diabetes is destined to become increasingly important, because diabetics are living so much longer and thus the time-risk of exposure is more than doubled, because diabetics are dying at an average age of sixty-five years instead of at forty-four and finally because the long duration of the disease exposes the patient still more to the sequelæ incident to it.

The diabetic, I regret to acknowledge, is vulnerable because of the nature of his ailment. He is apt to have more arteriosclerosis after some years' duration than the normal individual, a greater susceptibility to tuberculosis and to local infections of the skin, an increased liability to fractures, possibly sometimes related to deficient calcium in his bones, and is in danger of a certain degree of mental irresponsibility in consequence of diabetic coma or insulin reactions. All of these states in and of themselves constitute hazards which he must face and because he has these he is less able to protect himself from trauma.

The manifold opportunities for trauma in the course of insulin reactions and the medico-legal complications which may ensue have been enumerated by Adlersberg and Dolger.[1] The picture which they paint is far more vivid and the frequency of the instances cited appears far more common than I meet in my practice.

Direct Trauma.—The pancreas is so deeply situated in the abdomen, so well protected posteriorly by the backbone and the strong muscles of the back, and anteriorly by the stomach, intestines, the liver, and the overhanging chest wall, that it is sheltered from all save the severest injuries and almost absolutely excluded from

[1] Adlersberg and Dolger: Ann. Int. Med., 12, 1804, 1939.

selective and independent injury. The causation of diabetes directly by trauma, therefore, can only take place when the pancreas is injured to an extraordinary degree. To bring this about it is only conceivable when the injury is violent, productive of immediate symptoms of grave intensity accompanied by excruciating pain, and involves other surrounding vital structures of the body with prompt manifestations of damage to the same, and, indeed, generally the blow must be of so extreme a nature as to cause death instantly or within a few hours. Unquestionably if the blow or injury was not sufficient to warrant immediate medical attention it could not be assumed reasonably to be severe enough to cause diabetes.

To produce diabetes trauma must interfere with the secretion of the islands of Langerhans of the pancreas, but that it can do this except by actual physical injury to the same is not known. We know that the secretion of insulin is controlled chiefly if not wholly by the amount of sugar in the blood and that the blood sugar in turn is influenced by nervous stimuli originating in the sympathetic nerve tracts, connecting adrenal, thyroid, pituitary glands and regions of the brain adjacent to the latter, but trauma of these has never been proved experimentally, explained scientifically or, so far as my knowledge goes, been shown clinically to be the direct cause of diabetes. As yet the evidence for nervous control is conflicting and chiefly rests upon an experimental basis of an intricate nature. It is largely a question as to how much the liver enters into the problem. Recently even the interpretation of the Claude Bernard puncture is questioned.

Young's demonstration of the production of diabetes in dogs by the injection of an extract of the anterior portion of the pituitary gland suggested at first an extra-pancreatic influence, but the later finding of disease of the islands of Langerhans showed the pancreas was concerned with its development and thus maintained the unity of the disease. This also holds true for alloxan diabetes.

There are few cases of diabetes in the literature attributed to direct trauma which rest on as good a foundation as that reported by H. Gideon Wells[1] of Chicago. However, the diagnosis in his case depends upon one examination of the urine obtained after death, and Thomsen excludes it. Another case which we were privileged through the kindness of Professor Grafe of Würzburg to report for the first time is more complete, although even with this patient the urine had not been tested for some time prior to the accident.

A. K., aged fifty-seven years, married, merchant, supposedly free from diabetes, motoring to a bath cure on account of gall stones of several years' duration, May 19, 1934, while driving 50 miles an hour, was forced to put on his brakes sharply to avoid a motorcycle coming in the opposite direction around a curve, and hit a tree. The fender bore the shock fairly well, but the automobile went into the ditch. His abdomen and chest were pressed

---

[1] Wells: Am. Jour. Med. Sci., 164, 479, 1922.

against the steering wheel, but he had no pain following the accident and felt well. The automobile was righted and he resumed driving, but developed what was diagnosed as a gall stone attack in three hours, yet he continued the journey with a hired chauffeur on May 20. The attack persisting, he transferred to the train. Upon arrival at the Spa, May 21, he was somnolent, had an acetone breath, showed blood in the vomitus and stools, and had marked thirst. Glycosuria 4.7 per cent; blood sugar over 0.50 per cent. Not improving, he was sent to Professor Grafe May 21.

Upon entrance to the clinic acetone odor to breath, glycosuria 4.5 per cent, marked reactions for acetone and diacetic acid; blood sugar 556 milligrams; no vomiting; pallor; pulse good; hemoglobin 85 per cent; abdomen perfectly soft with no pain on pressure, and cautious palpation revealed indistinctly a sausage-shaped tumor. Leukocytes abundant in the urine, a few erythrocytes, no albumin or bile, temperature 38.8° C., pulse 120. Diabetes and acidosis were controlled during the night with insulin, 160 units, but although conscious in the morning with blood sugar 84 milligrams, he failed rapidly and died at 8.30 A.M.

The autopsy showed a beginning fat necrosis with local peritonitis near the pancreas. That organ was completely infarcted with blood and measured 15 to 20 cm. by 5 to 7 cm. In the pancreatic vein there was a large thrombus. Anatomical diagnosis: thrombosis of the splenic vein; extensive pancreatic apoplexy; thrombosis of a branch of the portal vein; fat necrosis of the omentum and mesentery; diffuse peritonitis; general congestion of the organs.

A third case is reported by Stern[1] to whom we are indebted for subsequent information regarding the patient.

The patient was hit in the left side and back by an automobile August 12, 1926, suffered with severe pain in the abdomen for six days, and when about to leave the hospital on the eighth day went into severe shock and collapsed with agonizing pain in the abdomen. Laparotomy revealed a hemorrhagic pancreatitis with diffuse peritonitis and fat necrosis. Recovery occurred after a ten months' stay in the hospital, during which time two large intraabdominal abscesses were opened. Later a subphrenic abscess developed which was drained. On August 21 her blood sugar was 0.128, on August 24, 0.140 and on August 27, 0.160 mg. per 100 cc. About November, 1929, severe diabetes developed, with a blood sugar of 308 mg. per 100 cc. and 4 per cent sugar in the urine which with dieting returned to normal. The father of the patient died of diabetes at the age of eighty-four years; a daughter at the age of thirty years had melituria, believed to be due to fructose, but the other three children were apparently free of diabetes. Insulin had been taken since March, 1930, at the last report, July, 1939.

A fourth case, subsequently recalled by Grafe,[2] from his days as a medical assistant, deserves mention, because of the presence of diabetes for a year or more after injury to the pancreas, with later recovery following subsidence of the suppurative pancreatitis. The case is as follows:

Case 143. "A man with a severe gunshot wound of the pancreas had a suppurative pancreatic fistula for a year. A severe diabetes developed, which lasted for a year following the closure of the fistula, and thereupon subsided. Although a great part of the pancreas was involved and destroyed at the time of the accident, yet, in this instance, infection played the chief

[1] Stern: Am. Jour. Surg., **8**, 58, 1930.
[2] Grafe: Med. Klin., **34**, 403, 1938; **34**, 430, 1938.

rôle, since it is known from experiments with animals that, as a rule, a tenth of the gland can maintain the function of the pancreas, provided, as Allen in his beautiful experiment showed, excessive carbohydrate alimentation is not administered. In favor of this explanation is the recovery from the diabetes as a result of the healing of the suppuration with closure of the fistula."

Geiger and Benson[1] and Lommel[2] have reported cases in which they believe the possibility of trauma having caused the diabetes should not be ignored. They concede the difficulty in reaching a decision, yet plead for an open-minded consideration of the facts even though scientific reasoning points against a traumatic etiology of the disease. Troëll,[3] in Stockholm, in a carefully prepared article, reports 10 cases in which glycosuria or diabetes was present with trauma, and even passed upon by the board of reparations. In only 2 of these was the trauma considered as a cause of the diabetes. The evidence by no means was as strong as in Grafe's case and, in one, followed an injury to the elbow, and the *post hoc propter hoc* argument was raised because the urine was said to be sugar free the day before the accident. These cases are carefully reported and the circumstances of each are clearly discussed. Troëll, like Lommel, is unwilling to concede that trauma to the pancreas alone can cause diabetes. He believes, as Naunyn emphasized, peripheral injury elsewhere *via* paths of the sympathetic nervous system could be a factor in bringing on the diabetes, disagreeing absolutely with Thomsen. His views seem to me to be biased by Swedish social accident insurance.

In this connection, a patient is recalled who had been himself an insurance salesman. He maintained in court action, directed against an insurance company, that he had sustained an accidental injury to one toe by stubbing it against a chair on a public excursion boat in Boston Harbor. This injury he claimed had led to infection, and the injury had resulted in diabetes followed by angina pectoris. It happened that he had a peculiar insurance policy which provided for triple indemnity in the event of injury occurring accidentally on a public carrier. If it could have been maintained successfully that this accident had caused not only the injury to the toe, but *via* the sympathetic nervous system, also the diabetes and angina pectoris, under the terms of his contract the total indemnity would have been about $80,000. Actually, in this case the records showed that his diabetes had existed prior to the accident. If such an interpretation as the claimant urged had been accepted by the courts and a precedent thus established, it is easy to see that insurance premium rates would eventually be greatly increased either generally or specifically in patients where diabetes could be established from hereditary family history. Therefore, actually, the acceptance of such a point of view while probably immediately profitable to the one person involved would have social consequences for a large number of people, which would be most costly.

In general the shorter the interval between the occurrence of the trauma and its alleged effect, the greater the likelihood of a relation between the

[1] Geiger and Benson: Am. Jour. Surg., **47**, 672, 1940.
[2] Lommel: Med. Welt, **13**, 836, 1939.
[3] Troëll: Der Chirurg., **12**, 113, 1940.

two. Each day which passes without diabetic symptoms or accentuation of diabetic symptoms lessens the probability or even the possibility of association of the trauma with the status found.

Transitory glycosuria after trauma, according to Thomsen, seldom persists more than seven days and it is unusual for the glycosuria to exceed 0.5 per cent; abnormal glucose tolerance curves were obtained in 34 of 100 instances following trauma, but as a rule these soon disappeared and in but 2 were found as late as thirty and forty-nine days after the accident, and in these two instances normal curves were later found. His data were similar to those of Davidson and Allen,[1] who performed sugar tolerance tests upon patients with concussion of the brain and skull fractures. Mock and deTakats[2] believe a head injury, if there is a diabetic tendency, may become a serious menace. Dr. deTakats writes as of March 18, 1946: "The conclusion reached in the study of head injuries which was undertaken with Dr. Harry Mock was that a temporary hyperglycemia occurred after any cerebral anoxia. However, we did not encounter a single case in which diabetes appeared after a head injury in a patient in whom there was no suspicion of a latent diabetes beforehand. . . . Since that time I have had very little contact with traumatic and industrial cases, but it has been the impression of our group that a latent or clinically not manifest diabetes might become more severe after head injury. I recollect one case of a known diabetic with a fasting blood sugar of 140 milligrams per cent who was sugar free without insulin. This rather obese woman developed a rather severe acute exacerbation of her diabetes. Six weeks later, however, her diabetic status was identical with what she had before the head injury." Compare Cushing, Eisenhardt and Horrax, see page 84, also Thomsen, page 87.

Indirect Trauma.—Indirectly trauma might cause diabetes if it could set in motion processes which would lead to the destruction of a sufficient number of the islands of Langerhans of the pancreas. One-tenth of the pancreas may suffice to prevent diabetes, but usually does not do so, so that we can say that diabetes will occur only when more than five-sixths, more probably nine-tenths, of the islands of Langerhans are destroyed or rendered inactive. This seldom happens as a result of disease, despite the comparative frequency of pancreatitis and of cancer of the pancreas.

For experimental pituitary diabetes, see page 120, and for alloxan diabetes, see page 178.

An infection makes diabetes worse. Could it bring on diabetes through involvement of the pancreas? In the opinion of our group infections are rare preceding the onset of diabetes and we note Lande,[3] writing from Umber's Clinic, holds the same view. However, recognizing that an infection makes diabetes worse it is reasonable to conclude that a diabetes latent, but almost having reached the stage of becoming frank, might be changed by an infection into a frank diabetes. Perhaps the best illustration of such an eventuality occurs in connection with carbuncles. It is not uncommon for a patient to be seen whose diabetes was not recognized before the carbuncle developed, yet during the active stage of the carbuncle it

[1] Davidson and Allen: Bull. Johns Hopkins Hosp., **37**, 217, 1925.
[2] Mock and deTakats: Ann. Surg., **90**, 190, 1929.
[3] Lande: Klin. Wchnschr., **101**, 359, 1931.

becomes marked or even alarmingly severe and controlled with the greatest difficulty, but following the subsidence of the carbuncle the diabetes retrogresses and insulin, which may have reached 50 or more units, can be omitted and the patient stay sugar-free upon a diet with 200 grams of carbohydrate. The diabetes may subside so completely after convalescence from the carbuncle that it is believed by the unwary to have been temporary.

Thus a hard working doctor, Case 14121, upon routine examination in September found his urine sugar-free. He was in health, but (1) he had a sister with diabetes, (2) he was sixty years old, and in the peak decade for onset of diabetes, (3) by being above normal weight, he was three steps on the road to the disease. It was the grape season and his friends laughingly said that he had eaten a bushel of grapes and (4) perhaps this excessive quantity of glucose calories advanced him a fourth step, while a carbuncle (5) of indefinite traumatic origin made a fifth, which took him over the line into the disease in October, 1935.

Occasionally an infection apparently of trifling nature in a diabetic may lead to dire, even fatal, consequences. This happened when a patient pulled out a protruding hair from the nose, and in another instance as a result of a simple paronychia. Very commonly trifling injuries to the feet lead to the loss of a toe, foot, leg or even the life of the patient. Infections of the biliary tract have been supposed to favor the onset of diabetes, but the experience of the Metropolitan Life Insurance Company, as studied by Dr. Louis I. Dublin[1] showed no particular relationship between gall bladder disease and the onset of diabetes.

Already we have summed up the prevailing view regarding the influence of the nervous system, physically or psychically, in the etiology of diabetes or upon its course, but we will cite a few examples.

Richard T., Case 5786, aged thirteen years, went fishing through the ice and fell in, but was rescued by his setter dog, Laddie. That night, January 2, 1927, for the first time polyuria began, and on January 14, I found 9 per cent of sugar in the urine. On January 26, the urine was sugar-free and the blood sugar normal both before and after meals, but the diabetes persisted. By contrast, I (E. P. J.), too, fell through the ice as a child and my Newfoundland dog, Major, played a rôle in the rescue, yet neither the dog nor I developed diabetes. Consider the number of boys who yearly have a similar escapade and never contract the disease.[2]

Carrasco-Formiguera[3] cites the following tragic case, No. 34, of his series, in which diabetes appeared to have arisen as a sequel to an extraordinary, psychical trauma. Diabetic symptoms, polydipsia, polyuria, physical and mental depression appeared suddenly and with extreme intensity in a man a few hours after suffering a double emotion. (1) He saw die on the seat beside him a fellow-worker whom he was accompanying from the shop

[1] Dublin, Jimenis and Marks: Proc. Assn. Life Ins. Med. Directors, **21**, 34, 1934.

[2] Rarely the symptoms of diabetes may follow a nervous shock as in an obese Italian, described by Root, but who can accept an etiologic relation, when the vast majority of cases begin without such shock? Root: Med. Clin. No. Am., **21**, 441, 1937.

[3] Carrasco-Formiguera: In Spanish edition of Joslin's Treatment of Diabetes Melitus, Barcelona, Montaner and Simon, 1925, p. 141.

because of sudden illness, and (2) he was held as the alleged slayer until the true circumstances were established a few hours later. The patient had suffered in his early childhood a serious traumatism with cerebral concussion. When the diabetes began he was aged eighteen years, and until then he had felt sound and strong. He died two years later in diabetic coma.

In contrast is cited Case 13332 who was in perfect health so far as he or his family knew on December 24, 1934. That night this fourteen-year old Jewish boy, with diabetic heredity, slept without rising from bed. On Christmas day there was no especial excitement or careless eating, yet that night he rose six times, and seventeen days later, when we first saw him, the urine contained 8 per cent sugar. He is doing well (in August, 1946) but the diabetes persists.

There was no accident here to cause diabetes. There was no heredity known at the time, although later it was learned his mother's cousin had diabetes. It was as if the thread which held the Damocles Sword had been cut. Suppose your automobile injured this lad while coasting on Christmas Day, or that for some reason you had severely reprimanded him and he had undergone an emotional reaction. I feel confident that abroad, if the case came into court, the acute onset of his diabetes would be put in evidence against you, and for social and insurance reasons he would have secured favorable consideration. In such a situation attention should be focused on the overwhelming number of similarly acute cases, which spring into being without any reason whatsoever to suspect physical or psychologic trauma.

All these considerations, therefore, show how essential it is to investigate the background of any case of trauma in which diabetes may be a factor.

There are approximately 10,000 (one per cent of 1,000,000) diabetics in the United States with the history of a sudden onset of diabetes. What opportunities they afford for traumatic, diabetic exploitation! This special group represents the *élite* corps from which recruits for the traumatic etiology of diabetes should be most easily obtained, but that I have recognized none with a traumatic basis among the more than 200 of this class I have personally studied, is of some import.

Our skepticism concerning the etiological significance of organic or functional brain disturbance as a forerunner of diabetes is shared by von Noorden and Umber and many others, but another group takes a different view. Among these is Schur[1] who cites Umber's notable case.

During a revolution a prisoner lived in a continuously well-grounded fear of death. Above all else he realized there was great danger in falling asleep. When his own brother, a fellow prisoner, dropped off to sleep, he was shot in his sleep. "From this moment, like a blow from the sky, symptoms of a severe diabetes set in." Previously a diabetes was said not to have existed. Could, Schur asks, one claim with any degree of definiteness that this man, without his trauma, would have become ill with a manifest diabetes, and, if so, when would it have occurred?

Injuries to the head quite frequently lead to glycosuria, but this is temporary in character. They are more prone to do this if there is a concussion as well. It is tempting at times to say diabetes results, but as yet I have not been satisfied to accept such an interpretation. Only too rarely is the case history as complete as that reported by Liniger.[2]

---

[1] Schur: Ztschr. f. klin. Med., **123**, 800, 1933.
[2] Liniger: Monatschr. f. Unfallheilkunde, No. 1. S. 2, 1896.

A young doctor following a fall from a horse had a fracture of the skull with concussion and showed glycosuria. However, it developed that before the accident he had examined his own urine and had found sugar clearly present, although in small amount. After the accident there was no increase in glycosuria. "Had the urine not by chance been examined before the accident we would have had another typical case of traumatic glycosuria."

A different point of view is brought out by the studies of Gissel.[1] Gissel observed hyperglycemia up to 270 milligrams per cent in all head injuries resulting in unconsciousness in the first three to four days after the injury. In all skull traumas even several days after the injury, the peak of the blood sugar curves following blood sugar tests with 50 grams glucose lay far above normal and did not return to those at the starting point, even at the end of three hours. They were diabetic curves, and in Isaac's[2] opinion, who quotes Gissel, indicated that a transitory injury to the function of the pancreas can occur. Isaac, therefore, believes that in rare cases injuries to the skull can reveal diabetes or set it loose, provided the constitutional tendency is present. How this is brought about he does not pretend to say, but he agrees with Stern,[3] Grote,[4] and Jacobi and Meythaler[5] that just because we cannot completely explain the anatomical connection between the brain and the pancreas is no reason to say it does not exist and thus totally discard traumatic diabetes. Grafe[6] writes in 1936: "The cerebral production of pure diabetes up until now has succeeded neither in our hands nor in those of others, but must be set down on the whole as possible or even probable." The work of Young does introduce a pituitary element, which, however, it should be easy to exclude by the absence of direct pituitary or indirect neighborhood symptoms.

Fractures.—Fractures, not alone of the skull, but elsewhere in the body, are frequently accompanied by glycosuria. Therefore it is necessary to apply to all cases of fractures in which sugar is shown in the urine the same rigid, critical, differential diagnostic criteria which should be applied to the diagnosis of diabetes at any time. Konjetzny and Weiland's conclusions, in 1915,[7] upon glycosuria, diabetes and fractures, although still often quoted, are invalidated by the modern studies of Timpe, supported by tests of the blood sugar. Timpe[8] investigated 500 fresh fractures on the first, second, fourth and seventh days. In only one case was there found a condition relating to diabetes.

[1] Gissel: Chirurg. H., **1**, 5, 6, 1933.
[2] Isaac: Monat. f. Unfallheilkunde, **40**, 181, 1933.
[3] Stern: Traumatische Entstehunginnerer Krankheiten, 3d ed., Jena, Gustav Fisher, 1930.
[4] Grote: Loc. cit., p. 88.
[5] Jacobi and Meythaler: Ergebn. d. inn. Med. v. Kindheilkunde, **45**, 189, 1933.
[6] Grafe: Handbuch der Biochemie des Menschen und der Tiere, Zweite Auflage, III, 702, 1936.
[7] Konjetzny and Weiland: Mitt. a. d. Grenzgeb. d. Med. u. Chir., **28**, 860, 1915.
[8] Timpe: Arch. f. Orthopäd. u. Unfall. Chir., **35**, 112, 1935.

Fractures are common in diabetic patients. It is the rule for the bone to heal promptly, and we recall but one instance in which this has not taken place, Case 14335, female, aged sixty-eight years, duration eight years, who sustained a broken hip which failed to unite despite many operative attempts. Now that diabetics live longer, there is more opportunity for fractures to occur, and we expect the incidence of fractures will show a considerable rise. Diabetics are older, and not actually older by chronological age, but also older because of their diabetes, and thus more susceptible to fractures. But there is another reason, namely, calcium deficiency. Possibly this will not be noted much in the future, but there have been seven notable instances in our experience. These occurred as spontaneous or nearly spontaneous fractures of the spine. In these cases the vertebræ showed deficient calcium. It is easy to understand that this could take place formerly when milk was so largely excluded from the diet and thus the main source of calcium removed. Likewise, formerly, there was more acidosis than today, and this would tend to remove calcium. A succession of fractures is not so very rare. Case 13906, onset of diabetes mellitus at 34.3 years, has sustained 7 fractures in the course of seven years.

Although the pituitary, thyroid and adrenal glands are intimately associated with the pancreas, experimental traumatic injury or disease of the same does not cause true diabetes. This statement still holds despite the work of Houssay and Young and Best on the pituitary and that of Long and Lukens and also Ingle upon the adrenal.

Trauma in Connection With the Use of Insulin.—Within a very few months after the use of insulin in human beings, instances of infection at the site of injection of insulin practically ceased. Among 1838 admissions to the George F. Baker Clinic during 1941 there were but 8 who entered for abscesses due to the injection of insulin. When one considers that only this small number of incidents occurred among many million injections in patients both inside and outside the hospital, it is evident both the manufacturers and patients use care. Needles broken in the skin during injection have never led to serious trouble in my experience, and such occurrences are even more rare than abscesses. A far more frequent, and infinitely more serious, opportunity for trauma is that incident to an insulin reaction. However, despite the thousands of insulin reactions occurring in the course of treatment of diabetes, I remember only two resulting in a fracture. This is in marked contrast to the incidence of fractures when insulin is employed to produce convulsions in non-diabetic neurologic patients. I did observe one case in which death appeared to result from the patient, while unconscious, having regurgitated food which plugged the trachea. Still more serious are those cases in which an insulin reaction has been mistaken for diabetic coma and, in consequence,

7

a dose of insulin has been given which resulted in death. Fortunately, such instances are few.

For a more detailed discussion of trauma in relation to diabetes with literature, see the author's article in Trauma in Relation to Disease[1] and also a paper published in the Annals of Surgery,[2] also Stern[3] in which the older literature is reviewed.

8. **Liver.**—(See pages 131, 211 and 543.)

9. **Various Endocrine Glands.**—The influence of the endocrine glands is discussed on pages 120 and 213 and also in Chapter XXVII.

10. **Gout.**—The number of cases of gout occuring in association with diabetes among our clientèle is trifling. However, even a single case is important, because in one instance under my care a bursa, which later proved to be inflamed because of gout, was incised, whereas with the correct diagnosis it would have been let alone. We are sure we have not seen more than 1 case of gout per 1500 true diabetics. Notable cases are 24640, 23799, 15798, 11844, 23042, 20777.

Diabetes and gout have many features in common. Among 56 patients with gouty arthritis Ishmael[4] found 42.8 per cent were from diabetic families. Obesity was a family characteristic in 71.4 per cent of his group.

D.   THE PREVENTION OF DIABETES.

Fortunately nearly everything that has been said thus far about the etiology of diabetes carries with it possibilities for prevention of the disease. The much higher incidence of glycosuria and diabetes among selectees (see page 42) than anticipated emphasizes the necessity of routine examinations of urine (the specimen voided after a meal) and blood to discover early cases. Only in this way can diabetes be attacked in its incipiency. The intervals between onset and diagnosis and diagnosis and the beginning of treatment must be shortened. In the section of this chapter devoted to heredity the means by which a diabetic may avoid transmission of the disease, namely, by marriage to a non-diabetic in a non-diabetic family, are set forth. (See page 66.) And as for obesity, the inference is so plain that it should be avoided generally, and particularly by the relatives of a diabetic, that no further comment is needed. However, these simple principles must be emphasized to the patient, in season and out of season. We doctors should remember that our struggle to prevent diabetes is largely wasted unless we concentrate our efforts upon diabetics themselves and their relatives.

[1] Joslin: Loc. cit., p. 66.
[2] Joslin: Loc. cit., p. 83.
[3] Stern: Trauma in Internal Disease, With Consideration of Experimental Pathology and Medico-legal Aspects, New York, Grune and Stratton, 1945.
[4] Ishmael: Jour. Oklahoma Med. Assn., 38, 415, 1945.

Focus on the diabetic family for the prevention of the disease, and focus on the patient for the prevention of its complications. These are the slogans. The relatives, and especially the obese relatives, are the susceptibles. One might even go further and say, focus on the diabetic family to prevent obesity in all its members, and then one is doing all that is possible to prevent new cases in the group. Relatives of diabetics must be instructed never to allow their weight to go above the normal standard and, in fact, after the middle of the fourth decade to keep the weight 5 to 10 per cent below such standards. Anyone thirty or more years old and 30 pounds overweight should be given a glucose tolerance test. When diabetes or diabetic heredity exists, the further transmission of the disease is only completely avoided when there is no progeny and there will be no transmission if the chosen partner in marriage is a non-diabetic of a non-diabetic family and in turn his descendants do not marry diabetics or diabetic carriers.

The announcement by Best *et al.*[1] that diabetes can be prevented in a dog receiving injections of anterior pituitary extract provided simultaneously insulin is administered, raised for the first time the possibility of a method by which diabetes can be attacked and stopped in its earliest stages or even avoided by prophylactic means. They suggested the prophylactic use of insulin experimentally in families with marked heredity. Lukens and Dohan[2] (see page 123) also prevented and reversed diabetes in a cat by maintaining the blood sugar at a normal level after injections of anterior pituitary extract.

In a study of our own cases,[3] although no cures of diabetes can be claimed, in certain patients early, vigorous treatment with either a restricted diet or insulin or both seems in retrospect to have brought about an amelioration in the diabetic condition of far greater degree than one would anticipate. However, many other patients, equally well treated, responded with only the expected amount of improvement. Are we on the brink of a new era? At any rate, no doubt exists about the wisdom of treating all the early cases and the mildest cases in the most vigorous fashion in the hope of overcoming the disease completely or at least halting its progress. (See also pages 325 to 327.)

E. LIFE INSURANCE.

Insurance companies have begun to insure diabetics. This is good news, because it is proof that insurance companies recognize the improved status of diabetics and, second, because of the effect it will have upon the diabetics themselves. The diabetic will

[1] Haist, Campbell and Best: New England Jour. Med., **223**, 607, 1940.
[2] Lukens and Dohan: Science, **92**, 222, 1940.
[3] McDaniel, Marble and Joslin: Conn. State Med. Jour., **4**, 710, 1940.

naturally ask: Who will be eligible? How must a diabetic live to secure insurance?

Insurance companies interested in the possibility of offering life insurance to diabetics have from time to time asked us for information which would help them establish criteria for the insurability of applicants. Accordingly, we submit below answers to specific questions received or, to save space, refer to pages where the various subjects have been treated.

I. Predisposing or Precipitating Factors.—To what extent do the following predispose to or precipitate diabetes?

1. *Q. Heredity?* A. From 25 to 40 per cent of diabetics admit a diabetic heredity, and the longer the passage of time since onset of the disease and the closer the knowledge of ancestors, the higher the percentage. Homologous diabetic twins show 49 per cent heredity. Fifty-five per cent of 249 cases with onset in childhood, who have survived the disease 20 or more years are hereditary. It is estimated that 1 individual in 4 in the United States has a diabetic relative. (See pages 54 to 68.)

2. *Q. Overweight?* A. Of increasing importance beginning with 32 per cent in the second decade and reaching 89–79 per cent from the fourth onward. (See Table 18 and pages 68 to 80.)

3. *Q. Lack of exercise?* A. Of considerable significance, although largely associated with obesity. Compare urban and rural mortalities, incidence among white collar workers and laborers. (See pages 43, 78 and 80.)

4. *Q. Use of alcohol?* A. Chiefly as predisposing to obesity.

II. Diagnosis.

1. *Q. What symptomatology, clinical and laboratory, warrants a diagnosis of diabetes?* A. The demonstration of glucose in the urine plus a fasting blood sugar of 130 mg. per 100 cc. or of 170 mg. or more at other hours of the day. Clinical signs—polydipsia, polyphagia, polyuria, loss of weight and strength—are suggestive but by no means essential. (See pages 306 and 313.)

2. *Q. Of what diagnostic value are analyses of urine specimens collected two hours after a full carbohydrate meal?* A. Few untreated diabetics two hours after a full carbohydrate meal will fail to show glycosuria, particularly if the specimen voided represents the entire quantity of urine secreted after the meal. Most will exhibit hyperglycemia, but only when glycosuria is present and the blood sugar is 170 mg. or more, is the diagnosis of diabetes justifiable.

3. *Q. Of what diagnostic value is the fasting blood sugar alone?* A. If the fasting blood sugar is 130 mg. or more, it is diabetes if glycosuria is present then or at some other time. However, many mild diabetics and especially children in the early months of their disease may have normal fasting blood sugar values.

4. *Q. Of what diagnostic value is the sugar tolerance test?* A. It is decisive of diabetes, but borderline and bizarre tests should always be repeated and all tests should be performed when the patient has been upon an unrestricted diet and free from infection.

(*a*) *Q. What quantity of glucose should be given?* A. 100 grams to an adult. (See pages 158–161.)

(*b*) *Q. How many determinations of the blood sugar should be made and at what intervals before and after administration of the glucose?* A. Our custom is to take four specimens—fasting, one-half, one and two hours. (See page 159.)

(c) Q. *What is the significance of each of the readings?* A. Diagnostic of diabetes are fasting values of 130 mg. or above and peak values of 170 mg. or above, in the presence of glycosuria. At two hours the value should have fallen to 120 mg. or below. (See page 161.)

(d) Q. *What is the significance of sugar in urine specimens voided at the time of determining the blood sugar before and after ingestion of glucose?* A. In each case positive glycosuria may mean diabetes, renal glycosuria (page 788) or unclassified glycosuria.

(e) Q. *Does the prior use of insulin destroy the diagnostic value of the sugar tolerance test?* A. It might do so.

(f) Q. *If the two-hour blood sugar is within range of 80 to 120 following the administration of 100 grams of glucose, can we disregard the fasting and the height of the half-hour or one-hour reading and rule out diabetes?* A. No. Certainly not with alimentary glucose tolerance tests. We do not have sufficient experience with intravenous tests. There might be an error in the two-hour test and this would be disclosed by evaluating the fasting, half hour and one hour percentages. Always be slow to trust a single, unsupported laboratory value.

5. Q. *To what extent may the occasional ("accidental") occurrence of sugar be disregarded?* A. The presence of sugar in the urine implies diabetes and unless proved to the contrary the patient should be watched for life.

6. Q. *Is it advisable to secure a sugar tolerance test in all cases of sugar in the urine regardless of number of times found?* A. In all cases of persistent or recurring glycosuria the presence of diabetes should be proved or disproved by a glucose tolerance test unless the diagnosis can or has been established by random positive blood sugar tests or if necessary by a glucose tolerance test.

7. Q. *What conditions warrant a diagnosis of lowered renal threshold for sugar?* A. Persistence of glycosuria with a blood sugar value under 170 milligrams per cent.

8. Q. *What is the significance of a low renal threshold for sugar?* A. A persistent normal blood sugar with constant glycosuria, including fasting, means renal glycosuria. We have had 76 such cases among 28,000 cases of diabetes and glycosuria. If less strict diagnostic criteria are used, the number of renal glycosurics increases accordingly.

III. Classification.

1. *What are the criteria for, and definition of, mild, moderate and severe diabetes?* A. There is no generally accepted classification. Before the use of insulin a severe case was said to have a tolerance for less than 10 grams of carbohydrate, a moderate case for 10 to 50 grams and a mild case for more. Classification with units of insulin employed is unsatisfactory, because the carbohydrate may vary from 100 to 200 grams or more and so involve the use of varying amounts of insulin.

A *mild* diabetic might be said to be one who is sugar free before and after meals with carbohydrate 150 grams in twenty-four hours and no insulin, or surgar free with carbohydrate 200 grams or more and 10 units or less of insulin daily.

A *moderate* diabetic might be considered one who is sugar free with 100 grams carbohydrate in twenty-four hours and no insulin or sugar free with 150 grams carbohydrate with 10 units or with more carbohydrate and 20 to 30 units daily.

A *severe* diabetic would be one with a tolerance for less than 50 grams carbohydrate without insulin and requiring 50 or more units of insulin to be sugar free with 150 grams carbohydrate.

IV. Duration of Life.

1. Q. *What is the difference in expectation of life in the three grades of severity of diabetes?* A. No one knows. One might estimate the average expectancy of life for mild cases as 90 per cent, for moderate cases 75 per cent and for severe cases 50 per cent of normal expectancies.

2. Q. *From your clinical experience or from overall figures on diabetes, what is the average duration of life after diagnosis is made?* A. Tables 39, 40 and 41 for duration of life of fatal cases and Table 42 for expectation of life of the living. This life expectancy table was computed in 1938. We hope to revise it before 1947.

3. Q. *Statistical or other evidence of the degree of increased longevity of diabetics from use of insulin?* A. (See Tables 39, 40 and 41.)

4. Q. *Does dietetic control or insulin control of the diabetic retard or accelerate the development of cardiovascular changes?* A. Both dietetic and especially insulin control retard the same. Before the use of insulin all diabetics, young or old, showed arteriosclerosis after a duration of diabetes of five years.

5. Q. *How important is the duration of diabetes?* A. Most important, because it could be compared with the diabetic life expectancy table. (See Table 42.)

6. Q. *Would a person with mild, easily controlled diabetes of thirty years' duration be a greater hazard from a mortality standpoint than an individual who had been diagnosed as a diabetic only two or three years before applying for insurance?* A. Yes. The thirty-year duration case, even if mild, would be at least fifty years old. The person with diabetes of thirty years' duration is as yet a rarity, assuming onset of diabetes at the age of twenty. Thus far we have no patient with onset under fifteen years of age who has yet lived over 35 years, although we have 249 who have lived twenty years or more, and 93 of these 25 years or more and 5 over thirty years.

Because of the relatively high incidence of complications, the diabetic with disease of twenty years' duration presents likewise a greater mortality risk than the individual of comparable age with diabetes of only two or three years' duration.

7. Q. *What are the facts regarding the life expectancy of diabetics at various ages or by age groups?* A. (See Tables 42 and 43 and page 320.)

V. Problems of Insurability.

1. Q. *Should the fact that a diabetic can be controlled by extremely rigid diet alone permit us to take a more liberal view in underwriting him for life insurance?* A. No. He is safer with 200 grams of carbohydrate and insulin than with 100 grams of carbohydrate without insulin.

2. Q. *If a diabetic is under control but has a past history of coma, acidosis, or severe infection, should we consider him for insurance?* A. Yes, provided the coma was accidental, due to inept treatment or occurred when the disease was undiagnosed. The diabetes is temporarily, but not permanently, impaired by an infection.

3. Q. *We see a large number of cases with a normal blood sugar curve, but a low renal threshold. What percentage of these individuals become diabetic?* A. We term these "unclassified glycosurics." We traced all but 1.5 per cent of 1946 of these over a period of years and found that in only 193 cases, or 9.9 per cent, true diabetes had developed and this in most instances was mild. (See page 806.)

4. Q. *Would you suggest rules for guidance in selecting diabetics for life insurance?* A. The following are suggested for consideration:

(1) Age: ten to sixty years.
(2) Age at onset: five to fifty-five years.

(3) Duration of diabetes: two to ten years or more but adding to the age of a diabetic 0–29 years old, $\frac{1}{2}$; between 30–50, $\frac{1}{3}$; and 60 years and above $\frac{1}{4}$, of the duration of the disease.

(4) Degree of financial security.

(5) Regularity at occupation.

(6) Adherence to treatment.

(7) History of diabetic coma or severe insulin reactions with information as to whether such were the result of ignorance, carelessness or accident.

(8) History of infections of skin or tissues.

(9) Diet. Learn his diet by asking specific replies to the following specific questions: (a) Bread, number of slices; (b) fruit, how much; (c) milk, quantity; (d) cereal; (e) potato, rice, macaroni; (f) desserts.

(10) Insulin: variety or varieties. Units in 24 hours and how distributed.

(11) Urine: (a) How often tested; (b) How often sugar free. Submit specimens.

(12) Blood sugar: Percentages, dates and time of day of last 4 tests with quantity of insulin at those times.

Date   Time of Day   Blood Sugar   Insulin in twenty-four hours

(13) Frequency of visits to a doctor or clinic for examination.

(14) X-ray of heart and lungs.

(15) Electrocardiogram.

(16) Examination of eyes with ophthalmoscope.

(17) Dorsalis pedis arteries.

(18) Usual physical examination for ordinary life insurance, including blood pressure and pulse rate.

(19) Alcohol: None, or almost none.

(20) Insulin: 80 units the maximum in 24 hours.

F. THE MARRIAGE OF DIABETICS.

With heredity playing such a predominant rôle in the etiology of diabetes, one may ask why marriage and the propagation of diabetics are allowed. You cannot indict a whole nation, the major portion of a nation or even 1 per cent of a people without causing a reverberation throughout the world. In this country of 140,000,000 we have probably 1,000,000 diabetics, and an estimated 4,000,000 who either have or will develop diabetes before they die. With their brothers and sisters the number concerned is easily raised to 12,000,000. One need add but few groups of more distant relatives to double or treble the total in order to show that approximately 1 citizen in 4 in the United States is an hereditary diabetes carrier (see page 54). This illustrates the extent of the social and medical aspect of the problem of heredity in diabetes in the abstract.

What should be done about it? Manifestly one cannot eliminate one-fourth of a nation. If we could only recognize who were carriers of diabetes the question would be simplified, but as it is we have great difficulty in deciding who is and who is not a diabetic. The number of borderline cases constantly grows and is likely to increase. Sterilization of brothers and sisters of diabetics would be unfair, because we cannot tell who are the carriers.

Wilder[1] writes, "It is not necessary to demand 'mass sterilization' or even to ask that members of diabetic families voluntarily remain childless. If such persons would limit their families to one child or even two, the same result would be accomplished, since for a family to survive the number of children in each generation must exceed three." I wonder if this is the solution. With the chances for survival far less in the past than in the future, diabetes has persisted over 2000 years and Bouchardat never saw a pregnant diabetic woman.

Now for the concrete. Let me cite a problem presented to me in 1935. An attractive young woman comes to my office and asks if she can get married. A moment's conversation suffices to disclose that she is unusually intelligent. She is evidently physically strong, because she is a champion tennis player, often rides to hounds for six hours at a time, has driven an automobile recently 300 miles in a day, and repeatedly dances all night. In the midst of city gaities she has learned stenography and typewriting and, what is more, secured and held a job. Physical examination reveals normal eyes, heart, blood vessels, lungs (the last three checked by x-ray) and abdomen. Catamenia are normal. The teeth, it is true, have exhibited unusual caries, although each tiny defect is now remedied. Sometimes there is sugar in the urine but her diabetes began two years before insulin was discovered at the age of seven years and eight months, and the patient is now twenty-one years old. Her diet is about carbohydrate 155 gm., protein liberal and enough fat to maintain weight at approximately 117 pounds (53 kg.). Her height is 63 inches (157 cm.). Insulin was injected four times daily for several years but is now in 1935 taken twice daily, 16–0–20 units, except upon unusual occasions. At one time the dose of insulin was 70 units daily. The cholesterol now is 185 mg. per 100 cc.

This young woman knows her disease. Once only in more than two years has she had an insulin reaction and that by mistake in Paris when she forgot to take her breakfast after injecting her insulin. She has never been so careless as to develop coma.

Now, what would you do under these concrete conditions? Perhaps you would like to learn what I did. I asked: (1) Is he a good boy? (2) Is he really in love, and are you, too? (3) Can I examine him physically and mentally and decide whether he is good enough for you, because you see I have known you fourteen years? (4) Are you sure neither he nor his relatives have diabetes? (5) Do his parents know you have diabetes? (6) Do your parents approve? (7) Are there funds enough to take care of you, if you are ill, and to provide exceptional attention in a hospital if you should become pregnant? (8) Does this young man realize that he must take unusual care of you and help you to keep your diabetes controlled and above all that you are a diabetic pioneer and that one cannot

[1] Wilder: P. 54, loc cit., p. 55.

guarantee what your future is, because literally you are exploring new paths? And only then, when all the examinations and answers were satisfactory, did I say—get married and God bless you.

The sequel to the above is that in 1946 one sees a family happy becasue the father has returned from overseas with many citations and the mother and two children are in excellent health, and she after twenty-six years of diabetes is pregnant for the fourth time, the first child being lost during a period of toxemia when not under our care. In the next pregnancy she received hormonal treatment and the baby was born by Cesarean section in the thirty-sixth week, being Dr. Priscilla White's third case of her 290 cases since January, 1936.

And what are the ideas floating around in my mind as I contemplate this young couple and think of the more than 1000 other diabetic girls and 1000 other diabetic boys who have consulted me in childhood and of whom 1774 are alive?

First of all, must I say that I do admire the backbone and the brains of the average diabetic and I truly believe on the whole they are superior to the common run of people and therefore their good qualities merit cultivation. Second, I think they are less apt to drink, far less likely to have syphilis or gonorrhea, and distinctly less to have, what is anathema to me, "nervous prostration and nerves." Third, my statistics of 29,000 diabetics and glycosurics studied with considerable care during forty-eight years indicate that the youthful individual contracting diabetes today has a life expectancy approaching forty years and, therefore, one should thoughtfully consider before sentencing a diabetic to a single life of forty years' duration. Fourth, I face the problem of heredity as follows: I acknowledge diabetes is an hereditary disease. Every child is born with or without an hereditary predisposition. The heredity is recessive in character and can skip a generation. Many predisposed to diabetes may go through life without developing it in its commonly recognized form, because the tendency is slight, either because they do not live to the age at which it would naturally appear, or because by chance or care they avoid precipitating causes such as obesity, lack of muscular development, and treat promptly disease of the gall-bladder or thyroid and remove sources of infection. People generally do not grasp the significance of the facts that from the fourth decade on, 79 to 89 per cent of diabetics at or prior to onset have been overweight.

The transmission of the disease, disclosed by studies of my cases by Priscilla White and Gregory Pincus, is along the definite lines known to be in force for a disease with recessive heredity. If two diabetics marry, all their descendants are destined to develop the disease, provided: (1) they escape death from all other causes, and (2) live beyond the eighth decade—to a ripe old age. However, it must be remembered that in each group of 100 children resulting from such unions, only 44 will develop the disease. Of these, about one-third will acquire it before the age of forty years, another one-third between forty and fifty-five years and the remainder between fifty-five and one hundred years. Moreover, at the age of forty and above, diabetes is controllable with relative ease.

When we speak of diabetic offspring we should not forget that in the whole history of the world as yet there have not been reported, so far as I know, half a dozen completely proved cases of congenital diabetes.

If a diabetic marries a non-diabetic, but in a diabetic family, the inheritance is cut in half. If two non-diabetics, but each with diabetes in their families, marry, theoretically one-fourth of the children are destined to the disease. If a diabetic marries a non-diabetic of a non-diabetic family, their children should escape unscathed, but of course all these children would be hereditary carriers and capable of transmitting the disease. However, unless they married persons who were also hereditary carriers, their own children would not develop diabetes.

Fifth, a considerable number of my diabetics have married and later died. As yet the one left behind, or the family of the survivor, in no instance has blamed me for allowing the marriage to have taken place and I have been told that despite the sadness a death caused (this held even before the discovery of insulin) all concerned were thankful that the marriage had occurred.

Sixth, what is the effect of diabetes upon a race? We do not need to look far. In Jews the incidence is two to two and a half times as great as in Gentiles. Has it injured or helped the Jewish race? Here is an experiment on a 15,000,000 scale. Suppose we watch it. Today the Jews are beginning to learn that they should not be fat. In consequence I wonder what the incidence of diabetes will be in Jews in the next decades. I suspect that intermarriage between cousins and between those of even closer relationship occurs less frequently among Jews today than formerly.

Seventh, in any crusade against diabetics no consideration appears to be given to possible advances in the treatment or prevention of the disease. Even a generation ago it was clear that progress in diabetes was imminent, because shortly before that time von Mering and Minkowski's discovery had been made and Opie's and Ssobolew's observation upon the relation of the islands of Langerhans to the disease had just been published. And what of today with the almost complete abolition of diabetic coma, the diminishing death rate in the young, the relative safety in operations, all of which have followed the discovery of insulin. Yet all of these past achievements seem significant when one realizes the better scientific weapons, the better fields for action in our laboratories and the greatly increased number of really skilled research workers, all now available for a successful attack on the disease. There was never a greater opportunity for the discovery of new methods of treatment of diabetes than today and he is certainly pessimistic who would exterminate diabetics upon the ground that advance in diabetic therapeutics had reached an impasse.

Eighth, the danger of a diabetic pregnancy to a mother today is almost non-existent. Insulin washed clean the slate of the old rules for pregnant diabetics. Cesarean section is permissible with practically the same freedom from worry as in a non-diabetic, provided it is performed by skilled obstetricians working in association with doctors skilled in the treatment of the disease. And as for the success of the pregnancy, whereas ten years ago survival of the fetus in the latter half of pregnancy was only 50 per cent, today we know it is 90 per cent and for patients under close observation 95 per cent.

Ninth, a Cesarean section is justifiable because it is unlikely that diabetic mothers will have many children and it is therefore important to do everything to save each one.

Tenth, sterilization is a last resort and in our experience does more harm than good.

On the twenty-fifth anniversary of the discovery of insulin the University of Toronto welcomed the annual meeting of the American Diabetes Association at Toronto on September 16–18, 1946. Nearly 500 physicians registered for the meeting which was designed to present the results obtained in the use of insulin together with those of investigations, both in the clinic and laboratory, stimulated by insulin. The chemistry and site of action of insulin were discussed and studies upon alloxan diabetes were described. These reports of progress to date stimulated hopes of important advances to come. Diabetic coma, pregnancy in diabetes, insulin mixtures, and diabetic statistics were among the topics discussed. The papers will be published in the Proceedings of the American Diabetes Association for 1946.

CHAPTER IV.

THE PHYSIOLOGY OF DIABETES.

REVISED BY ALEXANDER MARBLE, M.D.

A. INTRODUCTION.

DESPITE countless investigations in the laboratory and the clinic, the basic cause of diabetes mellitus in man remains obscure. Although insulin was first prepared by Banting and Best a full quarter of a century ago, its exact mode and site of action are still unknown. However, the realization of the inadequacy of our knowledge serves not to discourage but to stimulate continued efforts particularly since investigations to date have resulted in a tremendous body of useful data which point the direction for further studies. The outlook for the future appears bright and full of hope: (1) Since the fundamental studies of Claude Bernard a century ago, and particularly since the production of diabetes in 1889 by von Mering and Minkowski by pancreatectomy in dogs, probably no other disease has been so thoroughly, and over years of time so consistently, studied both by the physiologist and the clinician. Furthermore, interest is increasing rather than waning. (2) Enough time has elapsed to allow careful appraisal and interpretation of the results of the vast amount of work since the discovery of insulin in 1921, particularly in the field of endocrine interrelationships. (3) In the form of radioactive isotopes, new tools are available for intimate studies of intermediary metabolism, thereby opening up a whole new field. (4) A new and easily produced type of experimental diabetes may now be brought about by the injection of alloxan and related compounds. (5) Work, particularly by Cori and associates with enzymatic reactions *in vitro*, still in its beginnings, is yielding highly valuable and fundamental information as to the nature of the processes involved in the synthesis and breakdown of glycogen and other aspects of intermediary carbohydrate metabolism.

Three methods are now available for the production of permanent diabetes in susceptible species of animals: (1) removal of at least nine-tenths of the pancreas; (2) injection of extracts of the anterior pituitary (and in suitably prepared animals, by the administration of extracts of the adrenal cortex and of the thyroid); and (3) the administration of alloxan. Diabetic animals lend themselves well to the investigation of the many problems of the human disease. Although one must recognize and allow for differences between the experimentally produced and the naturally occurring disorder, the parallelism is close enough to make studies on diabetic animals of

(108)

the greatest value and in many instances of direct application. Indeed, in diabetes research one finds a most remarkable example of interdependence of laboratory and clinic. Even apart from the revolutionary influence of the discovery of insulin, the findings of the physiologist and the biochemist have often been of great benefit to the clinician in his understanding of, and care for, his patient. In turn, the worker in the basic sciences discovers his problems in the experience of the clinician and turns to the latter for application of laboratory data to human subjects.

The relative swiftness with which advances in knowledge have been made in the last twenty-five years warrants the hope that in the not too distant future the intriguing problem as to the factors responsible for the precipitation of diabetes in man may be solved, thus possibly opening the way for prevention of the disease in the predisposed. Prevention is already possible under some experimental conditions; permanent diabetes may be avoided in certain animals receiving anterior pituitary extract by the simultaneous administration of insulin, or by the feeding of fat, by fasting, or the giving of phlorhizin. These findings will be set forth in detail in the pages which follow.

B. PATHOGENESIS OF DIABETES

1. **Heredity and Precipitating Factors.**—Much evidence points to the validity of the Naunyn conception of the unity of diabetes with heredity as the common bond. It appears likely that in large part diabetes rests upon an hereditary basis. Upon this inherited tendency may well be superimposed a factor or factors which at a given time in the individual's life become prominent enough to precipitate the disease. As likely factors there come to mind obesity, hyperthyroidism, hyperpituitarism, overactivity of the adrenal cortex and other causative agents even less well defined. To this list in recent months speculation has added alloxan or some chemical precursor of this diabetogenic agent. Certain data from animal studies suggest that precipitating factors, if operative in man, have the common property of causing strain or overwork of the islets of Langerhans, which if sufficiently long-continued or severe, results in actual damage with inadequate production of insulin. There are obviously wide gaps in our knowledge both as to the existence, or the extent of the influence, of such precipitating factors in the human subject, and as to the even more fundamental problem regarding the exact nature of the metabolic defect which, presumably, diabetic individuals inherit. Indeed, certain workers maintain, with considerable basis, that diabetics do not inherit a functionally inadequate pancreas but that in most instances the characteristic insulin insufficiency is due primarily to increased destruction, increased utilization or inhibition of the hormone consequent to extra-pancreatic influences.

2. The Nature of the Metabolic Disorder in Diabetes.

—In what way does the diabetic differ from the normal individual? The outstanding difference may be expressed grossly by stating that the diabetic is unable to utilize glucose in the normal fashion. Normally, the monosaccharides, glucose, fructose and galactose, end-products of carbohydrate digestion, are carried by the portal blood to the liver, where to a large extent they are stored as glycogen. There is good evidence that fructose and galactose are first changed to glucose in the liver before such conversion. Following the absorption of monosaccharides, that portion not stored as glycogen in the liver is converted to muscle glycogen or oxidized directly to supply heat or energy. Glycogen stores are not static; they are constantly called upon to furnish glucose according to the requirements of the body. It must be emphasized that the synthesis and the breakdown of glycogen constitutes a reversible reaction (Glucose$\rightleftharpoons$Glycogen) which is continuously active, varying in the major direction of flow according to the availability of foodstuffs and the needs of the individual at any given moment.

In the diabetic, the metabolism of carbohydrate proceeds abnormally in that, depending upon the severity of the diabetes, the hexoses which result from the digestion of carbohydrate or from the breakdown of non-carbohydrate materials are, to a greater or less extent, not stored as glycogen or oxidized in the tissues in normal fashion, but instead, glucose tends to accumulate in the blood and to be lost in the urine. Hyperglycemia and glycosuria occur in the diabetic man or animal, even though fasting. Glucose is apparently formed from body protein (and probably fat) almost entirely in the liver, since the blood sugar falls rapidly after hepatectomy. The increased breakdown of protein is reflected in the high nitrogen excretion. The body prefers glucose as a source of energy but with impaired utilization of carbohydrate, protein and fat stores are called upon to an unusual extent to supply tissue needs. There is much evidence to indicate that whereas in the normal or diabetic individual ketone bodies which may result from the catabolism of fat in the liver are oxidized completely by the tissues as such, in the uncontrolled diabetic the amount of fat broken down may be so great that the quantity of ketone bodies produced exceeds that which can be used. Consequently these flood the organism; the end result is acidosis, which, if unchecked, leads to coma and death.

By the parenteral injection of the proper dose of insulin, this whole abnormal process may be corrected. It seems reasonable to suppose that if one could supply insulin day after day in exactly the correct amount throughout the twenty-four hours, as is done by the pancreas in the normal person, varying this secretion to meet the demands of activity, ingestion of food, infections, etc., the diabetic would be essentially a normal individual. In the diabetic patient, provided the diet is properly controlled, one can, with insulin, abolish glycosuria, lower the blood sugar and cause an accumulation of glycogen in the liver and muscles which approximates the normal.

3. "Overproduction" vs. "Underutilization."

—Since the beginning of modern thinking regarding the pathological physiology of diabetes there have been two conflicting views as to the nature of the disordered metabolism. Certain workers have held that in diabetes there is lost to a varying degree the ability to burn sugar in the tissues; in the completely diabetic animal, total inability to oxidize glucose is assumed. This underutilization theory was, quite naturally, championed by Minkowski. Opposed to this theory is that of overproduction, advanced by von Noorden, who felt that the disease represented increased glycogenolysis with overproduction of glucose in the liver from non-carbohydrate sources. Proponents of the underutilization theory have stated that it is the function of insulin to promote oxidation of carbohydrate in the tissues; those of the overproduction theory maintain that insulin acts to prevent overproduction of carbohydrate in the liver and that its action in the tissues to catalyze the oxidation of sugar is of minor importance.

According to the latter view which assumes that diabetic tissues retain the power of oxidizing carbohydrate,[1] carbohydrate metabolism represents a dynamic balance between blood sugar formation in the liver and its utilization in the body tissues. The starting point for this conception was the work of Mann and Magath[2] who showed that a steady fall in blood sugar following hepatectomy occurs in diabetic dogs as in normal animals. Mann's work established the liver as the source of blood sugar, since in his hepatectomized dogs during marked hypoglycemia appreciable quantities of glycogen in the muscles were incapable of sufficiently rapid conversion to glucose to play a significant rôle in maintaining the blood-sugar level. It has been established that known hyperglycemic agents, such as epinephrin, ether anesthesia, asphyxia, and anterior pituitary extracts, do not influence the falling blood sugar of hepatectomized animals.

The studies of Bridge and Winter,[3] in which they attempted to correlate the action of insulin with the blood sugar and respiratory quotient in diabetic patients, gave results in keeping with the view that the major aspect of the disturbance of metabolism in diabetes is centered in the liver. Bridge and Winter believe that insulin influences carbohydrate combustion in diabetes only indirectly by way of changes produced in the glycogen content of the liver.

Those who maintain that the completely diabetic animal cannot oxidize glucose base their argument on various findings, among

[1] Soskin: Endocrinology, **26**, 297, 1940.
[2] Mann and Magath: Arch. Int. Med., 31, 787, 1923.
[3] Bridge and Winter: Bull. Johns Hopkins Hosp., **64**, 213, 1939.

which are the following: (1) The supposedly constant ratio between the glucose and nitrogen content of the urine during fasting or during maintenance on a diet exclusively of protein after exhaustion of glycogen stores. The sugar found in the urine of depancreatized dogs is assumed to represent non-utilization of all glucose resulting from protein. The glucose:nitrogen ratio in the severest diabetes in man is approximately 3.65:1 and in depancreatized dogs, approximately 2.8:1. However, there is actually a wide variation in these values and many workers[1] regard them of questionable significance. Soskin[2] found that in diabetic animals the ratio tended to be high at the beginning of each experiment following the withdrawal of insulin and to show a progressive fall as the animals lost weight. (2) The failure of the respiratory quotient to rise when carbohydrate is fed to a diabetic animal. Soskin and Levine[3] believe that this does not necessarily indicate a failure of oxidation of carbohydrate. They state that the respiratory quotient cannot be regarded as the index of a single event but rather as a composite total effect of various metabolic processes. They cite the accepted fact that the brain derives its energy solely from carbohydrate and yields a respiratory quotient of about 1.0 at all times; when in any animal a figure, of say 0.7, is obtained this must represent an average or composite of values, on the one hand, for other tissues with respiratory quotients below 0.7 and, on the other hand, the 1.0 of the brain in order for the final figure of 0.7 to be obtained. The diabetic respiratory quotient, they state, can best be interpreted as a resultant of at least two factors, a low component due to formation of sugar from fatty acid and protein and a high component due to simultaneous oxidation of that carbohydrate.

There is as yet not complete agreement with regard to these matters, although in recent years more experimental data have seemed to support the "overproduction" theory. It is fair to state that most workers in the field of carbohydrate metabolism still believe that in diabetes the power of the tissues to oxidize glucose is impaired to some extent. In fact, it is not uncommon to find statements in published articles or books written by recognized authorities to the effect that the chief defect in diabetes is an inability to oxidize carbohydrate. In view of the evidence to the contrary, such statements are certainly unwarranted. However, it seems likely that carbohydrate oxidation does not proceed at a normal rate in the diabetic person or animal. It is probable that the difference between the normal and diabetic is a quantitative rather than a qualitative one, and that one of the actions of insulin

[1] Soskin and Levine: Carbohydrate Metabolism, Chicago, University of Chicago Press, 1946, Chapter IX.
[2] Soskin: Jour. Nutrition, 3, 99, 1930.
[3] Soskin and Levine: Ref. 1 above, Chapter XI.

is to speed up oxidative processes which the tissues themselves are capable of carrying out to a limited degree.

Yater, Markowitz and Cahoon[1] found that although the glucose consumption of *resting* muscle was the same in both the normal and the diabetic state, *during exercise* in the latter condition, muscular contraction did not involve an extra consumption of blood sugar. They concluded that the contracting diabetic muscle is unable to utilize glucose to obtain extra energy. Their findings were in agreement with the earlier results of Knowlton and Starling,[2] later confirmed by MacLean and Smedley[3] and by Cruickshank[4] to the effect that the isolated, perfused heart of a completely depancreatized dog has largely lost its power to obtain energy from glucose. Fazekas[5] *et al.* studied in a Warburg apparatus the metabolism of renal tissue excised from hypophysectomized, depancreatized dogs; no evidence for the combustion of glucose was obtained. In answer to these investigations, Shorr[6] kept excised cardiac tissue for ten hours at 37.5° in a Ringer-glucose-phosphate solution. Since at the end of this time it regained its capacity to oxidize carbohydrate, he concluded that this process is functionally independent of insulin.

From the data now available it seems logical to assume that in the depancreatized dog and in the human individual with spontaneous diabetes there exists not only an overproduction of glucose in the liver but also a diminished efficiency in the combustion of glucose in the tissues. The end-result is that the normal utilization of glucose is interfered with and proper storage as glycogen in the liver and muscles does not take place.

4. **Formation of Ketone Bodies.** Under ordinary conditions of normal living, carbohydrate is used chiefly and preferentially by the body as a source of energy. However, when carbohydrate is not available, as in starvation or in severe, uncontrolled diabetes, protein and fat are called upon to meet energy requirements. The catabolism of fat involves, at least in part, preliminary oxidation in the liver to ketone bodies. These ketone bodies may be utilized for energy in the peripheral tissues without the aid of insulin and without simultaneous oxidation of carbohydrate. However, when the production of ketone bodies is abnormally great, as in uncontrolled diabetes, body needs are exceeded and the excess accumulates in the blood and tissues and is excreted in the urine.

In recent years ideas have changed greatly as to the chemical steps by which ketone bodies are formed from fat. The Knoop theory of "successive beta oxidation" is now discredited by most

[1] Yater, Markowitz and Cahoon: Arch. Int. Med., **51**, 800, 1933.
[2] Knowlton and Starling: Jour. Physiol., **45**, 146, 1912.
[3] MacLean and Smedley: Jour. Physiol., **45**, 470, 1913.
[4] Cruickshank: Am. Jour. Physiol., **90**, 322, 1929.
[5] Fazekas, Campbell and Himwich: Am. Jour. Physiol., **118**, 297, 1937.
[6] Shorr: Science, **85**, 2210, 1937. Shorr, Barker, Cohen and Malam: Am. Jour Physiol., **129**, 463, 1940.

8

workers in favor of Hurtley's[1] suggestion of "multiple alternate oxidation" or the "beta oxidation acetic acid condensation" hypothesis of MacKay and co-workers.[2] According to this theory, all fatty acid chains, both odd and even numbered, are subjected to oxidation at each alternate carbon atom. Splitting then takes place at each keto group to form molecules of acetic acid except where a fragment made up of three carbon atoms forms propionic acid. Ketone bodies are then formed by the condensation of two molecules of acetic acid. That the last-named reaction can take place was shown by Friedmann,[3] Monguio[4] and others. (For further details see pages 423–425 and discussions by Stadie,[5] and Soskin and Levine.[6])

5. **The Formation and Breakdown of Glycogen.**—(*a*) **The Formation of Glycogen.**—The chemical steps thought to be involved in the formation of glycogen in the liver, muscles and other body tissues are outlined in Figure 3.

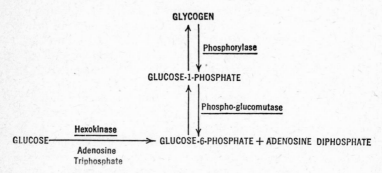

Fɪɢ. 3.—Chemical steps in the formation of glycogen.

In this figure are illustrated three of the features common to the processes by which the body on the one hand stores carbohydrate and on the other hand breaks down these stores to obtain energy: (1) The processes are enzymatic. For example, the first step, that of the formation of glucose-6-phosphate, is catalyzed by hexokinase. (2) The transfer of phosphate groups is of fundamental importance. In the chemical step just referred to, phosphate is supplied by adenosine triphosphate which reacts with glucose to form glucose-6-phosphate and adenosine diphosphate. (3) Most, though not all, of the reactions are reversible.

[1] Hurtley: Quart. Jour. Med., **9**, 301, 1916.
[2] MacKay, Wick and Barnum: Jour. Biol. Chem., **136**, 503, 1930. See also MacKay, Barnes, Carne and Wick: Jour. Biol. Chem., **135**, 157, 1940.
[3] Friedmann: Biochem. Ztschr., **55**, 436, 1913.
[4] Monguio: Klin. Wchnschr., **13**, 1116, 1934.
[5] Stadie: Jour. Clin. Invest., **19**, 843, 1940; Bull. New York Acad. Med., **19**, 778, 1943.
[6] Soskin and Levine: Ch. X, loc. cit., p. 112.

It will be noted in Figure 3 that the reversible reaction:

Glycogen $\leftrightarrows$ Glucose-1-phosphate ("Cori ester")

is catalyzed by phosphorylase. This enzyme, which is widely distributed in animal tissues, has been isolated and purified by Cori and Cori.[1] Of especial interest and significance was Cori's[2] demonstration in 1939 of the synthesis *in vitro* from glucose-1-phosphate of a polysaccharide indistinguishable from glycogen. The reaction took place under the influence of phosphorylase but in the absence of insulin.

More recent work from Cori's[3] laboratory has yielded results of equal or greater importance. It has been found that the activity of hexokinase in the reaction

$$\text{Glucose} + \text{adenosine triphosphate} \xrightarrow{\text{hexokinase}} \text{glucose-6-phosphate} + \text{adenosine diphosphate}$$

can be inhibited by anterior pituitary extract, either by injecting rats with anterior pituitary extract prior to the preparation of tissue extracts or by adding anterior pituitary extract to the enzyme preparation *in vitro*. The inhibition can be counteracted by insulin either in the living animal or in the test-tube. Rats with alloxan diabetes yield tissue extracts which give the same results as those previously injected with anterior pituitary extract. Because of the importance of the findings of Price, Cori and Colowick,[3] the following summary is taken directly from their paper: "The brain is an apparent exception, since brain extracts, prepared from rats injected with alloxan or with APE (anterior pituitary extract) do not show an inhibition of hexokinase activity. Brain extracts can, however, be inactivated by addition of APE *in vitro*.

"Insulin releases hexokinase from APE inhibition in all cases mentioned, but does not by itself enhance hexokinase activity under these experimental conditions. Within a certain range the release of inhibition is proportional to the amount of insulin added *in vitro*. That the *in vivo* action of insulin is of a similar nature is indicated by the fact that muscle extracts prepared from diabetic rats after the injection of insulin show normal hexokinase activity. When insulin is reduced by cysteine, it no longer exerts its antagonistic effect against APE inhibition of hexokinase activity." Special interest is attached to the last point mentioned, since insulin itself is a disulfide protein (S-S), and the activities of several enzymes are known to depend on their SH or S-S groups. It has been suggested[4] that both insulin and anterior pituitary extract exert their action by affecting the sulfhydryl balance of hexokinase.

[1] Cori and Cori: Jour. Biol. Chem., **72**, 615, 1927.
[2] Cori: Biological Symposia, **5**, 131, 1941.
[3] Price, Cori and Colowick: Jour. Biol. Chem., **160**, 633, 1945.
[4] Review article: Nutrition Reviews, **4**, 78, 1946.

Cori and his associates[1] regard the latent period exhibited by the hexokinase reaction in muscle extracts from rats with alloxan diabetes to be due to a preponderance of an inhibitory pituitary factor over insulin in such extracts. This view is supported by *in vitro* studies of the effect of adrenal cortical extract (unknown compounds in the amorphous fraction) on the hexokinase reaction in muscle extracts from normal and diabetic rats. Whereas cortical extract alone has no effect on hexokinase in normal extracts, it greatly intensifies the inhibitory effect of added or previously injected anterior pituitary extracts. Furthermore, with extracts from diabetic rats, cortical extract alone often produces a marked and prolonged inhibition. Whenever inhibition by cortical extract is observed, insulin invariably releases the inhibition, about 50 γ of insulin being required to counteract the effect of 0.1 cc. of Upjohn extract.

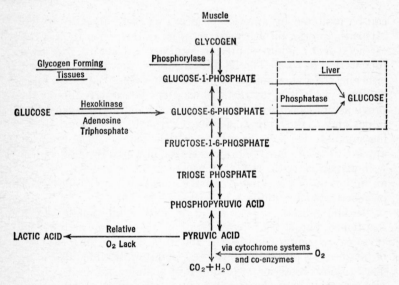

Fig. 4.—Formation and breakdown of glycogen and oxidation of carbohydrate. (From Best and Taylor.[2])

Cori, Price and Winston[3] have pointed out that their theory of the rôle of hexokinase in carbohydrate metabolism does not explain: (*a*) the insulin sensitivity of hypophysectomized animals; (*b*) the effect of anterior pituitary extract in promoting glycogen formation; and (*c*) the possible effect of insulin on pyruvate oxidation.

[1] Price, Slein, Colowick and Cori: Fed. Proc., **5**, 150, 1946.
[2] Best and Taylor: The Physiological Basis of Medical Practice, Baltimore, The Williams and Wilkins Co., 4th Edition, 1945, p. 571.
[3] Cori, Price and Winston: Jour. Industr. and Eng. Chem. (News edition), **24**, 895, 1946.

(b) **The Breakdown of Glycogen.**—The chemical processes concerned in the breakdown of glycogen either in the liver to supply glucose to the blood or in the muscles and other tissues to furnish energy are shown in Figure 4 which, it will be noted, consists of an elaboration of Figure 3.

As shown in Figure 4, under normal conditions the breakdown of glycogen proceeds through successive steps ending in carbon dioxide and water. The steps from glycogen to pyruvic acid can occur anaërobically but from then on, an adequate supply of oxygen is essential. When glycogen is broken down at an excessively rapid rate or there is a relative lack of oxygen, pyruvic acid tends to accumulate and is rapidly converted to lactic acid. If more favorable conditions are restored, the lactic acid may be oxidized back to pyruvic acid and then to carbon dioxide and water. However, the lactic acid not so reconverted diffuses out into the blood stream where it is carried to the liver and reconverted to glycogen. This latter chain of events ("Cori cycle") occurs only under conditions of strenuous exercise or relative anoxia.

It was formerly thought that the main source of energy of the contraction of muscle was furnished by the decomposition of phosphocreatine or phosphagen.[1,2] It seems likely now, however, that the breakdown of phosphocreatine serves merely to supply phosphate for the conversion of adenylic acid to adenosine triphosphate without the liberation of energy. The subsequent breakdown of the last-named compound actually supplies the energy for the resynthesis of both phosphocreatine and adenosine triphosphate.[3]

It should be brought out that the liver possesses a very active phosphatase which by action on the hexophosphates, diverts these compounds in large measure from the direct line of breakdown to carbon dioxide and water. Instead, phosphate is split off and glucose for blood sugar is formed.

Soskin[4] points out that at moments of stress or need, more energy is available to skeletal muscle from a certain amount of glycogen than from an equivalent amount of blood sugar. A certain amount of energy must be expended to bring the blood sugar into the metabolic system of the muscle (as hexose-6-phosphate) whereas the breakdown of glycogen to the same stage does not require the addition of energy (such energy had been previously expended in resting periods in order to form glycogen). It is likely for this reason that increased stores of glycogen are found in the muscles of animals trained to do prolonged work whereas low levels of muscle glycogen are found in individuals with poorly controlled diabetes and in those with hyperthyroidism. Soskin correlates the above with the fact that skeletal muscle must necessarily undertake

[1] Eggleton and Eggleton: Jour. Physiol., **63**, 155, 1927.
[2] Fiske and Subbarow: Jour. Biol. Chem., **81**, 629, 1929.
[3] Soskin and Levine: Ch. IV, loc. cit., p. 112.
[4] Soskin: Proc. Am. Diabetes Assn., **2**, 119, 1942.

bursts of activity, whereas in tissues such as those of the central nervous system, which characteristically work at more constant rates, the rôle of glycogen does not appear to be as important (and blood sugar is used preferentially). In this regard, heart muscle occupies a position intermediate between that of skeletal muscle and the central nervous system.

(c) **Rôle of Insulin.**—With the foregoing as a background, it is now pertinent to review present knowledge as to the precise rôle played by insulin in the various processes (its general effects have been outlined on page 110). First, in the living animal insulin greatly facilitates the transformation of glucose to glycogen. However, that glycogen synthesis, albeit at a lessened rate, proceeds in the total absence of insulin has been shown *in vivo* in diabetic animals and *in vitro* (see work of Cori referred to above). Second, as has been mentioned previously, insulin added to the test-tube or previously injected in diabetic rats, counteracts the inhibiting effect of anterior pituitary extract on hexokinase activity in the phosphorylation of glucose to glucose-6-phosphate. Third, although even the totally depancreatized animal can oxidize glucose to some extent, this action is far from normal and is greatly facilitated by insulin.

The exact site of action of insulin is not clear but the results of certain studies suggest that, as far as the chain of catabolic processes (see Fig. 4) is concerned, the site of action of insulin is higher than the pyruvic acid stage. It may be that the chief function of insulin is to facilitate the hexokinase reaction, thereby admitting glucose to the metabolic system. Whatever the truth may be in this regard, the known facts regarding insulin and pyruvic acid, supplied in part by the studies of Bueding, Wortis, Fein and Esturonne,[1] are as follows: Normally the ingestion of glucose is followed by a rise in blood pyruvate. Such a response is absent or decreased and delayed in diabetic subjects, human[2] or animal,[3] although if the blood sugar of depancreatized dogs is raised to extraordinarily high levels, there will be an increase in pyruvic acid. If, however, insulin also is administered to the diabetic subjects, the blood pyruvate is significantly elevated. On the other hand, the rate of removal of intravenously injected pyruvic acid is the same in the normal and depancreatized dog. Calling attention to the fact that thiamine pyrophosphate is important in the removal of pyruvic acid,[4] Bueding *et al.*[1] interpret their results as indicating that insulin is of

---

[1] Bueding, Wortis, Fein and Esturonne: Am. Jour. Med. Sci., **204**, 838, 1942.
[2] Klein: Jour. Biol. Chem., **145**, 35, 1942.
[3] Bueding, Fazekas, Herrlich and Himwich: Jour. Biol. Chem., **148**, 97, 1943.
[4] The removal of pyruvic acid is normally an oxidative process, dependent upon an enzyme, pyruvate oxidase, which cannot function in the absence of thiamine. Thiamine is thus considered to be a co-enzyme (actually not merely an activator but an integral part of the enzyme molecule) for pyruvate oxidase, acting in the enzyme system of the tissues as a hydrogen transporter. The accumulation of pyruvic acid inhibits in turn the removal of lactic acid. (Best and Taylor: P. 641, loc. cit., p. 116.)

importance in the formation of pyruvic acid following glucose administration. As the result of other studies in the same laboratory,[1] it was concluded that insulin has no direct influence upon the relationship between lactic and pyruvic acids.

In passing it may be noted that although marked fluctuations in blood pyruvic and lactic acid may occur in a variety of conditions such as excitement, exercise, anoxia, and different degrees of fasting, a strict relation between the two is maintained.[2]

Root, Stotz and Carpenter[3] in a study of 26 diabetic patients who had been without insulin for varying lengths of time, found that when the rise in respiratory quotient following the ingestion of 50 grams of glucose was 0.05 or above, there was usually a rise in the blood level of either pyruvic acid or lactic acid or both. In patients in whom the rise in respiratory quotient was less than 0.05, there was in general no significant rise in the pyruvic or lactic acid levels. When, however, insulin was given immediately preceding or immediately following the ingestion of glucose, most patients showed increases both in the respiratory quotient and in blood pyruvic and lactic acids. In fact, in some patients the rises were greater than would occur in the majority of normal subjects. These studies suggest that the action of insulin is to promote the formation of pyruvic acid and thereby an increase in the oxidation of carbohydrate. They support the idea that the metabolic defect in diabetes consists in part in diminished ability of oxidation of carbohydrate.

The oxidation of pyruvic acid in animal tissues involves a rather complicated mechanism regarding which very few of the details are known. Using chiefly minced pigeon breast muscle suspended in calcium-free Ringer-phosphate solution, Krebs and co-workers[4] carried out a long series of studies in an attempt to elucidate these reactions. According to the "Krebs citric acid cycle," pyruvate first of all reacts with oxaloacetate to form an intermediate compound which, upon oxidation and decarboxylation, yields citric acid. Citric acid then undergoes a series of reactions until finally oxaloacetic acid is again formed. This explanation has created much discussion. In general the evidence indicates that some sort of cycle of reactions does exist for the oxidation of pyruvate in muscle but reservation must be made with regard to the exact nature of the individual reactions. The biggest objection is to the inclusion of citric acid.

Ricketts and Stare[5] reported that insulin increased and prolonged the rate of *in vitro* oxygen consumption of minced skeletal muscle excised from patients whose severe diabetes was uncontrolled, but

1 Chesler, Himwich and Ferris: Jour. Biol. Chem., **155**, 413, 1944.
2 Stotz and Bessey: Jour. Biol. Chem., **143**, 625, 1942.
3 Root, Stotz and Carpenter: Am. Jour. Med. Sci., **211**, 189, 1946.
4 Krebs: Advances Enzymol., **3**, 191, 1943.
5 Ricketts and Stare: Jour. Lab. and Clin. Med., **30**, 594, 1945.

responsive to insulin therapy. Insulin was without effect on the *in vitro* respiration of skeletal muscle from a controlled insulin-sensitive diabetic or from 3 patients whose diabetes was uncontrolled and not readily responsive to insulin therapy.

Drury[1] has presented evidence to support the view that one of the important functions of insulin is to facilitate the formation of fat from carbohydrate and thus to store the latter in its most efficient form. The findings of Stetten and Boxer[2] are consistent with this view; these workers, using tracer elements in rats with alloxan diabetes, concluded that there is impairment of fatty acid synthesis from carbohydrate in the diabetic animal.

It seems probable that insulin, like other hormones, acts as an organic catalyst. Rather than initiating entirely new tissue reactions, it accelerates, or modifies activities which are the inherent property of living cells and in certain situations may oppose the contrary action of other hormones, as those of the anterior pituitary.

6. **The Influence of Other Glands of Internal Secretion.**—The pancreas has always held the center of the stage in any discussion regarding the basic defect in diabetes. This is rightly so, if for no other reason than the two central facts that extirpation of the pancreas in an experimental animal causes diabetes and that the supplying of an extract of the pancreas, namely, insulin, to a diabetic man or animal corrects the abnormalities of the disease, provided an adequate diet is supplied. From the very start of modern research, however, it was felt by many investigators that, whereas lack or lowered efficiency of pancreatic secretion was the basic abnormality, there must be influencing and modifying factors outside the pancreas. Indeed, many workers have ascribed to these extra-insular factors major rôles in the existence of the diabetic state. There is much evidence which can be marshalled in favor of this viewpoint.

(*a*) **Pituitary.**—*Pituitary Diabetes.*—The fact, long since pointed out, that overweight is a frequent forerunner of diabetes in adults, and that overheight is almost as consistent a predecessor of diabetes in children, suggests dysfunction of the pituitary gland.[3] In 1927, Davidoff and Cushing[4] reported that diabetes mellitus occurred in 12 per cent of 100 acromegalic patients. Coggeshall and Root[5] later reviewed these original 100 cases plus 53 cases of acromegaly subsequently studied at the Peter Bent Brigham Hospital. A total of 26 cases of diabetes were discovered in the 153 individuals, making an incidence of 17 per cent. Coggeshall and Root found 29 other patients in the series with glycosuria so that in all 55, or 36 per cent, of the 153 acromegalics were known to

[1] Drury: Am. Jour. Physiol., **131**, 536, 1940. See also Pauls and Drury: Jour. Biol. Chem., **145**, 481, 1942.
[2] Stetten and Boxer: Jour. Biol. Chem., **156**, 271, 1944.
[3] Young: Brit. Med. Jour., **2**, 897, 1941.
[4] Davidoff and Cushing: Arch. Int. Med., **39**, 751, 1927.
[5] Coggeshall and Root: Loc. cit., p. 86.

have had glycosuria. These findings are significant but one must confess that if there be an etiological relationship, it is surprising that diabetes is not even more common in acromegaly and that acromegaly is so rare in diabetics.[1]

More suggestive have been the results of the work initiated by Houssay and his associates.[2] At first with large South American toads and later with dogs they showed conclusively that following removal of the pancreas from a previously hypophysectomized animal, the resulting diabetes is extremely mild as compared with that which pancreatectomy produces in a normal animal. Hyperglycemia, glycosuria and ketonuria are much less in the doubly operated animals. The nitrogen excretion and the urinary D:N ratio are decreased. Hypoglycemic attacks are common, particularly if food is withheld, and the animals are hypersensitive to insulin. Diabetic acidosis and coma do not occur and the animals survive for much longer periods than do diabetic animals with an intact hypophysis. The injection of anterior pituitary extracts causes a return of the usual diabetic state.

In addition, Houssay showed that the injection of crude extracts of the anterior lobe of the pituitary gland into normal animals causes hyperglycemia and glycosuria. Similar results were reported at about the same time by H. M. Evans and associates,[3] E. I. Evans,[4] and by Barnes and Regan.[5] Although diabetes persisted for several months in the dogs of H. M. Evans, the possibility of producing the condition in permanent form in normal animals by this procedure was not fully realized until in 1937 Young,[6,7] working at the National Institute for Medical Research in London, announced that in normal dogs the daily intraperitoneal injection of fresh, crude extracts of anterior pituitary glands of oxen for a short period (eleven to twenty-six days in the first studies reported) causes diabetes, which then remains permanent, despite discontinuance of the injections. Once diabetes has developed, the amount of insulin required for control of the diabetes is, in general, a little larger than that needed for depancreatized dogs; however, if insulin is gradually withdrawn from the pituitary diabetic dogs, they will live for long periods whereas with gradual withdrawal of insulin from depancreatized animals, there soon comes a time when acidosis and coma intervene and death occurs.

Without altering experimental conditions, Young has been unable to produce diabetes of this type in animals of any species other than the adult dog. He found that during the period of natural

[1] Shepardson: Jour. Nerv. and Ment. Dis., **99**, 862, 1944.
[2] Houssay: New England Jour. Med., **214**, 971, 1936.
[3] Evans, Meyer, Simpson and Reichert: Proc. Soc. Exper. Biol. and Med., **29** 357, 1932.
[4] Evans: Proc. Soc. Exper. Biol. and Med., **30**, 1370, 1933.
[5] Barnes and Regan: Endocrinology, **17**, 522, 1933.
[6] Young: Lancet, **2**, 372, 1937.
[7] Young: Biochem. Jour., **32**, 513, 1938.

growth in the puppy, the administration of pituitary extract leads
not to diabetes but only to growth. When, however, the puppy
has reached adulthood under continuous pituitary treatment, it
becomes diabetic. In rabbits the injection of anterior pituitary
extract may set up a state of insensitivity to insulin, at least temporarily.[1] In rats hypertrophy rather than degeneration of the
islet tissue is seen; this proliferation of the islet cells may precede,
in the dog, the exhaustive or degenerative changes which accompany
the onset of permanent diabetes. Pituitary diabetes can be produced in cats[2] and rats[3] only by removal of part of the pancreas
before administration of anterior pituitary extract.

Young's[4,5] original work was confirmed by other investigators,
among whom were Campbell, Keenan and Best[6,7] at the University
of Toronto, and Dohan and Lukens[2] at the University of Pennsylvania. The Canadian workers found that in 2 of 3 dogs with experimental pituitary diabetes, total pancreatectomy produced little or
no aggravation of the diabetic state. In all 3 animals widespread
destruction of islet tissue was found and the insulin content of the
pancreases was extremely low or essentially lacking. Similar degenerative changes have been described by Richardson and Young.[8]

Richardson[9] found that injections both of crude anterior pituitary
extract and its globulin fraction cause initially degranulation and
hydropic degeneration in the beta cells of the islands of Langerhans.
This is, presumably, the first change in the production of a permanent diabetic condition. Similar observations were made by
Ham and Haist[10] who regarded the degranulation, hydropic degeneration and death of the beta cells to be due to excessive stimulation.
They suggested that anterior pituitary extracts may act in two
general ways to cause beta cells to overwork: (a) by acting on
body tissues in general so as to increase the body's need for insulin;
(b) by exerting a trophic effect on the pancreas, increasing secretion
as well as causing histological changes. Thus was attention temporarily diverted, again focused on the pancreas as the seat of the
disorder in diabetes.

A summary of the advances in knowledge of the rôle of the pituitary in carbohydrate metabolism during the twenty-five years
preceding 1942 has been prepared by Houssay.[11]

The production of permanent diabetes in dogs by anterior

[1] Ogilvie: Jour. Path. and Bact., 56, 225, 1944.
[2] Dohan and Lukens: Am. Jour. Physiol., 126, 478, 1939; Ibid., p. 125, 1939.
[3] Long: Trans. and Stud. Coll. Phys. Phila., 7, 21, 1939.
[4] Young: New England Jour. Med., 221, 635, 1939.
[5] Young: Brit. Med. Jour., 2, 393, 1939.
[6] Campbell, Keenan and Best: Lancet, 1, 1444, 1938.
[7] Campbell, Keenan and Best: Am. Jour. Physiol., 126, 455, 1939.
[8] Richardson and Young: Lancet, 1, 1098, 1938.
[9] Richardson: Proc. Roy. Soc. London, 128, 153, 1940.
[10] Ham and Haist: Am. Jour. Path., 17, 787, 1941.
[11] Houssay: Endocrinology, 30, 884, 1942.

pituitary extract can be prevented by the simultaneous administration of large doses of insulin which apparently protects the islet-cells from irreversible degenerative changes.[1] In partially depancreatized cats, the development of pituitary diabetes can be prevented by insulin, and, less effectively, by a diet low in calories or relatively high in fat. Furthermore, even though these measures are not introduced until diabetes has developed, "cure" of the condition can be accomplished provided the remedial measures are introduced early enough, *i. e.*, before irreversible changes have taken place in the pancreas.[2] Continuing their studies in this field, Lukens, Dohan and Wolcott[3] found that treatment of pituitary diabetes in the cat with phlorhizin, if begun before atrophy of the pancreatic islets has developed, is followed by morphological restoration of the islands and recovery of the animals. In an overall analysis of data, Lukens *et al.* point out that the only clear similarity of the action of insulin, low diet and phlorhizin is in abolishing hyperglycemia. They suggest therefore that the level of the blood sugar may play an important part in the pathogenesis of diabetes.

The influence of the pituitary has seemed so real that Hutton[4] employed irradiation of the skull of diabetic patients in an attempt to inhibit assumed hyperfunctioning of the pituitary. There has been no published confirmation of Hutton's work[5] and the experience of Selle, Westra and Johnson[6] was not encouraging. These workers found that in 5 of 7 diabetic (depancreatized) dogs the fasting blood sugar was not reduced after irradiation of the hypophysis by high dosage. In 3 animals the blood sugar was considerably higher after irradiation. There was no increased sensitivity to insulin and the insulin dosage necessary for control of the diabetes could not be reduced. Glucose tolerance tests were always typical of severe diabetes.

(*b*) **Adrenal Glands.**—1. *Medullary Secretion.*—Epinephrin causes a rise in the blood sugar by inducing glycogenolysis in the liver, thus opposing the action of insulin. Epinephrin increases the breakdown of muscle glycogen, but the product so formed is lactic acid and not glucose. Part of the lactic acid is carried by the blood to the liver, where it is reconverted to glycogen which in turn may later give rise to glucose. Thus, although the secretion of the adrenal medulla may exert a significant effect upon carbohydrate metab-

[1] Haist, Campbell and Best: Loc. cit., p. 99.
[2] Lukens and Dohan: Loc. cit., p. 99.
[3] Lukens, Dohan and Wolcott: Endocrinology, **32**, 475, 1943.
[4] Hutton: Arch. Phys. Ther., **20**, 287, 1939. Also Clin. Med. and Surg., **44**, 553, 1937.
[5] Dr. Herbert Pollack kindly gave us permission to quote his experience. On September 10, 1940, he wrote: "A selected series of 8 patients with diabetes mellitus were hospitalized for a period of ten weeks to insure supervised control of the diabetes. These patients were given an intensive course of *x*-radiation to the pituitary. No immediate effect was noted, nor has any appreciable effect been found in the follow-up of over three years."
[6] Selle, Westra and Johnson: Endocrinology, **19**, 97, 1935.

olism, this influence is confined to preformed glycogen stores, is of a relatively temporary nature and is not fundamental in the sense that the anterior pituitary hormone is. Diabetes has never been produced by the continued administration of epinephrin and removal of both adrenal medullæ does not ameliorate the diabetic condition of depancreatized animals.

DeTakats and Cuthbert[1] found that celiac ganglionectomy, denervation of the adrenals or section of the splanchnic nerves increased the response of the experimental animal to insulin, while atropine or section of both vagi did not decrease the sensitivity. Somewhat similar experiences were reported by Ciminata.[2] Because of their findings in animals, deTakats and co-workers carried out bilateral splanchnic nerve section in a girl, aged eighteen years, with severe diabetes. They reported that ten months after the operation the patient still showed an increased sensitivity to insulin. However, a second child operated upon was not so benefited. No other reports of operated cases have come to our attention. In the present state of our knowledge, it is unwise to advocate, for general use, surgical treatment of this type. Rogoff[3] described a patient who died of Addison's disease a little over a year after an adrenal denervation, having had little or no relief from the diabetic condition. He strongly objects to adrenal intervention for any condition except neoplasm.

2. *Cortical Secretion.*—The foregoing discussion has dealt only with the effect of epinephrin, the secretion of the suprarenal medulla, upon carbohydrate metabolism and diabetes. As pointed out above, however, although epinephrin stimulates glycogenolysis, it does not cause the breakdown of protein or produce ketonuria comparable to that seen in diabetes. Moreover, previous removal of the medullary portions of both adrenals does not prevent an animal from developing typical diabetes when the pancreas is subsequently removed. When, however, both adrenal glands are entirely removed, the diabetic condition of depancreatized cats is ameliorated in much the same fashion as hypophysectomy lessens the severity of diabetes of depancreatized dogs.[4] The administration of large quantities of adrenal cortical extract to adrenalectomized, depancreatized cats[5] or rats maintained with sodium salts increases the severity of the diabetes. Himwich and associates[6] have shown that ligation of the lumbo-adrenal veins produces the same effect.

Ingle, Sheppard and Kuizenga[7] produced diabetes in rats by the administration of adrenal cortical steroids to animals previously

[1] DeTakats and Cuthbert: Am. Jour. Physiol., **102**, 614, 1932.
[2] Ciminata: Klin. Wchnschr., **11**, 150, 1932.
[3] Rogoff: Jour. Am. Med. Assn., **106**, 279, 1936.
[4] Long: Harvey Lectures, **32**, 194, 1936–1937.
[5] Lukens and Dohan: Endocrinology, **22**, 51, 1938.
[6] Himwich, Fazekas and Martin: Am. Jour. Physiol., **123**, 725, 1938.
[7] Ingle, Sheppard and Kuizenga: Fed. Proc., **4**, 35, 1945; Endocrinology, **37**, 341, 1945.

subjected to partial pancreatectomy. In a comparison of adrenal steroid diabetes with pancreatic diabetes it was noted that the onset of glycosuria in each type was accompanied by an increase in urinary nitrogen, loss of weight and a temporary increase in the excretion of sodium and chloride. The two types of diabetes were unlike in that adrenal steroid diabetes was highly resistant to control by insulin. A second point of difference was that whereas in the depancreatized animals there was no increase in the level of urinary nitrogen until glycosuria had become severe, in the other rats a definite increase in urinary nitrogen preceded the onset of glycosuria.

In individuals with adrenal cortical hormone excess (Cushing's disease with or without adrenal tumor), the fasting blood sugar is usually normal but the glucose tolerance test shows impairment and the glucose-insulin tolerance test shows insensitiveness to insulin.[1]

(c) **Thyroid.**—The influence of the thyroid on carbohydrate metabolism is undoubted. Thus Burn and Marks[2] found that until the liver glycogen became depleted, thyroid feeding increased the hyperglycemia which followed adrenalin injections. Aszodi and Ernst[3] reported that following removal of the thyroid, dogs became markedly sensitive to insulin. The incidence of glycosuria and hyperglycemia, if not actual diabetes, among a large group of patients with thyrotoxicosis is high[4] By the administration of thyroid extract Houssay[5] was able to produce diabetes ("metathyroid diabetes") in dogs previously depancreatized to the extent that under ordinary conditions they still possessed sufficient islet tissue to maintain a normal blood sugar level. The production of diabetes was accompanied by lesions of the beta cells of the pancreas. It was shown that under these conditions the secretion of insulin was suppressed. The administration of insulin to such dogs protected them from diabetes in the early stages of the development of diabetes but was ineffective later on.

The giving of thyroid hormone in excess causes an increase of oxygen uptake, *i. e.*, of cellular activity, of all body tissues. Due to this, the carbohydrate, protein and fat stores of the body become depleted unless there is an adequate increase in the amount of food ingested. In consequence of this, slight elevation of the blood sugar, and not infrequently glycosuria, may occur particularly if, as in Houssay's dogs, the pancreatic reserve is already low.

No one, however, has assumed that the rôle of the thyroid may

[1] Fraser, Albright and Smith: Jour. Clin. Endocrinology, 1, 297, 1941.
[2] Burn and Marks: Jour. Physiol., 60, 131, 1935.
[3] Aszodi and Ernst: Arch. f. d. ges. Physiol., 215, 431, 1927.
[4] John: Jour. Am. Med. Assn., 99, 620, 1932. John: Jour. Clin. Endocrin., 2, 264, 1942.
[5] Houssay: Rev. Soc. Argent. de biol., 20, 179–198, 1944; Semana Med. (Buenos Aires) Tomo Cincuentenario, 1, 255, 1944.

be a primary and major one, such as that of the anterior pituitary. Thyroid feeding does not produce diabetes in animals with intact pancreases. The secretion of the thyroid hormone, thyroxin, is controlled by the thyrotropic hormone of the anterior pituitary. Houssay, in the experiments referred to above, could not produce diabetes in hypophysectomized or adrenalectomized animals; these died in hypoglycemia when given thyroid. Dohan and Lukens[1] found that although total removal of the thyroid both before and simultaneous with pancreatectomy in cats caused a diminution in the glucose, nitrogen, and acetone body excretion as compared with control animals, the changes were not striking and not comparable with those seen following removal of the pituitary or adrenal glands in similar animals.

Following the introduction in some clinics of the total ablation of the thyroid for long-standing and incapacitating heart disease, such complete removal was carried out for diabetes. Wilder, Foster and Pemberton[2] and Rudy, Blumgart and Berlin[3] published their results in such cases, one from each clinic. Although the severity of the diabetes and the requirement for insulin were somewhat lessened, the improvement so obtained did not compensate for the introduction of a new disease, myxedema.

(d) **Gonads.**—Although no direct and striking relationship between gonadal secretion and diabetes has been demonstrated, the influence of gonadotropic substances on both experimental and human diabetes has been the subject of considerable study and discussion. Since estrogens inhibit certain activities of the anterior pituitary, workers have studied the effect of such substances in depancreatized animals and diabetic persons with variable results. Barnes, Regan and Nelson[4] working with depancreatized dogs and Nelson and Overholzer[5] with depancreatized monkeys and dogs, reported a lessening of glycosuria but in some instances the effects seen were slight. On the other hand, Young[6] found that the administration of large doses of pure estrogen (estrone, estriol and diethylstilbestrol) to 4 dogs with pituitary diabetes and 1 depancreatized dog exerted no obvious antidiabetic action. It is true that Young used larger doses than the earlier investigators but, as he pointed out, one might reasonably expect these to suppress pituitary function more effectively than smaller amounts.

In a series of studies, Ingle obtained results which suggested that diethylstilbestrol exerts a diabetogenic effect in partially depancreatized and normal rats[7] and in partially depancreatized-adrenal-

[1] Dohan and Lukens: Am. Jour. Physiol., 122, 367, 1938.
[2] Wilder, Foster and Pemberton: Endocrinology, 18, 455, 1934.
[3] Rudy, Blumgart and Berlin: Am. Jour. Med. Sci., 190, 51, 1935.
[4] Barnes, Regan and Nelson: Jour. Am. Med. Assn., 101, 926, 1933.
[5] Nelson and Overholzer: Endocrinology, 20, 473, 1936.
[6] Young: Lancet, 1, 600, 1941.
[7] Ingle: Endocrinology, 29, 838, 1941.

ectomized rats receiving sub-diabetogenic amounts of adrenal cortical extract.[1] As to the mode of action, Ingle concluded[2] that diethylstilbestrol has some diabetogenic effect which is not mediated by either the pituitary or the adrenal glands but that its effect is less marked than in animals having these two glands intact. Findings opposed to those of Ingle were obtained by Janes and Dawson[3] working with rats with alloxan diabetes. Changes produced in those animals receiving diethylstilbestrol were, when compared with those of control animals, not marked and were interpreted as indicating that, under the conditions of the experiments, diethylstilbestrol was not diabetogenic.

Lack of agreement as to the effect of estrogens on diabetes is apparent also in clinical studies. Collens and co-workers[4] treated 7 diabetic patients with estrogenic substance and observed little or no effect upon the diabetic state. Lawrence and Madders[5] likewise obtained negative results even with large doses of diethylstilbestrol. However, Gessler, Halsted and Stetson,[6], Spiegelman,[7] Cantilo,[8] Sauer[9] and Morton and McGavack[10] reported improvement in the diabetic condition of certain women at or near the menopause with the administration of estrogens. Favorable results were noted also by Gitlow and Kurschner,[11] particularly in those women in whom diabetes had developed at about the same time as the menopause or those with aggravation of diabetes at this period. Large doses of estrogen, estrone (ketohydroxyestrin) or estradiol benzoate (dihydroxyestrin benzoate) were used. Improvement in the diabetes closely paralleled that of the menopausal symptoms.

In studies on partially depancreatized rats, dogs and toads, Souto-Maior and Foglia[12] found that the injection of testosterone produced little or no effect on the blood sugar and castration did not affect the development of diabetes in male rats with 95 per cent of the pancreas removed.[13] On the other hand, Malami[14] reported that testicular hormone increased the action of insulin in human diabetics while no influence was noted on the blood sugar of control subjects.

(e) **Clinical Application of Endocrine Interrelationships.**—Despite the remarkable influence of endocrine glands other than the pancreas

[1] Ingle: Am. Jour. Physiol., **138**, 577, 1943.
[2] Ingle: Endocrinology, **34**, 361, 1944.
[3] Janes and Dawson: Endocrinology, **38**, 10, 1946.
[4] Collens, Slo-Bodken, Rosenbliett and Boas: Jour. Am. Med. Assn., **106**, 678, 1936.
[5] Lawrence and Madders: Lancet, **1**, 601, 1941.
[6] Gessler, Halsted and Stetson: Jour. Clin. Invest., **18**, 715, 1939.
[7] Spiegelman: Am. Jour. Med. Sci., **200**, 228, 1940.
[8] Cantilo: Endocrinology, **28**, 20, 1941.
[9] Sauer: Schweiz. med. Wchnschr., **71**, 1577, 1941.
[10] Morton and McGavack: Ann. Int. Med., **25**, 154, 1946.
[11] Gitlow and Kurschner: Arch. Int. Med., **72**, 250, 1943.
[12] Souto-Maior and Foglia: Rev. Soc. argent. de biol., **20**, 79, 1944.
[13] Souto-Maior and Foglia: Rev. Soc. argent. de biol., **20**, 163, 1944.
[14] Malami: Boll. Soc. Ital. Biol. Sperim., **17**, 306, 1942.

upon experimental diabetes, the application of these findings to diabetes mellitus in man cannot be made automatically. The work of Houssay, Young, Long, Lukens and others suggests that in certain predisposed persons the onset of diabetes may be related to deranged functioning of the pituitary or adrenal glands, or both. So far, however, detailed and positive data in this regard have been lacking.

The problem has been attacked in various ways. For example, Mayer, Strouse and Soskin[1] carried out perimetric studies in 65 unselected diabetic patients in an attempt to obtain indirect evidence of pituitary enlargement. Although 7 patients had restricted visual fields, there was no correlation between the visual disturbance and the metabolic and endocrine characteristics of the patients. Then, too, there have been attempts to demonstrate a "diabetogenic hormone" in the blood and urine of diabetic patients; some workers have claimed positive results but the most that can be said is that with the urine of some normal and some diabetic persons it is possible to obtain extracts which will cause a transient increase in the blood sugar of animals into which such extracts are injected. Karelitz, Cohen and Deader[2] reported that the action of insulin injected into rabbits was inhibited if the insulin were previously mixed with the blood of diabetic patients. Control experiments in which the insulin was mixed with the blood of non-diabetic individuals also showed some inhibition of hypoglycemic action but to a lesser extent. DeWesselow and Griffiths[3] reported that when the blood plasma of certain elderly obese diabetic patients, chiefly women, was injected into rabbits, the hypoglycemic action of insulin was diminished. Others[4] have been unable to confirm this work, although it is true that in isolated cases Glen and Eaton[5] and Marble, Fernald and Smith[6] obtained a suggestion of an anti-insulin effect and Rushton[7] obtained a positive response with the plasma of 6 of 44 patients examined.

However, results of studies of this type by no means permit final judgment. There is ample reason for intelligent speculation as to the possible application to human diabetes of findings in experimental animals. There is abundant evidence to suggest that in animals the excessive activity of the anterior pituitary, adrenal cortex or, to a less extent, the thyroid, may by increasing the formation of glucose and inhibiting its utilization, cause hyperglycemia of such degree as to stimulate the pancreas to secrete additional insulin. The normal pancreas can presumably withstand

1 Mayer, Strouse and Soskin: Jour. Clin. Endocrin., **50**, 604, 1941.
2 Karelitz, Cohen and Deader: Arch. Int. Med., **45**, 690, 1930.
3 DeWesselow and Griffiths: Lancet, **1**, 991, 1936.
4 Dohan: Proc. Soc. Exper. Biol. and Med., **39**, 24, 1938.
5 Glen and Eaton: Quart. Jour. Med., **7**, 271, 1938.
6 Marble, Fernald and Smith: Endocrinology, **26**, 735, 1940.
7 Rushton: Proc. Staff Meet. Mayo Clinic, **15**, 417, 1940.

a great deal in the way of overwork. If, however, the hyperfunctioning of the other endocrine glands is sufficiently marked or prolonged, and particularly if the pancreatic reserve is low, then lasting damage to islet tissue and permanent diabetes may result.[1] This chain of events may well find its counterpart in man although positive proof is lacking.[2]

7. **Alloxan Diabetes.**—See Chapter V for a complete review of this form of experimental diabetes.

8. **Radioactive Isotopes.**—The use of radioactive isotopes as tracer substances in the body has already yielded valuable information regarding intermediary metabolism and may be expected to contribute greatly to our knowledge in the future. By virtue of identical chemical behavior, yet different physical properties due to the difference in atomic weight, an element in the diet, such as carbon, can be followed in metabolic processes in the body by incorporating a radioactive carbon isotope as C^{11} or C^{13} in substances fed or injected. The pathway of the carbon compound which has been introduced into the body can be traced by detecting the presence of the isotopic carbon in a particular site.

Throughout this monograph reference is made in appropriate places to investigations in which radioactive isotopes have been used. It is well here, however, to cite certain studies to illustrate the types of problems which have been attacked and the results secured. Workers at Harvard University,[3] continuing early work[4] on the metabolism of lactic acid containing radioactive carboxyl carbon, fed rats solutions of lactate containing C^{11} and measured the radioactivity of the expired CO_2 and liver glycogen. In 2.5 hours the CO_2 expired accounted for about 10 per cent, and the liver glycogen formed for 3.2 per cent, of the radioactivity. Another study[5] showed that although when radioactive bicarbonate ($NaHC^{11}O_3$) was injected into fasting rats which were fed glucose, the liver glycogen formed contained 13 per cent of the isotopic carbon, much lower amounts of C^{11} (0.17 to 0.45 per cent of the total C^{11} present) were incorporated in glycogen when the synthesis occurred *in vitro* with rabbit liver slices. The authors believe their results indicate that the formation of trioses is not a necessary step in the conversion of glucose to glycogen and are consistent with the findings of Cori and associates[6,7] that glycogen may be formed from glucose by

---

[1] Young: Brit. Med. Jour., **2**, 897, 1941.

[2] Shepardson: Loc. cit., p. 121.

[3] Vennesland, Solomon, Buchanan, Cramer and Hastings: Jour. Biol. Chem., **142**, 371, 1942.

[4] Conant, Cramer, Hastings, Klemperer, Solomon and Vennesland: Jour. Biol. Chem., **137**, 557, 1941.

[5] Vennesland, Solomon, Buchanan, and Hastings: Jour. Biol. Chem., **142**, 379, 1942.

[6] Sutherland, Colowick and Cori: Jour. Biol. Chem., **140**, 309, 1941.

[7] Colowick and Kalckar: Jour. Biol. Chem., **137**, 789, 1941.

9

phosphate transference and enzymatic action through the stages of hexose-6-phosphate and hexose-1-phosphate.

Continuing their studies in carbohydrate metabolism by the use of deuterium as an indicator, Stetten and Klein[1] obtained results which indicated that the glycogen appearing in the liver of a fasted rat after the injection of adrenalin is formed from blood lactate. The glycogen appearing in the muscle of rats after the administration of insulin is apparently formed largely from hexose directly. Likewise in rabbits[2] the glycogen deposited in muscle and in liver in response to insulin appeared to arise chiefly from dietary glucose by fairly direct processes. In rats and rabbits with alloxan diabetes, the rate of utilization of glucose in the synthesis of fatty acids is much reduced. Following the administration of insulin to both normal and diabetic rabbits there was a large increase in the rate of hepatic lipogenesis. Stetten and Klein[3] conclude that the rate of utilization of glucose in hepatic lipogenesis is dependent upon the level of circulating insulin.

Sacks[4] studied in cats the effect of insulin on phosphate turnover in striated muscle by means of radioactive phosphorus (P^{32}). In both fasting and post-absorptive animals given glucose, insulin increased in resting muscle the rate of turnover of phosphocreatine and the labile phosphate groups of adenosine triphosphate; it also increased the turnover rate of glucose-6-phosphate in the resting muscles of post-absorptive animals. However, insulin did not modify the extent of formation of glucose-6-phosphate on the cell membrane of resting muscle nor, in post-absorptive animals, did it increase the formation of glucose-6-phosphate on the cell membrane during recovery from muscular activity. Sacks concluded that insulin accelerates the rate of glucose oxidation within the muscle cell but that other factors are of greater importance in determining the rate of passage of glucose across the cell membrane.

9. **Nervous Regulation of Carbohydrate Metabolism.**—Although Claude Bernard's classical piqûre diabetique (production of glycosuria by puncturing the floor of the fourth ventricle) was performed in 1855, not a great deal in the way of exact and incontrovertible evidence has accumulated since then regarding the nervous regulation of carbohydrate metabolism. That a center (or centers) concerned with the behavior of sugar in the body exists in the hypothalamus seems likely, but there are differences of opinion as to the exact location and function of these regulatory areas. Morgan and Johnson[5] reported that the transient rise in blood sugar obtained following experimental lesions in the posterior

[1] Stetten and Klein: Jour. Biol. Chem., **159**, 593, 1945.
[2] Stetten and Klein: Jour. Biol. Chem., **162**, 377, 1946. See also Stetten, Boxer and Klein: Federation Proc., **4**, 106, 1945.
[3] Stetten and Klein: Federation Proc., **5**, 157, 1946.
[4] Sacks: Am. Jour. Physiol., **143**, 157, 1945
[5] Morgan and Johnson: Arch. Neurol. and Psychiat., **24**, 22, 1930.

part of the hypothalamus was apparently associated with hyperactivity of the adrenal glands and resulted in a depletion of the glycogen reserves of the liver. Morgan, Vonderahe and Malone[1] consider it possible, on the other hand, that a parasympathetic discharge from the anterior hypothalamus may influence the activity of the islets of Langerhans. Various workers have suggested that the extremely vascular paraventricular nucleus of the hypothalamus may be the center most concerned with carbohydrate metabolism. For example, Urechia and Nitescu[2] reported degenerative changes in this nucleus following pancreatectomy and Morgan and co-workers described degenerative lesions in the paraventricular nucleus in 15 consecutive cases of human diabetes. These findings, as yet, lack confirmation by other pathologists[3,4] who have made a special study of the problem. Brain[5] cited the work of Barris and Ingram[6] who noted mild, chronic hypoglycemia in 10 of 55 cats in which experimental lesions were produced in various parts of the hypothalamus. Hypoglycemia was most frequently encountered when the lesions were in the anterior portion.

10. **Lipotropic Substances and Experimental Diabetes.**—Lipotropic substances are those which prevent or remove an accumulation of excess fat in the liver. Three such factors are generally recognized: (1) choline and related compounds including precursors as methionine from which the body can synthesize choline; (2) lipocaic; and (3) inositol. The article by McHenry and Patterson[7] gives a comprehensive review of this subject and should be consulted by those with special interest.

A. **Choline.**—(*Ethylol-trimethyl-ammonium hydroxide*).—Shortly after the introduction of insulin, Allan, Bowie, Macleod and Robinson[8] reported that in order to keep completely depancreatized dogs in good condition or to maintain them for longer than eight months, it was necessary to give them not only insulin, lean meat and sugar, but also rations of raw pancreas. These workers noticed that at necropsy animals not given raw pancreas showed fatty infiltration and degeneration of the liver. Hershey and Soskin,[9] working in Best's laboratory, found that lecithin was able to supplant raw pancreas in this regard. From later experiments, Best, Hershey and co-workers reported that the active constituent of lecithin was choline. They stated further that a non-toxic oxidation product of

[1] Morgan, Vonderahe and Malone: Jour. Nerv. and Ment. Dis., **85**, 125, 1937.
[2] Urechia and Nitescu: Bull. de l'Acad. de méd., **93**, 188, 1925.
[3] Warren: Pathology of Diabetes Mellitus, 2d ed., Philadelphia, Lea & Febiger, Chap. XI, 1938.
[4] Davison, C.: Personal communication to Dr. Nathan Friedman.
[5] Brain: Recent Advances in Neurology, 4th ed., Philadelphia, The Blakiston Company, 1940.
[6] Barris and Ingram: Am. Jour. Physiol., **114**, 555, 1936.
[7] McHenry and Patterson: Physiol. Reviews, **24**, 128, 1944.
[8] Allan, Bowie, Macleod and Robinson: Brit. Jour. Exp. Path., **5**, 75, 1924.
[9] Hershey and Soskin: Am. Jour. Physiol., **98**, 74, 1931.

choline, betaine, also will prevent the fatty infiltration in the liver of normal rats. The amino acid, methionine, is of interest in this connection, because it may act as a source of methyl groups (which the body is incapable of synthesizing) to aid in the formation of choline in the body.[1]

Best[2] found that if raw pancreas, lecithin, choline, or betaine is not supplied to the depancreatized dogs, the diabetic condition, as far as glycosuria is concerned, is ameliorated. However, the animals do not seem well and die with much fat in the liver. If, before death, lecithin or choline be supplied, then the fat disappears from the liver, and along with this occurs an apparent increase in the severity of the diabetes. This is misleading, however, because the animal's general condition is very much improved and apparently, if insulin, meat and sugar are supplied in appropriate amounts, the animal can live a span of years approaching the normal.

Chaikoff and Kaplan[3] found that in depancreatized dogs maintained with insulin but without raw pancreas or choline, there occurs a reduction in the amount of all lipid constituents of the *blood;* this lowering was most marked in the ester cholesterol which in most of the animals had entirely disappeared from the blood. The *livers* of these animals were greatly enlarged and filled with fat. Most of the increase in liver lipids took place in the neutral fat fraction and very little in the phospholipid and cholesterol fractions.[4] The relative proportion of esterified cholesterol was greatly increased. When to such animals raw pancreas was given, there was a rise in all lipid constituents of the blood and particularly in the ester cholesterol fraction.[5]

Chaikoff and Kaplan were able to maintain depancreatized dogs for as long as four or five years on insulin and a diet containing meat, sucrose, bone ash and the necessary vitamins, but no pancreas and no dietary supplements such as lecithin or choline. Such dogs are not normal, however, possessing bilateral cataracts and the lipid changes in the blood and liver noted above.[6] However, it should be pointed out, as did Chaikoff and Kaplan[7] in a later publication, that although dietary supplements may not be necessary for survival of depancreatized dogs, it should not be concluded that the choline content of the diet itself is necessarily without significance in this regard. Furthermore attention must again be called to the fact that choline can be synthesized in the body provided that sufficient precursors are available. This synthesis may take place by a combination of methyl groups (from methionine) with

[1] duVigneaud: Biol. Symposia, **5**, 234, 1941.
[2] Best: Ann. Int. Med., **7**, 145, 1933.
[3] Chaikoff and Kaplan: Jour. Biol. Chem., **106**, 267, 1934.
[4] Kaplan and Chaikoff: Jour. Biol. Chem., **108**, 201, 1935
[5] Chaikoff and Kaplan: Jour. Biol. Chem., **112**, 155, 1935.
[6] Chaikoff: Proc. Soc. Exp. Biol. and Med., **33**, 211, 1935.
[7] Chaikoff and Kaplan: Jour. Nutrition, **14**, 459, 1937.

ethanolamine which the animal can produce. Chaikoff, Entenman and Montgomery[1] bring forth evidence to suggest that the anti-fatty liver factor of the pancreas acts to make available for lipotropic purposes the *bound* methionine contained in dietary protein.

Maclean, Ridout and Best[2] found that in rats choline favors the normal distribution of fat between the liver and the body depots and prevents the failure of certain functions of the liver. In rats with fatty livers it may accelerate the disappearance of fat from the liver during fasting.[3] Using deuterium as an indicator, Barrett, Best and Ridout[4] concluded that body depots are the source of the excess fat which accumulates in the liver during fasting, following the administration of certain extracts of the anterior pituitary gland, and following exposure to carbon tetrachloride vapor. Fat accumulating in the liver in animals on a diet low in protein and other lipotropic factors but rich in carbohydrate, comes probably from the carbohydrate of the diet.

As pointed out by McHenry and Patterson,[5] the simplest explanation of the lipotropic action of choline is that it promotes the formation of phospholipids which are essential for fat transport.

B. **Lipocaic.**—Dragstedt and associates[6] prepared fat-free alcoholic extracts of the pancreas to which they ascribed fat metabolizing properties and which they named lipocaic. They found that the oral administration of this substance to depancreatized dogs maintained with insulin permits their survival and prevents or reverses the abnormal accumulation of fat in the liver. They maintain that the beneficial effects of pancreas feeding in depancreatized dogs cannot be accounted for on the basis of its content of lecithin or choline.[7] Since the original announcement regarding lipocaic in 1936, there has been considerable discussion as to the existence of such a hormone and as to the possible identity of the potent influence with choline.[5]

The situation has been clarified to some extent by the recognition of the fact that there are several different types of experimental fatty livers with respect to method of production, character of the lipids, and response to lipotropic agents. In describing the action of a lipotropic substance it is essential, in the light of present knowledge, to give the method of production of the fatty liver.

A few years ago at a time when in our own clinic we had under observation a group of children with poorly controlled diabetes and gross hepatomegaly, we hoped to try the effect of lipocaic with them. However, protamine zinc insulin was introduced at just

[1] Chaikoff, Entenman and Montgomery: Jour. Biol. Chem., **160**, 489, 1945.
[2] Maclean, Ridout and Best: Brit. Jour. Exper. Path., **18**, 345, 1937.
[3] Best and Ridout: Jour. Physiol., **94**, 47, 1938.
[4] Barrett, Best and Ridout: Jour. Physiol., **93**, 367, 1938.
[5] McHenry and Patterson: Loc. cit., p. 131.
[6] Dragstedt: Am. Jour. Physiol., **117**, 175, 1936.
[7] Dragstedt: Jour. Am. Med. Assn., **114**, 29, 1940.

about that time and with better control of diabetes made possible with this preparation, the enlarged livers decreased in size and since then few or no suitable subjects have been available.[1,2] Reduction in the size of the liver in diabetic patients with the use of lipocaic has been reported by Rosenberg,[3] Snell and Comfort[4] and Grayzel and Radwin.[5] However, our own experience leads us to agree with Best and Ridout[6] that "the fatty liver of diabetic patients is much more likely to be due to inadequate insulin therapy than to a deficient supply of lipotropic factors." Dragstedt[7] likewise recognizes these two types of fatty infiltration of the liver in diabetes.

Dragsted[8] states that, as in human diabetes, the incidence of arteriosclerosis is greater in depancreatized than in normal dogs. He presents findings which suggest that the factors responsible for the primary deposition of lipids in the intima of arteries may be similar to those producing such deposits in the liver and discusses the possible rôle of lipocaic in the prevention of arteriosclerosis.

C. **Inositol** (*hexahydroxybenzene*).—Gavin and McHenry[9] found that the feeding of inositol to white rats prevents the "biotin type" of fatty liver (that caused by the administration of biotin along with thiamin, riboflavin, panthothenic acid and pyridoxine). Workers in Dragstedt's laboratory[10] found that inositol exerted some lipotropic effect in depancreatized dogs but not to the extent shown by lipocaic. They concluded that while lipocaic may contain inositol, the various effects produced by lipocaic are not given by inositol and that lipocaic probably contains a different, as yet unidentified, lipotropic factor. Rubin and Ralli[11] reached a somewhat similar conclusion. The exact rôle of inositol awaits clarification. McHenry and Patterson regard it likely that its lipotropic action is due, like that of choline, to the formation of phospholipids.

11. **Insulin.**—Thirty years prior to the discovery of insulin in 1921 by Banting and Best,[12] its production by the cells of the islands of Langerhans,first described in 1869,[13] had been suggested by Laguesse.[14] In the intervening period many workers tried with greater or less success to extract the active principle. We realize now that some almost succeeded but in the treatment of diabetic patients these researches found little or no practical application, largely for two

1 Marble, White, Bogan and Smith: Arch. Int. Med., **62**, 740, 1938.
2 White, Marble, Bogan and Smith: Arch. Int. Med., **62**, 751, 1938.
3 Rosenberg: Am. Jour. Digest. Dis. and Nutr., **5**, 607, 1938.
4 Snell and Comfort: Am. Jour. Digest. Dis. and Nutr., **4**, 215, 1937.
5 Grayzel and Radwin: Am. Jour. Dis. Child., **56**, 22, 1938.
6 Best and Ridout: Ann. Rev. Biochem., **8**, 349, 1939.
7 Dragstedt, Prohaska, Clark and Julian: Am. Jour. Physiol., **129**, 348, 1940.
8 Dragstedt: Biol. Symposia, **11**, 118, 1945.
9 Gavin and McHenry: Journ. Biol. Chem., **139**, 485, 1941.
10 Owens, Allen, Stinger and Dragstedt: Fed. Proc., **1**, 65, 1942.
11 Rubin and Ralli: Fed. Proc., **1**, 76, 1942.
12 Banting and Best: Jour. Lab. and Clin. Med., **7**, 251, 1921.
13 Langerhans: Inaugural Dissertation, Berlin, 1869.
14 Laguesse: Compt. rend. Soc. de Biol., **45**, 819, 1893.

reasons: (1) the administration of extracts by mouth—now recognized for practical purposes to be useless even with material of known potency—was often the method of trial; (2) extracts were so crude as to give rise upon injection to unpleasant symptoms of toxicity. Perhaps Zuelzer[1] came as close as any to the cherished goal. He even treated successfully several diabetic patients by injection of his extracts but he and other clinicians found the product too toxic for general use.

In the purification of their extract Banting and Best were aided by Collip,[2] Scott[3] and others. As time went on the market preparation became more and more highly purified. Scott and Parker[4] outlined a method employed at the Connaught Laboratories for securing highly purified insulin preparations. Insulin was first obtained in crystalline form by Abel and his co-workers[5] in 1926.

Scott[6] showed that insulin crystals represent the salt of some metal such as zinc, cadmium, cobalt or nickel, rather than the free substance. He demonstrated that the crystals occur in twins with the flattened surfaces of the rhombohedral plates in apposition. The melting point is 233° C., the molecular weight is about 35,000 (*i. e*, about that of egg albumin) and iso-electric point is at pH 5.2. Insulin is optically active and lævorotatory. Crystalline insulin gives all the reactions of a typical protein. It is precipitated by the usual protein precipitants and is denatured by strong acid or by boiling. It dissolves readily in dilute acid, dilute alkali and 90 per cent phenol. It is somewhat soluble in 80 per cent alcohol and insoluble in water-free organic solvents. It seems very unlikely that the active principle is merely adsorbed on the protein. Rather, it seems fairly certain that the protein is identical with the hormone, insulin.

Approximately 95 per cent of the constituents of the insulin molecule have been identified. The amino-acids, cystine, tyrosine, glutamic acid, leucine, arginine, histidine, lysine, proline, and phenylalanine have been isolated and identified as such. All of the sulphur, 3.2 per cent, is present as the disulphide linkage. Quite early Abel and co-workers noted a definite relationship between physiological activity and the so-called labile sulphur. Other groups which have been regarded as probably possessing especial activity are the amino and tyrosine groups.

Insulin crystals obtained from the pancreases of cattle, fish, pigs and sheep are identical in possessing the maximal physiological activity thus far obtained from insulin preparations, and all have

[1] Zuelzer: Berl. klin. Wchnschr., **33**, 415, 1907.
[2] Banting, Best, Collip, Campbell and Fletcher: Jour. Can. Med. Assn., **12**, 141, 1922. Banting, Best, Collip and Macleod: Trans. Roy. Soc. Can., **16**, 1, 1922.
[3] Best and Scott: Jour. Biol. Chem., **57**, 709, 1923.
[4] Scott and Parker: Trans. Roy. Soc. Can., **26**, 287, 1932.
[5] Abel, Geiling, Rouiller, Bell and Wintersteiner: Jour. Pharm. Exp. Ther., **31**, 65, 1927. See also Abel: Proc. Nat. Acad. Sci., **12**, 132, 1926.
[6] Scott: Endocrinology, **25**, 437, 1939.

the same sulphur content. The evaluation of the potency of a given insulin preparation is made by comparing its hypoglycemic action with that of the International Standard crystalline preparation (adopted in 1935) to which has been assigned the potency of 22 units per mg.

If the protein structure of insulin is affected by hydrolysis through chemical or enzymic means, the physiological activity is lost. In this fact undoubtedly lies the reason for the ineffectiveness of insulin given by mouth. (See page 142.)

Insulin is the product of the beta cells of the islands of Langerhans of the pancreas. Final and conclusive proof of this is afforded in the rare condition of carcinoma of the island (beta) cells; not only does the untreated condition result in profound chronic hypoglycemia, but insulin may be extracted in significant quantities from the tumor masses (as metastases in the liver) when removed from the body.[1] The granules in the beta cells are alcohol-soluble. The secretation of the islands leaves the gland by way of the blood stream and passes first to the liver. In a highly interesting microscopic study of the islet cells of living mice, O'Leary[2] observed that in response to the subcutaneous injection of dextrose, large vacuoles formed in a given islet cell and migrated to the periphery of the cell next the blood capillary where they were diminished in volume, presumably by diffusion of their contents through the cell membrane. Best[3] regards the production of insulin by any tissues other than the islands of Langerhans ("cellular insulin")[4] as not proved.

Nerve impulses affecting the islet cells are conducted by the vagus. A rich plexus of myelinated nerve fibers surrounds each islet[5] and both myelinated and non-myelinated fibers are said to invade the islet tissue itself.[6] Although some work such as that of Gayet and Guillaumie[7] with pancreatic grafts would suggest that the secretion of insulin can be stimulated by humoral influences alone, it is probable that the mediation of the vagus center is ordinarily an important link in the chain. From experiments involving crossed circulation in dogs, LaBarre *et al.*[8] conclude that the secretion of insulin is under the control of the vagus center which depends for its stimulation on an elevation of the blood sugar. The results of Clark[9] suggest the vagus may inhibit, as well as excite, the secretion of insulin.

[1] Wilder, Allan, Power and Robertson: Jour. Am. Med. Assn., **89**, 348, 1927. Power, Cragg and Linden: Staff Meet. Mayo Clinic, **11**, 97, 1936.
[2] O'Leary: Anat. Rec., **45**, 27, 1930.
[3] Best: Jour. Am. Med. Assn., **105**, 270, 1935.
[4] Tuttle: New England Jour. Med., **206**, 8, 1932; Jour. Am. Med. Assn., **99**, 985, 1932.
[5] Gentes and Pensa: Compt. rend. Soc. de biol., **54**, 202, 1902.
[6] deCastro: Rech. biol. de l'Univ. de Madrid, **21**, 422, 1923.
[7] Gayet and Guillaumie: Compt. rend. Soc. de Biol., **98**, 676, 1928.
[8] Zunz and La Barre: Compt. rend. Soc. de Biol., **96**, 421, 1400, 1927. La Barre and Destrée: Compt. rend. Soc. de Biol., **98**, 1240, 1928.
[9] Clark: Jour. Physiol., **59**, 466, 1925.

Geiger, Binder and Rusztek[1] report that electrical stimulation of the right or left vagus leads in dogs to definite lowering of the blood sugar which with nervous isolation of the pancreas changes over into an increase of the blood sugar. Rabbits show with vagotomy a lowered sugar tolerance; in dogs with right-sided vagotomy there is a lowering, and with left-sided vagotomy an increase, in sugar tolerance.

The studies of Meythaler and co-workers[2] suggest that it makes considerable difference as to how endogenous insulin reaches the circulation. If the pancreato-duodenal vein is anastomosed with the vena cava leaving the portal vein intact, abnormally low blood sugar values are the rule and the giving of glucose has a subnormal effect. Following carbohydrate, the blood sugar tends to fall very low and yet hypoglycemic symptoms are absent. The liver becomes pathologically filled with glycogen.

Monographs regarding insulin have been written by Staub,[3] Aubertin,[4] Jensen and Evans,[5] Hill and Howitt,[6] and Jensen.[7] The reader is referred to these and to the article by Scott[8] for further details.

12. Insulins With Prolonged Action.—Soon after the introduction of insulin in 1922 the relatively short duration of action of the preparation with the consequent necessity for repeated injections became apparent. Efforts were made to retard the action or to develop a preparation which would exert its effect over a longer period of time. Among the authors' patients attempts were made to delay the absorption of insulin by injecting it into thick fatty tissue instead of the subcutaneous spaces, but these trials were unsuccessful. Insulin was mixed with 20 per cent solution of gum arabic in 1923,[9] and in 1925 delayed absorption was sought by the addition of protein,[10] and, indeed, the combination of both gum arabic and protein yielded somewhat encouraging results. Bernhard in 1926 tried a mixture of insulin and fat. In 1929 Leyton[11] employed various oils to delay absorption with effect, and this was confirmed by others. A combination of lecithin and insulin was likewise used[12] but again without practical results. Combinations

[1] Geiger, Binder and Rusztek: Arch. f. exp. Physiol. u. Path., **176**, 355, 1934.
[2] Meythaler and Stahnke: Arch. f. exper. Path. u. Pharmakol., **152**, 185, 1930; also see Meythaler and Naegeli: Arch. f. exper. Path. u. Pharmakol., **172**, 630, 1933.
[3] Staub: Der Insulin, Julius Springer, Berlin, 1925.
[4] Aubertin: L'Insuline, Doin et Cie., Paris, 1926.
[5] Jensen and Evans: Physiol. Reviews, 14, 188, 1934.
[6] Hill and Howitt: Insulin, Hutchinson's Scientific and Technical Publications, London, 1936.
[7] Jensen: Insulin: Its Chemistry and Physiology, New York, The Commonwealth Fund, 1939.
[8] Scott: Loc. cit., p. 135.
[9] Burgess, Campbell, Osman, Payne and Poulton: Lancet, **205**, 777, 1923.
[10] DeJongh and Laqueur: Biochem. Zeit., **163**, 371, 1925.
[11] Leyton: Lancet, **216**, 756, 1929.
[12] Suranyi and Szalai: Klin. Wchnschr., **9**, II, 2159, 1930. Skouge and Schrumpf: Ztschr. f. klin. Med., **120**, 754, 1932.

of pituitrin and adrenalin were devised, but these, too, proved unsatisfactory.[1] Bischoff and Maxwell[2] reported prolongation of action of insulin in rabbits and rats by the addition of basic ferric chloride or tannic acid. The first real advance came in 1935 with the preparation and clinical trial of protamine insulin by Hagedorn and associates at the Steno Memorial Hospital, Gentofte, Denmark. The action of this preparation extended over some twelve to fifteen hours. With the addition of a small amount of zinc, the length of action was greatly prolonged. The present market protamine zinc insulin has a duration of effect of twenty-four to forty-eight hours. For details of this and other insulins with prolonged action, including histone zinc insulin, globin zinc insulin, and insulin mixtures, see page 368.

13. **Insulin Content of the Pancreas.**—Scott and Fisher[3] carried out analyses for insulin and zinc in the pancreases of 14 normal and 18 diabetic persons. They found that, whereas there were on the average 1.7 units of insulin per gram of non-diabetic pancreas, the corresponding value for diabetic pancreas was less than 0.4 unit. A similar, although not quite as striking, difference was noted as regards the zinc content, there being 0.14 mg. of zinc per gram of non-diabetic pancreas, as compared with 0.07 mg. per gram of diabetic pancreas. In a 35-page review of the literature in which 197 references are cited, Haist[4] includes a lengthy table summarizing the values obtained by various workers for the insulin content of the pancreas in different species. Although reported values in units per gram of pancreas are high for the rabbit (7.8 and 9.5) and chimpanzee (11.2) and low for the guinea pig (0.08 and 0.23), when calculated per kilogram of body weight of the animal, the values are more nearly uniform. Haist's article should be consulted for full coverage of the subject.

Haist, Best and associates[5,6] in a series of studies found that in rats, fasting, fat-feeding and the administration of insulin caused a reduction in the insulin content of the pancreas. Continuing their work with dogs, they found that fasting, fat-feeding and the administration of insulin prevented the reduction in the insulin content of the pancreas which results from administration of anterior pituitary extract. They concluded that in the studies both in the rat and the dog, the effects observed following the three procedures were due to resting the islets.

[1] Donath and Tanne: Arch. f. exp. Path., **119**, 222, 1927. Werner and Monguio: Klin. Wchnschr., **12**, I, 748, 1933. Clausen: Kliniske Underosgelser over Insulin resorptionens Paavirkeligbed af Adrenalin, Pituitrin og Ephetonin, Dissertation, Copenhagen, 1934.

[2] Bischoff and Maxwell: Am. Jour. Physiol., **112**, 172, 1935.

[3] Scott and Fisher: Jour. Clin. Invest., **17**, 725, 1938.

[4] Haist: Physiol. Reviews, **24**, 409, 1944.

[5] Haist, Ridout and Best: Am. Jour. Physiol., **126**, 518, 1939.

[6] Haist, Campbell and Best: Loc. cit., p. 99.

In this connection the findings of Latta and Harvey[1] are of interest. They noted that when albino rats are subjected to repeated injections of large or increasing doses of insulin, a selective reaction occurs in the beta cells of the islets of Langerhans, suggestive of a suppresion of secretory activity in these cells. Not only was there a shrinkage in cell volume, an almost complete disappearance of specific granules, a decrease in the size of nuclei and a condensation of chromatin but eventually in many beta cells the nuclei became pycnotic and the cytoplasmic outlines quite ragged. Following the discontinuance of insulin, the beta cells regained their normal appearance. Alpha cells remained unchanged throughout the course of the experiments. Prompt reversal of changes which may occur as the result of fasting was evident in the findings of Foglia,[2] who noted that the pancreas of dogs which had been fasted from two to three weeks, when grafted into the neck of a dog which had been depancreatized the day before, in 4 of 7 cases showed no impairment of its capacity to reduce blood sugar. Similarly, the pancreases of dogs which for thirty-seven days received 20 units of insulin and 30 gm. of sugar orally each day when grafted into the neck of depancreatized dogs still corrected the hyperglycemia in four hours like a normal pancreas.

14. **Insulin Requirement of Man.**—In the past there has been much speculation as to the amount of insulin required to maintain normal carbohydrate metabolism in man in the absence of the pancreas. Until recently only estimates, based on animal studies, were possible; these varied from 50 to 200 or 300 units daily.[3] However, within the past few years, total pancreatectomy has been carried out in several patients and direct information gained as to the insulin requirement. The first case reported was that of a man from whom Rockey[4] removed the pancreas because of carcinoma. On a glucose intake of 150 gm. daily, this patient required only about 27 units of insulin a day during the fifteen days he lived after operation. Autopsy disclosed, however, a pancreatic remnant weighing about 1 gm. In the two cases of Goldner and Clark,[3] the patients lived ten and eleven days respectively after total pancreatectomy because of carcinoma, and at autopsy no trace of pancreatic tissue was found. On daily glucose intakes of 150 to 200 gm., one of these patients required about 50 units, and the other 30 to 40 units, of insulin a day. In the patient of Priestley, Comfort and Radcliffe,[5] who recovered from total pancreatectomy performed because of hypoglycemia due to an islet cell adenoma, the insulin requirement was 30 units a day. A fifth patient was a woman

[1] Latta and Harvey: Anat. Rec., **82**, 281, 1942.
[2] Foglia: Compt. rend. Soc. de biol., **127**, 694, 1938.
[3] Goldner and Clark: Jour. Clin. Endocrinology, **4**, 194, 1944.
[4] Rockey: Ann. Surg., **118**, 603, 1943.
[5] Priestley, Comfort and Radcliffe: Ann. Surg., **119**, 211, 1944.

with cancer of the pancreas with extension to the stomach, left adrenal, omentum and lymph nodes, and studied by Brunschwig, Ricketts and Bigelow.[1] The patient's preëxisting diabetes was not aggravated by the operation which consisted of total pancreatectomy, total gastrectomy, total duodenectomy, splenectomy, left adrenalectomy and omentectomy. In fact, there were periods when the diabetic condition appeared less severe than before operation. With an intake of 400 gm. of carbohydrate and about 2500 total calories daily, the insulin requirement was 40 units a day. The patient died three and a half months after operation; autopsy revealed abdominal carcinomatosis but no remnant of pancreatic tissue.

More recently 3 cases have been reported by Waugh *et al.*[2] from the Mayo Clinic in addition to the patient studied by Priestley, Comfort and Radcliffe.[3] Their experience with the 4 cases may be summarized as follows: In two, operation was performed because of islet cell adenomata, in one because of carcinoma of the pancreas and in the fourth because of chronic pancreatitis and pancreatic lithiasis. At last report 3 patients had survived the operation for thirty-seven, eight and fifteen months respectively; the fourth died 2.5 months postoperatively following a severe hypoglycemic reaction. On diets furnishing daily from 243 to 272 gm. of carbohydrate, 75 to 124 gm. of protein and 70 to 103 gm. of fat, the approximate daily dose of insulin was, respectively, 30, 26, 40 and 38 units.

Striking in all these patients was the low insulin requirement of less than 50 units a day, an amount less than that needed by many diabetic patients. This is in keeping with the finding of Dragstedt, Allen and Smith[4] that the insulin requirement of partially depancreatized dogs is greater than that after total pancreatectomy. The experience bears out also the estimate of Bertram,[5] based on Holm's[6] experiments with depancreatized dogs, that a 60 kg. man with no insulin produced in his own body would require daily 7.8 units of insulin if fasting and 48 units if caloric needs were met exclusively by glucose.

As Ricketts[7] points out, the low insulin requirement of the completely depancreatized man raises the probability, already well supported by results of studies of experimental diabetes in animals, that in many patients with diabetes, extrapancreatic or anti-insulin factors must be prominently concerned. Total pancreatectomy in

[1] Brunschwig, Ricketts and Bigelow: Surg., Gynec. and Obst., **80**, 252, 1945.
[2] Waugh, Dixon, Clagett, Bollman, Sprague and Comfort: Proc. Staff Meet. Mayo Clinic, **21**, 25, 1946.
[3] Priestley, Comfort and Radcliffe: Loc. cit., p. 139.
[4] Dragstedt, Allen and Smith: Proc. Soc. Exper. Biol. and Med., **54**, 292, 1943.
[5] Bertram: Die Zuckerkrankheit, Leipzig, Georg Thieme, 2d ed., p. 78, 1939.
[6] Holm: Arch. f. exper. Path. u. Pharm., **121**, 368, 1927.
[7] Ricketts: Diabetes Abstracts, Editorial, **4**, 1, 1945.

man will afford an opportunity to reinvestigate, now for the first time in human subjects, fundamental problems regarding which data have been acquired since 1889 from studies of depancreatized dogs and other animals.

15. **Studies Regarding the Action of Insulin.**—Aubertin and Castagnon[1] studied the effect of small doses of insulin in lowering the blood sugar of depancreatized dogs before and after the pancreas was removed. A striking difference appeared. The effect of the same dose of insulin in the same animal was much greater in lowering the blood sugar of the dog after the pancreas was removed than it was beforehand. Thus 5 units might cause a fall of 43 mg. before the pancreas was removed and 167 mg. after the pancreas had been removed.

Several workers have pointed out that the activity of insulin might be expected to be different when injected subcutaneously, as is almost invariably done, than when delivered into the pancreato-duodenal vein which carries it first to the liver. Baodouin, Lewin, and Azerad[2] showed in dogs that the minimal dose of insulin necessary to produce a fall in blood sugar was 0.05 unit per kg. per hour if given into a peripheral vein, but it was only 0.01 unit per kg. per hour if given into the mesenteric vein or into an artery. Intradermal injections of a solution of crystalline insulin were shown to produce a more prolonged hypoglycemia and a greater incidence of convulsions in rabbits than subepidermal or subdermal injections. The lowering of blood sugar in fasting rabbits following the subdermal administration of insulin is more prompt when the reaction of its solution is at pH 7.0 than when it is at pH 2.9.[3] In studies of depancreatized dogs Greeley[4] found that the duration of action of a dose of insulin given intravenously depends upon its size. For doses of physiological magnitude the duration of action is proportional of the logarithm of the size of the dose. The intensity of the activity at any instant after a given dose of insulin is dependent upon the amount of insulin remaining in the body at that time. Brouha, Cannon and Dill[5] showed that in sympathectomized dogs a dose of only 1 unit of insulin per kg. of body weight produces a more marked drop in the blood sugar than a dose four times as large in a normal animal.

Tyler[6] found that the survival period of rabbits receiving lethal doses of insulin was prolonged by cooling the animals to temperatures below 30° C. The duration of insulin action in the cooled rabbits was greatly prolonged, the blood sugar returning to normal

[1] Aubertin and Castagnon: Compt. rend. Soc. de biol., **118**, 697, 1935.
[2] Baodouin, Lewin and Azerad: Compt. rend. Soc. de biol., **127**, 772, 1938.
[3] Sahyun: Jour. Lab. and Clin. Med., **25**, 619, 1940.
[4] Greeley: Am. Jour. Physiol., **129**, 17, 1940.
[5] Brouha, Cannon and Dill: Jour. Physiol., **95**, 431, 1939.
[6] Tyler: Proc. Soc. Exper Biol. and Med., **42**, 278, 1939.

after six to ten hours instead of after three to five hours in non-cooled animals.

Meythaler and Schroff[1] observed that in patients with disease of the liver, particularly in cancer and cirrhosis, the duration of action of insulin was more than double that in normal individuals and there was a more marked hypoglycemic effect, whereas in acromegaly "the action intensity" was much below normal. It was increased in Cushing's disease, Addison's disease and particularly in Simmonds' disease with marked cachexia.

16. **Methods of Administration of Insulin.**—Insulin is a protein and as such is broken down by the digestive juices of the stomach and intestine. When this happens, potency is lost. Preparations on the market claiming to control diabetes when taken orally are, by and large, quack medicines and advertisements of such products are barred from reputable medical journals. To date insulin administered parenterally is the only agent available which affords treatment specific for diabetes.

Although attempts to date to secure absorption of insulin from the gastro-intestinal tract have been unsuccessful from a practical point of view, much has been done in the way of investigation with this in mind. Murlin[2] and his associates for years carried out studies with the object of finding some way in which to protect the insulin molecule from the destructive action of the digestive juices and to facilitate its absorption through the intestinal wall. These and other workers found that in general there are three classes of substances which are effective: (1) alkyl derivatives of resorcinol; (2) glycol derivatives; and (3) sapogenins. Favorable effects seem to depend in part on surface action (the resorcinols and the sapogenins lower surface tension) and in part on the presence of hydrophylic and hydrophobic groups. Calcium reduces intestinal permeability; consequently agents such as sodium hexametaphosphate which combine with calcium, favor absorption. In a report[3] of the Rochester workers published in September, 1940, describing their results with an insulin-hexylresorcinol mixture given to 20 human patients with diabetes, they characterize their findings as "only mildly encouraging."

Wilson, Sappington and Salter[4] have shown that the inactivation of insulin by proteolytic enzymes *in vitro* may be reversed in whole or in part. Under the conditions of their experiments, the oral administration of insulin preparations caused hypoglycemic coma or convulsions in mice within two hours after administration. The effective oral dose for "undigested" insulin was about 90 times, and for "digested" insulin about 45 times, the subcutaneous dose. Iron

[1] Meythaler and Schroff: Klin. Wchnschr., **14**, 893, 1935.
[2] Driver and Murlin: Am. Jour. Physiol., **126**, 480, 1939.
[3] Murlin, Gibbs, Romansky, Steinhausen and Truak: Jour. Clin. Invest., **19**, 709, 1940.
[4] Wilson, Sappington and Salter: Endocrinology, **23**, 535, 1938.

salts increased the effectiveness of insulin preparations given orally. Cutting and Robson[1] treated 10 ambulatory diabetic patients with insulin orally, using quinine sulfate and insulin in capsules which were insoluble in gastric juice. Quinine was selected with the idea that it might allow absorption by inhibiting enzymatic action and by local effect on the cell surface. The results were not encouraging.

Insulin is effective when injected subcutaneously, intravenously, intraperitoneally or into the liver or spleen.[2] Absorption from the rectum, vagina and skin is incomplete and uncertain. It has been reported that intratracheal application produces hypoglycemia though not so regularly as do hypodermic injections. The literature regarding unusual modes of administration was summarized by Jensen[3] and in an editorial in the British Medical Journal.[4]

17. **Rate of Absorption of Insulin.**—The rate of absorption of three types of insulin injected subcutaneously was studied by Reiner and co-workers,[5] by using radioactive insulin preparations. As might be anticipated, the rate of absorption was most rapid in the case of unmodified insulin, next with globin (zinc) insulin and slowest with protamine zinc insulin. The differences in rates of absorption were correlated with the differences in intensity of hypoglycemic action of the preparations studied.

Root and associates[6] injected insulin-4-iodo-azobenzene containing radioactive iodine subcutaneously into selected diabetic patients and normal controls and studied the rate of absorption. This occurred rapidly during the first two hours and more slowly thereafter in both normal controls and in cases of uncomplicated diabetes but was delayed in patients with idiopathic insulin resistance, although the absorption rate became normal during recovery from insulin resistance. In such cases, intravenously injected insulin produced a more definite effect on the blood sugar and the respiratory quotient than subcutaneously injected insulin. Insulin absorption was retarded in indurated areas but was restored to normal on disappearance of the induration. The authors conclude that the cause of delayed insulin absorption is resident in the tissues at the site of injection and is unrelated to long duration of diabetes. It tends to be corrected by the use of insulin in sufficient amount to control hyperglycemia and glycosuria.

18. **Sensitivity to Insulin.**—It is a common clinical finding that diabetic patients vary greatly in their sensitivity to insulin. In certain patients, particularly those with the severe juvenile type of diabetes, the blood sugar tends to respond quickly and markedly to

[1] Cutting and Robson: Endocrinology, **28**, 375, 1941.
[2] Mark and Lewis: Bull. Johns Hopkins Hosp., **72**, 246, 1943.
[3] Jensen: Loc. cit., p. 137.
[4] Editorial: Brit. Med. Jour., **1**, 585, 1942.
[5] Reiner, Lang, Irvine, Peacock and Evans: Jour. Pharm. and Exper. Therap., **78**, 352, 1943.
[6] Root, Irvine, Evans, Reiner and Carpenter: Jour. Am. Med. Assn., **124**, 84, 1944.

an injection of insulin and in these patients insulin reactions are common. On the other hand, in middle-aged or elderly individuals with mild diabetes, relative insensitiveness is the rule rather than the exception, and with such individuals insulin reactions are less common. Various workers[1,2] have attempted to determine the sensitiveness of patients to insulin by more accurate methods.

Radoslav Test.—In the Radoslav test the effect of a definite amount of insulin on the capillary blood sugar of a fasting subject is determined over a period of four or five hours. It is assumed that a large decrease in the capillary blood sugar shows a weak, and a small decrease a strong, hepatic counter-regulatory mechanism. Since, however, the capillary blood-sugar curve tells nothing regarding the degree of sugar uptake by the tissues, workers in Falta's clinic[3,4] elaborated the Radoslav experiment by the simultaneous determination of the venous blood-sugar curve. The size of the plotted surface between the capillary and venous blood-sugar curves gives an idea of the strength of counter-regulatory factors in the tissues. With the aid of this elaborated test it is said to be possible to differentiate two types of insulin resistance: (1) hepatogenous and (2) peripheral or tissue resistance. These two types of insulin resistance are differentiated also through their clinical manifestations; whereas in cases of hepatogenous resistance hypoglycemic reactions occur with difficulty, even though enormous doses of insulin are given, in cases of tissue resistance there is an easy tendency to hypoglycemic reactions in the presence of a liberal In this connection, see discussion of Holm's work on pp. 140 and 362.

Himsworth Test.[5]—In this procedure a fasting subject is given glucose by mouth and insulin by vein simultaneously and capillary blood samples are taken at frequent intervals for the following ninety minutes. In insulin-sensitive persons the blood-sugar rise which would ordinarily follow the giving of glucose is wholly or partly prevented by the insulin, whereas in insulin insensitive subjects, the injection of insulin appears to have had little or no effect.

The test of Himsworth is valid in that all individuals, diabetic or non-diabetic, can be divided in two groups, those who are insulin-sensitive and those who are insulin-insensitive. However, in our own work[6] in which some 30 patients of varying ages and severity of diabetes were carefully studied, it became apparent that the results often cannot be correlated with clinical facts so that from a practical standpoint such tests are of no great assistance. DeWesselow and Griffiths[7] likewise found that the type of response could

[1] Radoslav: Wien. Arch. f. inn. Med., **8**, 395, 1924.
[2] MacBryde: Arch. Int. Med., **52**, 932, 1933; Jour. Clin. Invest., **15**, 577, 1936.
[3] Falta: Renaler und Insulärer Diabetes, Berlin and Vienna, Urban & Schwarzenberg, p. 7, 1939.
[4] Decaneas and Uiberrak: Klin. Wchnschr., **19**, 347, 1940; Ibid., **19**, 366, 1940.
[5] Himsworth: Lancet, **1**, 127, 1936.
[6] Marble, Smith and Fernald: Unpublished data.
[7] DeWesselow and Griffiths: Quart. Jour. Med., **12**, 17, 1938.

not be correlated with the initial blood-sugar level, sex, age, blood-pressure, body weight, or other clinical features of the patient. Klatskin[1] found no significant relationship between the sensitivity of 50 diabetic patients to a test dose of insulin and their clinical characteristics or their response to high-carbohydrate diets. Studying non-diabetic patients with dementia præcox, Harris[2] found some to show normal, others decreased, and others increased sensitivity to insulin.

On the other hand, Himsworth and Kerr[3] maintained that insulin-sensitive diabetics react favorably to an increase in carbohydrate in the diet, whereas insulin-insensitive diabetics suffer an impairment of sugar tolerance. Conceding that the correlation between the results of the insulin-glucose test and the clinical response of patients is not a precise one, they insist that classified according to the test, "insulin-sensitive diabetics tend to be younger, thin, to have a normal blood-pressure and healthy arteries; in them the disease is sudden and severe at onset; they easily develop ketosis and react to a slight excess of insulin with a hypoglycemic attack. The insulin-insensitive diabetics, on the other hand, tend to be older, obese, to have hypertension and to exhibit arteriosclerosis; in them the onset of the disease is insidious; they rarely develop ketosis and can tolerate overdosage of insulin without showing symptoms of hypoglycemia." Himsworth and Kerr[4] found that among 13 healthy individuals from eighteen to sixty-four years of age, insulin insensitiveness occurred more frequently in the higher than in the lower age groups.

According to Himsworth, in the insulin-sensitive diabetic the disease is due primarily to lack of insulin, whereas in the insulin-insensitive diabetic it is due primarily to impairment of insulin action. In the insulin-sensitive diabetic the removal of sugar from the blood by peripheral tissues under the influence of insulin is at a normal rate, while in the insulin-insensitive diabetic it is impaired. Soskin and Levine,[5] however, produced both insulin-sensitive and insulin-insensitive types of diabetes in the same completely depancreatized dog at different times. They found the significant difference between the two types to depend upon the functional capacity of the liver.

As suggested by Himsworth the glucose-insulin test may be elaborated by taking samples of venous and arterial (capillary) blood throughout the period of the test. The arteriovenous differences may then be used as an index of the degree and rate of utilization of sugar in the tissues. Griffiths[6] carried out such studies in a

[1] Klatskin: Jour. Clin. Invest., 17, 745, 1938.
[2] Harris: Arch. Neurol. and Psychiat., 48, 761, 1942.
[3] Himsworth and Kerr: Clin. Sci., 4, 119, 1939.
[4] Himsworth and Kerr: Clin. Sci., 4, 153, 1939.
[5] Soskin and Levine: Jour. Am. Med. Assn., 110, 768, 1938.
[6] Griffiths: Clin. Sci., 3, 91, 1938.

group of normal and diabetic subjects. He found that in spite of the differences in effect of insulin on the arterial blood sugar of diabetics of sensitive and insensitive types, there was no corresponding differences in the peripheral action of insulin; in both types it was less than in the normal subject.

Chen, Anderson and Maze[1] found birds (canary, pigeon, duck and rooster) to be less sensitive to insulin than mammals (mouse, rabbit and dog). The duck was about 30 times as tolerant of insulin as the rabbit. Among the birds studied, the rooster was the least sensitive and failed to develop convulsions even with lethal doses of insulin. In further studies,[2] horned owls were likewise found insensitive to insulin and did not develop convulsions even with extreme prolonged hypoglycemia. Intravenous injections of 1000 to 4000 units per kilogram caused death in only 4 of 11 tests. This experience with birds brings out the fact that insensitiveness to insulin may be reflected in lack of symptoms even though the blood sugar is low. It is common in the treatment of schizophrenia to find that certain persons require large doses of insulin to produce the desired effect. The case of Rivers and Elliott[3] was extreme in this regard; this patient received doses of insulin up to 1200 units intramuscularly and up to 2500 units intravenously without going into deep stupor despite an associated fall in blood sugar equal to that in other patients who went into stupor.

(For a discussion of patients with "insulin resistance," requiring large amounts of insulin daily, see pages 223 and 379.)

19. **Tests of Pancreatic Function.**—Various special tests have been devised in order to evaluate the functional efficiency of the pancreas. These may be summarized as follows:

(a) **The Hamman-Hirschman[4] (Staub-Traugott) Effect.** — Hamman and Hirschman[5] and later Staub[6] and Traugott[7] showed that the administration of sugar in two divided portions separated by a definite space of time (thirty to ninety minutes) produces a different effect on the blood sugar in the normal as compared with the diabetic. In the normal healthy individual the administration of sugar by mouth usually produces, first, a rise in the blood-sugar curve, but after one or two hours a fall, until eventually a value even lower than the initial one is reached. If at the time the descending limb of the curve occurs, one gives a second dose of sugar of the same or a larger amount, then in normal individuals the blood-sugar curve in the following one or two hours either rises only slightly or not at

1 Chen, Anderson and Maze: Jour. Pharm., **84**, 74, 1945.
2 Scott and Chen: Fed. Proc., **5**, 201, 1946.
3 Rivers and Elliott: Jour. Lab. and Clin. Med., **29**, 55, 1944.
4 Dr. F. M. Allen kindly called to our attention the fact that Hamman and Hirschman in 1919 demonstrated beautifully the effect commonly designated by the names of Staub and Traugott.
5 Hamman and Hirschman: Johns Hopkins Hosp. Bull., **30**, 306, 1919.
6 Staub: Biochem. Ztschr., **118**, 93, 1921.
7 Traugott: Klin. Wchnschr., **1**, 892, 1922.

all, while in diabetic individuals following the second administration of sugar there is a further and definite rise in blood sugar. The less severe the diabetes the more nearly does the Staub-Traugott curve approach the normal.

These relationships are brought out even more clearly if one gives, as Grote[1] suggested, at intervals of every half hour, 10 grams of glucose by mouth. Such administration causes the blood sugar of the diabetic, at least for a certain period, to continue to rise. With the normal person, however, after the second or third dose of sugar, the peak of the blood-sugar curve is reached. Then follows a fall and a more or less horizontal course from then on. Grote concluded that with diabetic patients who are not receiving injected insulin it is best to give food, particularly carbohydrate, at intervals throughout the day rather than concentrating it in three meals. In this connection, see discussion of Holm's work on pp. 140 and 362.

(*b*) German authors have written a good deal concerning the value of the determination of the blood-sugar curve throughout an entire day ("Tagesblutzuckerkurve" or "Tagesprofil") in giving a good idea of the tolerance of the patient and the severity of the diabetic condition.[2]

(*c*) Among others, Depisch and Hasenöhrl, in Falta's Clinic,[3] ascribed the hypoglycemic phase which follows the overloading of the body with sugar as in a tolerance test, to overstimulation of the pancreas and the overproduction of insulin. This view has been attacked by Soskin.[4] Depisch and Hasenöhrl determined both the capillary and venous blood sugar following the giving of glucose. They found, as others have, that whereas in the fasting state capillary and venous blood-sugar values were always the same or nearly so, following the giving of sugar the venous blood sugar fell below the level of the capillary- blood sugar, so that there was a definite difference at the peak of the curve. This was taken to mean that because of the influence of the overloading with sugar the pancreas was made to secrete insulin and the avidity of the tissues for sugar was raised. The arterial venous difference may be slight or lacking in severe diabetes, whereas in the normal person it is always present. This is held to indicate that in the normal person sugar is taken out by the tissues, thereby making the venous blood sugar lower than the capillary. In the diabetic this does not properly take place. This abnormality may be corrected in the diabetic by the administration of an appropriate dose of insulin.

(*d*) **Triangle d'Hyperglycémie.**—In differentiating between normal individuals and patients with non-diabetic glycosuria (obese

[1] Grote: Ergebn. d. ges. Med., **18**, 301, 1933.
[2] Schöne and Zimmer: Klin. Wchnschr., **14**, 1672, 1935.
[3] Falta: Renaler und Insulärer Diabetes, Berlin and Vienna, Urban and Schwarzenberg, p. 7, 1930.
[4] Soskin, Allweiss and Cohn: Am. Jour. Physiol., **109**, 155, 1934.

patients, patients with liver disease and patients with hyperthyroidism) and true diabetes, Labbé[1] measured the area of the triangle of hyperglycemia which is formed by the blood-sugar curve obtained following the giving of 50 grams of glucose, taking blood sugars fasting, at one-half hour and one, two and three hours after the giving of the sugar.

20. **Duodenal Extract.**—Duncan, Shumway, Williams and Fetter[2] reported in 1935 concerning the effect upon diabetic patients of the oral administration of an extract of the duodenal mucosa (Laughton and Macallum[3]). They were unable to reduce marked hyperglycemia or to benefit certain severe diabetics with the extract but stated that in most of their patients it prevented noteworthy hyperglycemia and glycosuria. Taken all in all, the results were inconclusive, and since in the years since the report of Duncan and co-workers, duodenal extract has not received clinical trial generally, it is to be assumed that failure to report upon it implies lack of promising results. It is true that in a privately printed monograph, Flint,[4] in 1939, reported further studies regarding the action of "The Macallum-Laughton Synergist," but to date, insofar as we are aware, published data confirming his views are lacking.

21. **Preparations of Vegetable Origin.**—In 1938 Large and Brocklesby[5] reported that extracts of roots of the Devil's club (Fatsia horrida), a wild plant growing along the coast of British Columbia, possess hypoglycemic properties. Hyperglycemic extracts could also be produced. Somewhat similar findings were obtained by MacDonald and Wislicki,[6] who made extracts of large quantities of raw cabbage. More recently reports have appeared regarding the hypoglycemic action and possible therapeutic value of extracts from two other plants: (1) "cundeamor," made from Momordica charantia and investigated by Rivera[7] in Puerto Rico; (2) "amellin," isolated from Scoperia dulcis Linn. and studied by Nath and associates[8] in India. In interpreting results obtained with these and similar preparations, it is necessary to keep in mind that a substance may lower the blood sugar without being able to correct the faulty metabolism of diabetes. Thus, the preparation synthalin used some years ago for clinical trial had some slight effect in reducing hyperglycemia and glycosuria in patients with mild diabetes; it was later demonstrated, however, that these effects were in reality due to toxic action upon the liver.

[1] Labbé: Leçons Cliniques sur le Diabète, Paris, Masson et Cie, p. 16, 1932.
[2] Duncan, Shumway, Williams and Fetter: Am. Jour. Med. Sci., **189**, 403, 1935.
[3] Laughton and Macallum: Canad. Med. Assn. Jour., **23**, 348, 1930.
[4] Flint: Further Observations on Hypophyseal Diabetes Mellitus and the Action of The Macallum-Laughton Synergist, Canada, A. B. Macallum, 1939.
[5] Large and Brocklesby: Canad. Med. Assn. Jour., **39**, 32, 1938.
[6] MacDonald and Wislicki: Jour. Physiol., **94**, 249, 1938.
[7] Rivera: Am. Jour. Pharm., **113**, 281, 1941; Ibid., **114**, 72, 1942.
[8] Nath and others: Ann. Biochem. and Exper. Med., **3**, 1943, in 5 parts: I, pp 55–62; II, pp. 63–84; III, pp. 107–120; IV, pp. 121–130; V, pp. 147–156.

22. Factors Influencing the Accumulation of Glycogen.—Although glucose is the form in which carbohydrate is present in the body fluids and, through transportation in the blood stream, the form in which it is made available for energy, by far the largest amount of carbohydrate in the body is in the form of glycogen stored in the liver, muscles and skin. In a diabetic, with the administration of appropriate doses of insulin, amounts of glycogen approaching the normal accumulate in the liver and muscles. In normal animals, however, as shown by Bridge,[1] the effect of insulin is not to increase liver glycogen but, rather to deplete it by transferring it to the muscles. Much the same experience was reported by Bretano.[2] It is true that Goldblatt[3] and Corkill[4] succeeded in obtaining an increase in liver glycogen with insulin when young rabbits (and later young kittens) were used, but it seems likely that this increase in young animals is a secondary effect, due to liberation of epinephrin.[5]

Bodo and Neuwirth[6] carried out continuous infusions of sugar into normal dogs, obtaining thereby a rise in liver glycogen. If, however, in addition, relatively large amounts of insulin were given in single injections, the liver glycogen fell. With continuous slow infusion of insulin in small but effective amounts, storage of glycogen was prevented. In depancreatized animals, if the pancreas was removed at the time of the experiment, the liver glycogen fell regardless of whether sugar alone or sugar and insulin were infused. If, however, pancreatectomy was performed at least forty-eight hours before the experiment, the administration of insulin with sugar caused a gradual rise in liver glycogen from the very beginning of the experiment.

In the experiments of Greeley, Martin and Hallman[7] on diabetic patients and depancreatized dogs and rabbits, the blood-sugar level was controlled by the administration of glucose intravenously. It was found that under the action of insulin, more glucose disappeared from the blood at high than at physiological levels of blood sugar. The glucose which disappeared at high blood-sugar levels could not be fully accounted for by increased liver or muscle glycogen or by oxidation. The liver glycogen in the depancreatized animals actually fell at the high blood-sugar levels.

The liver of a completely depancreatized animal becomes free of glycogen if neither sugar nor insulin is given for forty-eight hours. If sugar is administered alone, storage of glycogen occurs up to a

[1] Bridge: Bull. Johns Hopkins Hosp., **62**, 408, 1938.
[2] Bretano: Klin. Wchnschr., **18**, 42, 1939.
[3] Goldblatt: Biochem. Jour., **23**, 83, 1929.
[4] Corkill: Biochem. Jour., **24**, 779, 1930.
[5] Cope and Corkill: Jour. Physiol., **82**, 407, 1934.
[6] Bodo and Neuwirth: Am. Jour. Physiol., **103**, 5, 1933.
[7] Greeley, Martin and Hallman: Jour. Clin. Endocrin., **2**, 590, 1942.

maximum of about 1 per cent. If insulin is given along with the sugar, a greater degree of glycogen formation occurs.[1]

It is generally accepted that fructose is more readily transformed into glycogen than is glucose. Use has been made of this fact in the treatment of conditions of liver impairment, supplying a high-carbohydrate diet made up to a certain extent from fructose.

Dann and Chambers[2] found in dogs that a fast sufficiently long (three weeks or more) to suppress almost all oxidation of carbohydrate did not seriously derange the process of glycogen formation from ingested glucose. At least 35 per cent of the glucose was deposited as glycogen in the liver and muscles. Glycogen in the heart was found to be unusually high, comparable to the values characteristic for pancreatic diabetes.[3] Although the experiments of Cori[4] and Major and Mann[5] present evidence that insulin is not necessary for the formation of small amounts of glycogen in muscle, it seems certain that its action is to increase greatly the rate at which sugar and lactic acid are converted into muscle glycogen. Marks[6] showed that in the spinal eviscerated cat, the peripheral action of insulin in favoring the deposition of glycogen in the muscles, is diminished by the previous administration of anterior pituitary extracts (prolactin preparations). The studies of Long and Horsfall[7] suggest that insulin promotes the formation of glycogen in the recovery of muscle exercise.

23. **Rhythmic Variations in Carbohydrate Metabolism.**—For years, certain workers, particularly those in Scandinavian countries, have been interested in the problem of possible rhythmic variations in carbohydrate metabolism apart from those dependent upon nutritional differences. Forsgren[8] from work on rabbits concluded that glycogen storage in the liver exhibited daily rhythmic changes with a maximum at night and a minimum in the daytime. Forsgren's results were confirmed by Holmgren[9] and by Agren, Wilander and Jorpes.[10] Petrén[11] described a morning minimum and an afternoon maximum in the liver glycogen content of the guinea-pig.

American investigators have, in general, been skeptical that such rhythmic changes take place in animals independent of food intake, outside stimuli, as noise and disturbance from handling, age and physiological factors related to sexual activity. Thus Higgins

[1] Bodo, Tui and Farber: Am. Jour. Physiol., **103**, 18, 1933.
[2] Dann and Chambers: Jour. Biol. Chem., **95**, 413, 1932.
[3] Fisher and Lacket: Am. Jour. Physiol., **72**, 43, 1925. Evans and Bowie: Proc. Soc. Exper. Biol. and Med., **35**, 68, 1936.
[4] Cori: Physiol. Rev., **11**, 143, 1931.
[5] Major and Mann: Am. Jour. Physiol., **102**, 409, 1932.
[6] Marks: Jour. Physiol., vol. **87**, Proc. Physiol. Soc., March 14, 1936.
[7] Long and Horsfall: Jour. Biol. Chem., **95**, 715, 1932.
[8] Forsgren: Klin. Wchnschr., **8**, 1110, 1929; Acta med. Scandinav., **73**, 60, 1930.
[9] Holmgren: Ztschr. f. mikr. anat. Forsch., **24**, 632, 1931; Acta med. Scandinav., **88**, Suppl. 74, 1936.
[10] Agren, Wilander and Jorpes: Biochem. Jour., **25**, 777, 1931.
[11] Petrén: Morph. Jahrb., **83**, 256, 1939.

Berkson and Flock,[1] Deuel and collaborators[2] and Marble, Grafflin and Smith[3] have reported findings which in general do not support the contention of Scandinavian investigators. Furthermore, despite the carefully presented observations of Möllerström,[4] one hesitates to agree entirely with his conception of an endogenous periodicity of carbohydrate metabolism in many diabetic patients and his conclusion that in these cases insulin should be administered with due regard for the endogenous rhythm rather than in relation to meals.

24. **Sugar Content of Tissues.**—Trimble and Carey[5] found that the average true sugar content of skin and muscle in non-diabetic subjects was 56 and 28 milligrams per cent, respectively, whereas for diabetics the corresponding average values were 144 and 51 milligrams per cent, respectively, but the average true sugar of the whole blood was 226 milligrams per cent. Thus, the elevation of sugar concentration in the blood was accompanied by a marked absolute increase in the quantity of sugar in the skin, while the elevation in muscle was much smaller. Power and Clawson[6] found the free-sugar content of the normal liver to be as low as 100 to 125 milligrams per 100 grams of tissue (non-fermentable fraction, 30 milligrams), thus corresponding closely with the blood sugar. The corresponding value for normal muscle was 45 to 60 milligrams of sugar (total reduction) for each 100 grams of tissue of which approximately one-half was non-fermentable. The fermentable fraction was, therefore, much lower than that of the blood sugar. (See also pages 588 and 599.)

C. THE BLOOD SUGAR.

1. **The Blood Sugar in Health and Diabetes.**—The blood sugar of normal individuals after an overnight fast is remarkably constant, averaging about 100 mg. per 100 cc. or slightly lower. This fasting blood-sugar value may vary from 70 to 120 mg. per cent. A value of 130 mg. per cent is regarded by practically all workers as sufficiently abnormal to warrant the diagnosis of diabetes. The fasting blood sugar may vary in the same individual at different times. Reports upon percentages of sugar in the blood vary also according to the method used in the determination. Methods in common use in America are those of Folin, of Hartman, Shaffer and Somogyi, and of Benedict. In Europe the most popular methods are the microprocedures devised for capillary blood by Bang, Hagedorn and Jensen and McLean.

[1] Higgins, Berkson and Flock: Am. Jour. Physiol., **102**, 673, 1932; Ibid., **105**, 177, 1933.
[2] Deuel, Butts, Hallman, Murray and Blunden: Jour. Biol. Chem., **123**, 257, 1938.
[3] Marble, Grafflin and Smith: Jour. Biol. Chem., **134**, 253, 1940.
[4] Möllerström: Arch. Int. Med., **52**, 649, 1933; Acta med. Scand., Supplement No. 147, 1943.
[5] Trimble and Carey: Jour. Biol. Chem., **90**, 655, 1931.
[6] Power and Clawson: Proc. Staff Meet. Mayo Clinic, **4**, 46, 1929.

For years European workers have used almost universally capillary blood for the determination of sugar, and in this country likewise such methods have now come into wide use. Microprocedures are of especial help in dealing with children and with patients from whom it is desirable to take blood for examination at frequent intervals. It must be noted, however, that the use of capillary methods requires that not only the laboratory technician, but also the person who withdraws the blood, must be a careful worker, trained in the manipulation involved. This is not so much the case when venous blood is used, for then the main requisite is to get a sufficient quantity of blood into a suitable container. It may then later be examined in the laboratory by a trained technician.

By excluding, to a greater extent, the non-glucose-reducing substances, newer methods of blood analysis give in general lower values for sugar than do older procedures. Benedict's method[1] and Folin's colorimetric ferricyanide method[2] give results averaging about 20 mg. less than those by older methods in the literature. By most of the methods in common use, however, one still determines, particularly by the copper-reduction methods, a small and relatively constant non-glucose fraction. This is made up of glutathione, ergothionine, cysteine, creatinine and undetermined substances. This non-glucose fraction usually has reducing ability equivalent to that of about 10 to 30 mg. of glucose per 100 cc. of blood, although Mosenthal[3] found that in 38 per cent of 200 consecutive determinations, the upper limit of 30 mg. was exceeded and in 4 instances the non-glucose fraction amounted to 70 mg.

In diabetes the increase in the percentage of sugar in the blood varies widely, depending upon the severity of the disease, upon the previous treatment and upon complicating conditions. Thus, the blood sugar in the postabsorptive state may be normal, although a common diabetic value is that of two times the normal, namely, 200 mg. per 100 cc. In patients with severe diabetes, particularly in children, the fasting blood sugar may be 300 mg. per cent or higher. High fasting values are almost invariably accompanied by marked glycosuria. In diabetic coma, values from 300 to 600 mg. per cent are the rule, but at times one finds values of 1000 mg. per cent or over. In our series of 651 consecutive cases of diabetic coma there were 24 such cases.

Mosenthal and Lauber[4] remind us that the fasting blood sugar is not a fixed quantity. In 70 fasting diabetics, there was a significant change in the blood sugar as fasting continued over a period of three hours. In 48 per cent there was a drop and in 15 per cent, a rise in the value.

[1] Benedict: Jour. Biol. Chem., **76**, 457, 1928.
[2] Folin: Jour. Biol. Chem., **77**, 421, 1928; Ibid., **81**, 231, 1929.
[3] Mosenthal: Quart. Bull., Northwestern Univ. Med. School, **20**, 99, 1946.
[4] Mosenthal and Lauber: New York State Jour. Med., **44**, 1555, 1944.

In the normal individual, within the first thirty to sixty minutes following the intake of food, the blood sugar rises and then falls to normal within two hours. It is difficult to say how high the post-prandial blood sugar may rise without being abnormal. Consequently it is helpful to set up definite, reliable standards in order to make the matter of diagnosis systematic and to avoid confusion. It is our rule to regard a blood sugar of 170 mg. per 100 cc. following a meal as indicative of diabetes. This value applies to venous blood; for capillary blood, since postprandial capillary values are in the normal individual higher than venous values, we have arbitrarily accepted 200 mg. per 100 cc. as the lowest value on which to make the diagnosis of diabetes. When diabetes and hyperthyroidism coëxist, then it is helpful to raise the postprandial value for venous blood from 170 to 200 mg. per 100 cc., thus excluding certain thyrotoxic individuals in whom slight hypergycemia may not indicate diabetes. Althausen, Lockhart and Soley[1] demonstrated that in some patients with hyperthyroidism the blood-galactose curve following the oral administration of the sugar is usually abnormally high, whereas a normal response is obtained in the same person after intravenous administration. They attributed the difference to abnormally rapid absorption from the gastro-intestinal tract probably due to an increase in tissue (mucosal) phosphatase in hyperthyroidism.

2. **Sugar in Venous and Arterial Blood.**—In the normal individual, although the concentration of sugar in venous and arterial (capillary) blood in the fasting state is essentially the same, after a meal the arterial blood sugar rises on the average 20 to 50 or more milligrams higher than the venous blood sugar. In 200 consecutive tests Mosenthal[2] found the difference to vary widely from -26 to $+102$ mg. This arteriovenous difference reflects the oxidation or storage of glucose in the tissues. In the untreated diabetic the arterial and the venous blood-sugar curve following a meal or following the giving of sugar may be almost identical, indicating that very little sugar is taken up by the tissues. Indeed, at times, as in the diabetic patient described by Grott,[3] the sugar of venous blood may throughout a tolerance test remain at a higher level than that of capillary blood. With the giving of insulin, however, and control of the diabetic state, an arteriovenous difference approaching the normal may be achieved. One must record, however, Mosenthal's finding in 200 consecutive determinations that the arteriovenous difference was about the same whether or not the subject was fasting, whether or not he was diabetic and if diabetic, whether or not he was being treated with insulin. He found that the difference

[1] Althausen, Lockhart and Soley: Am. Jour. Med. Sci., **199**, 342, 1940. See also Althausen and Stockholm: Am. Jour. Physiol., **123**, 577, 1938.
[2] Mosenthal: Loc. cit., p. 152.
[3] Grott: Arch. mal. de l'App. dig., **25**, 140, 1935.

might vary widely in the same individual on different days under like conditions of diet and insulin dosage.

Because of variable and unpredictable capillary-venous differences, all would agree with Langner and Fies[1] that if only capillary blood-sugar values are obtained, the interpretation of glucose tolerance curves is frequently difficult. This applies not only to the Exton-Rose but also the standard one-dose procedure.

3. **Sugar in Plasma and Erythrocytes.**—Some observers[2] have attempted to explain the occurrence of supposed hypoglycemic symptoms in the presence of blood-sugar levels higher than normal by suggesting that whereas the sugar content of the whole blood was normal, the erythrocytes were impoverished ("cytoglycopenia"). On the other hand, Olmsted[3] reported that *in vivo*, even under normal conditions, the red blood corpuscles contain no sugar whatsoever; after blood is shed, changes take place swiftly and sugar passes quickly into the erythrocytes. Olmsted's findings were not confirmed by Neuwirth[4] and Klinghoffer.[5]

4. **Factors Affecting the Blood Sugar.**—Endocrine influences affecting the blood sugar such as those arising from the pituitary, adrenal and thryoid, have been discussed earlier in this chapter in connection with experimental diabetes. Soskin[6] has recently presented his views in this field.

Aside from endocrine factors and from the giving of food or glucose there are many influences which may cause a rise in the sugar content of the blood. Most, if not all, of these factors cause their effect by the breakdown of glycogen in the liver and the release of glucose into the blood. As an example of a purely physical influence may be mentioned the experience of Samaras[7] who lowered the body temperature of rats swiftly to under 22° C. by plunging them into ice water. This led to a transient rise of the blood sugar, to an almost complete disappearance of the liver glycogen and to almost a 50 per cent decrease in the muscle glycogen. Creatinuria of two to three days' duration resulted.

Kirstein and Bromberg[8] found slight increases in the blood sugar and slight decreases in the blood phosphorus during fever therapy. They believe the blood sugar increases to be due not to concentration of the blood but to breakdown of glycogen stores in the liver in response to increased utilization of glucose in the tissues.

From studies on normal individuals Meyer[9] concluded that the intake of fluid has no constant influence on the blood-sugar level.

[1] Langner and Fies: Am. Jour. Clin. Path., **12**, 95, 1942.
[2] Foshay: Am. Jour. Physiol., **73**, 470, 1925.
[3] Olmsted: Am. Jour. Physiol., **111**, 551, 1935.
[4] Neuwirth: Am. Jour. Physiol., **117**, 335, 1936.
[5] Klinghoffer: Am. Jour. Physiol., **118**, 431, 1937.
[6] Soskin: Clinics, **1**, 1286, 1943.
[7] Samaras: Ztschr. f. d. ges. exper. Med., **106**, 510, 1939.
[8] Kirstein and Bromberg: Jour. Lab. and Clin. Med., **25**, 7, 1939.
[9] Meyer: Ztschr. f. d. ges. exper. Med., **106**, 409, 1939.

McKittrick and Root[1] have shown that during anesthesia produced by ether or nitrous oxide and oxygen, the blood sugar rises. This is true to a lesser extent with ethylene, and still less with spinal anesthesia. In experiments on rabbits Lauber and Bersin[2] stated that the liver glycogen sank 50 per cent during ether narcosis. Incidentally, they reported that the administration of vitamin B_1 for several days before the anesthesia reduced greatly the glycogenolytic effect. Larson[3] found that neither pentobarbital nor evipal in the doses he used, had any appreciable effect on the blood-sugar level of rats or on hypoglycemia induced by insulin. Oelkers and Schultze[4] found that cocaine produces a rise in blood sugar in normal individuals and that in rabbits treated with cocaine, sugar tolerance curves exhibited a higher rise and longer extent than in control studies.

5. **Absorption of Sugar.**—From experimental data it has been assumed that sugar is not absorbed in significant quantities from the stomach.[5] Therefore, in conditions of pyloric obstruction or when for any reason the emptying of the stomach is interfered with, it has seemed reasonable that food or liquid given by mouth may not be absorbed. This is of practical importance to the physician who is treating an unconscious patient suffering from hypoglycemia due to insulin. Under such conditions one often obtains little or no relief from orange juice or other carbohydrate-containing solutions given by mouth and only after glucose has been injected intravenously does recovery take place. One must, however, call attention to the works of Morrison, Shay, Ravdin, and Cahoon[6] who concluded that glucose is absorbed from the stomach to some extent when introduced in concentrations over 40 per cent. Absorption was slight when solutions of 15 per cent glucose were introduced and negligible or absent when concentrations below 7 per cent were used. These findings suggest that in severe hypoglycemia in which delay in gastric emptying is suspected, the use of syrup by mouth might be more efficacious than that of fruit juices. On the other hand, Goldfarb and Golden[7] found that in patients with hypoglycemic coma due to insulin, the ingestion of glucose in 5 per cent solution produced a more rapid recovery than when a 30 per cent solution was administered.

Trimble, Carey and Maddock[8] found that the average rate of absorption of dextrose from the gastro-intestinal tract was about 1 gram per kilogram per hour. No definite relationship was detected

[1] McKittrick and Root: Diabetic Surgery, Philadelphia, Lea & Febiger, p. 76, 1928.
[2] Lauber and Bersin: Klin. Wchnschr., 7, 232, 1939.
[3] Larson: Fed. Proc., 5, 189, 1946.
[4] Oelkers and Schultze: Klin. Wchnschr., 25, 871, 1938.
[5] Maddock, Trimble and Carey: Jour. Biol. Chem., 103, 285, 1933.
[6] Morrison, Shay, Ravdin and Cahoon: Proc. Soc. Exper. Biol. and Med., 41, 131, 1939.
[7] Goldfarb and Golden: Proc. Soc. Exper. Biol. and Med., 51, 134, 1942.
[8] Trimble, Carey and Maddock: Jour. Biol. Chem., 100, 125, 1933.

between the average rate of absorption and variations in certain other factors, such as the concentration of dextrose ingested, the length of the absorption period, the weight of the animals used and the excitement occasioned by experimentation.

Pijoan and Gibson[1] injected intravenously 50 cc. of a 50 per cent solution of glucose into 5 normal human subjects and determined the blood volume and blood sugar at frequent intervals after the injection. They found in a representative experiment that 87.5 per cent of the added glucose was removed from the circulating plasma within four minutes of the time of injection. Studies of the respiratory quotient showed no significant rise until thirty-six minutes had elapsed since the injection. The studies emphasize the capacity of the organism to store glucose. Pijoan and Gibson observed, as have others, a depression of inorganic phosphate of the serum following the administration of dextrose.

The problem as to whether or not glucose administered rectally is absorbed has been studied by various workers, with variable results. Carpenter's[2] results suggested that from 55 to 90 per cent might be absorbed with the greater part of the absorption taking place within the first two hours. Scott and Zweighaft[3] were unable to demonstrate a rise in the blood-sugar curve as a result of administering dextrose in retention enemata. Absorption increases, of course, if by reverse peristalsis the sugar solution is carried through the ileo-cecal valve into the lower ileum. Eberling[4] found that glucose solutions were absorbed very slowly when placed in the entire colon of a dog, and that 10 per cent solutions were absorbed only slightly better than isotonic solutions. He observed, however, that with hypoglycemia prevailing, the absorption of glucose from the colon can be as rapid as that from a low ileal loop of a non-insulinized dog. Retardation of absorption of water takes place when glucose is added to the solution introduced into the colon.

6. **Renal Threshold for Glucose.**—The glucose or renal threshold, that is, the percentage level of sugar in the blood above which sugar appears in the urine, has been carefully investigated. Campbell, Osgood and Haskins[5] found the renal threshold for "true sugar" to vary from 99 to 228 mg. per cent, 80 per cent of the cases having values that ranged from 140 to 190 mg. per cent. The glucose threshold may be taken on the average to lie between 160 and 180 mg. per cent sugar for whole blood (venous) but there is much variation from individual to individual, and it is not possible to designate any figure as "normal."

In certain species, as in the domestic fowl, the renal threshold

[1] Pijoan and Gibson: Am. Jour. Physiol., **121**, 534, 1938.
[2] Carpenter: Human Metabolism with Enemata of Alcohol, Dextrose and Levulose, Washington, Carnegie Institution of Washington, Pub. No. 369, 1925.
[3] Scott and Zweighaft: Arch. Int. Med., **49**, 221, 1932.
[4] Eberling: Am. Jour. Med. Sci., **183**, 876, 1932.
[5] Campbell, Osgood and Haskins: Arch. Int. Med., **50**, 952, 1932.

for glucose is said to be relatively high; values ranging from 260 to to 310 mg. per 100 cc. of blood have been reported.[1] Robinson and co-workers[2] have demonstrated that with a given individual the threshold varies with the amount of sugar administered. In determining the glucose threshold, reliance should not be placed on a single examination, but rather on repeated tests. It makes a difference as to whether the threshold is determined on the basis of a rising or a descending curve of sugar concentration in the blood since with a falling blood sugar glycosuria often occurs at a level of glycemia unassociated with urinary sugar on the ascending limb of the curve.

Steinitz[3] points out that the appearance of glucose in the urine depends upon three factors: blood sugar level, glomerular filtration and renal threshold. The renal threshold in turn is dependent upon the capacity of the kidney tubules to reabsorb sugar from the glomerular filtrate.[4] This capacity may be overtaxed by the excessive amounts of sugar presented, as in diabetes mellitus; it may be paralyzed, as in phloridzin poisoning;[5] or it may be deficient, as in spontaneously occurring renal glycosuria in man, possibly because of a defect in the phosphorylating mechanism. In the renal glycosuria of pregnancy, the effect on the tubules has been thought by some to be of pituitary origin. Factors influencing the renal threshold have been discussed by Roch and collaborators.[6]

There are conflicting reports in the literature as to the renal threshold in diabetes. The data may be summarized by stating that in diabetic patients as in normal persons the level of the threshold is an individual matter and may be high or low, but in general the threshold in diabetics tends to be higher than in normals. This is true particularly in elderly diabetics and especially in the presence of arteriosclerosis and hypertension or chronic nephritis; Steinitz[3] states that in these patients the high threshold may be explained on the basis of kidney disease. For further discussion, see the article by Marble.[7]

7. **Food Tolerance Tests.**—Since even in the diabetic the fasting blood sugar may be normal, various food and sugar tolerance tests have been devised to aid in diagnosis. Food tolerance tests, and particularly sugar tolerance tests, are often fallacious.[8] The results may be as unfair to the patient as to the doctor or insurance company. The previous diet of the subject is a definite factor and will

[1] Batt: Am. Jour. Physiol., **129**, 307, 1940.
[2] Robinson, Derivaux and Hewell: Am. Jour. Med. Sci., **189**, 795, 1935.
[3] Steinitz: Jour. Clin. Invest., **19**, 299, 1940.
[4] Nelson and Mirsky: Am. Jour. Physiol., **129**, 429, 1940.
[5] Govaerts and Muller: Jour. Clin. Invest., **18**, 25, 1939.
[6] Roch, Martin and Sciclounoff: Acta med. Scandin., **88**, 1, 1936.
[7] Marble: Med. Clin. North America, **21**, 427, 1937.
[8] Meyers and McKean: Am. Jour. Clin. Path., **5**, 299, 1935. Leyton: Brit. Med. Jour., **2**, 536, 1935.

be discussed at some length in the next section. If an individual lives upon a rigid, low-carbohydrate diet for some days and a liberal carbohydrate meal is then taken, hyperglycemia may develop to such an extent that a diagnosis of diabetes is warranted.

This phenomenon has been emphasized by Odin,[1] Malmros,[2] Adlersberg and Porges[3] and Sweeney.[4] The last-named writer found that there was a delayed postprandial rise in blood sugar in hydrated animals, a definite decrease in tolerance after a fat diet and starvation, a slight decrease in tolerance on a protein diet, but an increase in tolerance on a carbohydrate diet.

Every meal is a food tolerance test. A simple way in which to determine whether or not a patient has diabetes is to make the examination without previous notice after a dinner of meat, potato, bread, pie, and coffee with sugar. The urine should be essentially free from sugar before, at one hour and at two hours, after the meal. (See Table 21.) It can be tested immediately, and if sugar-free, the probabilities are that the patient has not diabetes, but for more conclusive evidence simultaneous tests for sugar in blood and urine should be performed. For nearer 100 per cent proof, a sugar-tolerance test with 100 grams of glucose is essential.

TABLE 21. FOOD TOLERANCE TEST.

Time.	Urine sugar, per cent.	Blood sugar, per cent.
Four hours after breakfast	0.1	0.10
Lunch: Baked beans, potato, 1½ rolls, apple pie, ice cream		
One hour after lunch	trace	0.23
One and a half hours after lunch	3.0	0.27

Wishnofsky and Kane[5] carried out tolerance tests on 21 diabetics, comparing the effect of 100 grams of dextrose with 90 grams of starch in the form of potato, barley, rice and bread (90 grams of starch on hydrolysis yield 100 grams of dextrose). They found that the blood sugar curves which resulted did not differ significantly.

8. **Sugar Tolerance Tests.** — (a) **Type and Amount of Sugar.** — Although sugar tolerance tests are widely used, interpretation of them varies greatly. Some workers depend most on the height to which the blood sugar rises, others on the rate of fall, and still others on both features. The last attitude is undoubtedly safest, but even then we regard formal sugar tolerance tests as often unsatisfactory. In order for results to be valid for diagnosis of diabetes, the glucose tolerance test must be done under carefully controlled conditions. Otherwise various factors may cause a normal

[1] Odin: Acta med. Scand., Suppl. **18**, pp. 1–573, 1927.
[2] Malmros: Zentralbl. f. inn. Med., **48**, 244, 1927.
[3] Adlersberg and Porges: Klin. Wchnschr., **5**, 1451, 1926.
[4] Sweeney: Arch. Int. Med., **40**, 818, 1927. See also Sweeney, Tunnell and Tunnell: Am. Jour. Clin. Path., **14**, 437, 1944.
[5] Wishnofsky and Kane: Am. Jour. Med. Sci., **189**, 545, 1935.

person to exhibit a diabetic type of response.[1] The subject must have been on an unrestricted diet for at least three days prior to the test and should not have taken insulin during this time. He should be free from infection and fever. He should be free from disease states known to lower carbohydrate tolerance, such as hyperthyroidism or acromegaly, or due allowance should be made for such. Due regard must be had for the effect of conditions altering absorption from the gastro-intestinal tract (if glucose is administered orally), for the age of the patient, previous physical activity, and liver function. Even in the same non-diabetic individual variable results may be obtained.[2] However, in ordinary clinical work the tolerance test, if carefully done and intelligently evaluated, is consistent enough to be of great value in the diagnosis of diabetes.[3]

For a few years we used as a tolerance test 75 grams of cane sugar but in 1935 returned to the use of glucose. Schmidt, Eastland and Burns[4] carried out both glucose and sucrose tolerance tests on 57 hospital cases; they found the general pattern of the glucose and sucrose curves to be the same, but the average blood-sugar values following the ingestion of sucrose were slightly lower than those obtained using glucose. The authors concluded that clinically sucrose is as satisfactory as glucose both for the detection of diabetes and for the demonstration of lesser abnormalities in carbohydrate metabolism.

However, because of the abundance of literature with the easy availability of comparable values, the giving of glucose is preferable and in dosage of 100 grams to adults. To individuals under 100 pounds in weight the test dose may well be 50 grams, and to children 1.9 gm. per kg. body weight are given. It has been stated that tolerance curves satisfactory for diagnostic purposes can be obtained as readily with the use of 50 grams of glucose as with 100 grams, even in adults of average size. This is undoubtedly true to a large extent. However, in the normal person, the larger amount of sugar may be expected to prolong the hyperglycemia obtained and in the diabetic, both a higher level and a prolongation of the hyperglycemia may be produced.[5] In our practice it is the custom to take urine and blood samples fasting and at one-half, one hour and two hours after the giving of the sugar. Occasionally it is worth while to prolong the test to three hours. Blood may be taken either from a vein or from the ear or finger. If capillary blood is used, due regard must be given for the higher values which are usually secured on such samples. Whereas we ordinarily make the diagnosis of diabetes if a venous blood sugar rises to a height of 170 mg. per 100

[1] Corkill and Marks: Med. Jour. Australia, 1, 577, 1943.
[2] Freeman, Looney and Hoskins: Jour. Clin. Endocrin., 2, 431, 1942.
[3] Sevringhaus: Proc. Am. Diabetes Assoc., 4, 119, 1944.
[4] Schmidt, Eastland and Burns: Jour. Lab. and Clin. Med., 21, 13, 1935.
[5] Exton and Rose: Proc. Assn. Life Ins. Med. Dir. Am., 18, 252, 1931. Hansen Acta med. Scand., Supp. IV, 1, 1923.

cc. or more, we do not feel that the diagnosis of diabetes is justified unless the capillary blood sugar rises at least to 200 mg. per 100 cc. These values for both venous and capillary blood are lower than those chosen by certain other clinicians for the diagnosis of diabetes. Indeed, certain authorities pay little or no attention to the height of the tolerance curve, but classify a curve as a normal one if at the end of two hours the blood-sugar value has returned to 120 mg. per 100 cc. or lower. We consider this latter point to be of great value, but we believe that one cannot disregard the height to which the curve goes.

McKean, Myers and von der Heide[1] devised a "micro interval glucose clearance test" which involves the intravenous injection in one and one-half minutes of 0.2 gram of glucose per kilogram of body weight and the removal of venous blood specimens at exactly three, four, five, ten and fifteen minutes after the end of the injection. In the procedure described by Tunbridge and Allibone[2] the capillary blood sugar is determined at intervals of one and a half to seven and a half minutes for at least one hour after the intravenous injection of 92 cc. of a 30 per cent solution of glucose. In this article is an excellent summary of papers published regarding intravenous glucose tolerance tests. The intravenous administration of glucose has much to commend it, particularly in that it avoids errors arising from abnormal rates of absorption from the gastro-intestinal tract,[3] but the procedure has the disadvantage of not lending itself well to the carrying out of tolerance tests except by especially trained workers.

The Hamman-Hirschman effect (see page 146) has been utilized by some workers, among them Exton and Rose[4] as means of diagnosis. Patients are given 50 grams of glucose after the fasting blood sugar has been determined. At the end of one-half hour a second blood sugar is taken and another 50 grams of glucose are given. When another half-hour has passed a third blood sample is obtained. In the case of the diabetic individual, the third blood sugar will be definitely higher than the second, in the case of the non-diabetic person the third blood sugar will be lower or only negligibly higher than the second. Matthews, Magath and Berkson[5] of the Mayo Clinic reported their results with the Exton-Rose test in a group of 117 persons considered clinically to have a normal tolerance for carbohydrate, 304 diabetic patients who had been graded clinically as to severity, and 70 persons regarded clinically as having renal glycosuria. Using this test, they believe the most effective criterion for differentiating diabetic and non-diabetic persons to be the hour value of the blood sugar. They take 158 mg. per cent as the dividing

[1] McKean, Myers and von der Heide: Am. Jour. Med. Sci., 189, 702, 1935.
[2] Tunbridge and Allibone: Quart. Jour. Med., 9, 11, 1940.
[3] Gildea, McLean and Man: Arch. Neurol. and Psychiat., 49, 852, 1943.
[4] Exton and Rose: Am. Jour. Clin. Path., 4, 381, 1934.
[5] Matthews, Magath and Berkson: Jour. Am. Med. Assn., 113, 1531, 1939.

line. They state that by using the Exton-Rose test the number of cases of doubtful laboratory diagnosis is smaller than by any other method employed. The findings of Wayburn and Gray[1] were much the same as those of the Mayo Clinic workers. With the two-dose test they believe that the one hour value is the best single aid in the diagnosis of diabetes. They add another test at two hours which they believe offers a means of differentiating the severe classes of diabetes. Wayburn and Gray found that the two-dose test was relatively free from the influence of fairly marked changes in the composition of the preceding diet.

(b) **The Normal and the Diabetic Respose Compared.**—In the fasting state the blood sugar of the normal individual varies from 80 to 120 mg. per cent; after an overnight fast, values between 110 and 130 mg. must be regarded with suspicion. Following the administration of 100 grams of glucose by mouth the blood sugar rises quickly, reaching a maximum within thirty or sixty minutes. Usually the value does not exceed 140 mg. per cent, although the diagnosis of diabetes would in the average case not be justifiable unless a value of 170 mg. per cent or more was attained. Within two hours the blood sugar should have fallen to 120 mg. per 100 cc. or lower. The data collected and analyzed from the literature by Gray[2] in 1923 showed that following 100 grams of glucose, the blood sugar of 40 diabetic patients with a normal fasting blood sugar rose to 0.18 per cent in one-half hour, 0.20 per cent in one hour, 0.15 per cent in two hours and 0.10 per cent in three hours. With 54 diabetic patients whose fasting blood sugar was 0.12 per cent or more the values were distinctly higher. These values are compared with normal values in Table 22.

In normal persons the blood sugar rises less after the mid-day meal than after breakfast if the interval between is three hours. This difference is not constant in normals and still less so in diabetics. In the latter the greater the severity, the greater the advantage in separating the meals instead of approximating them.[3] Maclean[4] found that the blood-sugar curve following the administration of 50 grams of glucose to fasting diabetics might be high and prolonged. After feeding the patient for a time, though starting at the same blood-sugar level, the same amount of glucose produced a reaction which was not so high or lasted so long, and to this extent indicated improvement of the patient. Sakaguchi[5] explains the above phenomena on the basis that at breakfast-time glycogen formation by the liver is at a low ebb. The indication,

[1] Wayburn and Gray: Am. Jour. Med. Sci., **204**, 823, 1942.
[2] Gray: Arch. Int. Med., **31**, 241, 1923.
[3] Sakaguchi and Sato: Mitt. d. med. Fakultät d. Kais. Universität zu Tokyo, **23**, 373, 1920. See also Petrén: Compt. rend. Soc. de biol., **93**, 380, 1925.
[4] Maclean: Modern Methods in the Diagnosis and Treatment of Glycosuria and Diabetes, London, Constable & Co., 1922.
[5] Sakaguchi: Mitt. d. med. Fakultät d. Kais. Universität zu Tokyo, **20**, 439, 1918.

11

therefore, would be not only to make the carbohydrate at breakfast less than at the other meals, but to precede breakfast with a small amount of carbohydrate. Gray's[1] experience with divided meals in our clinic was a practical confirmation of these observations.

TABLE 22.—GLUCOSE-TOLERANCE TESTS IN DIABETICS AND NORMALS COMPARED (GRAY[2]).

Individuals.	Glucose given, gm.	Blood sugar (fasting), per cent.	Average percentage of blood sugar.				
			Fasting.	½ hour.	1 hour.	2 hours.	3 hours.
Diabetics.							
40 . . .	100	0.11 or less	0.09	0.18	0.20	0.15	0.10
54 . . .	100	0.12 or more	0.17	0.25	0.27	0.25	0.21
Normals							
300 . . .	100	....	0.09	0.14	0.12	0.11	0.09

(c) **Changes in Blood Elements Other Than Sugar Following the Administration of Glucose.**—Sunderman and Williams[3] found that after the ingestion of 75 grams of glucose in 200 cc. of water by 18 fasting diabetic individuals there occurred an increase in glucose concentration, a decrease in chloride concentration, an increase in the osmotic pressure, and an increase in the total quantity of glucose, chloride and water. The authors point out from their experiments that the change in concentration induced with respect to a single component, such as glucose, tends to disturb the concentration of other components of the serum and to induce transfers of some of them to or from the serum. In the course of tolerance tests on 87 individuals including normal persons as well as those with various diseases, Schmidt and Eastland[4] found an appreciable decrease in the amino-acid nitrogen and the urea nitrogen of the blood. They report that except for individual variations, there was no change in the blood volume or hemoglobin concentration.

(d) **Factors Influencing the Sugar-tolerance Curve.**[5]—1. *Previous Diet.*—As has been mentioned earlier, the sugar-tolerance curve is greatly influenced by the previous diet.[6] Thus, with normal individuals or animals who have either been starved[7] or kept on a low-carbohydrate diet or on a diet high in fat, a diabetic type of curve may be obtained following the giving of the usual dose of dextrose.

[1] Gray: Boston Med. and Surg. Jour., **186**, 763, 1922.
[2] Gray: Loc. cit., p. 161.
[3] Sunderman and Williams: Jour. Clin. Invest., **14**, 245, 1935.
[4] Schmidt and Eastland: Jour. Lab. and Clin. Med., **21**, 1, 1935.
[5] John: Southern Med. Jour., **36**, 624, 1943.
[6] Chabanier, Lobo-Onell and Lelu: Presse méd., **39**, 1133, 1931. Boller and Ueberrack: Klin. Wchnschr., **11**, 511, 1932. Sweeney: Arch. Int. Med., **40**, 818, 1927. Himsworth: Jour. Physiol., **81**, 29, 1924. Malmros: Acta med. Scand., Suppl. 27, 1928.
[7] Aubertin, Lacoste, Soric and Castagnon: Compt. rend. Soc. de biol., **120**, 1107, 1935.

The same individual if placed on a higher carbohydrate diet will later be found to have a normal tolerance curve. For example, Bowman and associates[1] studied the sugar tolerance in 18 alcoholic patients admitted to the wards of the Bellevue Hospital in New York City. They found that on admission there was a marked diminution in the sugar tolerance as measured by glucose tolerance tests. This improved after one week in the hospital on a normal diet, suggesting that the diminution was due to an undernourished state previous to admission. It is of interest that Gounelle, Marche and Bachet[2] found that in 9 patients with edema due to starvation, glucose tolerance tests gave very irregular results.

Conn[3] advises that for at least three days before a test is done a diet providing at least 300 grams of carbohydrate, 80 grams of protein, and calories sufficient for maintenance be used. He states that diabetics who have taken the standard preparatory diet for three to five days have not appeared to be harmed.

If doses of dextrose are given to normal men or animals on successive days the rise of the blood-sugar curve becomes less and less day by day, or if on the same day successive doses of glucose are given, the second curve reaches its peak at a lower level than the first and the third lower than the second, and so on. With rabbits it is possible eventually to produce severe hypoglycemia with convulsions by this method.[4] Ellis[5] found that hourly doses of insulin and glucose produced a temporary improvement in the carbohydrate tolerance of severe diabetics.

As increasing quantities of carbohydrate are given in a preparatory diet the fasting normal individual oxidizes increasing amounts of glucose. The response of the diabetic is qualitatively similar but quantitatively smaller, the ability to oxidize glucose being directly related to the severity of the disease. When given in excess of the ability of the diabetic patient to oxidize it, carbohydrate is of no benefit.

A common explanation for the above findings[6] is that the carbohydrate given stimulates the pancreas so as to produce more insulin. Another explanation has been offered by Soskin and coworkers[7] who, from studies of depancreatized dogs receiving a constant intravenous injection of glucose and insulin, concluded that the pancreas is not essential for the production of a normal dextrose-tolerance curve. On the other hand, the presence of a normal liver

[1] Bowman, Wortis, Orenstein and Goldfarb: Proc. Soc. Exper. Biol. and Med. **42**, 37, 1939.
[2] Gounelle, Marche and Bachet: Compt. rend. Soc. de Biol., **136**, 725, 1942.
[3] Conn: Am. Jour. Med. Sci., **199**, 555, 1940.
[4] Lennox: Jour. Biol. Chem., **73**, 237, 1927; Jour. Clin. Invest., **4**, 331, 1927.
[5] Ellis: Quart. Jour. Med., **3**, 10, 137, 1934.
[6] Sweeney: Loc. cit., p. 158. Macleod: Lancet, **2**, 512, 1930.
[7] Soskin, Allweiss and Cohn: Am. Jour. Physiol., **109**, 155, 1934. Soskin and Allweiss: Am. Jour. Physiol., **110**, 4, 1934. Soskin, Mirsky, Zimmerman and Heller: Am. Jour. Physiol., **114**, 648, 1936.

was necessary. They postulate that the normal liver, as one of its responses to administered dextrose, decreases the output of blood sugar which it has been supplying from its own stores. They maintain that the hypoglycemia which follows the cessation of prolonged sugar administration does not depend upon an increased mobilization of insulin from the pancreas, but rather represents another aspect of a homeostatic liver mechanism.

With especially prepared dogs Soskin, Essex, Herrick and Mann[1] studied by means of a thermostromuhr the rate of blood flow through the liver and the arterial and venous components of the total hepatic blood flow. They found that the administration of glucose was followed invariably by cessation of excretion of sugar by the liver and by retention of a portion of the incoming sugar. With inhibition of the output of sugar noted following the giving of doses of sugar the level of arterial blood sugar temporarily fell below original control values and remained low until resumption of secretion of sugar by the liver restored it to its previous levels.

Best and Taylor[2] and Ricketts,[3] while recognizing the significance of the experiments of Soskin and co-workers, cite as evidence of chemical control of insulin liberation through action of dextrose on the pancreas the finding that the injection of small amounts of dextrose into the artery supplying a pancreas grafted into the neck of a depancreatized dog[4] or into the pancreatic artery in a decerebrated cat[5] causes a prompt lowering of blood sugar, whereas (in the decerebrated animal) the effect was not obtained when the splenic or portal vein was used.

2. *Infections and Toxemias.*—With a diabetic an infection, even a non-febrile coryza, exerts a profound effect upon sugar tolerance. The same tendency is evident in non-diabetic individuals, who, however, have a greater ability to compensate. Hence, under no circumstances should diagnostic significance of final nature be attached to blood-sugar values unless the element of an infection is absolutely excluded at the time of the test. Therefore, it is desirable to record the body temperature of patients routinely at the beginning and end of a sugar tolerance test.

Much has been written regarding this effect of infections and toxemias on carbohydrate tolerance. Relevant papers are those of Corkill,[6] Long and Downie,[7] Schmidt, Eastland and Burns,[8]

[1] Soskin, Essex, Herrick and Mann: Am. Jour. Physiol., 124, 558, 1938.
[2] Best and Taylor: P. 578, loc. cit., p. 116.
[3] Ricketts: Jour. Clin. Invest., 17, 795, 1938.
[4] Houssay, Lewis and Foglia: Compt. rend. Soc. de biol., 100, 140, 142, 1929.
[5] LaBarre: Compt. rend. Soc. de biol., 106, 1247, 1931.
[6] Corkill: Jour. Physiol., 75, 381, 1932.
[7] Long and Downie: Med. Jour. Australia, 1, 647, 1932.
[8] Schmidt, Eastland and Burns: Arch. Int. Med., 54, 466, 1934.

Strauss,[1] Williams and Dick,[2] Brems and Nissen,[3] and Soskin and Mirsky.[4]

3. *Insulin.*—Previous insulin administration has been shown to cause a temporary loss of tolerance for carbohydrate in normal men[5] and animals.[6]

4. *Physical Inactivity.*—Blotner[7] compared the glucose tolerance of normal active adults and children with that of 86 non-diabetic patients, 70 adults and 16 children, who had been confined to bed for periods of time ranging from one month to thirteen years because of various pathologic conditions. He found the sugar tolerance diminished in those patients who had been bedfast for considerable periods. In some who later became ambulatory, the tolerance returned to normal. Although various disease conditions may in themselves lower sugar tolerance, Blotner concluded that in his studies hypertension, vascular disease, obesity and infection were not responsible for the abnormalities noted.

5. *Age.*—Spence[8] showed that sugar tolerance tends to become less as age advances. Curves were obtained on 5 men over sixty years of age; 4 of these showed a marked diminution of sugar tolerance. Included in the study of glucose tolerance by Hale-White and Payne[9] were 4 persons between the ages of fifty and seventy and 10 over seventy years of age. Of the 10 over seventy, 5 gave curves with peaks of blood sugar over 0.21 per cent. Most of the 14 cases showed some delay in returning to the fasting level.

The higher rise and slower fall in blood sugar in old age after the administration of glucose were confirmed by Marshall[10] who studied 50 men aged sixty-five to ninety-four years with an average age of seventy-two years. Of the 28 healthy subjects, only 6, or 21 per cent, showed normal ("normal adult" and "flat" types) blood sugar curves. The remaining 22 men all showed curves classified as "lag," "storage defect" and "typical diabetic;" in all but 4 of these the peak blood sugar (capillary) was 200 mg. per cent or above. Thus 18, or 64 per cent, of the 28 healthy men had a capillary blood sugar of 200 mg. per cent or higher after the giving of 50 grams of glucose. However, of especial interest was the finding that in these 18 cases, only 7 showed glycosuria during the tolerance test and in 3 of the 7 instances only traces of sugar were exhibited.

[1] Strauss: Bull. Johns Hopkins Hosp., **44**, 459, 1929.
[2] Williams and Dick: Arch. Int. Med., **50**, 801, 1932.
[3] Brems and Nissen: Ugesk. f. Laeger, **94**, 1203, 1932; Abst., Jour. Am. Med. Assn., **100**, 706, 1933.
[4] Soskin and Mirsky: Am. Jour. Physiol., **112**, 649, 1935.
[5] Wilder, Smith and Sandiford: Ann. Int. Med., **6**, 724, 1932. Blotner: Arch. Int. Med., **53**, 153, 1934. Clark, Gibson and Paul: Jour. Lab. and Clin. Med., **20**, 1008, 1935. Rosenbaum, DeKruif and Lavietes: Jour. Clin. Invest., **23**, 45, 1944.
[6] Opdyke: Proc. Soc. Exper. Biol. and Med., **55**, 119, 1944.
[7] Blotner: Arch. Int. Med., **75**, 39, 1945.
[8] Spence: Quart. Jour. Med., **14**, 314, 1921.
[9] Hale-White and Payne: Quart. Jour. Med., **19**, 393, 1926.
[10] Marshall: Quart. Jour. Med., **24**, 257, 1931.

The conclusion was reached that in healthy old age the renal threshold is generally raised and may be taken to be in the neighborhood of 200 mg. per cent. The 22 other men included in the study had various conditions such as senility, chronic bronchitis, cardiac disease, rheumatoid arthritis, carcinoma, etc. In this group the incidence of "typical diabetic" curves was 50 per cent and actually 14 of the 22 had peak capillary blood-sugar values of 200 mg. per cent or higher. Twelve of the 14 had sugar in the urine during the test; in 6 cases this amounted to only a trace.

Porter and Langley[1] studied 50 normal individuals, 10 in each of 5 decades starting with that of thirty to forty years. Using 50 grams of glucose, the following average results were obtained for the capillary blood sugar:

Age.	Before.	½ hr.	1 hr.	1½ hrs.	2 hrs.	2½ hrs.
30–40 . .	105	184	174	153	150	140
40–50 . .	120	192	207	165	155	152
50–60 . .	146	225	218	195	166	155
60–70 . .	145	225	238	245	205	185
70–80 . .	115	175	190	185	165	130

John[2] found abnormal glucose tolerance curves (venous blood samples used) in 18 per cent of 192 children (up to twenty years of age) and in 38 per cent of 1535 adults. The following summary of his results has been made to bring out the influence of age.

Age of subjects by decades:	1	2	3	4	5	6	7
Diabetic curves, per cent of total curves	8	9	9	12	22	39	51
Pre-diabetic plus diabetic curves, per cent of total curves . . .	8	13	18	23	41	51	62

John's 1727 subjects were unselected patients in varying degrees of health who were being examined in the clinic. He states that among 52 children and 337 adults with glycosuria, 33 and 37 per cent respectively showed a diabetic type of tolerance curve.

Blotner's[3] findings, previously referred to, suggest that at least part of the decreased sugar tolerance found in elderly persons may be due to relative inactivity.

6. *Race and Dietary Habits.*—A study of blood-sugar curves in 24 Jewish and 25 non-Jewish patients with no apparent glycogenic disturbance indicated that race is not a factor, even though the Jew is also endowed with a nervous or emotional temperament.[4] Apparently it may vary according to the country or rather the dietary habits of a particular country. Concepcion[5] found that in 30 Filipinos the blood sugar was 123 mg. per cent, but in American

1 Porter and Langley: Lancet, 2, 947, 1926.
2 John: Endocrinology, 18, 75, 1934.
3 Blotner: Loc. cit., p. 165.
4 Morrison and Ohler: Boston Med. and Surg. Jour., 188, 852, 1923.
5 Concepcion: Philippine Is. Med. Assn. Jour., 3, 285, 1923; Abstr. Jour. Am. Med., 82, 580, 1924.

residents of long standing in the Philippines it was 134 mg. per cent and in Europeans of long residence in Batavia it was 154 mg. per cent.

7. *Diseases and Abnormal States Other Than Diabetes.*—Conditions other than diabetes are at times accompanied by abnormal blood-sugar percentages or diminished tolerance for carbohydrate. Of these, hypertension, nephritis,[1] pregnancy, hyperthyroidism,[2] hypothyroidism, diseases of the liver, of the pituitary and of the adrenals are the most common. In 1923 Gray[3] summarized the data in the literature up to that time.

In a study of 1100 glucose-tolerance tests, John[4] found that diabetic curves were shown in 40 per cent or more of cases having the following conditions: diabetic history in the family, obesity, hyperthyroidism, acromegaly, hypertension and pregnancy. The percentage of sugar in the blood may also be increased in apoplexy, pneumonia, typhoid, tuberculosis in the presence of fever, and in some cases of cancer. A high incidence of lowered dextrose tolerance was found in chronic ulcerative colitis by Bercovitz and Page.[5]

That disturbed gastro-intestinal absorption plays an important rôle in abnormal glucose tolerance curves which may be obtained with organic or functional gastro-intestinal disorders is suggested by the findings of Goldner and Haerem.[6] These workers subjected dogs to resections of various parts of the gastro-intestinal tract and then carried out glucose tolerance tests. Following the administration of glucose intravenously, the curves were normal. Following oral administration, blood-sugar curves were abnormally high in the case of gastrectomy, high and delayed in the case of jejunectomy and normal in ileectomy.

Ohler[7] analyzed the results in 160 cases studied by means of glucose-tolerance tests and found that a very large percentage of the abnormal reactions were associated with the following pathological conditions (arranged in order of frequency): gall-bladder disease, cirrhosis of the liver, bronchial asthma, arteriosclerosis, carcinoma, obesity, endocrine disturbances, chronic nephritis, chronic arthritis.

In arthritis, Pemberton, *et al.*[8] and in cases of high blood-pressure, O'Hare[9] and John,[10] have recorded hyperglycemia, which in O'Hare's cases was at times sufficient to suggest the diagnosis of diabetes. Nissen and Spencer[11] found that 57 per cent of 222 arthritic patients

[1] Oefelin: Klin. Wchnschr., **15**, 407, 1936.
[2] John: Jour. Am. Med. Assn., **99**, 620, 1932; Jour. Clin. Endocrin., **2**, 264, 1942.
[3] Gray: Arch. Int. Med., **31**, 259, 1923.
[4] John: Endocrinology, **13**, 388, 1929.
[5] Bercovitz and Page: Ann. Int. Med., **20**, 239, 1944.
[6] Goldner and Haerem: Proc. Soc. Exper. Biol. and Med., **52**, 186, 1943.
[7] Ohler: Personal communication.
[8] Pemberton, Cajori and Crouter: Jour. Am. Med. Assn., **85**, 1793, 1925.
[9] O'Hare: Am. Jour. Med. Sci., **160**, 366, 1920.
[10] John: Ann. Clin. Med., **5**, 340, 1926.
[11] Nissen and Spencer: New England Jour. Med., **210**, 13, 1934.

showed abnormal tolerance curves. Serial tests covering one to nine years on a group of 33 patients showed, however, that even a markedly low sugar tolerance did not *per se* indicate a future diabetic. Pemberton *et al.* found that interference, through posture, with the blood flow in the limbs of normals and arthritics favored a lowered sugar tolerance. They thus explain the benefits which accrue to such patients by measures which improve the circulation.

Tyson, Otis and Joyce[1] found that of 92 epileptic patients, 56.4 per cent showed subnormal fasting blood-sugar levels as compared with only 12.5 per cent of a non-epileptic controlled group. This was true despite the fact that 85 of the epileptic patients were on phenobarbital therapy which may in itself cause a rise in the fasting blood-sugar level. Glucose tolerance tests were made on 7 epileptic patients. The authors interpret the results obtained as demonstrating a correlation between abnormal glucose tolerance and the frequency of the seizures experienced by the patient, both during the test and during the patients' institutional life. However, the seizures that occurred during the tolerance test were as likely to occur at medium as at low blood sugar values.

Shay and associates[2] carried out three-hour glucose tolerance tests in 50 patients with anacidity and 50 others with normal and hyperacidity. Forty-eight per cent of the anacid patients showed an abnormal glucose tolerance curve while only 16 per cent of the control group showed such a disturbance. They believe that the higher incidence of abnormal glucose tolerance curves in advancing years is related to the higher incidence of anacidity in those age groups.

In an analysis of 500 obese subjects Embleton[3] found abnormal glucose tolerance curves in 70 per cent of the males but in only 35 per cent of the females. This sex difference was found chiefly in the older age groups. He, unlike Ogilvie,[4] found that the percentage of abnormal glucose tolerance curves did not parallel the degree of obesity; if a patient was overweight at all, and it did not matter how much, there was the same chance of having an abnormal glucose tolerance curve. Oglivie stated that tolerance was in most cases normal in the early stages of obesity but steadily diminished after obesity had persisted for several years.

(*e*) **Galactose-tolerance Tests.**—Pollak and Selinger[5] reported that galactose-tolerance tests produced in diabetic patients a considerable increase in the dextrose content of the blood, which they took to indicate production of sugar by the liver.

On the other hand, Roe and Schwartzman[6] carried out galactose-

---

[1] Tyson, Otis and Joyce: Am. Jour. Med. Sci., **190**, 164, 1935.
[2] Shay, Gershon and Fels: Am. Jour. Dig. Dis., **5**, 4, 1938.
[3] Embleton: Brit. Med. Jour., **2**, 739, 1938.
[4] Ogilvie: Quart. Jour. Med., **4**, 345, 1935.
[5] Pollak and Selinger: Ztschr. f. klin. Med., **124**, 321, 1933.
[6] Roe and Schwartzman: Jour. Biol. Chem., **96**, 717, 1932.

tolerance tests with 10 normal and 10 diabetic subjects and found no essential difference between the response obtained with the two groups, except in the case of 3 of the diabetic subjects who showed slightly greater total blood-sugar increases following galactose ingestion, than was obtained with the normal subjects. Roe and Schwartzman conclude that diabetics have practically as good a tolerance for galactose as normal subjects and that insulin is not involved in the anabolism of galactose.

Furthermore, Kosterlitz and Wedler[1] have reported that galactose fed to diabetic patients in doses of from 10 to 20 grams, from two to four times daily, is antiketogenic, is protein-sparing and results in less glycosuria than occurs when corresponding amounts of dextrose are fed. The conclusions of Deuel, Gulick and Butts[2] are essentially the same.

9. **Extreme Hyperglycemia.**—It is remarkable that the human body can at times withstand successfully marked variations in the sugar content of the blood. The highest blood sugar value on record of a patient who recovered was that in the case of Dillon and Dyer,[3] a colored woman, aged twenty-one years, who entered the Philadelphia General Hospital in diabetic coma with a blood sugar of 1.85 per cent. Eight hundred and ten units of insulin were given during the first twenty-four hours. Dillon and Dyer report also 15 other cases from the same hospital with blood sugar values on admission of 1 per cent or more. Five of the 16 recovered. The highest percentage observed in our own series, 1.68 per cent, was in a patient with diabetic coma who survived.[4] We have had, in all, 24 cases with values of 1 per cent or above; of these 19 recovered. High blood sugar values in cases resulting fatally have been reported by others. Lawrence's[5] case had a value of 2.06 per cent, Argy's[6] 1.71 per cent, Pitfield's[7] 1.7 per cent, and Olmsted's[8] 1.4 per cent. See also page 436.

10. **Effect of Nicotine Upon the Blood Sugar.**—Lundberg and Thyselius-Lundberg[9] made detailed studies regarding the effect of tobacco-smoking on the blood sugar of both normal and diabetic individuals. By taking samples at intervals of one minute they found that immediately after the beginning of smoking the blood sugar rises sharply. The highest value obtained may be as much as 50 per cent above the initial value and is usually reached during the smoking of two cigarettes, one after the other, at an ordinary rate. The subsequent fall to normal is accomplished usually within

[1] Kosterlitz and Wedler: Klin. Wchnschr., **11**, 553, 1932.
[2] Deuel, Gulick and Butts: Jour. Biol. Chem., **98**, 333, 1932.
[3] Dillon and Dyer: Am. Jour. Med. Sci., **190**, 683, 1935.
[4] Curtis and Dixson: Jour. Am. Med. Assn., **90**, 1115, 1928.
[5] Lawrence: Brit. Med. Jour., **1**, 377, 1934.
[6] Argy: Boston Med. and Surg. Jour., **103**, 1236, 1925.
[7] Pitfield: Med. Jour. and Record, **120**, 433, 1924.
[8] Olmsted: Personal communication.
[9] Lundberg and Thyselius-Lundberg: Acta med. Scand., Suppl. 38, pp. 1–65, 1931.

one-half hour. With diabetic patients, a more marked hyper-glycemic effect is seen than in normal persons, and this is even more pronounced in diabetics who are excreting sugar and acetone. In common with other investigators, Lundberg and Thyselius-Lundberg ascribe the blood-sugar-raising effect described above to the stimulation of the suprarenal glands by the nicotine which the smoker absorbs.

The results of Haggard and Greenberg[1] agreed with those of Lundberg and Thyselius-Lundberg, except that, in as far as their tests (on normal individuals) went, they observed the hyperglycemic effect only when the blood sugar was below 0.13 per cent and the respiratory quotient below 0.85. More recently, Scheer[2] reported that smoking produced a change in the blood sugar level in 85 per cent of men. He found most curves to have a biphasic pattern. The response started usually between one and three minutes after the beginning of smoking and seldom lasted more than fifty minutes.

Contrary to the above, Dill, Edwards and Forbes[3] found that smoking one cigarette produced no change in blood sugar, lactic acid or respiratory quotient. They did find that in some individuals the metabolic rate was increased 5 to 15 per cent and suggested, there-fore, that subjects for basal metabolic rate determination not smoke on the morning of the test before it is made.

11. **Glycogen in Blood.**—The concentration of glycogen in the blood was determined by Brummer[4] in 125 individuals. In both healthy persons and in those with certain chronic diseases including diabetes, the amounts found were very small and were not increased by the administration of insulin or the ingestion of glucose. The only high values noted were in 21 patients with pneumonia; this increase was thought possibly to be due to the presence of polysac-charides of bacterial origin.

D. BLOOD LIPIDS.[5]

(SECTION ORIGINALLY PREPARED BY HAZEL HUNT, A.B.)

1. **Blood Lipids in Health.**—Blood lipids or fats include: (a) neutral fat, triglycerides of fatty acids; (b) phosphatids or phospho-lipids, a lecithin, cephalin and sphingomyelin; and (c) cholesterol. Cholesterol occurs in the blood in the free state and in ester combina-tion with fatty acids. Under normal conditions about 60 to 70 per cent of the total cholesterol of the blood is in the latter form. Average values of lipids in the blood plasma of normal individuals after a sixteen-hour fast are given in Table 23.

[1] Haggard and Greenberg: Science, **79**, 165, 1934.
[2] Scheer: Ztschr. f. d. ges. esper. Med., **113**, 356, 1943.
[3] Dill, Edwards and Forbes: Am. Jour. Physiol., **109**, 118, 1934.
[4] Brummer: Acta med. Scand., **114**, 373, 1943.
[5] See Bloor: Biochemistry of the Fatty Acids, New York, Reinhold Pub. Co., 1943, for a full discussion.

	Mg. per cent.
Total lipid	589
Neutral fat	154
Total fatty acid	353
Total cholesterol	162
Combined cholesterol	115
Free cholesterol	47
Phospholipid	196

Although cholesterol is not chemically related to the fats, it is intimately associated with them physiologically. Its level in the blood is a fairly accurate index of the level of total lipids and because of its comparative ease of determination it has been studied more than the other lipid constituents of the blood. Total cholesterol in the blood of a given individual was found to be remarkably constant by Sperry,[2] although wide variations in the cholesterol of a single individual had been reported earlier by various workers.[3,4,5] In some of these studies it is possible that the differences may have been due to hemoconcentration,[6] although the variations up to 31 per cent found by Man and Gildea[7] were not explainable on this basis.

The total cholesterol content of the plasma of normal individuals varies from 110 to 230 mg. per cent with most values in the range of 150 to 200 mg. per cent. It may be increased in uncontrolled diabetes, xanthomatosis, nephrosis, anesthesia and narcosis, myxedema, alcoholism, pregnancy and jaundice. It may be markedly decreased in anemia, tuberculosis, toxic hyperthyroidism and acute infections. Race or sex has little effect on the level of the blood lipids, except for the cyclic variation noted in women at catamenia.[8] Age has an effect on blood cholesterol chiefly in that infants up to one year of age have very low values, approximately 50 to 70 per cent of adult values. The level gradually rises after the first year to the normal adult value. In 4 of our newborn babies of diabetic mothers the cord blood cholesterol has ranged from 50 to 65 mg. per cent. Gordon and Cohn[9] reported a value of 89 mg. per cent in cord blood.

The mere addition of an unusually large amount of fat to an otherwise normal diet does not necessarily cause hyperlipemia, except immediately after a meal. Fat is delivered to the blood mainly by way of the chyle as a suspension of fine droplets of what is largely pure fat. Reports are variable but it is doubtful that a

[1] Boyd: Jour. Biol. Chem., **101**, 323, 1933.
[2] Sperry: Jour. Biol. Chem., **117**, 391, 1937.
[3] Bruger and Somach: Jour. Biol. Chem., **97**, 23, 1932.
[4] Bruger and Poindexter: Jour. Biol. Chem., **101**, 21, 1933.
[5] McEachern and Gilmour: Canad. Med. Assn. Jour., **26**, 30, 1932.
[6] Man and Peters: Jour. Clin. Invest., **13**, 237, 1934.
[7] Man and Gildea: Jour. Biol. Chem., **119**, 769, 1937.
[8] Okey and Boyden: Jour. Biol. Chem., **72**, 261, 1927.
[9] Gordon and Cohn: Am. Jour. Dis. Child., **35**, 193, 1928.

characteristic increase in blood cholesterol occurs after fat feeding.[1] The greatest degree of hyperlipemia occurs in persons with a tendency to ketosis.[2,3,4,5] Campbell[6] has suggested that durable increases of blood fat result not when more fat enters the body to be burned or conveyed to storage centers, but when there is a continuously greater demand for fat as fuel, because of the absence of available carbohydrate. The liver takes an active part in fat transport as well as acting as a place for temporary storage.

One to three hours after a fat meal the blood fat rises distinctly, usually reaching a peak at the end of six or seven hours. In patients with diabetes the blood fat curves may be somewhat prolonged. Fat tolerance tests have been suggested as having importance in determining the nutritional state of the diabetic patient; the blood fat curves of the obese patient with and without insulin following a fat meal are reported to differ from corresponding curves of the normal individual.[7] The increase in concentration of fat in the blood may become so extreme that the serum or plasma becomes visibly milky and fat separates out. Such alimentary hyperlipemia is a transient condition and disappears very rapidly. The visibility of lipoids in the serum is not entirely dependent upon their concentration but also upon their physical state.

2. **Blood Lipids in Diabetes.**—In our experience today the blood lipids of the well controlled diabetic are, in general, normal. With the better control which has been possible since the introduction of protamine zinc insulin, abnormal values have become relatively infrequent so that in the last few years estimations of blood cholesterol have seemed worthwhile only in especially selected cases. How different is this picture than formerly when, in the pre- or early-insulin days, values near or well above 300 mg. per cent were commonly encountered (see Table 24).

TABLE 24.—TRENDS IN CHOLESTEROL VALUES IN AUTHORS' DIABETIC PATIENTS.

Year.	Investigator.	Analyses.	Cases.	Cholesterol, mg. per cent (avg. values).
1916	Bloor	36	Adults	360
1917	Bloor and Gray	131	Adults	385
1924	Gray	1062	Adults and children	290
1927	Hunt	335	Adults and children	257
1930	Hunt and White	110	Children	211
1932–1939	Hunt	5496	Children and adults	214

The accompanying table gives an incorrect picture of cholesterol values for the years since 1927 in that the average figures listed were, no doubt, actually well above the true averages for all patients,

[1] Oppenheim and Bruger: Am. Jour. Med. Sci., **205**, 77, 1943.
[2] Bloor: Jour. Biol. Chem., **49**, 201, 1921.
[3] Blix: Acta med. Scandinav., **64**, 142, 1926.
[4] Lieb and Tolstoi: Proc. Soc. Exp. Biol. and Med., **26**, 324, 1929.
[5] Fenz: Klin. Wchnschr., **15**, 46, 1936.
[6] Campbell: Quart. Jour. Med., **18**, 393, 1925.
[7] Blotner: Medical Papers dedicated to Henry A. Christian, Baltimore, Waverly Press, Inc., p. 450, 1936.

because for some years we have selected for cholesterol determinations only those patients in whom we suspected the values might be abnormal.

Disordered fat metabolism was first associated with diabetes when phlebotomy disclosed a creaminess of the blood of diabetic patients. Severe diabetes was, and is, the only disease in which lipemia is frequent enough to be of special significance. The percentage of fat found in such lipemic bloods may be extreme. Frugoni and Marchette[1] reported 27 per cent and Klemperer[2] found 26 per cent; figures of 15 to 24 per cent were not unusual. Among our cases the highest value was 19.9 per cent found in Case 9629, a patient in diabetic coma in 1930.

The origin of the fat in diabetic lipemia appears to be mainly the fat of the food. Although an increase in the blood lipids as a result of the ingestion of fat has been repeatedly demonstrated,[3,4,5,6,7] visible lipemia does not normally appear in the postabsorptive period, even though large amounts of lipid material may be present in the blood. Bloor obtained a value of 4.35 per cent total lipid in Case 310 with clear plasma. Such cases of "masked lipemia" have been frequently observed. The "masking may be an unstable condition, since on standing for a time, twenty-four to forty-eight hours, milkiness may develop in a plasma which was clear when drawn." This is due probably to a change only in the physical condition of the fat present. Milkiness may develop, upon standing, in plasmas which do not contain an excess of lipid material. Of the 5 per cent of our cases in whom visible lipemia was shown when the blood was first drawn it is striking to note that the cholesterol values varied from 75 mg. per cent to 1600 mg. per cent.

3. **High Values in Diabetes.**—Of 2200 selected diabetics whose blood was studied for cholesterol content during 1935–1939, there were only 93 whose values exceeded 400 mg. per cent, and of these, in 68 cases the cholesterol was high, wholly apart from coma or acidosis.

An extremely high cholesterol, when it occurs during coma, does not carry any worse prognosis than holds for all cases of coma.

Diabetic patients who show a cholesterol above 400 mg. not associated with coma, however, present a problem which is of graver import than similar cases in coma, perhaps because they represent a permanent rather than transient state of high blood fat. Of the 68 cases mentioned there were 22 instances with diabetes beginning in childhood, and only 1 of 13 cases studied carefully

---

[1] Frugoni and Marchette: Berl. klin. Wchnschr., **45**, 1844, 1908.
[2] Klemperer: Deutsch. med. Wchnschr., **36**, 2373, 1910.
[3] Bloor: Jour. Biol. Chem., **24**, 447, 1916.
[4] Hiller, Linder, Lundsgaard and Van Slyke: Jour. Exp. Med., **39**, 931, 1924.
[5] Hejda: Am. Jour. Med. Sci., **180**, 84, 1930.
[6] McClure and Huntsinger: Jour. Biol. Chem., **76**, 1, 1928.
[7] Man and Gildea: Jour. Biol. Chem., **99**, 61, 1932.

failed to exhibit some serious complication of diabetes, such as cataracts, arteriosclerosis, retinitis, abscess or lipemia retinalis. The diabetes in these children was uncontrolled and these complications demonstrate what is likely to happen to the carelessly treated diabetic. Seventeen of the 22 patients were girls.

There were 3 adolescents with high cholesterols above 400 mg. per cent. One of these died of lipoid nephrosis, another has xanthoma, and the third (6593) appeared in good condition but his cholesterol was high, 325 mg. per cent in November, 1934; he was reported alive in February 1946 although he had developed tuberculosis in 1942.

Forty-three adults had cholesterol values apart from coma which were above 400 mg. per 100 cc. of blood. Among these the complications have been as follows: arteriosclerosis, retinitis or cataracts, xanthoma, and a variety of other conditions, such as gangrene, carbuncles, jaundice and gall stones. In other words, for practical purposes a cholesterol consistently above 400 mg. per cent in a diabetic implies that serious complications exist or are imminent.

4. **Low Values in Diabetes.**—Strange to say, the low cholesterol, apart from those in patients under one year of age, is the serious cholesterol. Patients with values of 90 mg. per 100 cc. of blood or under have shown the shortest duration of life after the test and the highest mortality. There were but 25 among 2200 diabetics in this group with so low a cholesterol. This means much, because during the entire life of the investigations, 1926 to December, 1939, probably 14,000 diabetics were under observation, and the 2200 cases whose blood was examined for cholesterol were selected from this number because they appeared unusual. Therefore, a cholesterol under 90 mg. per cent in a diabetic is a rare finding.

Approximately 40 per cent of the patients with cholesterol of 90 mg. per cent or below died on the average within five weeks after the test was done. Five of the 25 patients had tuberculosis also, 5 had severe sepsis, 3 had pernicious anemia, 2 had endocrine disturbances, pituitary in character, 1 had hemochromatosis, 1 a calcified pancreas, and 1 had cirrhosis of the liver. Among the 12 others were included 2 with tuberculosis, 1 with pernicious anemia, 3 with other endocrine disorders, and 3 cases of severe juvenile diabetes. Without diabetes a low-cholesterol content of the blood could occur with most of these conditions, particularly tuberculosis or sepsis. Nevertheless, pernicious anemia, endocrine disturbances, and a calcified pancreas are neighborhood diseases to diabetes, and one knows that tuberculosis and sepsis thrive in diabetes. Although it is likely that the low cholesterol in diabetic patients with such diseases is associated with the response of the body to the complications rather than to diabetes itself, the rôle of the latter is difficult to assay.

5. **Acidosis and Blood Fat.**—The influence of acidosis upon blood lipids deserves attention, because it is from abnormalities in the fat metabolism that so great a percentage of our patients formerly died. In 75 per cent of the first 1000 cases seen in this practice, an increase of body fat preceded the onset of diabetes, and in 61 per cent of the earliest cases abnormal fat metabolism resulting in acidosis caused death. Of 137 coma cases whose blood lipids were studied at the New England Deaconess Hospital from 1926 to December, 1939, only 24 showed a marked increase of blood cholesterol. The highest blood lipid value we have ever found in coma was in Case 9629 whose total lipid was 19.9 per cent and whose cholesterol was 1.42 per cent. This patient did not recover.

Acidosis and coma are not always associated with high blood lipid values. In our series 50 per cent of the coma cases had cholesterol values which were normal or only slightly above normal at the height of the acidosis. Only 5 per cent of the cases had markedly elevated cholesterol values which did not return promptly to normal with therapy.

The height of the cholesterol does not seem to be dependent upon the severity of the acidosis. Thus in 5 cases of coma in which the plasma CO_2 was 2 volumes per cent, the cholesterol values ranged from 200 to 425 mg. per cent, with an average of 321 mg. per cent, whereas in 14 cases of coma in which the CO_2 values averaged 19 volumes per cent the cholesterol range was 147 to 658 and the average 311 mg. per cent. Man and Peters[1] found that the concentration of cholesterol in their 15 coma cases when corrected for hemoconcentration was seldom above the normal limit at the height of acidosis and was often below these limits at the end of the recovery period.

6. **Blood Sugar and Blood Fat.**—There is no close parallelism between blood sugar and blood cholesterol values. Especially is this true in extreme cases. Case 12383 with a blood cholesterol of 1600 mg. per cent and lipemia retinalis had a blood sugar of 0.21 per cent, whereas the 2 patients who have had the highest blood sugar of our group, Case 4099 and Case 6884, with blood-sugar values of 1600 and 1580 mg. per cent, respectively, had cholesterol values of 370 and 348 mg. per cent. Both of these patients recovered. Case 4099 lived six years and Case 6884 nine years after this attack of coma (see pages 394, 545 and 573). In a group of 43 cases with abnormally high blood cholesterol, the average value for the cholesterol was 557 mg. per cent, but the average blood sugar was only 0.24 per cent.

7. **Insulin and Blood Fat.**—Insulin has made the diabetic so nearly a normal individual from a metabolic point of view that today we do not see many patients who show gross abnormalities of fat metabolism. By administration of insulin, hyperlipemia in

[1] Mann and Peters: Loc. cit., p. 171.

diabetes can be reduced with great rapidity. In the case reported by Rabinowitch,[1] extreme lipemia was eliminated in the course of a few hours by intensive insulin therapy (a pound of fat overnight and a pound the next day). Similar rapid, although not as striking, decreases in total blood fat occurred in our Cases 9629, 12383 and 12384. In insulin-sensitive cases blood cholesterol values are reduced very promptly by insulin therapy. If insulin is omitted the hypercholesteremia returns.

The studies of Nitzescu et al.[2] indicated that insulin, which, except in large doses,[3] does not affect the cholesterol content of normal blood, reduces the hypercholesterolemia of both experimental and clinical diabetes. Bruger and Mosenthal[4] found, however, that single doses of insulin produced no significant change in plasma cholesterol of diabetics. It is our experience that it is usually the uncontrolled diabetic who has the high blood cholesterol and that normal cholesterol values are associated with well-controlled diabetes regardless of the dosage of insulin required to keep the diabetes controlled. However, Case 6767, a juvenile with onset of diabetes in May 1925, showed a high blood-cholesterol value over a period of three years when her daily insulin dosage averaged 30 units. When her carbohydrate was raised and her daily insulin dosage was increased to 70 units, her blood cholesterol promptly dropped to a level of approximately 170 mg. per cent. She was well in December 1944 except that she had areas of necrobiosis lipoidica diabeticorum over both shins. On the other hand, Case 12383, who came to us with lipemia retinalis, and whose blood cholesterol was 1600 mg. per cent, showed a spectacular drop to 175 mg. per cent in two months with no increase in insulin dosage.

8. **Diet and Blood Cholesterol.**—The diet of diabetics has altered greatly in the past twenty-five years. As the carbohydrate of the diet has risen and the amount of fat fallen, the average cholesterol value of our patients has dropped. Although there is evidence to suggest that higher carbohydrate, lower fat diets in themselves favor lower blood cholesterol values,[5] the relationship is probably more chronological than causal and the fall in average cholesterol values is most likely due chiefly to better general control of diabetes with insulin.

The experience of Curtis, Sheldon and Eckstein[6] and of Freyberg, Newburgh and Murrill[7] suggests that when carbohydrate

[1] Rabinowitch: Am. Jour. Med. Sci., **176**, 489, 1928.

[2] Nitzescu, Popsecu-Inotesti and Cadarin: Compt. rend. Soc. de biol., **90**, 538, 1924.

[3] Lewin: Ztschr. ges. exp. Med., **96**, 532, 1935.

[4] Bruger and Mosenthal: Jour. Clin. Invest., **13**, 399, 1934.

[5] Geyelin: Jour. Am. Med. Assn., **104**, 1203, 1935.

[6] Curtis, Sheldon and Eckstein: Am. Jour. Med. Sci., **186**, 548, 1933.

[7] Freyberg, Newburgh and Murrill: Arch. Int. Med., **58**, 589, 1936

metabolism is controlled with insulin, high-fat diets may be borne without increase in blood lipids.

9. Prognosis and Blood Cholesterol.—In the past a bad prognosis has always been associated with abnormally high blood lipids. Actually one needs be just as much concerned over the low cholesterol as the high cholesterol, since the former usually indicates serious disease apart from diabetes. Patients with values of 90 mg. per 100 c. of blood or under have shown the shortest duration of life after the test and the highest mortality. Blood cholesterol values above 400 mg. per cent do not necessarily present a grave prognosis as to life, but the prognosis for, and as the result of, complications may be grave.

The blood cholesterol, whose response to insulin is not so prompt or so spectacular as the blood sugar, is in some respects, a more reliable index of the fundamental clinical condition than is the blood sugar, which reflects a temporary state. Particularly is this true if one is dealing with single, isolated values. Normal blood-cholesterol values are as important in diabetics, particularly juvenile diabetics, as are satisfactory blood sugar values. Glycosuria and hyperglycemia, which respond so promptly to insulin therapy, do not always suggest the gravity of an uncontrolled diabetic condition, whereas a high blood cholesterol is, in general, reliable evidence that the disease is uncontrolled. Fortunately, with the better control of diabetes made possible by the slowly acting insulins, definitely abnormal blood cholesterol values have become relatively uncommon.

12

CHAPTER V.

ALLOXAN DIABETES.

By C. Cabell Bailey, M.D.

A. Introduction.—*The discovery by Dunn that a chemical could cause the destruction of the islands of Langerhans was so unexpected and so startling, and introduced such a new element into the etiology of diabetes that the authors believe readers will welcome its presentation as a separate entity in detail, rather than its inclusion in the chapter of Physiology. It is particularly appropriate that this summary be made by our colleague, Dr. C. Cabell Bailey, because it was he who concurrently with the Chicago group first demonstrated that alloxan would produce permanent diabetes.*

History.—The injection of alloxan into rabbits,[1] rats,[2] dogs,[3] monkeys,[4] pigeons,[5] or turtles[6] is followed in twenty-four hours by the development of diabetes mellitus. Thus, three methods are now available for the production of experimental diabetes in animals:

(1) By the removal of the pancreas, first described by von Mering and Minkowski in 1889; (2) by the repeated injection of anterior pituitary extract, finally accomplished by Young in 1937 but based on the work of Houssay, Evans, and others; and, (3) by the injection of the chemical alloxan.

In 1937 Jacobs[7] found that alloxan injected intravenously into fasted rabbits in doses greater than 70 mg. per kg. produces a transitory hyperglycemia followed in three to four hours by hypoglycemia and convulsions. The hypoglycemia was relieved with glucose but recurred at intervals of two to three hours. No histological sections were reported.

Widespread interest in alloxan developed when Dunn, Sheehan, and McLetchie,[8] apparently unaware of Jacobs' work, injected alloxan intravenously into rabbits in attempting to elucidate the pathogenesis of the renal lesion of the crush syndrome and reported that the animals died during the first day or so with "distinctive symptoms which were not related to renal disease." On histological examination they discovered a selective necrosis of the islets of

---

[1] Bailey and Bailey: Jour. Am. Med. Assn., **122**, 1165, 1943.
[2] Dunn and McLetchie: Lancet, **2**, 384, 1943.
[3] Goldner and Gomori: Endocrinology, **33**, 297, 1943.
[4] Banerjee: Lancet, **2**, 658, 1944.
[5] Goldner and Gomori: Proc. Soc. Exp. Biol. and Med., **58**, 31, 1945.
[6] Garcia Ramos: Revista de la Sociedad Mexicana de Historia Natural, **5**, 25, 1944.
[7] Jacobs: Proc. Soc. Exper. Biol. and Med., **37**, 407, 1937.
[8] Dunn, Sheehan, and McLetchie: Lancet, **1**, 484, 1943.

(178)

Langerhans. The same lesion was detected in the albino rat injected subcutaneously with similar doses.

In a letter to the Journal of the American Medical Association, Brunschwig, Allen, Goldner, and Gomori[1] reported that they had observed rabbits "which survived injections of alloxan and exhibited only transitory hyperglycemia." In five dogs they reported "hyperglycemia sustained for two to three weeks."

Permanent diabetes produced with alloxan was reported by Bailey and Bailey[2] in rabbits and soon afterwards by Dunn and McLetchie[3] in rats and by Goldner and Gomori[4] in dogs.

Animals Sensitive to Alloxan.—In addition to the rabbit, rat, and dog, Banerjee[5] has shown that three of six monkeys developed diabetes when given 300 mg. of alloxan per kilogram. The pigeon, as reported by Goldner and Gomori,[6,7,8] not only develops diabetes but also a profound disturbance in uric acid metabolism with the development of visceral gout. The cat and guinea pig although reported "sensitive in various degrees" to alloxan parenterally do not develop diabetes. Recently, however, Ruben and Yardumian[9] produced diabetes in cats by feeding 0.5 to 1 gram per kg. of alloxan mixed with food. In the duck, according to Mirsky,[10] the islets are destroyed but diabetes does not develop. Owls and chickens likewise fail to develop diabetes when given alloxan.[11]

Dosage.—For intravenous or subcutaneous injections, a 5 per cent solution of alloxan is satisfactory. Although a water solution has been used,[2,4] when large quantities are injected intravenously, a saline solution is preferable to avoid hemolysis.

The optimum diabetogenic dose varies with the animal. With rabbits, 150 to 200 mg. per kilogram of alloxan is effective whereas doses as small as 100 mg. per kilogram usually produce diabetes.[12]

In dogs, a dose of 50 to 75 mg. per kilogram produces typical diabetes without renal lesions,[4] whereas a larger amount produces a diabetic-uremic syndrome from which the animals die. Doses of 25 mg. per kilogram are ineffective.

Rats usually develop diabetes with the subcutaneous injection of

[1] Brunschwig, Allen, Goldner, and Gomori: Jour. Am. Med. Assn., 122, 966, 1943.
[2] Bailey and Bailey: Loc. cit., p. 178.
[3] Dunn and McLetchie: Loc. cit., p. 178.
[4] Goldner and Gomori: Loc. cit., p. 178, ref. 3.
[5] Banerjee: Loc. cit., p. 178.
[6] Goldner and Gomori: Loc. cit., p. 178, ref. 5.
[7] Goldner: Bull. New York Acad. Med., 21, 44, 1945.
[8] Goldner and Gomori: Proc. Am. Diab. Assn., 4, 89, 1944.
[9] Ruben and Yardumian: Science, 103, 221, 1946; Am. Jour. Clin. Path., 15, 230, 1945.
[10] Mirsky: Proc. Soc. Exp. Biol. and Med., 59, 35, 1945.
[11] Scott, Harris and Chen: Endocrinology, 37, 201, 1945.
[12] Leech and Bailey: Jour. Biol. Chem., 157, 525, 1945.

150 to 200 mg. per kilogram of alloxan[1] although some workers[2] prefer the same dose intraperitoneally. Dunn and McLetchie[3] used doses of 300 to 400 mg. per kilogram subcutaneously or intramuscularly. Turtles given 400 mg. per kilogram intrapulmonarily develop diabetes.[4]

Monkeys develop diabetes with the intravenous injection of 300 mg. of alloxan per kilogram,[5] whereas pigeons need only 125 to 200 mg. per kilogram intravenously.[6]

Kass and Waisbren[7] have shown that rats starved for forty-eight to sixty hours are more susceptible to the diabetogenic action of alloxan than non-fasted animals.

Use of Alloxan in Man.—Human subjects were first given alloxan by Brunschwig, Allen, Owens, and Thornton,[8,9] who administered it to patients with carcinomata. The first was a case of islet cell carcinoma of the pancreas with metastasis to the liver, who had previously had a subtotal pancreatectomy. He received several series of alloxan injections with individual doses varying from 25 to 350 mg. per kilogram. After each series of treatment, the attacks subsided for several days and, on one occasion, twenty-one days passed without a hypoglycemic reaction. The patient finally died from "a complication at laparotomy" but histologic sections of the malignant nodules in the liver and of the pancreas revealed no evidence of necrosis that could be attributed to the alloxan. It must be remembered, however, that death occurred twenty-two days after the last injection of alloxan and earlier changes might not be apparent. On three occasions reactions to the intravenous injections of alloxan occurred consisting of *chills, nausea, vomiting, anemia, icterus* and in one instance, *coma.*

Four other patients with carcinomatosis of other types were likewise injected with alloxan by Brunschwig *et al.* In two of these, no effect was noticed, while the third developed a chill, nausea, and cyanosis for several hours. No significant blood sugar change occurred. The fourth patient died six hours after termination of the injection of 600 mg. per kilogram in 1200 cc. of saline. The blood sugar fell to 16 mg. per cent, and there was improvement after 50 per cent dextrose was administered intravenously. He died suddenly, however, a few hours later. Microscopic study of the pancreas revealed "questionable evidence of injury to a number of cells in some of the islets, although many islets were not affected." The liver showed rather diffuse degenerative changes in the hepatic cells. The adrenals were normal. Degenerative changes were

[1] Bailey, Bailey and Leech: New England Jour. Med., **230**, 533, 1944.
[2] Gomori and Goldner: Proc. Exp. Biol. and Med., **54**, 287, 1943.
[3] Dunn and McLetchie: Loc. cit., p. 178.
[4] Garcia Ramos: Rev. de la Soc. Mex. de Hist. Nat., **5**, 25, 1944.
[5] Banerjee: Loc. cit., p. 178.
[6] Goldner: Loc. cit., p. 179.
[7] Kass and Waisbren: Proc. Soc. Exp. Biol. and Med., **60**, 303, 1945.
[8] Brunschwig, Allen, Owens and Thornton: Jour. Am. Med. Assn., **124**, 212, 1944.
[9] Brunschwig and Allen: Cancer Research, **4**, 45, 1944.

noted in the renal tubules which the authors hesitated to attribute to alloxan in view of chronic progressive deterioration of the patient from the carcinoma.

Recently a nine-month-old girl with hypoglycemia apparently due to hyperinsulinism was admitted to the Children's Medical Service of the Massachusetts General Hospital.[1] This case is reported through the courtesy of that service. At laparotomy no adenoma of the pancreas could be found and it was decided not to perform a subtotal pancreatectomy. Fasting blood-sugar values were below 30 mg. per cent and frequent hypoglycemic convulsions occurred.

In such an extreme case, it was felt justifiable to try alloxan. Daily injections starting with 20 mg. per kilogram were begun, and the dose slowly increased to 100 mg. per kilogram for a period of seven days. The fasting blood sugar steadily rose to normal and the tendency to hypoglycemia disappeared.

After three weeks without symptoms, the blood sugar gradually decreased to 50 mg. per cent and one hypoglycemic attack occurred. Accordingly, a second series of 8 injections of 100 mg. per kilogram of alloxan was administered. The symptoms again promptly disappeared and the child has remained symptom-free, with a normal blood sugar to the present time—eight months later.

In view of the known tendency for occasional spontaneous remissions in cases of hyperinsulinism, one must be cautious in attributing the benefit in this case to alloxan; nevertheless, the improvement with its use was very striking.

Certainly the routine use of alloxan in cases of hyperinsulinism is to be condemned both because of the dangerous toxic effect of the drug and because its use may allow time for malignant changes to develop in an otherwise removable islet cell adenoma.

B. Chemistry. — Alloxan is the ureide of mesoxalic acid with the structural formula

$$
\begin{array}{cc}
\text{HN} & \text{CO} \\
| & | \\
\text{OC} & \text{CO} \\
| & | \\
\text{HN} & \text{CO}
\end{array}
$$

It can be produced by oxidation of uric acid or from barbituric acid and is a colorless powder easily soluble in water or alcohol. In solution, it is distinctly acid and cannot be neutralized without inactivation. Neutralized alloxan or alloxan dissolved in either rabbit or human blood plasma is not diabetogenic when injected into rabbits.[2] Chemically, it is a very reactive substance with ability to act either as a strong oxidizing or as a strong reducing agent. Acting as an oxidizing agent it is itself reduced to dialuric acid whereas acting as a reducing agent, it is oxidized to parabanic acid. Despite its structural similarity to uric acid, alloxan has not

[1] Dr. Nathan Talbot gave permission to report this case.
[2] Leech and Bailey: Loc. cit., p. 179.

been found in the human body,[1] although Tipson and Ruben[2,3] using their pyrrole test and "purple" test state that their results suggest that alloxan may be a normal constituent of certain human and animal tissues.

Archibald[4] suggests that when alloxan is injected into circulating blood that it is rapidly converted "(a) to alloxanic acid by the alkali, (b) to alloxantin, thence to dialuric acid by the thiol groups of plasma proteins, circulating cysteine and any small amounts of glutathione which may be present in plasma; a slower reaction with the NH_2 groups of circulating amino acids with formation of dialuric acid (or alloxantin or purpuric acid) would be anticipated, (c) part, (although a small part) of the alloxan probably combines with urea." He further states that "the possibility that circulating blood normally contains small amounts of alloxan should not be over-looked, especially in view of the report by Ascoli and Izar and Preti that dog liver or blood contains an enzyme system capable of splitting uric acid to dialuric acid in the presence of oxygen and of synthesizing uric acid from dialuric acid in the absence of oxygen." "If dialuric acid is formed in blood, it would not be surprising if minute amounts of alloxan were formed by action of molecular oxygen carried by the hemoglobin." He described six methods for the determination of alloxan.

Leech and Bailey,[5] using their method for the determination of blood alloxan, showed that alloxan reaches its highest concentration in the blood at the end of the injection and rapidly decreases during the next five minutes. Using a modification of this method, alloxan was detected also in the pancreas in quantities of 24 to 56 mg. per cent at the end of the injection. Following the injection of alloxan there is a sudden and profound reduction in the blood reduced glutathione suggesting an interaction of these two substances. The injection of the molecular equivalents of reduced glutathione immediately before and during the time alloxan is injected does not prevent the diabetogenic action of alloxan upon the pancreas. However, Lazarow[6] demonstrated that the intravenous injection of much larger doses of glutathione (2500 mg./kg.) or of cysteine (912 mg./kg.) immediately before the injection of alloxan protects the rat from the diabetogenic action of alloxan. The injection of these compounds one minute after alloxan affords only partial protection, whereas their injection three or more minutes after alloxan does not prevent diabetes. Labes and Freisburger[7] had previously shown that alloxan has an especial affinity for the sulf-hydryl (S-H) group.

[1] Karrer, Koller and Sturzinger: Helvet. chim. acta, 28, 1529, 1945.
[2] Tipson and Ruben: Arch. Biochem., 8, 1, 1945.
[3] Ruben and Tipson: Science, 101, 536, 1945; Ibid., 103, 634, 1946.
[4] Archibald: Jour. Biol. Chem., 158, 347, 1945.
[5] Leech and Bailey: Loc. cit., p. 179.
[6] Lazarow: Proc. Soc. Exper. Biol. and Med., 61, 441, 1946.
[7] Labes and Freisburger: Arch. exp. Path. u. Pharmakol, 156, 226, 1930.

Banerjee, Dittmer, and duVigneaud,[1] using a microbiological and a fluorometric test which involves the conversion of alloxan to riboflavin, detected quantities of alloxan as small as 0.05 to 0.4 mg. but thus far this method has not been applied to blood or biological extracts.

Weinglass, Frame and Williams[2] found that the injection of either 3, 4 diaminotoluene, orthophenylenediamine or sodium bisulfite in large amounts into a rabbit within five minutes before the injection of alloxan chemically neutralized the alloxan and prevented its action upon the pancreas. The injection of adrenalin[3] (1 : 1000) intraperitoneally in a 0.1 cc. dose immediately before the injection of alloxan has also been shown to prevent the diabetogenic effect of alloxan in rats.

Lehmann[4] has shown that alloxan inhibits the formation of the Robison and Cori esters.

Price, Cori and Colowick[5] have recently reported that tissue extracts from rats made diabetic with alloxan or with anterior pituitary extract show an inhibition of hexokinase, the enzyme needed in the reaction glucose + adenosine triphosphate = glucose-6-phosphate + adenosine diphosphate. Insulin *in vivo* or *in vitro* releases this inhibition. Later Price, Slein, Colowick and Cori[6] showed that whereas adrenal cortical extracts have no effect upon hexokinase in muscle extracts from normal rats, it greatly intensifies the inhibitory effect in muscle extracts from diabetic rats.

Specificity of Alloxan.—Until recently many substances with structural formulas similar to alloxan have failed to produce diabetes when injected into animals. However, Koref *et al.*[7] have produced diabetes with the injection of alloxantin into rabbits and this has been confirmed.[8] They overcame its low solubility by injecting solutions at 50° C.

Bruchmann and Wertheimer[9] report that besides alloxan, methyl alloxan,[10] alloxantin, dimethyl alloxantin, methyl dialuric acid and dialuric acid will produce diabetes in rats if injected intravenously. Bailey, Bailey and Leech[11] also have demonstrated the diabetogenic action of dialuric acid.

Styrl Quinolin No. 90 was earlier reported[12] to destroy the islets of Langerhans but diabetes thus far has not been produced with this chemical.

[1] Banerjee, Dittmer and duVigneaud: Science, **101**, 647, 1945.
[2] Weinglass, Frame and Williams: Proc. Soc. Exp. Biol. and Med., **58**, 216, 1945.
[3] Kass and Waisbren: Loc. cit., p. 180.
[4] Lehmann: Biochem. Jour., **33**, 1241, 1939.
[5] Price, Cori and Colowick: Loc. cit., p. 115.
[6] Price, Slein, Colowick and Cori: Loc. cit., p. 116.
[7] Koref, Vargos, Rodriguez and Telchi: Endocrinology, **35**, 391, 1944.
[8] Bailey, Bailey and Leech: Bull. New England Med. Center, **7**, 59, 1945
[9] Bruchmann and Wertheimer: Nature, London, **155**, 267, 1945.
[10] Also reported by Hidy: Jour. Biol. Chem., **163**, 307, 1946.
[11] Bailey, Bailey and Leech: To be reported.
[12] Dunn, Sheehan and McLetchie: Loc. cit., p. 178.

Goldner and Gomori[1] injected several ureides including violuric acid, barbituric acid, dialuric acid, alloxantin, N dodecyl-barbituric acid; several oxidizing substances including sodium nitro-ferricyanide, sodium molybdate, ceric acid, quinine, persulfate and two quinoline substances, quinoline and cinchophen, none of which produced diabetes.

Jacobs,[2] before the discovery of alloxan diabetes, discovered that rabbits injected with alloxan developed a transitory hyperglycemia and then a fatal hypoglycemia. He was unable to detect a similar effect, however, when he gave alloxanic acid, dialuric acid, isodialuric acid, barbituric acid, isobarbituric acid, alloxantin, murexide, mesoxalic acid, parabanic acid, oxaluric acid, formyloxaluric acid or formylurea. Kennedy and Lukens[3] injected nitrates, methylene blue and sodium tartrate but none produced diabetes. Dunn *et al.*[4] reported negative results with oxalic acid, uranium, guanidin and uric acid. Bailey, Bailey and Leech,[5] in addition to several chemicals listed above, found no diabetogenic effect from ninhydrin, alloxan-6-phenylhydrazone-p sodium sulfonate, cytosine, isocytosine, glyoxal or styryl quinoline.

C. Mode of Action.—The triphasic blood sugar curve consisting of initial transitory hyperglycemia lasting fifteen minutes to one hour in rabbits, followed by profound hypoglycemia within two to eight hours after injection and finally permanent hyperglycemia in twenty-four to thirty-six hours has provoked considerable interest and discussion.

Dunn, Sheehan and McLetchie[6] suggest that the first phase may be due either to excessive mobilization of glucose through the adrenosympathetic system or to diminished combustion due to lack of insulin and the second or hypoglycemic phase due to overstimulation of the islets of Langerhans. Bailey and Bailey[7] suggested that the initial hyperglycemia was a non-specific effect and that the hypoglycemic phase might be due to the escape of a large amount of insulin from necrosis of many of the islets.

The initial hyperglycemia and subsequent hypoglycemia were closely duplicated by Hughes, Ware and Young[8] when they injected into a normal rabbit adrenalin and 10 units of protamine zinc insulin, the amount of insulin estimated that might be extracted from the pancreas of a 1 kg. normal rabbit. Corkill *et al.*[9] found that ergotoxine, which blocks sympathetic nerve action, abolishes the initial hyperglycemic phase in rabbits injected with alloxan.

[1] Goldner and Gomori: Loc. cit., p. 179, ref. 8.
[2] Jacobs: Loc. cit., p. 178.
[3] Kennedy and Lukens: Proc. Soc. Exp. Biol. and Med., **57**, 143, 1944.
[4] Dunn, Kirkpatrick, McLetchie and Telfer: Jour. Path. and Bact., **55**, 245, 1943.
[5] Bailey, Bailey and Leech: Unpublished data.
[6] Dunn, Sheehan and McLetchie: Loc. cit., p. 178.
[7] Bailey and Bailey: Loc. cit., p. 178.
[8] Hughes, Ware and Young: Lancet, **1**, 148, 1944.
[9] Corkill, Fantl and Nelson: Med. Jour. Australia, **31**, 285, 1944.

· Goldner and Gomori[1] showed that adrenalectomized rabbits or rabbits with their adrenal medullæ destroyed with formalin did not show an initial transitory hyperglycemia when given alloxan. Hence, they attributed this phase to adrenalin secretion. Further, the administration of alloxan to depancreatized dogs and to rabbits previously rendered diabetic with alloxan failed to lower the blood sugar in either which supported the theory that insulin released from necrosed islet cells was responsible for this phase. Kennedy and Lukens[2] obtained similar results by reinjecting rabbits previously made diabetic with alloxan, and Foglia[3] *et al.* by reinjecting rats. Goldner and Gomori[4] further showed that the initial hyperglycemia could be prevented with insulin and the subsequent hypoglycemia with glucose yet islet necrosis occurred and diabetes developed. If this hypothesis is correct, bio-assay of the insulin content of the pancreas at repeated intervals following the injection of alloxan should reveal a steady decline. This was precisely the observation of Ridout, Ham and Wrenshall[5] in rats and dogs, and of Goldner and Gomori[6] in dogs.

The speed with which alloxan acts was shown by Gomori and Goldner[7] who found that if part of the pancreas is deprived of blood by temporary blood vessel ligatures for the first six minutes after alloxan is injected, the islets in that part of the pancreas are not damaged. This coincides with the finding of Leech and Bailey[8] that alloxan can be detected in the blood and pancreas for only five minutes after its intravenous injection into rabbits.

Kirschbaum, Wells and Molander[9] showed that in rats, adrenalectomy abolished the initial hyperglycemia and Goldner and Gomori obtained similar results with rabbits. Houssay and his associates,[10,11] however, challenge these findings.

In Houssay's laboratory the initial hyperglycemic phase was observed in five dogs and six toads given alloxan after adrenalectomy. There was an absence of the initial hyperglycemia in both hepatectomized dogs or toads and in eviscerated dogs given alloxan. Houssay *et al.* challenge the suggestion that the cause of the hypoglycemia phase lies in the sudden release of large amounts of insulin from the pancreas, for they found marked hypoglycemia in nine dogs totally depancreatized half an hour before the injection of alloxan, but in seven dogs depancreatized twenty-four to forty-

[1] Goldner and Gomori: Endocrinology, **35**, 241, 1944.
[2] Kennedy and Lukens: Loc. cit., p. 184.
[3] Foglia, Orias and Sara: Rev. Soc. Argent. Biol., **20**, 440, 1944.
[4] Goldner and Gomori: Proc. Soc. Exp. Biol. and Med., **55**, 73, 1944.
[5] Ridout, Ham and Wrenshall: Science, **100**, 57, 1944.
[6] Goldner and Gomori: Endocrinology, **35**, 241, 1944.
[7] Gomori and Goldner: Proc. Soc. Exp. Biol. and Med., **58**, 232, 1945.
[8] Leech and Bailey: Loc. cit., p. 179.
[9] Kirschbaum, Wells and Molander: Proc. Soc. Exp. Biol. and Med., **58**, 294, 1945.
[10] Houssay, Orias and Sara: Rev. Soc. Arg. Biol., **21**, 30, 1945; Jour. Am. Med. Assn., **129**, 145, 1945.
[11] Houssay, Houssay and Sara: Rev. Soc. Arg. Biol., **21**, 74, 1945.

eight hours previously, no hypoglycemia occurred when alloxan was given. Hence, they surmise[1] that (1) the initial hyperglycemia can be attributed to the direct action of alloxan upon the liver, and (2) the secondary hypoglycemia is not due to the liberation of insulin but to an extrapancreatic effect, probably to lack of glucose production by the liver. The final hyperglycemia is attributed to destroyed beta cells in the islets of Langerhans. Carrasco-Formiguera[2] found the initial hyperglycemia and hypoglycemia following the injection of alloxan in the dog slower in appearance and of smaller magnitude than in the rabbit.

Since the injection of crude anterior pituitary extract produces diabetes in dogs, it was considered important to ascertain if alloxan exerted its diabetogenic action through the pituitary. Bailey et al.[3] have shown that hypophysectomized rats given alloxan develop islet necrosis and diabetes. Kirschbaum et al.[4] showed that hypophysectomy or adrenalectomy prevented the initial hyperglycemia in rats given alloxan.

Rats made diabetic with alloxan and later adrenalectomized have been shown by Janes and Friedgood[5] to have a marked reduction or complete disappearance of diabetic symptoms, which is similar to the amelioration of the diabetes by adrenalectomy in pancreatectomized animals. Later reports,[6] however, have indicated that the apparent amelioration is associated with a lowered food intake rather than with adrenalectomy *per se*.

Alloxan has no direct effect on the utilization of glucose according to Corkill, Fantl, and Nelson[7] who injected it into an eviscerated cat without affecting the blood sugar.

Lackey et al.[8] found a significant increase in the glycogen content of the heart muscle and a decrease of glycogen in skeletal muscle and liver in rats made diabetic with alloxan. If glycosuria has been present, glycogen may be demonstrated in the tubular epithelium of the kidneys, especially in Henle's loop.[9] Burn, Lewis and Kelsey[10] found that rats made diabetic with alloxan had little or no glycosuria when given a high fat, carbohydrate-free diet containing 80 to 90 percent margarine and 10 to 20 per cent casein.

Alloxan injected intravenously into pregnant rats passes through the placenta into the fetal circulation within one to two minutes.[11] Nevertheless, diabetes was not produced in the fetus although the

[1] Houssay, Orias and Sara: Science, **102**, 197, 1945.
[2] Carrasco-Formiguera: Jour. Lab. and Clin. Med., **29**, 510, 1944.
[3] Bailey, Bailey and Leech: Loc. cit., p. 183.
[4] Kirschbaum, Wells and Molander: Loc. cit., p. 185.
[5] Janes and Friedgood: Endocrinology, **36**, 62, 1945.
[6] Janes, Dawson and Myers: Am. Jour. Physiology, **145**, 538, 1946.
[7] Corkill, Fantl and Nelson: Loc. cit., p. 184.
[8] Lackey, Bunde, Gill and Harris: Proc. Soc. Exp. Biol. and Med., **57**, 191, 1944
[9] Duff and Starr: Proc. Soc. Exp. Biol. and Med., **57**, 280, 1944.
[10] Burn, Lewis and Kelsey: Brit. Med. Jour., **2**, 752, 1944.
[11] Friedgood and Miller: Proc. Soc. Exp. Biol. and Med., **59**, 61, 1945,

mother rat developed diabetes and the fetal blood sugar paralleled that of the mother until parturition. Bailey and Bailey[1] found the islets in the offspring of diabetic rabbits unusually large apparently as the result of an attempt of the fetus to offset the mother's insulin deficiency. No evidence of either diabetes or hyperinsulinism was apparent in the offspring despite the enlarged islets.

The repeated injection of 25 mg. per kilogram of alloxan intravenously into rats produces a progressive decrease in carbohydrate tolerance as demonstrated by the glucose tolerance test.[2]

Orias[3] reports the remarkable finding that rats with only 5 per cent of their original pancreatic tissue present are more resistant than normal controls to the diabetogenic action of single doses of alloxan. Thyroidectomy also decreases sensitivity to alloxan.[4]

Thorogood and Zimmermann[5] found that following pancreatectomy the insulin requirement in dogs made diabetic with alloxan decreased to approximately one-third. Dogs made diabetic with alloxan were more resistant to acidosis than depancreatized dogs though the diabetes following alloxan was more severe.

D. Pathology.—Changes in the islet cells can be detected as early as five minutes after the injection of a single diabetogenic dose of alloxan.[6,7] From the beginning the changes are degenerative in nature. Bailey, Bailey and Hagen[7] took serial biopsies from anesthetized rabbits at varying intervals after the injection of alloxan. At the five-minute interval they describe slight but definite changes in the nuclei of the beta cells with a suggestion of some diminution of the specific granules in the cytoplasm. At ten and fifteen minutes the alpha cells appear normal, but most of the granules have disappeared from the cytoplasm of the beta cells at the center of the islets. At thirty and forty-five minutes the central cells appeared closely packed. Their nuclei were shrunken but the chromatin was still granular. The cytoplasm was still intact with a further loss of granules. At one and one and a half hours the nuclei were further shrunken and showed definite pyknosis. Early cytoplasm degeneration was apparent. At two hours those processes had extended and distortion of the general architecture of the islets was more clearly indicated. Similar changes have been described in the rat by Hughes, Ware and Young[6] and by Gomori and Goldner.[8]

Between three and six hours many cells undergo degeneration and coalesce and apparently some cells disappear entirely with the result that the islets sometimes appear smaller. The peripheral alpha cells are well preserved in most cases.

[1] Bailey and Bailey: Unpublished data.
[2] Shipley and Rannefeld: Endocrinology, **37**, 313, 1945.
[3] Orias: Rev. Soc. Argentina Biol., **20**, 199, 1944.
[4] Martinez: Rev. Soc. Argent. de biol., **21**, 254, 1945.
[5] Thorogood and Zimmermann: Endocrinology, **37**, 191, 1945.
[6] Hughes, Ware and Young: Loc. cit., p. 184.
[7] Bailey, Bailey and Hagen: Am. Jour. Med. Sci., **208**, 450, 1944.
[8] Gomori and Goldner: Loc. cit., p. 180.

These changes continue until at the twenty-four hour period the centers of the islets are occupied only by pale staining granular débris in which the outlines of nuclei and occasional degenerated cells can scarcely be recognized. Often a collar of well preserved peripheral alpha cells remain. At three days most of the débris has been removed and the center of the islet contains only a few stroma cells. No inflammatory cells are visible at any time. It is likely that some islets have disappeared entirely since the islets at this stage seem to be less numerous than in normal control animals.

In one rabbit sacrificed two months after the development of alloxan diabetes, the islets appeared normal except that they were definitely reduced in size. Using Gomori staining technic these islets were found to consist wholly of alpha cells; no demonstrable beta cells could be identified.[1]

The alpha cells generally appear unaffected, although Dunn et al.[2] state that the alpha cells may be enlarged with apparent increase of granules when the beta cells are necrosed or exhausted. Duff and Starr[3] found a marked increase in mitotic figures in the acinar cells reaching a peak at seventeen hours and returning to normal in twenty-four hours following the injection of alloxan into hooded rats. Goldner and Gomori[4] observed extreme vacuolation or hydropic degeneration of the intralobular pancreatic duct epithelium in dogs sixteen to eighteen days after the injection of alloxan.

Organs other than the pancreas show slight or no changes in the rabbit following alloxan. With the usual diabetogenic dose of 150 to 200 mg. per kilogram, the only changes found were slight fatty metamorphosis in the liver and mild degeneration of the tubular epithelium in the kidney.[1] Dunn et al.[5] state that the suprarenal cortex and thymus have sometimes shown congestion and petechial hemorrhages in the rabbit while minor cytological changes have been observed histologically in the thyroid. Adrenal changes are stressed by Hard and Carr[6] who describe marked fragmentation and shrinkage of the cells in non-localized areas of the adrenal medulla in rabbits given 300 mg. per kilogram of alloxan, although with smaller doses these changes are minimal.

Duffy[7] described areas of necrosis in all layers except the zona glomerulosa of the adrenal cortex in one rabbit, whereas Kendall et al.[8] detected in 7 rabbits diffuse and focal necrosis in the adrenal cortices accompanied by infiltration of polymorphonuclear leukocytes, mononuclear and eosinophilic cells. Necrotic areas in the

[1] Bailey, Bailey and Hagen: Loc. cit., p. 187.
[2] Dunn, Duffy, Gilmore, Kirkpatrick and McLetchie: Jour. Physiol., **103**, 233, 1944.
[3] Duff and Starr: Proc. Soc. Exp. Biol. and Med., **57**, 280, 1944.
[4] Goldner and Gomori: Loc. cit., p. 178, ref. 3.
[5] Dunn, Sheehan and McLetchie: Lancet, **1**, 484, 1943.
[6] Hard and Carr: Proc. Soc. Exp. Biol. and Med., **55**, 214, 1944.
[7] Duffy: Jour. Path. and Bact , **57**, 199, 1945.
[8] Kendall, Meyer, Lewis and Victor: Proc. Soc. Exp. Biol. and Med., **60**, 190, 1945.

zona fascicularis layer of the adrenal cortex in rats has been reported.[1]

Using the relatively large dose of 300 mg. per kilogram, Thomas and Emerson[1] found severe degenerative changes in the basophils of the pituitary of rabbits. With the smaller 200 mg. per kilogram dose the pituitary changes were less but still striking. Others[2,3] have found no changes in this gland.

The thymus was congested and showed minute hemorrhages in three rabbits described by Dunn *et al.*[3] No abnormality has been reported in the thyroid or parathyroid glands.

In the usual diabetogenic dose of 150 to 200 mg. per kilogram in rabbits the changes in organs other than the pancreas seem slight and probably insignificant.

The pathology in the rat closely simulates that in the rabbit although there is a definite tendency to more extensive tubular damage in the kidneys.[2,4] Dunn and McLetchie[4] found no macroscopic or microscopic changes in the liver, thyroid, thymus or pituitary of the rat.

The dog shows the same general pathology as the rabbit. Goldner and Gomori[5] describe hyperlipemia and fatty degeneration of the liver ten to twelve days after the injection of alloxan into dogs. They feel that the extreme fatty infiltration of the liver represents a specific effect of alloxan poisoning. They further point out the extreme vacuolation of the epithelium of all intralobular ducts in the pancreas.

In all species it must be stressed that the larger the dose employed, the more toxic changes will be found.

The production of diabetes in the rabbit by the repeated injection of small (40 to 50 mg. per kilogram) doses of alloxan causes islet cell changes not seen with a single overwhelming diabetogenic dose.[6] After 7 to 18 daily injections the blood sugar values gradually reach a diabetic level. Rabbits sacrificed at this point and studied histologically, revealed unique lesions in the islets of Langerhans. Some of the islet cells, especially those at the periphery, appeared normal; in other cells the nucleus and ground substance of the cytoplasm was well preserved, but the granules were markedly decreased or absent. Some cells presented the typical picture of hydropic degeneration and a few showed irreversible nuclear changes. Mitotic figures were seen in several islets but in no case was there more than one mitosis in a single islet. Kennedy and Lukens[7] described hydropic degeneration in beta cells in 2 rabbits forty-eight and fifty-eight days re-

[1] Thomas and Emerson: Texas Rep. Biol. and Med., **3**, 142, 1945.
[2] Bailey, Bailey and Hagen: Loc. cit., p. 187.
[3] Dunn, Kirkpatrick, McLetchie and Telfer: Jour. Path. and Bact., **55**, 245, 1943.
[4] Dunn and McLetchie: Lancet, **2**, 384, 1943.
[5] Goldner and Gomori: Loc. cit., p. 178, ref. 3.
[6] Bailey, Bailey and Leech: Loc. cit., p. 180.
[7] Kennedy and Lukens: Loc. cit., p. 184.

spectively after the administration of alloxan, and Duffy[1] found similar changes at one hundred ninety-four days. These changes were attributed by them to the effect of hyperglycemia on beta cells that had escaped destruction by alloxan.

Hughes and Hughes[2] repeatedly injected rats with doses of alloxan varying from 25 to 125 mg. per kilogram. Although none developed diabetes, degranulation and pyknotic nuclei were found in the beta cells. They present evidence to show that the older larger beta cells are more susceptible to alloxan and are destroyed first. Duff and Starr[3] produced transitory diabetes in hooded rats with the repeated daily injection of 100 mg. per kilogram of alloxan, but the blood sugar returned to normal despite continued injections. On histological section, these animals revealed only slight pyknosis of some of the central cells in the islet.

The pathology in alloxan diabetes has been completely summarized in a splendid article by Duff[4] and the new reports on alloxan each year have been abstracted by Joslin.[5,6]

E. Complications.— Diabetic cataracts have been reported by Bailey, Bailey and Leech[7] in rabbits and rats made diabetic with alloxan. The onset usually occurs between four and eight weeks after the onset of the diabetes in severely diabetic rabbits and the lens changes appear to be similar to the cataracts reported by Foglia and Cramer[8] in depancreatized rats. The cataracts appear earlier and develop much more rapidly in rabbits with poorly controlled diabetes as compared with those receiving insulin. In one rabbit with moderately early cataracts there was no progression of the lens changes over a period of two years during the administration of adequate doses of insulin daily. Other groups of investigators in Cleveland,[9] Philadelphia,[10] New Jersey,[11] Chicago,[12] and England[1] have observed similar lens changes.

Diabetic acidosis and coma have been reported in both rabbits and rats[13] with alloxan diabetes. Bailey *et al.*[14] reported pronounced lipemia reaching 14 per cent, elevated blood acetone to 144 mg. per 100 cc. and lowered carbon dioxide content of the blood in rabbits with coma.

[1] Duffy: Loc. cit., p. 188.
[2] Hughes and Hughes: Brit. Jour. Exper. Path., **25**, 126, 1944.
[3] Duff and Starr: Loc. cit., p. 188.
[4] Duff: Am. Jour. Med. Sci., **210**, 381, 1945.
[5] Joslin: New England Jour. Med., **230**, 425, 1944.
[6] Joslin: New England Jour. Med., **232**, 219, 1945.
[7] Bailey, Bailey and Leech: Loc. cit., p. 180.
[8] Foglia and Cramer: Proc. Soc. Exper. Biol. and Med., **55**, 218, 1944.
[9] Schneider, Lewis, Moses and McCullagh: Proc. Cent. Soc. Clin. Res., **17**, 17, 1944.
[10] Lukens: Personal communication.
[11] Chesler and Tislowitz: Science, **101**, 468, 1945.
[12] Gomori: Personal communication.
[13] Franks, Friedgood and Kaplan: Proc. Amer. Fed. Clin. Research, **2**, 41, 1945.
[14] Bailey, Bailey and Leech: Loc. cit., p. 183.

A transitory period of hypercholesteremia and hyperlipemia may accompany the early stages of severe diabetes produced in rabbits with alloxan and Kendall *et al.*[1] report this in 29 of 32 rabbits receiving 125 mg. per kilogram doses.

This type of experimental diabetes provides excellent opportunities by which many of the unknown or debatable questions in diabetes may be studied. Recently Stetten and Boxer[2] using alloxan diabetic rats and deuterium as a tracer substance, showed that on a 60 per cent carbohydrate diet about one-fourth of the urinary glucose was synthesized *in vivo* and about three-fourths was derived from the carbohydrate in the diet. They further demonstrated the failure of diabetic rats to utilize glucose in the synthesis of fatty acids. Lowry and Hegsted,[3] making use of rats made diabetic with alloxan, showed that diabetic animals develop thiamine deficiency at approximately the same rate, or perhaps slightly less quickly, than non-diabetic controls and once the deficiency has developed, the diabetic rats respond to thiamine as readily, if not more so, than the control animals.

Comparison With Other Types of Experimental Diabetes.—The production of experimental diabetes with alloxan has several definite advantages in comparison with other methods, namely, (1) pancreatectomy and (2) the injection of crude anterior pituitary extract.

In comparison with pancreatectomy, alloxan, (1) requires no operation; (2) does not remove the structures connected with the external secretion of the pancreas; (3) is applicable to animals with diffuse pancreases, such as the rabbit; (4) is much simpler, and (5) usually produces a more severe diabetes.[4,5]

Alloxan has the following advantages over the injection of crude anterior pituitary extract: (1) It requires only one injection; (2) It is applicable to many more animals especially the small laboratory animals such as the rat, thereby making mass experiments feasible; (3) it produces diabetes more responsive to insulin therapy; (4) alloxan is much more easily obtainable than pituitary extract, less expensive, requires less handling and is much more stable at room and ordinary refrigeration temperatures.

D. Relation to Human Diabetes.—Besides providing a splendid method for the production of diabetic animals simply and quickly in the laboratory with which to study many of the problems of diabetes, one cannot help but wonder if alloxan is in any way related to human diabetes. As yet no one has been able to answer this question conclusively.

There are several facts which have been raised against this relationship: (1) It is claimed that alloxan is so reactive a substance

[1] Kendall, Meyer, Lewis and Victor: Loc. cit., p. 188.
[2] Stetten and Boxer: Jour. Biol. Chem., **156**, 271, 1944.
[3] Lowry and Hegsted: Jour. Lab. and Clin. Med., **30**, 839, 1945.
[4] Dragstedt, Allen and Smith: Proc. Soc. Exp. Biol. and Med., **54**, 292, 1943.
[5] Thorogood and Zimmermann: Loc. cit., p. 187.

that it could not be expected to exist as such in the body, especially since an acid medium is necessary for its stability; (2) Alloxan has not as yet been definitely isolated from human tissues, although in 1862 Liebig[1] reported its detection in human intestinal mucus from an intestinal catarrh and Lang[2] claimed its detection in urine from a cardiac patient. Recently Tipson and Ruben[3] have detected an alloxan-like substance in animal and human tissue extracts; (3) Alloxan is not known to be an intermediate product in the break-down of any substance in the human body; (4) The pathology after a single diabetogenic dose of alloxan is not similar to the pathology of human diabetes.

Points, on the other hand, that suggest a possible relationship between alloxan and human diabetes are: (1) The remarkable specificity which alloxan has for the islets of Langerhans and particularly for the insulin-forming beta cells; (2) Since alloxan joins with 1,2-dimethyl-4-amino-5(d-1-ribitylamino)-benzene to form riboflavin,[4] the question has been raised as to whether the reverse reaction may occur under certain conditions; (3) The pathology of slowly produced diabetes with the repeated small injections of alloxan more closely simulates the pathology of pituitary diabetes and of human diabetes than the mass islet necrosis described with the single diabetogenic dose; (4) It has been shown that dog livers contain an enzyme capable of splitting uric acid to dialuric acid in the presence of oxygen. The latter is readily converted to alloxan on standing *in vitro* and it has been suggested that the action of molecular oxygen carried by hemoglobin might do the same.[5]

Despite the apparent weight of evidence against such an association, the relationship of alloxan to human diabetes remains unknown.

[1] Liebig: Liebig's Ann., **121**, 80, 1862.
[2] Lang: Wien. med. Wchnschr., **16**, 1513, 1866.
[3] Tipson and Ruben: Loc. cit., p. 182.
[4] Banerjee, Dittmer and duVigneaud: Loc. cit., p. 183.
[5] Archibald: Loc. cit., p. 182.

Addendum.—Lazarow recently pointed out that Wiener in 1899 administered alloxan to rabbits, apparently by mouth, and reported that convulsions developed. See Lazarow: Loc. cit., p. 182, and Wiener: Arch. f. exp. Path. u. Pharm., **42**, 375, 1899.

CHAPTER VI.

THE PATHOLOGY AND CAUSES OF DEATH IN DIABETES.

Revised by Howard F. Root, M.D.

A. THE PANCREAS AND DIABETES.

The degenerative and destructive lesions in the pancreas, and especially in the islands of Langerhans, have been the center of pathological study since their discovery. In recent years investigations in experimental diabetes have directed attention to reversible lesions in the pancreas and to the capacity for regeneration of the pancreas with a consequent emphasis on the hope of improvement and even a cure of the disease. The last half century has seen the transfer of diabetes from a symptom associated with multitudinous clinical states to a disease with a definite pathological basis in the pancreas and notably in the islands of Langerhans. Beginning with Cawley[1] in 1788, the connection between gross lesions of the pancreas and diabetes was noted and similar observations were repeated with increasing frequency as time went on. The removal of the pancreas from dogs by von Mering and Minkowski[2] in 1889 with resulting diabetes established the relation between the gland and the disease and opened a field for experimental study. It was not, however, until Opie[3] in 1901 and Ssobolew[4] in 1902 localized the essential morbid process in the islands of Langerhans, and Weichselbaum and Stangl[5] described the hydropic degeneration and vacuolation of the island cells, that the pathologist hoped to diagnose the disease without the help of the clinical records. The experiments of Young and Best show that even diabetes produced by anterior pituitary extract produces changes in the pancreas, but degeneration of the islands can be prevented if insulin is injected simultaneously, or if the animal is fasted or fed with fat,[6] during the injections of anterior pituitary extract. Likewise the remarkably specific action of alloxan, by which it causes diabetes, results in necrosis of the islands of Langerhans. The pathology of the pancreas in the various forms of experimental diabetes has been summarized recently by Duff.[7] Experiments with rats and rabbits have disclosed the existence of a pancreatropic factor, derived from the

---

[1] Cawley: London Med. Jour., **4**, 289, 1788.
[2] von Mering and Minkowski: Arch. f. exp. Path. u. Pharm., **26**, 371, 1889–1890.
[3] Opie: Bull. Johns Hopkins Hosp., **12**, 263, 1901.
[4] Ssobolew: Virchow's Arch. f. Path. Anat., **168**, 91, 1902.
[5] Weichselbaum and Stangl: Wien. klin. Wchnschr., **14**, 968, 1901. Weichselbaum: Ibid., **24**, 153, 1911.
[6] Haist, Campbell and Best: Loc. cit., p. 99.
[7] Duff: Loc. cit., p. 190.

13

anterior pituitary, which is not identical with either the diabetogenic or growth-promoting principle.[1] Increases in the number and
the volume of islet cells can be produced. Who can foresee the
next step in demonstrating the influences which stimulate the
islands to improve functionally under appropriate conditions?

The pancreas is man's protection against diabetes. Destroy it by
disease, by means of the chemical alloxan or remove it by experiment, and diabetes results. Organic or functional injury of the gland
is the essential feature; the means by which this is produced is
immaterial. Pathologists, however, would not have been baffled
so many years did not another factor enter into consideration.

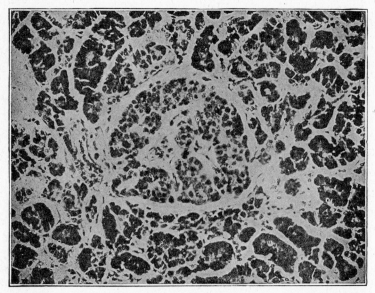

Fig. 5.—Normal island of Langerhans whose cells produce the insulin required by
the body.   × 250.   (Mallory.)

A small remnant of healthy pancreas will suffice to prevent
diabetes. This explains why fairly extensive destruction of the
gland by necrosis, infection, or the inroads of malignant disease
frequently is unaccompanied by diabetes. Minkowski's extirpation
experiments proved this point when he showed the disease was
averted if the remnant amounted to one-tenth of the gland. This
would be equivalent to 5 or 10 grams. These pathological and
experimental observations, however, almost added to the difficulty
of explaining diabetes in the presence of an apparently normal
pancreas until Opie's discovery.

The weight and estimated size of the pancreas are misleading

[1] For convenience the physiology and pathology of alloxan diabetes are discussed
in a single section. See Chapter V.

criteria of its state, whether normal or abnormal, because of the great variation in connective tissue and fat, chiefly interlobular, which are present in the organ. Thus of two pancreases, both of which contained but little pancreatic tissue, the one weighed 30 grams and the other 240 grams. This variation is not altogether dependent on the weight of the individual from which the organ came, as both women weighed over 200 pounds. The smallest pancreases in adult diabetics in our series weighed 15 grams and 12 grams in Cases 3194 and 11558 respectively, aged 62 and 73 years, with durations of 12 and 8 years.

The islands of Langerhans (Fig. 5), embedded in the pancreas, and constituting about 3 per cent of its weight, Opie showed to be the seat of its protective agency against diabetes. They are particularly well supplied with blood vessels. Ogilvie[1] found that the average weight of the pancreas increased from 2.6 grams at birth to 66 grams for those over twenty-one years of age, while the average total weight of the islands increased from 0.12 grams at birth to 1.07 grams for those over twenty-one years of age. The number of islands varied greatly from 117,226 in a one-year old female to 2,325,123 in an eight-months-old male. Gomori[2] has compared the number of islets in human pancreas of diabetics and non-diabetics. Normally the total number of islets lies between 250,000 and 2,500,000, the majority of pancreases having about 500,000. He regards as more significant the total area of the islets expressed in percentages of the total since this includes both size and number of the islets. The average normal value for man is from 1 to 3.5 per cent.

Substantial differences in the insulin content of pancreas of different species are shown in the following table (see Marks and Young).[3]

TABLE 25.—INSULIN CONTENT OF PANCREAS OF DIFFERENT SPECIES

Species	Weight of pancreas (gm./100 gm. body weight).	Insulin content of pancreas	
		Units/gm. pancreas	Units/100 gm. body weight.
Chimpanzee	0.09	11.2	1.01
Dog	0.23	3.3	0.76
Cat	0.21	2.2[4]	0.47[4]
Rabbit	{ 0.15	9.5	1.42
	{ 0.13	7.8[5]	1.17[5]
Guinea pig	{ 0.37	0.08	0.028
	{ 0.31	0.23[5]	0.070[5]
Rat	0.48	1.3	0.62
Mouse	1.10	1.7	1.87
(Methods are those of Marks and Young (1939) unless otherwise indicated.)			
Human diabetic		0.4[6]	
Human non-diabetic		1.7[6]	

[1] Ogilvie: Quart. Jour. Med., **6**, 287, 1937.
[2] Gomori: Bull. New York Acad. Med., **21**, 99, 1945.
[3] Marks and Young: Nature, **146**, 31, 1940.
[4] *Cf.* Scott and Fisher: Amer. Jour. Physiol., **121**, 253, 1938.
[5] Picrate insulin extraction method of Dodds and Dickens: Brit. Jour. Exp. Path., **5**, 115, 1924.
[6] Values reported by Scott and Fisher: Loc. cit., p. 138.

At least three types of cells are present in the islands. The alpha cells tend to be arranged toward the periphery and contain acidophilic granules, while the more numerous beta cells make up the bulk of the islands.[1] The D cells described by Warren[2] and later named by Bloom,[3] are scattered irregularly. The function of the alpha and D cells is unknown unless the alpha cells may be proven to be the source of lipocaic. The beta cells are probably concerned with insulin production, although the evidence as yet is not conclusive.[4] In a few diabetic pancreases, a reduction in the ratio of beta to alpha cells was found by Gomori.[5] The origin of the islands has been disputed, the generally accepted view being that the island cells are derived from the epithelium of the ducts, although the claim has been made that insular epithelium may be derived from the acinus and even that transition forms may be present.

The origin and differentiation of the alpha and beta cells in the pancreatic islets of the rat from the twelfth day of gestation to the third postnatal weeks may be from three and perhaps four sources, according to Hard.[6] These are: (1) islets arising from the solid pancreatic lobe, few in number and appearing the thirteenth day; (2) islets formed from the pancreatic tubules very actively from the sixteenth to eighteenth days, and resulting in the majority of the so-called embryonic islands; (3) postnatal islets developing from the duct systems. (4) There is some evidence of a secondary duct system contributing to added formations as described by Bensley.[1] The beta cell is the only cell type differentiated during fetal life and first appears on the eighteenth day. The alpha cell is first identified by its granular content and on the second day postpartum, and possibly becomes an active secretory type.

That the pathological signs in the diabetic pancreas are by no means confined to the islands of Langerhans all are agreed, although this does not prove that any part of the pancreas save the islands is involved in the disease. The acinar tissue shows definite changes and perhaps the outstanding feature in the diabetic pathology of the pancreas in the last few years is the demonstration, largely suggested by the work of physiologists and clinicians, that in diabetes the external as well as the internal secretory activity of the pancreas is impaired.[7]

The independence of the islands of Langerhans is of importance from the point of view of their regeneration. Obviously the greater the supply of tissue which can lead to the development of new

[1] Bensley: Am. Jour. Anat., 12, 297, 1911.
[2] Warren: P. 33, loc. cit., p. 131.
[3] Bloom: Anat. Rev., 49, 363, 1931.
[4] Gomori: Arch. Path., 36, 1, 1943.
[5] Gomori: Am. Jour. Path., 17, 395, 1941.
[6] Hard: Am. Jour. Anat., 75, 369, 1944.
[7] Dubnova and Izigson: Klinidus. Medits, 5, 531, 1927.

islands, the better. However, the weight of evidence leads us to believe that the islands are not derived from acinar tissue. For details, the reader should consult the monograph by Warren.[1]

The arguments in favor of the integrity of the islands, which appear to us as most convincing are: (1) Demonstration of the principal islet in certain species of fish, later to be described, from which insulin could be prepared, whereas it is not obtainable from the pancreas itself; (2) the persistence of islands in cases where practically all the acinar tissue and the duct system have been destroyed by carcinoma or other lesions; (3) the special blood supply of the islands; (4) the improbability that acinar cells, which do not secrete insulin but, indeed, have specific zymogenous function, could later acquire so specific a function as to produce that complicated hormone; (5) Wilder's[2] patient from the Mayo Clinic, without diabetes and with hypoglycemia so intense that to prevent collapse he was compelled for weeks to take food every two hours and for a time every half-hour, and as much as 1000 grams cane sugar daily, all because, as proved by autopsy, a cancer of the islands had metastasized in the liver. An extract of the metastatic nodules in the liver lowered the blood sugar of rabbits, while that of the surrounding tissue did not.

As congenital anomalies, aberrant pancreatic tissue[3] is found in the liver and in the mucosa of the small intestine and this aberrant tissue is capable of secretion. Pancreatic tissue with islands has been found in dermoid cysts.[4]

During the past six years we have had 5 cases of hyperinsulinism due to tumors of the islands of Langerhans. All 5 were operated upon by Dr. L. S. McKittrick and Dr. T. C. Pratt, and will be reported by Marble and McKittrick. (See pages 408 to 412.)

Twenty instances of adenoma of the islands of Langerhans were collected by Warren[5] up to 1926, although their clinical significance was not then appreciated. These tumors are characterized by resemblance to the islands in the arrangement of their cells and in the appearance of the individual cells, by absence of mitotic figures, by the presence of a definite capsule, and by compression of the adjacent tissue. Since then, the clinical signs of hyperinsulinism[6] have been associated with adenoma of the islands and our understanding of the disease process well established.

Murray and Bradley[7] have cultivated *in vitro* two adenomas of the

[2] Warren: P. 29, loc. cit., p. 131.
[2] Wilder, Allan, Power and Robertson: Jour. Am. Med. Assn., **89**, 348, 1927.
[3] Seyfarth: Klin. Wchnschr., **3**, 1085, 1924.
[4] Warren: Personal communication.
[5] Warren: Am. Jour. Path., **2**, 335, 1926.
[6] Harris: Endocrinology, **16**, 29, 1932; Annals Int. Med., **10**, 514, 1936. Whipple and Frantz: Ann. Surg., **101**, 1299, 1935. Liu, Loucks, Chou and Chen: Jour. Clin. Invest., **15**, 249, 1936.
[7] Murray and Bradley: Am. Jour. Cancer, **25**, 98, 1935.

islands of Langerhans from two human adults, for periods of five and six weeks.

Heiberg[1] described an adenoma, 6 x 5 mm. in the pancreas of a white female, aged sixty-four years, dying in diabetic coma. West and Kahn[2] report 2 first cousins with islet cell adenomas and similar symptoms. One in the head of the pancreas could not be palpated or seen at operation and was only found at autopsy.

Successful surgical removal of adenomata of the pancreas in 4 women, aged 24 to 67 years, are reported by Walker and Boger,[3] Isaacs, [4] and Clyne, Leeds and Cowdery.[5] A review of the literature up to January 1, 1944, by Clyne, Leeds and Cowdery gives a total of 127 benign adenomata among 176 islet tumors, and includes a listing by Whipple[6] of 105 tumors found at 158 operations. Tumors were found at autopsy in 29 cases. Benign adenomata occurred in 101 cases.

Fairly extensive removal or destruction of the pancreas does not produce diabetes provided the islands of Langerhans or a sufficient number of them are left intact. This is shown by the absence of diabetes following experimental removal of less than a certain minimum amount of tissue and by partial destruction of the gland, but not of the islands, in infections and other lesions and by ligation of the ducts which results in atrophy of the acini, but not of the islands, a procedure utilized by Banting in his preparation of insulin. Fortunately Banting did not know that only partial atrophy of the acini took place as a result of the ligation of the duct. In a positive way it is proved by Macleod's[7] experiments with the angler fish and the sculpin. In these fish the islands are collected in a principal islet distinct from the balance of the pancreas. Extracts of the principal islet act powerfully in lowering the percentage of sugar in the blood in contrast to extracts of the remaining zymogenous tissue which are inert.

When Opie[8] first described the hyalinization of the islands of Langerhans in diabetes it was naturally hoped that this would prove to be a lesion distinctive in this disease. While it is still the classic lesion associated with diabetes, it is none the less not a distinctive one. Hyalinization may be considered as due to production of intercellular substance by fibroblasts and possibly by endothelial cells. In Warren's[9] series of 484 diabetic pancreases,

[1] Heiberg: Centralbl. f. allg. Path. u. path. Anat., 22, 532, 1911.

[2] West and Kahn: West. Jour. Surg., 47, 364, 1939.

[3] Walker and Boger: Arch. Int. Med , 75, 75, 1945.

[4] Isaacs: Jour. Am. Med. Assn., 130, 404, 1946.

[5] Clyne, Leeds and Cowdery: New York State Jour. Med., 45, 405, 1945.

[6] Whipple: in Nelson's Loose Leaf System of Surgery, New York, Thomas Nelson & Sons, 5, Chapter VIII, p. 397, 1945; New England Jour. Med., 226, 515, 1942.

[7] Macleod: Jour. Metab. Res., 2, 149, 1922.

[8] Opie: Jour. Exp. Med., 5, 397, 1901.

[9] Warren: P. 39, loc. cit., p. 131.

200 (41 per cent) showed hyaline change, more than any other lesion However, this change occurs rarely in non-diabetics,[1] but one wonders whether in time they might have become diabetic.

Actually in 4 cases among 200 non-diabetic autopsies moderate or marked hyaline change occurred in the islands of Langerhans. Such an infrequent occurrence of lesions in the islands of non-diabetic individuals similar to those found in diabetics is a prerequisite if we consider insular changes the cause rather than the result of diabetes. Gellerstedt[2] regards the hyaline change in the islands of diabetics as identical with amyloidosis. His report is based upon study of 181 autopsies, including only 3 diabetics. Amyloid deposition, determined by differential staining, was found in the islands of Langerhans in 67 out of 105 middle-aged and older diabetic persons (64 per cent), and in 5 out of 50 consecutive non-diabetic patients over fifty years of age by Ahronheim.[3] Warren found in hyalinized islands typical staining reactions for amyloid in 14 out of 51 cases.[4] Hyaline areas in the islands gave positive methyl violet reaction in all of 48 cases reported by Arey.[5]

The diagnosis of diabetes from the examination of the pancreas alone, even though obtained soon after death, is not possible in any large percentage of the cases, according to most pathologists. Herxheimer,[6] however, emphasizes the constancy of pancreatic lesions. In 97 autopsies performed by himself, 89, or 92 per cent, showed changes in the pancreas. He holds that diabetes caused by disease of other organs than the pancreas is not anatomically demonstrable.

Diabetic patients rarely die of diabetes today. In a compilation of 8384 deaths, only 2.9 per cent were ascribed on death certificates to "diabetes" alone in the period from 1898 to 1946. (See page 229.) Uncomplicated diabetes is responsible for death in only 12 per cent of Wilder's 81 cases on whom a postmortem was performed. We believe that clinicians and pathologists must continue to correlate their findings and that both should study the case during life.

No single distinctive lesion of the islands in diabetes mellitus was encountered in the 484 cases studied by Warren, which included both adults and children. This is to be expected in light of the work by Allen,[7] Opie,[8] and Cecil.[9] This was true even of the young uncomplicated cases of diabetes among whom, as among any group, one might expect uniformity in pathological appearance, if there

[1] Warren: Arch. Int. Med., **44**, 663, 1929.
[2] Gellerstedt: Beitr. z. path. Anat. u. z. allg. Path., **101**, 1, 1938.
[3] Ahronheim: Am. Jour. Path., **19**, 873, 1943.
[4] Warren: P. 33, loc. cit., p. 131.
[5] Arey: Arch. Path., **36**, 32, 1943.
[6] Herxheimer: Verhandl. d. Gesell. f. Verdauungs. u. Stoff., **11**, 112, 1933.
[7] Allen: Glycosuria and Diabetes, Boston, W. M. Leonard, 1913.
[8] Opie: Disease of the Pancreas, 2d ed., Philadelphia, J. B. Lippincott Co., 1910.
[9] Cecil: Jour. Exp. Med., **11**, 266, 1909.

was one definite causal agent giving rise to the disease. Heiberg[1] compared the number of islands of Langerhans in the tail of the pancreas in 75 diabetics with the number in non-diabetics. Fifty-three of the non-diabetics had from 76 to 150 islands, whereas 51 of the diabetics had less than 50 islands per 50 mm. of area. Warren believes that the reduction of insular tissue in many cases of diabetes in children is congenital rather than the result of disease. Uniformity in reduction, however, is so lacking that it hardly could represent the *anlage* of Naunyn.

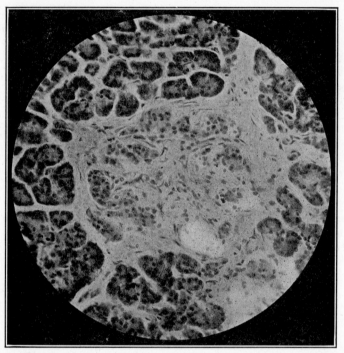

Fig. 6.—Fibrosis of island of Langerhans. U23–8. Aged fifty-nine years. Duration of diabetes seventeen years. Eosin-methylene blue stain. × 170.

Fibrosis of the islands is nearly as common a finding as is hyalinization, 129 cases in Warren's series showing this lesion. (Fig. 6.) Evidence of hypertrophy of the islands was seen in 38 cases, sometimes associated with other lesions. Hydropic degeneration of insular epithelium was encountered twenty-two times, although in most of the cases it was merely suspected and postmortem change could not be ruled out. The most extreme hydropic degeneration that we have seen was found in the pancreas of a man dying of fulminating diabetes sent to Dr. F. B. Mallory by Dr. Willard S.

[1] Heiberg: Nord. Med. Ark. avd. 2, 50, Stockholm, 1918.

Hastings. Conroy[1] found hydropic degeneration in only 1 of his 12 cases. This change, so strongly emphasized by Allen and Weichselbaum,[2] although one of the rarest lesions occurring in the islands and not pathognomonic of the disease, deserves fresh investigation. A lesion frequently encountered in children is lymphocytic infiltration of the islands. This was encountered nine times in Warren's series. However, as stressed by Page and Warren,[3] the islands in the pancreases of children are usually without definite pathological change. This is of utmost importance in estimating the probable course of the disease in diabetic children.

That structural pathology cannot give a complete answer to the problem of diabetes, at least with the methods at present available, is evidenced by the fact that practically one-fourth of Warren's cases (127) showed essentially negative insular tissue. Labbé[4] came to a similar conclusion, while giving an excellent description of the pathological findings in the pancreas, and especially the islands of Langerhans. Robbins and Tucker[5] found pancreatic lesions in only 42.5 per cent of 184 diabetic autopsies.

The acinar tissue of the pancreas presented varying degrees of sclerosis in some cases independent of pathology in the islands. The acinar sclerosis was not apparent in any case much under two years' duration, even though the islands showed considerable change. Fibrosis may at times be due to chronic passive congestion. There is enough reason for such congestion and often evidence of it in other organs.

Primary tuberculosis of the pancreas has never been described. However, secondary tuberculosis of the pancreas, particularly miliary processes, is by no means rare in the course of generalized tuberculosis. (See page 640.)

Only 23 cases (5 per cent) of Warren's series of 484 autopsies showed marked sclerosis of the pancreatic vessels. Arteriosclerosis as a factor in the production of diabetes, while it cannot be ruled out, is hardly of great importance.

Zinc is constantly found in the pancreas of normal and diabetic persons. Eisenbrand, Sienz and Wegel[6] found the content to be 18.5 and 30.4 mg./kg. fresh gland tissue for diabetics and non-diabetics respectively.

Vartiainen[7] compared the results of postmortem examination in 166 diabetic patients with a similar number of non-diabetic patients used as controls of similar age. Eighteen diabetic patients had a pancreas weighing less than 30 grams and the causes of death in these patients were pulmonary tuberculosis, diabetic coma and

[1] Conroy: J. Metab. Res., **2**, 367, 1922.

[2] Weichselbaum: Wien. klin. Wchnschr., **24**, 153, 1911.

[3] Page and Warren: New England Jour. Med., **200**, 766, 1929.

[4] Labbé: Bull. et mém Soc. Méd. d. Hôp. de Paris, February 18, 1910 and April 25, 1913.

[5] Robbins and Tucker: New England Jour. Med., **231**, 865, 1944.

[6] Eisenbrand, Sienz and Wegel: Med. u. Chem., **4**, 259, 1942.

[7] Vartiainen: Acta Med. Scand., **118**, 539, 1944.

bronchial pneumonia. None of the control cases had pancreases of such small size. Cirrhosis of the pancreas was present in 30 diabetics. The liver of the diabetic patients weighed on the average of 100 grams more than the liver of the control cases.

When F. M. Allen[1] applied intermittent clamping or ligation to the arterial supply of the pancreas, diabetes resulted and he postulated a vascular neurosis as a possible cause of diabetes.

1. **Hydropic Degeneration.**—The important place of hydropic degeneration in the development of diabetes was emphasized by F. M. Allen as a result of his epoch-making studies of experimental diabetes in dogs. Most recently hydropic degeneration has been observed in the islands of Langerhans of animals made diabetic by injections of alloxan. (See page 189.) Lukens and Dohan[2] have shown the same development of hydropic degeneration in the islands of Langerhans of cats made diabetic by partial removal of the pancreas and then the injection of extract of anterior pituitary. Just as Allen showed that recovery might occur from this stage, so Lukens has shown that hydropic degeneration characterizes a period in the development of diabetes in the dog and the cat produced by extract of anterior pituitary which may last from one to four months in the cat and is reversible. Thus, the use of insulin during this period will bring about a disappearance of the evidences of degeneration and the return of the islands to normal. The prevention of diabetes in man, therefore, will depend upon a knowledge of the duration and the occurrence of this period of reversibility and on our ability to diagnose the disease during this period. Allen says that hydropic degeneration can be shown experimentally when dogs have been rendered diabetic by the removal of the larger portion of the gland. In sequence the changes are: disappearance of the granules in the cells of the islands, swelling of the cells with fluid, and eventually disappearance of the islands. These changes are the result, not the cause, of the diabetes. These susceptible animals, according to Allen, develop diabetes if overfed. This takes place irrespective of the quality of the food, carbohydrate, protein, or fat, only the time required for the effects of fat feeding is longer. The dogs are potentially diabetic, but free from symptoms on limited diets. Overfeeding causes active diabetes, which in turn causes the hydropic changes.

Recently Lukens[3] has obtained data which suggests that it is the level of glucose in the blood which may itself be the determining factor in the production of hydropic degeneration. (See page 123.)

2. **Regeneration of Islands.**—Species differences appear when the response to partial depancreatization in animals is compared. Thus

[1] Allen: Jour. Urology, **49**, 512, 1943.
[2] Lukens and Dohan: Loc. cit., p. 99.
[3] Lukens: Yale Jour. Biol. and Med., **16**, 301, 1944.

Friedman and Marble[1] found that the dominant reaction on the part of the islands of Langerhans in the partially depancreatized rat is hyperplasia, with degenerative changes playing a minor rôle. In the dog, however, the dominant changes are those of degeneration. The demonstration by Lukens that recovery from the diabetes produced by anterior pituitary injections in the cat is a result of regeneration of the islands of Langerhans has led to a review of the cases of unusual improvement in diabetes.

In 7 cats, after recovery from experimental diabetes, 5 had normal and 2 had diabetic glucose tolerance curves. Cases of remission in diabetes have been reported by Root[2] and Lukens and Dohan.[3] The duration of remission varied from one month to ten years. Of 19 patients described by Lukens and Dohan, 9 relapsed following gross neglect of diet. Bliss,[4] working at the Physiatric Institute in 1922, noted that the pancreatic remnant in a partially depancreatized dog had doubled in size by the end of a year. "Copp and Barclay[5] at the Physiatric Institute . . . have shown that in dogs in which a diabetic status was induced by the ablation of a large portion of the pancreas, and by overfeeding, if the damage to the islands of Langerhans had not progressed beyond the stage of hydropic degeneration of the beta cells, the process could be reversed by a proper dietetic treatment or with insulin if necessary."

Friedländer[6] described a case of pancreatic lithiasis with severe diabetes and pulmonary tuberculosis in which, during the course of the disease, an improvement of the diabetes bordering on recovery appeared. Cytological examination showed an atrophy of the excretory apparatus and an hypertrophy of the islands of Langerhans. Graner,[7] working in Bensley's laboratory, tied or otherwise obstructed the duct of the pancreas and after sufficient time had ensued to allow for the destruction of the acinous and some of the islet tissue, restored the connection of the pancreas to the bowel. In 4 cases the second operation was successful and regeneration of the pancreas took place, and in 2 the regeneration was complete. Regeneration begins first in the islets, but when the occlusion of the duct has been removed, is fairly complete in the acini. If the occlusion is permanent, diabetes may result.

Warren and Root[8] found evidences of the power of the pancreas, and of the island tissue in particular, to regenerate after acute injury. "Thus in a pancreas from a non-diabetic patient dying of lobar pneumonia (A15–16) we found numerous mitotic figures in the island cells, as high as seven mitoses in a single island. Mitotic figures can

[1] Friedman and Marble: Endocrinology, **29**, 577, 1941.
[2] Root: Philadelphia Med., **36**, 1238, 1941.
[3] Lukens and Dohan: Pa. Med. Jour., **48**, 24, 1944.
[4] Bliss: Jour. Metab. Res., **2**, 385, 1922.
[5] Copp and Barclay: Jour. Metab. Res., **4**, 445, 1923.
[6] Friedländer: Zeit. klin. Med., **128**, 184, 1935.
[7] Graner: Proc. Inst. Med. of Chicago, **6**, 80, 1926.
[8] Warren and Root: Am. Jour. Path., **2**, 69, 1926.

occasionally be found in the island cells of cases dying of diphtheria and of lobar pneumonia. At times necrotic cells are found. This injury and subsequent repair not only indicate the regenerative power of the pancreas, but perhaps explain the transient glycosuria occasionally encountered in acute infections."

The same transient injury to the islands may explain the severe drop in sugar tolerance noted in diabetic patients during acute infections. The rapid reëstablishment of the former level of sugar tolerance following recovery from the acute process may well represent the result of the rapid regeneration of the island cells.

In one of our cases, Case 896, whose diabetes had lasted for fourteen years and who had been under insulin treatment for five months, receiving 15 to 100 units daily with a gradual decrease of the insulin requirement, there was evidence of regeneration of the islands. No functioning acinar tissue was present. The bulk of the pancreas was occupied by a carcinoma from which the patient died, but the tail was not invaded by the tumor. Here the islands were closely packed. Some showed a moderate degree of hyalinization, but most were entirely free from hyaline or other degenerative changes. Columns of cells extended out from the islands into the surrounding stroma, and in places entire low-power fields were made up of island tissue. There were more islands than could be accounted for by their concentration due to contraction of the stroma of the pancreas following destruction of the acinar tissue.

The regenerative capacity of the islands of Langerhans is again emphasized by von Bakay,[1] who compared the unusually large size of the islands of Langerhans in a newborn infant, who died during the delivery of a diabetic mother, with specimens from adults. In the islands of the infant polymorphism of the nuclei was striking, and a large number of giant nuclei were present in the adult. He felt that regeneration occurred even under pathological conditions involving the entire pancreas as in cases of true diabetes and regarded the absence of symptoms of diabetes as explained by the compensating effect of the intense regenerative process. This capacity was not reduced even in advanced age.

The influence of the pituitary upon hypertrophy of the islands of Langerhans was studied by Krichesky.[2] In rats, the ratio of island tissue to body weight increased by 63 per cent after hypophysectomy. If, however, pituitary extract was administered hypodermically after hypophysectomy, the increase in the island tissue was largely prevented.

3. **Effect of Insulin Upon the Pancreas.**—The extraordinary effect of insulin in preventing degeneration of the islands of Langerhans under the influence of injections of anterior pituitary extract in dogs, together with its power to allow regeneration of the islands

[1] von Bakay: Virchow's Arch. f. Path. Anat. u. Physiol., **310**, 291, 1943.
[2] Krichesky: Proc. Soc. Exp. Biol. and Med , **34**, 126, 1936.

of Langerhans even after the stage of hydropic degeneration has begun, are outstanding discoveries. On the other hand, in patients dying after long periods of chronic diabetes Warren and Root found no difference in the pancreases of those patients given insulin and those on dietary treatment alone, with one exception. In Case 263, treated with insulin for thirteen months there were more apparently normal islands than would ordinarily be the case.

4. Pathology in Infants or Fetuses of Diabetic Mothers.—Helwig[1] has studied the occurrence of enlarged islands of Langerhans in 9 premature or full-term infants born of diabetic mothers, of whom 7 were patients of the George F. Baker Clinic and 2 of the Boston Lying-In Hospital. The islands of Langerhans in the infants of diabetic mothers exhibited a variable degree of hypertrophy and hyperplasia, most marked in those infants nearing full term. The nuclei were frequently enlarged and occasionally hyperchromatic. The stroma and occasionally the islands were infiltrated with eosinophilic granulocytes. Splanchnomegaly involving liver, spleen and heart, glycogen infiltration in the heart, hematopoiesis in liver and spleen, advanced bone and gonad development and a film in the pulmonary alveoli are discussed on page 773. von Bakay[2] describes the islands of an infant who died during the delivery of a diabetic mother as enlarged with a diameter of 500 to 800 microns. Vix[3] found 19.3 per cent of 192 diabetic mothers to have abnormally large children. Kraus[4] tabulated the weights of 608 infants of 155 diabetic women and found that 10.8 per cent of the children weighed from 5 to 6 kilograms and actually 35 per cent of the children weighed 4 kilograms or more. Kraus, in analyzing the development of the organs in relation to the size of the babies, suggests that the anterior pituitary lobe is an important factor. Autopsies showed no striking lesions. The size of the islands varied from average (200 micra) to large (650 micra) in diameter. It is tempting to believe that this hyperplasia represents an effort to compensate for the mother's pancreatic deficiency. Gordon[5] reported 3 cases of fetal hypoglycemia due to hyperinsulinism. However, the pathologist not used to seeing the normal fetal or infantile pancreas may misinterpret the striking size of its islands. Okkels and Brandstrup[6] hold that the enlargement of the islands of Langerhans as well as the increased signs of activity in thyroid and anterior pituitary in fetuses of diabetic mothers are secondary to the hyperglycemic condition in the fetus. The assumed large size of diabetic infants at term is of marked interest and deserves careful investigation. Babies of diabetic mothers have been of more nearly normal size when the

[1] Helwig: Arch. Int. Med., **65**, 221, 1940.
[2] von Bakay: Loc. cit., p. 204.
[3] Vix: Med. Klin., **29**, 50, 1933.
[4] Kraus: Handb. d. Gyn., 3d ed., München, **9**, 865, 1936.
[5] Gordon: Jour. Michigan Med. Soc., **34**, 167, 1935.
[6] Okkels and Brandstrup: Acta path. et microbiol. Scandin., **15**, 268, 1938

blood hormones of the mothers have been controlled. (See Chapter XXIX.)

5. **Acute Pancreatitis Preceding Diabetes.**—Warfield[1] found 7 cases in the literature and added 4 of his own in which diabetes developed after acute pancreatitis. Two of his own cases followed influenza and 2 occurred as apparently primary acute pancreatitis. The diabetes began during or soon after the attack in 6 cases, but an interval of 6 years intervened in another. Warfield explains the absence of diabetes in hemorrhagic pancreatitis on the ground that the patients live for too short a period for it to develop. The diabetes was permanent in the 5 cases in which the subsequent history was known, although its later mildness in one of the cases which survived the acute pancreatitis suggested a recovery from the diabetes. Quite rightly Warfield emphasizes the importance of the explanation of pain in the epigastrium in the beginning of diabetic coma. He considers that in some instances it may be related to an acute pancreatitis. That coma is occasionally associated with appendicitis is well-known and it is useful that Dr. Warfield has called attention to a possible pancreatitis, so that all can be alert to diagnose such an instance.

Limper and Miller[2] describe an infant, aged three weeks, in coma, with a blood sugar of 0.952 per cent and gangrene of the left leg. The pancreas showed scarring of the islets and in the tail portion there was moderate pyknosis with acute degeneration and small groups of dead cells in the islets. The mother had had mumps at the time of delivery and possibly the virus of mumps had involved the pancreas.

Rodriguez[3] also reports a case of acute pancreatitis preceding the onset of diabetes and Dunn, Vatcher, and Woodwork[4] 2 others. Grott's[5] case developed acute diabetic symptoms during acute pancreatitis, which subsided under treatment only to return some months later in the usual chronic form. Only once, in a previously healthy man with normal blood sugar, has Umber[6] seen diabetes develop in 38 cases of widespread infectious necrotic destruction of the pancreas even after several years of observation. In 16 cases of the series, who later became diabetic, a pre-existing diabetic tendency was probable. In the remaining 21 cases, despite extensive necrosis of the pancreas, no sign of disturbed carbohydrate metabolism occurred. He considers the insular tissue more resistant than the non-insular tissue. Therefore, Umber believes that diabetes can develop only if there exists an hereditarily inferior insulin mechanism.

[1] Warfield: Jour. Am. Med. Assn., **89**, 654, 1927.
[2] Limper and Miller: Am. Jour. Dis. Child., **50**, 1216, 1935.
[3] Rodriguez: Jour. Am. Med. Assn., **82**, 203, 1924.
[4] Dunn, Vatcher and Woodwork: Lancet, **1**, 595, 1926.
[5] Grott: Medycyna, Nr. 21, 649, 1936.
[6] Umber: Med. Welt, **9**, Nr. 25, 889, 1935.

Two cases of acute pancreatitis in males, thirty-three years of age, are reported by Sobel.[1] One had beginning diabetic coma and required 165 units of insulin; both recovered. A statistical study of hemorrhagic necrosis of the pancreas is given by Weiner and Tennant.[2] Fourteen cases of acute pancreatitis at the Worcester City Hospital are discussed by Dunlop and Hunt.[3] Six out of 7 cases with blood sugar determinations showed hyperglycemia.

The diabetic patient may be more subject to acute pancreatitis than the non-diabetic. Warren found acute pancreatitis in 4 cases, apoplexy of the pancreas in 2 and subacute pancreatitis in 6 cases in 484 diabetic autopsies. This incidence of 2.4 per cent is eight times the incidence of pancreatitis in 20,000 autopsies found by Hamperl.[4] Shumacker[5] found 78 instances of glycosuria in 700 reported cases of acute pancreatitis. Twenty-eight of 55 cases had blood sugar levels above 200 mg. per cent. Four cases, or 15 per cent of 26 cases of diabetic coma studied at autopsy and reported by Root[6] showed acute pancreatitis, together with fatty change in and enlargement of the liver.

Gangrenous pancreatitis may occur in the course of diabetes. Case 3267 developed diabetes in December, 1922, when she was forty years of age, without diabetic history, and was first seen in August, 1923, with 6.6 per cent sugar and blood sugar 0.27 per cent. With 15 units of insulin she became sugar-free with a tolerance for 78 grams of carbohydrate. During the summer of 1925 diet was broken and on September 22, 1925, she developed nausea, vomiting, pain in the abdomen, and labored breathing, but under the treatment of her physician, Dr. Coulson of Lawrence, came out of coma. On account of unusual symptoms she was referred to the Deaconess Hospital on September 25, three days later, when the blood sugar was 0.44 per cent, the non-protein nitrogen 98 mg. per 100 cc., the plasma CO_2 8 volumes per cent. With insulin the patient at first improved, but she gradually failed and the next day was unresponsive. The autopsy revealed atheroma of the coronary arteries, and calcified plaques in the abdominal aorta, numerous small stones in the gall-bladder, an infectious pancreatitis with areas of fat necrosis in the peritoneum.

Since then 3 other cases (9987, 10115, 14370) of acute pancreatitis with coma have occurred.

6. **Pancreatic Calculi.**—According to Reginald Fitz, Thomas Cawley[7] recognized the first case of diabetes during life in which a lesion of the pancreas was noted later at postmortem examination,

[1] Sobel: Med. Rec., **11**, 38, 1938.
[2] Weiner and Tennant: Am. Jour. Med. Sci., **196**, 167, 1938.
[3] Dunlop and Hunt: New England Jour. Med., **218**, 376, 1938.
[4] Hamperl, quoted by Böse: Zentralbl. f. Chir., **63**, 261, 1936.
[5] Shumacker: Ann. Surg., **112**, 177, 1940.
[6] Root: Jour. Am. Med. Assn., **108**, 777, 1937.
[7] Cawley: Loc. cit., p. 193.

and this pancreas was filled with small calculi. In 1667 pancreatic lithiasis was reported by deGraff[1] without mention of glycosuria. Pancreatic calculi preceding diabetes are rare. The patient of Dr. Hackney in March, 1923, had cholelithiasis and chronic appendicitis. Within six months diabetes developed. Four years later, following many lapses of diet and irregularities in the use of insulin, the patient succumbed to hypoglycemia, 0.013 per cent, despite the intravenous injection of 90 grams of dextrose. At the autopsy the pancreas weighed 190 grams; it was ovoid, constricted near the middle, the greatest diameter 12 cm., the lesser diameter being 4.5 cm., and the diameter of the constricted portion 2.5 cm. The part of the organ corresponding to the head of the pancreas had a smooth

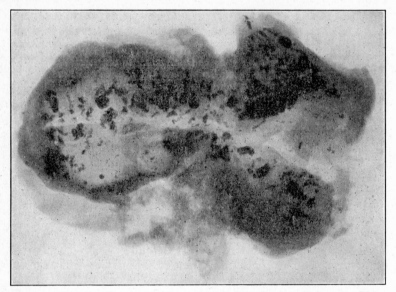

Fig. 7.—Calculi in Pancreas. (Courtesy of J. S. Hackney of Uniontown, Pa.)

rounded surface and on incision was found to consist of a fibrous wall having an average thickness of about 5 mm. containing approximately 15 cc. of cloudy, white liquid, in which about 100 irregularly-shaped calculi, less than 5 mm. in diameter, were found. The other half of the organ had an irregular, nodular surface, and on dissection was found to consist of solid white tissue in which ducts having diameters up to 3 mm. and encrusted with concretions were seen. (Fig. 7.)

Later Dillon's[2] reprint disclosed that in 2800 autopsies at the Pennsylvania Hospital there were but 2 cases of pancreatic calculi and in but 1 of these was glycosuria observed.

[1] Rockwern and Snively: Arch. Int. Med., **65**, 878, 1940.
[2] Dillon: Ayer Clin. Lab. Pennsylvania Hospital, Bull. No. 8, p. 35, 1924.

A third instance of diagnosis of pancreatic calculi (6359) during life was discovered by Dr. Bogan in a routine roentgenogram taken of the chest. The patient's diabetes developed five years before, at the age of eighteen years, and when she came under our supervision, in September, 1927, she required 45 units of insulin to metabolize carbohydrate 74 grams, protein 54 grams, fat 88 grams, and even then frequently showed traces of sugar. Despite the relatively high calories per kilogram body weight she lost $3\frac{1}{2}$ kilograms in twenty days. She died of coma and pyonephrosis on March 25, 1936.

Multiple calcified areas outlining the pancreas were observed in Case 17162, aged thirty-two years, whose diabetes was so resistant to insulin that he developed diabetic coma in the hospital even while taking 400 units of insulin a day and later, for a number of weeks, required 1900 units of insulin a day. Six months later, however, in September 1939, his insulin requirement had fallen to 100 units a day. In March 1940 his diabetic condition was poorly controlled on 60 units of insulin daily. He died December 31, 1943. At autopsy extreme atrophy and fibrosis of both acinar and insular tissue was found, probably the result of acute or subacute pancreatitis in the past. Fatty cirrhosis of the liver also was present. Case 17685 with pancreatic lithiasis, on the contrary, has quite mild diabetes.

Among 527 diabetic autopsies, pancreatic calculi were encountered only three times by Warren.[1]

Seeger[2] summarized 104 cases of pancreatic lithiasis from the literature. Mayo[3] states that 25 cases, proven, of pancreatic calculi have been found at the Mayo Clinic. Lüdin[4] made an x-ray examination of each pancreas removed in 542 autopsies and found stones in 28 cases, or about 5 per cent. The stones varied in size from the head of a pin to a hazelnut.

Pancreatic lithiasis is of two types: (1) true stones, found in the ducts, and (2) false stones or calcifications of fat or parenchyma resulting from pancreatitis. In 70 cases of Oser,[5] 24 showed diabetes or glycosuria. In 26 cases operated upon, 1 developed fatal diabetes subsequent to the operation. In Phillips's[6] case stones were not found at operation. Jaundice persisted, sugar appeared in the urine and the patient died in diabetic coma. At autopsy the duct of Wirsung was packed with stones. Mason's[7] case with pancreatic calculi was extremely resistant to insulin, as was Case 17162.

[1] Warren: P. 61, loc. cit., p. 131.
[2] Seeger: Radiology, **10**, 126, 1928.
[3] Mayo: Proc. Staff Meet. Mayo Clin., **11**, 456, 1936.
[4] Lüdin: Arch. f. Verdauungskrankh., **63**, 273, 1938.
[5] Oser: Diseases of the Pancreas, in Nothnagel's Encyclopedia of Practical Medicine, Philadelphia, W. B. Saunders Company, pp. 11–303, 1903.
[6] Phillips: Trans. Clin. Soc. of London, **37**, 96, 1904.
[7] Mason: Jour. Clin. Invest., **9**, 31, 1930.

14

7. **Effect of Coma.**—Coma causes no distinctive pathology in the pancreas. In 53 cases of uncomplicated coma studied by Warren there was no essential difference in the pancreatic findings from those in diabetics dying from other causes.

Immunity to infection in diabetes has seemed to be peculiarly specific in that the resistance of diabetic patients to infections with Staphylococcus aureus and the tubercle bacillus is strikingly low. The phagocytic power of the leukocytes of diabetic patients and depancreatized cats was studied by Richardson.[1] Phagocytosis was not different from normal in diabetic patients with reasonably satisfactory blood chemistry, but in the presence of acidosis or uncontrolled diabetes this power was significantly decreased.

Dillon, Riggs and Dyer[2] studied the brains of 8 patients dying in uncomplicated coma. The lesions found resembled those seen in acute asphyxia. The primary changes were in the cerebral capillary bed. As a result of cerebral edema, proliferation of neuroglia and acute degenerative changes in the ganglion cells were found. They felt that cerebral anoxia due to the reduced blood volume, and the hemoconcentration were the chief causes. See page 447 for further discussion.

8. **Pathological Evidence Concerning the Etiology of Diabetes.**— The variation and inconstancy of the pancreatic lesions are against an infectious origin for the disease, and the character of such lesions as may be present does not suggest the result of invasion by organisms. While it is true that in a few relatively early cases of diabetes we[3] found lymphocytes about the islands, this can hardly be considered as evidence for infectious origin of the lesion.

The experimental production of diabetes by alloxan suggests the possibility that some such substance may be an etiologic agent in human diabetes. The close chemical relationship between alloxan and uric acid is well known. (See page 181.)

Whatever the cause may be, it seemingly acts over a long period of time, perhaps throughout the duration of the disease. The pathology which we find in the pancreas at autopsy rarely represents the initial damage to the organ, but rather the result of a long struggle between the regenerative activity of the pancreas and the degenerative changes caused by the diabetogenic factor. The pancreas is not a static organ like the brain or myocardium, unable to repair itself after injury.

For some reason this static conception of the pancreas has become firmly established in spite of clinical and anatomical evidence to the contrary, probably because the diabetic patient cannot be cured and frequently goes steadily down hill in spite of treatment. We believe that this unfavorable course of the disease is

---

[1] Richardson: Am. Jour. Med. Sci., **204**, 29, 1942.
[2] Dillon, Riggs and Dyer: Am. Jour. Med. Sci., **192**, 360, 1936.
[3] Warren and Root: Loc. cit., p. 203.

not due to failure of the pancreas to regenerate, but to continued injurious action on the organ by the causal agent, eventually overcoming the regenerative efforts.

In any disease as insidious in onset and as chronic as diabetes, with pathological changes largely restricted to one portion of a single organ, one cannot expect any striking evidences of either destruction or regeneration. It is not unnatural that the conception of the diabetic pancreas as an inert organ, passively submitting to gradual destruction, has been firmly established.

We may assume that the lesions in diabetes are not infectious but toxic in origin. Their course is extremely chronic, and consequently the attempts at regeneration are slow. Mitotic figures would hardly be expected under the circumstances.

Practically all toxic lesions of the same age in the same organ resemble one another, as in toxic myocarditis or central necrosis of the liver. But in the islands of the pancreas showing either hyalinization or sclerosis, practically every stage from masses of hyaline or dense connective tissue embedded in the stroma to apparently normal islands can be found. It is difficult to conceive a toxic substance of very chronic action or a long-continued functional strain totally destroying one island and completely sparing the next. Much more logical is the assumption that we are dealing with a gradual destruction of islands, a formation of new islands to replace them, exposure of these to the toxic substance with consequent pathological change and still more islands formed to take their places. The apparently normal cells found represent those most recently formed. Eventually the destructive process wears down the regenerative powers of the organ producing diabetes of severest type.

B. OTHER ORGANS AND DIABETES.

1. **The Liver.**—The pathological changes found in the diabetic liver do not always accord with its known functional importance. Joynt[1] reports a case of primary carcinoma of the liver combined with tuberculosis and diabetes mellitus. This rare association of diseases could easily result in severe hypoglycemia because of variations in glycogenetic function of the liver. Enlargement of the liver with fatty infiltration of the parenchymal cells occurs in uncontrolled cases, especially with acidosis, as in 4 cases reported by Labbé, Boulin and Balmus.[2] The presence of glycogen in the liver cell nuclei and relative absence in the cytoplasm is of diagnostic importance in denoting diabetes. Alternate storage of glycogen and secretion of bile at varying periods during the day, indicated by pathological examination in animals, was considered to be of clinical

[1] Joynt: Canad. Med. Assn. Jour., **50**, 529, 1944.
[2] Labbé, Boulin and Balmus: Jour. de Med. de Paris, **55**, 277, 1935.

importance in diabetic treatment, by Möllerström.[1]   Boulin,[2] in
reporting 70 cases of clinical hemochromatosis among 4266 diabetics
states that ten years or more may be required for the development
of the complete syndrome of diabetes, melanoderma and cirrhosis.
Hemochromatosis has been proven in 24 cases at the Deaconess
Hospital. (See pages 223 and 547.)

An analysis of diabetic livers at autopsy by Warren divided the
cases treated prior to January 1, 1930, from cases treated between
1930 and 1937 on the basis that the early group would include the
pre-insulin cases and those of the early Banting Era, whereas those
in the second group received more insulin and a much higher carbohydrate diet.   However, the weights of the liver were strikingly
similar in the two series.   Although a slight trend towards heavier
livers in the diabetic patients occurred, actually it was far from
striking.   An analysis of the fat in the livers of diabetic and non-
diabetic patients by Dr. Halliday at the Deaconess Hospital showed
the total fatty acid to range from 2.2 to 4.3 per cent net weight in
the non-diabetics and from 4.1 to 10.8 per cent in the diabetic cases.
Large amounts of fat do not preclude the presence of normal or even
large amounts of glycogen and, indeed, fatty infiltration may occur
in von Gierke's disease.   A biopsy of the liver of Case 6884 disclosed
glycogen 12 per cent and fat 10 per cent.   (See pages 394 and 545.)

Meythaler and Naegeli[3] show that if the portal vein is attached to
the vena cava so that the liver is completely deprived of venous
blood, there arise definite changes in carbohydrate metabolism.
The fasting blood sugar level is usually subnormal.   The temporary
rise after glucose tolerance test by mouth in contrast to the normal
is somewhat delayed.   On the other hand, if the portal vein without
the pancreatic duodenal vein is anastomosed with the vena cava,
then no disturbance in carbohydrate metabolism results.   In other
words, with the Eck fistula the disturbance in carbohydrate metabolism results because there is no direct transfer of endogenous insulin
to the liver cells; undisturbed direct hormonal relation between liver
and pancreas is a necessary prerequisite for the normal course of
carbohydrate metabolism.

Dragstedt, Prohaska and Harms[4] studied 45 dogs from whom the
pancreas had been removed.   All but one of these developed fatty
livers.   They describe a method for the preparation of a fat-free
alcohol extract of pancreas, lipocaic, which on oral administration
to depancreatized dogs treated with insulin permits their survival
and prevents or relieves the fatty degeneration and infiltration of
the liver of these animals.   According to Sergeyeva,[5] the predominating influence of the abdominal sympathetic nerves increases the

---

[1] Möllerström: Loc. cit.; p. 151.
[2] Boulin; Presse Med., **53**, 326, 1945.
[3] Meythaler and Naegeli: Arch. f. exp. Path. u. Pharm., **172**, 630, 1933.
[4] Dragstedt, Prohaska and Harms: Am. Jour. Phys., **117**, 175, 1936.
[5] Sergeyeva: Rev. Canadienne Biol., **2**, 495, 1943.

content of alpha cells in the rat pancreas. Dragstedt suggests that lipocaic is made by the alpha cells. Lagerlof and Hultquist[1] describe a woman forty-five years of age who suffered for eighteen years with attacks of pain in the upper part of the abdomen. Operation showed calcified areas in the tail of the pancreas. Two years later at autopsy the pancreas aas cirrhotic and contained several jagged stones. The liver was large. Microscopic examination showed sclerosis and atrophy with perhaps some areas of proliferation of islands. The relative number of the alpha cells was reduced to 70 to 75 per 1000 cells of the islands as compared with normal of 200 to 300 alpha cells. For a discussion of lipocaic and related topics, see page 133.

2. **The Involvement of Pituitary, Thyroid, Adrenals, and Ovaries.** —The frequency of diabetes among acromegalic cases, together with the demonstration by Young that an extract of the anterior lobe of the pituitary when injected in large amounts will produce degeneration of the islands of Langerhans and permanent diabetes in dogs, have left no doubt as to the influence of the anterior pituitary upon carbohydrate metabolism, but as yet the rôle of this gland in human diabetes is obscure. The earlier demonstration by Johns, O'Mulvenny, Potts and Laughton[2] in 1927 that they had produced hyperglycemia, glycosuria and polyuria in dogs by the injection of an anterior lobe extract was followed by the experiment of Houssay and Biasotti in 1930, who showed that diabetes produced in animals by removing the pancreas could be ameliorated in turn by removing the pituitary gland. Ham and Haist[3] studied the histological changes which follow the injection of anterior pituitary extract in dogs. They described the progressive degranulation, hydropic degeneration and death of the beta cells as due to stimulation of these cells to excessive function. The anterior pituitary extract may act in two ways to cause the beta cells to overwork: (*a*) by acting on tissues and organs other than the pancreas, such as the thyroid gland, the parathyroid gland and the adrenal cortex so as to increase the body's need for insulin; such effect includes increasing the amount of carbohydrates to be metabolized and also making insulin relatively ineffective; (*b*) by exerting a trophic effect on the pancreas which was indicated by mitotic figures in various elements including the beta cells. The injections of these extracts produced prompt decline in the amount of insulin retained in the pancreas as shown by Best, Campbell and Haist.[4] A low carbohydrate diet also reduces the insulin content of the pancreas, but there is no associated degenerative change in the islets of Langerhans. Actually Best[5] also showed that fasting, apparently by reducing the strain

---

[1] Lagerlof and Hultquist: in Papers from St. Erik's Hospital, Stockholm, Ed. H. Berglund, 1945.

[2] Johns, O'Mulvenny, Potts and Laughton: Am. Jour. Physiol., **80**, 100, 1927.

[4] Ham and Haist: Am. Jour. Path., **17**, 787, 1941.

[4] Best, Campbell and Haist: Jour. Physiol., **97**, 200, 1939.

[5] Haist, Campbell and Best: Loc. cit., p. 99.

on the islands of Langerhans, made it possible for them to resist the effect of the injections of anterior pituitary extract. Best showed that in the dog the injection of insulin at the same time with an enormous amount of anterior pituitary extract would actually protect the islands of Langerhans against the degenerative effect of the injections. One may well ask whether in human beings such a relatively enormous amount of anterior pituitary substance is ever secreted for a long period of time. If a comparatively small amount of insulin will protect the dog against this large amount of injections, may it not be true that in human diabetes a primary defect in the insulin producing islands must first be present before the islands of Langerhans will lose their resistance against the diabetogenic substance produced in the anterior pituitary?

Colwell[1] collected 15 cases of acromegaly showing a variety of pancreatic changes, including hyalin change, diminution in number of islands, pancreatitis, but no one distinctive lesion was detected. Dr. Louise Eisenhardt has examined in serial sections the pituitary gland from 18 of Warren's series of diabetic autopsies and random sections from 26 additional cases. In this group in which a fair cross-section of the diabetic population was sampled, the pancreas showed a wide range of appearances such as are usually found in diabetic patients. However, the pituitary glands showed no constant or significant change. Certain cases showed invasion of the posterior lobe by basophilic cells and slight vacuolization of those basophilic cells in the anterior lobe. Only 1 case showed the diminution of acidophiles that Kraus had reported, as described below. Crooke[2] failed to find any hyalin change in the basophilic cells in 20 cases of diabetes. Parsons[3] studied 107 pituitary glands, including 7 cases of diabetes and 1 of hemochromatosis, and found no significant changes.

The association of disturbances in other endocrine glands with diabetes was described by Root[4] in Cases 4289 and 13172, who entered the hospital with acute thyroid "storm" and diabetic coma. With Lugol's solution and insulin Case 4289 recovered from both these complications to succumb in two weeks to septicemia arising from a furuncle. Her diabetes was of recent onset and was preceded by goiter and symptoms of hyperthyroidism. At autopsy a hyperplastic thyroid gland containing 0.9 mg. iodine per 100 grams gland was found by R. B. Cattell. The adrenals were enlarged, weighing 19.5 grams, and small ovarian cysts were present. The liver contained 5.5 per cent fat, or a total of 99 grams, and no glycogen by either chemical or pathological tests. The insulin content of various tissues per 100 grams of tissue was as follows: pancreas, 25 units;

[1] Colwell: Medicine, **6**, 1, 1927.
[2] Crooke: Jour. Path. and Bact., **41**, 339, 1935.
[3] Parsons: Medical Papers Dedicated to Dr. Henry A. Christian, p. 366, 1936.
[4] Root: Trans. Am. Clin. and Climat. Soc., p. 1, 1935.

liver, 3; kidneys, 10; heart, 3; thyroid, 9.[1] The pancreas weighed 30 grams. The islands were larger than normal, but the usual number were present. Several islands showed a slight degenerative change, with nuclear pyknosis and rounding of the cytoplasm.

The pancreatic changes in diabetes associated with hyperthyroidism are indefinite.

Long and Lukens[2] have shown that cats and dogs after combined adrenalectomy and pancreatectomy may be kept alive for considerable periods (eight to thirty-five days) with only slight glycosuria. Moreover, ketonuria does not appear. In such animals, administration of cortical hormone may lead to increased glycosuria. These observations suggest that the adrenal is one medium through which the pituitary acts on the pancreas. (See page 123.) Studies of the adrenal glands removed from cases of diabetes at autopsy have thus far failed to provide morphological evidence of adrenal changes.

Multiglandular syndromes involving the pituitary have special interest. Calder's[3] review would indicate 70 cases of Simmonds' pituitary cachexia in the literature, but Silver's[4] critical analysis accepts but 41 cases on the basis of autopsy data. Weinstein[5] reports a non-diabetic man, aged twenty-seven years, with typical emaciation, secondary anemia, eosinophilia, hypoglycemia, and basal metabolism 35 to 40 per cent below normal. At autopsy a tumor, probably ependymal glioma, had invaded the hypophysis, leaving only 30 to 35 per cent of the anterior hypophysis. Atrophy of the testes, prostate and thyroid with reduction in size of the viscera generally were noted, but the pancreas weighed 65 grams and appeared normal microscopically.

Lukens, Flippin and Thigpen[6] describe a woman with typical Cushing syndrome, including the obesity, the striæ, with a proven adrenal cortical adenoma at autopsy. The patient had an absence of the opposite adrenal and this explains the fatal result. The fasting blood sugar was 113 mg. per 100 cc., but a glucose tolerance test showed a definite diabetic curve with blood sugars rising to 330 mg. per 100 cc. and a large amount of sugar in the urine. At autopsy there was no pituitary tumor, but the basophilic cells showed the hyaline change of Crooke. They summarize 55 cases of proven tumors or hyperplasia of the adrenal cortex in which 49 per cent of the cases had some impairment of carbohydrate tolerance. (See page 739.)

The unusual frequency of diabetes in persons shown at autopsy to have cortical adenomas is well brought out by Russi, Blumenthal and Gray.[7] They found in 9,000 autopsies, 131 patients with cortical

[1] Analyses secured through courtesy of Charles H. Best.
[2] Long and Lukens: Proc. Soc. Exp. Biol. and Med., **32**, 392, 1934; Proc. Soc. Exp. Biol. and Med., **32**, 743, 1935.
[3] Calder: Bull. Johns Hopkins Hosp., **50**, 87, 1932.
[4] Silver: Arch. Int. Med., **51**, 175, 1933.
[5] Weinstein: Am. Jour. Med. Sci., **189**, 245, 1935.
[6] Lukens, Flippin and Thigpen: Am. Jour. Med. Sci., **193**, 812, 1937.
[7] Russi, Blumenthal and Gray: Arch. Int. Med., **76**, 284, 1945.

adenoma, or 1.45 per cent. Possibly some much smaller adenomas were missed. In the 9,000 cases were 270 diabetics, an incidence of 3 per cent. However, among the 131 patients with cortical adenomas there were 21 with proved diabetes, or an incidence of 16 per cent. Of these 21, 16 were also in the group with both clinical and pathological evidence of hypertension. Certain adrenal cortical hormones increased the rate of glyconeogenesis and thus increased the blood sugar level.

Cluston, Bennett, Power and Kepler's[1] case of Cushing's syndrome with adenomatous or hyperplastic changes in the pituitary body or adrenal cortices was complicated by alkalosis. This is the fourth instance of low blood potassium level in Cushing's syndrome from the Mayo Clinic.

Belozerov[2] found that denervation of the liver had no essential effect on carbohydrate metabolism; denervation of the suprarenals increased insulin sensitivity; and denervation of both organs caused flattening of alimentary glucose curves for from two to three months. The advisability of using such surgical methods in the treatment of diabetes is questionable.

Duncan, Semans and Howard[3] report a case in which a large adrenal medullary tumor (pheochromocytoma) in a diabetic patient was removed with apparent cure of the diabetes.

Warren found in female autopsies varying degrees of atrophy of the ovaries and uterus largely proportional to the duration and severity of diabetes. Whether the effect is a direct one or indirect by way of the pituitary or due to malnutrition alone is not certain.

3. **Cardio-renal-vascular System.**—With arteriosclerosis in its various forms responsible for 67 per cent of the deaths in diabetes today, and with its demonstration in life by x-ray in approximately 90 per cent of the cases of ten or more years' duration, it is not surprising that only 4 diabetics of five or more years' duration have failed to show arteriosclerosis at autopsy. In the diabetic atheromatosis is the characteristic vascular lesion, although medial change is often present, particularly in the muscular arteries of the legs and arteriolosclerosis is frequent both in the kidneys and the pancreas. Rarely do other forms of arterial disease occur. Case 16353, age forty-five years with diabetes of eight years' duration, had periarteritis nodosa (see page 522), and a second case in a diabetic is reported by Logue and Mullins.[4]

The ages at death of the diabetic patients imply the existence of arteriosclerosis. Among 484 autopsies arteriosclerotic deaths number 143. To justify its recognition as a sequel of diabetes, therefore, the pathologist must demonstrate its appearance in youthful dia-

[1] Cluston, Bennett, Power and Kepler: Jour. Clin. Endocrin., **5**, 61, 1945.
[2] Belozerov: Med. exptl., **4**, 33, 1940.
[3] Duncan, Semans and Howard: Ann. Int. Med., **20**, 815, 1944.
[4] Logue and Mullins: Ann. Int. Med., **24**, 11, 1946.

betics and must show that it is peculiar in type. These questions have been discussed clinically in later pages.

Hart and Lisa,[1] in an analysis of 2,798 autopsies with special consideration for the sex ratio in arteriosclerosis found that in non-diabetic patients there was a male predominance, and the ratio between arteriosclerosis in the two sexes with diabetes changed to unity.

In comparing 166 diabetic autopsies with the same number of non-diabetic cases Vartiainen[2] found that gangrene occurred in 13 diabetics and in only 2 of the controls.

Warren's series of diabetic autopsies, including all age groups, showed coronary occlusion or infarction in 72 of 440 cases. In contrast to this number of cases, Benson and Hunter[3] found only 72 cases of infarction among 1750 medico-legal autopsies. For even more convincing data, see page 509.

In Warren's series an arteriosclerosis of the aorta generally ran fairly parallel with that of coronary arteries, though in a few cases the aortic changes were either more or less marked than those in the coronaries. Thus the frequency of severe myocardial damage and of sclerosis of the coronary arteries and the aorta is much greater than would be expected for similar age groups of non-diabetics.

Page and Warren found 6 cases of atherosclerosis and atheromatosis in 11 young diabetics. In 1 boy, aged sixteen years (Case 1305), there were found at autopsy atheromatous plaques on the aorta. He had a high blood fat, and it seems quite possible that this was related to the arteriosclerosis. In addition, large numbers of lipid-filled cells were present in the spleen.

Pariente, Present, and Ralli[4] report a man, aged forty-five years, with carotinemia. The blood carotene rose from 0.24 to 0.688 mg. per cent after taking carotene. At autopsy the aorta and mesenteric artery showed orange-yellow plaques some of which contained much carotene. The liver contained an excessive amount of carotene and fat. The arteries of the legs also showed an excessive amount of arteriosclerosis.

Intercapillary glomerulosclerosis in its advanced forms[5] occurs much more frequently in diabetics than non-diabetics, and especially is this true in young diabetics of long duration. (See pages 500-502). Intercapillary glomerulosclerosis occurred in 20 per cent of the series of 184 autopsies reported by Robbins and Tucker,[6] whereas in the series of 124 diabetics analyzed by Laipply, Eitzen and Dutra,[7] 63.7 per cent (79 cases) showed this lesion. In 19 of

[1] Hart and Lisa: Clinics, **3**, 196, 1944.
[2] Vartiainen: Acta Med. Scan.. **118**, 575, 1944.
[3] Benson and Hunter: Northwest. Med., **24**, 606, 1925.
[4] Pariente, Present and Ralli: Am. Jour. Med. Sci., **192**, 365, 1936.
[5] Kimmelstiel and Wilson: Am. Jour. Path , **12**, 83, 1936.
[6] Robbins and Tucker: Loc. cit., p. 201.
[7] Laipply. Eitzen and Dutra: Arch. Int. Med., **74**, 354, 1944.

the 79 cases the glomerular lesion consisted of focal fibrosis but no characteristic spherical hyaline masses. They regarded this latter lesion as an early stage of the condition and describe intercapillary glomerulosclerosis as a most reliable criterion for the postmortem diagnosis of diabetes. The reports of Siegal and Allen,[1] and Herbert[2] also emphasize its specificity. Horn and Smetana[3] found similar lesions in non-diabetics. Bell[4] stated that there are no definite clinical features by which to distinguish diabetes with this lesion from diabetes without it. We wish that each group of authors could have exchanged sections, studied the same and then compared their conclusions.

Arteriosclerosis in the legs implies its existence in the heart. Case 3210 died two hours before operation for gangrene and Case 4108 died at the very beginning of operation for gangrene. If the surgeons only realized how the hearts of these patients looked they would hardly be persuaded to operate at all. While all types of arteriosclerosis are found in the legs, the intimal type, commonly found only in vessels of elastic type in non-diabetics, occurs very frequently in the muscular arteries in the legs of diabetics, either with or without the accompaniment of medial calcification. Leary[5] has produced coronary atherosclerosis in rabbits by feeding cholesterol.

The most remarkable example of arteriosclerosis in a diabetic in association with deposits of fat and cholesterol which we have seen is the case reported by Gordon, Connor and Rabinowitch.[6] The patient was a mild diabetic, a familial diabetic, a gall-stone diabetic. For thirteen years this mild diabetic, with the onset at the age of forty-five years, was conscientiously treated and studied, but throughout most of the period lived on a diet low in carbohydrate with an excess of fat and his weight rose in the five years before his death from $97\frac{1}{2}$ to 174 pounds at autopsy.

Sections from the vertebral, basilar and internal carotid arteries showed marked fatty infiltration. The media of some of the vessels were almost completely replaced by calcium and fat. The aorta showed marked fatty changes beneath the intima and irregular thickening, by fibrosis, of the intima. In places the media was encroached upon by fat-laden cells, and small amounts of calcium were present between intima and media. Chemical analyses of the bright yellow portions of the vessels suggested the presence of vegetable lipochromes in that they had high cholesterol content. A section of the coronary artery showed moderate intimal thickening and marked fatty infiltration beneath the intima. Many large fat-

[1] Siegal and Allen: Am. Jour. Med. Sci., **201**, 516, 1941.
[2] Herbert: Arch. Path., **31**, 501, 1941.
[3] Horn and Smetana: Am. Jour. Path., **18**, 93, 1942.
[4] Bell: Am. Jour. Path., **18**, 744, 1942.
[5] Leary: Arch. Path, **17**, 453, 1934; Ibid., **32**, 507, 1941.
[6] Gordon, Connor and Rabinowitch: Am. Jour. Med. Sci., **175**, 22, 1928.

laden cells were present, partly encroaching upon the media of the vessel.

This patient did not live in vain. He became one of Woodyatt's so-called pedigreed diabetics and as celebrated as his own cases and "Cyril K." and "Bessie B." With this portrayal before us we doubt if ever again any one will expose a diabetic to a low carbohydrate-high fat diet for so long a period.

Arteriosclerosis has been suggested by some as a cause of diabetes. If that is true, why is it that as the diabetes progresses in duration and the arteriosclerosis increases the diabetes becomes less severe? Pancreatic arteriosclerosis may be practically absent in diabetics with severe damage elsewhere. Many cases of non-diabetic arteriosclerosis show more pathology of the pancreatic vessels than do cases of diabetes. Arteriosclerosis is a sequel rather than an antecedent of diabetes, and this opinion was strengthened by the demonstration that the incidence of onset of diabetes began to decrease in the sixth decade.

Arteriosclerosis of the aorta was observed in 10 completely and 1 partially depancreatized dogs, an incidence of 13 per cent, by Dragstedt, Clark, Julian, Vermeulen and Goodpasture.[1] Similar lesions but less extensive were observed in normal dogs in only 5 per cent. The animals received insufficient amounts of lipocaic and the possible rôle of this deficiency in arteriosclerosis is suggested.

4. Glycogen.—Owing to its diffusibility, sugar cannot be histologically demonstrated in diabetic tissues. However, glycogen can be, and for over fifty years the glycogenic infiltration of Henle's loops of the kidney and the peculiar vacuolization of the liver cell nuclei, combined with absence of glycogen from the liver cell cytoplasm, has been known. Robbins and Tucker emphasize the finding of glycogen nephrosis as important in the diagnosis of diabetes, but this is a variable finding, varying with treatment. Glycogenic infiltration of the heart muscles is marked in many cases of diabetes and is particularly striking in fibers at the margins of the infarcts. The chief normal storehouses of glycogen are the liver, the skeletal muscles and the skin. In the diabetic, the normal glycogen store tends to be depleted and abnormal deposits appear in the liver cell nucleus, the cardiac muscle and the renal epithelium. Administration of insulin leads to a reëstablishment of the normal distribution of glycogen.[2]

Changes in glycogen concentration occur during fasting and hypoglycemia. Chesler and Himwich[3] found that the glycogen content of the most recent phyletic parts, the cerebral cortex, caudate nucleus of the cat and dog increased with age. On the contrary, the percentage of glycogen in the oldest parts, the cere-

[1] Dragstedt, Clark, Julian, Vermeulen and Goodpasture: Surgery, **8**, 353, 1940.
[2] Warren: Am. Jour. Med. Sci., **179**, 482, 1930.
[3] Chesler and Himwich: Arch. Biochem., **2**, 175, 1943.

bellum, the medulla and cord fell progressively with age both in the cat and dog. Cerebral glycogen is an additional source of carbohydrate during hypoglycemia or during anoxemia and, therefore, protects the central nervous system in these emergency states.

Glycogen storage disease with hepatomegaly presents unusual features. Unshelm[1] described a case with 14 per cent liver glycogen. Although death in this condition usually occurs in childhood and in the absence of diabetes, cases have been reported which might be explained by diabetes developing in glycogen storage disease, such as cases of Gjuric[2] and Stetson and Ohler.[3]   The liver of Case 6884, aged twenty-five years, showed 12 per cent glycogen in a biopsy specimen after twelve years of uncontrolled diabetes.   See page 212.

5. **Abnormal Deposits of Fat in the Diabetic.** — (a) **Obesity.** — For discussion, see pages 68–80.

(b) **Gall Stones.** — The frequency of gall stones in diabetes will be discussed on pages 552 and 708.   They were present in 139 of 453 diabetics over thirty years of age in Warren's series and 28 more showed cholecystitis.   This is over triple the incidence (10.9 per cent) found in Kaufmann's series of 16,025 autopsies in a general hospital population at Basle.   Aschoff has pointed out how such stones encourage secondary infection of the gall-bladder and this by extending to the pancreas may play some part in the etiology of diabetes.

(c) That blood of uncontrolled diabetics may contain large amounts of lipid substances has long been known.   Following a fatty meal, even in normals, the blood contains minute fat droplets for a time.   These chylomicrons are increased in a diabetic dog. Zon and Warren[4] compared their frequency in diabetics and non-diabetics.   Abnormally high counts occurred only in diabetic patients not well controlled by treatment.

The trail of the harmfulness of an excess of fat in the diabetic can be seen: (1) In his obesity; (2) in the deposits of fat in his arteries, whether large or small; (3) in the formation of gall stones; (4) in the fat in the liver, which in animals experimentally may reach 25 per cent; and, in addition (5) in the reticulo-endothelial system, most noticeably in the spleen.[5]

6. **Lipid-containing Cells in the Reticulo-endothelial System.** — The significance of large numbers of lipid-holding cells in the reticulo-endothelial system is not clear, but their presence in the diabetic in conjunction with other abnormal deposits of fat deserves mention. In the average spleen removed at autopsy there is no evidence grossly of lipid content and very little microscopically.   There are, however, scattered cases in which a marked accumulation of lipid appears in the reticulo-endothelial cells.   These cases are commonly asso-

---

[1] Unshelm: Jahrb. Kinderh., **137**, 257, 1932.
[2] Gjuric: Cited by Brian, Schechter and Persons: Arch. Int. Med., **59**, 685, 1937.
[3] Stetson and Ohler: New England Jour. Med., **217**, 627, 1937.
[4] Zon and Warren: Proc. Soc. Exp. Biol. and Med., **33**, 236, 1935.
[5] Warren and Root: Loc. cit., p. 203.

ciated with diabetes with lipemia. The first instance of this striking change in the spleen was mentioned by Coats,[1] in 1889. The patient suffered from diabetes with lipemia and died in coma.

In the reticulo-endothelial system, so far as can be judged from the staining reactions, the lipid is present in various forms and sometimes even varies in the same case, though cholesterol esters or related substances predominate. Oppenheimer and Fishberg[2] have stressed this involvement of the reticulo-endothelial system in lipemia and regard this group of cells as very important in relation to lipid metabolism. Very similar changes to these in the human cases were produced in rabbits by Anitschkow[3] and Leary[4] through feeding cholesterol.

In the discussion of their cases Warren and Root point out that there is another element of interest. Vascular lesions are very common. Whether these are merely xanthomas occurring in the intima of the vessels instead of the skin or definite atheromatous plaques is not easily decided. The case reported by Oppenheimer and Fishberg was a girl, aged six years, in whom yellowish patches occurred in the intima of the aorta and in the endocardium. Both patients reported by Lutz,[5] aged fifty-three and thirty-six years, respectively, showed atheromatous patches in the aorta. The aorta in Smith's[6] case, a man, aged twenty-two years, contained atheromata. Atheromata were found in the aorta of our Case 1305, aged sixteen years. Our Case 1794 died of a cardiac infarct resulting from coronary sclerosis at the age of thirty-three years. The aorta also was markedly sclerosed. The lipid present in the endothelial cells in the vascular lesions gave the same staining reactions as that in the cells in the spleen. Case III of Root and Warren, aged twenty-one years, showed numerous yellowish, raised patches in the intima of the aorta.

7. The Duration of the Disease and the Effects Upon Its Pathology.—Sixty-one out of 527 cases of diabetes in Warren's series of autopsies were of fifteen years' duration or longer, an incidence of 12 per cent, as compared with 18.6 per cent of all fatal cases.

Advanced atherosclerosis was present in all 61 cases of long duration. The median age was sixty-six years. All but 7 showed very severe arteriosclerosis of the aorta. Infarction of the heart had occurred in 21 cases and rupture of the heart occurred in 2. Gangrene occurred in 15 cases, or 25 per cent; coma, on the other hand, occurred in only 2 of the 61. One-half of these cases showed some degree of hyalinization or fibrosis of the islands. However, one-fourth of the cases showed no definite pancreatic pathology.

[1] Coats: Glasgow Med. Jour., **32**, 95, 1889.
[2] Oppenheimer and Fishberg: Arch. Int. Med., **36**, 667, 1925.
[3] Anitschkow: Beitr. z. path. Anat. u. z. allg. Path., **59**, 306, 1914.
[4] Leary: Loc. cit., p. 218.
[5] Lutz: Beitr. z. path. Anat. u. z. allg. Path., **58**, 273, 1914.
[6] Smith: Bull. Johns Hopkins Hosp., **36**, 203, 1925.

Neighborhood lesions such as peptic ulcer are not rare (see page 540). Lesser[1] studied all patients observed between 1924 and 1933 for the frequency of gastric and duodenal ulcer. In autopsies upon patients between thirty-five and eighty-four years of age, ulcers or scars of ulcer were found in 20.5 per cent of 444 non-diabetic men but none in 10 diabetic men. Among 438 non-diabetic women, ulcers or scars occurred in 18.5 per cent, but only 1 case (4.1 per cent) was found among 24 diabetic women. Explanation may be that less adrenalin is produced in diabetics and less vasomotor spasm is present. Dublin did not find that diabetes develops frequently in patients who have had gall stones.

8. **Hypoglycemia.**—The effects of lethal insulin doses may be seen either in experimental animals or at autopsy in cases of fatal accidents. Diffuse changes in the central nervous system have been described by Wohlwill[2] and Terplan.[3] Loubatiers and Broussy[4] produced fatal hypoglycemia in a dog and after its death with convulsions they observed congestion of the cerebellar capillaries, together with some chromatolysis in the Purkinje's cells. In Case 12882, aged twenty-seven years, with diabetes for six years, death followed forty hours after the accidental administration of 200 units of insulin. In spite of repeated convulsions, the examination of the brain and other tissues showed only cerebral edema. In Dahl's case, a woman, aged fifty-two years, with death following 15 units of insulin, the autopsy also showed nothing of importance. Grayzel[5] found experimentally that in rabbits insulin convulsions produced changes in the central nervous system largely according to the frequency and severity of the convulsions.

A variety of lesions may cause hypoglycemia. A white male, aged nineteen years, had hypoglycemia twice in one day and then died. The report of his case by Margolin[6] included an autopsy report showing acute necrosis of the adrenals. In this instance, insulin hypoglycemia was fatal probably because of the Addison's disease. A white male, aged thirty-one years, whose record was kindly provided by Dr. H. B. Anderson, of Johnstown, Pa., died in hypoglycemia, and at autopsy a large carcinoma of the adrenal was found. Terbrüggen[7] describes the anatomical findings in a case of multiple adenomata of the pancreas. Primary carcinoma of the islands of Langerhans with metastasis, as in the famous case of Wilder, Allan, Power and Robertson,[8] or primary liver cell carcinoma, as in Elliott's case, may cause hypoglycemia.[9] The remarkable diabetic woman,

[1] Lesser: Arch. Klin. Chir., **182**, 143, 1935.
[2] Wohlwill: Klin. Wchnschr., **7**, 344, 1928.
[3] Terplan: Arch. Path., **14**, 131, 1932.
[4] Loubatiers and Broussy: Arch. Soc. Science. Med., **8**, 399, 1938.
[5] Grayzel: Arch. Int. Med., **54**, 659, 1934.
[6] Margolin: Nebraska State Med. Jour., **23**, 92, 1938.
[7] Terbrüggen: Beitr. z. path. Anat., **88**, 37, 1932.
[8] Wilder, Allan, Power and Robertson: Loc. cit., p. 197.
[9] Elliott: Trans. Assn. Am. Phys., **44**, 121, 1929.

aged forty-three years, described by Judd, Kepler and Rynearson,[1] required 500 units of insulin daily at one time and then gradually changed, so that without any insulin severe spontaneous hypoglycemia occurred. A section of liver removed at operation showed severe fatty metamorphosis possibly with slight portal cirrhosis.

Perhaps the commonest cause is the adenoma of the islands, usually either of pure beta cell type or rich in beta cells. These are sometimes not readily demonstrable, but found only after the removal of a mass of pancreatic tissue.[2] (See also page 407.)

9. **Insulin Resistance.**—Pathological findings in such cases have included lesions causing extensive destruction of the pancreas, disturbance of liver function, or lesions interfering with the nervous control of the islet mechanism. (See pages 379–386.) Pollack and Long's[3] diabetic patient had thrombosis of the hepatic artery with sudden resistance to insulin.

After complete pancreatectomy in dogs, from 2 to 3 units of regular insulin per kg. body weight per day were required to limit the glucose excretion to less than 2 grams per day in Dragstedt's[4] animals. From 90 to 94 per cent of the pancreas was removed from 9 adult male dogs, the pancreas remnant being left in connection with the duct system. On the same diet, these dogs required more insulin to control glycosuria than did similar animals after complete pancreatectomy, and 2 animals were observed that required 10 and 11 units of regular insulin respectively per kg. body weight per day. This would come within the range of so-called insulin resistance in man. Yet in 2 men who underwent total pancreatectomy for malignant disease, Goldner and Clark[5] reported unexpectedly low insulin requirements and great insulin sensitivity. In the diabetic patient of Ricketts, et al.,[6] who underwent total excision of the pancreas together with the duodenum, stomach, left adrenal and omentum, the insulin requirement fell from 50 to 65 units to 40 units daily, but after six days without insulin and three days without food, death occurred in typical diabetic coma.

10. **Hemochromatosis.**[7]—Hemochromatosis or bronzed diabetes, as stated by Warren and Root, gives us an excellent opportunity to test the assumption made on pages 210 and 211. In this disease we are dealing with a known injurious agent, hemofuscin. This is a breakdown product derived from hemoglobin and is deposited in various cells of the body, where it very slowly changes to hemosiderin. Eventually the accumulated pigment causes necrosis of

[1] Judd, Kepler and Rynearson: Am. Jour. Surg., **24**, 345, 1934.

[2] Derick, Newton, Schulz, Bowie and Pokorny: New England Jour. Med., **208**, 293, 1933.

[3] Pollack and Long: Arch. Path., **13**, 530, 1932.

[4] Dragsted, Allen and Smith: Proc. Soc. Exp. Biol. and Med., **54**, 292, 1943.

[5] Goldner and Clark: Loc. cit., p. 139.

[6] Ricketts, Brunschwig and Knowlton: Proc. Soc. Exp. Biol. and Med., **58**, 254, 1945.

[7] Mallory: Am. Jour. Path., **1**, 117, 1925.

the cell containing it.   The liver is the first site of deposit, but as its cells become filled, the pigment overflows, one might say, to other organs.   The pancreas is one of these.

In those cases of hemochromatosis where the pancreas has become seriously involved before death, diabetes occurs. (See page 547 for clinical data.) If the pathology referable to the pigment cirrhosis of other organs be disregarded, this diabetes differs in no whit from diabetes mellitus, except that the course is more rapid.

Here then we have an ideal means of studying diabetes, with a known etiology and a fairly rapid course.

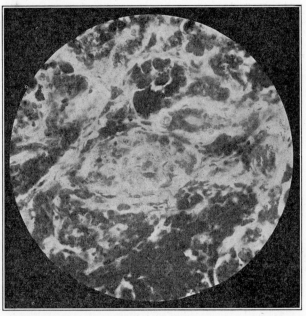

Fig. 8.—Hemochromatosis. Section of pancreas showing one island heavily loaded with pigment and another nearly pigment free, suggesting new formation. × 500 (Warren).

Warren and Root had the opportunity of studying several cases of bronzed diabetes in the laboratory. They found the same variations in involvement of the islands as have been mentioned in cases of diabetes mellitus, ranging from the remains of islands represented by clusters of pigment-loaded endothelial leukocytes and fibroblasts in the stroma to islands without pigment and apparently normal. The conclusion is inevitable that new islands are being formed to take the place of those destroyed by the pigment deposits.   In further substantiation of this evidence, occasional mitotic figures (in Case A 17-8) can be found in the cells of the younger, pigment-free islands.   (Fig. 8.)

The pigment is not restricted to the island cells, but affects the acinar tissue as well. The same evidence of regeneration is offered by the acinar cells as by those of the islands.

The well-established evidence of destruction and regeneration of parenchymal cells in the liver offers a striking parallel to the changes in the pancreas in hemochromatosis. Just as in the liver the parenchymal cells show every stage from newly-formed pigment-free cells through those containing hemofuscin and those containing hemosiderin to necrotic cells, the same steps can be traced in the acinar and island cells of the pancreas. If we substitute diabetes mellitus for hemochromatosis and hyaline formation in the islands for pigment deposit in the island cells, the analogy is complete.

There is no reason to doubt that the increased fibrous tissue noted in the pancreas in some cases of diabetes mellitus accumulates in the same way as the fibrous tissue in cirrhosis of the liver. The parenchymal cells, sometimes of the islands, sometimes of the acinar tissue, or of both, are killed and disappear. Their stroma remains behind. The parenchymal cells regenerate and new stroma forms to support them. In this way the fibrous tissue gradually increases in amount. The increased fibrous tissue noted in the pancreas in some cases of diabetes is therefore not due to a simple proliferation of the interacinar and interlobular connective tissue. Probably in most cases there has been damage to and regeneration of the acinar tissue as well as the islands. The inability of depancreatized dogs to live more than eight months without trypsin, as shown in Toronto[1] and Montpellier,[2] and the clinical evidence of disturbed external secretion of the pancreas in diabetic patients, as shown by Jones[3] and confirmed by Labbé,[4] proves the entire gland to be involved. The recent work of the Toronto school of workers by which choline is shown to be a factor along with insulin in the prolongation of the lives of depancreatized dogs reopens this question,[5] as does the later work of Dragstedt.[6]

In our series fibrosis of the pancreas was not found in those cases whose diabetes had existed less than two years. However, some of the cases of fairly long duration do not show any great increase in fibrous tissue.

11. **Need for Autopsies.**—Autopsies upon diabetic patients should be more numerous. One should never be content with a diagnosis of coma as a cause of death. What caused the coma?

Any physician who knows that his method of treatment will be checked up by an autopsy will unwittingly take more pains with his patient. It is human nature to do better work when one is under

[1] Macleod: Fuel of Life, Princeton, Princeton Univ. Press, p. 58, 1928.
[2] Hédon: Jour. d. physiol. et de path. gén., **25**, 1, 1927.
[3] Jones, Castle, Mulholland, and Bailey: Arch. Int. Med., **35**, 315, 1925.
[4] Labbé et Réchad: Arch. d. mal. de l'app. digest., **16** 865. 192€.
[5] Best: Loc. cit., page 132.
[6] Dragstedt: Loc. cit., page 133.

supervision, if only his own supervision. Doctors make mistakes, but in general the doctors who have the most autopsies are the ones who err the least. It is insurance for the best sort of treatment during life to stipulate that after death an autopsy shall be performed.

Patients are far more ready today than formerly to grant permission for autopsies and the hereditary element in the disease is a good reason for a request. On its part, the medical profession should do more than it has in the past to conform to proprieties and customs, and to protect the serious responsibilities laid upon undertakers.

A postmortem examination should be performed with as much delicacy and decorum as a surgical operation in an operating room. Hitherto this has not been the case largely because of lack of funds. The room for such examinations should be modernized, more adequately equipped, and should resemble an operating room. A nurse should be in charge and thus provide for the autopsy all the refinements a woman can lend to any medical procedure.

12. **Medico-legal Aspects of Diabetes.**—(See pages 82–98.) The medico-legal aspects of diabetes may be considered under four headings: (1) the etiology of the disease in relation to trauma; (2) special hazards of diabetes; (3) the effect of insulin, particularly in overdoses; and (4) diagnoses of diabetes from postmortem material.

1. The usual onset of diabetes is so insidious that it is difficult in most cases to establish the date of onset very accurately. Rigid standards of diagnosis must be maintained and control of blood and urine tests required in order to avoid the errors of mistaking transient glycosuria for diabetes or failing to recognize diabetes in the absence of glycosuria when hyperglycemia is present.

Among the etiological factors in diabetes, trauma is extremely rare. The analysis of statistics upon the incidence of diabetes in the United States, England, France and Germany during World War I gave no evidence that trauma was an etiological factor. Actually, trauma to the pancreas itself must be grave and extensive for trauma to be considered a direct cause of diabetes. Yet it is not impossible to consider that a person hereditarily exposed to diabetes in whom obesity was present, a serious accident which confined the patient to bed, disturbed his usual habits of exercise and diet, might advance the date of onset of diabetes. It is strikingly true, however, that as yet no evidence exists that head injuries or surgical operations upon the brain or the pituitary gland or its neighborhood have resulted in diabetes mellitus.

2. The special dangers of diabetes are acidosis and coma, infection and arteriosclerosis. Case 22733, a boy eight years of age, came for treatment May 1, 1943, with 8.7 per cent sugar in his urine, 3 plus diacetic acid, and acetone odor to his breath and early

Kussmaul respiration. Both father and mother were told the child was in early coma and that he should go to the hospital. The family physician in New Hampshire was called by telephone and joined in urging the parents to send the child to the hospital. Nevertheless, this advice was disregarded, the child was taken home to another doctor and died in six days. Shall the parents of such a diabetic child in acidosis be held responsible and be brought to trial should their refusal to accept competent medical advice with respect to the use of insulin and hospital treatment result in the child's death? The fact that a child with diabetes, unlike the child with diphtheria, does not endanger others prevents action by Boards of Public Health.

The existence of unrecognized or untreated diabetes may have important legal relations with regard to accidents and insurance benefits. A woman stepped from the curbstone and walked directly in front of an approaching automobile. Serious injuries were found upon her admission to the emergency room of a nearby hospital, together with 4 plus sugar and diacetic acid tests in her urine. Her diabetes was not produced by the trauma. Upon study it appeared that actually her blurred vision, due to unrecognized diabetes, was responsible for her failure to recognize the speed of the approaching car as well as its nearness. A man, age thirty-six, hard at work, stubbed his toe against a truck wheel. The result was necrosis of the end of the toe, requiring amputation due to deficient blood supply in the foot. In this instance, although the trauma was so slight that in a non-diabetic patient healing would undoubtedly have occurred, the evidence that an accident had occurred led the insurance company to take a position of responsibility for his hospital expenses. In diabetes not under proper control, especially when it has not as yet been diagnosed, infections with organisms of low pathogenicity, such as the Staphylococcus aureus or albus and E. coli may be highly dangerous to diabetics.

A diabetic boy, age twenty-one years, shot a jeweler who resisted robbery. His diabetes had begun five years previously when he did casual work on a race course, sleeping in the barn and living away from his family. Diabetic symptoms were severe and uncontrolled for two years until with its discovery the use of insulin was begun. During the two years prior to the crime he had suffered from occasional insulin reactions. As a child he had shown sadistic traits and had been a state ward in foster homes and a state school. Parents were separated in his infancy. His school record was poor but did not indicate feeble-mindedness. Having in mind the abnormal cortical function shown by electroencephalograms in diabetic patients with sensitiveness to insulin, the evidences shown in his early life of constitutional inferiority and the unfortunate lack of normal family training, it was difficult to form an opinion as to his actual responsibility. He was found guilty of first degree murder. Later sentence was commuted to life imprisonment.

3. Insulin reactions are common and seldom serious if treated promptly. Nevertheless, dangerous reactions may occur under unusual circumstances when treatment is delayed. During hypoglycemia patients may be confused, obstinate or wildly belligerent. A diabetic woman was jailed as an alcoholic. After twelve hours, she was transferred to the hospital in coma and died. The presence of a bottle of insulin in her handbag was not noted until too late. The use of insulin with suicidal intent is known, but actually has been surprisingly rare. A man, a few days after discharge from the Deaconess Hospital, was bending over to tie his shoe when he complained of faintness, lay down on the bed and died. Death from an insulin reaction was suspected, but an autopsy done within two hours showed advanced coronary disease and a fresh small thrombus causing the occlusion of one coronary artery. No death should be ascribed to insulin without a postmortem examination and blood sugar determination.

4. In the postmortem diagnosis of diabetes, examination of the blood taken from the left side of the heart is of great importance. Owing to postmortem discharge of glucose from the liver glycogen, the sugar content of the blood from the right side of the heart is not dependable. The absence of sugar in the urine is not to be relied upon, especially if the urine is contaminated with bacteria, or if there has been a terminal renal shut-down. In diabetic patients the fall of the blood sugar after death may be very slow, hence the blood sugar from the left side of the heart, if it is abnormally high, may remain as an evidence of diabetes for some hours after death, as shown particularly well in the table of Warren.[1] For the diagnosis of diabetes mellitus from histological study of postmortem material, the most valuable evidence consists of the following: (a) changes in the islands of Langerhans; (b) deposits of glycogen in the liver cell nuclei; (c) presence of glycogen in the renal tubules; (d) characteristic lesions of intercapillary glomerulosclerosis.

C. CAUSES OF DEATH IN DIABETES.

The disappearance of coma as a cause of death and the great prolongation of life of patients whose diabetes begins in early life have so altered the causes of death that it is necessary to be governed almost entirely by data assembled since the introduction of insulin. Coma and arteriosclerosis, however, are so important and so frequently preventable, the latter particularly when it takes the form of gangrene, that they merit all the emphasis laid upon them in the past. A more detailed treatment of these complications will be found in later pages.

[1] Warren: P. 229, loc. cit., p. 131.

TABLE 26.—THE CAUSES OF DEATH OF 8384 DIABETICS.*

Cause of death.	Naunyn Era, 1898 to May 31, 1914.		Allen Era, June 1, 1914 to August 6, 1922.		Banting Era, August 7, 1922 to December 31, 1936.		Hagedorn Era, January 1, 1937 to December 31, 1943.		Charles H. Best Era, January 1, 1944 to date.	
	Deaths.	Per cent of all cases.	Deaths.	Per cent of all cases.	Deaths.	Per cent of all cases.	Deaths.	Per cent of all cases.	Deaths.	Per cent of all cases.
All causes	326	100.0	836	100.0	3988	100.0	2583	100.0	651	100.0
A. Coma present	208	63.8	347	41.5	336	8.4	87	3.4	20	3.1
B. Coma absent:										
1. Cardio-renal-vascular	57	17.5	206	24.6	2162	54.2	1663	64.3	439	67.4
Arteriosclerotic	57	17.5	203	24.3	2146	53.8	1655	64.0	434	66.6
(a) Cardiac	20	6.1	83	9.9	1186	29.7	1041	40.3	290	44.5
(b) Nephritic	11	3.4	32	3.8	185	4.6	107	4.1	40	6.1
(c) Apoplexy	9	2.8	41	4.9	371	9.3	309	12.0	74	11.4
(d) Gangrene	12	3.7	35	4.2	322	8.1	133	5.1	19	2.9
(e) Site unassigned	5	1.5	12	1.4	82	2.1	65	2.5	11	1.7
Other circulatory and rheumatic heart diseases	0	0.0	3	0.4	16	0.4	8	0.3	5	0.8
2. Infections, total	24	7.4	106	12.7	542	13.6	298	11.5	51	7.8
Pneumonia and respiratory	14	4.3	64	7.7	275	6.8	156	6.0	27	4.2
Throat and ear	0	0.0	6	0.7	21	0.5	3	0.1	0	0.0
Gall-bladder	0	0.0	4	0.5	20	0.5	13	0.5	2	0.3
Appendicitis	2	0.6	3	0.4	24	0.6	17	0.7	2	0.3
Carbuncle	6	1.8	13	1.6	38	1.0	16	0.6	0	0.0
Kidneys, acute	0	0.0	1	0.1	35	0.9	25	1.0	8	1.2
Abscesses	0	0.0	7	0.8	56	1.4	27	1.0	0	0.0
Other infections	2	0.6	8	0.9	73	1.9	41	1.6	12	1.8
3. Cancer	5	1.5	32	3.8	350	8.8	227	8.8	58	8.9
4. Tuberculosis	16	4.9	41	4.9	166	4.2	66	2.6	16	2.5
5. Diabetes	8	2.5	56	6.7	115	2.8	63	2.4	11	1.7
6. Accidents	0	0.0	7	0.8	82	2.0	52	2.0	16	2.4
7. Inanition	1	0.3	18	2.2	6	0.2	0	0.0	0	0.0
8. Suicides	1	0.3	2	0.2	27	0.7	17	0.7	3	0.5
9. Insulin reactions	0	0.0	0	0.0	7	0.2	8	0.3	4	0.7
10. Other diseases	6	1.8	21	2.5	195	4.9	102	4.0	33	5.0

* Deaths reported through May 15, 1946. Prepared by the Statistical Bureau of the Metropolitan Life Insurance Company.

By May 15, 1946, 8384 of our diabetic patients had died. Their causes of death are recorded in Table 26 an are grouped into five periods, each representing a transition in treatment. First was that of Naunyn, which extended from 1898 until June, 1914; second, that of Allen, with emphasis laid upon undernutrition, lasting until August, 1922; the third began with Banting and the use of insulin, lasting until December 31, 1936; the fourth, that of Hagedorn, extending from January 1, 1937 to December 31, 1943; the fifth, that of Charles H. Best, from January 1, 1944 to May 15, 1946.

In the Naunyn era coma was all-important, and the habit was then established of dividing all diabetic deaths into those with coma present, meaning acidosis, and those without coma.

So protean in character have the causes of death in diabetes become that real danger exists that diabetes itself may disappear largely from the death certificate. This omission of diabetes from the death certificate will confuse public statistics, but it should not occur in statistics privately compiled.

1. **Deaths With Coma.**—Among 651 deaths in the Charles H. Best era, up to May 15, 1946, only 3.1 per cent were due to coma and in 0.6 per cent the coma was incidental to other causes. Formerly the deaths of all the children, 87 per cent of the deaths during the first year of diabetes, and in the Naunyn era as high a percentage as 63.8 per cent of the 326 deaths, were due to coma.

Coma is still needless and today is universally so regarded although in June, 1922, when this statement was made in public,[1] it was received here with incredulity and in Germany with criticism. If deaths from coma can be abolished in the hospital, they should be abolished in the home. When one sees the word coma on a death certificate, there is reason for hope for other diabetics, because coma is curable, whereas many complications of diabetes are not.

2. **Deaths Without Coma.**—(a) **Cardiorenal and Vascular.**—When patients ceased to die of coma, they lived to die of arteriosclerosis. In the Naunyn era the average age at death was forty-four and eight-tenths years; in the Charles H. Best era it is sixty-four years. It is not surprising that arteriosclerosis has advanced to first place as a cause of death, because the average diabetic is growing old. If one includes all the cases classified as cardiorenal-vascular and gangrene under this heading, it is responsible for 66.6 per cent of the total deaths now in contrast to 17.5 per cent in the Naunyn era. Fortunately in diabetes there is more chance of preventing excessive arteriosclerosis than has been usually supposed. (See page 496.) Irrespective of the possibility of the prevention of arteriosclerosis as a whole, there is a certainty that it can be prevented as a cause of death to large degree in the form in which it has been so fatal to diabetics in the past, namely, gangrene.

The most usual form for the arteriosclerosis to take is that which

[1] Joslin: Shattuck Lecture, Boston Med. and Surg. Jour., **186**, 833, 1922.

affects the heart. More than one-third (2517) of all the non-coma deaths since August, 1922 were due to heart disease. Coronary thrombosis is the common type and symptoms of angina pectoris are the most frequent. Next to the heart stands the brain as a site of arteriosclerosis. Under apoplexy, a total of 371 is reached in the Banting era, 309 in the Hagedorn era and 74 in the Charles H. Best era. Nephritis caused 40, or 6.1 per cent, of deaths since January 1, 1944. The gradual reduction in the percentage of deaths from gangrene since 1922 is due to improved prophylaxis, better surgery, and insulin, we believe, perhaps coincidental with a lessening of arteriosclerosis.

(*b*) **Infections.**—The advent of an infection lowers the tolerance of a diabetic for carbohydrate and this increases the severity of the disease. Since 1922 one new type of infection which has attained prominence is acute infection of the kidneys, due in its fatal form usually to blood-borne pyogenic infection. Sixty-nine such deaths are recorded. (See page 229.) The incidence of pneumonia and respiratory infections has declined in recent years. Carbuncles and abscesses, including mediastinal, as well as multiple superficial abscesses, caused 132 deaths. Diabetic patients do astonishingly well following operations upon tonsils and the mastoid. Other instances of infection undoubtedly occurred often during coma.

(*c*) **Cancer.**—Six hundred and thirty-five patients have died of cancer between 1922 and 1946. The per cent of all deaths due to cancer has increased from 1.5 in the Naunyn era to 8.9 in the Charles H. Best era, proving that the diabetic is living long enough to acquire diseases common to the community as a whole. The figure is high, partly because the cancer clinic at the Palmer Memorial (adjacent to and a part of the New England Deaconess Hospital) attracts many diabetics with cancer.

(*d*) **Tuberculosis.**—Since August, 1922, pulmonary tuberculosis has been responsible for the death of 248 cases. The medical profession has too pessimistic a view about this complication. When the treatment of the diabetes is faithfully carried out, these patients do quite well. The trouble in the past has been that consumption was usually advanced when diagnosed.

(*e*) **Inanition.**—Inanition first appeared as a cause of death in our mortality tables in 1916, but it has vanished as a cause of death since 1930.

(*f*) **Miscellaneous.**—Deaths from cirrhosis of the liver have increased to 60, and hemochromatosis caused 14 deaths. Pernicious anemia caused 13 deaths. Suicides, with 47 deaths, and accidents with 150 deaths, have increased most of all since the use of insulin, owing largely to the greater activity and longer duration of life. Diabetes alone appeared on the death certificate in 189 cases. The possible existence of tuberculosis, coronary disease or even coma in these cases, can only be surmised.

(*g*) **Needless Diabetic Deaths.**[1]—It is not customary in the tabulation of causes of death to include what is quite as important, namely, imperfect medical supervision, but we believe almost as many deaths to be chargeable to this deficiency as to any single factor. The needless mortality in diabetes is unfortunately greater than we realize. Diabetics seldom die of their disease *per se*, but of complications which are largely preventable, coma, gangrene, infections. Coma still is the chief preventable complication. Outside of the hospital it still occurs, but it rarely develops in a hospital, and patients who enter with it usually recover.

Deaths resulting from the omission of insulin can be traced to the advice of the laity or irregular practitioners and often to the patients themselves. For all such deaths one feels regret, but not the keen concern excited by deaths under supervision, trained, yet not quite free from errors of judgment. These deaths most commonly occur when the diet of a patient is suddenly changed. When the carbohydrate is restricted and protein and fat simultaneously increased, death from coma may take place the same week unless resort is had to insulin. How many such cases! Nearly all of us have one or more such sorrowful deaths to our discredit. It is, therefore, well to hold to the rule in severe, long-standing, complicated, obese and elderly cases, as well as in all cases with acidosis, to make changes in the diet gradually, not suddenly or radically.

Infections precipitate coma. It not infrequently happens that the infection is not recognized. Better statistics upon this point and in general about the circumstances attending coma should be accumulated. Early treatment of acidosis makes possible diagnosis of the accompanying pneumonia or renal infection before coma obscures the clinical picture. The use of penicillin or streptomycin will then save many a patient. Examples of latent infections are described in the section on Surgery. Appendicitis is one of the most important.

All cases of coma can be traced to increased metabolism, endogenous or exogenous, and in that metabolism fat and protein take an excessive share, because insulin is not available to lay its restraining hand on their catabolism. Sometimes the fat is taken in obvious excess, as happened when a diabetic, Case 1511, of long duration, living with little dietetic restriction, went to a fashionable hotel, suddenly decreased carbohydrate and made up by indulging to the limit in larded mushrooms. Remember that a little carbohydrate, utilized, goes a long way toward preventing coma in a mild or moderately severe case of diabetes. The diabetic dog, whether fat or fat-fed, is prone to coma. Beware before you expose a diabetic to a high-fat diet, whether endogenous or exogenous.

Omission of insulin is a most frequent cause of coma, but fortunately the patient usually escapes death. Not so with Case 4665,

---

[1] Joslin: Loc. cit., p. 230.

who took up Christian Science. Contrary to the Christian Science healer's advice she gave up insulin, and coma with death promptly ensued. A boy, Case 6033, omitted insulin and upon a layman's advice took herbs; the next he remembers was the attention of a doctor at the Deaconess Hospital.

Autopsies are necessary if a doctor wishes to have his case reports rated valid. It is altogether too easy to credit deaths to coma.

Gangrene stands next to coma as a preventable cause of death. This is the reason for our Beauty Parlor for Diabetics' Feet at the Deaconess Hospital. In the first place, injuries to the feet should not occur. A diabetic should keep his feet as clean as his face and protect them with equal care. Never allow one of your diabetic patients to develop gangrene ignorantly. Warning and admonition should penetrate so deeply the minds of your cases that if such a catastrophe should ever occur the unhappy patient will feel compelled to say: "Doctor, you warned me about injury to my feet, about the dangers in cutting corns, toe nails, about blisters from new shoes or old shoes with poor linings, about nails in my shoes, flat-foot plates and hot-water bags. You are not to blame for my present condition."

But what I consider of far more importance is the number of procrastinating cases of mild infections in mild diabetics, chiefly in their lower extremities, which frequently prove fatal. These conditions develop at a time of life when diabetes is mild. Why should they so frequently be fatal? Consider with what these mild cases of diabetes have to contend. Handicapped by a lingering infection, which only too often is allowed to continue for months, with kidneys less efficient for throwing off the attack of acidosis, deprived of exercise—that proved stimulus to sugar consumption—these pitiful patients used to meet a fourth enemy in ether anesthesia, unprotected by insulin. Is it any wonder that a formerly innocent disease became virulent and that the victim died of coma?

D. SUMMARY OF DIAGNOSES AT AUTOPSY.

The causes of death as *disclosed at autopsy* in 429 cases emphasize by their variety the many-sided problems of treatment. The complications were many; space forbids listing all the associated conditions. In Table 27 only diagnoses of genuine importance or interest are given. Thus, slight degrees of arteriosclerosis, bearing apparently little relation to the clinical condition of the patient, have not been counted. It is not the treatment of diabetes itself but rather the treatment of the complications which engrosses the time of the doctor.

In Table 27 a prime distinction has been made between cases who entered the hospital with diabetic coma, numbering 42, and cases in whom coma was not at any time present. Thus, among 42 cases with coma, 12 died without complications, whereas 30 recovered from coma but died of the complications. Among these complications it is evident that 20 were acute infections. Other complications present in these coma cases numbered 44. Among the infections, first place has been given to carbuncles, causing 14 deaths, because of its standing as a remediable condition under early treatment. Septicemia, arising in abscesses, renal foci, otitis media, caused 19 deaths, all in the period before the use of penicillin. Acute pulmonary infections caused 18 deaths in 84 cases.

TABLE 27.—CAUSES OF 429 DIABETIC DEATHS AND CHIEF COMPLICATIONS AT AUTOPSY. (George F. Baker Clinic—1923–1945.)

	Cause of death	Present as complication
I. *Coma*	12	30
II. *Alkalosis*	1	
III. *Hypoglycemia*	1	2
IV. *Inanition*	1	
V. *Infections:*		
A. Acute:		
1. Carbuncles	14	1
2. Abscesses	..	14
3. Cellulitis	6	6
4. Septicemia	19	13
5. Phlebitis	..	8
6. Osteomyelitis	1	2
7. Meningitis	1	3
8. Sinusitis	3	2
9. Appendicitis	5	
B. Chronic:		
1. Tuberculosis	7	12
2. Syphilis	1	5
VI. *Diseases of respiratory tract:*		
A. Abscess of lung	4	2
B. Pulmonary infections, acute	18	66
C. Empyema	..	12
D. Asthma	1	
VII. *Tumors:*		
A. Carcinoma of pancreas	9	1
B. Carcinomata	36	10
C. Sarcomas	3	1
VIII. *Diseases of blood:*		
A. Pernicious anemia	..	1
B. Leukemia	2	
C. Purpura hemorrhagica	1	
IX. *Diseases of bones and joints:*		
A. Paget's disease	..	1
B. Atrophic arthritis	..	2
C. Fractures	..	2
X. *Diseases of circulatory system:*		
A. Coronary sclerosis	6	137
B. Coronary occlusion with infarction	87	26
C. Myocardial failure	18	68
D. Cardiac hypertrophy	..	180
E. Pericarditis	5	15
F. Endocarditis	1	4
G. Rheumatic valvular disease	2	11
H. Mesenteric thrombosis	2	1
I. Pancreatic apoplexy	1	
J. Pulmonary embolus	15	23

TABLE 27.—CAUSES OF 429 DIABETIC DEATHS AND CHIEF COMPLICATIONS AT AUTOPSY. (George F. Baker Clinic—1923–1945.)—(*Continued.*)

	Cause of death	Present as complicatiou
K. Emboli, misc.	1	2
L. Gangrene	53	15
M. Cerebral thrombosis, hemorrhage	20	8
N. Arteriosclerosis	1	287
O. Periarteritis nodosa	1	
XI. Thyroid disease:		
A. Adenomas	..	30
B. Primary hyperthyroidism	1	4
XII. Pregnancy	1	
XIII. Diseases of digestive system:		
A. Cirrhosis of liver	3	19
B. Hepatitis, acute	1	2
C. Hemochromatosis	5	3
D. Cholecystitis	7	84
E. Perforation of gall-bladder	1	1
F. Intestinal obstruction	2	1
G. Duodenal ulcer	2	6
H. Acute pancreatitis	3	2
I. Ulcerative colitis	1	
J. Hernia incarcerated	2	
XIV. Genito-urinary disease:		
A. Intercapillary glomerulosclerosis	3	8
B. Pyelonephritis	15	35
C. Hydronephrosis	1	3
D. Nephritis, all other forms	15	107
E. Perinephritic abscess	4	2
F. Urinary calculi	1	12
G. Benign prostatic hypertrophy	2	28

Carcinomata of various organs, including 10 instances involving the pancreas, were present in 56 cases. The two largest groups of causes of death consist of conditions consequent upon coronary disease, 93, and gangrene, which was present in 53 cases. Chronic degenerative diseases of the kidneys have steadily increased as a cause of death in recent years. Comparison between the frequency of certain lesions and their incidence of actual causes of death has been noted. Pulmonary embolism caused 15 deaths but occurred in another 23 cases. Intercapillary glomerulosclerosis was recorded in 11 cases.

CHAPTER VII

THE EXAMINATION OF THE URINE AND THE BLOOD IN DIABETES.

Revised by Alexander Marble, M.D.

A. THE EXAMINATION OF THE URINE.

1. **The Importance of Routine Examinations of Urine.**—An early diagnosis in diabetes is as important as in tuberculosis. The diagnosis is made largely from the examination of the urine and since the disease usually begins insidiously, its prompt detection depends upon the routine testing of the urine not only of all patients regardless of whether or not symptoms of the disease are present, but also of the supposedly healthy.

In all illnesses urine examinations should be made for albumin and sugar, and invariably at the last medical visit of a series the doctor should secure a specimen of urine for the patient's and his own protection. Never allow a new patient to leave the office without obtaining a specimen of urine. Do not trust to the patient's sending a twenty-four-hour sample. It is especially desirable to secure a specimen of urine within two hours after a hearty meal since it is not uncommon for this sample to contain sugar, while one obtained fasting or two or three hours later may be sugar-free. The importance of securing several samples, particularly in doubtful cases, cannot be overemphasized; the specimen voided on rising may be sugar-free when specimens voided later contain sugar.

Neglect in examining the urine of any case coming for treatment may bring embarrassing or even disastrous results. The wealthy parents of Case 1123 built a hospital for their community, but two doctors failed to examine the urine of their child and diabetes was diagnosed by a nurse. Similarly, the parents of Case 2568 took the precaution to send their children for medical inspection prior to an European trip, but examinations of the urine were omitted and the diagnosis of diabetes postponed for a year, to the sorrow and chagrin of the doctor. The physician who was called to see Case 12139 failed to examine the urine, failed to recognize the condition of on-coming acidosis, and the patient died in diabetic coma thirty-six hours later, four hours after he was brought to the hospital in a moribund state. The physician of Case 18373, seen for the first time in diabetic coma, had told the patient one week previously that the abnormal thirst was due to hard work. Case 17523, an eighteen-year-old student nurse in a hospital in a neighboring city, was sent home from training school because of weakness, but no physical examination or examination of the urine was made. She was admitted the next day to the New England Deaconess Hospital

(236)

in diabetic coma and died twenty-three hours after admission of pneumonia and an abscess of the right labium with septicemia and involvement of heart, kidneys, and right adrenal.

Examination of the urine should cost the patient little. Recognized essentials alone should find place in the report, which in turn should be expressed in the simplest terms and not be designed to impress patients. When one sees two or even four full pages covered with a single urine report and padded printed matter, yet at times showing on the face of it that modern analytical methods were not employed, one blushes for the profession. When a urine report was shown for which a boy's father had paid $10 it was with considerable satisfaction that the child was taught to do the qualitative Benedict test for sugar, the materials for which can be purchased for 1 cent.

Coöperative laboratories should be established even in small communities so that routine urine and blood tests can be performed near the homes of patients. Such laboratories can be branches of larger ones in which the more unusual and complicated tests can be done. A laboratory may be life-saving, because with its help a patient in diabetic coma may receive insulin more promptly and a patient in hypoglycemia may be spared a death-dealing dose of insulin. It is imperative that a hospital laboratory furnish service in emergencies at any hour, nights, Sundays and holidays. A competent technician, not a poorly trained substitute, should be constantly on call to do thoroughly reliable work at times of real need.

2. **The Volume of Urine in Twenty-four Hours.**—The average normal quantity of urine is 1200 to 1500 cc. (40 to 50 ounces) a day. In diabetic patients the amount frequently parallels the quantity of sugar eliminated, but the relationship between volume, specific gravity, and sugar percentage is by no means invariably close. Moreover, the volume of urine voided in twenty-four hours may give but little index of the severity of diabetes. Cases of "diabetes decipiens" are common. The twenty-four-hour quantity of urine may be normal and yet contain a large amount of sugar. Case 8 showed 5 per cent of sugar in 1030 cc. of urine, Case 340 5.8 per cent in 1860 cc. of urine, and Case 356 5.8 per cent of sugar in 1035 cc. of urine. Therefore, although it is unusual for the urine to be normal in quantity, unless the patient is sugar-free this is by no means always the case and such a history is no excuse for the neglect of a urine examination.

The greatest volume of urine in twenty-four hours, in comparison to the weight of the patient, was voided by Case 1151, who developed diabetes at the age of three years, and came at the age of ten years, weighing 18.6 kilograms, in October, 1916. During the first sixteen hours in the hospital the volume of urine was 7200 cc. and for the following twenty-four hours 7000 cc. Case 2448, a seventeen-year-old boy, weighing 50.5 kilograms, voided 8800 cc. of urine during the first twenty-four hours in the hospital. Since the percentage of sugar was 7.5, a total of 660 grams, or 22 ounces, of sugar was excreted during this period.

The volume of urine should be expressed in cubic centimeters. This enables the amount of sugar in the twenty-four-hour quantity of urine to be most readily calculated. An ounce of urine is actually 29.6 cc., but in clinical work one may reckon it as 30 cc. because the errors in collection of urine more than offset the trifling error in the equivalent. Likewise 1 quart of urine is equivalent to 946 cc., but sufficiently accurate figures are obtainable, except for scientific experiments, if we consider 1 quart of urine 1000 cc. Naturally, such methods are absolutely barred when careful investigative work is being done. To facilitate measurement of the volume of the urine, wide-mouthed, stoppered bottles, of 2000 cc. capacity graduated at intervals of 50 cc., may be employed. If at all possible, the container for collection of the twenty-four hour amount should be kept in the cold; if left at room temperature, the addition of a few cubic centimeters of xylol as a preservative is desirable.

3. **The Specific Gravity.**—The normal average specific gravity of the urine is about 1.017 to 1.020. The specific gravity of the urine in uncontrolled diabetes is usually high, and in Case 18477 a value of 1.054 was found in a specimen containing 14 per cent sugar. On the other hand, Case 38 showed sugar in the urine with a specific gravity of 1.007; Case 1673 had 0.34 per cent sugar with a specific gravity of 1.006; and Case 1151, 0.3 per cent, with a specific gravity of 1.004. In a series of 147 routine examinations of diabetic urine specimens selected for study because the specific gravity was 1.010 or below in each case, John[1] obtained a positive test for sugar in 72.5 per cent. A low specific gravity, therefore, is no more excuse for neglecting to examine the urine than is a normal quantity of urine.

4. **Sugars of Normal Urine.**—It has long been known that the urine of presumably normal individuals gives the usual copper reduction tests characteristic of sugar if sufficiently sensitive reagents are used; the amount of these substances is found to vary between 0.01 and 0.1 per cent. The nature of these reducing substances (non-nitrogenous) was a subject for controversy for years. S. R. Benedict[2] observed that in normal people there is often a greater excretion of reducing substances following ingestion of carbohydrate, if a sufficient amount be given; to this he gave the name "glycuresis." He maintained that the factors which lead to this excretion of a small amount of sugar following a meal are usually the same as those which lead to the concomitant elevation of blood sugar and regarded the sugar in the urine of diabetics as

[1] John: Jour. Am. Med. Assn., **81**, 1939, 1923.
[2] Benedict, Osterberg and Neuwirth: Jour. Biol. Chem., **34**, 217, 1918; **55**, 769 1923.

representing only a quantitative exaggeration of a preëxisting normal excretion. On the other hand, Folin and Berglund[1] maintained that the sugar of normal urine has no relation to the main carbohydrate metabolism and that it consists of foreign unusable carbohydrate materials found in grains, vegetables and fruits, and in decomposition products resulting from the preparation of foods. Folin believed that "glycuresis" is independent of the blood-sugar level.

In 1931, Peters and Van Slyke,[2] in concluding a discussion of this subject, stated: "The available data taken together indicate that the actual glucose content of ordinary human urine, of the order of magnitude of 0.001 per cent, is not increased by variations in food intake within ordinary limits. Conditions that have been found to cause melituria detectable by the ordinary qualitative tests appear to cause excretion of genuine glucose. Apparently until the glucose threshold of the body is reached, only a minimal amount of glucose passes into the urine. Then an entirely different mechanism is set in order, and glucose is excreted at a rate exceeding many fold its ordinary physiological excretion. It is as though the flood gates were kept almost tightly closed until a certain pressure opened them, but that when they were opened glucose poured out in relatively large amounts. The rate of output is variable, but altogether of greater order than the ordinary leakage of questionable traces. There occurs a true glycosuria, a phenomenon altogether different from the usual slight excretion of almost entirely non-glucose-reducing substances."

5. **Glucose in Urine.** (Dextrose, $C_6H_{12}O_6$).—The quantity of sugar in the urine should be recorded in per cent and in grams for the twenty-four hours. The clinic upon diabetes given by Friedrich Muller at the Boston City Hospital, in which he illustrated the total amount of sugar voided by the patient by exhibiting an equivalent amount of cane sugar, was most impressive to patient and student. One may to advantage employ this method in teaching; it never fails that some in the audience appear astonished at the pound of sugar, more or less, which has been excreted in twenty-four hours. The pound, not the percentage, leaves the desired indelible impression.

In most chronic diseases there is no criterion by which the success or failure of treatment can be readily estimated. Fortunately, in diabetes, one can tell when treatment is successful, for the patient should be free from sugar and diacetic acid and be happy and vigorous. While the twenty-four-hour quantity of sugar in the urine is not an absolute measure of the degree of control of diabetes, still in the vast majority of cases it is an accurate index.

The sugar in the urine of diabetic patients usually varies directly

---

[1] Folin and Berglund: Jour. Biol. Chem., **51**, 213, 1922.

[2] Peters and Van Slyke: Quantitative Clinical Chemistry, Baltimore, Williams & Wilkins Company, **1**, 132, 1931.

with the quantity of carbohydrate-forming material in the diet, to a lesser extent with the protein, still less with fat, except as that influences the total caloric intake. A change of diet is shown in the urine within a few hours and sugar may appear within a few minutes after food.

(*a*) **Qualitative Tests.**—Many of the qualitative tests for glucose are excellent, and nearly all have the advantage that although mere traces of sugar may be present in the urine of normal individuals, they fail to demonstrate its presence unless the sugar exists in an amount greater than normal. The Benedict test is the one most generally useful. It requires a single solution, keeps indefinitely, and the reaction offers less chance of error in that it is so adjusted as to be rather more sensitive to glucose than Fehling's solution and is not reduced by creatinine or uric acid, or by chloroform which is at times used as a urine preservative.

Benedict's Test.—The test is carried out as follows: Four (not more) drops of the urine to be examined are placed in the test-tube and to this are added 2.5 cc. (an ordinary teaspoon holds about 5 cc.) of Benedict's solution. Eight drops of urine and 5 cc. of Benedict's solution are often employed, but the use of half-quantities is just as satisfactory and more economical. The tube is shaken to mix the urine and solution and then placed in water that is already boiling. If a number of tests are to be made at once, time may be saved by use of a large water-bath and a wire test-tube rack. After being in the boiling water for five minutes, the tube or rack is removed and examined for evidence of reduction. In the presence of glucose the entire body of the solution will be filled with a precipitate, which may be greenish, yellow or red in color, according to whether the amount of sugar is slight or considerable. Particularly, if 4 drops are used with 2.5 cc. of Benedict's solution, the test should be carried out in bubbling boiling water rather than over a free flame, because of evaporation of the solution. If 5 cc. of Benedict's solution and 8 drops of urine are employed, as in the original test, the solution may be boiled over a free flame for two minutes in which case a Pyrex test-tube should be used.

As used with urine the test is sufficiently delicate to detect quantities as small as 0.08 or 0.1 per cent sugar, in which case a faint pea-green change in color takes place. This green color changes to a yellowish-green when the urine contains about 0.5 per cent sugar. When the solution loses the greenish tint entirely and becomes yellow or brown, the urine contains over 1 per cent sugar. Above this percentage the color of the solution gives very little aid in estimating the amount of sugar in the urine, although large amounts of sugar will produce an orange or a brick-red test. The entire amount of copper in the 2.5 cc. of solution may be reduced (as determined by allowing the test to stand and observing a water-clear supernatant fluid) by a urine of approximately 1.5 per cent glucose content or greater. Rarely urines are tested which give a fluorescent appearance, due to a very fine, brick-red precipitation of the copper oxide. This seems to occur with severe diabetics who show sugar after eating certain fruits, are on low diets and void large quantities of urine. Its appearance is related to the rapidity of reduction. It is so slight in amount that one is thrown off guard as to the amount of glucose present in the urine. On titration it is often found that there may be as much as 1 per cent sugar in a urine which tested qualitatively might be estimated as 0.2 per cent.

The presence of a large amount of phosphate in the urine may produce a flocculent precipitate upon boiling with the copper reagent, but such a falsely positive test is very easily distinguished by the fact that it is not green but blue and also that it is coarsely flocculent and not in the fine suspension that the oxide of copper exhibits. Another source of falsely positive tests occurs when the urine is concentrated, amounting in twenty-four hours to less than 1000 cc.; under such circumstances creatinine is probably the disturbing factor. It should also be remembered that lactose will reduce Benedict's reagent, and positive tests during the latter months of pregnancy are not at all infrequent. Fermentation of such a urine will help to differentiate lactose from glucose but, as Castellani and Taylor[1] have pointed out, many samples of baker's yeast ferment lactose with gas production, so that this test cannot by any means be taken as infallible. Levulose and pentose reduce Benedict's solution even at room temperature if the test is set up and allowed to stand for a few hours or at 50° to 60° C. for ten minutes. (See pages 244 and 801.)

From time to time various modifications of Benedict's test have been devised. One of these is the "Clinitest"[2] in which a reagent tablet is dropped into a measured amount of diluted urine. Heat is generated within the test-tube, causing boiling which lasts a few seconds. The colors produced by varying amounts of sugar are those of the standard Benedict test and interpretations are made accordingly. A color scale allows for the estimation of approximate percentages of sugar.

In addition to the procedures which depend upon the reduction by sugar of copper in alkaline solutions (Benedict's, Haines', Trommer's and Fehling's tests), there are other methods such as that of Nylander. This test depends upon the reduction of bismuth in alkaline solution. A modification of this is to be had in the "Galatest"[3] in which is used a gray alkaline powder containing bismuth. A drop or two of urine is placed on a small mound of the powder;

[1] Castellani and Taylor: Jour. Am. Med. Assn., **86**, 523, 1926.

[2] The Clinitest apparatus and tablets are made by the Ames Company, Inc., Elkhart, Indiana.

[3] "Galatest": The "Galatest" powder is made by the Denver Chemical Manufacturing Company, 163 Varick Street, New York, N. Y.

16

the presence of sugar in the urine is indicated by the production of a gray or black color (reduction of the bismuth). The reaction is complete in less than thirty seconds.

(b) **Quantitative Tests.**—The more accurate of the quantitative procedures require a laboratory, but methods sufficiently correct for clinical work can easily be performed by the general practitioner, the nurse, or by more intelligent patients in the home. In fact, a reasonable approximation of the percentage of sugar in the urine may be obtained with the "Clinitest" apparatus described above and the Sheftel method mentioned later. Simplification of the treatment of diabetes means everything to the practitioner and to the patient.

The highest percentage of sugar found in the urine of our patients was with Cases 2292 and 18477. When Case 2292 first came for treatment on July 23, 1921, the urine had a specific gravity of 1.045 and contained 14 per cent sugar. The quantitative analyses were checked twice by Dr. H. F. Root. This patient, now taking insulin, was reported to be alive and well in October, 1945. At the first visit of Case 18477 on December 6, 1939, the first specimen of urine had a specific gravity of 1.054 and contained 14 per cent sugar. A second specimen had a specific gravity of 1.053 and contained 13.2 per cent sugar. This patient was reported alive and well in November, 1944.

The quantitative tests listed below are those which we have found to be most practical. These various methods are described in the original articles and in standard books on laboratory procedures; accordingly, for the most part they are given brief mention here.

1. *Original Method of Benedict.*[1] This original method is the one from which the various modifications have been devised. It is now used very little in our laboratory or in the laboratory of the New England Deaconess Hospital, but it is regarded as the method of choice when definitely accurate determinations are desired. The method is based on the fact that in alkaline solution a given quantity of glucose reduces a definite amount of copper, precipitating it as cuprous sulphocyanate, which, being snow-white, is an aid to accurate observation of the disappearance of the last trace of color.

2. *The Micro-modification of Benedict's Test.*—This method, devised by Millard Smith,[2] is the one which we use routinely. The test can be performed in a minimum of time, is simple, and if carefully carried out furnishes sufficiently reliable data. It is not necessary to calculate the final percentage of sugar, for this can be read directly on the special pipette used for titrating. The method is described in detail below.

---

[1] Benedict: Jour. Am. Med. Assn., **57**, 1193, 1911.
[2] Smith: Jour. Lab. and Clin. Med., **7**, 364, 1922.

The apparatus[1] needed consists of a small ring stand with test-tube clamp, a micro-Bunsen burner or small alcohol lamp, a pyrex test-tube (18 by 160 mm.), a Millard Smith pipette No. 2 and one 1-cc. Ostwald pipette.

With the Ostwald pipette transfer 1 cc. of Benedict's original quantitative solution into the test-tube (held in the ring-stand clamp) and then add 0.2 to 0.7 gram of anhydrous sodium carbonate. A small well-dried pebble, a piece of quartz, or a pinch of talcum powder should also be added to prevent bumping.

Heat the mixture to boiling and add the urine from the Smith pipette until reduction is complete, as evidenced by the disappearance of the blue color. Read the percentage of sugar directly from the pipette. Urine specimens expected to contain 1 per cent or less of sugar may be titrated directly, while those containing over 1 per cent are diluted (1 to 10 or 1 to 20) before titration. All dilutions of the urine reduce, of course, the accuracy of the results obtained, due to lowered concentration of the urinary salts.

For *rapid* reduction of the reagent vigorous boiling is essential, which may result in too rapid evaporation. This is avoided by allowing more time for reduction between additions of urine.

The best results are obtained if the urine is added slowly and if the solution is kept at the boiling-point by manipulation of the flame. A very small flame should be employed. *The tendency in the titration is to go past the end-point, since the reduction does not take place as rapidly as in many titrations to which one is accustomed. When nearing the end-point the urine must be added slowly.* In urine of low sugar content the boiling should be rather vigorous at first in order to maintain a constant volume, while 1 to 2 cc. of urine necessary to give complete reduction are being added. With a moderate amount of practice the regulation of the volume of the boiling solution becomes quite simple.

3. *Sheftel's Method.*—Sheftel[2] has devised a method in which the colors produced by the reduction of a copper reagent are compared with those of a semi-permanent color chart. It is simple to carry out and may be used by the patient in the home.

4. *Polariscopy and Fermentation.*—One may determine the amount of sugar by polariscopy or by fermentation but these methods are by no means as accurate or satisfactory as chemical methods and are now seldom used.

6. **Tests for Other Sugars.**—Sugars other than glucose are found in urine sufficiently often to make it imperative that one ascertain the type of sugar excreted in all cases of non-diabetic melituria. This can be done most conveniently by taking advantage of the

[1] This may be purchased from many surgical supply houses or from the manufacturers, Emil Greiner Company, 55 Vandam St., New York City.

[2] Sheftel: Med. Jour. and Rec., **126**, 663, 1927. See also Rhodehamel, Rose and Chen: Med. Rec., **145**, 324, 1937. Apparatus and reagents may be purchased from Eli Lilly & Co., Indianapolis, Ind.

fact that sugars found in urine reduce copper solutions[1] and the di-sodium-di-nitro-salicylate reagent of Exton[2] at differing rates and temperatures. For further discussion consult Chapter XXX on Non-diabetic Glycosuria.

(a) **Lactose.** $(C_{12}H_{22}O_{11})$.—Lactose in the urine may give rise to confusion in the performance of Fehling's or Benedict's tests. Fortunately, the condition in which it characteristically occurs, namely, lactation, is usually known to the physician, and it is then not considered of significance. It has also been found in the urines of nurslings. Lactose, like glucose, reduces copper, is dextro-rotatory, but it yields a characteristic osazone with phenylhydrazine and is not fermented by pure yeast. However, the osazone is very difficult to obtain from the urine and ordinary yeast is not to be depended upon for the fermentation test. Rubner's test and the mucic acid test for lactose are described in texts of laboratory procedures.

(b) **Pentose.** $(C_5H_{10}O_5)$.—Pentoses are occasionally present in the urine and possess along with levulose the property of reducing Benedict's solution at room temperature over a period of a few hours or at 50° to 60° C. in ten minutes. At boiling temperature the reduction by pentose begins within one minute of the time the tube is placed in the water-bath. It is well to note that urine containing large amounts of dextrose may also give a positive Benedict's test which slowly develops without heating. Pentose is not fermented by yeast and is not optically active. It may be detected by the Bial test.

Orcinol— Hydrochloric Acid (Bial) Test.—Bial's reagent has the following composition:

Orcinol	1.5 grams
Fuming HCl	500 grams
Ferric chloride (10 per cent)	20 to 30 drops

To 5 cc. of the reagent in a test-tube add 2 to 3 cc. of urine and heat the mixture gently until the first bubbles rise to the surface. Immediately or upon cooling, the solution becomes green and a flocculent precipitate of the same color may form.

To date we have recorded only 9 cases of essential pentosuria despite a constant search for such among patients with normo-glycemic melituria. (See page 802.)

(c) **Fructose (Levulose)**, $C_6H_{12}O_6$.—Fructose is said to be present frequently in the urine of patients with severe diabetes. It is levorotatory, but so is β-oxybutyric acid, which is found under similar conditions. Levulose is fermented by yeast; like pentose, gives a positive Fehling and Benedict test after several hours even without heating or within ten minutes at 50° to 60° C.; and yields the same osazone as does

---

[1] Lasker and Enklewitz: Jour. Biol. Chem., **101**, 289, 1933.

[2] Exton: New York State Jour. Med., **36**, 1545, 1936. Exton, Rose and Roehl: Proc. Am. Life. Insur. Med. Dir. America, **22**, 288, 1935.

dextrose with phenylhydrazine. With methyl-phenylhydrazine it gives a characteristic osazone, however. Levulose can be differentiated by the Seliwanoff reaction, provided the test is carefully performed and certain precautions followed. This test is carried out as follows:

Place in a test-tube equal quantities (2 or 3 cc.) of urine and 25 per cent hydrochloric acid. Bring to boiling over a free flame. Add a few crystals of resorcinol and boil actively for ten seconds. If levulose is present, almost immediately the solution becomes red and a dense reddish-brown precipitate forms. This precipitate is entirely soluble in alcohol.

We have recognized only four instances of essential fructosuria. (See page 805.)

(*d*) **Maltose** ($C_{12}H_{22}O_{11}$).—Maltose very rarely occurs in human urine, and has not been shown to be of clinical significance.

(*e*) **Sucrose** ($C_{12}H_{22}O_{11}$).—The finding of sucrose, or cane-sugar, in the urine has been reported only rarely except, of course, following the injection of this sugar intravenously, in which case it is promptly excreted, since under these conditions there is no provision for hydrolyzing it to simpler sugars. Spontaneous sucrosuria has no clinical significance. Elmer[1] reported 2 cases and cited the relevant literature. A striking feature of his patients was the high specific gravity of the urine, reaching values as high as 1.070.

(*f*) **Mannoheptulose.**—Following the ingestion by 10 normal persons of 136 to 214 gm. of avocado, mannoheptulose (a non-fermentable sugar which reduces Benedict's solution in the cold as do pentose and fructose) appeared in the urine in amounts from 0.06 to 0.32 per cent.[2]

(*g*) **Substances Found in the Urine Which Give Rise to Confusion in Testing for Sugar.**—Very few substances interfere with the accuracy of the Benedict test, although Fehling's test may be misleading in more instances. Of those met with in normal urine, creatinine and uric acid are the most common.

Glycuronic acid as such is not found in fresh urines, but conjugated glycuronic acids occurring in the urine spontaneously decompose and may cause confusion. Such conjugated glycuronic acids only appear after the ingestion of chloral hydrate, camphor, menthol, turpentine or phenol in large enough quantities to be of significance. If this point is borne in mind confusion will not arise. Glycuronic acid reduces copper and bismuth, but is not fermented by yeast. It may be difficult to detect in the presence of pentose, although one can rely on the characteristic osazone of pentose if differentiation becomes necessary.

Alcaptonuria deserves mention because the homogentisic acid (dihydroxyphenyl acetic acid) which is present in the urine of such cases reduces alkaline copper solutions, giving thus a falsely positive

[1] Elmer: Pol. Arch. Med., Wown., **16**, 449, 1938; Pol. Gaz. Lek., **17**, 491, 1938
[2] Blatherwick, Larson and Sawyer. Jour. Biol. Chem., **133**, 643, 1940.

test for sugar. Urine containing this oxyacid turns dark brown or black if it is allowed to stand exposed to the air and if alkali be added or if the urine becomes alkaline through ammoniacal putre-faction. The urine may frequently be dark even when voided. We have not encountered alcaptonuria.

7. Methods for the Determination of the Urinary Acids.—At the present time, in our experience both with hospitalized and ambulant diabetic patients, acidosis as demonstrated by a positive Gerhardt or Rothera test is relatively infrequent.

(a) **Qualitative Tests.**—1. *Diacetic Acid.* (CH_3COCH_2COOH).— The simplest method for the detection of acidosis by urine exam-ination is Gerhardt's ferric chloride reaction for diacetic acid (aceto-acetic acid). This test may be performed as follows: To 5 or 10 cc. of freshly voided urine carefully add a few drops of a 10 per cent aqueous solution of ferric chloride. A precipitate of ferric phosphate first forms, but upon the addition of a few more drops is dissolved. The depth of the Burgundy-red color obtained is an index to the quantity of diacetic acid present. The intensity of the reaction may be roughly recorded as 1, 2, 3 or 4+. Benedict and Joslin[1] have pointed out the unreliability of such a designation in a quanti-tative way.

Diacetic acid occurs in the urine in the same conditions as acetone and rarely is found except associated with acetone. The latter represents diacetic acid from which in the process of decompo-sition one molecule of CO_2 has been removed. If very little diacetic acid is formed it may be entirely transformed into acetone, whereas if a larger quantity is produced both acetone and diacetic acid may be present in the urine.

It should not be forgotten that if a patient is taking salicylates, antipyrin, cyanates, or acetates, the foregoing test will give a somewhat similar reaction, but one that cannot be mistaken if the solution is boiled for two minutes. Diacetic acid is unstable and any color it causes will disappear upon boiling, whereas the red color caused by any of the above substances does not disappear upon boiling. Diabetic patients often take salicylates for pain of one kind or another, and, therefore, one must always be on the watch for this possibility.

As a routine procedure the sodium nitroprusside test should be performed on all urine specimens which give a red color with the Gerhardt test which does not fade upon boiling. In this way acetone bodies masked by the "drug reaction" can be detected.

2. *Acetone.* (CH_3COCH_3).—Folin[2] called attention to the fact that in strictly fresh urines containing "acetone bodies," the quantity of diacetic acid is nine or ten times that of acetone. The older the

[1] Benedict and Joslin: Metabolism in Diabetes Mellitus, Carnegie Inst. of Washington, Publ. 136, 1910, p. 25.

[2] Folin: Laboratory Manual of Biological Chemistry, 5th ed., New York, D. Appleton-Century Company, Inc., p. 211, 1934.

urine, the greater becomes the relative proportion of acetone, because of the spontaneous decomposition of the acetoacetic acid. The Rothera test given below is much more sensitive for acetoacetic acid than for acetone.

The simplest and most reliable test for acetone plus diacetic acid is a modification of Rothera's test. The reagent is prepared as follows: Dry sodium nitroprusside is ground to a fine powder and mixed with dry ammonium sulphate in the proportions of 5 grams of sodium nitroprusside to 200 grams of ammonium sulphate. The resulting mixture has a pale pink color; it is stable and may be kept indefinitely, thus being much more satisfactory than the usual 5 per cent solution of sodium nitroprusside which should be prepared fresh nearly every time it is used.

To perform the test for acetone proceed as follows: Place 2 or 3 cc. of urine in a test-tube, saturate with the nitroprusside mixture described above and overlay with a small quantity of strong ammonia water. In the presence of diacetic acid and acetone a strong purple color is rapidly developed at the juncture of the two liquids. At the end of two or three minutes the maximum color appears and the test may be read. Since the color slowly turns into a muddy brown, one should read the test before this occurs. A little practice enables one to tell the point of maximum color formation. A positive test is evidenced by a range of color from a faint purplish-pink to a very dark purple and may be recorded as 1, 2, 3 or 4+.

If preferred, the test may be done in the following way: Add 1 to 2 cc. of 10 per cent acetic acid and a small crystal of sodium nitroprusside to 5 cc. of urine in a test-tube. Shake, add 2 to 3 cc. of strong ammonia water, and shake again. A purple color indicates diacetic acid and acetone and the reaction is read as described above.

There are available certain especially prepared nitroprusside reagents in powder or tablet form which permit the rapid detection of acetone in the urine.[1]

3. *β-oxybutyric Acid.* ($CH_3CH(OH)$ CH_2COOH).—There is no simple qualitative test for β-oxybutyric acid.

(*b*) **Quantitative Tests.**—The determination of the extent of the acidosis is of prime importance in the treatment of any case of severe diabetes. Fortunately, comparatively simple methods are at hand which are quite satisfactory in routine treatment, but even most of these simple methods are too complicated for a physician with a large practice who has only a few cases of diabetes in the course of a year.

1. *Reaction of Urine.*—The most easily performed of the urine tests is concerned with its reaction. The total titratable acidity is a good index of the amount of acidosis and runs parallel with the

---

[1] Such preparations are made by the Ames Co., Inc., Elkhart, Indiana; Brewer and Co., Inc., Worcester, Mass., and Denver Chemical Mfg. Co., Inc., New York, N. Y.

ammonia excretion. For details of the determination, consult standard laboratory texts.

2. *Ammonia.*—The quantity of ammonia in the urine is a measure of the reaction of the body to counteract the acidosis produced in it. To this extent its estimation gives a more accurate idea of the acid production of the body than any other of the urine tests at our disposal, which simply show the quantity of acid leaving the body. The test, however, becomes of less value as soon as extraneous alkali is administered, because under such conditions the ingested alkali is used by the body in preference to ammonia. The normal amount of ammonia nitrogen in the urine varies between 0.5 and 1 gram per day, and the ratio between the ammonia nitrogen and the total nitrogen in the urine is fairly constant at 1 to 25 (4 per cent). In severe diabetes the ammonia may gradually increase, and in Case 344 it amounted to 8 grams in one day. The total nitrogen upon this same day was 19.2 grams, giving an ammonia nitrogen-nitrogen ratio of 34.3 per cent. On another day this ratio reached 44.4 per cent, but the absolute quantity of ammonia was only 4.4 grams and the nitrogen 8.7. Case 208 had an ammonia nitrogen-nitrogen ratio of 53 per cent when the total nitrogen excretion was 9.2 grams and the ammonia nitrogen amounted to 4.9 grams. These high ammonia nitrogen-nitrogen ratios are ordinarily obtained only when the total quantity of nitrogen in the urine is small. The two procedures which we have employed for the determination of ammonia are the aëration method and the permutit method, as described by Folin.[1]

3. *β-oxybutyric Acid.*—The tests for β-oxybutyric acid are all complicated, because they depend upon the extraction of the acid. However, in urine containing significant amounts of ketone acids, β-oxybutyric acid makes up about two-thirds of the total "acetone bodies" and may be determined along with the other ketone acids by a modification of Nanavutty's[2] blood acetone method. For further details, reference is made to original articles and standard laboratory texts.

8. **Nitrogen.**—The determination of the nitrogen in the urine is valuable because it furnishes an index to the quantity of protein which the patient is metabolizing. Incidentally, this is the easiest way to determine the quantity of protein in the diet, provided the calories utilizable are adequate. Since nitrogen constitutes 16 per cent of the protein molecule, one can multiply the quantity of nitrogen obtained in the urine by $6\frac{1}{4}$ to obtain the protein which it represents. One will not be far wrong if to this one adds 1 gram of nitrogen per day to offset the nitrogen of the feces, and considers this total quantity as representing the protein in the food. The determination of the nitrogen is also valuable because it is often

---

[1] Folin: Pp. 127 and 141, loc. cit., p. 246.
[2] Nanavutty: Jour. Biol. Chem., **26**, 1391, 1932.

useful to know the ammonia nitrogen-nitrogen ratio as well as the dextrose-nitrogen ratio. Formerly large quantities of nitrogen were obtained in the urines of diabetic patients, but improved treatment and modern diets make these excessive amounts rare, because abnormal tissue breakdown is prevented.

A daily analysis for nitrogen is time-consuming, but it is a simple matter to aliquot specimens of urine for a week and then obtain the average nitrogen excretion per day. If albumin is present in the urine, to be tested quantitatively for nitrogen, it must be removed before the nitrogen determination is made.

Simple methods by which the nitrogen in the urine may be determined may be found in Folin's Manual[1] and other laboratory texts.

9. **Albumin.**—The test for albumin in the urine should be performed at frequent intervals during the care of diabetic patients. The diagnosis of diabetes should not lead to neglect of the general treatment of the case.

We formerly employed two tests for albumin in the urine: that with sulphosalicylic acid (2 per cent in 0.5 per cent acetic acid) and that with Roberts' reagent (1 volume concentrated HNO_3 and 5 volumes of a saturated solution of $MgSO_4$). More recently we have routinely carried out a quantitative estimation of the amount of albumin by a simple, rapid technique described by Kingsbury, Clark, Williams and Post.[2] This method consists of adding 4.5 cc. of 3 per cent sulphosalicylic acid to 1.5 cc. of clear, centrifuged urine in a specially marked tube, mixing, letting stand for ten minutes, and comparing the turbidity produced with that in standard tubes. It is much more satisfactory to express the amount of albumin in terms of milligrams per 100 cc. of urine rather than in the indefinite terms of a slightest possible trace, very slight trace, etc.

10. **Casts.**—From the time of Külz the irritation of the kidneys in the first stages of diabetic coma has been observed. Repeatedly we have seen typical "showers" of granular casts in the urine of patients in diabetic coma. They may occur at times when the amount of albumin in the urine is small and by no means necessarily indicate a poor prognosis. Usually the appearance of casts during coma is the expression of acute temporary damage to the kidneys and is not necessarily an indication of an underlying nephritis.

11. **Chlorides.**—The remarkable changes in weight of diabetic patients which are in part related to the excretion and retention of sodium chloride are discussed under "Influence of Sodium Chloride Upon the Weight." (See page 293.) For the determination of

[1] Folin: P. 145, loc. cit., p. 246.
[2] Kingsbury, Clark, Williams and Post: Jour. Lab. and Clin. Med., **11**, 981, 1926. The necessary apparatus may be purchased from R. P. Cargille, 118 Liberty St., New York, N. Y.

chlorides in urine, Folin's simplified method[1] or any of the simplified methods found in standard laboratory tests may be used.

12. **Tests of Renal Function.**—We make use routinely of three tests for the efficiency of the kidneys: (1) The level of non-protein nitrogen in the blood; (2) the phenolsulphonephthalein test; and (3) the "two-hour renal" test. We have perhaps not used the urea-clearance test as extensively as we should. The two-hour renal (concentration and dilution) test, as originally devised by Mosenthal, required a special diet for the day of the test together with care to force fluids during part of the day and to restrict them at others. In this way a varying load is placed upon the kidneys and their ability to meet these demands can be estimated. In practice we have found it more convenient and almost as satisfactory to allow the patient his regular diet and his choice as to the amount and time of taking fluids. The urine is collected from 7 A.M. to 7 P.M. every two hours and the night amount passed between 7 P.M. and 7 A.M. is collected in one container. If the specific gravity of the different specimens does not show a variation of at least 6 points or if the night volume exceeds the day volume, the finding is regarded as abnormal. The test is best performed with a minimum of glycosuria because of the effect of sugar itself in raising the specific gravity. The importance of this factor in confusing results may be minimized if the amounts of sugar are small and do not vary appreciably from specimen to specimen. If albumin is present, correction should be made for its influence on the specific gravity.

B. THE EXAMINATION OF THE BLOOD.

1. **Collection of Blood.**—Although we make extensive use of micro methods of analysis on capillary blood, we still employ venous blood on certain occasions. Such specimens have two distinct advantages over capillary samplings: (1) The only essential in the drawing of venous blood is that a sufficient quantity be put into a container where it is adequately mixed with an anticoagulant. With capillary blood considerable skill and care are required to measure with a capillary pipette exactly 0.1 cc. of blood with sufficient celerity to avoid clotting. (2) When a larger quantity of blood is drawn as from a vein, determinations of more than one constituent of blood are possible on a single sample.

Blood is ordinarily drawn from a vein in the antecubital space with the use of a 5- or 10-cc. syringe and a 21-gauge needle. Two to 10 or more cc. are withdrawn, depending upon the determinations which are desired. The blood is best placed in 1-ounce, widemouthed bottles in the bottom of which has been placed a small amount of a mixture of 5 parts sodium fluoride to 2 parts powdered potassium oxalate in the approximate amount of 7 milligrams of the

---

[1] Folin, P. 179; loc. cit., p. 246.

mixture per cc. of blood. A neutral salt of sodium fluoride is essential. Blood which has been mixed with sodium fluoride will retain its sugar content at room temperature for at least several hours and for several days if kept in the ice-box. When blood is withdrawn for a determination of the carbon dioxide content of the plasma (blood taken under oil) or for a determination of blood cholesterol or fat, a satisfactory anticoagulant is potassium oxalate. In this instance the blood should be analyzed promptly, particularly if the sugar content is desired. For special determinations there are special indications as to the drawing of the blood.

In those determinations of blood constituents in which colorimetric comparisons are employed, the photoelectric colorimeter is recommended for accuracy and speed. This instrument is particularly well suited for determinations of hemoglobin, non-protein nitrogen and cholesterol. Blood-sugar estimations present some difficulty because with methods in common use, the depth of color obtained in the final stage of the procedure is not in all concentrations a straight-line function of the amount of sugar present. However, the use of the photoelectric colorimeter is entirely feasible if suitable calibration curves are prepared.

2. **Units of Measurement of Blood Electrolytes.**—It is preferable to express values for electrolytes in the blood in terms of chemical equivalence, *i. e.*, milliequivalents per liter, rather than as milligrams per 100 cc., since only in this way can their relative magnitude and interrelationship be evaluated properly. The figure for milliequivalents per liter is obtained by use of the following formula:

$$\frac{\text{No. of mg. per 100 cc.} \times \text{valency}}{\text{Atomic wt.}} \times 10 = \text{milliequivalents per liter}$$

Thus, to convert a plasma chloride value of 355 mg. per 100 cc. to milliequivalents, one proceeds as follows:

$$\frac{355 \times 1}{35.5} \times 10 = 100 \text{ milliequivalents per liter}$$

In Table 28 is shown the normal range of blood electrolytes expressed in milligrams per 100 cc. and as milliequivalents per liter. In Table 29 illustrative values for acid and base constituents of normal human plasma are shown and in Figure 13, page 438, one of the electrolyte patterns illustrated is that for normal plasma.

3. **Blood Sugar.**—Without a knowledge of the blood sugar both the diagnosis and the treatment of a patient with sugar in the urine have an unsteady foundation. Case 11680 was regarded for several years as a diabetic because of abundant glycosuria and for months had been taking enormous doses of insulin which had been supplied by a welfare society at public expense. When blood-sugar determinations showed that he was not a diabetic, but rather a renal

glycosuric, he was relieved of the inconvenience of repeated injections of insulin and the welfare society relieved of the expense. Non-diabetic, doubtful, or borderline cases of glycosuria are not as uncommon as is sometimes thought. In 1937 a survey was made of 14,000 patients who had come for diagnosis or treatment of diabetes. Among this group it was found that 14.8 per cent had glycosuria of a non-diabetic type as shown by determinations of the blood sugar. In diagnosis, particularly in mild cases, blood sugar determinations one hour after a meal are of the greatest aid.

TABLE 28.—COMPARISON OF NORMAL VALUES FOR BLOOD ELECTROLYTES EXPRESSED AS MILLIGRAMS PER 100 CC. AND AS MILLIEQUIVALENTS PER LITER.

Blood constituent.	Normal range in	
	Mg./100 cc.	M.eq/liter.
Sodium	313–333	136–145
Potassium	16–22	4.1–5.6
Calcium	9–11	4.5–5.5
Magnesium	2–3	1.7–2.5
CO_2 content	50–65	22.5–29.3
	(Vols. per 100 cc.)	
Chloride	350–390	95–105
Phosphorus	3–4	1.7–2.3
Sulfate	0.9–1.5	0.6–1.0
Protein	6.0–8.0	14.6–19.4
	(Grams per 100 cc.)	

Values refer to serum or plasma except that in the case of calcium, for technical reasons serum must be used in the determination and that, due to the loss of fibrinogen in clotting, the protein content of serum is slightly lower than that of plasma.

CO_2 volumes per cent are converted to milliequivalents per liter by dividing by 2.22. The base equivalence of protein is obtained by multiplying grams per 100 cc. by 2.43.

TABLE 29.—VALUES FOR ACID AND BASE CONSTITUENTS OF NORMAL HUMAN PLASMA.

Acid.	M.eq./liter.	Base.	M.eq./liter
HCO_3^-	27	Na^+	142
Cl^-	103	K^+	5
HPO_4^{--}	2	Ca^{++}	5
SO_4^{--}	1	Mg^{++}	3
Organic acids	6		
Protein	16	Total	155
Total	155		

It is not only in matter of diagnosis, however, that blood-sugar tests are of tremendous value to the physician. Determinations, particularly of the fasting blood sugar, at intervals of months or years, give a splendid index of the increasing or decreasing severity of the condition. Furthermore, in patients using regular or crystalline insulin exclusively, the level of the fasting blood sugar will indicate whether or not a bedtime dose of insulin would be beneficial. For patients taking protamine zinc insulin once daily before breakfast, the fasting blood sugar gives an index as to the amount of insulin to prescribe. Blood-sugar determinations made just before lunch or before supper serve as a valuable guide as to the amount of insulin which can be safely given before breakfast and before lunch, respectively. In this way hypoglycemia and consequent insulin reactions may be foreseen and patients be spared the inconvenience caused by them. In the treatment of diabetic coma a knowledge of blood-sugar values is almost imperative.

Ideally, blood-sugar methods should eliminate entirely the effect of non-glucose substances, chiefly glutathione.

The methods which we have continued to use have been in large part those devised by Folin and his co-workers. The macro-method for blood sugar is the original one published in 1920, except for minor modifications. Precipitation of the blood protein is accomplished by tungstic acid.[1]

The use of capillary blood often is desirable, particularly in children, in patients such as those in diabetic coma from whom frequent samples of blood for sugar determination are helpful and in those patients whose veins, either because of nature or because of medication, are difficult to puncture. If care is used in taking the blood samples and in performing the analyses, results which can be readily duplicated may be easily obtained. In interpreting results obtained on capillary blood, it must be remembered that whereas in the fasting state, the sugar content of capillary and venous blood is approximately the same, after a meal or after glucose the capillary values are (in the normal person) 20 to 50 milligrams higher than the corresponding figures on venous blood. (See page 153.) The micro-method which we have routinely used is that of Folin[2] on laked blood.

4. **Non-protein Nitrogen.**— —In recent years, as the number of patients with diabetes of long duration has increased, the incidence of chronic nephritis has become greater. From January 1, 1944 to May 15, 1946, of 434 deaths due to arteriosclerosis, the chief cause of death was chronic nephritis in 40 cases or 9.2 per cent. For a discussion of chronic nephritis, including intercapillary glomerulosclerosis, see p. 500. For methods of analysis of the blood for non-protein nitrogen content, see Folin's *Manual*[3] and other standard laboratory texts.

5. **Chlorides.**—As in the case of urine, the determination of the chlorides in the blood gains importance from the fact that the water content of the body in diabetes may vary rapidly and widely. This is in addition to the value which such determinations have in the diabetic management of cases of nephritis and hypertension in connection with diabetes. The method used in our office laboratory is a modification of the method of Wilson and Ball[4] carried out on

[1] Folin, P. 301; loc. cit., p. 246.   Folin: Jour. Biol. Chem., **82**, 83, 1929.
[2] Folin, P. 245; loc. cit., p. 246.
[3] Folin, P. 265; loc. cit., p. 246.
[4] Wilson and Ball: Jour. Biol. Chem., **79**, 221, 1928.

blood serum. The method of Schales and Schales[1] has been recommended as simple and accurate.

A low plasma chloride is seen chiefly in diabetes in connection with acidosis when chloride is lost from the body through vomiting or through excretion in the urine. Despite liberal administration of normal salt solution parenterally, hypochloremia (? hyponatremia) may persist, and anuria result. In suitable patients this may be strikingly relieved and the secretion of urine provoked by the intravenous injection of hypertonic (10 per cent) sodium chloride solution (50 to 130 cc.) as reported by Root.[2]

6. **Total Protein.**—In the last few years a knowledge of the total protein and albumin and globulin content of the blood plasma has become of increasing and practical importance in the treatment of certain diabetic patients, particularly those patients with onset of diabetes in childhood or adolescence who have had the disease for fifteen or twenty years. With these patients chronic intercapillary glomerulosclerosis with marked albuminuria, azotemia, edema, hypertension and retinitis, has presented a difficult problem. Edema is often accompanied by low serum protein values with reversal of the albumin-globulin ratio. In the determination of the serum protein we have used the method of Kingsley[3] with success, although it has seemed important that the plasma or serum used be clear and not turbid as with blood containing large amounts of lipid material. In the laboratory at the New England Deaconess Hospital, the Kagan[4] falling drop technic is used for the determination of total protein.

7. **Total Base, Sodium and Potassium.**—Not infrequently, particularly in patients in diabetic acidosis, a knowledge of the total base, sodium and potassium of the blood is of value. In the laboratory of the New England Deaconess Hospital the method of Sunderman[5] for total base is used.

For the determination of sodium and potassium we have recently begun to use the method of Berry, Chappell and Barnes[6] in which an improved flame photometer is said to provide for the rapid and accurate determination of these elements. The method is applicable to high dilutions of blood and urine. The solution to be analyzed is atomized into the base of a gas burner, whereupon the vapor is carried into the flame and ignited. The light arising from the flame characteristic of the element being determined is filtered free of other radiation and is brought to fall upon a photocell. By measur-

[1] Schales and Schales: Jour. Biol. Chem., **140**, 879, 1941.
[2] Root: Jour. Am. Med. Assn., **103**, 482, 1934; **108**, 947, 1937.
[3] Kingsley: Jour. Biol. Chem., **133**, 731, 1940.
[4] Kagan: Jour. Biol. Chem., **17**, 369, 1938; Ibid., **17**, 373, 1938.
[5] Sunderman: Jour. Biol. Chem., **143**, 185, 1942.
[6] Berry, Chappell and Barnes: Ind. and Eng. Chem., **18**, 19, 1946. We are indebted to the American Cyanamid Co. for furnishing the apparatus with which to carry on this work.

ing the intensity of the light produced with solutions of known concentration and preparing a calibration curve of intensity versus concentration, the metal content of other solutions may subsequently be determined by making use of the curve.

Shinn[1] found no significant difference in the mean quantities of serum potassium or in the sodium-potassium ratio between diabetic children and normal adults. The mean sodium level of uncontrolled diabetics was significantly lower than that in controlled cases and that in normal adults.

8. **Carotin.**—Certain diabetics retain ingested vegetable pigments to a greater extent than do normal individuals and a characteristic yellow discoloration of the skin is thus produced. One finds in such cases a marked increase in the carotin content of the blood. Using the method of Connor,[2] values for blood carotin up to 0.07 mg. per cent were found. Values as high as 0.85 mg. per cent have been obtained in some of the writers' patients showing a yellowish discoloration of the skin. Connor found values up to 0.16 mg. per cent in a group of patients in whom no pigmentation was seen.

Heymann[3] carried out carotin tolerance curves in 10 diabetic and 12 non-diabetic children determining the content of carotin in the blood serum at intervals after the oral administration of carotin in oil. His results indicated that carotin metabolism is interfered with in diabetes. From studies involving the daily feeding of carotin in oil to 3 normal and 3 diabetic individuals, Ralli and co-workers[4] came to the same conclusion. They explain the hypercarotinemia in diabetes as due to an inability of the liver to convert it to vitamin A. In continuation of this work, Stueck, Flaum and Ralli[5] studied 13 patients with signs of carotinemia, as shown by pigmentation of the palms, soles, or subconjunctival fat. Whereas the average value for normal subjects three hours after breakfast (method of White and Gordon) was 0.109 milligrams per 100 cc. and for diabetic patients 0.262 milligrams, the average for the group with carotinemia was 0.392 milligrams per 100 cc. of blood.

Mosenthal and Loughlin[6] determined the carotin content of the plasma of 24 normal and 32 diabetic individuals. They conclude that the majority of diabetics today, in contrast to a decade or more ago, have plasma carotin and vitamin A levels that are within normal limits; this agrees with our own impression although we have made no systematic observations in recent years. However, they found a tendency for the carotin to be elevated (24 per cent of cases) and the vitamin A to be depressed (11.6 per cent of cases).

[1] Shinn: Bull. Pittsburgh Univ., **39**, 405, 1943.

[2] Connor: Jour. Biol. Chem., **77**, 619, 1928.

[3] Heymann: Jour. Am. Med. Assn., **106**, 2050, 1936.

[4] Ralli, Pariente, Brandalione and Davidson: Jour. Am. Med. Assn., **106**, 1075, 1936. See also Ralli, Brandalione and Mandelbaum: Jour. Lab. and Clin. Med., **20**, 1266, 1935.

[5] Stueck, Flaum and Ralli: Jour. Am. Med. Assn., **109**, 343, 1937.

[6] Mosenthal and Loughlin: Jour. Mt. Sinai Hosp., **12**, 523, 1945.

Lembrechts, Leleux and Thomas[1] found that the somewhat elevated values for blood carotin of diabetics studied prior to World War II fell to normal levels during the period of food rationing. From this they concluded that the carotinemia of diabetes must be of alimentary origin and not due to an inability to convert carotin to vitamin A (which was present in normal amounts during both periods).

9. **Lipids.**—Accurate analyses of the fat of the blood and particularly partitive studies of the various lipid fractions are time-consuming, and for that reason by most physicians cannot be made a part of the routine investigation of a patient. Nor would such seem to be necessary, because only 93 of 2200 patients studied during the ten years ending December, 1939 showed blood cholesterol values of 400 mg. per cent or more; this was all the more significant because the determinations had, for the most part, been done only in instances in which it was thought possible that abnormal values might be revealed.

We have continued to employ the methods of lipid analysis designed by Bloor[2] and his associates in which the determination of total fat is made by iodometric titration following oxidation by dichromate in the presence of concentrated sulphuric acid. Fortunately the amount of cholesterol in the blood ordinarily gives a good index as to the status of fat metabolism. Consequently, one may carry out this determination alone. In clinical work we employ a modification of Bloor's colorimetric method for cholesterol, using 0.2 cc. of plasma and omitting saponification. In cases of suspected liver damage particularly, estimation of the ester cholesterol may be of distinct advantage. Whereas normally the ester cholesterol represents 65 to 75 per cent of the total cholesterol,[3] in cases of hepatic insufficiency the percentage may be reduced considerably even to complete disappearance of the ester fraction.[4]

10. **Acetone in the Blood.**—It sometimes occurs that acidosis is present, yet is not disclosed by the simple ferric chloride test for diacetic acid in the urine. Under such circumstances the test for acetone in the urine may be made, or, better still, a qualitative test for acetone in the blood. The description of such a test follows:

Wishart Method for Detection of Aceto-acetic Acid and Acetone in the Blood.—The blood is drawn into a syringe or tube containing a few crystals of potassium oxalate, then centrifuged for five minutes at medium speed. The test is made on the plasma with as little delay as possible, as there may be some loss of acetone on standing.

To 4 drops of plasma add solid ammonium sulphate until the plasma is thoroughly saturated and the protein precipitated; then

[1] Lembrechts, Leleux and Thomas: Acta med. Scandinav., **116**, 11, 1943.
[2] Bloor: Jour. Biol. Chem., **77**, 53, 1928.
[3] Sperry and Schoenheimer: Jour. Biol. Chem., **110**, 655, 1935.
[4] Epstein: Arch. Int. Med., **50**, 203, 1932.

add 2 drops of a freshly made 5 per cent solution of sodium nitro-prusside and 2 drops of concentrated ammonium hydroxide. Thoroughly mix. (One may instead overlay with the ammonium hydroxide and then without shaking the tube, observe any color reaction at the junction of the two liquids.) If the test is positive, in from one to ten minutes a color develops which varies from a pale lavender to a deep permanganate hue, in this way indicating whether little or much acetone is present. This is an adaptation to the plasma of the Rothera nitroprusside reaction ordinarily used for urine. It is said to be sensitive to 1 part in 20,000.

The acetone reagent described on page 247 may be used in this test and is recommended because of its stability. The plasma is saturated with the reagent and a few drops of strong ammonia water are added.

Quantitative Estimation of Acetone in Blood.—We have found satisfactory Nanavutty's[1] titrimetric modification of Van Slyke's gravimetric method for the determination of "total acetone bodies" in the blood and urine. This method is applicable to quantities of blood as small as 0.5 cc. but cannot be used with accuracy for amounts of acetone under 5 milligrams per 100 cc. The highest value that we have found so far in diabetic coma has been 198 mg. per cent. In normal individuals values approaching zero are found.

11. **Carbon Dioxide in Blood Plasma.**—Whether in health or in disease, the reactions of the body remain nearly constant and the blood not only conforms to this general law but helps to enforce it. This end is accomplished in the presence of acidosis: (1) By removing the CO_2 from the blood by way of the lungs; (2) by neutralization of the acid through buffer action; and (3) by saving of alkali through the excretion of acid phosphate through the kidneys.

The blood plasma normally contains a certain amount of bicarbonate ($NaHCO_3$). An idea of the amount can be obtained by measuring the quantity of CO_2 which is set free when a stronger acid, such as sulphuric acid or lactic acid, is added to the blood. The CO_2 thus obtained ("CO_2 content") is expressed as milliequivalents (m.eq.) per liter or, less desirably, as volumes of CO_2 per 100 cc. of blood (volumes per cent). Normal venous blood contains from 22 to 29 milliequivalents per liter (50 to 65 volumes per 100 cc.) of CO_2.

Despite the introduction of an acid, the blood preserves its normal degree of alkalinity to a certain point through the buffer action of the alkali (chiefly sodium bicarbonate) of the plasma and the proteins, especially hemoglobin. Just how much reserve in alkalinity a given blood plasma may possess is comparatively easily learned by exposing the blood to an atmosphere of CO_2 until it has become saturated and then measuring the amount of CO_2 which has been taken up. This gives the alkali reserve capacity (combining-power) of the blood for CO_2; normal values vary between 25 and 34 milli-

---

[1] Nanavutty: Loc. cit., p. 248.

17

equivalents per liter (55 and 75 volumes per cent). Both the CO_2 content and the CO_2 combining-power of the blood are measures of alkalinity. We routinely use the standard method of Van Slyke[1] for determination of the carbon dioxide content of the plasma, collecting blood samples under oil.

12. **The Hydrogen-ion Concentration of the Blood.**—Human blood is slightly alkaline, having an hydrogen-ion concentration a little less than that of pure water. The hydrogen-ion concentration—pH—of oxalated normal blood is 7.35. In clinical acidosis the values for oxalated blood may fall to pH 7.1, and Bock *et al.*[2] found them as low as pH 7.03 in diabetic coma. In artificially produced acidosis in dogs the pH may fall as low as pH 6.9. A reaction of pH 7.6 or higher is obtained only after the administration of alkalies. The buffer action of the carbonates of the plasma and the protein of the whole blood enables the blood to take up considerable amounts of acids or alkali without appreciable change in hydrogen-ion concentration. Until practically all the plasma bicarbonate is taken up by acid, little or no change occurs in the pH of the blood. After this point rapid changes in pH occur. In the determination of the pH of the blood one may use electrometric, colorimetric, or gasometric methods, as described in laboratory texts. For the colorimetric method of Hastings and Sendroy[3] reference is made to the original article.

Shock and Hastings[4] described an ingenious method by means of which, with a specially designed capillary pipette, the pH of the blood serum, the total CO_2 content and the percentage of cells are determined on the same 0.1 cc. sample.

[1] Van Slyke: Jour. Biol. Chem., **30**, 347, 1917. Van Slyke and Stadie: Jour. Biol. Chem., **49**, 1, 1921.
[2] Bock, Field and Adair: Jour. Metab. Res., **4**, 27, 1923.
[3] Hastings and Sendroy: Jour. Biol. Chem., **61**, 695, 1924.
[4] Shock and Hastings: Jour. Biol. Chem., **104**, 565, 575, 585, 1934.

CHAPTER VIII.

THE DIET IN HEALTH AND DIABETES.

A. INTRODUCTION.

THE diet of the diabetic not only should be equal but superior to the diet in health. Its components of carbohydrate, protein and fat should be selected from the best of their class, properly balanced in relation to one another, and of such a nature as to provide a full complement of amino-acids, of salts such as calcium to protect the bones, phosphorus which is so intimately associated with calcium, of potassium, and also of carbohydrate and fat, of iron and above all of vitamins. It will not suffice for the diabetic diet to contain vitamins adequate for a normal individual to escape avitaminosis; it should contain more of each specific kind. We are still in the dark as to whether the diabetic, both at the onset and in the course of his disease, is deficient in any of the vitamins, can absorb or utilize them fully even if offered in the food, or requires a super-abundance of the same to maintain or regain vitamin equilibrium. He may need an excess to prevent and surmount infections, acute or chronic, and to ward off complications as, for example, the various neuropathies to which the diabetic is liable.

B. A STANDARD DIABETIC DIET.

The diet outlined in Table 30 fulfills most of these requirements. If the patient fails to utilize it, the use of insulin can be assumed to be indicated.

In simple terms, it is represented by three slices of whole-wheat bread, a saucer of cereal, 3 oranges, 4 portions of 5 per cent vegetables, ¼ pint of milk, ¼ pint of cream, 1 egg, 2 moderate portions of meat and 1 ounce of butter. The diet contains approximately 1600 calories and is composed of carbohydrate 150 grams, protein 70 grams and fat 80 grams.

Practically all published values for carbohydrate, protein and fat in foods, save such pure foods as sugar, starch and oil, represent the average of many analyses with wide individual variations. Thus the carbohydrate in one slice, one ounce or 30 grams, of white bread may vary between 15 and 18 grams. It is therefore absurd to calculate diets in fractions of a gram. (Table 33 see also Tables 44, 45, and 46.)

The diet shown in Table 30 would be deficient in calcium for a child and should be increased by 1 pint of milk. It is deficient in vitamin B, which can be rectified for adults by the addition of liver once or twice weekly. The deficiency in vitamin D for children is offset by the addition of cod-liver oil, 1 tablespoonful daily, or its equivalent.

All doctors, dietitians and nurses should know simple dietetic values and should become intimately acquainted with them by calculating what they eat themselves before attempting to teach others.

TABLE 30.—A BASIC DIABETIC DIET.

Carbohydrate 150 grams; protein 70 grams; fat 80 grams; calories 1600.

Food.	Unit portion.	Grams in each portion.				Total daily portions.	Total grams.		
		Weight.	C.	P.	F.		C.	P.	F.
Bread	1 slice	30	18	3	..	3	54	9	
Oatmeal	1 large	30, dry	20	5	2	1	20	5	2
Orange	1	150	15	..	..	3	45		
Vegetables, 3–5% . .	1 cup	150	5	2½	..	4	20	10	
Milk	¼ pt.	120	6	4	4	1	6	4	4
Cream, 20%	¼ pt.	120	4	4	24	1	4	4	24
Egg	1	60	..	6	6	1	..	6	6
Meat	1 small	60	..	16	10	2	..	32	20
Butter	1 square	10	..	..	8	3	..	..	25

Grand total grams (approximate) C150 P70 F80

Calories per gram . . . . ×4 ×4 ×9

Total calories—1600 . . . . . . 600 280 720

C. THE METABOLISM OF THE DIABETIC.

A Discussion of Certain Features of Metabolism Pertinent to the Diet in Diabetes.—The caloric needs of the diabetic are the same as those of a normal individual, no more and no less. However, the term normal individual is to be interpreted literally and therefore the diet should be planned for the patient with the age, sex, weight and activity always in mind. Since longevity goes with substandard weights in middle life, the weight of the patient should be slightly below that for recognized standard weights. This is all the more important in diabetes, because overweight, except for heredity, is the factor not only chiefly contributing to the onset of the disease but is also one of the most disturbing factors in its satisfactory control.

We can assume that the digestion, assimilation and utilization of food in the controlled diabetic is the same as in the non-diabetic, save for the non-utilization of more or less of the carbohydrate derived from carbohydrate, protein and the glycerol moiety of the fat and for the tendency to excessive production of ketone acids. The loss of carbohydrate, nitrogen and fat in the feces is, as in the normal, due more to excretion into the digestive canal than from the residue of food itself and seldom would be as much or more than 5 per cent of the intake. The dried feces amounts to not far from 30 grams per day.

1. *Carbohydrate.*—Carbohydrate in the normal is stored in the body almost entirely as glycogen, the glucose in the blood seldom amounting to more than 5 grams and, even when the blood sugar is four times the normal, to 20 grams. The total quantity of carbohydrate stored in health ranges between 200 and 500 grams. Of this, 40 to 60 per cent will be found in the muscles as glycogen, although the percentage in them seldom rises over 2 per cent, 35 to 40 per cent as glycogen in the liver, in which the percentage

is usually between 5 and 10 per cent. The glycogen both in the muscles and liver is greatly reduced during prolonged fasting or in severe, uncontrolled diabetes. Another 7 to 10 per cent of the carbohydrate may be found as glycogen in the skin and other tissues, and the balance occurs as other forms of carbohydrate.

Glucose is the circulating form of carbohydrate and glycogen the storage form. Glucose is a monosaccharide with the simple formula $C_6H_{12}O_6$; whereas starch and glycogen are complicated $(C_6H_{10}O_5)_x$, representing a dehydrated form of glucose. The conversion of carbohydrate into glucose and its rapid passage out of the alimentary tract is explained not wholly by diffusion or absorption, but rather by its association with phosphoric acid (phosphorylation), the phosphoric acid playing here an intimate part in the process, as it also does in the muscle in the breakdown of glycogen through the stage of pyruvic acid and lactic acid to furnish energy. See page 117.

The other monosaccharides and disaccharides are either interchangeable or converted into glucose as a rule in the course of assimilation and combustion by the tissues. Differences in the utilization of various carbohydrates by the diabetic or non-diabetic are insignificant, although such exist. Levulose is readily interchangeable with glucose. Lactose is less sweet and soluble and less subject to fermentation than glucose. The other monosaccharides are of minor importance. It makes little difference whether the carbohydrate is taken in vegetables and in unripe fruits largely in the form of starch or in the ripened fruits as sugar.

2. *Fat.*—The fat in the body is derived largely from the fat in the food. The fatty acids of the food may be deposited in identical form and readily identified, particularly with the aid of deuterium (heavy hydrogen) as an indicator. If a dog is fed on mutton fat, the dog's fat may resemble the fat of the sheep. Body fat is also formed from the dehydration of carbohydrate of the diet and also can be manufactured out of protein. Notwithstanding the formation of fat to a large extent in the body from changes in the food consumed, it would appear that one or more of the fatty acids, which are necessary for normal functions, cannot be manufactured by the body *de novo*, although the information regarding these is less definite than concerning the amino-acids of the protein molecule. There is a certain fat minimum as well as a carbohydrate minimum for the best utilization of foods.[1]

Fat-free diets produce degeneration of the kidneys in rats. Rats with the low-fat diseases are not cured by saturated fatty acids but are cured by linoleic acid (either isolated or in olive oil, lard, corn oil, poppy seed oil, linseed oil or egg lecithin). High grade butter fat does *not* cure the disease, thereby indicating that the kidney damage is not due to lack of vitamin A and vitamin E. The need of the animals is not for fat in general but for specific unsaturated fatty acids. Warm-blooded animals cannot synthesize linoleic, linolenic, or arachidonic[2] acids. Apparently there are necessary features about fatty acids with curative powers. There must be at least two double bonds and these double bonds must occupy certain positions (9:10 and 12:13).

The fats form an essential part of the structure and cells of the body. They also play an intimate part in its functional processes. Just as phosphorus is important in the transfer of carbohydrate to glucose from the alimentary canal and in the intricate metabolism of glycogen in the muscles, so, too, phosphorus has an essential rôle in the distribution of fats in the body. Thus phospholipids represent the form of fat in active fat tissues

[1] Krogh and Lindbard: Jour. Biol. Chem., **14**, 290, 1920.
[2] Hume, Nunn, Smedley, Maclean and Smith: Biochem. Jour., **32**, 2162, 1938; Ibid., p. 2178.

of the body in contrast to the inactive adipose tissue. Furthermore, the phospholipids are omnipresent and, in fact, are constantly found in association with proteins in protoplasm. Lecithin and cephalin are the best known of the phospholipids and are especially important in the formation of nerve tissue.

Cholesterol and ergosterol are the best known of the sterols in the body. The former is an essential element in the cell membranes of the various cells of the body. The importance of the sterols in the skin has been recognized, because through the action of the ultra-violet rays of light upon the skin calciferol is formed, and this is similar to vitamin D.

3. *Protein.*—Proteins are the prime essential constituents of all cells with life. As a rule, animals cannot build them up but must depend upon obtaining them from plants or other animals. Therefore, proteins are necessary ingredients of the food of all animals, and because of this important source being animal food, are correspondingly expensive. Proteins are anhydrides of amino-acids of which more than twenty have been identified, each different from the others.

Each tissue of the body has its specific amino-acids and, therefore, the proteins ingested must be of such a wide variety that these amino-acids will be available.

Amino-acids are to proteins as glucose is to starch; and proteins, like starch, have a high molecular weight. The protein molecule contains a large number of amino-acid molecules. All of the proteins contain carbon, hydrogen, oxygen, nitrogen, sulphur, and usually phosphorus. A very few proteins can be obtained in crystalline form, but most of them are of a colloidal nature. Just as vitamins are specific and if totally lacking an essential process of nutrition will cease, so, too, with the amino-acids. The essential amino-acids include threonine, valine, leucine, isoleucine, arginine, lysine, methionine, phenylalanine, tryptophane, histidine, and to a certain extent cystine. The last-named apparently can be formed from methionine in the body except for the regeneration of plasma protein. Arginine can be synthesized in the body but not in adequate amounts for normal growth. Tyrosine can be formed from phenylalanine. Glycine can be formed in the body and there is also experimental evidence that alanin can be made either from lactic or pyruvic acid, which are constantly appearing in the intermediary metabolism of carbohydrate. These are the links which show the close connection between all the foodstuffs, carbohydrate, protein and fat. Minerals and vitamins, and one might add also hormones and enzymes, similarly are intimately involved in reactions between the foods and each other in the metabolism of the body. It is natural that the milk proteins which are rich in lysine and tryptophane are the ones which are especially useful for growth. (See page 282.)

In general, animal proteins are of greater value than the vegetable proteins.

4. The Basal Metabolism of Diabetics Upon High and Low Diets.— Before entering upon a discussion of the caloric needs of the diabetic, reference to the studies of the metabolism of diabetes carried on in three American laboratories will explain the confusion which existed between 1900 and 1920 and how the truth came to the surface.

The metabolism of the mild and moderately severe diabetic was early recognized to be essentially normal, but at one time Benedict and Joslin concluded that the metabolism of the severe diabetic was increased. As years passed on, however, it developed that the same patient with severe diabetes might exhibit a metabolism at one time distinctly above normal and at another time far below normal, not from intrinsic causes as with the thyroid patient but from extrinsic causes of which the diet was foremost. Thus in the Naunyn era, prior to June, 1914, Benedict and Joslin[1] found the average basal metabolism of 27 of 29 diabetics to be +13, but during the undernutrition of the subsequent Allen era the metabolism of 57 of 76 diabetics was −7.

A notable case studied with infinite pains by Geyelin and DuBois[2] illustrated much of what is described above; so, too, did a patient of Wilder, Boothby and Beeler.[3] Finally it was driven home to us all that it was the hand of man that made the diabetes severe, just as later the hand of man made it mild.

L. Hédon[4] also noted an increase of metabolism of severe diabetics who lost weight on a diet poor in carbohydrate, but liberal in protein and fat. In severe acidosis it even exceeded 30 per cent. But if these patients were first fasted and then given a limited amount of food the basal metabolism became −40 per cent.

The fundamental change in treatment of my diabetics began about June, 1914, and it promptly exerted an influence upon the metabolism. The cause for a marked alteration in the aspect of the diseased patient was surely adequate. Prior to 1914, diabetic patients were overfed, all cases being treated with a low-carbohydrate and high-protein-fat diet. Excess of calories was encouraged, and to guard against coma, instead of limitation of fat and undernutrition, sodium bicarbonate was employed in large doses and continued for periods of months. Fat was given *ad nauseam*, and even such fatty foods as cheese and eggs were served, mixed with about equal proportions of butter. The good results of fasting days were overlooked; Naunyn's observation, von Noorden's recommendation, and Weintraud's proof that diabetic patients could subsist upon remarkably few calories, were known but unappreciated and considered more of scientific interest than of therapeutic significance. Hodgson, however, had grasped the principle and with it attained unusual success in practical treatment. It was at this time that Guelpa's conceptions of fasting and of the waning severity of diabetes in the presence of an emaciating disease were recognized, utilized and enlarged by Allen[5] into a system of treatment based upon a reduced caloric intake.

Patients given the fasting treatment when this procedure was first used were almost invariably underfed to a marked degree,

[1] Joslin: Diabetic Metabolism With High and Low Diets, Washington, Carnegie Institution of Washington, 1923. Publication No. 323.

[2] Geyelin and DuBois: Jour. Am. Med. Assn., **66**, 1532, 1916; Arch. Int. Med., **19**, 908, 1917.

[3] Wilder, Boothby and Beeler: Jour. Biol. Chem., **51**, 312, 1922.

[4] Hédon: Paris méd., **63**, 446, 1927; Arch. internat. de phys., **29**, 175, 1927.

[5] Allen: Jour. Am. Med. Assn., **63**, 939, 1914.

because the hospital period was spent in securing quick results and these were most readily obtained by extreme dietetic restriction.

In 1915, Joslin recognized that fat was largely responsible for acidosis, and its omission at the beginning of treatment was emphasized. Sodium bicarbonate was abandoned in September, 1915, and has never been resumed.

The wide divergence which may be found in the metabolism of diabetics is strikingly shown in Table 31, which presents the 6 cases with the highest and the 7 cases with the lowest metabolism in the entire series, as indicated by the percentage variation from standard. With all of these cases the diabetes was severe. For the cases with high metabolism the percentage variation ranged between +26 per cent and +33 per cent. Perhaps the best idea of the gravity of the conditions under which the subjects were living is obtained from the duration of life following the recorded observations. Case 1412 succumbed to the disease within three days; Cases 549, 210 and 246 lived from one to six months; Case 220 lived nearly a year and a half; but Case 983 died twelve years later. The observations upon this woman were most instructive and of enormous importance to Joslin at that time, 1916, because they showed that a marked increase in metabolism and acidosis could be temporary and not necessarily of bad prognostic import.

In contrast to the cases with high metabolism are 7 patients with an exceptionally low metabolism, these averaging 32 per cent below standard, the lowest being −40 per cent. Despite this extraordinary decrease in metabolism, the life of these patients was evidently not in as great jeopardy as those with high metabolism, although all succumbed within the following two years and five months. Evidently, therefore, a diabetic patient whose metabolism is far below normal is, on the whole, in a safer condition than the diabetic patient whose metabolism is exceptionally high, though either extreme in metabolism may be dangerous but not necessarily of fatal significance.

5. **The Respiratory Quotients of Diabetics.**—The respiratory quotients were strikingly different, according to the method of treatment. With the omission of Case 983, the 5 remaining patients with the highest metabolism on the low carbohydrate high caloric diet had an average quotient of 0.7, while with the 7 patients with the low metabolism on the undernutrition regime the average quotient was 0.84.

6. **Relation Between Loss of Weight and the Metabolism.**—The average loss in weight from maximum of 5 of the 6 patients with the high metabolism was 21 per cent. The average loss in weight of the 7 patients with the low metabolism was 37 per cent. Three patients were 46 to 49 per cent below normal weight! The low metabolism was evidently connected with an exceptional loss of body weight, but this was not the only factor.

TABLE 31.—HIGHEST AND LOWEST POSTABSORPTIVE METABOLISM OF SEVERE DIABETICS AS EXPRESSED BY VARIATION FROM STANDARD.—A TRAGIC TABLE, BUT IT ILLUSTRATES THE RESULTS OF AGGRESSIVE TREATMENT OF SEVERE DIABETICS IN THE NAUNYN AND ALLEN EPOCHS.

Case No.	Date.	Variation of metabolism from normal standard, per cent.	Loss from maximum body weight, per cent.	Variation from normal standard of body weight.	Acidosis.	Sugar in blood, per cent.	Urinary nitrogen per kg. of body weight per 24 hours.			Sugar in urine on preceding day, gm.	Respiratory quotient.	Duration of life after this observation, years.
							For days preceding observation.		On observation day, gm.			
							Number of days.	Nitrogen.				
		HIGHEST METABOLISM.										
210	Aug. 2- 3, 1910	+26	24	-27	+++	..	7	0.325	0.315	268	0.71	0.3
220	Mar. 13-14, 1909	+32	24	-25	+++	..	..	..	..	..	0.69	1.4
246	June 8- 9, 1909	+28	15	+1	++	..	1	0.210	..	104	0.67	0.5
549	Nov. 5- 6, 1912	+30	18	-14	++++	..	2	0.370	..	185	0.69	0.1
983	Feb. 2- 3, 1916	+28	..	+43	++++	0.30	1	0.145	0.125	72	0.73	12.0
1412	Oct. 18-19, 1917	+33	22	-23	++++	0.37	..	..	0.380	170	0.72	} 3 days
	Oct. 19-20, 1917		22	-23	+++	..	..	..	..	167	0.76	
		LOWEST METABOLISM.										
765	Feb. 9-10, 1916	-27	23	-31	++	0.23	7	0.180	0.110	14	0.76	0.8
821	Apr. 3- 4, 1916	-30	25	-17	+	..	7	0.260	0.225	0	0.81	} 0.5
	Apr. 10-11, 1916		26	-19	+	0.20	7	0.285	0.210	+	0.82	
1011	Nov. 23-24, 1917	-37	49	-49	0	0.29	7	0.285	0.260	42	0.94	0.8
1085	Oct. 11-12, 1916	-40	50	-43	0	..	..	..	..	0	0.81	} 0.1
	Oct. 31-Nov. 1, 1916		54	-46	++	0.35	7	0.275	0.165	..	0.81	
1196	Dec. 15-16, 1916	-27	29	-22	++	0.15	6	0.255	0.115	15	0.80	} 1.0
	Jan. 6- 7, 1917		34	-27	0	..	3	0.415	0.380	35	0.80	
1233	Feb. 19-20, 1917	-33	30	-23	0	0.13	1	0.280	0.210	0	0.86	1.3
1378	Nov. 13-14, 1917	-29	31	-46	0	0.24	..	..	..	..	0.88	2.4

7. **Acidosis in Relation to Metabolism.**—With one exception the cases with the highest metabolism had an extreme degree of acidosis, but of the 7 cases with the lowest metabolism 3 showed no acidosis, while with the other 4 cases acidosis was either absent in some of the tests or not more than moderate in degree in others. The rôle of acidosis in the metabolism of a diabetic is "extremely complicated, and I doubt if it will ever be definitely settled. At the present time it seems as if a severe acidosis might cause a moderate increase in metabolism in some cases of diabetes."[1]

8. **Urinary Nitrogen in Relation to Metabolism.**—The nitrogen excretion per kilogram body weight for a normal adult is about 0.165 gram. For the cases with *high* metabolism (omitting Case 983) the average urinary nitrogen per kilogram body weight for the days preceding the observation and also for the day of the test was 0.320 gram, and the average urinary nitrogen for the patients with low metabolism approached it, being 0.255 gram per kilogram body weight. The highest value for urinary nitrogen per kilogram body weight was encountered with Case 1196, whose metabolism was −27 per cent. The significance of a high urinary nitrogen is twofold. A high urinary nitrogen implies the disintegration of much protein, usually superabundant in the diet, and this leads to a high metabolism under ordinary conditions, as is universally recognized. On the other hand, a high urinary nitrogen due to disintegration of body protein and loss of body nitrogen is an entirely different situation, because it represents the last resort of the body to preserve existence and occurs when the metabolism is at its lowest ebb.

These extreme losses in body protein by the undercontrolled or miscontrolled diabetic are similar to what is recognized today to occur as a result of burns, infections or major surgical procedures (See Case 513, p. 279.)

D. CALORIC REQUIREMENTS.

It is not as fashionable now as at the turn of the century to count the calories and record carbohydrate, protein and fat, but it is just as practical and as desirable as ever for the diabetic to do so. A calorie is a calorie exactly as it was in the Naunyn Era, and if it is lost in the urine it must be subtracted from the calories of the diet to learn the net caloric intake. Friedrich Müller drove this home in a clinic at the Boston City Hospital a generation ago by exhibiting to the students the equivalent in cane sugar of carbohydrate unutilized by the patient, the needless protein metabolized and the fat wasted in the formation of ketone bodies. It is true today we need not worry about excessive metabolism of protein, as shown by a nitrogen elimination of 30 grams more or less to make up for lack

[1] DuBois: Basal Metabolism in Health and Disease, 3d ed., Philadelphia, Lea & Febiger, p. 277, 1936.

of total calories, because insulin changed all this, and needless destruction of protein is avoidable. So, too, lost calories in acidosis are for the same reason avoidable and only temporary. Not so formerly. Case 344 excreted 25 to 50 grams β-oxybutyric acid daily for weeks, representing about 5 calories per gram if allowance is also made for other ketone bodies. At present both the doctor's and the diabetic's dietetic problems are lightened. In 99 cases out of 100 today they need to watch for lost calories in carbohydrate alone. Now as always it has been the diet of the untreated diabetic which is expensive.

The total caloric value of the diet for adults during hospital life ranges between 25 and 30 calories per kilogram or 1500 to 1800 calories for a weight of 132 pounds, 60 kilograms. Often elderly people, men or women, complain this is too much, and few wish more than 1800 calories before they leave or ask for more following discharge, when they report a few weeks later. Diabetics require more calories now than formerly because their health is better and they are more active. Even if the weight is 70 kilograms (154 pounds) the figures rise little and proportionately still less with an added 10 kilograms, thus bringing the body weight to 80 kilograms (176 pounds), because the excess weight proportionately is more likely to be inert fat. Children sometimes wish more food, but usually they are satisfied with 40 to 50 calories per kilogram, save those children who are under ten years of age. For these, figures rise to 70, 80, 90 or even 100 calories in infancy or the first two years of life and likewise for undernourished children and those with retarded development. *Benedict*[1] *is convinced that the basal metabolism of normal women above sixty-six years of age is about 1000 calories.* I know that the metabolism of a diabetic patient, Case 1541, amounted to 20 calories per kilogram body weight for twenty-four hours. She was confined to her bed with hemiplegia for a year, remained sugar-free, held her weight. Her diet was accurately weighed by a trained nurse for the entire period. The 40 calories per kilogram body weight, supposedly required by individuals at moderate work, are certainly not consumed today. Such figures are based on working men's hours of ten and more out of the twenty-four and upon labor without the aid of machinery. In fact, my Metropolitan Life Insurance Company friends attribute in no small measure the increase of diabetes to the lessened muscular activity both of men and women.

We are convinced people eat far less than one would think from dietary tables. Recent carefully conducted studies show this. One will wait a long time to meet in the office the 100 kilogram (220 pound) man or woman who has enough active protoplasm in contrast to adipose tissue to make the ingestion of 4000 calories a day desirable.

[1] Benedict: New England Jour. Med., **212**, 1111, 1935.

1. **Variation in Caloric Requirements in Daily Life.**—The caloric needs of the body vary not only from day to day and hour to hour, but from moment to moment. It is convenient to remember that 1 calorie per kilogram body weight per hour represents the metabolism of normal individuals while at rest in a horizontal position and 1.2 calories while sitting in a chair. In other words, 20 per cent more energy is required to sit in a chair than to lie on a couch. At the Nutrition Laboratory normal men at rest eliminated on the average 25.5 calories per kilogram body weight per twenty-four hours, and normal women 24.9 calories, an almost negligible difference.

Mental activity plays little part in the metabolism of the body, because the total weight of the brain and nerve substance constitutes only about 2 per cent of the body weight. Intense mental work, according to experiments by Benedict and Benedict, may raise the basal metabolism some 4 per cent, a trifling factor when compared with the effect of muscular work.

A group of college students who underwent an average loss of weight of 12 per cent showed lowering of the basal metabolic rate of 18 per cent in contrast with underweight school children in whom there is an increase in the basal metabolic rate of 16 to 25 per cent. However, in fasting, the total metabolism of adults is maintained at about the normal rate, thus showing that the body burns up its own food approximately at the same rate as it does food ingested.

Too often in dietetic computations it is assumed that the caloric needs of the body can be accurately estimated. As a matter of fact, the error in such computations is considerable, and it is absurd to expect to compute the needs of the individual when up and about, whether normal or diabetic, more closely than within 10 to 20 per cent of the real value. The reason for this is apparent if one observes the attitudes and motions of individuals in a trolley car. The one is quiet, the other restless, the one avoids exertion, the other is all activity. In disease these differences of habit and disposition are accentuated. I suspect one will not err greatly if for each mile of walking one allows 1 calorie per 1 kilogram body weight. Sewing and knitting require about 9 calories per hour more than that for the same subject sitting quietly in a chair, whereas washing, sweeping and scrubbing floors require 50 calories additional for the actual period of work; but who washes, sweeps and scrubs floors today? (This was written half a generation ago and we know our wives would resent it today.) Carpenter[1] found 30 calories per hour additional were required by a typist when writing at the rate of 50 words a minute, compared with sitting still and reading. Farmers in various parts of the United States have been shown to consume on an average 3500 calories.

One is apt to forget that an individual doing heavy work requires

[1] Carpenter: Jour. Biol. Chem., **9**, 231, 1911.

additional calories only for the actual period of that work and not for the entire twenty-four hours. With the cessation of work the metabolism falls abruptly. Furthermore, the actual period of heavy work is short and represented by minutes rather than hours. If of a pessimistic nature one has only to watch street laborers to be convinced, though a far more enjoyable and as scientific a proof is furnished by the minutes spent in actual play by two football teams. In two entire games the minutes in which the ball was in play actually numbered, respectively, eleven minutes and eleven minutes and twenty-three seconds, instead of the supposed four quarters of fifteen minutes each.

2. Calories Consumed by Healthy Dietitians and Technicians. —A doctor who treats diabetics will never treat them understandingly unless he knows what he himself eats in calories and, indeed, in carbohydrates, protein and fat. Diabetics simply do not require, save in rare instances, more food than the ordinary individual living under similar conditions. I am more than grateful to Miss Rosina Vance, formerly head dietitian at the New England Deaconess Hospital, and to the group of dietitians and technicians, who volunteered estimates of their caloric intake for two successive days.

The diets of 9 dietitians and technicians were computed by Miss Vance and analyses of nitrogen excretion made under the supervision of Miss Hazel Hunt. Ages averaged 25.3 years, weights 55.5 kilograms (122 pounds), heights 159.5 cm. (63.7 inches). For such an average woman the basal metabolism (H. & B.) would be 1365 calories or 24.6 per kilogram. The food calories varied from 1173 to 2213, the average being 1687 or 30 calories per kilogram body weight. Carbohydrate varied from 130 to 254 grams, average 181 grams, protein about 64 grams. It is true that one of the days included a Friday ("fish day"), which accounts for the protein being low in a few instances. The calcium was far too low with 3 dietitians, due to lack of ingestion of milk. The lowest calcium was 0.22 gram and the highest 1.54 grams, the average being 0.78. Phosphorus varied between 0.60 and 1.56 grams. The lowest value for iron was 6.4 milligrams and the highest 13.3 milligrams, the average being 8.5 milligrams. Of the vitamins, the lowest value for vitamin A was 3000 I.U. and the highest 11,000 I.U., the average being 7000 I.U.; of vitamin B_1 the lowest value was 125 I.U. and the highest 460 I.U. Ascorbic acid ranged between 435 I.U. and 4960 I.U. Of the 9 individuals, ascorbic acid was below 1000 in 6, 1400 in 1, between 4000 and 5000 in 2. The high values were due to oranges and the lowest value to the fact that the only fruit ingested was in the form of cantaloupe and pineapple juice.

3. Caloric Value of 1 Kilogram Body Weight.—The caloric value of 1 kilogram of body weight is problematical but most important. Patients are constantly referring to their gains or losses in weight and the doctor should have clearly in mind what these mean. Bene-

dict's[1] normal subject for the last twenty-seven days of his fast of
thirty-one days lost an average of 0.7 per cent of his body weight
daily, the equivalent of 3258 calories per kilogram or approximately
1500 calories per pound body weight. For comparison Joslin[2] has an
experiment with a healthy nurse who in 1916 volunteered to go
through the exact procedure to which diabetics were subjected at
that time. Her loss of weight in twenty days represented the equivalent of 3170 calories for each kilogram of her body weight lost, and
this agrees quite closely with Benedict's fasting subject. Therefore, one must assume that a patient will not lose or, conversely,
gain a pound of actual body tissue unless he receives at least 1500
calories less or more food than he requires for his standard metabolic
need computed for rest and exercise. Bearing in mind this fact,
many fantasies of gains and losses in weight of diabetics and non-
diabetics are explained.

E. COMPOSITION OF THE NORMAL DIET AND CALORIES CONSUMED.

Men whose work is in office or store are those most frequently
seen by the urban doctor and by no means all of the rural population are engaged in heavy labor. Their diet would consist of 25–35
calories per kilogram body weight, while for women a median figure,
we suspect, would be more nearly the truth. The composition of the
diet undoubtedly varies, but we believe is seldom less than carbohydrate 150 grams, protein 60 grams, fat 60 grams, or more than
carbohydrate 350, protein 125, fat 120 grams, respectively.

TABLE 32.—THE PROPORTION OF CARBOHYDRATE, PROTEIN AND FAT IN THE NORMAL DIET.

Food.	Quantity, grams.	Calories, per gram.	Total calories.
Carbohydrate	150–350	4	600–1400
Protein	60–125	4	240– 500
Fat	60–120	9	540–1080

In estimating calories one allows for carbohydrate and protein
each 4 calories, fat 9 and for alcohol 7 per gram, instead of the actual
calories, 4.1, 4.1, 9.3 and 7.1, respectively.

For diabetics, save at the extremes of life, no less or more are
needed unless an increase or decrease in body weight as a part of
the treatment is indicated.

1. **A Comparison of the Food Ingested With the Food Burned.**—
Before entering upon the detailed discussion of the components of
the diet in health and diabetes, we would call attention to the chart
of DuBois and Richardson, which to us has been of inestimable

---

[1] Benedict: A Study of Prolonged Fasting, Carnegie Institution of Washington,
Pub. 203, p. 251, 1915.

[2] Joslin: Loc. cit., p. 263.

value and deserves far more consideration than it has received. It portrays in vivid fashion that the diets we give our patients are not the diets upon which they actually live. When we contemplate the carbohydrate, protein and fat of the diet, by no means is it identical with the carbohydrate, protein and fat which the patient burns during the same twenty-four hours. Instead he may fall back upon his reserves of these various foods in his own tissues. Unless we realize this, our conception of the results of our alterations in the diet are entirely wrong.

CALORIES OF CARBOHYDRATE, PROTEIN AND FAT IN DIET AND METABOLISM COMPARED. (DUBOIS AND RICHARDSON.)

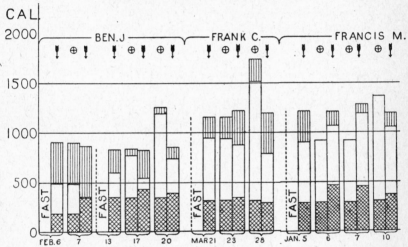

FIG. 9.—The columns indicate calories per twenty-four hours; the lowest portion indicates protein; the middle, fat; the upper, carbohydrate. The circles ⊕ indicate calories in diet; the arrows (↓), calories metabolized. The diet was given, divided into two-hour intervals, and the calorimeter observations were made after the last meal. In the chart comparison may be made between calories metabolized on different days under different conditions of diet, or between the calories of the diet and those metabolized on any given date. Ben. J. was a boy with severe emaciation and a high respiratory quotient.

This is graphically shown in Figure 9. Thus, although Ben. J. on February 6 was deprived of all fat, yet, as demonstrated in the calorimeter, he burned a liberal quantity of fat along with carbohydrate and protein. On the following day when fed exactly the same number of calories and similarly distributed, he burned half again as much protein, practically no fat at all and one-third more carbohydrate. This table of DuBois and Richardson should be taken to heart because otherwise results of temporary changes in diet will seem astounding. The table proves that far more time than a few days is essential in order to reach a proper conclusion about the efficacy of a dietary prescription.

2. **Carbohydrate.**—Approximately one-half the calories of the normal diet are made up of carbohydrate. This leaves no doubt as to how large a place sugar and starch occupy in the daily ration. What percentage of carbohydrate is furnished by sucrose is problematical. One estimate is one-seventh of the total caloric ration. For the years 1930–1937, however, it is estimated that the average individual in the United States consumed 95 pounds of cane sugar yearly. This would amount to 118 grams daily or about one-third of the total carbohydrate calories. In tropical countries the proportion of carbohydrate rises materially, but in colder regions similarly falls, although probably far less than to the 50 grams per day which formerly may have been the average amount.

The total carbohydrate in the diet of diabetic patients under treatment varies with the physician, but we believe should not be less than 100 grams or much over 200 grams. We suspect our present average is between 150 and 165 grams, with 25 or rarely 75 grams additional for children. (See Table 47.) This quantity is rendered possible with insulin. Such a diet lowers the carbohydrate ration probably not more than one-quarter to one-third for the average individual, and only rarely as much as one-half for any one. So far as the utilization of the form of carbohydrate given is concerned, there is little variation provided allowance is made for the time element. Thus the utilization of 100 grams of pure sugar would be less in a diabetic compared with 100 grams of starch in the form of coarse vegetables if taken approximately in the same interval of time. However, Wishnofsky and Kane[1] found that glycosuria and increase in blood sugar following the giving of glucose did not differ significantly from that following a meal, containing the molecular equivalent of 90 grams of starch, of 100 grams of glucose in the form of potato, barley, rice and bread. Of the sugars themselves, apparently glucose is especially desirable, particularly because of its prevention of the accumulation of lactic acid due to exercise. Levulose sometimes failed, whereas lactose and sucrose have no inhibiting effect on the rise in the level of exercise-fixed acid in the subjects studied.[2]

Bertram[3] has little use for dietary tables—"Die Nährmittel Tabellen sind ein Unsinn"—because he finds such great variations in the same. If he should visit our clinic and study our charts we are sure he would alter his opinion. The average analyses for foods in this country are based upon such extensive data that they are trustworthy, although not to the decimal point. When accurately calculated diets are used they meet scientific computations when checked with metabolic determinations. Compare the calculated ingestion of foods and minerals and the excretion of nitrogen and

[1] Wishnofsky and Kane: Loc. cit., p. 158.
[2] Schultz: Am. Jour. Dis. Child., 53, 960, 1937.
[3] Bertram: P. 68, loc. cit., p. 87.

iron in the metabolic experiment of Marble and Smith[1] upon a patient with hemachromatosis.

3. The Estimation of the Carbohydrate in the Diabetic Diet.—The quantity of carbohydrate in the various foods is easily calculated and far more simply than is usually thought. This is not true if one desires scientific accuracy, for in that event analyses of the food given the patient must be made. In any estimation of carbohydrate in the diabetic diet one must not overlook the possibility of 58 grams of carbohydrate being formed out of 100 grams of protein and 10 grams out of the glycerol of 100 grams of fat. The "total glucose" value of the three foodstuffs would be, therefore, 100 grams C. $\times$ 100 per cent $+$ 100 grams P. $\times$ 58 per cent $+$ 100 grams F. $\times$ 10 per cent. Such calculations, of course, are based upon the assumption that the D to N ratio of 3.65 to 1 is a reliable index of the carbohydrate-forming power of protein and that only the glycerol of the fat turns to sugar. Bertram[2] gives 50 to 64 grams as the quantity of sugar formed from 100 grams protein.

TABLE 33.—FOOD VALUES IMPORTANT IN THE TREATMENT OF DIABETES.[3]

30 grams, 1 oz., contain approximately:	Carbo-hydrate, grams.	Protein, grams.	Fat, grams.	Calories.
Vegetables, 5 per cent	1	0.5	0	6
Vegetables, 10 per cent	2	0.5	0	10
Potato	6	1	0	28
Bread	18	3	0	84
Uneeda Biscuits, 2[4]	10	1	1	53
Oatmeal, dry weight	20	5	2	118
Shredded Wheat, 1[4]	23	3	0	104
Milk	1.5	1	1	19
Meat, cooked, lean	0	8	5	77
Fish, fat-free	0	6	0	24
Chicken, cooked, lean	0	8	3	59
Egg, 1	0	6	6	78
Cheese	0	8	11	131
Bacon	0	5	15	155
Cream, 20 per cent	1	1	6	62
Cream, 40 per cent	1	1	12	116
Butter	0	0	25	225
Oil	0	0	30	270

4. Important Food Values.—The quantity of carbohydrate, protein and fat found in an ordinary diet must be known by a physician if he wishes to treat a case of diabetes successfully. If he cannot calculate the diet he will lose the respect of his patient. The values of the different foods in the diet can be calculated easily from Table 33. This is purposely simple, because a diet chart, to be useful, must be easily remembered. With these food values as a basis it is possible to give a rough estimate of the value and

[1] Marble and Smith: Ann. Int. Med., **12**, 1592, 1939.
[2] Bertram: Loc. cit., p. 87.
[3] I consider Table 33 the chief dietary table in this book.
[4] Values for biscuits and prepared foods vary from time to time. A constant weight would be desirable.

composition of almost any food. Various foods are also classified according to the content of carbohydrate (see page 275) in 5, 10, 15 and 20 per cent groups, and the lists are so arranged that those first in each group contain the least, those at the end the most. This is a practical and sufficiently accurate arrangement, because except in the most exact experiments the errors in the preparation of the food are too great to warrant closer reckoning.

The only safe way for diabetic patients at the commencement of their training is to weigh their food. Today the average level of education in this country has advanced, and we doctors should take cognizance and advantage of it. After a few days of weighing, patients select utensils which conform to the size of the portions of their own special diets and use these almost exclusively. As a matter of fact, practically all of our patients use scales at one time or another in the course of treatment. The 500-gram scale manufactured by John Chatillon and Sons, New York City, has been of such great service to us in the treatment of our diabetics that it is a matter of sentiment as well as of duty that we express our indebtedness to that firm for assistance during nearly half a century. It is true today there are also other excellent varieties. Scales are more accurate than the eye, and we do not give them up.

5. **Carbohydrate.**—In teaching diabetic patients their diet, we lay emphasis first on carbohydrate values, and only to a few patients attempt to teach the values for protein and fat. As a rule, we find that patients do not eat too much meat, and as for the fat in the diet, it can be regulated largely by body weight. If a patient will grasp the carbohydrate values of six types of food and use his common sense, he will seldom make egregious errors. (See Table 30.)

(*a*) **Carbohydrate in Vegetables.**—It would appear perplexing to determine the amount of carbohydrate in each of the various vegetables which the patient eats in twenty-four hours. Diabetic patients have too much to do in their daily work to be encumbered with unnecessary details of arithmetic. An attempt to force accuracy to the extent of a gram may result in loss of accuracy to the extent of an ounce by the patient giving up weighing entirely.

For convenience we have classified the vegetables which enter into the diabetic diet under four headings—those containing approximately 5 per cent, 10 per cent, 15 per cent and 20 per cent carbohydrate. (See Table 34.)

The range of carbohydrate is so great in these different groups, *e. g.*, lettuce contains 2.2 per cent carbohydrate and summer squash may contain 3.4 per cent (squash ranging between 3.6 to 12.8 per cent), that in clinical work it is safe to count a mixture of vegetables in the 5 per cent class as averaging 3 per cent carbohydrate or approximately 1 gram to the ounce, in the 10 per cent group at 6 per cent. Since in the 15 per cent and 20 per cent groups the cellulose is less, the variations are less marked and it is safer to hold to the actual figures of 15 per cent and 20 per cent. As a matter of fact it is seldom that patients will take as much and practically never eat more than 20 grams of carbohydrate in vegetables of the 5 per cent group. Considering that the total carbohydrate content of the diet of the diabetic averages 150 grams, the errors introduced in these approximate calculations in vegetables are trifling, and to this extent I heartily agree with Bertram. In fact, it is not uncommon in Europe for the 5 per cent vegetables and perhaps even the 10 per cent vegetables to be given freely to diabetics without any allowance for them at all in the diet, but to that plan we will not assent.

TABLE 34.—FOODS ARRANGED APPROXIMATELY ACCORDING TO CONTENT OF CARBOHYDRATE. VEGETABLES FRESH OR CANNED (WITHOUT ADDED SUGAR).

5 per cent (net average 3 per cent).		10 per cent (net average 6 per cent).	Calculate average as 1 per cent.	Calculate average as 20 per cent.
Lettuce	Sea kale	String beans	Green peas	Potatoes
Cucumbers	Cauliflower	Brussels sprouts	Jerusalem	Shell beans
Spinach	Egg plant	Pumpkin	artichokes	Baked beans
Asparagus	Cabbage	Turnips	Parsnips	Lima beans
Rhubarb	Radishes	Squash	Lima beans,	Green corn
Endive	Leeks	Okra	young	Boiled rice
Marrow	String beans,	Beets		Boiled macaroni
Sorrel	young	Carrots		
Sauerkraut	Broccoli	Onions		
Beet greens	French arti-	Green peas,		
Dandelions	chokes	very young		
Swiss chard	Green peppers			
Celery				
Mushrooms	Summer squash			
Tomatoes	Kohlrabi			
Water cress				

The vitamins vary even more in vegetables than does the carbohydrate content. In 100 grams of iceberg lettuce these are approximately Vit. A, I.U. 90; Vit. B, I.U. 18; Vit. C, I.U. 80; and as contrasted with those of green lettuce, Vit. A, I.U. 2855; Vit. B, I.U. 18; Vit. C, approximately the same strength.

Potatoes contain approximately 20 per cent carbohydrate. The variation in the percentage of carbohydrate in potatoes before and after cooking is negligible, *save with potato chips, in which it is more than double.* If the potatoes are boiled with the skins on, the loss in protein and mineral matter is slight, but if soaked in cold water before boiling, the loss of protein may reach 25 per cent and mineral matter 38 per cent. Sweet potatoes contain 42 per cent carbohydrate.

Eggplant not only is an agreeable vegetable for diabetics with its total carbohydrate content only 5.1 per cent, protein 1.2 per cent and fat 0.3 per cent, but it has another favorable quality. According to Roffo[1] it induces both in man and in animals a reduction in the cholesterol of the blood. This amounted to more than 50 per cent in some cases. It also acted as a diuretic.

[1] Roffo: Yale Jour. Biol. and Med., **18**, 25, 1945.

(*b*) *Nuts.*—The utilizable carbohydrate in nuts containing 15 and 20 per cent carbohydrate is probably far less than most other foods with a similar carbohydrate content. This is due to the fact that in such nuts as almonds a larger part of the carbohydrate is in the form of pentosan, galactan or other hemicelluloses, some of which probably do not readily form glucose.

The usefulness of nuts in the diabetic dietary furnishes an interesting problem for investigation. Since the carbohydrate is slowly absorbed they serve as a preventive of a reaction and in fact I have often given them to patients upon retiring as a protection from hypoglycemia during the night. One ounce, 30 grams, of peanuts contains about carbohydrate 6, protein 8 and fat 10 grams or the equivalent of a graham cracker and an ounce of cheese.

Pollack[1] has used this idea in a slightly different manner by giving at the evening meal or even upon retiring, the major quantity of protein of the day. The danger of nuts to the diabetic exists not in the content of carbohydrate, but rather in their high percentage of protein and fat. Ignorant diabetics often eat nuts as freely as they would 5 per cent vegetables and wonder why they develop glycosuria or, in the pre-insulin days, serious acidosis.

(*c*) *Fruit.*—Fruit offers carbohydrate and vitamins in about the most pleasant form. The taste is agreeable, it serves instead of a dessert, and so relieves the patient of the embarrassment of sitting idly at the table when others are eating. Grapefruit, 6.6 to 8.2 per cent, strawberries, 6 per cent, and oranges, 10.6 per cent carbohydrate, are the most desirable. As for apples, there are few more graphic illustrations of the change in the dietetic treatment of diabetes than my attitude toward them. In the Naunyn and Allen Eras, I never dared to give them to a child, because they were such a temptation and, unlike oranges, they left no residue. The diabetic catechism even included the question, "What are you to do with an apple?" and the answer, "Give it away." Today the carbohydrate in the diet is so great that they can be included with allowance for their content of sugar. Apples not only vary very greatly in size, but the range in carbohydrate is from 7 to 16 per cent. However, apples still carry the same temptation as did that early one in the Garden of Eden. Diabetics in this country have no idea of the palatability of their diets as compared with those in Europe where fruits, and especially tropical fruits, are less available because of climate and cost.

The vitamin content of a small orange weighing peeled 100 grams is considerable[2]—vitamin C 440–1780 units, or ascorbic acid 22–89 mg. Apples are to be compared to *peeled* oranges and then reduced $\frac{1}{3}$ in size because oranges contain 10 per cent carbohydrate

---

[1] Pollack: Modern Diabetic Care, New York, Harcourt, Brace & Co., p. 151, 1940.

[2] See page 294 for discussion of vitamins.

and apples 15 per cent, and in comparing the sizes of each a diabetic often forgets he does not eat the thick skin of the orange.

TABLE 35.—EQUIVALENT OF 10 GRAMS CARBOHYDRATE IN VARIOUS FRUITS.

Food.	Carbo-hydrate, 10 grams.	Food.	Carbo-hydrate, 10 grams.
Grapefruit pulp	150	Apricots	80
Strawberries	150	Honeydew melon	75
Watermelon	150	Pineapple	70
Blackberries	120	Apple	70
Cantaloupe	150	Cherries	60
Orange pulp	100	Blueberries	70
Pears	90	Banana	50
Peaches	90	Ice cream	50
Plums	80	Prunes	50
Raspberries	80		

(d) *Bananas.*—Bananas are useful for diabetic patients not because the content of carbohydrate is low, for in reality it is equivalent to that in potato, 20 per cent, but because of their comparative uniformity in size. It is safer for a patient to be told that he can have a banana of moderate size than a slice of bread unless commercially sliced, though each should contain about the same amount of carbohydrate. For the same reason they are safer than potatoes.

(e) *Milk.*—The carbohydrate in milk is in the form of lactose and can be reckoned at 5 per cent, or 1.5 grams per 30 cc., or 1 ounce. It is the same in skimmed milk and whey; but cream and koumyss contain about 3 per cent, or 1 gram carbohydrate to the ounce. Buttermilk contains essentially the same quantity of carbohydrate and protein as milk, but only a trifling amount of fat. Fermented milk may contain 3 per cent sugar. In the last generation the good results of a "skimmed milk cure" in mild diabetics are easily attributed to the undernutrition which it represented. One quart of milk contains between 600 and 700 calories and skimmed milk one-half as much.

Milk contains so many valuable food elements that it is essential to insert some of it as milk, cream, or cheese into the diet. Without milk or milk products it is practically impossible to provide an adequate calcium intake. One gill (120 grams) of milk contains carbohydrate 6 grams, and 1 gill of 20 per cent cream carbohydrate 4 grams; thus ½ pint of equal parts milk and cream contains 10 grams of carbohydrate—a useful figure to use in substitutions. Vitamins A, B, D are found to an appreciable extent in milk.

(f) *Oatmeal.*—Oatmeal is two-thirds carbohydrate. In calculations one should always be guided by the dry weight, because the different preparations vary greatly in bulk and weight when cooked. Formerly it was by far the most desirable cereal for the diabetic, because it contained the least amount of carbohydrate and was bulky. Even today the diabetic who needs a carefully chosen diet and wishes to simplify estimations will find it advantageous to take cereal in the form of oatmeal. Thirty grams of dry oatmeal, 240 grams cooked or a large portion contains carbohydrate 20 grams, protein 5 grams, fat 2 grams. A discussion of the oatmeal treatment of diabetes appears on page 352.

(g) *Bread.*—The carbohydrate in white wheat bread amounts to about 53 per cent. If the bread is dry or toasted, enough water is lost to raise the percentage of carbohydrate in the toast to about 60 per cent. If the bread is made without sugar and with water instead of milk the carbohydrate content is lowered and may amount only to 45 per cent. Coarse breads if made without sweetening or milk would contain slightly less carbohydrate. An error in weight of 1 ounce of 3 to 5 per cent vegetables amounts to 1 gram carbohydrate, of potato to 6 grams, but of bread to 18 grams. Crackers, zwieback, shredded wheat and many dry cereals contain still less water than toast, and in consequence the percentage of carbohydrate may rise to 80 per cent. In general carbohydrate in breads and bread-like preparations varies with the moisture and thus the range is between 40 and 80 per cent.

Breads and cereals made from whole grains have had many advantages over white bread, but today artificially they are made nearer alike. The vitamin content, the calcium and phosphorus and iron are doubled. In refined cereals vitamin B is negligible, whereas in whole-grain products it varies between 150 and 300 I.U. per 100 grams and yet the cost is the same. The annual per capita consumption of wheat bread alone in the United States is over 80 pounds, and of all types almost 90 pounds (4 slices a day). Bread is a concentrated food and one of the cheapest sources of energy. The nutritive value of the protein of whole wheat is superior to that of various flours milled from it. The removal of wheat bran and wheat germ in the preparation of wheat flour effects a reduction in mineral content to about one-half for calcium, one-fourth for potassium, one-fifth for phosphorus and one-fifth for iron. Wheat flour contains an insignificant amount of provitamin A, but its content of the B group is not inconsiderable. White bread contains only about one-fourth to one-sixth as much thiamin as whole-wheat bread and whole-wheat flour contains a higher percentage of vitamin B complex. Whole-wheat grain contains an appreciable amount of vitamin A, carotene, but this gives a yellow color to the flour.

6. **Protein.**—Advances in the knowledge of proteins in the last fifty years, and particularly in the recent decade, are so great as to be almost bewildering. These are discussed in their special application to surgical problems on page 673 and to diseases of the kidneys on page 502. Suffice it to say here that the emphasis of modern thought is the desirability of giving more rather than less protein to normal individuals and we may assume that this would apply also to diabetics.

Protein present in blood plasma is not static but reflects stores of protein in the tissues. Moreover, there is a constant interchange between plasma protein and hemoglobin. Following tissue injury by infections, burns or trauma, the loss of protein is very material. Almost lamentably I report that Case 513,[1] male, onset diabetes at age thirty-three in 1911, with a carbuncle in 1915, excreted an average of 32.5 grams of nitrogen daily for eight days and his weight fell 17 pounds in the same period. A minus nitrogen balance, due to a low diet and inability to retain food, of 111 grams which he showed, represented a loss of (111 x 6.25) 694 grams protein, not counting that lost in the feces, or approximately 7 pounds of muscle protoplasm. Such a deficiency in protein can lead to edema, as it did in the above patient prior to the above period of observation, delay healing and interfere with digestion, and favor the production of peptic ulcers and damage to the liver. Recent work points to the advantage of a liberal protein diet in hepatic disease. And we all recognize the spectacular effect of the giving of liver proteins to patients with pernicious anemia. The quantity of protein required by diabetic patients varies with the age, weight and activity of the individual. It is a safe rule at the beginning of treatment to increase the protein gradually up to the same quantity as that required by a normal person. Safety lies not far from 3 grams protein for each kilogram body weight for children and decreases to 1 gram or even 0.66 gram for the aged. According to Professor Cannon,[2] the average daily excretion of nitrogen during four days for 46 students was 12.8 grams. If we allow for that eliminated in the feces, the total elimination of nitrogen would be 14 grams, and this would represent the equivalent of (14 × 6.25) 88 grams protein. A group of nine dietitians and technicians excreted an average of 7.1 grams per day, of nitrogen in the urine. Lusk[3] states that even if no protein were given an individual for a year he would survive providing carbohydrate and calories were furnished in liberal quantities. The protein metabolism is easily brought to less than 50 grams per day, and Karl Thomas by these means and frequent feeding lowered the same to that represented by 2 and 3 grams of nitrogen, but this is no proof that it is desirable to do so.

Data upon the average ingestion of protein and excretion of nitrogen per kilogram body weight in countries like the Argentine in which meat is more freely consumed would be desirable. I feel sure their diabetic patients eat far more protein than do ours. Whether a high protein intake in South American countries is

[1] Joslin: The Treatment of Diabetes Mellitus, Philadelphia, Lea and Febiger, p. 269, 1916.

[2] Cannon: Personal communication.

[3] Lusk: The Science of Nutrition, 4th ed., Philadelphia, W. B. Saunders Co. p. 361, 1928.

confined to the well-to-do or spreads to the masses of the population is obviously important.

With an excess of protein in the diet the protein metabolized may rise to 150 or 200 grams. A liver well stored with glycogen protects the body protein of a fasting man for a day equally as well as does carbohydrate in the diet. On the second day, since the glycogen is nearly exhausted, the protection is distinctly less.

The influence of the available supply of body fat upon the protein metabolism of fasting, as stated by Sherman,[1] is shown by the observations of Falck, on the protein metabolism of 2 fasting dogs— the one lean, the other fat. The fat dog was healthy thirty-five days after the lean dog died.

Half a century ago protein values were extremely high in diabetic diets, because of the restriction of carbohydrate and at that time the large quantity of carbohydrate which could be formed from protein was overlooked. This explains why gluten breads were so frequently a delusion and a snare even though the protein being in vegetable form might be less assimilated.

The restricted allowance of carbohydrate with an unrestricted allowance of protein and fat must be held responsible for many untimely diabetic deaths. Indeed, it was not until von Mering and Minkowski with their depancreatized dogs, and Lusk with his phlorizinized dogs, established a dextrose-nitrogen ratio in total diabetes that the profession fully appreciated the carbohydrate-forming qualities of protein. Even if both the theory and the accuracy of the dextrose-nitrogen ratio are supplanted, they have been of the greatest service both scientifically and practically in the every-day treatment of patients.

Protein stimulates the metabolism more than any other kind of food, favors acidosis both experimentally and clinically and can lead to the formation of 58 grams of glucose for every 100 grams metabolized. Case 550, an Italian, before treatment began excreted 48.1 grams urinary nitrogen in twenty-four hours and, if we allow 4.8 grams nitrogen for that lost in the feces, he must have consumed $(48.1 + 4.8) \times 6.25 = 331$ grams protein. A coma case with a carbuncle, in 1915, lost between 31.6 and 37.8 grams urinary nitrogen daily for a period of six days. In extreme inanition Case 1011, weighing 26.4 kilograms, or 52 per cent below normal, excreted 0.515 gram urinary nitrogen (3.2 grams protein) per kilogram body weight.

Vegetable proteins are said to give rise to less carbohydrate in the diabetic organism than do animal proteins. As a matter of fact, carbohydrate may be formed out of any protein.[2] On the other hand, animal protein has a higher biologic value than vegetable

[1] Sherman: Chemistry of Food and Nutrition, 7th ed., New York, The Macmillan Company, p. 198, 1946.
[2] Janney: Arch. Int. Med., 18, 584, 1916.

protein and, according to Bertram, one-half of the protein in the diabetic diet, which he places at 75–80 grams, should come from animal sources. Gelatin is lacking in the amino-acids, tryptophane, tyrosine and cystine, and thus is not as adequate a protein as is found in meat, milk, and fish. Moreover, gelatin is poor in vitamins; it will yield sugar like any protein, but it will never build up new tissue. In any plan for the diet of the diabetic, one must not lose sight of the inherent qualities in protein and fat, not only as nutritive, but in their content of vitamins. The former diet of Eskimos demonstrates this, but scientifically it was proved by McClellan and DuBois.[1] By maintaining two men upon an exclusive meat diet for a year, the protein content varied from 100 to 140 grams, the fat from 200 to 300 grams, the carbohydrate, derived entirely from the meat, from 7 to 12 grams, and the fuel value from 2000 to 3100 calories. Vitamin deficiencies did not appear. In these trained subjects the clinical observations and laboratory studies gave no evidence that any ill effects had occurred from the prolonged use of the exclusive meat diet.

Diabetic breads and also patent diabetic foods may contain a small quantity of carbohydrate, yet the protein in them may be high and capable of furnishing a large amount of glucose. The result is that such commercial products may actually lead to the production of as much glucose in a diabetic as does ordinary bread. However, one must not be wholly governed by analytical conditions, as Janney[2] has pointed out, for although vegetable and animal proteins yield glucose according to their content of amino-acids, it is quite possible that the vegetable proteins will be less well digested, owing to the form in which they are eaten, and thus less protein is assimilated, and in consequence less glucose formed.

Fish differs from meat chiefly in the small quantity of fat. Even salmon, which contains more fat than most other fish, showed in its analysis only 12.8 per cent fat, shad, 9.5 per cent, and herring and mackerel, 7.1 per cent. In general, other kinds of fish show 6 per cent or less of fat. Halibut steak, for example, contains 5.2 per cent, and cod, 0.4 per cent. Preserved fish, however, is quite rich in fat; thus sardines contain 19.7 per cent.

Shell-fish make agreeable additions to the diet: (1) They are desirable because they are palatable; (2) they are usually bulky foods and so are satisfying; (3) they furnish a separate course at a meal. The edible portion of a medium-sized oyster on the shell weighs on the average ½ ounce, and one-half dozen oysters would amount to 90 to 100 grams. The 6 would contain about 6 grams protein, 1 gram fat and 4 grams carbohydrate—the equivalent of 50 calories. One-half dozen clams on the shell (edible portion)

[1] McClellan and DuBois: Jour. Biol. Chem., **87**, 651, 1930.
[2] Janney: Loc. cit., p. 280.

weigh 35 grams and contain 0.7 gram carbohydrate, 3 grams protein and a negligible quantity of fat.

Broths in the days of undernutrition were a real factor in the diet. As a rule broths do not contain more than 2.2 per cent protein, even if all the nitrogen in the broth is in the form of protein, which, of course, is never the case. The fat in broths varies according to whether it is skimmed off before serving, and may be as low as 0.1 per cent. The amount of carbohydrate is negligible, 0.2 per cent or less. For practical purposes calorically, therefore, broths are allowable, but in metabolism experiments and in the presence of edema they should be excluded. In coma they may be utilized with advantage, because of their content in salt and the desirability of giving hot liquids. The salt varies greatly, from 2 per cent to 0.1 per cent, in samples analyzed under our direction.

The amino-acids in protein are classified according to their ketogenic and antiketogenic properties as follows: *ketogenic* (-oxybutyric acid formers), leucine, tyrosine, phenylalanine, histadine; *antiketogenic* (glucose formers), glycine, alanine, aspartic acid, glutamic acid, arginine, proline, cystine, serine.

The fate of lysine, valine, histadine and tryptophane is obscure. Tryptophane is the one amino-acid we must all have to maintain nitrogen equilibrium. (See also page 262.)

7. **Fats.**—The changes in the conception with which the metabolism of fat is now regarded compared to the early days of our practice are very great. At present we know that ketone bodies derived from fat normally enter into the metabolism and are of great importance unless their production is extreme. We are only entering the era of the understanding of enzymatic action in the various transformations and decompositions not only of fat but of protein and carbohydrates.

The quantity of fat in the normal diet varies, partly from choice and partly from economic reasons. In general, in those cases where the carbohydrate in the diet is high the fat is low, and *vice versa*. The average in a series of 1300 dietary studies among different races and in different climates was about 135 grams fat per person per day, the variation being from 45 to 390 grams. The more agreeable varieties of fat, such as butter, cream and eggs are expensive foods, counterbalanced to some extent, it is true, by little waste in them, but more especially by the high vitamin content. The oils commonly used are very poor in vitamins, except such medicinal oils as from the livers of cod and halibut. The heat required in the preparation of lard may be largely responsible for its lack of vitamins, also a characteristic of vegetable oils. Fat is also concentrated food, not only because it has twice the caloric value of either carbohydrate or protein, but because it occurs more frequently in pure form. Oil, butter and lard contain little water, whereas, except for pure sugar and starch, most carbohydrates and proteins are diluted five to ten times with water.

The chief source of error in calculating the total caloric value of the diet, and especially of the diabetic diet, is in the estimation of fat. We know that some diabetic patients assigned high-carbohydrate and low-fat diets do not keep the fat at the prescribed low level. Thus for many years we have considered that, on an average, lean meat and fish contained 10 per cent fat and have taught patients to reckon 3 grams of fat to each ounce of lean meat or fish. This figure is unquestionably correct for poultry and very lean meat, and is very high for most varieties of fish, such varieties as cod, haddock and flounder containing only 1 per cent; but an analysis of a mixture of 10 portions of cooked meat exactly identical with similar portions about to be served patients at the New England Deaconess Hospital was made at the Nutrition Laboratory and showed 14.4 per cent fat. It is, therefore, better to reckon 5 grams of fat to the ounce of cooked meat when the patient is taking several varieties. The fat of cooked bacon varies from 37 to 79 per cent and we have adopted 50 per cent as an average value.

Eggs in some cities by law must weigh 1½ pounds a dozen, and average 60 grams (2 ounces) apiece. Such eggs contain approximately 6 grams of protein and 6 grams of fat. How gross our caloric reckonings are is obvious if a collection of eggs is weighed and the minimum and maximum weights noted. The weight of the heaviest egg in a collection of 56 was 72 per cent more than that of the lightest. The weight of egg-shells is usually about 7 grams.

The cholesterol in one egg amounts to 0.38 grams, according to Professor Bloor, but we do not yet banish them from the diabetic's table, out of fear that they might cause arteriosclerosis, although we often reduce the number to one egg daily for patients over fifty years of age. Brain (cattle), liver, kidney (mutton), pancreas (calf) contain in decreasing values from 3.7 to 3.1 per cent cholesterol; thymus (calf), salmon roe and egg-yolk, 2.3 to 2.2 per cent, a whole egg, 0.45 to 0.24 per cent; chicken, 0.5 per cent; lard and suet, 0.35 to 0.1 per cent; dried beef, 0.23 per cent; butter, 0.22 per cent.

(*a*) **The Value of Fat to the Diabetic.**—In the past fat has formed the bulk of the diabetic patient's calories. In the normal diet it furnishes less than one-third of the total calories and today in the diabetic diet it often forms less rather than more than one-half.

It is surprising how readily in the past double and even treble the quantity of fat ingested by normal individuals was borne by the stomach of the diabetic patient. Frequently we see patients who have taken large quantities of fat with obvious benefit for long periods. Case 8 (pp. 286, 288) outlived most of her family and, as has been said, her own life expectancy. It is, however, unwise to push the administration of fat too energetically for fear of causing a dislike for it, or even indigestion.

One-half pint of 20 per cent cream contains approximately 48 grams of fat, and but little over 8 grams carbohydrate and 8 grams of protein. Thirty grams of butter contain 25 grams of fat. Margarine contains no sugar and has about the same percentage of fat as butter and the cost is approximately one-half that of first-class butter. Lard is nearly 100 per cent fat. A vegetable fat, also nearly 100 per cent fat, is often more welcome than lard, because of its lack of flavor.

Vegetable fats (margarines), reinforced as they now usually are with vitamins A and D, are equivalent to butter.[1] Oil is an ideal diabetic food, because it is a pure fat and Italian patients naturally bear olive oil unusually well. An Italian diabetic patient under my care at the Boston City Hospital with typhoid fever not only passed through the disease uneventfully about thirty-five years ago upon oatmeal gruel and olive oil, but incidentally became sugar-free and developed no acidosis.

Next to the role played by glycogen is that played by fat, and there are many mysteries connected with it. Stadie's work has revolutionized our thoughts. Today we realize that the ketone bodies derived from fat have a place in the normal metabolism of fat. We know that acidosis comes through the fat molecule, but why it is that in marked acidosis, diabetic coma, the percentage of cholesterol in the blood has no relation to the prognosis of coma is an enigma. However, Bertram[2] has seen no diabetic coma patient recover whose total acetone in the blood exceeded 70 mg. per cent, although he has observed total acetone 135 mg. per cent and β-oxybutyric acid 213 mg. per cent. So, too, we are in a cloud about the relation of fat to arteriosclerosis. (See pages 218 and 293.) We do know that tolerance for carbohydrate is less when the patient is on a low-carbohydrate high-fat diet, and yet how important this may be in the ultimate course of the disease is still a subject of discussion.

(*b*) **The Danger of Fat to the Diabetic.**—Fat is the chief source of the dreaded acidosis, though to this in lesser degree the amino-acids of the protein molecule contribute as well. One of the most potent agencies in the prevention of acidosis is the withdrawal of fat from the diet. Fat dogs are more susceptible to acidosis than thin dogs. As soon as undernutrition was introduced into treatment the mortality from diabetic coma fell from 60 per cent to 40 per cent, and fresh cases of coma almost ceased to arise in hospitals. One must remember that fat forms a part of the diet even if it is not ingested unless sufficient calories are furnished in protein and carbohydrate. A diabetic always eats (!) even if compelled to eat his own body fat.

We think it is unreasonable to give less fat than in health or more

[1] Cowgill: Phys. Rev., **25**, 664, 1945.
[2] Bertram: P. 51; loc. cit., p. 87.

than the patient can take without developing acidosis. Probably an amount sufficient to bring the weight up to 10 per cent below normal is adequate, except in younger individuals who should be of normal weight.

Enormous quantities of fat were given formerly; thus, Case 344 took 372 grams of fat on an oatmeal day, September 15–16, 1910. The acidosis on this day was extreme, as shown by the excretion of 27.6 grams β-oxybutyric acid. Many diabetic patients took 100 grams fat in the form of cream in addition to that in bacon, butter, eggs and fat meat. Von Noorden's oatmeal cure called for 200 to 300 grams butter. The fact, as we now know, that one molecule of a fat like palmitic acid can yield as many as 4 molecules of aceto-acetic acid instead of one as by the old Knopp theory, emphasizes the enormous quantities of ketone bodies these patients metabolized.

Weeks, Renner, Allen and Wishart[1] in studies upon the effects of fasting and diets in epilepsy observed a remarkable hyperglycemia which developed in every case on a high-fat diet, but not with any of the other diets. This has been confirmed by Odin,[2] noted also in depancreatized dogs as a consequence of which the insulin must be increased, and extensively studied by Sweeney.[3]

Allen[4] made us all his debtors by a series of experiments upon diabetic dogs which show the insidious way in which fat is harmful in the manner in which it was at one time employed in the treatment of diabetes. "Fat unbalanced by adequate quantities of other foods is a poison." And Shaffer, Woodyatt, Newburgh and Marsh, Petrén, Campbell, Strouse, Ladd and Palmer all contributed formulæ to show the adequate quantities of other foods. Newburgh and Marsh and Petrén courageously demonstrated that patients did not die in the hospital while living upon a high-fat, but low-carbohydrate and very low-protein diet, even before the explanation therefor was perfectly plain.

Fat in any form is absorbed by the diabetic patient very well, but probably in more cases than supposed it has escaped absorption due to a deficiency in the external secretion of the pancreas as Chester Jones[5] has demonstrated. It also escapes absorption in those rare cases of diabetes with general pancreatic involvement. One such case (Case 670) was seen by me a few days before coma. In this instance diabetes occurred after partial loss of the gland from acute pancreatitis. The case was reported in detail by Jurist.[6]

Fat, however, is not well absorbed by the dog made diabetic by the removal of the pancreas. This fact explains one of the difficulties experienced in producing acidosis in dogs. When Allen[4] succeeded in making a dog with severe diabetes gain or even hold his weight by forced feeding of fat, increasing acidosis occurred.

[1] Weeks, Renner, Allen and Wishart: Jour. Metab. Res., **3**, 317, 1923.
[2] Odin: Acta med. Scandin., Suppl. 18, pp. 1–573, 1927.
[3] Sweeney: Arch. Int. Med., **41**, 420, 1928.
[4] Allen: Am. Jour. Med. Sci., **153**, 313, 1917.
[5] Jones, Castle, Mulholland and Bailey: Loc. cit., p. 225.
[6] Jurist: Am. Jour. Med. Sci., **138**, 180, 1909.

Depancreatized dogs treated with insulin also show defective fat metabolism which must be protected by administration of the pancreatic gland in some form in order to prolong life beyond eight months or, as Dragstedt has pointed out, by the administration of lipocaic. (See page 133). Apparently this is not due merely to defective fat absorption, but to defective fat metabolism in the liver, and this is caused not by lack of feeding pancreas or even its component lecithin, but by absence of the choline portion of the lecithin molecule.

(c) **Choline.**—The importance of this constituent in the diet of depancreatized dogs (and presumably in that of human diabetics) has been demonstrated by Best and his associates.[1] Fletcher, Best and Solandt[2] analyzed animal and plant tissues for choline using a method of biological assay. Beef liver, beef pituitary, beef pancreas, dog liver and pig pancreas contained about the same amount of choline (from 217 to 270 mg. per cent). Among foods, potato starch, cane sugar, corn oil, vegetable oils and olive oil were found to contain little or no choline. Wheat flour, meat extract, rice, milk powder, and particularly yeast contained relatively large amounts.

For a discussion of the rôle of choline, its synthesis[3] from methionine, and lipocaic in metabolism, see pages 131, 134.

F. THE CARBOHYDRATE BALANCE AND GLUCOSE BALANCE.

1. **The Carbohydrate Balance.**—The carbohydrate balance represents the difference between the total quantity of carbohydrate as such ingested in the diet and the sugar excreted in the urine during the same period. When the quantity of carbohydrate in the diet is greater than the quantity of sugar in the urine the patient is said to have a positive carbohydrate balance. When the carbohydrate in the diet is less than the quantity of sugar in the urine the carbohydrate balance is said to be minus or negative. Under the latter circumstances it is evident that the sugar in the urine is derived either from sugar stored in the body or is being formed out of protein or fat. If it simply represents stored-up sugar, within a few days the negative carbohydrate balance will promptly change to zero and perhaps eventually to a positive balance. Case 8, in Table 36, will illustrate this, but Case 2095 shows it also and illustrates how we treated diabetes before the advent of insulin. (See Table 37.) These cases are inserted for their historical interest and because they proved that faithful diabetics can live.

This moderate case of diabetes, Case 8, first came under observation June 28, 1899, and she lived out her full expectation of life after the onset of diabetes, and constitutes my standard case of the efficacy of the Naunyn diet. Heredity was not disclosed until six months after death, when her

---

[1] Best: Loc. cit., p. 132.
[2] Fletcher, Best and Solandt: Biochem. Jour., **29**, 2278, 1935.
[3] Chaikoff, Entenman and Montgomery: Loc. cit., p. 133.

oldest sister, maximum weight at least 205 pounds, developed diabetes (5 per cent sugar) at the age of eighty-three years. She died at eighty-seven years of pneumonia following a hemiplegia, having acquired a carbohydrate tolerance of at least a liberal slice of apple pie and "ice cream on top" at her Sunday dinner, thus constituting a standard example of gain in tolerance if a diabetic will only live long enough. A great, great nephew developed diabetes at the age of five years in 1934.

TABLE 36.—THE CHANGE IN THE CARBOHYDRATE BALANCE FROM NEGATIVE TO POSITIVE. CASE 8. AGE AT ONSET, SIXTY YEARS.

(Maximum weight, 185 pounds. An older sister developed diabetes in 1914 and a great grandchild of an older brother in 1934.

Date.	Diacetic acid, grams.	Sugar in urine, grams.	Carbohydrate intake, grams.	Carbohydrate balance, grams.	Weight, pounds.	Remarks.
1899						
June 28 . .	0	61	?	?	161	Diabetes discovered
30 . .	0	65	0	−65		
July 1 . .	0	13	10	− 3		
2 . .	0	0	10	+10		
1900						
Jan. 1		4	45	+41	174	
1909						
Oct. 12 . . ++	19	54	+35	. .		Carbuncle.
17 . . +	0	76	+76			
21 . . 0 .	0	70	+70	146		
1911						
May 18 . .	0	42	65	+23	. .	Pneumonia.
1912						
Sept. 11 . .	0	10	30	+20	143	
1913						
April 20		21	?	. .	140[1]	Hemiplegia.
June 17		2.4%	?	. .	. .	Pneumonia; died.

[1] March 23.

TABLE 37.—CHANGES IN CARBOHYDRATE AND GLUCOSE BALANCES. CASE 2095. AGE AT ONSET, TWENTY-SEVEN YEARS, DECEMBER, 1920.

Date.	Urinary sugar.		Diet, grams.			Carbohydrate balance, gm.	Glucose balance, gm.	Weight, pounds.	Blood sugar, per cent.	Insulin, units.	Remarks.
	Per cent.	Gm.	C.	P.	F.						
1921											
Feb. 21	9.0	54	53	25	0	−1	+14	131			
22	3.7	37	99	57	0	+62	+95	132	0.20		
25	0	0	16	6	4	+16	+20	131			
28	0	0	61	33	9	+61	+81	132	0.08		
Mar. 7	0	0	131	67	22	+131	+172	131			
14	0	0	205	74	52	+205	+253	130	0.08		
1922											
Feb. 7	0	0	175	74	85	+175	+227	132	0.11		
Apr. 26	0.5	8	88	37	43	+80	+113	115	0.17	. .	Temperature, 102°; jaundice in March.
May 19	0	0	140	60	68	+140	+182	115	0.11		
Sept. 13	0	0	175	75	85	+175	+227	122	0.18		
1923											
Mar. 14	0	0	148	64	72	+148	+194	124	0.12	2	
21	0	0	147	73	121	+147	+209	126	0.18	2	
April 2	0	0	171	77	133	+171	+230	125	0.08	3	
1934											
Sept. 26	1.9	−	129	76	102	. .	. .	160	0.14	48	
1939											
Sept. 9	1.5	26	149	80	91	+123	+178	160		48	
1946											
Feb. 10	0	0	185	100	115	. .	. .	162	0.05	42	

For the first twenty-four hours during which the urine of Case 8 was collected the intake of carbohydrate was not known. Upon the following day no carbohydrate at all was administered, but sugar had existed for so considerable a period in the body that time was necessary for its excretion. The minus carbohydrate balance of 65 grams, therefore, was simply due to retained sugar in the body. This is plainly shown because upon the following day, when 10 grams carbohydrate were allowed, the sugar in the urine decreased to 13 grams, constituting a minus carbohydrate balance of 3 grams; but a day later upon the same diet the urinary sugar completely disappeared and the carbohydrate balance was +10 grams. Six months later the tolerance for carbohydrate had risen to 41 grams. It rose somewhat during the subsequent years, persisted during a carbuncle, fell with an attack of pneumonia, then again fell as intermittent claudication appeared and restricted exercise, and in 1913 the patient died of a second attack of pneumonia, three months after a cerebral hemorrhage, in the fourteenth year of the disease. With insulin the carbohydrate could have been increased and I believe her arteriosclerosis could have been deferred and life prolonged with comfort.

Case 2095, a minister, married three years, aged twenty-seven years, developed symptoms of diabetes in December, 1920, and came for treatment February 21, 1921. He followed the scheduled régime employed at that time, the negative carbohydrate balance changed to positive, and with a high-carbohydrate, low- rather than high-fat diet he remained sugar-free and held his weight for one year. He then returned to see if insulin would put him back into the pulpit. It did, and at the same time it put him into mine, for his case preaches that (1) 9 per cent of sugar is consistent with mild diabetes when treatment, based upon a high-carbohydrate, moderate-protein and low-fat diet, is begun early; (2) tolerance can be maintained when the diet is faithfully followed with (a) preservation of weight, (b) absence of glycosuria, (c) a normal percentage of blood sugar, (d) a gain in strength, mental vigor, and weight, which have persisted to date, February 20, 1946. His diet is now approximately 185 grams of carbohydrate, protein 100 grams, fat 115 grams. The weight is 162 pounds, insulin CI 14 and PZI 28. His blood sugar was 50 mg. in the forenoon, but he reported and orange test on retiring. He has an active parish.

2. The Glucose Balance

—The term "glucose balance" or the "total glucose" of the diet is usually employed in reckoning the glucose equivalent of insulin. But what is the glucose equivalent of the diet? Here in the United States we obtain it by multiplying the carbohydrate by 100 per cent, the protein by 58 per cent and the fat by 10 per cent and adding the products. In Europe it is estimated otherwise by Falta[1] and by Priesel and Wagner.[2] The term "glucose balance" also is not wholly satisfactory aside from the doubt as to the accuracy of the percentages, because it implies that all the protein and fat consumed are immediately oxidized and that the carbohydrate, which can be formed out of them, has at once entered into the metabolism which the DuBois-Richardson chart clearly demonstrates not to be the case. (See page 271.)

To the total glucose and the glucose balance of the diet Woodyatt[3] attached great weight. His classic paper should be read, because

[1] Falta: Wien. klin. Wchnschr., **38**, 577, 1925.
[2] Priesel and Wagner: Loc. cit., p. 56.
[3] Woodyatt: Arch. Int. Med., **28**, 125, 1921.

it represented a progressive step in the dietetic treatment of diabetes. Also the searching but friendly criticism of it by Allen[1] is worth perusal.

G. ALCOHOL.

In no disease would the employment of alcohol appear to be more useful or more justifiable, but I very rarely give it to diabetics, because of (1) the pathetic cases, relatively few I acknowledge, of protracted neuritis which I have seen among diabetics, (2) the liability of a patient with a chronic disease contracting a dangerous habit, (3) the great danger, and the very real mistake repeatedly made by lay people, of a diabetic being considered drunk when in insulin shock, (4) the heart-breaking letters and interviews I have had with the relatives of patients who used it in excess and (5) my personal disapproval. Finally, (6) there are no vitamins in alcohol.

A diabetic, taking insulin, should never venture on the street with an alcoholic breath. According to Newman and Cutting[2] insulin accelerates the metabolism of ethyl alcohol 50 per cent in therapeutic doses in man. Alcohol is not convertible directly into glucose or fatty acids: *i. e.*, neither ketogenic nor anti-ketogenic. Higgins, Peabody, and Fitz[3] from tests upon themselves when upon a carbohydrate-free diet found that alcohol did not show any anti-ketogenic action.

Few of our cases have taken alcohol and still fewer take it now than in years gone by. In former days with our crude notions about diet 15 to 30 cc. of alcohol were often useful, when the patients were given excessive quantities of fat. Though Allen originally suggested its use in fasting at the beginning of treatment, he discarded it so soon that I doubt if a dozen of our patients received it under such circumstances. Diabetic patients require no alcohol and as yet we have not found it necessary or desirable to prescribe it. Thirty cc. of alcohol are to be found in approximately 60 cc. of whisky, brandy, rum or gin or 300 cc. of most sugar-free wines. Thirty cc. of alcohol furnish 210 calories and this is of some moment.

The results of studies of Allen and Wishart[4] on the effect of alcohol upon two diabetics indicated that the assimilative power of the diabetic organism is limited not only in respect to carbohydrate (preformed or potential) but also in respect to total calories as such. They found that alcohol, which is clearly recognized as not convertible into sugar or acetone in the body, produces a return of glycosuria and other symptoms when added to the diabetic diet in quantities exceeding caloric tolerance. Leclercq[5] likewise demonstrated on 2 patients with severe diabetes the production of hyper-

[1] Allen: Jour. Metab. Res., **3**, 61, 1923.
[2] Newman and Cutting: Jour. Clin. Invest., **14**, 945, 1935.
[3] Higgins, Peabody and Fitz: Jour. Med. Res., **34**, 263, 1916.
[4] Allen and Wishart: Jour. Metab. Res., **1**, 304, 1922.
[5] Leclercq: Jour. Metab. Res., **1**, 307, 1922.

19

glycemia in consequence of adding excessive calories to the diet either in the form of fat or alcohol. It is readily conceivable that replacing a certain amount of fat might lower glycosuria and acidosis, and Fuller[1] found this true in most cases of mild and moderate diabetes, but lacking in diabetic cases of great severity.

Fortunately chemical methods are giving us more and more accurate data about the effects of alcohol upon the nervous system. Thus in Sweden[2] an individual in whom the percentage of alcohol in the blood is less than 0.5 milligram per 100 cc. is considered sober. Apparently between the range of 0.5 and 1.5 milligrams per 100 cc. not only individuals react differently but the same individuals react differently under special conditions. Above 1.5 milligrams per 100 cc. everyone is definitely affected and is so recognized by all.

It is said to be conclusive evidence that a person is under the influence of intoxicating liquor sufficiently to affect his ability to drive safely if it is shown by chemical analysis that within one-half hour after he has ceased operating a motor vehicle his blood contains 0.5 mg., or more, of alcohol per 100 cubic centimeters.

The conclusion reached is that "60 cc. (2 oz.) of whiskey (a highball), somewhat less of gin (a Martini cocktail), or 1000 to 1500 cc. (1 to 1½ qts.) of beer may be taken on an empty stomach without the concentration of alcohol in the blood exceeding 0.5 milligram per 100 cubic centimeters. With, or soon after a meal, double these quantities can be taken with the same effect."[3]

H. LIQUIDS, EDEMA, LOSS OF WEIGHT AS INFLUENCED BY SODIUM CHLORIDE.

Save in connection with coma, it is exceptional for a diabetic to take too little or too much liquid if the diabetes is under control. Prior and subsequent to operations the same rules for liquids hold as in the non-diabetic. Often uncontrolled diabetes in an old man simulates disease of the prostate. Clear up the diabetes and the polyuria and pollakiuria disappear. Rapid retention of water, thus overcoming the dehydration of untreated diabetes, may seriously impair vision by producing myopia although only temporarily.

It is seldom if ever necessary to restrict the liquids at the beginning of treatment in diabetes. The diminution of the carbohydrate in the diet usually leads to a corresponding diminution in the thirst and quantity of urine. The latter is not always a guide to the liquids needed, because the sudden utilization and storage of carbohydrate may lead to the retention of several liters of water by the emaciated and desiccated patient in twenty-four hours. I hesitate to restrict liquids in severe diabetes for fear too little liquid will be available

[1] Fuller: Jour. Metab. Res., **1**, 609, 1922.
[2] Haggard, Greenberg and Cohen: New England Jour. Med., **219**, 466, 1938
[3] Henderson: Alcohol and Accidents, Connecticut Motorist, April, 1939.

for the body with which to eliminate the acids that may have been formed. Particularly is this essential in diabetic coma, because so often vomiting and lack of retention of liquids or their collection in a dilated stomach have depleted the patient.

The metabolism increases 3 per cent according to Benedict and Carpenter[1] when large quantities of liquids are drunk. The increase has amounted to 16 per cent. Liquids also impose a demand upon the metabolism if they are taken cold. The quantity of heat required of the body to raise the temperature of a glass of ice water to body temperature is not negligible. Patients on the verge of coma often upset the digestion by drinking large quantities of cold liquids rapidly. Seldom is it safe to allow in coma more than $\frac{1}{2}$ or at the most 1 glass of liquid at a time and that not oftener than every hour. The rest of the liquid administered, and this usually amounts to 2 liters and may reach 11 liters, is best given subcutaneously or intravenously.

Polyuria persists in certain cases of diabetes. Usually a cause can be found in some peculiarity of diet such as an excess of salt. This happened with Case 1196 who continually voided large quantities of urine. Upon investigation it was found that he ingested 20 or more grams of salt, bouillon cubes in variable number, and 21 half-grain saccharin tablets a day.

Graphic charts of the liquids ingested and excreted are often seen on hospital rounds. These are very crude affairs. In recording the intake, even if everything that flows is regarded as intake, there are amusing inconsistencies. While an egg, in an egg-nog is liquid, it escapes being recorded if boiled to the point of coagulation; cream is liquid, ice cream solid; vegetables and fruits are solid, though they contain 85 per cent, more or less, of water; potatoes are 75.5 per cent water and meat 77 per cent. The retained water of an enema is forgotten. Errors also creep into the estimation of the quantity of liquids excreted. The urine in whole or in part is lost. The water in the feces is seldom estimated, the excretion of water by the skin is more variable, depending largely on the amount of exercise.

The insensible perspiration includes both the invisible water vapor and carbon dioxide eliminated from the lungs and skin. Benedict and Root[2] found the amount of insensible perspiration per hour closely related to the twenty-four-hour heat production of patients with diabetes or with hyperthyroidism.

After operations, according to Coller and Maddock,[3] the loss by the skin may reach 2000 cc. in twenty-four hours. The excretion by the lungs is often entirely neglected and this amounts to about

---

[1] Benedict and Carpenter: Carnegie Institute of Washington, Publ. No. 261, p. 247, 1918.
[2] Benedict and Root: Arch. Int. Med., **38**, 1, 1926.
[3] Coller and Maddock: Internat. Clin., **3**, 190, 1934.

300 cc., Dr. Carpenter tells me. Finally, as DuBois pointed out to members of the Interurban Club, in the combustion of each 60 grams of sugar there are 5 cc. of water formed, of 100 grams of p otein 41 cc. of water, of 100 grams of beef fat 107 cc. of water.

Already on page 270 it has been mentioned that a gain in weight of 1 pound of actual tissue by a diabetic can take place only when some 1500 calories above ordinary metabolic needs are ingested. This is of great importance in the practical management of the diabetic patient.

1. **Edema.**—Perhaps no one gross observation made during the course of his disease is of greater significance and causes greater alarm than the persistent loss in body weight. Slight changes in body weight which may accompany dietetic alterations or the ingestion of sodium chloride and sodium bicarbonate are looked upon as material gains and are thus liable to be misunderstood. Few realize that the normal individual is continually undergoing changes in body weight throughout the twenty-four hours. Even during sleep a man of 85 kilograms lost 30 grams per hour, and a woman of 65 kilograms 29 grams per hour. With exercise this is, of course, greatly increased and may amount to 6.4 kilograms for a football player during one hour and fifteen minutes of active exercise. Since about 60 per cent of the body is water, a relatively small change of water in the body may produce a change in body weight of 1 kilogram. Skelton[1] points out that approximately one-half of the water in the body is in muscles, one-fifth in the skin and only one-fourteenth in the blood.

Edema is a common source of error and it is important to recognize it as a cause of gain in weight in diabetes. Patients may seem to be gaining when in reality they are losing weight because of insufficient diet. Edema occurred most frequently in former years following oatmeal days and the administration of alkalis, while later it was common with fasting diabetics of severe type and was partly, although not always, related to the large quantity of salt which they ingested with broths and vegetables. In these days of insulin it is quite likely the result of carbohydrate storage which simultaneously implies water storage.

The edema may become extreme, and one of my patients (Case 922), whom I had not seen for months, called in a laryngologist and barely escaped tracheotomy for edema of the larynx in pre-insulin days. This quickly disappeared with the omission of salt and a diet of water and a few oranges. Case 3739 during coma developed edema following the removal of an intubation tube inserted on account of laryngeal obstruction, and reinsertion of the tube was necessary. She is now thirty-four years of age, with diabetes of twenty-two years' duration, and is a most efficient trained nurse.

---

[1] Skelton: Arch. Int. Med., **40**, 140, 1927.

A sudden gain in body weight in the latter weeks of pregnancy is a premonitory symptom to toxemia. (See p. 772.)

Fluctuations in the water content of the body are the first factor in changes of body weight. The average man at rest without food oxidizes per day about 75 grams of protein, 25 grams of glycogen and 200 grams of fat—a total of 300 grams of water-free organized body tissue. It can readily be seen, therefore, that with subjects at rest, large and rapid changes in weight must be due not to the oxidation of organic material, which amounts to only 300 grams per day, but to the retention or excretion of water. Thus dehydration is a constant factor in coma and gain in weight an almost inevitable accompaniment of recovery, and it is by no means unusual for a patient under such conditions to increase his weight 7 pounds in twenty-four hours. In an exceptional instance in which dehydration was extreme, Root and Riseman[1] brought about recovery by the administration by mouth, subcutaneously and intravenously of 11 liters of liquid in twelve hours without any hint of circulatory failure on the part of the patient and with gratifying recovery.

The laying down of protein in the body involves the retention of water to the extent of approximately 3 grams of water per gram of solid. Fat and glycogen, however, are accompanied by a relatively small water storage. Water retention occurs following a change from a high fat to a high carbohydrate diet; on the other hand, water is lost from the body when the diet is changed from carbohydrate to fat. These facts are difficult to explain but they are probably not due, as was thought by Zuntz[2] to a large volume of water being bound to glycogen.[3] Bridge and Bridges,[4] in questioning the statement that with every gram of glycogen 3 grams of water are stored in the body, suggests that the controlling mechanism is more likely to be found in the metabolism of fats rather than of carbohydrates.

2. **Influence of Sodium Chloride Upon Weight.**—The quantity of sodium chloride in the diet also affects the weight. For example, in the study by Goodall and Joslin[5] of a medical student upon a salt-free diet, consisting of the whites of 18 eggs, 120 grams olive oil and 200 grams crystallized sugar, total 2096 calories, or 30 calories per kilogram body weight, the weight fell from 70.2 kilograms on the first day to 64.9 kilograms on the thirteenth day, and upon an unrestricted diet three days later was 69 kilograms. The chlorine in the urine fell to 0.17 gram and the P_2O_5 to 0.86 gram. The administration of sodium bicarbonate was frequently followed by a gain in weight. Thus in Case 220 with 20 grams of sodium bicarbonate daily the body weight rose in five days from 49.3 to 53.3 kilograms. To

[1] Root and Riseman: Jour. Am. Med. Assn., **110**, 1730, 1938.
[2] Zuntz: Biochem. Ztschr., **44**, 290, 1912.
[3] Best and Taylor: P. 17, loc. cit., p. 116.
[4] Bridge and Bridges: Jour. Biol. Chem., **93**, 181, 1931.
[5] Goodall and Joslin: Arch. Int. Med., **1**, 615, 1908.

demonstrate that this gain in weight was not directly due to the alkali, but rather to the retention of salt, the weights of another diabetic patient, Case 135, were taken while on a salt-free diet. With bicarbonate of soda while upon this salt-free diet, the weight fell in four days, from 40.1 to 39 kilograms. In the following four days he was given, respectively, 25, 25, 37 and 52 grams of sodium bicarbonate, and the weight continued to fall to 37.2 kilograms, at which time, in the year 1910, he went into coma and died! This unfortunate termination taught me not to lower but to raise the sodium chloride in coma or in near-coma. Apparently the administration of sodium bicarbonate, by favoring the excretion of large quantities of retained acid bodies, leads to irritation of the kidneys, resulting in their inability to excrete salt in the normal manner. If at the same time the salt in the diet is restricted, there is less to be retained and consequently no gain in weight results. This observation has been confirmed by Levison.[1] Falta[2] has shown that if sodium bicarbonate is replaced by potassium bicarbonate the edema will disappear, although the salt in the body and in the diet is low. Labbé[3] explains the edema by the retention of the sodium and not of the chlorine. McQuarrie, Thompson and Anderson[4] found that where potassium and sodium salts were given simultaneously 1 part of potassium antagonized the effect of at least 3 parts of sodium. Atchley, Loeb and Benedict[5] have removed the edema of a diabetic with the daily use of 20 to 35 grams of calcium chloride.

I. VITAMINS.

Vitamins are organic substances, insignificant calorically or in weight, but without which no diet or healthy life can be complete.

The diet of the diabetic is rich in vitamins since it contains liberal portions of vegetables and fruit in addition to meat, eggs, milk, cereal and bread. The diabetic is fortunate in being denied granulated sugar, which is computed to provide one-seventh of the total calories in the diet of the non-diabetic, for sugar contains no vitamins.

When the commonly used diabetic diet, 165 grams of carbohydrate, 82 grams of protein and 97 grams of fat, was computed with the help of Miss Rosina Vance, former head dietitian New England Deaconess Hospital, it was found to contain thiamin, chloride 1.5 mg., riboflavin 1.9 mg., ascorbic acid 250 mg. and vitamin A 16,000 U.S.P. units. In comparison with the daily individual vitamin intake recommended by the Food and Nutrition Board of the National Research Council[6] the diabetic diet contained

[1] Levison: Jour. Am. Med. Assn., **64**, 326, 1916.

[2] Falta: Wien. Arch. f. inn. Med., **5**, 581, 1922–1923.

[3] Labbé and Cumston: A Clinical Treatise on Diabetes Mellitus, London, W. Heinemann, p. 115, 1922.

[4] McQuarrie, Thompson and Anderson: Jour. Nutr., **11**, 77, 1936.

[5] Atchley, Loeb and Benedict: Jour. Am. Med. Assn., **80**, 1643, 1923.

[6] Recommended Dietary Allowances: Reprint and Circular Series No. 115, Food and Nutrition Board, National Research Council, Washington, 1943.

approximately three times the recommended amount of vitamin A and C, adequate thiamin and almost optimal riboflavin content.

For children especially, the addition of vitamin D in the form of cod liver oil is advisable and the prescription of liver once a week is probably desirable for all because of its high content of B complex.

What are the vitamin requirements of a diabetic patient? Are they the same as for a non-diabetic patient? Can the vitamins be absorbed and utilized as efficiently in the diabetic as in the normal individual? These questions are difficult to answer specifically but in our opinion the diabetic patient, especially the severe diabetic, is safer with a little more vitamins than his non-diabetic brother.

Consider what the untreated diabetic represents. As a rule, he is a middle-aged or elderly patient suffering from a chronic disease of long duration with a digestive apparatus often handicapped by loss of teeth, commonly involving a low intake of meat, and by achlorhydria, partial or complete, thus leading to destruction or interference with absorption of thiamin, a liver overburdened with fat, susceptible to infection and known to have complications resembling the signs of avitaminosis such as neuritis, hemorrhages in the eyes, cataracts, a dry skin, occasionally a dry, red tongue, emaciation, weakness and low vitality. Perhaps his vitamins have been depleted by glucose or salt infusions prescribed in the treatment of surgical complications or coma or even by therapeutic roentgen-rays. Such was the former diabetic, but this description does not apply to the well-treated diabetic today.

Vitamins play an essential part in the metabolism of carbohydrate. Deficiency of thiamin (B_1) interferes with the normal metabolic interplay between glycogen, lactic and pyruvic acid. In thiamin deficiency the blood pyruvic acid level is elevated, especially after glucose feeding.[1] It is believed that thiamin acts as a co-enzyme with pyruvate oxidase in the oxidation of pyruvic acid. (See p. 118.)

Vitamin D, the anti-rachitic factor, is similar in chemical structure to the sex hormones, and undoubtedly there are other instances, *e. g.*, the association of ascorbic acid and the adrenal cortex, in which vitamins and hormones work together. We know that in their chemical constitution vitamins and enzymes are closely related, *e. g.*, nicotinic acid and cozymase, thiamin and cocarboxylase. Unfortunately, most vitamins are not readily stored.

The vitamin question in diabetes is a disturbing one. After getting rid of most quack diabetic remedies as a result of the patient's learning the Benedict test and the use of insulin, it would be a shame if, disguised in scientific paraphernalia, vitamins replaced them. It is so easy to say the patient requires more vitamins and give him a shot-gun prescription for them instead of intently studying his dietary and insulin needs and his employment of exercise in relation to the details of his daily life. It is

[1] Bueding, Stein and Wortis: Jour. Biol. Chem., **140**, 697, 1941.

almost unfortunate for accurate prescribing that so often a deficiency of one vitamin is accompanied by lack of another. Just as an order for a teaspoonful of soda to combat acidosis, extra carbohydrate to favor the combustion of oxybutyric acid, and a pious look have covered up a multitude of sinful diabetic coma deaths, I fear we doctors will be tempted to give vitamins and unfortunately will not know when to stop. It must be admitted that although an excess of soda can cause nausea, vomiting, anuria, alkalosis, thus far there is comparatively little evidence of any harm from an excess of vitamins save to deplete the pocketbook.

The Council on Pharmacy and Chemistry[1] compared the vitamin content and cost of twenty-five leading multivitamin preparations on the market. The low content of B complex components and the ridiculously high cost of some stress the need for closer inspection of the contents of vitamins prescribed.

In recent years laboratory procedures have become available whereby certain vitamin deficiencies may be measured chemically. Ascorbic acid determinations upon blood plasma[2] are used frequently. Although it has been shown that the niacin content of blood may remain normal in pellagra,[3] further investigation suggests that the determination of trigonelline excretion after a test dose of 500 mg. of nicotinic acid amide[4] may be used to help ascertain niacin deficiencies.

Melnick and Field[5] consider the determination of the thiamin excreted by a patient in the fasted state four hours after the intramuscular test dose of 0.35 mg. of thiamin per square meter of body surface a reliable measure of thiamin nutrition.

Although the vitamin A content of plasma can be measured and at times may prove useful, many conditions, such as liver disease, obstructive jaundice, increased blood lipids, infections and nephritis may produce marked changes in this determination.

The requirements of the body for vitamins vary according to circumstances. In general they rise in the presence of infections and disease, pregnancy and lactation, and during physical exertion, in the latter instance especially for vitamin C, just as the demand for thiamin chloride rises with the quantity of carbohydrate ingested.

The recognized minimum daily requirements of the individual vitamins have been reported by the Food and Drug Administration[1] as follows:

Vitamin.	Minimum requirement for an adult
A	4000 USP units
D	400 USP units
B₁ (thiamin hydrochloride)	1 mg.
B₂ (riboflavin)	2 mg.
C (ascorbic acid)	30 mg.

The minimum requirement of niacin was not established, but there appears to be general agreement that 10 mg. is approximately the minimum daily requirement of this vitamin.

The recommended daily dietary allowance of the vitamins and minerals has been estimated and reported by the Food and Nutrition Board of the National Research Council.[6]

[1] Council on Pharmacy and Chemistry: Jour. Am. Med. Assn., **126**, 29, 1944.
[2] Bessy: Jour. Biol. Chem., **126**, 771, 1938.
[3] Field, Melnick and Robinson: Jour. Clin. Invest., **20**, 379, 1941.
[4] Perlzweig, Sarett and Margolis: Jour. Am. Med. Assn., **118**, 28, 1942.
[5] Melnick and Field: Jour. Nutrition, **24**, 131, 1942.
[6] Food and Nutrition Board, National Research Council: Loc. cit., p. 294.

1. **Vitamin A.**—$C_{20}H_{29}OH$, fat soluble, isolated in crystalline form. Source: The green leafy and yellow vegetables are rich sources of vitamin A. A single serving of greens, carrots or squash provides more than the daily recommended requirements of 4000 U.S.P. units. Since the carotene in green vegetables and carrots is transformed in the liver to vitamin A, liver itself is a rich food source of this vitamin and contains approximately 5000 U.S.P. units of vitamin A per 100 grams. The content of cod liver and halibut oil varies with the sample, and the minimum standard is 850 I.U. per gram, but in some preparations it is more than double this amount. Milk, cream, butter, eggs and cheese are also valuable sources of this vitamin. Vitamin A has one-half the molecular weight of carotene. Bile and pancreatic juice are essential for its absorption. Mineral oil, being a fat solvent, prevents absorption of carotene to a considerable degree.

Lack of vitamin A in animals leads to decreased appetite and decreased growth, may interfere with reproduction and lactation, brings on xerophthalmia and certain types of night blindness; the last-named occurs because vitamin A is a constituent of the retinal pigment, visual purple. It is one of the vitamins whose adequate supply may lead to prevention of certain types of infections in man. Vitamin A deficiency during the formative period of teeth outranks in the human being all other deficiencies in importance.

Vitamin A influences epithelial tissues, particularly those of the respiratory passages, glands and their ducts and the alimentary tract, as does vitamin C those tissues with collagen as a base. No instances of hyperkeratosis of the skin relieved by administration of vitamin A have been recognized by us, and I know of no work in diabetics upon the relation of the lack of vitamin A to cataracts, such as has been observed in animals.

2. **Vitamin B Complex.**—This is made up of at least three vitamins especially important in the human dietary. These are thiamin (vitamin B_1), or thiamin chloride (vitamin B_1 hydrochloride, $C_{12}H_{17}ON_4SCL.HCl$); niacin and riboflavin (vitamin B_2 or G). The vitamin B complex is composed also of other less well understood factors including pyridoxine, pantothenic acid, para aminobenzoic acid, inositol, biotin, choline and folic acid. Deficiencies in these components have been studied extensively in animals but their relation to human nutrition is yet not clearly defined.

(a) **Vitamin B_1.**—Thiamin, water soluble, thermolabile, can be prepared synthetically, Source: Whole wheat and enriched breads, whole grain cereals, yeast, legumes, milk, eggs, meat and especially pork. Pork holds a unique position for a single large pork chop may supply nearly the entire thiamin requirement for a whole day. In refined cereals vitamin B_1 is negligible. In whole-grain products vitamin B_1 varies between 60 and 300 I.U. per 100 grams and yet the cost of whole-wheat bread is no more than of white bread. A century ago, before the refinement of grains, it is said our ancestors had ten times as many vitamins as we.   There is increasing evidence that more vitamin B_1 in the diet may be desirable, and that in certain parts of the country there is, in general, a low intake of all the members of the vitamin B complex.   Vitamin B_1 is stored only to a limited extent and the symptoms due to its lack are common.

The symptoms and signs of thiamin deficiency in humans was strikingly shown by Williams et al.,[1] who induced their deficiency in 11 women on diets containing only 0.45 mg. of thiamin a day. General symptoms including irritability, depression, easy fatigue and inefficiency developed.   Anorexia with episodes of nausea and vomiting with marked constipation also appeared.   Cardiovascular signs included vasomotor instability, hypotension and bradycardia at rest with tachycardia on moderate exertion of the 11 patients. Five developed macrocytic anemia, three achlorhydria, eight decreased serum protein and all a lowered basal metabolic rate.   Elevation of the glucose tolerance curve and blood pyruvate was found. Strikingly enough, none lost weight.

Two other women placed on a daily intake of only 0.1 mg. of thiamin per 1000 calories supplemented once every two weeks by 1.0 mg. of thiamin intramuscularly to relieve gastro-intestinal complaints, for a period of one hundred and twenty days, developed definite neuritis showing that polyneuritis is a late manifestation of severe thiamin deficiency.   Several months of treatment with thiamin were required to cure the neuritis.[2]

In animals a high-carbohydrate diet deficient in thiamin leads more rapidly to the production of the symptoms of B-avitaminosis than does a high-fat diet.   This is sometimes expressed by the statement that the requirement of thiamin for human beings varies with the non-fat calories.   It is believed that biologic oxidative mechanisms are involved.[3]

The point of action of cocarboxylase (thiamin pyro-phosphate), according to the work of Peters and others lies in the enzymic activation of oxidation of pyruvic acid.   When thiamin, and hence cocarboxylase, are absent, carbohydrate metabolism stops with its formation.   When thiamin is deficient, the products of carbohydrate metabolism, namely, pyruvic acid, accumulate in the blood and tissues.   Give thiamin and this is remedied and then the abnormal metabolism of the tissues is brought to normal.   The pyrophosphoric acid ester of the vitamin is the enzyme cocarboxylase which is indispensable to the metabolism of the products of carbohydrate breakdown through the oxidation of pyruvic acid.   Thiamin may also be instrumental in the formation of fat from carbohydrate.

[1] Williams, Mason, Smith and Wilder: Arch. Int. Med., **69**, 721, 1942.
[2] Williams, Mason, Power and Wilder: Arch. Int. Med., **71**, 38, 1943.
[3] Cowgill: Jour. Am. Med. Assn., **110**, 805, 1938.

Styron *et al.*[1] at the New England Deaconess Hospital showed that there was no significant difference in the length of time required by diabetic (depancreatized) and non-diabetic rats on a thiamin free diet, to develop signs of marked thiamin deficiency. Carbohydrate tolerance in both the diabetic and non-diabetic rats as judged by glucose tolerance tests, showed little change until signs of marked deficiency appeared when there was impairment of tolerance.

Richter[2] has studied rats on a McCollom diet and self-selected diets before and after pancreatectomy. He found that normal rats make beneficial selections of purified substances including carbohydrates, fats, proteins, minerals and vitamins. Rats made diabetic by removal of the pancreas select low carbohydrate, high fat diets which help to alleviate or even to eliminate the diabetic symptoms. Furthermore, he has observed the effect of various components of the B complex upon the selection of diets. In the absence of vitamin C complex, the rat chooses large amounts of fat, little or no carbohydrate and no protein. When thiamin is added, they eat carbohydrate, little fat and still avoid protein. When all components of the B complex are available they thrive on a diet of very little fat, high carbohydrate and moderately high protein.

The effect of B complex upon 3 depancreatized dogs maintained with insulin, lipocaic, yeast, pancreatic enzymes and a basic diet was reported by Gaebler and Ceszewski.[3] When the yeast was omitted, glycosuria appeared in two weeks in 2 animals in amounts about equivalent to the carbohydrate intake. Ketosis and lipemia were negligible but weight and nitrogen losses occurred. Resumption of yeast feeding abolished glycosuria in twelve days and restored nitrogen balance. The third dog, however, failed to develop glycosuria when yeast was withdrawn.

In human diabetes published observations upon the effect of vitamins are still scanty and not sufficiently controlled. Vorhaus, Williams and Waterman[4] state that diabetes was ameliorated in 6 out of 11 patients by the use of vitamin B_1. Biskind and Schreier[5] report that among 94 diabetics studied every one showed signs and symptoms of deficiency of factors of the B complex. They believe that improvement in general health and often marked improvement in carbohydrate metabolism frequently follows B complex therapy. Labbé noted improvement in 8 of 11 diabetics with vitamin B_2 and B_3. Aszodi and Mosonyi[6] published a similar result with vitamins B_1 and C, and Wilson concluded that B_1 increased the action of insulin. Beckert[7] reports favorably upon his experience with the

[1] Styron, Tucker, Rhodes, Smith and Marble: Proc. Soc. Exp. Biol. and Med., 50, 242, 1942.
[2] Richter: Essays in Biology, Berkeley, Univ. of California Press, 1943.
[3] Gaebler and Ceszewski: Endocrinology, 36, 227, 1945.
[4] Vorhaus, Williams and Waterman: Jour. Am. Med. Assn., 105, 1580, 1935.
[5] Biskind and Schreier: Exp. Med. and Surgery, 3, 299, Nov., 1945.
[6] Aszodi and Mosonyi: Klin. Wchnschr., 16, 1214, 1937; Mosonyi and Aszodi: Ibid., 17, 337, 1938.
[7] Beckert: Münch. med. Wchnschr., 86, 1078, 1939.

use of baker's yeast (20 grams two or three times daily) in 120 cases of diabetes over a period of six months to two years. In 27 per cent he noted a lowering of blood-sugar values and an increase in the carbohydrate tolerance. There was no effect in 62 per cent and in 11 per cent the treatment was discontinued because of gastrointestinal disturbances. In another series of 20 cases a preparation of brewer's yeast was given and the improvement was more marked. However, no specific figures are given in the paper. One hesitates to accept the conclusions without further substantiation, and in general one must say that the basis for the conclusions reached regarding the favorable effect of vitamin B_1 in all these publications is open to question.[1]

At the New England Deaconess Hospital thiamin chloride has been given to many patients, in large and small doses, but none of us has observed any notable effect on the blood sugar or insulin requirement. Thiamin, even in enormous doses, has produced no dramatic relief of patients with diabetic neuritis. (See page 566.) One cannot say whether its prolonged use has or has not hastened recovery.

Detailed studies upon the effects of vitamin B deficiency upon a normal individual have been carried on by Elsom, Lukens, Montgomery and Jonas.[2] Evidences of disturbance of carbohydrate metabolism while the subject was on the deficiency diet were noted by the failure of the blood sugar to return to normal within three to four hours after glucose, but this was relieved as soon as yeast was given. No increase in the bisulphite-binding substances or in pyruvic acid was noted in the fasting state; abnormalities were not noted until after giving glucose, but there was a return to normal with the administration of thiamin. The respiratory quotient was not altered during the period of deficiency. The response to insulin decreased as the deficiency increased but returned when thiamin was given and when riboflavin was added to the thiamin, the subject was supersensitive. Their work showed the symptoms of vitamin B deficiency in an elderly woman who had lived on such a diet for five to eight weeks were relieved best of all by brewer's yeast and only slightly with thiamin and riboflavin. At first, the edema and later loss of weight were observed, but ultimately the weight was maintained when yeast was given.

(b) **Niacin.**—$C_6H_5NO_2$. Water soluble, thermo-stable. Source: Similar to that of thiamin. Meats especially pork and liver provide its richest sources. Whole wheat bread, and whole wheat cereals are good sources. Milk and milk products, however, are comparatively poor sources of niacin. It is a relatively simple organic compound and is closely allied to various enzymes. It is nearly specific in the prevention and treatment of pellagra. Its deficiency may be asso-

[1] Smith and Mason (Proc. Staff Meet. Mayo Clinic, **15**, 529, 1940) made special studies in two diabetic patients who were fed diets deficient in thiamin but adequate in other respects. They found that in these two patients the intake of vitamin B_1 did not influence either the intensity of diabetes or their sensitivity to insulin.

[2] Elsom, Lukens, Montgomery and Jonas: Jour. Clin. Invest., **19**, 153, 1940.

ciated with stomatitis, and a swollen, sore, indented tongue, for some time preceding its red character. Symptoms of vitamin deficiency may be observed in pneumonia, and DuBois[1] voiced the thought that the large diets fed typhoid fever patients years ago by Coleman and himself were valuable, not from calories alone, but from their content of nicotinic acid. Gobell[2] claims that the injection of 100 mg. of nicotinamide subcutaneously in children produces a regular but slow fall in blood sugar of 10 to 45 mg. per cent, averaging 21.3 mg. per cent. He further found that niacin intensified the action of insulin in experiments in which both were administered intravenously. Niacin alone seems to have no curative effect in either pernicious anemia or sprue, although it is curative in pellagra. The importance of niacin and riboflavin, both components of the vitamin B complex, is recognized in that they are both active in enzyme formation after phosphorylation and combination with specific proteins. These enzymes, of which cozymase in yeast is an example, are required for the proper oxidation and reduction processes of the body. Without these our most fundamental processes cannot proceed.

(c) **Riboflavin.**—$C_{17}H_{20}N_4O_6$ (vitamin G or B_2) water soluble, represents a thermostable component of vitamin B complex. Source: Liver and milk are the most important sources. Meat, yeast, legumes and eggs contain significant amounts. It has also been prepared synthetically. The natural and synthetic forms apparently have the same biologic activity. The compound has also been called vitamin B_2, lactoflavin, ovoflavin, and in some of the literature simply "flavin." It combines with protein to yield an oxidation enzyme which is present in every living cell, is concerned with the reaction involved in cell respiration and the oxidation of hexose monophosphate in the tissues. A deficiency of riboflavin may produce cheilosis, a shark skin appearance of the skin covering the nose, a smooth tongue with a magenta color, and ocular lesions consisting of congested vessels at the periphery of the cornea leading to vascularization of the cornea with associated photophobia and lacrimation. In rats cataracts may develop if they are denied it.

Folic acid, the L. casei factor, however, has recently been shown by Spies[3] when administered parenterally or orally to be effective in producing a significant hematopoietic response in humans with nutritional macrocytic anemia, or with the macrocytic anemias of pellagra, pernicious anemia, sprue or pregnancy.

3. **Vitamin C.**—$C_6H_8O_6$. Vitamin C is ascorbic acid, synonym: cevitamic acid, water soluble and heat labile. It is necessary for maintenance of all tissues whose base is collagen. It was the first vitamin to be synthesized (1933) and can be made at less cost than

---

[1] DuBois: Jour. Am. Med. Assn., **113**, 301, 1939.
[2] Gobell: Z. ges. exptl. Med., **109**, 96, 1941.
[3] Spies: Jour. Am. Med. Assn., **130**, 474, 1946.

by extraction from oranges. It can be estimated in blood and urine. Rats and most species of animals can synthesize it. Source: Fresh fruits and vegetables, expecially lemons, oranges, grapefruit, tomatoes, strawberries, fresh non-pasteurized cow's milk, because in the pasteurizing process most of the vitamin C is lost. The vitamin C content of cow's milk is much below that of human milk. An orange or one-half a grapefruit supplies approximately 75 mg. of ascorbic acid, the recommended daily intake. Wolbach[1] states, "Vitamin C is necessary for the formation of all intercellular substances having collagen as their basis, and its absence prevents the formation of the matrices of white fibrous tissue, cartilage, bone and dentine."

Lack of this vitamin causes scurvy and the principle of its application dates back to 1747, when James Lind, a British Navy surgeon, proved that orange and lemon juice prevented and cured this disease, formerly so common in long sea voyages.

Sebesta, Smith, Fernald and Marble[2] determined the vitamin C status of 77 adult patients with diabetes. Patients with uncomplicated diabetes, whose vitamin C intake had been adequate, showed normal levels of plasma ascorbic acid (above 0.80 mg. per cent in the fasting state) and showed a normal excretion in the urine of more than 400 milligrams of ascorbic acid in response to a 1000 milligram dose given intravenously. Only those patients confined to bed with surgical lesions tended to show low normal or subnormal values. In 4 normal individuals in good vitamin C nutrition no effect on the blood sugar was observed after the intravenous injection of either 300 or 1000 milligrams of ascorbic acid. Their findings, therefore, did not support the idea of a specific relationship of vitamin C to diabetes. Mosenthal and Loughlin[3] studied the plasma vitamin C level in 114 diabetic children in a summer camp and found values above 0.8 mg. per cent in 57 per cent, between 0.8 and 0.4 mg. in 39 per cent and less than 0.4 mg. in only 4 per cent.

The administration of ascorbic acid does not affect the severity of the diabetic state as shown by Owens[4] *et al.* who gave large doses of this vitamin to 16 diabetic patients in various stages of vitamin C nutrition.

Since fruits are prescribed for desserts and large quantities of vegetables are given, the patient on a diabetic diet usually receives even more vitamin C than the non-diabetic.

4. **Vitamin D.**—$C_{28}H_{43}OH$. This represents a dozen or more similar compounds. The two forms of prime importance are activated ergosterol (calciferol) and activated 7-dehydrocholesterol. Fat-

[1] Wolbach: Am. Jour. Path., **9**, 689, 1933.
[2] Sebesta, Smith, Fernald and Marble: New England Jour. Med., **220**, 56, 1939.
[3] Mosenthal and Loughlin: Arch. Int. Med., **73**, 391, 1944.
[4] Owens, Wright and Brown: Am. Jour. Med. Sc., **201**, 636, **1941**.

soluble; the anti-rachitic factor. The average daily minimal requirement for adults is probably about 400 I.U., nearly twice this amount during infancy and is increased during pregnancy and lactation. Source: halibut- and cod-liver oil, and the short ultra-violet rays of the sun which convert 7-dehydrocholesterol of the skin into the active form which is then absorbed and is as effective as vitamin D fed and absorbed through the intestine. The keto form of cholesterol is thought to be produced by the action of ultra-violet ray upon the enol form. It is associated with the metabolism of calcium and phosphorus and can be isolated from irradiated ergosterol in pure crystalline form. Aside from the treatment of rickets it is claimed to reduce the susceptibility of the teeth to decay. Uses: vitamin D is specific in prevention as well as in the treatment of infantile rickets, spasmophilia (infantile tetany) and osteomalacia. Of the vitamins, vitamin D has the most limited distribution.

5. **Vitamin E.**—Sources: Whole wheat, wheat germ, rolled oats, lettuce. It is so widely distributed in the human dietary that one can eliminate it as a factor to consider here. Lack of it is associated with sterility in animals.

6. **Vitamin K.**—Widely distributed in Nature but confined almost entirely to the photo-synthetic portion of plants. It is present in alfalfa, kale, cauliflower, cabbage, spinach, dried carrot tops and tomatoes. It can be prepared from fish meal, rice, bran or casein following putrefaction. It is essential for the formation of prothrombin, and thus for proper clotting of the blood. In hemorrhagic states where a prolonged prothrombin clotting time can be demonstrated, the administration of vitamin K brings about a prompt return to normal. It is of value in obstructive jaundice and in disease of the parenchyma of the liver, due in part to a failure of absorption of fat-soluble substances when bile is excluded from the intestinal tract, or when the secretion of bile salts in the liver is reduced.

J. MINERALS.

Gradually the importance of the mineral salts in diabetes has forced its way to attention. Already reference has been made to the abrupt alterations in body weight according to the ingestion of sodium chloride. Frequent reference has likewise been made to the intimate rôle of phosphorus in the metabolism of fat and carbohydrates. Perhaps the discovery of the influence of almost insignificant quantities of zinc in prolonging the action of insulin is the most striking illustration of our dependence upon inorganic ions.

1. **Sodium Chloride.**—Salt is of great service to the diabetic patient.[1] If it is withdrawn from the diet the weight falls, due to

[1] For papers dealing with the effect of salt ingestion upon diabetes see McQuarrie, Thompson and Anderson: Proc. Soc. Exper. Biol. and Med., 31, 90, 1934; Wilder: Arch. Int. Med., 57, 422, 1936; Adlersberg and Wachstein: Klin. Wchnschr., 16, 85, 1937. See also page 292.

excretion of water, and the skin and tissues of the patient become obviously dry. In the early days of the fasting treatment patients often lost much weight because water alone was allowed, and I learned of one case who lost 13 pounds in four days. Conversely, when broths are freely given during fasting, it is not uncommon, particularly in the presence of acidosis, to see a patient gain weight, and invariably such patients feel better than those who lose.

Salt is used very freely by diabetic patients. I do not remember having ever seen a diabetic patient who took too little salt of his own volition. One of my fasting cases was accustomed to shake it into his hand to eat. In the early days of treatment I remember a boy, Case 707, who once carried a saltcellar to the midst of a garden planted with tomatoes and regaled himself with 40 in an afternoon.

Case 982, a young man with onset of diabetes at the age of twenty years, excreted 40.3 grams of sodium chloride on February 15, 1916, and a few days later the aliquoted urine of two days contained 89.6 grams. Upon inquiry I learned from his nurse that in addition to the ordinary amount of salt in the food, as it was prepared, the young man filled a saltcellar each morning and emptied it before night.

The quantity of sodium chloride in 30 grams of cooked bacon at one hospital amounted to 3.3 grams and at another hospital to 7.3 grams.

An oatmeal cure is accompanied by the use of much salt. In the preparation of the standard 240 grams dry oatmeal a cook would employ about 10 grams salt, which in part explains the edema that often accompanied the oatmeal cure.

Butter contains approximately 2.5 per cent salt.

Vegetable foods are rich in potassium and, as any farmer's child knows who salts the cattle Sunday mornings, are deficient in sodium. It is not strange that with our free use of vegetables the diabetic patients, like cattle, crave salt. But there is still another reason, because when an excess of potassium is eaten, it is quickly discharged and along with the potassium goes sodium as well. A meat diet requires little salt.

Attention may be called to the low excretion of salt in coma. In one case (1053) two days before death the quantity of salt was 1.28 grams, and in the twenty-four hours preceding death amounted to but 0.44 gram. Magnus-Levy's[1] series of cases of severe acidosis showed a low-salt excretion particularly in those which were fatal. It is possible that under such conditions renal insufficiency may enter in, but more probably the sodium ions are retained to offset the acidosis.[2]

Sodium ions in combination with carbonate and lactic acid ions increase the sugar in the blood in contrast to calcium ions which cause hypoglycemia when given in the form of chloride or lactate.[3] Hypochloremia is a very real factor in diabetic coma, because it may result in anuria. (See page 441.)

[1] Magnus-Levy: Die Oxy-Buttersäure, Leipzig, F. C. W. Vogel, 1899.
[2] Peters, Bulger, Eisenman and Lee: Jour. Clin. Invest., 2, 167, 1925.
[3] Labbé, Nepveux and Rohacek: Arch. d. mal. de l'app. digestif., 17, 601, 1927.

2. **Calcium.**—Acidosis if prolonged depletes the stores of alkali in the body and this process extends even to the bones. In coma the pathway for the excretion of calcium and magnesium is altered and the greater proportion passes out through the renal tract. This in itself would not be harmful if the diet replenished the calcium and magnesium so lost, but in this respect it may fail, because milk, the great source of calcium, is often prohibited. Such deprivation may result in decalcification of the bones to such a degree that a slight trauma may lead to a fracture. If such a fracture occurs in the spine of an elderly, feeble patient, the resulting pain may be so slight at the time that it will be unnoticed and later can be looked back upon as a spontaneous fracture. The incidence of fractures in our cases of diabetes is considerable, although possibly not greater than among non-diabetic persons of comparable ages. (See page 711.) Adults require 0.7 gram and children 1 gram calcium in the daily diet. An ordinary hospital diet without milk and eggs or their products contains about 0.4 gram calcium, but milk 90 cc., cream 120 cc., American cheese 10 grams, or 3 eggs each contain 0.1 gram, so that it is easy to bring the calcium up to a proper figure. Beet greens, broccoli, cauliflower, chard, dandelion greens, kale, turnip tops are rated "excellent" in content of calcium.

3. **Potassium.**—See pages 399, 401 and 425.

4. **Phosphorus.**—If the calcium is adequate in the diet, so far as I am aware one need not prescribe phosphorus. The daily amount of phosphorus required by the adult averages 1.3 grams. In the blood the calcium is 10 milligrams per 100 cc. and the phosphorus 2 to 3 milligrams. The daily excretion of the calcium and phosphorus in the urine of normal individuals in a state of equilibrium depends upon the intake; the daily loss from the body by all sources equals the intake.

Phosphorus is a component of the nucleus of all cells, is especially abundant in nerve tissues, and most of all in the carrier of fats, lecithin. It exists in active rather than inactive fat tissues, is a component of the amino acids and even is associated with carbohydrate in the metabolism of the starch molecule.

5. **Iron.**—In the Naunyn era few patients were anemic, because they were supplied so much iron in the form of meat and vegetables. Even in the Allen era anemia was not a marked symptom, but obviously the patients presented a less healthy appearance, largely due to cachexia. In diabetics today anemia is noted with about the same frequency as in non-diabetics. (See page 601.) The daily requirement for iron is between 5 and 15 milligrams. Iron is especially abundant in liver, meat, navy beans, lima beans, eggs, beef, prunes, whole wheat. Unfortunately, molasses, which is rich in iron, finds no place in the diabetic diet.

20

CHAPTER IX.

THE DEFINITION, DIAGNOSIS, CLASSIFICATION, SYMPTOMATOLOGY AND PROGNOSIS OF DIABETES

A. DEFINITION.

DIABETES is an hereditary disease, characterized by an increase of glucose in the blood and the excretion of this sugar in the urine; it is dependent upon the deficient formation or diminished effectiveness of insulin secreted by the islands of Langerhans of the pancreas and is functionally interrelated with conditions arising in the liver and in endocrine glands other than the pancreas, particularly the pituitary, but also the adrenal and thyroid.

B. THE DIAGNOSIS OF DIABETES.

If a patient has sugar in the urine, it is a safe rule to consider the diagnosis to be diabetes until the contrary is proved. The use of the term glycosuria begets indifference and may lead to disaster. Patients with glycosuria whose venous blood sugar is either 130 milligrams per cent fasting or 170 milligrams per cent at any other time of the day are diagnosed as diabetics. If capillary blood is used, the fasting value remains the same, but the other value is raised to 200 milligrams per cent. Prior to July, 1939, our fasting diagnostic level was 140 milligrams per cent, but as a result of the continuous tracing of diabetics and glycosurics, we have felt warranted in adopting 130 milligrams per cent. At the other end of the field 170 milligrams per cent may seem a low value: it is less reliable than the 130 milligrams fasting but only slightly less so than 180 milligrams after food. However, after much thought, we decided to hold to this value for two reasons, first, because all our cases up to now have been so diagnosed, and second, because errors in diagnosis with the use of this value have been remarkably few, as judged by information obtained by means of an intensive follow-up program over many years of time. Many clinicians depend upon the value at the end of two hours after a meal, but such a value is unreliable. Its significance depends upon its comparison with the value before the meal and also upon the rapidity of absorption of the meal, and other factors which are not to be overlooked, namely, confusion as to the time spent in taking the meal and whether the period should be reckoned from its beginning or its close. Even the time itself often is inaccurate.

(306)

But we warn here, as elsewhere in this book, that dependence upon blood-sugar tests must be subject to cautious and critical analysis. Doubting the accuracy of a reported value of 200 milligrams per cent, we were able to protect a girl from the diagnosis of diabetes, because recalculation showed the true value to be 100 milligrams per cent. One swallow does not make a summer, particularly if there is possible doubt about the identification of the swallow. For a discussion of normal blood-sugar values and blood-sugar tolerance tests, see pages 151–170.

As *true diabetics* are classified all patients whose venous blood sugar on an unrestricted diet is 130 milligrams per cent or more fasting or 170 milligrams per cent or more after a meal with simultaneous glycosuria which is plainly related to diet. Glycosuria is considered essential for the diagnosis of diabetes. By holding to this principle one avoids snares which hyperglycemia alone, in the form of a high renal threshold, as in certain aged people or in individuals with certain chronic diseases, often sets. *Potential diabetics* are those with glycosuria closely related to the diet who easily become sugar-free with slight restrictions, but whose blood sugar is below 130 milligrams per cent fasting, never quite reaches 170 milligrams per cent after a meal and may or may not fall to 120 milligrams or below at two hours after a 100 gram glucose tolerance test. The authors often have been tempted to give up the group of potential diabetics and for some years have classified very few as such, but recent work indicates they exist. Hence fresh zeal to recognize them and new hope to avert frank diabetes are aroused. An explanation of their small number of late is that we have more assiduously tried to force new cases into the diabetic or unclassified glucosuric groups and have often postponed a diagnosis for this purpose for a few days, weeks or even months. *Renal glycosurics* are individuals who have shown a constant glycosuria, irrespective of diet, for years, are symptomless, and have a blood sugar which is invariably normal. The *unclassified glycosurics* form a heterogeneous class and undoubtedly include many cases of so-called alimentary glycosuria, cases with a low renal threshold, chance glycosurias in the course of infections, incipient, potential diabetics and others associated with organic disease of the pituitary and hypothalamic regions, thyroid, adrenals, liver, biliary tract and pancreas. These cases form a dangerous group. One never rests easy with an "unclassified" glycosuric. Such a diagnosis worries the doctor, annoys the patient, and exasperates insurance agents.

A positive Benedict test may be shown by patients other than those above mentioned, and it is only treating them fairly to prove, if the blood sugar is normal, that the copper-reducing agent in the urine is glucose and not pentose or fructose. The glycosurias due to drugs, cerebral trauma and emotional instability, are almost invariably temporary, whereas diabetes, levulosuria and pentosuria are permanent. Resort to a glucose-tolerance test is unavoidable at times, but routine reliance solely upon such a test for the differential diagnosis of the glycosurias is undesirable. Confidence in the diagnosis is gained if symptomatology and physical examination support the laboratory findings.

It is not always wise or just to the patient to complete the diagnosis at the first visit, although we usually attempt to do so. He may have been living upon a restricted diet and in consequence the results of a glucose tolerance test may give a false indication. However, we often give the patient 50 grams of glucose and the tests of urine and blood in an hour may suffice, if they are outstandingly abnormal. If doubt remains, a routine sugar-tolerance test with 100 grams glucose can be performed subsequently. A sugar-tolerance test is by no means to be considered as law and gospel in and of itself. The previous diet or the presence of an infection may invalidate it. (See pages 162 and 164.) Umber[1] emphasized the need of discrimination in evaluating such tests. He added that a high fasting blood sugar can exist under various circumstances apart from diabetes and in one instance of carbon monoxide poisoning it reached 350 milligrams per cent.

If another physician has diagnosed diabetes in the past, but urine and blood are normal at the time of the first visit to us, we are loath to perform a glucose-tolerance test unless and until it appears necessary to substantiate the diagnosis. First of all, the insulin is gradually reduced and omitted, then the diet enlarged, and only when these procedures fail to disclose diabetes is a glucose-tolerance test employed. In all cases when dealing with patients diagnosed diabetic by other doctors it is well to follow the golden rule and to avoid statements to the contrary until time and study have yielded unequivocal data.

Two methods of control of the diagnosis, as made in our group of cases, are available, and these depend upon the element of time. Thus, the outcome of those cases not considered diabetic, *i. e.*, errors of omission, were studied in 1937. This is discussed in detail on page 806. It showed that between the years 1900 and 1935, 9.9 per cent of 1946 patients originally thought non-diabetic were subsequently found to have developed diabetes. Obviously a certain percentage of individuals, not actually showing diabetes upon the day of examination, will develop it in the course of ten to thirty years, and so the error represented by this percentage is above rather than below the true value. Diagnostic errors of commission also have been studied. The death certificates of our patients originally diagnosed by us as diabetics but dying under the care of other doctors have been examined.[2] Among 746 true diabetics so

---

[1] Umber: München. med. Wchnschr., **22**, 878, 1936.
[2] Lombard and Joslin: Loc. cit., p. 23. A detailed report of the second series will soon be published.

investigated, there were found to be only 567 certificates of death, 62.9 per cent, with the diagnosis diabetes. In a subsequent series of 1000 of our cases also studied by Lombard and myself, the percentage was 64.9 per cent. The record of each one of these cases was then compared with our own data. This showed to our satisfaction that in only 6 instances in the first series was our diagnosis wrong or questionable and that the omission of the word diabetes was not due to the doubtful character of the diabetes, but simply because the doctor considered diabetes only a minor factor. The query might arise as to whether these diabetics represented cured diabetics, but we are loath to admit such a possibility, because over and over again we have seen patients sugar-free for long periods and with normal blood sugars, and yet their true diabetes would be disclosed when they lived upon a free diet for some weeks or after taking a sugar-tolerance test.

If diabetes is detected early, it is far more susceptible to treatment. The fact that the development of diabetes in a dog as a result of injections of anterior pituitary extract can be prevented by the administration of insulin[1, 2] emphasizes the need for prompt and energetic treatment of a case so soon as the diagnosis is made. Naunyn firmly believed in this, and so do we. Unfortunately the interval between onset and diagnosis is far too great, and this will be lessened only by more frequent routine examinations of the urine. The only way in which an early diagnosis of diabetes will ever be made is to search for it. It is far easier to diagnose than tuberculosis or cancer.

Blotner's[3] surveys of selectees at the Boston Induction Center show how many diabetics, largely symptomless, can be brought to light. (See page 42.) Only the persistent examination by physicians of all patients coming to them will reveal the disease, and these examinations during periods of supposed health must be made at regular and stated intervals (yearly) for the relatives of diabetics and for all adults overweight above the age of forty years. Particularly should these be instituted in schools, colleges, all public institutions, transportation units of all kinds, and manufacturing plants, in police and fire departments, just as such examinations are carried out by insurance companies, and one cannot emphasize too strongly the advantage of the latter following up their policy-holders by a yearly examination of those who are susceptible to diabetes. Everyone should have the urine examined on his or her birthday. Start the custom with the children and it will persist to old age. The urine should be tested before departure from a hospital as well as at entrance, and no physician should discharge a patient

[1] Haist, Campbell and Best: Loc. cit., p. 99.
[2] Lukens and Dohan: Endocrinology, **30**, 175, 1942. See also ref. 2, p. 99 and ref. 3, p. 123.
[3] Blotner and Hyde: Loc. cit., p. 42. Blotner: Loc. cit., p. 43.

following acute disease or childbirth without making an examination of the urine for albumin and sugar.

March 30, 1920, there came to my office a woman with diabetes. She was given the usual examination with suggestions for treatment, and as it was impracticable for her to enter the hospital, she was taught on the spot to examine her urine. She went home and shortly after contracted pneumonia and died. But in the intervening days amid her household cares she found time and took enough interest to examine the urines of 10 others in her boarding house, and in so doing discovered the presence of diabetes in a boy. She gave him sound advice and sent him to his own physician, who also subsequently died, and eventually the boy came to me, telling this story. At the time she learned the Benedict test and made these urinary examinations for her friends, Louisa Drumm, Case 1796, was seventy-nine years and four months old.

The physician should take pride in prevention of diabetes in his practice. Obese patients should be frankly told that they are voluntary candidates for the diabetic army just as those hereditarily predisposed may enter it as diabetic conscripts. The physician should consider it as important to prevent his patients acquiring diabetes as he feels it incumbent on himself to vaccinate them against smallpox, diphtheria, typhoid fever and tetanus, or to protect them from exposure to tuberculosis.

C. METHODS OF CLASSIFICATION OF DIABETES.

No method for the classification of diabetics to my mind is satisfactory. This must of necessity be so if the conception of the unity of diabetes is correct. No sooner are the boundary lines drawn than one case after another like sheep breaks through the fence. The severe case with advancing years grows mild, the mild case in childhood as it passes through puberty may become severe only in turn in later adolescence to change to diabetes of moderate degree. The functional derangement of the diabetic outweighs the organic and he becomes a prey to many influences. We know that a diabetic is mild, moderate, or severe largely as the doctor with his diet, insulin, and exercise makes him. Moreover it is not true that the patient necessarily need progress through the stages of mild, moderate and severe diabetes. Various methods of classification frequently have been useful, because they have suggested different viewpoints from which to regard the disease.

1. **The French Methods.**—The older French clinicians divided their cases into two classes: (*a*) Diabète gras and (*b*) Diabète maigre, and immediately the picture of the old, mild, fat individual and the young, severe, thin patient come to mind. Yet time and treatment destroy the grouping because on the one hand the thinnest of the severe thin may have been at one time the fattest of the

mild fat, and the uncontrolled fat girl of severe type in her middle teens may have been a slim, mild diabetic when first seen at seven years and change back to a much less severe diabetic at twenty years of age.

Labbé[1] established two categories, (1) les diabètes sans dénutrition azotée, in which the error of metabolism is concerned exclusively with carbohydrate and the glycosuria of carbohydrate origin, and (2) les diabètes avec dénutrition azotée, in which the fault of metabolism is dependent upon all three foodstuffs, carbohydrate, protein and fat and in which glycosuria is simultaneously of alimentary and tissue origin. The patient loses in urine and feces more nitrogen than is furnished by the diet. The closer interrelation of carbohydrate, protein and fat accepted today upsets such a division, but it shows the view of an astute clinician only a decade ago.

2. **Tolerance for Carbohydrate.**—Early in this century the basis of classification of diabetics was their tolerance for carbohydrate. Severe diabetics were those who showed glycosuria with less than 10 grams of carbohydrate in the diet, moderately severe diabetics, those between 10 and 50 grams, and other cases were considered mild. Gradually in the last twenty years the number of the severe cases has dwindled, and today one seldom finds severe diabetics of the old school. Benedict and Joslin[2] agreed with von Noorden that no diabetes was complete.

3. **Units of Insulin Required.**—The units of insulin employed in the treatment of a case and division according to those who take and those who do not take insulin have also been employed for classification, but here too there are many difficulties, because few doctors use identical diets, and few doctors have the same rules for the use or non-use of insulin. Falta[3] determined the glucose equivalent of insulin by placing his patients upon a standard diet. He used the quotient of sugar excretion on this diet as compared with the insulin requirement to arrive at the glucose value of a unit. When the patient was sugar-free, insulin was omitted and the effect noted on that and succeeding days. MacBryde[4] described these methods and reported upon 200 observations in Falta's Clinic. He distinguished patients relatively sensitive to insulin from those relatively resistant by noting the effect produced upon the blood sugar by injecting 1 unit of insulin per 10 pounds body weight. Degree of sensitivity is also shown by the "tolerated overdose," meaning the amount of insulin the diabetic can tolerate above his ordinary requirement without symptoms. The "sensitive" case tolerates little or none, the "resistant" case may tolerate considerable, even as much as 60 units. John R. Williams[1] also

[1] Labbé: Précis de pathologie médicale, Paris, Masson et Cie, **6**, 995, 1934.
[2] Joslin: Arch. Int. Med., **16**, 693, 1915.
[3] Falta: Extrait du Volume Jubilaire en l'Honneur du Professeur G. Marinesco.
[4] MacBryde: Arch. Int. Med., **52**, 932, 1933. See also Southern Med. Jour., **29**, 488, 1926.

employed the dextrose equivalent of insulin as compared with the total endogenous and exogenous insulin requirement in classifying his cases.

4. Acidosis.—The presence, absence, or intensity of acidosis affords an unsatisfactory basis for classification. The mildest case of diabetes by restriction of carbohydrate and increase in the amount of fat can be made to develop an acidosis which will be mild, moderate, or severe in degree. According to Bertram[2] the person with mild diabetes is continuously free from ketone bodies on an adequate caloric diet containing at least 100 grams of carbohydrate; the patient with moderate diabetes is not ketone free on such a diet save with the use of insulin; but the patient with severe diabetes is not ketone free on such a diet, even with insulin.

TABLE 38.—ASTHENIC AND STHENIC TYPES OF DIABETES. (LORANT–SCHMIDT.)

"Asthenic" or "Unterdruck" diabetes.	"Sthenic" or "Überdruck" diabetes.
Age, usually under thirty years.	Age, older individuals.
Blood-pressure, usually normal or subnormal.	Blood-pressure, usually elevated.
Tendency to ketonuria.	No tendency to ketonuria.
Weak muscles, slender, without energy.	Muscular, often obese, energetic.
	Tendency to gangrene, arthritis, neuralgia.
	Tendency to formation of stones.
Pigment, poor (blue iris).	Pigment, rich.
Patellar reflexes usually diminished.	Patellar reflexes often increased.
Diabetic coma, frequent, typical, easily influenced by insulin.	Diabetic coma, infrequent, atypical and fatal outcome despite insulin.

5. Asthenic and Sthenic Types.—The division into asthenic and sthenic types as suggested by Lorant[3] and Schmidt[4] does not appeal to us, because there is no sharp boundary line between the two forms, and the two sets of characteristics, as outlined in Table 38, merge one into the other. Certainly there are many young diabetic patients who are overweight and of the sthenic type and likewise many older diabetic patients with normal or subnormal blood pressure, weakness, and sensitivity to insulin. Many European writers, however, including Bertram,[5] find this classification useful. Himsworth[6] divided diabetics into two groups according to their sensitivity to insulin. In some respects his insulin-sensitive patients would fall into the asthenic group and his insulin-insensitive patients would fall in the sthenic group.

Umber[7] refers frequently to insular and extra-insular diabetes, but in general he uses the terms to differentiate between true dia-

---

[1] Williams: Ann. Int. Med., 5, 264, 1931.
[2] Bertram: P. 37, loc. cit., p. 87.
[3] Lorant and Adler: Wien. Arch. inn. Med., 7, 137, 1924.
[4] Schmidt: Klin. Wchnschr., 9, 1969, 1930.
[5] Bertram: Ergebn. d. inn. Med. u. Kinderh., 43, 258, 1932.
[6] Himsworth: Loc. cit., p. 144.
[7] Umber: Handbuch der gesamten Unfallheilkunde, Stuttgart, Ferdinand Enke, vol. 1, 1932.

betes and the glycosurias. We agree with Marañon[1] that one cannot draw a sharp distinction along these lines. Sometimes the hypophysis, thyroid, adrenals are primary and the pancreas secondary and so the pancreas may compensate for the others.

6. **Mild, Moderate, Severe Diabetes.**—There is therefore no generally accepted classification for mild, moderate, and severe diabetes. Classification with units of insulin employed is unsatisfactory, because the carbohydrate may vary from 100 to 200 grams or more and the total calories as well, and so involve the use of varying amounts of insulin. "Nevertheless," as Lukens and Dohan[2] state, "the amount of insulin required is the best clinical indication of the severity of diabetes." With these considerations in mind, diabetics might be grouped in three types.

A *mild* diabetic might be said to be one who is sugar-free before and after meals with carbohydrate 150 grams in twenty-four hours and no insulin, or sugar-free with carbohydrate 200 grams and 10 units of insulin daily.

A *moderate* diabetic might be considered one who is sugar-free with 100 grams carbohydrate in twenty-four hours and no insulin or sugar-free with 150 grams carbohydrate with 10 units or with more carbohydrate and 20 to 30 units daily.

A *severe* diabetic would be one with a tolerance for less than 50 grams carbohydrate without insulin and requiring 50 or more units of insulin to be sugar-free with 150 grams carbohydrate.

For attempts to distinguish various types of diabetics according to their reactions to insulin and to evaluate hepatogenous and tissue resistance, see pages 143–148. Also see pages 121 and 124, for the milder types of diabetes in animals following the removal of the pituitary or adrenal cortex.

See Chapter XXX for a discussion of other types of melituria.

D. THE SYMPTOMS OF DIABETES.

1. **Onset.**—The date of onset of diabetes is usually indefinite, particularly in adults, whereas in children the diagnosis far more often can be assigned to a definite month, week or even day. My associates and I have zealously investigated this point, first with 500 cases, and subsequently Dr. White studied 1009 adults and 489 children. In addition, the records were searched for cases with "*sudden*" onset (*i. e.*, within twenty-four hours) in seven other groups of approximately 1000 patients each and the percentage varied per group between 1 and 1.6 per cent, the average being 1.3 per cent.

The time of onset was considered "*indefinite*" if it could not be located within any two months' period, and 86 per cent of the adults fell into this indefinite classification, but only 35 per cent of the children. If the onset appeared to be within an interval of two

[1] Marañon: Med. Klin., **31**, 42, 1935.
[2] Lukens and Dohan: Loc. cit., p. 203.

months to one week it was considered *"gradual,"* and this group claimed 9.4 per cent of the adults and 44 per cent of the children. The onset was considered *"rapid"* if it appeared to occur during a period of six days; in this group are 2.7 per cent of the adults and 18 per cent of the children. In fact, this percentage holds for all the 2191 children. An onset developing in the course of twenty-four hours was considered *"sudden"* and in this category are found 1.9 per cent of the adults and 3 per cent of the children, but I consider even these percentages far too high.

The reason for statements in the literature that diabetes is of sudden onset may be due to imperfect histories, based more upon impressions or upon death certificates, but for such a purpose both are unreliable. The diabetic patient a generation ago lived so short a time and his career was so tragic, particularly in childhood, that it was very natural to record the onset as "acute" and the end as "acutely fatal." It may be said that "acutely fatal" diabetes is a diabetic ghost which, like another of its kind, "complete diabetes," has vanished from medical nomenclature.

The latency of diabetes is illustrated by its development in a parent, or even a grandparent, after it has appeared in a child, and in obesity in which one can observe the disease in its stage of incubation. A mother may have a series of big babies and not until the third or fourth 10-pound baby appears is the explanation of the others disclosed by her showing diabetes. In cases in which it came on almost as an apoplectic stroke the circumstances were varied.

Of examples of acute onset which stand out in my memory are Case 7, the man who was injured by a bull, Case 10, the Boston bank clerk, whose diabetes came on during an important and unaccustomed mission while turning a corner in New York City, Case 5786, the boy who fell through the ice and was rescued by his dog. Yet I could not take oath that these patients were free from sugar even a few days before the assigned date. Moreover, the records of these cases were taken by me in 1898, 1899 and 1927 respectively, when my experience in diabetic history taking was of a less critical character. The most reliable of all amoung the 29,000 cases is 13332 described on page 95. Sprague[1] cites a similar case observed by Wilder.

It will be worth while to endeavor to learn more accurately the type of onset of diabetes. It will furnish assistance in a search for the etiology and will raise queries in the minds of the pathologists; it should indicate the character of the methods which must be adopted for prevention; it may be of value in classification and prognosis, and even treatment.[2]

The symptoms of the latent period, corresponding to the pro-

[1] Sprague: Diabetes Mellitus, *in* Tice's Practice of Medicine, Hagerstown, Md., W. F. Prior Co., Inc., vol. 9, 1945, p. 85a.
[2] Smith and Grishaw: Arch. Int. Med., **66**, 465, 1940.

dromal period in an infectious disease, in contrast to the symptoms of the clinical period at onset, are instructively discussed by Marañon.[1] He emphasizes that this latent period should be utilized for preventive treatment, and how important this may be has been mentioned. In addition to the etiological factors mentioned above, such as obesity and heredity, he includes hypertension and itching of the skin as of much importance. Escudero[2] seeks to determine the prodromal stage by slight alterations in the blood-sugar curves. Colwell[3] goes so far as to say its course may be half run before it is even recognized, basing his argument on the comparison of the amount of insulin required with the length of time the disease existed in comparable groups of diabetic subjects. Priscilla White[4] has noted the flattened type of blood-sugar curve after tolerance tests in the relatives of diabetics. (See page 63.) We are altogether too much in the dark about the prodromal symptoms of diabetes. We should learn how to recognize its approach and not simply suspect it because of heredity and obesity.

Irrespective of the type of onset, whether fulminating or slow, as soon as the diagnosis of diabetes is made the profession has come to regard the active stage of the disease, the progressive stage, completed and to feel that all the damage has been done. This is contrary to common sense and analogy. Even in hemiplegia the first few hours of the illness show rapid changes taking place about the embolus or the hemorrhage and in an acute infectious disease there is no sharp line between pathological degeneration and regeneration. During the beginning stage of diabetes the patient should be considered as in a labile condition and we should hold ourselves expectant to observe whether the disease is to become mild, moderate, or severe. Quite likely it receives its stamp of severity at its very inception and is severe or mild largely as the diet and the doctor decree. If an established diabetes of moderate severity of long standing can be made to become severe by improper treatment, such as sudden restriction of carbohydrate and excessive administration of protein and fat, how much more easily may the diabetes in its nascent stage suffer increase in severity; conversely, what an opportunity exists for active prophylactic and therapeutic effort.

2. **Symptoms.**—As a rule the approach of the disease, like that of the complication coma, is insidious. Loss of strength, polyuria, polydipsia, and polyphagia are the commonest symptoms. Polyuria is the most frequent symptom, being present in 73 per cent of the cases; polydipsia in 67 per cent and loss of strength in 64 per cent stand next in importance. Symptoms and signs referable to the skin existed in 31 per cent of the cases. Pruritus vulvæ is frequent

[1] Marañon, Carrasco and Soler: Arch. d. med. cirugia y especialidades, 1924.
[2] Escudero: Diabetes Aglucosurica, Barcelona, Manuel Marin, 1930.
[3] Colwell: Arch. Int. Med., **70**, 523, 1942.
[4] Pincus and White: Loc. cit., p. 63, ref. 2.

and always demands exclusion of the diagnosis of diabetes. Loss of weight is common, not always noted by patients, and occasionally a gain in weight occurs. Blurring of vision is not uncommon. Pain in the extremities was noted in 20 per cent. Polydipsia is a very important symptom and much more so than polyuria which follows it. Often the patients report that they have been water drinkers since early childhood. Polydipsia frequently precedes coma and not rarely is associated with a dilated stomach.

Most of the symptoms which we involuntarily attribute to diabetes are really symptoms caused by complications and will be discussed under such heads. These complications are far more common now than formerly, because diabetics live so long that they have an opportunity to develop. Thus neuritis, once thought by my colleagues and me to be exceptional in diabetics, proved to be very frequent when Dr. W. R. Jordan, who worked with us for two and one-half years, carefully examined patients with this in mind.

It is far more difficult to determine the interval between onset and diagnosis in diabetes than in cancer. The average interval between what my associates and I consider to be the date of onset and the date of diagnosis, demonstrated by the finding of glycosuria, was three months in one series of 500 cases and, five and four-tenths months in a similar series, but it is true that these are figures which in more than 80 per cent are acknowledged to be indefinite. In children such delays occur less frequently and intervals between onset, diagnosis and the beginning of treatment are much shorter. This may account for the favorable course of the disease in many cases in children.

The fall in weight from maximum to first visit, based on the recent 500 cases mentioned in the preceding paragraph, shows an average loss of 30.7 pounds. Four hundred twenty-six were adults. For those under twenty years of age at examination, the 45 cases for whom the data were available show an average loss of 6 pounds— again evidence that diagnosis is far more prompt in young than in older people.

Impotence is rarely a complaint. It very likely could be more often elicited, but has been neglected purposely in the anamnesis, because with general improvement under treatment it may disappear, or if not, the less the attention of the patient is directed to it, the better.

In closing this section we would warn against depending upon symptoms for diagnosis. Diabetes will not be found without search.

E. THE DURATION OF LIFE AND THE PROGNOSIS IN DIABETES.

1. **Duration.**—I measured the length of life of my first diabetic children in days; a few years later I could change to months, but

this duration held for what I have termed the Naunyn era of my practice (1898-1914). F. M. Allen and undernutrition and Wood-yatt and others helped me to double the duration so that I was just barely able to reckon it in terms of years, two years, in the Allen era (June, 1914 to March 16, 1922). By the last Banting era (January 1, 1935 to December 31, 1936) children almost ceased to die, because of 793 deaths, only 8 were in patients who had contracted diabetes under ten years of age and these lived 7.9 years. In the Charles H. Best era (January 1, 1944 to May 15, 1946) there were 651 deaths, of whom 15 were those with onset under ten years, but their duration was 16.7 years. Children with diabetes now live so long that we are forced to depend upon their calculated life expectancy. (See Tables 42 and 43.) At present among our 2191 children with onset under fifteen years of age, we have 749 who have had the disease more than fifteen years, 249 who have had it more than twenty years, 93 over twenty-five years, 5 over thirty years. Of 301 diabetic deaths in Boston during 1935 there was no death under the age of nineteen years,[1] and but 3.4 per cent of the patients were less than forty years old at death. The average age was 64.3 years.

In 1913 I[2] reported 8 diabetics, whom I considered standards, who had lived from three years and eleven months to twenty-one years, but by 1927 insulin had raised the number of diabetics living ten or more years to 934 and forced us to adopt new criteria and to be content only when a diabetic patient lives longer with his disease from the time it begins than he or she would be expected to live without it.[3] To these we give a medal (see illustration on page 327).

The percentage of fatal cases who survived twenty years of diabetes in the Naunyn era (1898–1914) was 1.8 per cent of the total deaths, but of deaths in the Charles H. Best era between January 1, 1944, and May 15, 1946, they now aggregate 22.1 per cent. (I never could have had the courage to treat diabetics between 1898 and 1922 unless I knew I had in my notebook in my pocket irrefutable proof that some progress was being made. At the commencement, of course, it seemed as if it might prove to be a Cyrano de Bergerac experience and there was so much of a thrill in the thought that today I feel almost guilty to reap the rewards of insulin and still more from protamine zinc insulin.—E. P. J.)

Tables 39, 40 and 41, as well as 26 in the chapter on Pathology, present the result of treatment of diabetes between 1898 and May 15, 1946, in the group of patients cared for by my associates and myself. The tables represent literally years of work of secretaries, assistants and the coöperation of doctors throughout the United States and Canada and even beyond the seas. Of the 657 cases

---

[1] Lynch: New England Jour. Med., **215**, 822, 1936.
[2] Joslin: Am. Jour. Med. Sci., **145**, 474, 1913.
[3] Joslin: Ann. Clin. Med., **5**, 1061, 1927.

seen in the Naunyn era, 326 have died; of 1740 in the Allen era, 836 have died and 12 are untraced.   In the first part of the Banting era, August 7, 1922 to December 31, 1929, there were 5004 cases, and of these, 1455 have died and 336 are untraced.   From this date onwards all the known deaths are reported, but because of the large number the complete follow-up ends with December 31, 1929 except for special groups hereinafter mentioned.

TABLE 39.—AVERAGE DURATION OF LIFE SUBSEQUENT TO ONSET OF DIABETES AMONG 8385 DECEASED EX-PATIENTS IN EACH OF THE IMPORTANT ERAS OF TREATMENT.   BY AGE GROUP AT ONSET.*

(Experience of Elliott P. Joslin, M.D., 1898–1946.)

Age groups of onset.	Naunyn era. Before June 1, 1914.		Allen era. June 1, 1914, to Aug. 6, 1922.		Banting era. Aug. 7, 1922, to Dec. 31, 1936.		Hagedorn era. Jan. 1, 1937, to Dec. 31, 1943.		Chas. H. Best era. Jan. 1, 1944, to date.‡	
	No. of cases.	Dura-tion, yrs.	No. of cases.	Dura-tion, yrs.	No. of cases.	Dura-tion, yrs.	No. of cases.	Dura-tion, yrs.	No. of cases.	Dura-tion, yrs.
All ages . .	326	4.9	836	6.1	3989	9.6†	2583	12.9	651	14.1
0–9 . .	24	1.3	61	2.9	45	5.2	35	10.2	15	16.7
10–19 . .	39	2.7	84	2.7	112	5.5	71	11.1	31	13.2
20–39 . .	85	4.3	215	4.9	464	12.2	299	17.4	70	17.9
40–59 . .	126	7.0	351	8.0	2175	11.0	1373	14.4	328	16.2
60 and over .	51	4.4	117	6.4	1173	6.6	804	9.0	200	9.3
Unknown .	1	..	8	..	20	..	1	..	7	

* Deaths reported through May 15, 1946.
† Based on cases with known duration.
‡ Prepared by the Statistical Bureau of the Metropolitan Life Insurance Company.

TABLE 40.—DURATION OF LIFE SUBSEQUENT TO ONSET OF DIABETES AMONG DECEASED EX-PATIENTS IN EACH OF THE IMPORTANT ERAS OF TREATMENT.*

(Number and Per Cent of Cases Classified According to Duration.)
(Experience of E. P. Joslin, M.D. and Associates, 1898–1946.)

Duration, yrs.	Naunyn era. Before June 1, 1914.		Allen era. June 1, 1914, to Aug. 6, 1922.		Banting era. Aug. 7, 1922, to Dec. 31, 1936.		Hagedorn era. Jan. 1, 1937, to Dec. 31, 1943.		Chas. H. Best era. Jan. 1, 1944, to date.‡	
	No. of cases.	Per cent.	No. of cases.	Per cent.	No. of cases.	Per cent.	No. of cases.	Per cent.	No. of cases.	Per cent.
All cases .	326	100.0	836	100.0	3989	100.0	2583	100.0	651	100.0
Less than 5 .	217	66.8	463	55.9	1162	29.4	390	15.1	99	15.5
Less than 1 .	63	19.4	72	8.7	173	4.4	61	2.4	21	3.3
1 . .	51	15.7	108	13.0	227	5.7	68	2.6	20	3.1
2 . .	53	16.3	121	14.6	230	5.8	80	3.1	14	2.2
3 . .	23	7.1	97	11.7	264	6.7	90	3.5	19	3.0
4 . .	27	8.3	65	7.9	268	6.8	91	3.5	25	3.9
5–9 . .	58	17.8	210	25.4	1171	29.4	550	21.3	119	18.5
5 . .	18	5.5	49	5.9	242	6.1	106	4.1	27	4.2
6 . .	10	3.1	51	6.2	239	6.0	103	4.0	21	3.3
7 . .	9	2.8	46	5.6	250	6.3	115	4.5	22	3.4
8 . .	16	4.9	36	4.3	220	5.5	109	4.2	25	3.9
9 . .	5	1.5	28	3.4	220	5.5	117	4.5	24	3.7
10–14 . .	32	9.8	89	10.7	832	21.0	710	27.5	133	20.7
15–19 . .	12	3.7	40	4.8	493	12.4	538	20.8	150	23.2
20 or more .	6	1.8	26	3.1	311	7.8	394	15.3	143	22.1
Unknown .	1	..	8	..	20	..	..	..	7	
Average . .	4.9		6.1		9.6†		12.9†		14.1	
Median . .	2.9		4.3		8.4†		12.6†		14.0	

* Deaths reported through May 15, 1946.
† Based on cases with known duration.
‡ Prepared by the Statistical Bureau of the Metropolitan Life Insurance Company.

The compilation of the data outgrew our capabilities several years ago, and for their present form we are profoundly grateful to the Metropolitan Life Insurance Company, Dr. August I. Knight, Dr. Charles Christiernin, and Dr. Earl C. Bonnet, Medical Directors, and especially to Dr. Louis I. Dublin, second Vice-president and Statistician, and above all, to Mr. Herbert H. Marks.

TABLE 41.—THE CHANGING AVERAGE AGE AT DEATH AND AVERAGE DURATION OF DIABETES IN THE NAUNYN, ALLEN, BANTING, HAGEDORN AND BEST ERAS.[1]

(Experience of E. P. Joslin, M.D., and Associates, 1898–1946.)[2]

Era.	No. of deaths.	Average age at death, yrs.	Average duration of diabetes, yrs.
Naunyn, 1898 to June 1, 1914	326	44.5	4.9
Allen, June 1, 1914, to August 6, 1922 . .	836	46.7	6.1
Banting:			
August 7, 1922, to December 31, 1925 .	537	54.3	7.5
January 1, 1926, to December 31, 1929 .	918	60.0	8.4
January 1, 1930, to December 31, 1934 .	1741	62.7	10.0
January 1, 1935, to December 31, 1936 .	793	63.9	11.6
Hagedorn:			
January 1, 1937, to December 31, 1939 .	1229	64.8	12.4
January 1, 1940, to December 31, 1943 .	1354	65.0	13.3
Charles H. Best, January 1, 1944, to May, 15, 1946	651	64.5	14.1

[1] Prepared by the Statistical Bureau of the Metropolitan Life Insurance Company.
[2] Includes deaths recorded up to May 15, 1946.

The average duration of life to their death according to the ages of onset of their diabetes among my patients is shown for the Naunyn, Allen, the four Banting epochs, the two Hagedorn epochs and the Charles H. Best era in Table 39. For all ages the average duration of life has risen steadily from 4.9 years in the Naunyn era ending in 1914 to 14.1 years in the present Charles H. Best era. The gain in duration has been relatively the most among those with onset in the first decade, from 1.3 to 16.7 years, quintupled in the second, but quadrupled, 4.3 to 17.9 years in the combined third and fourth and more than doubled both in the fifth and sixth and even from sixty years onwards. Recognizing the inconsiderable number of deaths to total cases under twenty years of age and the 17.9 years' duration for those between twenty and forty, who have died, it is not unreasonable to conclude that the (average) total span of life for diabetics developing the disease in 1940 will average twenty years. The percentage of deaths in the first decade to total deaths in the Naunyn era was 8.4 but in the current Charles H. Best era is 2.3, and for deaths 40 and 59 was 39 per cent and now 50 per cent, and for above sixty years of age has changed from 15.6 per cent to 30.0 per cent.

The duration of life subsequent to onset of diabetes among fatal patients in each of the important eras of treatment, the Naunyn, Allen, Banting, Hagedorn, and Charles H. Best periods, is shown in

Table 40, classified by number and per cent according to duration. Whereas in the Naunyn period 19.4 per cent died in less than a year, in the Charles H. Best era the per cent has fallen to 3.3 in contradistinction to the twenty-year and more duration cases where the percentage has risen from 1.8 per cent to 22.1 per cent. At present 15.5 per cent of our diabetics die in the first five years of their disease, 18.5 per cent in the second five years, 20.7 in the third five-year period, 23.2 per cent in the fourth, leaving 22.1 per cent, as stated above, to live for more than twenty years. The average duration of life has risen from 4.9 years in the Naunyn period to 14.1 years in the Charles H. Best era, and of still more significance, the median age from 2.9 years to 14.0 years.

The average age at death of diabetics in the various epochs above described is shown in Table 41. In the Naunyn era it was 44.5 years, rose twenty years ending in the Hagedorn era and has remained constant since. This table likewise shows the steady increase in average duration for all cases from 4.9 years in the Naunyn era to 14.1 in the Charles H. Best era (to date). Therefore, any patient today who dies under the age of 64.5 years or without having had diabetes 14.1 years lowers our present standard. Today we are caring for a group of patients who have had the disease nearly three times as long and more than twenty years older than a generation ago. What a change this represents in the social aspects of the disease for patient, doctor and society.

The duration of life of diabetics in the Naunyn era was based upon the deaths occurring in those patients dying in it or between 1898 and 1914, but that was not the true duration for the entire group. Thus the total number of patients in the group was 657, and 326 died in the Naunyn era and it is their average duration which was 4.9 years. There are known to have been 317 deaths subsequently and living in 1946, 14 patients, and the duration of life for the combined fatal and living cases to date is 9.6 years.

Applying this same statistical study to cases dying in the Allen era, the duration of life of that group rises from its original 6.1 years to 12.1 years. Again applying it to the Banting era, ending December 31, 1929, the duration of life of the combined fatal and living cases to date (1946) is 14.9 years. "It is important to note that these comparisons fall short of the whole truth. The story is almost complete for the Naunyn era cases because only 14 or a little over 2 per cent were living at the beginning of this year, whereas 12 per cent of the Allen era cases and 34 per cent of the early Banting cases were still living." (H. H. M.)

The expectation of life of our diabetics at specified ages has been computed by the Statistical Department of the Metropolitan Life Insurance Company on data available in 1938. This table should be recomputed, but it necessitates sampling and following up 25 cases out of each 100 seen since January 1, 1930, and we were forced to postpone the task. We are indebted to them for Tables 42 and 43. Table 43 is based upon death-rates at each age, subsequent to the first observation of the patient, regardless of the duration of diabetes. At ten years of age the normal child has an expectancy of fifty-seven years, but the diabetic child has an expectancy of forty years, in contrast to a scant two years a half generation ago. This is 70 per cent of the life expectancy of the general population and really represents a shortening of the life's span by fifteen years. At the age of sixty-five years, the normal expectancy is twelve years and the diabetic expectancy is eight years. These tables, the first of their sort with which we are familiar, give a clearer idea of the outlook for the diabetic than tables based alone upon diabetic mortality. We are sure they are the precursors of many others.

TABLE 42.—EXPECTATION OF LIFE FOR THE GENERAL POPULATION AND FOR DIABETICS.[1]

Age.	White persons, U. S.*	Diabetics, Joslin.†
10	57	40
20	48	33
30	39	28
40	31	21
50	23	14
60	16	10
65	12	8

[1] Prepared with the coöperation of the statistical bureau of the Metropolitan Life Insurance Company.
* United States, 1935.
† Based on death-rates of each age, subsequent to first observation, regardless of duration of diabetes.

TABLE 43.—EXPECTATION OF LIFE AT SELECTED AGES.[1, 2]
(Death-rate per 1000.)

Age.	Naunyn Era. 1897–1914.	Allen Era. 1914– Aug. 6, 1922.	Early. Aug. 7, 1922– 1925.	Middle. 1926–1928.	Late. 1929–1938.
10	1.3	2.6	14.3	31.7	39.8
30	4.1	6.3	16.8	22.7	27.6
50	8.0	9.5	12.3	13.2	14.4

[1] Excludes deaths within one week of first observation or hospital discharge.
[2] Prepared by the Statistical Bureau of the Metropolitan Life Insurance Company.

(a) **Children.**—Here again reference may be made to the group of 249 children who have had their disease twenty years or more. Of these, 237 were alive in 1946. There are 93 children who have already survived more than twenty-five years and 5 more than thirty years of diabetes, and it is obvious that the number will grow very rapidly because insulin began to be used quite generally in 1923. See Chapter XXVIII.

(b) **Early Insulin Cases.**—A second collection of our cases, namely, the first 83 treated with insulin between August 7, 1922 and January 25, 1923, gives a hint of prognosis of diabetics in general. On the whole these first 83 cases were selected because they were severe

21

diabetics and therefore one has a right to conclude that for diabetics *en masse* the prognosis would be somewhat more favorable. Thus, of the original 83 patients, 54 have died at an average age of 47.8 years with a duration of diabetes of 11.5 years. On January 1, 1945, we knew that the remaining 29 cases in the group were alive, and the average duration of the diabetes in these 29 cases at that time was 24.2 years. I might add that of the 22 recent deaths there were 8 from coronary thrombosis, 2 from cerebral hemorrhage, 2 from tuberculosis, 3 from hemiplegia, 1 from diabetic coma, 1 from gangrene, 1 with multiple abscesses of both kidneys, 1 with nephritis and furunculosis while pregnant, 1 of pneumonia, 1 of Parkinson's disease and 1 of cardio-renal disease.

(*c*) **Cases With Onset Under Forty Years.**—In 1930 H. C. Shepardson,[1] now of San Francisco, studied the effects of diabetes upon the vascular system of 50 of our patients then under the age of forty years who had already survived the disease five or more years. Fortunately it has been possible to check the condition of all these patients up to January 1, 1945. Seventeen of the 50 have died, and the duration of their diabetes has been 16.4 years. The causes of death of these cases were cerebral thrombosis 1, chronic nephritis 2, coronary thrombosis 2, myocardial insufficiency associated with nephritis 1, coma associated with tuberculosis 1, meningitis originating in the mastoid 1, carbuncle 1, coma 1, renal infection and coma 1, pulmonary tuberculosis 2, appendicitis 1, pulmonary embolism 1, paranephric abscess and septicemia 1, and automobile accident 1. Of the remaining 33 cases living, the duration of the diabetes was 23.5 years.

(*d*) **Physicians.**—Information concerning the incidence of diabetes among physicians came as an outgrowth of the Arizona study. Thus, in Arizona 334 physicians replied to my query as to whether they had diabetes, 8 in the positive and 326 in the negative, or 1 physician in 42. For comparison similar data were obtained in Rhode Island in response to an exactly similar number of letters. The replies numbered 393, 11 positive and 382 negative, or 1 in 36. Another means of inferring the incidence of diabetes among physicians in the United States is furnished by the 44 doctors who are reported to have died in the United States during 1945.[2] Since the number of doctors in the United States is reported as 191,689 for 1945, 1 doctor in 4357 died of diabetes, and allowing a duration of disease of fifteen years, 1 doctor in 290 had the disease, or if one allows a duration of twenty years of diabetes, 1 doctor in 218. However, if errors occurred to the same extent with physicians as with all patients (see page 23) the number of doctors reported as dying with the disease would have been only two-thirds of the total, and using the enlarged figure, the frequency of the disease on the basis

[1] Shepardson: Arch. Int. Med., **45**, 674, 1930.
[2] Editorial: Deaths of Physicians in 1945, Jour. Am. Med. Assn., **130**, 148, 1946.

of 15 and 20 years' duration would be 1 in 193 and 1 in 145 respectively, which comes nearer to the figures obtained in Arizona, 1 in 42, and Rhode Island, 1 in 36. Personally, I think this lower ratio shows how unsatisfactory mortality statistics are in determining the morbidity of diabetes.

The duration of diabetes in doctors also affords information for prognosis. Thus, 522 physicians prior to January 15, 1946 have consulted us for glycosuria and of the number 432 (405 men and 27 women) have had true diabetes, 67 unclassified glycosuria, 20 potential diabetes, 2 renal glycosuria and 1 pentosuria.

The average age at death of the 225 fatal cases of true diabetes in physicians was 65.5 years, and in the corresponding 207 living physicians already the average age has reached 59.7 years. The average age at death of the diabetic doctors has been rising. In the pre-insulin period it was 57.5 years; it rose to 66.0 in the Banting era and in the Charles H. Best era it has reached 66.3 years.

The onset of diabetes in the medical profession runs true to form, because the greatest number developed the disease in the sixth decade. In no instance was the onset in the first decade; there were 4 cases in the second, 39 in the third, making it probable that a considerable number of students entered medical schools when they were diabetics, 78 in the fourth, 102 in the fifth, 112 in the sixth, 77 in the seventh, 19 in the eighth, 1 in the ninth.

Among 225 fatal diabetic doctors, deaths were apportioned as follows: cardio-renal-vascular disease, including gangrene and apoplexy 144, coma 17, infections 19, cancer 19, tuberculosis 10, and miscellaneous 16.

For years we have preached that diabetic coma is needless and this our diabetic doctors exemplify. Deaths due to diabetic coma among physicians in the Naunyn era numbered 40 per cent[1] and in the Allen era 5.6 per cent.[2] In the Hagedorn era there were no deaths among doctors due to coma and in the Best era there was one. When we report to our patients the paucity of deaths from coma among physicians, someone in the audience often will ask, "But why do the doctors let us die of coma if they are not willing to die of it themselves?"

(e) **The Diabetic Coma Group.**—The number of cases of diabetic coma treated at the New England Deaconess Hospital by us between May, 1923 and January, 1946 has been 651 (in 495 patients). The average duration of diabetes of the 61 cases dying in the hospital has been 4.0 years, of 67 cases who have died since discharge 9.2 years, and the average duration of the 246 living cases, who developed coma prior to January 1, 1940 is already 15.5 years. It seems now as if the coma group ultimately as a whole would live more than ten years. (See Chapter XIII.)

---

[1] Includes 1 classified as diabetes.
[2] Includes 2 classified as diabetes.

(*f*) **War Veterans.**—Matz,[1] former Chief, Research Subdivision, Veterans' Administration, performed an important service by making an analysis of data relating to diabetes among ex-service men. This group is particularly valuable because it can be followed with so much ease to death. The average age of the group of veterans at the onset of diabetes was 33.7 years. Eighty-four per cent were being treated with insulin. The average survival period of this group of insulin-treated diabetic patients to date of the study was 9.1 years. With the increasingly greater attention being paid to Veterans we can look forward to expanding and valuable data.

2. **Prognosis.**—The prognosis of diabetes depends first of all upon the general physical condition of the patient entirely apart from the existence of the diabetes; second, upon his disposition, intelligence and *savoir faire*, his willingness and opportunity to carry out faithful treatment; third, upon the disease as registered by the possibility of its control, as is shown by the condition of the blood and urine on the one hand, and by the strength and weight of the patient on the other; and fourth, upon your zeal, doctor, to provide for him the best treatment which modern medicine affords.

The presence of obesity, a favorable heredity, an early diagnosis, followed by prompt treatment, the history of benign diabetes of several years' duration with gain rather than loss in tolerance, the retention of body weight, are good prognostic signs. Carelessness and coma have ended the life of many a diabetic, and, of course, will continue to do so. Therefore, for careless cases cut the life expectancy one-third. Will the average diabetic live more or less years than have the average fatal cases for his age group thus far? (See Table 40.) The chances are, so far as the diabetes is concerned, he will live longer.

Postpone a Prognosis.—Never hazard a prognosis upon the severity of the diabetes at the first visit. Cases often appear severe when first seen, but upon further acquaintance it is found that this is due to some temporary and alleviable circumstance, such as the presence of acidosis brought on by an infection, by the sudden institution of a fat-protein diet or simply lack of knowledge in the use of diet and insulin. One cannot too strongly emphasize the mild character of most cases of diabetes. Therefore, we repeat the above in other words. Do not rest a prognosis upon the quantity of sugar in the urine, the percentage of sugar or fat in the blood, or even upon acidosis. These signs are transient.

The diabetic dies of his complications and not of his disease. If he has diabetic coma and is under the age of twenty years, the chances are 97.4 per cent that he will recover, but if the patient is above the age of twenty years and has coma, the chances for recovery

[1] Matz: Jour. Am. Med. Assn., **106**, 2214, 1936.

are 86.7 per cent. If he has a carbuncle, instead of every other patient dying as formerly, the chances of recovery today are almost 100 per cent. For 3551 operations of all types between January 1, 1923 and December 31, 1941 the mortality was 7.3 per cent, but for 1453 operations between January 1, 1942 and December 31, 1945 fell to 2.2 per cent. Twenty-nine per cent of 380 cases of gangrene treated between 1923 and 1939 were alive January, 1939. Should the patient be pregnant and ask for a prognosis, it is probably conservative to say that the number who will go through the pregnancy safely closely approximates that of non-diabetics. If the patient has pulmonary tuberculosis along with the diabetes, and even if there is a cavity, the chances for recovery are nearly as good as in non-diabetics no matter whether the patient is young or old. If he has symptoms of angina pectoris, his prognosis for duration of life has been less favorable than for the non-diabetic, although at least 2 cases survived their first symptoms by fifteen years.

F. REMISSIONS, CURABILITY OF DIABETES AND CRITERIA FOR CURES.

It is an error to speak of a cure of diabetes. The tendency to diabetes is inborn and must remain so for life. In many it will never become manifest, in others only some exciting cause will disclose it, such as the acquirement of obesity, the presence of an infection, general or local, hyperactivity or organic disease of the thyroid, pituitary, adrenal, liver or pancreas (hemochromatosis, cancer). We have sought zealously for cures and have not found them and one of our best possible examples of subsidence or even cure of the disease (see Ed. 7, page 336) later proved to be false, just as did the case recently described by Conn *et al.*[1]

Remissions of the disease are common when the exciting cause for onset is removed and prompt aggressive treatment, soon after the onset of the diabetes is recognized, is instituted particularly in children, and this often drives it into hiding. We should expect this from the results of animal experimentation as observed by Haist, Campbell and Best,[2] and Lukens and Dohan[3]. The more I see of diabetes, the more strongly I think we should speak of remissions rather than of cures. My Aunt Lydia had diabetes and eventually could eat blueberry pie and ice cream on top without glycosuria but I never considered her a "cure" even though she was then eighty-five years old.

A cure of diabetes should last for life. Therefore, I think we should always look up the life expectancy of a diabetic at the onset

---

[1] Conn, Johnston and Conn: Ann. Int. Med., **24**, 487, 1946.
[2] Haist, Campbell and Best: Loc. cit., p. 99.
[3] Lukens and Dohan: Loc. cit., p. 99.

of his disease and then compare with the number of years of life expectancy the number of years he has actually lived free from evidences of diabetes. (See Tables 40, 43 and 44.)

It is most dangerous to hint to a patient that he may be cured. One can speak of a remission[1] because that implies the possibility of a relapse. As my son says, it is safer for the patient to prick himself daily and be reminded of his diabetes than to tell him to omit insulin, because then he may forget diet, body weight and exercise as well.

Remarkable remissions occur and such have been reported and in recent years more often as remissions than as cures. Space forbids inclusion here. In general in these series the diabetes has come into the open because of obesity, an infection ("infection is nature's sugar-tolerance test"[1]), a diabetic glandular complication with subsidence after removal of the exciting cause, or it has been in an individual who early received prompt and energetic treatment. Even in the latter and most important group we have encountered no actual cure as measured by the standards we have set for ourselves. Today we would increase rather than reduce the severity of these criteria. Quite arbitrarily, therefore, the writer proposes the following standards to which cures from diabetes should conform and by which they should be classified.

1. **Criteria for Cures in Diabetes.**—(a) **Diagnosis.**—The diagnosis of diabetes shall be based upon a glycosuria of 0.5 per cent or more accompanied by a fasting blood sugar of at least 130 milligrams per cent or a venous blood sugar after a meal on a glucose-tolerance test of at least 170 milligrams per cent.

(b) **Duration of Proved Diabetes.**—The duration of proved diabetes, by repetition of the tests described under diagnosis, shall be recorded in months. By this plan the individual can be classified as a proved diabetic of one or more months' duration. The longer the duration of the proved diabetes, the greater the respect which will be attached to its cure. Chance glycosurias and hyperglycemias resulting from errors in the laboratory, from operative procedures, from temporary infections, and abnormal diets preceding glucose tolerance tests, thus would be ruled out. Hyperthyroidism and hyperpituitarism would not be excluded and, therefore, a statement upon these conditions should be included in the report of the case.

(c) **Test for Recovery.**—Glycosuria and hyperglycemia should be absent, while the patient is without diabetic medication, both before and an hour after a meal. This meal must contain at least two-fifths of the carbohydrate for the day. The carbohydrate for the twenty-four hours shall comprise at least two-thirds of the calories

[1] Lukens and Dohan: Loc. cit., p. 203.

necessary to provide 30 calories per kilogram body weight. Better still, the carbohydrate tolerance shall be unimpaired as judged by a normal glycemic curve following the oral administration of 100 grams of glucose to the patient in the post-absorptive state.

(*d*) **Establishment of Recovery.**—A proved case of one or more months' duration, which conforms to the test for recovery at the beginning and end of an interval of five or more years, shall be considered cured.

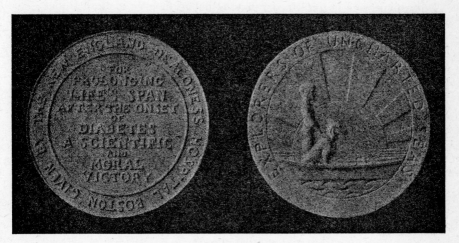

AT THE GEORGE F. BAKER CLINIC

NEW ENGLAND DEACONESS HOSPITAL

A MEDAL IS GIVEN

TO THOSE WHO HAVE CONQUERED DIABETES

BY LIVING LONGER WITH IT

THAN THEY WERE EXPECTED TO LIVE WITHOUT IT

CHAPTER X.

THE TREATMENT OF DIABETES.

A. INTRODUCTION.

Diabetics fall into three categories, first those with complications of a diabetic or non-diabetic nature necessitating hospital care, second, those ambulatory cases requiring the inauguration or readjustment of treatment who can be housed advantageously in less expensive hospital beds, nursing homes or even in the families of trained diabetics and, third, the largest group of all, those who can be cared for through visits to the doctor's office. Intensive education is needed by all diabetic patients and especially so by this third group. It demands more time than the doctor can spare. Consequently he must utilize the services of others, and, as nurses are not available, it means he must depend upon a secretary, technician, a member of his own family, or a trusted and trained diabetic patient to do the teaching.

Diabetic patients must be taught the nature of diabetes, how to take advantage of diet, insulin and exercise in its treatment and how to prevent or combat the common complications of the disease. They can live almost indefinitely, when once taught, if they will follow the rules of the game and give their doctors an opportunity to examine them completely three or four times a year. Such frequent health examinations put them in an advantageous position compared with that of non-diabetics because latent and serious diseases bearing no relation to diabetes should be discovered earlier.

The first visit of a diabetic demands all the resources of the doctor at his best. He must learn the personal and family background of the patient and its relation to his constitution at the moment. There will be plenty of psychological problems to be met, but fascinating as these are and easy to elicit they must not divert the physician from acquiring a complete knowledge of the patients' physical status. Only when the physician realizes that he is practicing general medicine on a diabetic basis will he be alert enough to discern the non-diabetic along with the diabetic complications which beset the patient. The standard, diagnostic rule that all symptoms and signs in the individual case should be explained by one diagnosis does not hold in diabetes. The patients are not immune to any disease. With these considerations in mind we attempt to carry out the following procedures.

During the first visit in the course of the history taking and the physical and chemical examinations the endeavor is made to secure data which will establish an absolute diagnosis or confirm an existing one. In case of doubt, particularly if the patient comes from a dis-

(328)

tance, we are apt to give 50 grams glucose and secure a specimen of urine and blood at the end of an hour. This may save the patient a visit and make unnecessary a formal glucose tolerance test. At the same time, an estimate of the diet upon which the patient is living is made. This diet can be continued, cautiously simplified or modified, so that the carbohydrate content can be easily reckoned and amount to 150 to 200 grams in twenty-four hours. Details of protein and fat are left to instructions in a letter or another visit.

To gain a knowledge of the previous diet it is more expeditious to ask specific questions than to let the often forgetful patient haltingly describe it. Thus, ask (1) Do you eat 1, 2 or 3 slices of bread at each meal?—remembering most of his carbohydrate will always be in the form of bread, and 3 slices contain about 50 grams. (2) Do you have fruit one, two, three or more times daily?—each portion contains about 15 grams. (3) Cereal for breakfast?—a large bowlful of oatmeal contains about 20 grams. (4) Potato for lunch and dinner?—one portion is about equal to one slice bread, 18 grams carbohydrate. (5) How many portions of 5 per cent vegetables?—four represent approximately 20 grams carbohydrate. (6) How much milk? How much cream in the twenty-four hours? (See Tables 30, 33, 44, 45 and 46.)

If one knows the amount of bread, fruit, cereal, 5 per cent vegetables, milk and cream the patient consumes one will be quite well oriented as to what he eats.

By this time one has determined in which category the patient belongs, whether he must or should enter a hospital, go into a nursing home for training, or return the next day or soon thereafter alone or with another patient for further education by a doctor, nurse, dietitian or secretary who can devote a whole hour for this purpose.

If insulin obviously is to be needed, give the first injection of protamine zinc insulin immediately, even if it is only a token dose of 8 units, erring on the side of too little rather than too much. If the patient is apprehensive, try to bring it about that he injects the first dose himself. Naturally, if diacetic acid is present, this would be supplemented by crystalline insulin in similar dosage, with definite arrangements for adjustment for further dosages in a few hours in the hospital, nursing home, at the office or by a doctor.

Treat the patient promptly so that he can leave the office with the assurance that treatment has begun and that immediate improvement in his symptoms will follow.

The three following diet sheets will meet the needs of most adult patients. The carbohydrate ranges from 150 to 200 grams and can easily be raised or lowered by changes in bread, milk or fruit, the protein between 70 and 100 grams subject to increase or depletion with egg (1 = P6, F6 grams), meat, cooked, cheese (1 oz. or 30 grams = P8, F5–8 grams) and fat 80 to 125 grams by the use of

Name _____　　　　　　　　　　　　　　　　Date _____

TABLE 44.

	BREAKFAST CRYS. INSULIN ___ UNITS. PROT. INSULIN ___ UNITS.		DINNER CRYS. INSULIN ___ UNITS.		SUPPER CRYS. INSULIN ___ UNITS.		TOTAL DAILY DIET. C. 150 - P. 71 - F. 81 - CAL. 1613
	Grams.	Portions.	Grams.	Portions.	Grams.	Portions.	Grams.
Eggs . . .		1					(One)
Meat, cooked .	15	or	60	small serving 2 oz.	60	2 oz.	120
Bacon . .		2 strips					15
5% Veg. .			150	1 cup	150	1 cup	300
10% Veg. .			75	½ cup	75	½ cup	150
Oat., dry .	(15)						(15)
Oat., cooked .	120	½ cup					120
Uneedas .							(Two)
Butter .	5	1 tsp.	10	2 tsp.	10	2 tsp.	25
Cream, 20% .	60	¼ cup	30	2 tbsp.	30	2 tbsp.	120
Milk .	120	½ cup					240
Orange .	100	Small	150	Medium	150	Medium	400
Cheese .							—
Potato .							—
Bread .	30	1 slice	30	1 slice	30	1 slice	90

Bedtime 2 uneedas + 120 milk (½ cup)

TABLE 45

Name _____   Date _____

| | BREAKFAST | | DINNER | | SUPPER | | TOTAL DAILY DIET |
| | CRYS. INSULIN —— UNITS. PROT. INSULIN —— UNITS. | | CRYS. INSULIN —— UNITS. | | CRYS. INSULIN —— UNITS. | | C. P. F. CAL. 168 - 85 - 98 - 1894 |
	Grams.	Portions.	Grams.	Portions.	Grams.	Portions.	Grams.
Eggs . . .		1					(One)
Meat, cooked .		or	75	2½ oz.	75	2½ oz.	150
Bacon . .	15	2 strips					15
5% Veg. .			150	1 cup	150	1 cup	300
10% Veg. .			75	½ cup	75	½ cup	150
Oat., dry .	(15)						(15)
Oat., cooked .	120	½ cup					120
Uneedas .							(Two)
Butter . .	10	2 tsp.	10	2 tsp.	10	2 tsp.	30
Cream, 20% .	60	¼ cup	30	2 tbsp.	30	2 tbsp.	120
Milk . .	120	½ cup					240
Orange .	100	Small	150	Medium	150	Medium	400
Cheese .							—
Potato .					90	Large	90
Bread . .	30	1 slice	30	1 slice	30	1 slice	90

Bedtime 2 uneedas + 120 milk (½ cup)

TABLE 46.

NAME _____   DATE _____

CRYS. INSULIN ____ UNITS.
PROT. INSULIN ____ UNITS.

	BREAKFAST.		DINNER.		SUPPER.		TOTAL DAILY DIET.
	CRYS. INSULIN ____ UNITS.		CRYS. INSULIN ____ UNITS.		CRYS. INSULIN ____ UNITS.		C. 180 - P. 95 - F. 103 - CAL. 2027
	Grams.	Portions.	Grams.	Portions.	Grams.	Portions.	Grams.
Eggs		1 or					(One)
Meat, cooked			90	3 oz.	90	Large	180
Bacon	15	2 strips					15
5% Veg.			150	1 cup	150	1 cup	300
10% Veg.			75	½ cup	75	½ cup	150
Oat., dry	(15)						(15)
Oat., cooked	120	½ cup					120
Uneedas							(Two)
Butter	10	2 tsp.	10	2 tsp.	10	1 pat	30
Cream, 20%	60	¼ cup	30	1 oz.	30	2 tbsp.	120
Milk	120	½ cup					240
Orange	100	Small	150	Medium	150	Medium	400
Cheese							—
Potato			75	2½ oz.	75	Medium	150
Bread	30	1 slice	30	1 slice	30	1 slice	90

Bedtime 2 uneedas + 120 milk (½ cup)

If your physician wishes to increase the diet to approximately C. 200, P. 102, F. 123, Cal. 2315
ADD THE FOLLOWING:
15 grams (2 strips) bacon at breakfast or an egg
120 grams (½ cup) oatmeal at breakfast
5 grams (1 teaspoonful) butter at each meal
75 grams (½ cup) 10% vegetable at dinner and supper

bacon (4 strips or 1 oz. or 30 grams= P 5, F 15, grams), butter (1 oz. or 30 grams= F 25 grams), cream 20 per cent (1 oz. or 30 grams= P 1, F 6 grams).

Within twenty-four hours of the first visit the patient should be well started on his diet erring on the side of too little rather than too much. Seldom when inactive should calories rise above 30 per kilogram body weight.[1] In general, the diet should be prescribed so that it can be increased rather than decreased as time goes on with breakfast early and evening meal late. It should be planned to suit the digestive capabilities of the young and strong, the old, feeble or toothless. Moreover, the exact division of meals and food must not be arbitrary but individualized.

Protamine zinc insulin 8 to 16 units would be repeated the following morning, if sugar persists, supplementing it with crystalline insulin in half or the same amount if the glycosuria is considerable.

The urine should be tested at first four times each day—morning, afternoon, evening, night—as well as collecting the twenty-four hour quantity when practicable to determine the effect of the diet and insulin. Exercise should be limited to an amount consistent with the diet; and the diabetic education continued with the expectation that the patient remain in the hospital, nursing home or come frequently to the office during the first six or ten days of treatment. During this early period in the hospital or at the office we would treat the patient aggressively, and the more so the younger the patient and the shorter the interval from the onset of his disease, hoping thereby to prevent further damage to the pancreas. Patients can be treated in their homes or at the doctor's office, but such treatment is more time-consuming for the physician, and the patient misses class instruction and what can be gained from contact with other patients.

If the blood sugar, fasting, did not reach 0.13 per cent, or after a meal 0.17 per cent, insulin would be withheld until the diagnosis was confirmed (not forgetting to exclude pentosuria and levulosuria, see pages 244 and 805) either by increasing the carbohydrate in the diet or by a test with 100 grams glucose. (For performance and interpretation of test, see page 158.)

If the glycosuria should not decrease materially and the blood sugar, fasting, not approach normal, we should raise the insulin daily until they did or until 40 units of protamine zinc insulin are injected daily before breakfast. If progress is slow, despite increasing the protamine zinc insulin, we would temporarily supplement its slow action with the quickly-acting crystalline insulin in small

[1] Calories allowed in the literature often greatly exceed this figure, but are they not based on the gross food allowed the kitchen for a group rather than on the net actual food calories which the individual eats?

doses before one or more meals. The reaction of individual specimens of urine with the Benedict test would be the criterion:

red	*orange*	*yellow*	*green*
12	8	4	0

The effect of the protamine zinc insulin is determined by the presence or absence of sugar in the urine voided the following morning or more accurately, by a second specimen thirty minutes later. The full power of its action does not become manifest for three, four or more days, and consequently one must be cautious in the size of supplementary doses of crystalline insulin. By contrast, the response to crystalline insulin is shown by tests of specimens of urine and blood obtained in the late forenoon and afternoon. Eventually protamine zinc insulin and crystalline insulin, if also needed, are to be administered exclusively before breakfast. Even if crystalline insulin is employed with protamine zinc insulin before breakfast, the aim is ultimately to eliminate the crystalline insulin and to depend upon one dose of protamine zinc insulin daily.

In Table 47 are summarized the amounts of carbohydrate and the quantities of crystalline or protamine insulin administered on the average to our patients treated in the George F. Baker Clinic at the New England Deaconess Hospital during 1941.

TABLE 47.—SUMMARIES 1691 PATIENTS, 1831 ADMISSIONS, GEORGE F. BAKER CLINIC, NEW ENGLAND DEACONESS HOSPITAL, 1941.

Age at admission.	Average duration of D.M. (years).	Average carbo- hydrate at discharge (gms.).	Insulin at discharge.					
			C. I.		P. Z. I.		C. I.+P. Z. I.	
			No.	Av. dose units.	No.	Av. dose units.	No.	Av. dose units.
0 to 14 . .	3.3	175	1	120	17	20	123	14+33
15 to 24 . .	7.1	180	1	36	17	24	242	26+48
25 to 34 . .	7.8	167	4	38	30	14	92	12+35
35 to 44 . .	6.8	165	2	88	64	19	90	11+36
45 to 54 . .	6.7	158	4	30	144	18	114	12+34
55 to 64 . .	8.5	156	5	25	219	19	132	11+32
65 to 74 . .	9.3	152	3	20	191	16	73	11+33
75 or over .	10.3	149	7	33	46	19	9	10+32
Total . .	7.6	162	27	49	728	19	845	13+35

It will be observed that the average carbohydrate for the 1619 patients was 162 grams in general falling from 175 and 180 grams before twenty-five years of age to about 150 grams from sixty-five onward. Both crystalline and protamine zinc insulins were given to nearly all patients under the age of twenty-five years, but to only 24 per cent above sixty-five years of all in those groups requiring insulin. Before twenty-five years of age for 1 unit of CI approximately 2 units of PZI were injected and for the remaining patients one of CI to 3 units of PZI.

The preliminary diet above described is one designed to take advantage of moderate undernutrition; the diet toward the close of the hospital stay should be sufficient for maintenance at quiet occupation, but that at discharge should be adjusted to support the patient at his regular duties and, if he is much below weight, to enable him to gain gradually or, if above weight, to reduce gradually. Repeatedly soon after admission we plan the discharge diet and then adjust the insulin to it as recommended by R. D. Lawrence. Under such circumstances we must see to it that the patient is securing in the meantime exercise somewhat comparable to what he takes ordinarily in his daily life. Certainly at first 10 to 20 grams of the total carbohydrate should be reserved for lunches in the late forenoon, afternoon and upon retiring to counteract any tendency to an insulin reaction, and the greater the tendency the larger the quantity of carbohydrate. Upon retiring, the carbohydrate could be matched with fat to delay its absorption and with protein from which more than half by weight of carbohydrate can be formed. It is exceptional for the carbohydrate to exceed 200 grams and still more rarely 225 grams and practically never does it fall under 150 grams.

Protamine zinc insulin acts during every hour of the day, "acts while you sleep," and therefore the body should have in store carbohydrate-forming material to offset it and prevent hypoglycemia. Protamine zinc insulin is particularly useful in controlling endogenous carbohydrate metabolism and crystalline insulin especially that of exogenous carbohydrate metabolism.

Protamine zinc insulin controls the diabetes during the sleeping part of the day; crystalline insulin controls it during the eating part of the twenty-four hours.

Meals in a hospital come too closely together (8 A.M., 12 noon, 5 P.M.) for a diabetic. If spread over a longer period (7 A.M., 1 P.M., 7 P.M.) and lunches given in the intervening hours, they are better tolerated. Moreover, a late evening dinner, supplemented if necessary by a lunch upon retiring, usually will prevent an insulin reaction due to protamine zinc insulin during the night or upon rising. Occasionally, if the patient is dependent upon both crystalline insulin and protamine zinc insulin, for the same reason the breakfast fruit should be taken when the insulin is injected. Rarely, to guard doubly against a reaction during the night, both protein and fat can be added to the retiring lunch in the form of a biscuit with cheese or, instead, 15 to 30 grams of nuts. These little additions of food may make all the difference between joy and sorrow, success and failure in treatment. Another measure, advocated by Pollack,[1] is to make the evening meal by far the heaviest in the day and especially rich in protein.

Everyone knows that diets are better utilized if spread out through the twenty-four hours and likewise that in preventing reactions a few grams of carbohydrate given at the first symptoms are worth more than many times the quantity when the reaction

[1] Pollack: P. 64, loc. cit., p. 276.

is well established. Taking advantage of these two features patients most exposed to reactions are often given a little carbohydrate— 3, 4 or 5 grams—*every hour on the hour* between meals such as found in various biscuits or some other form of carbohydrate. If exercise is considerable, then the quantity can be increased or protein and fat added in the form of butter, peanut butter or cheese.

The nearer to the onset of the disease that treatment begins, the more quickly and the higher the carbohydrate can rise while maintaining satisfactory urine and blood tests. It is natural to expect and it is true in practice that changes in the quality and quantity of the diet in the young can be made more rapidly than with the old. Often one can see the trend the case is taking in becoming sugar-free under treatment with diet and insulin and advance carbohydrate even though the urine is not sugar-free.

Exercise will lower the glycosuria and the blood sugar by the utilization of sugar in the muscles provided that insulin is available either as in health or by injection. Good treatment of the diabetic always takes advantage of exercise whether the patient is in the hospital or at home. However, if the blood-sugar lowering properties of insulin and unusual exercise are combined, one must be alert and usually advise taking a little food, a piece of fruit, a few crackers or a small glass of milk, or else a reaction may terminate ingloriously a game of golf, a mountain climb or a day of hard work; at times the reaction may not be experienced until the following day.

Home life, therefore, should be easier for the diabetic than hospital life for two reasons: first, it allows for an appropriate division of meals and lunches, and second, enables the patient to take exercise. Consequently, as a rule the diet can be increased and the insulin lowered when the patient is discharged home and to a more active life.

Vitamins in full complement are another adjuvant in treatment and are indicated for any patient with a chronic disease, especially if he is susceptible to infections, has digestive impairment, and liability to complications of nerves or eyes proverbially associated with lack of vitamins or is confined indoors or is at bed rest. (See page 294.)

B. DIABETIC CREED.

For our own practical guidance in 1923 we adopted a diabetic creed, but it has undergone revision. My associates and I believe:

1. That the *diagnosis* of diabetes mellitus should be considered so probable in any person who has a clearly positive test of sugar in the urine that it should be immediately investigated and diabetes proved or disproved. If it is determined that the patient does not have diabetes, but must be classified as an "unclassified glycosuric" or especially as a "potential diabetic" he should be watched for life. Glycosuria plus a fasting venous blood sugar of 0.13 per cent

and above or of 0.17 per cent or more at any time is proof of the existence of the disease. (See page 151.)

2. That the potentiality for developing diabetes is *hereditary* and therefore one should concentrate upon the families of diabetics for the detection of the disease.

3. That the *prevention* of diabetes should be undertaken aggressively, first, by the avoidance of its hereditary transmission—two diabetics should not marry and have children, and a diabetic or child of a diabetic should not marry into a diabetic family—and second, by the recognition that moderate undernutrition is a powerful aid in the prevention or postponement of diabetes and a foundation-stone of diabetic treatment. Hence, normal weight or less should be insisted upon in each diabetic, suspected diabetic, or relative of a diabetic. Therapeutic loss of weight should be extremely gradual, and thus not accompanied by loss of strength or the creation, even temporarily, of an endogenous high-fat-low-carbohydrate diet with its attendant lowering of carbohydrate tolerance. Treatment always should be vigorous.

4. That *mildness* of the diabetes should be assumed, a duration at least of four decades in young adults and five or more in children expected, and the life of the patient planned accordingly.

5. That the nearer *normal* the proportions of carbohydrate, protein and fat in the diabetic diet, always seeking to avoid glycosuria, hyperglycemia and hyperlipemia, as well as avitaminosis and deficiency in minerals, the better it will be for the patient.

6. That diabetes of itself is *not fatal*, but that death ensues from other diseases or complications; that coma is an accident, usually inexcusable, more easily preventable in 99 cases than treated in 1, and, therefore, diabetics when ill from any cause should (1) go to bed, (2) keep warm, (3) take a glassful of hot liquid—water, tea, coffee, broth, orange juice, gruel—every hour, (4) empty the bowels with an enema, (5) call a doctor, who, if he finds acidosis the dominant factor, will give insulin, may wash out the stomach and counteract dehydration if fluid is not retained orally by the injection subcutaneously or intravenously of salt solution. A diabetic under treatment with insulin should not omit it unless sugar-free and under medical supervision. He should carry an identification card suggesting possibility of coma or an insulin reaction.

7. That the diabetic is unusually *susceptible* to arteriosclerosis and tuberculosis and should be treated with these complications in view. Gangrene can generally be avoided by washing the feet daily and by reporting promptly the discovery of any lesion to the physician. Tuberculosis can be prevented or controlled, if tuberculosis contacts are avoided and diagnosis is sought diligently by frequent roentgen-ray examinations, preferably yearly for life but surely up to the age of thirty-five years.

22

8. That all patients should be taught how to test the urine, and if it cannot be kept sugar-free with diet and exercise, protamine zinc insulin alone or in combination with crystalline insulin should be employed.

9. That the immediate aim of diabetic practice should be to provide *facilities* for treatment and to encourage physicians to develop laboratories in their own offices or immediate neighborhood, and to provide opportunities in clinics and camps where they can treat, or, if they wish, refer their patients for a diabetic education.

10. That *adherence* to treatment with diet, insulin and exercise finds ample justification in the good health, comfort and longevity of those who obey the rules as contrasted with the poor health, suffering and shortened lives of those who are careless.

C. NOTES UPON THE INAUGURATION AND PRINCIPLES OF TREATMENT.

Whether treated in a hospital, at home or at a doctor's office, at the beginning there should be daily lessons. The patient is at school to learn how to save his life and live it. Education can be carried out by classroom instruction, by supervised study of books and pamphlets, by example through observation of other patients, or by all three methods combined, but education in one way or another the patient must have and of a sort suited to his comprehension. Time should be taken at the beginning of treatment to describe thoroughly to the patient the plan of procedure to get control of his diabetes and the necessity of his being under close observation until the urine is sugar-free and until he understands how to keep it so. The diabetic patient should be made to realize that he has lessons to learn and that if he will learn them he need not worry about coma, reactions, gangrene, carbuncles or intercurrent infections.

The reasons for the treatment prescribed should be made real to the patient from the very start. It should be visibly demonstrated to him, for example, that the quantity of sugar which he is excreting amounts to a pound, more or less, in twenty-four hours, and that this waste of food accounts for his loss of strength and weight, his unusual appetite, thirst, frequency of urination, and his liability to complications. He should be shown that, with rearrangement of diet and the aid of insulin, the sugar in the urine decreases.

Throughout the period of the inauguration of treatment, daily contact between patient and doctor is essential, the day's duties must be simplified and somewhat curtailed and an extra hour provided for sleep.

Should the above plan of treatment be begun in a hospital or nursing home in contact with a group of other diabetics, the patient will profit so much that he will never regret it.

The treatment of a case of diabetes is a problem which should be undertaken seriously, because it should last for the lifetime of both patient and doctor. One must not discourage the patient at the start, yet he must face the facts and realize that successful treatment will be achieved only if he and the doctor work whole-heartedly and painstakingly together. It is as important for the doctor as for the patient to understand that treatment pays and that the patients who survive with comfort are those who follow the rules and secure a thorough examination by their physican at first frequently and later several times a year. The patients who neglect treatment are the ones who develop complications and die prematurely, often in a distressing manner. Constantly we are comparing results of treatment in those who follow advice with those who disregard it. We believe and we know that the diabetic who carries out treatment faithfully under the care of a skilled and devoted doctor will avoid most of the complications of the disease. Should such non-diabetic complications arise, as cancer, tuberculosis, or appendicitis, the intimate contact of doctor and patient should insure an early diagnosis. Whereas one can be optimistic for dura-tion of life and usually for an ultimate lessening severity of the disease and an increasing liberality in diet, it is only fair, when the appropriate moment comes, to point out to the patient or his family the dangers of coma, premature hardening of the arteries with its localization chiefly in the legs and heart, susceptibility of the skin and urinary tract to infection, the nerves to neuritis, com-plications in the eyes and vulnerability of the lungs to tuberculosis.

The responsibility for the management of the diet of a diabetic patient should always rest upon one individual, preferably the patient, but at times another member of the household. Children who are above the age of ten years should be taught to plan their own diet. They readily learn to do this and in so doing make their elders blush. In fact it is more important for diabetic children to learn what and how much to eat than all the knowledge which their schools afford, for upon this information their life depends. A child at five years should be familiar with the Benedict test and some one of the other tests which require no heat and so can be performed anywhere and at any time. Perhaps it is because this personal responsibility is so deeply felt in the management of little children that the treatment of diabetes in them proceeds so uni-formly and always produces results so much better than are ex-pected. Conversely, the failure of diabetic patients to do well in the open wards of large hospitals has been due not so much to the alleged dishonesty of the patient as to the division of responsibility among several nurses. Errors in the diet or in the collection of the urine must be promptly traced to their source.

The treatment of diabetes is so successful today that when unsat-isfactory results are obtained, the whole situation should be investi-gated anew to determine the cause. One cannot standardize treatment. Each case must be individualized, but rules of treatment are so well established, that if success is not secured, one must remember that diabetes is a good disease which often had bad companions whose medical identity must be sought and fought. More than once we have discovered the existence of advanced tuberculosis or malignant disease which had previously escaped attention. Once we saw the removal of a substernal thyroid abolish the need for 32 units of insulin and necessitate a tolerance test to prove that the patient still had diabetes. Patients with diabetes often come to the physician in a state which is endurable. It is the function of the physician to improve upon this state. In the past far too frequently treatment has done the patient more harm than good, the fault lying not in the principles of treatment, but rather in their application. The physician who undertakes to treat the patient with diabetes, whose condition is comfortable, resembles the surgeon, who, operating for an interval appendix, assumes a responsibility far greater than when acute symptoms make such an operation imperative. The one outstanding and useful fact I learned about the treatment of diabetes as a medical house officer in 1895 was that a diabetic might enter the wards in tolerably good condition and yet within a few days could be *in extremis* consequent upon abrupt changes in his diet.

In further illustration of this point I will cite the following instance which has left an indelible impression upon me.

Case 473, aged forty-eight years, buried her diabetic child at the age of fifteen years. During November, 1911, she began to lose weight, and though 2 quarts of urine were voided daily, no sugar was found in two morning specimens of urine. On December 5, 1911, a little sugar was discovered. January 24, 1912, she consulted a "specialist." The quantity of urine per day was then 6 quarts, the percentage of sugar 7 per cent, making the total quantity of sugar for the day nearly a pound.

The "specialist" radically restricted the carbohydrate in the diet and three days later, in consultation with her family physician, I found her in coma. This is one of the cases which led me to consider the first year following the detection of the disease to be the diabetic's danger zone. It is one of the cases which formerly would have gone down in the literature as "acute diabetes." How needless a death! If a specimen of urine after a meal instead of a fasting specimen had been examined, the diagnosis might have been made earlier. Under no consideration should the diet have been altered suddenly, particularly by extreme curtailment of carbohydrate which inevitably must lead to ketonuria. Moreover, a high percentage of sugar is usually a favorable sign in that it is seldom accompanied by advanced acidosis and is evidence that the patient has not been living on a low-carbohydrate, high-protein, high-fat diet and thus injuring his tolerance, and often that the disease is of recent origin, untreated, and thus particularly amenable to improvement.

Case 14756 is a replica of 473, but more shocking, because of recent date and with insulin available.

The older the patient the more gradually should treatment begin. By this means sudden changes in the body fluids are prevented. Sugar disappears slowly from the urine of elderly people and of diabetic cases of long duration, and it is seldom advisable to attempt to hasten the process by rigid dieting or large doses of insulin. Time will effect the same result with less danger or annoyance to the patient. The striking effect of faithful but prolonged dieting is well exemplified by a table for 7 cases of gangrene compiled by Root long before the discovery of insulin. Here the average fasting blood sugar with prolonged hospital supervision fell from 0.27 per cent to 0.13 per cent in seven weeks.

One is always happy when the weight of the patient is constant for the first week unless one is overcoming the dehydration of coma and in that event a gain in weight is welcomed. Likewise the older the patient the more thoroughly should the condition of other organs such as the heart, the arteries, the lungs, gastro-intestinal and genito-urinary tracts, as well as the neurologic and endocrine systems, be investigated—in short, the entire body.

Week-end treatment for diabetics is quite satisfactory. Repeatedly patients have entered the hospital for a week-end treatment. Most of the patients who have jobs are clever enough to gain a great deal of information in this short period. One day in a hospital spent in contact with other diabetics, seeing patients with gangrene, a patient with a carbuncle, perhaps another with diabetic coma or in hypoglycemia, will do more to instill a knowledge of what diabetes really is than any amount of textbook teaching. The shocking examples are easily offset by the cases who are doing extraordinarily well. Frequently, however, cost of hospital care forces a short hospital stay and the doctor can aid his patient by making a shrewd guess that the glucose in the urine is decreasing and that it will decrease despite slight increase of carbohydrate in the diet. On the other hand, the sudden removal of sugar from the urine, when it has been persistent for long periods, is undesirable because the procedure often upsets the water balance. As a result changes in refraction occur with temporary blurring of vision. These usually right themselves within a few days. The patient should be warned not to be fitted for glasses because a week or two hence they would be worthless. He should wait for nearly a month after the reduction of marked glycosuria to zero.

Office visits are sufficient for the treatment and education of the patient, but they are time-consuming and it is hard to instill the spirit of the game into a patient when alone. The urine should be examined at the visit, preferably a twenty-four-hour specimen, and in addition a specimen obtained at the time and corresponding to each blood-sugar test. Thus a specimen may be loaded with sugar at 11 A.M. but by 11.30 A.M. sugar-free, the former specimen simply registering the non-utilization of carbohydrate at breakfast. The results of the urinary tests should be reported before the patient leaves the office and then their value for purposes of treatment is doubled. Similarly, records of the tests of the blood sugar should be given the patient, and it is often not a disadvantage if this is done later by letter, because then the patient will have received double advice, written as well as oral. We must not forget that the overwhelming majority of diabetics are old and forgetful and they do not grasp the advice given them. Nevertheless I shall welcome the day when the blood sugar can be reported half an hour after the sample has been taken.

Patients weary of testing the urine, but any modern patient knows that without urinary examinations a diabetic cannot secure the best results. Only under very exceptional circumstances should they be allowed to omit making tests. A daily negative Benedict reaction gives confidence and, on the other hand, in the presence of danger, it is never wise to follow the habits of the ostrich. Advice to omit tests because they affect the psychology of the patient hastens the approach of death. Rarely is there an exception to this rule. Of course meticulousness must be avoided, but a knowledge of the state of diabetic control is essential for a patient. The new heatless tests for sugar should save many lives and, incidentally, they destroy the alibi that opportunity was not afforded for doing a test.

Diabetes is an out-and-out chronic disease, but it must not be forgotten that the first years of diabetes following the discovery of the disease truly are the diabetic's danger zone. It is a triumph of modern medicine that the greatest mortality from diabetes has been transferred from the first years following its onset to later years. The first years of a diabetic's life obviously should be his safest and not the most dangerous, as was true a generation ago, and deaths in the early years should be regarded as preventable accidents which interfere with the diabetic securing an average duration of thirty or more years.

There is nearly enough knowledge today for the adequate treatment of diabetes, but it needs more general and more intense application and the development in the patient of a deeper sense of his own responsibility for his care. Coma should be abolished, gangrene halved, tuberculosis prevented. pregnancy in suitable cases made safe, insulin reactions avoided and the average duration of the disease raised above twenty years, the ultimate goal being the avoidance of death in any way due to the disease.

Undernutrition and particularly its corollary—avoidance of overnutrition—widened the horizon for the diabetic and wiped out one-third of the deaths from diabetic coma, but insulin has given him life and protamine zinc insulin has added comfort and happiness. Without what was learned from undernutrition a large share of the wonders attributed to insulin would not have been forthcoming. The simplicity of undernutrition and the incidental avoidance of overnutrition showed its worth and the increasing duration of life of all diabetics and pre-diabetics since its introduction, to a considerable degree, is to be explained by it.

Insulin, including protamine zinc insulin, makes even more necessary the education of the diabetic. It is his accident insurance policy, and he cannot acquire its use too early. If he does not need it permanently, so much the better. His favorable acquaintance with it may rescue him in an emergency. Incidentally, insulin introduces the diabetic to medical science, creates respect for medical research, and thus builds up among the laity a group of individuals in sympathy with medical aims. An understanding of the properties of insulin will make clear the value of the different components of the diet, of exercise, and the harmful effect of an infection.

The improvement brought about today in the condition of diabetic patients during their hospital stay is almost too rapid to be desirable. They hardly realize what discomforts they are spared. Examination of the charts of diabetic patients at entrance and after an interval of a week or ten days at discharge shows the gain in the chemical status of the patients to be astounding. The metamorphosis of the physical, mental and psychical condition of the patient is less rapid than the chemical recovery.

Details of diet will now be discussed and later details relating to the use of the various insulins.

D. DIET.

1. **Preliminary and Permanent Diets With Adjustments to Insulin.**—The diabetic diet is far simpler than often thought or taught. It should be a positive and not a negative diet. One tells the patient what to eat instead of what to avoid. In the doctor's mind there must be a clear conception of the proportion of carbohydrate, protein and fat which is to be prescribed, but there are any number of ways in which this can be conveyed to the patient. The fundamental dietetic principle is to avoid overfeeding. It matters little what measures for food are adopted. Scales and the metric system are the best in the end, but if the patient is averse to the same, lacks funds or is ignorant one can use a slice of bread, a standard biscuit or a tablespoon as a measure.

The diets usually employed are those outlined in Tables 30, 44, 45 and 46. Computations of the diets can be made from the food values in Tables 33, 34, 35 and 112. Adjustments may be necessary. All too often elderly patients and patients with heart disease are upset, because they are given unaccustomed amounts of coarse vegetables, which their toothless mouths cannot masticate or the inadequate secretion of their alimentary tract digest. In general, patients require far less food than the books imply.

As soon as it is evident by the diminishing glycosuria at any one of the periods (morning, afternoon, evening, night) in the day that the diabetes is coming under control, one can revise and rearrange the diet and insulin dosage in order to bring the patient to a more nearly normal status.

Two methods are available for the determination of the ultimate diet. The first, and I think preferable, is to begin with a diet of carbohydrate 150 grams, protein 70, fat 80 grams, as is shown in Table 30, and then progress to higher values gradually and, as a rule, except with children, ending with carbohydrate 165 to 180, protein 82 to 90 and fat 97 to 100 grams. These diets provide sufficient calories for an individual, at work in an office, whose weight is 60 to 70 kg., 132 to 154 pounds. By the second method one decides on the final diet at once and then adjusts the patient to it with the help of insulin. Actually one combines both methods when patients remain but a week in the hospital.

As a practical rule it is best not to make changes in the diet oftener than every other day, because this allows more time to disclose the effects of the diet and insulin and further saves work for dietitians, nurses, and patients. The exigencies of the case, however, may demand a change daily, or at each meal, because patients often improve with unexpected rapidity and it is wasteful not to adapt the diet to their gain in tolerance.

When the adult patient is sugar-free or shows only a few tenths per cent of sugar in the urine and is receiving a nearly maintenance diet, which ordinarily is about 30 calories per kilogram body weight, he can be sent home. It is always well to discharge a patient upon a ration somewhat too low rather than too high, because in home cooking caloric equivalents are plus rather than minus those in the hospital. On the other hand usually it is desirable to increase the carbohydrate by a few grams as a safeguard against insulin reactions.

The dosage of insulin may change from day to day in the hospital. but in order to avoid reactions it is well to lower it upon discharge, Particularly is this the case with combinations of crystalline and protamine zinc insulin unless the patient has been upon a constant diet and quantity of insulin for several successive days. Even then trouble may ensue because of additional exercise due to its blood-sugar lowering value. Constantly one aims at reduction in the number of daily injections and thus endeavors to depend upon the use of protamine zinc insulin alone before breakfast or, if additional crystalline insulin is employed, gradually to dispense with it by rearrangement of the carbohydrate in the diet and the timing of the meals and lunches and the utilization of exercise.

If dependence must be placed on a quick-acting insulin alone, crystalline or regular, almost always one can get along with two injections, one before breakfast and one before the evening meal, but if a third is required that is most conveniently administered upon retiring. The retiring dose is small, usually 2 or 4 units, and almost never as much as 10 units. It may be given with food and is prescribed so that the patient in the eight hours or more at night will be protected and thus wake up sugar-free and with a satisfactory blood sugar. If a patient is sugar-free on rising it implies he has glycogen stored in his liver and under such conditions the day is sure to progress more favorably than if he begins it with hyperglycemia and glycosuria. These are the conditions which protamine insulin prevents.

If a patient does not become sugar-free with 40 units of protamine zinc insulin or a combination of crystalline and protamine zinc during twenty-four hours, upon a diet of 30 calories per kilogram body weight and carbohydrate approximately 150 grams, seek (1) for errors in diet, (2) infections of any sort, whether general or local, acute or chronic, (3) acidosis, (4) hyperthyroidism or hyperpituitarism, (5) cancer, (6) hemochromatosis. The last named condition is not nearly so rare as has been thought and the skin may show little of the typical brown pigmentation. (7) Last but not least, recheck the basis for the diagnosis of diabetes and (8) only as a last resort concede insulin resistance. (See page 379.)

If a diabetic does not do well, there is a reason, and one must not blame insulin or the diet but discover what it is.

2. **Carbohydrate.**—Occasionally one can give even more than 200 grams of carbohydrate, but we believe that a diet below 150 grams or over 200 grams is still an experimental diet. Under no circumstances do we countenance diets containing less than 100 grams carbohydrate in twenty-four hours and seldom under 150 grams. Many normal adults do not care for more than 200 grams carbohydrate. The effect of such higher diets or uncontrolled carbohydrate diets upon diabetic children at the end of twenty years, we are just beginning to learn. Among our 249 patients, 12 fatal and 237 living, who acquired diabetes in childhood and have lived this length of time, the complications are considerable in number and variety. The evidence is not yet conclusive as to whether a diet of carbohydrate 150 to 200 grams is preferable to one of 200 to 250 grams, because it cannot be based on data which are concrete. Other elements than carbohydrate have entered into the picture. Too often the treatment of the diabetes has been grossly neglected. Our impressions are recorded on page 338. It is our opinion that the average patient, even if allowed originally a high-carbohydrate diet, later restricts it at least to the neighborhood of 200 grams,

and we must say that those who fail to do so usually likewise fail to control their diabetes and present a sorry picture. Similarly, patients started on less than 150 grams carbohydrate often fail to follow that and therefore the number is small representing either type of treatment. Time alone can solve the question of optimal diet, and there is little prospect for a decision to be reached before the year 1950. Sansum,[1] one of the first to advocate these high diets, reported in 1933 that his average carbohydrate was 180 grams. That seemed high, but today we look upon it as a desirable diet if the patient will control his diabetes with insulin. Indeed, in any appraisal of the diet employed by any physician of repute with a large number of diabetic patients under his care, one should remember that good physicians always individualize their cases and combine common sense with dietary formulæ. My many vists to diabetic clinicians, treating their patients in ways distinctly different from what we follow, have taught me to be open-minded and to recognize that each doctor may have and usually does have a type of clientèle which requires a special type of treatment, and that this is one of the reasons why different methods are adopted. It is vitally important for any doctor to remember this and not destroy the confidence of a patient in the medical profession by condemning off-hand those methods which are different from his own.[2] Each case has its own peculiarities and there are many cheerful surprises, in fact, more cheerful than discouraging are encountered in the inauguration of the treatment of diabetes at any stage of the disease. The doctor must keep his mind alert and expectant to note the mildness of the disease and to take advantage of a growing tolerance for carbohydrate. It is absolutely impossible to predict which cases will be unusually mild or severe, and I say this after the experience of a lifetime.

3. **Protein and Fat.**—The protein in the diet of a diabetic is practically the same as would be advised for a similar non-diabetic individual. It varies not only according to age, but also according to the patient's activity and the condition of the renal and digestive tracts; an increase of 10 per cent above normal might be allowable, but we believe few clinicians particularly interested in the treatment of diabetes would increase the protein 25 per cent. Undoubtedly in countries like the Argentine, where meat is abundant, far more protein is consumed by the normal, and I suspect by the diabetic individual, in the more prosperous ranks of society. Added light on the diabetic's diet should come from such sources. The

[1] Gray and Sansum: Jour. Am. Med. Assn., **100**, 1580, 1933.

[2] But I will acknowledge it is difficult to be reticent when parents state their child was to eat four slices of bread at a meal and failing to do so at one meal is to take eight at the next. Probably the doctor never made this statement. Rats made diabetic by pancreatectomy, when allowed to select the ingredients of their diet, take only small amounts of carbohydrate.[3]

[3] Richter, Schmidt and Malone: Bull. Johns Hopkins Hosp., **126**, 192, 1945.

fat in the diet raises the calories to a sufficient level. Only under extraordinary circumstances has it been permanently below 50 grams or often over 125 grams. A diabetic likes fat almost more than carbohydrate, or at least craves more than a minimum of fat. He will gladly renounce carbohydrate in order to have the fat in the diet raised from a total of 50 grams to 70 grams or more. In fact, I believe few patients prescribed a diet containing only 50 grams fat keep it down to that level. One egg contains 6 grams fat; meat 6 oz., (180 grams) cooked, even if lean meat, contains 30 grams and it is almost inconceivable for the individual to escape receiving over 14 grams more through milk, cream, butter, oil salads, cheese, nuts. Even if he does hold down his fat ration to 50 grams the chances are he would consume enough of his own body fat to increase the fat he metabolizes.

A tendency to undernutrition rather than overnutrition underlies all diabetic therapy. No one wishes a diabetic to be above normal weight. Few wish the weight to be much below normal, save in early middle life and later when a minus weight of 20 pounds or more is conducive to longevity and to the prevention of the onset of diabetes. We fear underweight in young people and especially in those patients who have had coma, because of the danger of tuberculosis. In boys and girls during adolescence the weight may increase far above normal. This is quite unnecessary and only to be condoned when a previous excess of undernutrition, either because of lack of control of the disease or from misguided design, has made the diabetic retarded in development. In such instances one must tolerate overweight temporarily in order to promote growth in height.

4. **Comment in Retrospect.**—The dietetic principles thus far enunciated seem almost too simple, but they represent decades of experiment and study by many men. In the Naunyn era, 1898 to 1914, overfeeding was the rule and protein and fat particularly were given *ad nauseam.* As a result, the ketogenic-anti-ketogenic balance was disturbed and patients in comparative comfort were suddenly changed into patients at death's door with acidosis. Newburgh[1,2] and his school have shown the harmful effects of obesity and the subsidence—or what might be termed "cures" (?)—of diabetes by its removal.

Then came the Allen era of undernutrition. The gains were so great by its adoption that undernutrition was overdone; tolerance could have been regained more rapidly than was then supposed. Never forget, therefore, these two eras in which great curtailment in carbohydrate in order to make the urine sugar-free not only often led to acidosis but at the same time lowered the tolerance of the severe case. Remember, too, all the unintentional harm done to the patient in the days of undernutrition by failure to recognize

[1] Newburgh and Conn: Jour. Am. Med. Assn., **112**, 7, 1939.
[2] Sheldon, Johnston and Newburgh: Jour. Clin. Invest., **16**, 933, 1937.

that it was not the carbohydrate, protein or fat in the food which we gave the patient that did the harm, but rather the fat in the food derived from his own tissues when we did not feed him. During the early days of undernutrition when I saw a patient with a carbuncle show for days a minus nitrogen balance of 35 grams, I learned extreme undernutrition hastened death. Gradually it dawned upon me that restriction of the total diet, largely by the diminution in fat, made many a patient sugar-free without fasting and this preserved the carbohydrate tolerance of those whose diabetes was mild. Evidently it is this same experience which led Newburgh to treat many of his fat adults without insulin.

The onset of diabetes is slow and it is rational to take advantage of this and to correct the disturbed metabolic balance of the body as quickly as possible, always with the purpose in mind to restore pancreatic function as much as to dispel diabetic symptoms. The preceding sentence, first written in 1928 had even greater meaning in 1940 because of the work of Best, Lukens and associates, who have shown that the simultaneous administration of insulin or maintenance of a normal blood sugar prevents the development of permanent diabetes in dogs and cats injected with anterior pituitary extract.

Objectives in the treatment of diabetes are the maintenance of comfort, vigor, a reasonable weight within the normal zone or slightly below, and control of glycemia and glycosuria, although all agree that chemical meticulousness is to be avoided to prevent the exposure of the patient to hypoglycemic reactions. The guide in treatment is the total glucose excreted in the twenty-four hours and this makes determinations of the whole day's urine essential. A yellow, orange or even a red test in a single specimen may be just a flash in the pan and to alter a day's total of carbohydrate or insulin because of it, when only a rearrangement of the two is indicated, would be unfortunate. John[1] has recently emphasized this point. Having determined the total loss of glucose, one compares it with the carbohydrate in the diet. If the diet contains 150 grams carbohydrate, the glucose excreted should certainly not exceed 10 grams daily, better less or, best of all, none, and with any diet not over 10 per cent of the total ingested. With children, we would fight to prevent a loss of any sugar in the early months of the disease and would never capitulate to an amount which was more than 20 grams in the twenty-four hours. These objectives correspond closely with Mosenthal's[2] practice.

The urine should be kept sugar-free always upon rising, or in the specimen voided one-half hour later, (thus obviating confusion from sugar voided during the early part of the night and collecting in the bladder), nearly always upon retiring, and if possible and practicable

[1] John: Southern Med. Jour., **39**, 60, 1946.
[2] Mosenthal: New York Medicine, **11**, 4, 1946.

throughout the day. The aim should be to keep the percentage of sugar in the blood normal before and after meals, but exceptions will arise in cases with infections, hyperthyroidism, pituitary involvement, and upon occasion in nephritis, heart disease, hypertension, arteriosclerosis, cancer of the pancreas, and almost always for the first few days following operations. During pregnancy a renal glycosuric element enters into the picture and glycosuria is out of proportion to the glycemia.

5. **Reasons for Control of Hyperglycemia and Glycemia.**—Why is so much effort expended to make the urine sugar-free and the blood sugar normal? (1) Because normal values are obviously the best and, as a rule, indicate a blood normal in other respects as well. (2) Because a high blood sugar is a constant stimulus for insulin secretion and the islands of Langerhans should be spared overwork. Time should be allowed for recuperation such as the pancreas of the healthy individual enjoys between meals and at night. (3) Because the removal of the glycosuria proves utilization of the diet. Hyperglycemia and glycosuria involve accessory annoyances such as polydipsia and polyuria, the attendant necessity for extra food to make up for the loss of calories in the urine and the obvious wear and tear on the system for ingestion, assimilation and excretion of this unutilized extra food. Even in experimental anterior pituitary diabetes in a dog one finds intercapillary glomerulosclerosis[1] after some years. A fourth (4) reason is customarily given: namely, that a high percentage of sugar in the blood implies the same in the tissues and that this conduces to lack of tissue repair and resistance to infection, causes degenerative phenomena in arteries and nerves, leads to weakness, weariness, and impotence. Concerning this fourth reason we have some doubt. The sugar in the tissues in diabetes (pages 151 and 599) is not especially high, wounds heal well in the presence of a high blood sugar (pages 527 and 670), and there is little reason to suspenct that a high blood sugar causes arteriosclerosis (page 492). We prefer to say that the blood sugar should be normal because the blood sugar is an index of the disease and if normal it is one assurance that the whole disease is being treated well. It is the red light which we should no more disregard, although we cannot always explain its significance, than we should fail to heed the red signal at the railroad crossing because we cannot see the train around the corner.

Bertram[2] assigns few diabetic symptoms to the blood sugar but instead relates them to acidosis. In our cases, however, one encounters those symptoms just described far more frequently than one encounters even mild acidosis, and, therefore, we cannot agree with his view. (However, we must confess that the average CO_2 combining power of the blood of a small, unselected group of diabetics before breakfast was slightly lower than that of normal individuals.)

[1] Lukens and Dohan: Arch. Path., **41**, 19, 1946.
[2] Bertram: P. 37, Loc. cit. p. 87.

Breaking the diet and cheating the doctor are infrequent episodes today. Seldom if ever do we charge a patient with either, but together with the patient review the diet and insulin; in this way what has happened becomes unmistakably evident, and then we simply let the patient draw his own conclusion. If breaking the diet is quite wilful, then bed rest is prescribed for the patient, whether child or adult, because when he is in bed there is far less opportunity to deceive. Nothing is said to him about the reason for his going to bed, but after the urine clears, the situation is discussed and wonder expressed that without the aid of exercise and with little insulin the urine became sugar-free upon the same diet on which it showed sugar when he was up and about.

The mild case of diabetes is the case which demands the most energetic treatment but hitherto has received the least. These cases are analogous to the cases of incipient tuberculosis. As in tuberculosis, a "cure" is not effected, but the disease is held in check. Emphasis should be placed on freedom from glycosuria. Naunyn's dictum that "many a severe case was originally mild, but neglected," should not be forgotten.

The education of the diabetic and his family is fundamental for success in treatment. The diet may be perfect, the quantity of insulin prescribed ideal, and exercise suited to the needs of the patient, but unless the patient and his family are taught how to harmonize these three elements under various conditions of life, the whole structure of treatment is likely to collapse during a trifling emergency. The reasons that one patient goes to one doctor and not to another are that one doctor takes the time to teach the patient how to examine his urine, explains about the diet, the insulin, the value of exercise, the adjustment of the three to daily life and tells him little by little of complications which he can avoid and shows him how to protect not only himself but his family. From each visit the patient makes to that doctor he draws a dividend and is willing to go back, because he expects to have another dividend declared. While he is learning something new about diabetes himself, at the same time he discovers that the doctor is trying to learn something new on his own part, and is taking pains to make the effort to secure fresh information that will be helpful to his patients. Such are the doctors who get the diabetic patients and keep them. This is the reason why a diabetic straying into a young doctor's office becomes that young doctor's golden opportunity, because the young physician has the time to educate the patient and, incidentally, himself; the occasion is instant and, if young Æsculapius takes advantage of it, the patient is his for life.

Teaching diabetics is almost a fine art, because it requires so much ingenuity. One must not only instruct, but train so that one's precepts will be followed to the letter. It not only demands medical knowledge, but a knowledge of human nature. If successful, the life of a man or woman, a boy or a girl is saved and who knows but what another diabetic genius like Edison, who firmly believed that he had had the disease for sixty-two years, or like Minot, who shared a Nobel prize for his part in the discovery of liver in the treatment of pernicious anemia, may be provided for humanity?

6. **Follow-up Methods.**—Almost any physician can get his diabetic patients sugar-free, but to keep these patients sugar-free and in good health requires skill and zeal. A doctor's ambition should be not to see how large a number of diabetic patients he can have, but how long they remain alive and are free from complications. His estimate of his success or failure will be the number and status of his patients after they have had the disease twenty years.

Patients must be taught that the preliminary treatment represents only a beginning of treatment; that treatment lasts for life; that whenever sugar or acidosis returns or unusual loss of weight occurs they must report to a physician. The physician, too, must do everything in his power to keep in touch with his patient at regular intervals. Of course, this is quite difficult, because he is laid open to the suspicion of seeking practice, but it is better to run the chance of a misunderstanding on this score in 1 case than to let 10 other cases perish. Hitherto we have almost specialized in the follow-up of fatal cases, but from now onwards the purpose of the tracing will be to protect the patients during life and to learn from their physical condition in the later years of their disease how treatment can be improved, rather than simply to record the lessons learned by their deaths.

The 4,000,000 pre-diabetics and 1,000,000 diabetics in this country should be looked upon as a trust placed in the doctors' hands for conservation and development. The lives of these people must be preserved, but they must yield dividends of health for all. These patients are under constant supervision. Here is the opportunity for health examinations and health studies on a vast scale. What other such select group of adult individuals exists which can demonstrate better the efficacy of preventive medicine, the success of prompt surgical intervention in acute and chronic surgical affections including cancer, the effect of early diagnosis of tuberculosis, and especially arteriosclerosis which eventually claims a half of our diabetics, usually prematurely, and, in fact, all other medical ills which can be thwarted or cured? What a trust! The public and the patients, too, will watch our administration of it with critical eyes.

7. **High-carbohydrate Diets.**—The normal diet for an adult of 60 kilograms (132 pounds) with moderate activity per kilogram body weight consists approximately of carbohydrate 4 to 5 grams (240–300 grams), protein 1.25 to 1.5 grams (75 to 90 grams), and fat 1 to 1.25 grams (60 to 75 grams), making 30 to 37 calories or a total of 1800 to 2235 calories. The minimum diet for diabetic patients consists approximately of carbohydrate 2.5 grams, protein 1.25 grams, and fat 1.5 grams, or in other words for an

individual weighing 60 kilograms, carbohydrate 150 grams, protein 75 grams, and fat 90 grams, 1810 calories. Up to 1927 most of our diets contained even less than 100 grams carbohydrate. There is no question but that the change to carbohydrate 150 grams has been beneficial, but as to diets with over 200 grams we are hesitant save with children and under exceptional circumstances. This transition is due largely to the effectiveness of insulin and also to the publications of Adlersberg and Porges abroad, and to Sansum, Geyelin and Rabinowitch in this country, and others in various lands who have expressed a favorable opinion of the higher-carbohydrate and low-fat diet. These physicians recommend a diet essentially normal, tending toward one which contains rather more carbohydrate and less fat per kilogram body weight or actually, as expressed by Rabinowitch, carbohydrate 275 grams, protein 80 grams, fat 45 grams, Calories 1800.

When von Noorden[1] published his oatmeal diet in 1903 he upset dietetic notions which had been in vogue for more than a century, but the greatest contribution of the oatmeal diet to the treatment of diabetes was not the diet itself, but the stimulus which it gave to the imagination and to scientific workers throughout the world to explain it. Everywhere the opinion was prevalent that the pancreas should be rested and spared from work and thus permitted to regain some of its lost efficiency. The oatmeal diet challenged this view because it introduced a revolutionary principle and investigators both in the laboratory and in the clinic were filled with wonder as to how and why it worked.

In earlier years Mossé[2] and von Düring[3] had introduced their potato and rice cures and skimmed milk had been recommended by Donkin.[4] It was recognized that sometimes these diets acted favorably, but on the whole it was seen that their general adoption was not practical and they did not yield favorable results in most cases.

A direct outgrowth of the work of von Noorden was what we recognize in its present form as the high-carbohydrate low-fat diet. Taking advantage of all the knowledge which had been accumulated as a result of the investigation of the oatmeal cure and appreciating the therapeutic value of the Staub-Traugott effect, already described on page 146, as well as the deleterious effect of fasting or a high-fat low-carbohydrate diet upon sugar tolerance, as shown by their use as compared with a high-carbohydrate low-fat diet preceding glucose tolerance tests, Adlersberg and Porges[5] formulated their plan for the treatment of diabetes. The first articles by Porges and by Adlersberg and Porges appeared in 1925 and almost simultaneously (1926) appeared an article in this country by Sansum[6] to be followed by others by Geyelin[7] and by Rabinowitch.[8] The free diets of

[1] Von Noorden: Berl. klin. Wchnschr., **40**, 817, 1903.

[2] Mossé: Rev. de méd., **22**, 107, 279, 371, 620, 1902; cited by Naunyn.

[3] Von Düring: Ursache und Heilung des Diabetes melitus, 4th ed., Hannover, 1852.

[4] Donkin: Brit. Med. Jour., **1**, 838, 1874.

[5] Adlersberg and Porges: Klin. Wchnschr., **5**, 142, 559, 1926; **5**, 1451, 1926; **6**, 2371, 1927; **7**, 1503, 1928. Die Behandlung der Zuckerkrankheit mit fettarmer Kost, Berlin, Urban & Schwarzenberg, 1929.

[6] Sansum, Blatherwick and Bowden: Jour. Am. Med. Assn., **86**, 178, 1926; Colorado Med., **24**, 307, 1927.

[7] Geyelin: Atlantic Med. Jour., **29**, 825, 1926. Cecil: Text Book of Medicine, 2d ed., Philadelphia, W. B. Saunders Company, 1927. Jour. Am. Med. Assn., **104**, 1203, 1935.

[8] Rabinowitch: New England Jour. Med., **204**, 799, 1931; Canad. Med. Assn. Jour., **26**, 141, 1932; Diabetes Mellitus, Toronto, The Macmillan Company of Canada, Ltd., 1933.

Stolte,[1] and Enklentz[2] and Lichtenstein[3] whose recent article contains a summary of the literature and also his own experience, in reality are high-carbohydrate diets without the scientific qualifications introduced by the writers already quoted. As yet neither these authors nor others who favor the "free diet," have reported their results in a large series after twenty years of treatment of diabetic children or even of adults so far as we are aware. The twenty year diabetic child is the crux of the problem.

There is little mystery today in the use of the high-carbohydrate-low-fat diet. If the patient has been underfed and then is placed upon a maintenance ration and assimilation of the same guaranteed by insulin he will improve. The utilization of the glucose value of the diet will be promoted if the introduction of the diet is preceded by definite undernutrition.

The fat in the high-carbohydrate low-fat diet is restricted by some even to 40 grams, usually about 50 grams, and never allowed to reach 100 grams. In our experience it is extraordinarily difficult to maintain the fat at 40 grams and the danger is that the patient not only eats carbohydrate in superabundance, but almost innocently raises the fat and thus secures excess of calories which defeats the entire program.

Gray and Sansum[4] in 1933 stated that 180 grams was the average quantity of carbohydrate prescribed to their patients. They were far ahead of their times and I am only too ready to acknowledge it. Russell Richardson[5] has shown that one could replace advantageously gram for gram of fat with carbohydrate to a moderate degree without materially increasing the quantity of insulin required.

Among the advantages of the high-carbohydrate, low-fat diet are claimed to be a greater sense of well-being on the part of the patients (one must be cautious in accepting such proof because the diabetic in the Naunyn era when first placed upon the low-carbohydrate high-fat diet felt he was on top of the wave and this often lasted until he was engulfed by coma), a lessened susceptibility to diabetic coma and even to infections, little if any increase in insulin, no increase in the blood sugar and a tendency to a lowering of the percentage of cholesterol in the blood. As concomitant features the patient becomes less conspicious in his selection of food, the food itself is cheaper, and finally the patient is less tempted to break his diet. The diet is said to have an especially favorable effect on cardio-vascular conditions.

But all these claims are largely based upon comparisons between former diets of less than 100 grams carbohydrate with diets above 200 grams. Today comparisons between diets containing from 150 to 200 grams carbohydrate and those with 200 to 300 grams are more to the point, bearing in mind the attempt and, indeed, success in controlling the total glycosuria in the former instance with considerable indifference to its control in the latter.

The effect of any diet is to be judged by those who follow it, not by those who break it. Patients who are under the direct supervision of the physicians who prescribe a special form of treatment, adhere to the plan he proposes more closely than those of his patients who are away from him. Consequently it is almost unfair for anyone who does not use these high-carbohydrate diets to criticize them sharply. It is our belief that our average diabetic with onset under fifty years who develops the disease in 1946 will live more than twenty years with the methods of treatment which are generally in vogue in this country with carbohydrate 150 to 175 grams

[1] Stolte: Med. Klin., **27**, 831, 1931.

[2] Enklentz: Deut. med. Wchnschr., **61**, 1911, 1935.

[3] Lichtenstein: In *Opera Pædiatrica*, Jundell, Lichtenstein and Wallgren, Eds., Upsala, Almquist & Wiksells, pp. 370–391, 1945.

[4] Gray and Sansum: Loc. cit., p. 346.

[5] Richardson: Am. Jour. Med. Sci., **177**, 426, 1929.

and fat in the neighborhood of 80 to 100 grams daily, but whether he would live as long or longer with carbohydrate raised to 200 or 300 grams and fat lowered to the neighborhood of 50 grams, no one can say. We can only express the opinion that we believe more insulin is required on a high-carbohydrate low-fat diet than upon a diet containing 150 grams carbohydrate, that it is easier for a patient to live upon a diet containing 150 grams carbohydrate, and fat 80 to 100 grams, and that he is less apt to break such a diet and that, if he does, he is more likely to raise it proportionately in grams of carbohydrate, protein and fat than if he lived upon a diet with more than 200 grams of carbohydrate and supposedly 50 grams of fat. And as for the cholesterol in the blood of patients living upon the one or the other of these two types of diet, we must wait for further evidence, because the cholesterol now is seldom high, although it is perfectly clear that individuals who break their diet in any direction are apt to have a high cholesterol value. Therefore, while welcoming experiments with this type of diet, we think it safer for the average doctor in the country today to utilize a diet in which the carbohydrate ranges between 150 and 200 grams. With our children the carbohydrate approaches the upper limit and at times exceeds it by a small margin.

8. **Fasting Days and Undernutrition.**—Only those who treated diabetics in the decades before and after the turn of the century can appreciate the advance which Allen gave to diabetic therapy with his introduction in 1914 into general practice of fasting and undernutrition. Naunyn, several years before, had strongly urged the use of starvation days in the treatment of diabetes. He emphasized the value of a low-caloric intake. Hodgson, too, was precise upon this point. He writes, "Again it should be stated that the quantity of all food, even if it is carbohydrate-free must be greatly restricted. The number of calories that the body ordinarily requires is no safe criterion of the amount of food that should be given a diabetic. It is not the quantity of food that should be metabolized, but the amount that can be metabolized that should determine the quantity given to the patient." Hodgson[1] should be given the credit of having published this article in 1911. Guelpa[2] in 1910 reported his success in the treatment of diabetes by the employment of several days' fasting combined with purgation. Von Noorden preceded his oatmeal "cure" with several days of undernutrition.

Others had employed fasting, but Allen[3] proved prolonged fasting efficacious. The recent work of Best throws light upon its possible action. (See page 123.) Before Allen treated any human patients by fasting, he demonstrated that his method gave good results with animals!!!

Fasting saved the life of many a patient, but the principle of undernutrition and the possibility of keeping the urine sugar-free, as demonstrated by the Benedict test, and thus knowing whether the disease was at least partially controlled saved far more. Many children, who were kept sugar-free with painstaking adherence to the principles of undernutrition, preserved for years the spark of life and lived to benefit from insulin. The children who were fed for comfort died. The principle of undernutrition still underlies the methods we use. Excess of food, at least in the hereditarily predisposed, favors the onset of diabetes; excess of food makes the diabetes worse; the normally nourished or slightly undernourished patient does the best.

The method which we eventually found preferable to immediate fasting follows. We have not used actual fasting for years, but occasionally restric-

[1] Hodgson: Jour. Am. Med. Assn., **57**, 1187, 1911.
[2] Guelpa: Brit. Med. Jour., ii, 1050, 1910.
[3] Allen: Jour. Am. Med. Assn., **63**, 939, 1914. See also Allen, Stillman and Fitz: Loc. cit., p. 54.

tion of food for a few hours will drive home a lesson to a patient such that nothing else does. In severe, long-standing, complicated, obese, and elderly cases, as well as in all cases with acidosis or in any case if desired, without otherwise changing habits of diet, omit fat, after two days omit protein, and then halve the carbohydrate daily until the patient is sugar-free or taking only 10 grams; then fast. In other cases begin fasting at once. The majority of diabetic patients show little acidosis because they gain carbohydrate tolerance in the process, and actually seldom reach the fasting day. During such a period they remain strictly abed. If acidosis has been present it will decrease while following this rule. With this plan of treatment many patients were treated in the Allen era, 1914 to 1922, and the average duration of life rose 25 per cent and deaths from coma dropped from 60 per cent to 40 per cent.

Fasting untangled many complexities of diabetes, but it was dreadful to see the patients. The best description of fasting and of the advent of insulin was written by the Prophet Ezekiel. Ezekiel 37: 1 to 10.

9. **Low-carbohydrate and Low-protein and High-fat Diets.**—Newburgh and Marsh[1] in this country, and Petrén[2] in Sweden pushed ahead our knowledge of treatment and their methods, although not applicable today, deserve recognition. While most of us feared fat, they demonstrated how it could be used safely by combining with it, perhaps unwittingly, the principle of undernutrition.

The courage of Newburgh and Marsh, and of Petrén in giving a diet of high fat, with low carbohydrate and protein deserves praise. They demonstrated that diabetic patients protected by a diet of undernutrition even largely composed of fat will not develop coma. They showed empirically the advantage of low-carbohydrate and protein, made possible by adequate calories in the form of fat, in the prevention of acidosis. Their diabetic creed was sound in essentials. They believed the urine should be sugar-free, they endeavored to keep the blood sugar normal, and they gave no alkalis. The patient who breaks over only in carbohydrate, pays an immediate penalty and is warned by increased urination; the patient who breaks over only in fat and protein is not warned and dies.

Petrén[3] was an enthusiastic advocate of an extremely low-protein diet in diabetes and he employed an excess of fat for this purpose. He certainly improved the treatment of diabetes, although his views of the harmfulness of protein did not gain credence. He treated his severe diabetics (blood sugar 0.24 per cent or more) with a diet consisting almost exclusively of fat and vegetables with protein so low that the nitrogen in the twenty-four-hour urine fell to 2 or 3 grams or even less. He used sufficient 5 per cent vegetables so that I suspect the carbohydrate never fell below 20 grams in twenty-four hours and usually was more, employed the inulin group freely and fruits containing the lowest carbohydrate. His clientèle contained few children.

Fat was furnished by butter and lard, and the amount seldom exceeded 300 grams! In addition he gave wine. Interspersed with the diet were one or more fast days a week if the blood sugar did not fall below 0.12 per cent, which he considered pathological. Also butter days were given. All patients received opium.

[1] Newburgh and Marsh: Arch. Int. Med., **26**, 647, 1920; Ibid., **27**, 699, 1921 (Blood Sugar); Ibid., **29**, 97, 1922 (Urinary Nitrogen); Ibid., **31**, 3, 1923 (Fat Lipemia); Ibid., **31**, 455, 1923.

[2] Petrén: München. Med. Wchnschr., **74**, 1123, 1927.

[3] Petrén: Verhandl. d. XXXIV Kong. d. Deutsch. Gesell. f. inn. Med., 1922; Acta med. Scand., Suppl. 3, pp. 101, 112; Verhandl. Verdau. u. Stoff.-Krank., **8**, 5, 1923; Ergebn. d. inn. Med. u. Kinderh., **28**, 92, 1925; Verhandl. Verdau. u. Stoff.-Krank., 2d ed., vol. **8**, No. 5, 1927; Studies on Diabetes, Jour. Metab. Res., **5**, 1, 1924; Handb. d. gesampt. Therap., Jena, Gustav Fischer, **1**, 827, **1926.**

Petrén liked to have the blood sugar normal for fourteen days before any increase in carbohydrate was made, and then such increases were very gradual, not more than 10 grams of bread every fourth day. His treatment of coma was without alkalis or glucose, but he gave carbohydrate in the form of vegetables and fats in large quantity. Among 75 attacks of coma occuring in 49 patients, there were 3 deaths.

10. **Levulose, Its Clinical Use.**—Levulose (fructose) behaves differently from the other sugars both in normals and diabetics. Its unusual utilization by diabetics vanishes, however, when given continuously. In normal individuals only a slight increase in the blood sugar occurs when levulose is administered. In diseases of the liver the blood-sugar curve after injection of 45 grams of levulose was high in 43 cases reported by King.[1] Levulose is less effective than glucose in relieving hypoglycemic convulsions after insulin or in relieving the hypoglycemia which follows hepatectomy. At the Carnegie Laboratory the unusual degree to which levulose raised the respiratory quotient in normals as compared with other sugars was demonstrated by Benedict and Carpenter.[2] From their observations the conclusion seemed justified that levulose instead of being burned wholly as carbohydrate was, particularly in the diabetic, to some extent first transformed into fat.

For several years the usefulness of levulose, and its polymer inulin, was tested on patients clinically and by respiratory experiments at the New England Deaconess Hospital. The daily administration of levulose in small quantities for prolonged periods was studied in 4 patients. At first the levulose appeared to be well utilized but later hyperglycemia and glycosuria usually followed its use.

We suspect Minkowski's observation that levulose, in contrast to dextrose, when given to depancreatized dogs led to the formation of glycogen in the liver, encouraged clinical attempts to prescribe levulose for diabetics. Since honey may contain, when inulin-forming plants are available for the bees, approximately 39 per cent levulose along with 35 per cent dextrose, it was often allowed diabetics, but, we now know, without justification.

11. **Dihydroxyacetone.**—This ketone triose, one of three trioses considered to be products of normal carbohydrate metabolism, seems to affect the metabolism somewhat as does levulose. In experiments on rats and mice some workers have found a greater proportion of glycogen in the liver than was obtained after glucose. Testing the utilization of dihydroxyacetone Rabinowitch[3] gave the same patient dihydroxyacetone one day and glucose the next and found the blood sugar rose less after dihydroxyacetone and less sugar was excreted in the urine than after the glucose.

12. **Inulin and Jerusalem Artichokes.**—Inulin, the chief carbohydrate constituent of artichokes, yields levulose by hydrolysis. Other polysaccharides, including polymers of levulose more readily hydrolyzable than inulin, as well as small amounts of sucrose, were also found in artichokes by Jackson et al.[4] The analyses of Thaysen, Bakes and Green[5] also show that in the ripe Jerusalem artichoke lower and more soluble polymers of levulose occur than the relatively insoluble inulin. During the winter months the artichokes when stored change and the concentration of sugar and lower polymers increase.

Inulin itself is not hydrolyzed and absorbed in the raw condition although

[1] King: Lancet, i, 385, 1927.
[2] Benedict and Carpenter: Carnegie Institution, Washington, Pub. No. 261, 1918.
[3] Rabinowitch: Jour. Biol. Chem., 65, 55, 1925.
[4] Jackson, Silsbee and Proffit: Scientific Papers of the Bureau of Standards, Washington, D. C., No. 519, 1926.
[5] Thaysen, Bakes and Green: Biochem. Jour., 23, 444, 1929.

certain students have shown a rise in the respiratory quotient and metabolism after its administration and Okey[1] recovered from the stool an inulase and observed hydrolysis by the acid of the stomach. Root and Baker[2] found no significant change in the respiratory quotient after giving pure inulin, but the respiratory quotient, as well as the blood sugar, rose after the taking of cooked Jerusalem artichokes. The absorption of some carbohydrate was clearly proved but further demonstration of the utilization of large quantities of carbohydrate derived from artichokes was made possible through the coöperation of Dr. Carpenter of the Nutrition Laboratory of the Carnegie Institution and Professor X, Case 1500, aged fifty-two years, who had used dried artichokes for a period of three years.[3] Metabolism experiments carried out at the Carnegie Nutrition Laboratory clearly showed that the patient absorbed fully 100 grams of carbohydrate from the artichokes. Furthermore, when an equivalent amount of carbohydrate in the form of potato was substituted for artichokes, glycosuria and hyperglycemia occurred within two hours and disappeared only after the potato was discontinued and artichokes resumed.

For several years Jerusalem artichokes were used freely in the diet of patients at the Deaconess Hospital. At present insulin and the use of more liberal carbohydrate diets have lessened the indication to use artichokes.

E. EXERCISE IN TREATMENT OF DIABETES.

Exercise tends to lower the blood sugar in the diabetic in whose body there is an adequate supply of insulin whether this be of endogenous or exogenous origin. This effect is so striking and so beneficial that exercise along with diet and insulin is now accorded a definite and prominent place in the everyday treatment of diabetes. Patients themselves recognize and make use of the principle. Unless an accompanying condition contraindicates activity, diabetic patients should not be kept in bed, but rather must be encouraged to take regular, daily exercise. Through muscular activity food tolerance improves and higher diets with smaller dosages of insulin are possible. This is most strikingly shown in the much lower insulin requirement of diabetic children while in summer camps as compared with the larger need during the winter when they are in school and relatively inactive. The "insulin reaction" which may follow unusual or strenuous exercise in the well-controlled diabetic is a matter of common knowledge. Patients in bed are aided with exercise and the lack of it always raises difficulties in the management of diabetes. The patient crippled with rheumatism requires large doses of insulin, and if his joints can be limbered and he can move about, the insulin can be lowered. A game of golf, Case 632 often said, was the equal of 5 units. But exercise is harmful, even lethal to a severe diabetic, if diabetes is uncontrolled and conversely if over controlled and he becomes hypoglycemic. Exercise to be helpful must always be supported by endogenous or exogenous insulin and carbohydrate.

[1] Okey: Jour. Biol. Chem , **38**, 33; 1919, **39**, 149, 1919.
[2] Root and Baker: Arch. Int. Med., **36**, 136, 1925.
[3] Carpenter and Root: Arch. Int. Med., **42**, 64, 1928.

Before insulin became available in 1922, clinicians had recognized that whereas patients with milder grades of diabetes profited by exercise, those with severe or poorly controlled diabetes were made worse.[1] This is undoubtedly correlated with the fact that when, at the time of the exercise, the diabetic is deficient in insulin, muscular activity causes a rise and not a fall in blood sugar. This can readily be demonstrated by allowing a patient with moderately severe or severe diabetes to exercise in the morning before insulin or breakfast has been given. Determinations will show that the immediate effect is a definite rise in blood sugar.[2] If a small dose of insulin then be given, further exercise causes a greater fall in blood sugar than would be expected from the insulin itself.

Richardson[3] found that the effect of exercise in diabetic patients depended upon the initial level of the blood sugar. In patients who had been given neither food nor insulin for sixteen hours, when the fasting value was below 175 mg. per 100 cc., exercise caused a decrease, and when the fasting value was above 300 mg. per 100 cc., exercise caused an increase in the blood sugar. Exercise after food or after even small doses of insulin was accompanied by a decrease in blood sugar even in patients in whom the same exercise, without previous food or insulin, caused either no change or an increase in blood sugar.

The practical application of such studies is clear. Exercise helps a mild diabetic, because he has enough of his own insulin; it will similarly help a severe diabetic if he recives an accessory supply of insulin. The exercise should be systematic and at regular hours. The insulin dosage must be large enough to maintain the diabetes well controlled in order for the exercise to produce the maximal benefit.

The favoring effect of exercise upon the utilization of carbohydrate and the lowering of the blood sugar must be borne in mind whenever insulin is prescribed. As a rule the dose of insulin outside of the hospital should be less than that in the hospital and it is *usually wise to reduce the insulin allowance of a patient when he is discharged*. Patients receiving protamine insulin may require more carbohydrate in repeated feedings to counteract exercise than do patients upon regular insulin. Lawrence[4] found the effect of exercise in increasing the action of insulin was greatest at the maximum period of insulin activity. This is why exercise plus insulin so frequently cause insulin reactions and particularly do so if the next meal is postponed. Protamine zinc insulin simulates endogenous insulin, transforms the patient to a milder type of diabetes and thus enables him to profit by exercise.

[1] Allen, Stillman and Fitz: P. 468, Loc. cit., p. 54.
[2] Marble and Smith: Arch. Int. Med., **58**, 577, 1936.
[3] Richardson: Jour. Clin. Invest., **13**, 699, 1934.
[4] Lawrence: Brit. Med. Jour., **1**, 648, 1926.

Exercise for diabetic patients has a very practical bearing, because it raises the question of their ability to support themselves. The results of a survey of a group of 100 consecutive patients in England made by Lawrence and Madders[1] showed that with an average duration of five years of employment no time was lost by 39 per cent; time was lost only at initial stabilization by 38 per cent, for restabilization by 8 per cent and through diabetic illnesses by 15 per cent. In a study of 653 patients of our own group between twenty and sixty-five years of age, full time capacity for work was reported by 63 per cent of the men and by 46 per cent of the women, and two-thirds capacity by an additional 27 per cent of the men and 34 per cent of the women. At the Mayo Clinic,[2] of a group of 60 patients of either school or working age taking insulin for at least a year, nearly three-quarters were continuing their previous employment, and 17 per cent had simply made some adjustment in their working habits. Ponteva,[3] in his survey of 266 patients under treatment in Finland, found 63 per cent capable of performing their usual occupation, 29 per cent could do a lighter kind of work and only 8 per cent who were completely incapacitated. Yet one must bear in mind that during exercise the tendency to hypoglycemia is increased and that 4 in 42 observations, carried out by Brauch and Schultz[4] at Garz on exercising patients with hypoglycemia, showed significant changes in the electrocardiogram as evidenced by a lowering of the T wave.

Miss H. B. McKay was the first nurse to tell me that she regulated her patient's insulin by the exercise he intended to take. In 1928 she wrote: "I have to vary his insulin according to the exercise he gets. When he does not have a chance to play golf he takes 30 units, 16 in the morning and 14 in the afternoon, but when he has a chance to play golf, 14 in the morning and 10 in the afternoon keep him sugar-free." The patient, Case 2419, developed diabetes at the age of fourteen and six-tenths years in 1920; he is now happily married and has 3 lovely children. He is in good health, height $72\frac{3}{4}$ inches, weight 155 pounds, and at important work in June, 1946. His present diet is approximately carbohydrate 155 grams, protein 100 grams, fat 125 grams, and insulin, CI 12+PZI 64 units.

Exercise out of bed and in bed is essential for the diabetic. His muscles live on sugar and help him utilize it. Our hospital cases suffer from lack of exercise, even though a gymnasium is theoretically available for them and supplements our School Room, Dentists' Office, and "Beauty Parlor for Diabetic Feet" in their care. Lack of exercise in hospitals often makes a diabetic appear worse than he really is. The disarrangement of a patient's routine when transferred to a hospital often makes it extremely difficult to determine

[1] Lawrence and Madders: Brit. Med. Jour., **2**, 1076, 1938.
[2] Peterson: New England Jour. Med., **211**, 397, 1934.
[3] Ponteva: Acta med. Scandin., Suppl., **88**, 84, 1938.
[4] Brauch and Schultz: Klin. Wchnschr., **18**, 642, 1939.

his true state. Even before the discovery of insulin the value of exercise was appreciated by one of my wisest and mild diabetics. Case 352, Major W., wrote: "First, it is very hard to start the exercise, and the less one feels inclined to start the more one needs it. Second, it is neither necessary nor desirable that it should be violent. I found a quiet ride of an hour, walking or jogging after taking something on the stomach, started up my old metabolism for the whole day. If I rode hard I got tired out." Various patients on mountain hikes have tolerated unusual quantities of carbohydrate. I was always impressed in former days with the better results frequently obtained by ambulatory as compared with hospital treatment, provided the same degree of attention was given to the details of the diet and hygiene of the patient.

F. THE INSULINS.

1. **Introduction**—All of us require insulin, and if we cannot manufacture what we need in our own pancreases, we are fortunate if we can secure it by purchase or gift. None of us, the normal or the diabetic, know the quantity required to maintain health and strength. Fortunate it is that Nature regulates the supply with surprising accuracy, balancing its production with the carbohydrate consumed, whether this be for prompt utilization or for storage, and adjusting its output to the momentary demands of exercise or rest. This normal regulatory mechanism rarely may go awry and too much insulin be produced and, in fact, so much that at times death may result from hypoglycemia. Probably at other times all of us experience symptoms from an increased production of lesser degree which we recognize in ourselves by hunger and fatigue and our friends suspect by our altered disposition. But it is difficult to decide whether these states are actually due to too much insulin or to deficient carbohydrate through lack of body glycogen.

2. **Insulin Susceptible to Many Influences.**—The efficiency of insulin may be impaired by the overaction of the pituitary, thyroid or suprarenals. The lowering of the alkalinity of the blood, infections, starvation or an excessively high-fat diet also affect its action adversely, but not strikingly enough to prove that any of these brings on diabetes. The development of diabetes in the obese focuses attention on the possible effect upon insulin production of the constant stimulation of the insulin-producing function of the pancreas in order to assimilate the luxus carbohydrate consumed, but it seems hardly likely that the pancreas would be injured in this way, because there is no analogy to this in the field of other ductless glands. Although it is true that a diet high in fat and low in carbohydrate lowers insulin production, as shown repeatedly by many, nevertheless the effect of such a diet when carried out in the Du Bois laboratory for over a year on two human beings, and recently by

Best,[1] although it temporarily lowered carbohydrate tolerance, did not do so permanently. It is remarkable that whatever agency injures the pancreas, it practically never wholly destroys the ability of the gland to make insulin, save experimentally. Diabetes is not complete. Obviously this complicates the problem of the therapeutics of insulin enormously, because one never knows how much insulin the active pancreatic remnant yields and therefore how much must be supplied. Just as in health we are reasonably certain that the production varies under different conditions, so too we can infer it varies in diabetes. Therefore, in the administration of insulin we must always recognize that we are dealing with a *variable* and interpret results cautiously and with extreme deliberation.

3. **Insulin Requirement by Severe Diabetics**—Miss P., Case 3194, a diabetic of twelve years' duration with onset at fifty years of age, bedridden with rheumatoid arthritis, took daily for years approximately carbohydrate 180 grams and Calories 1600 with insulin 80 units to maintain weight and aglycosuria. She died of endo- and pericarditis. Her pancreas, which weighed 15 grams, is one of the smallest encountered by Shields Warren in 585 autopsies upon diabetic adults. How many units of insulin Miss P.'s pancreas produced daily is useless to conjecture, but presumably not many. This patient ate 4 eggs daily for many years. Her cholesterol was 182 milligrams. At postmortem, twelve years after the onset of the disease, the circulatory system was particularly free from arteriosclerosis. (See page 195.)

Miss M., Case 1542, was considered to be my severest diabetic, and on August 7, 1922, was my first patient to receive insulin. Her tolerance was estimated at about 7 grams carbohydrate. In January, 1946, at sixty-five years of age with diabetes of twenty-eight years' duration she weighs 125 pounds instead of her erstwhile 69 pounds, to which her weight had fallen from 155 pounds when she began insulin, leads an active, useful life, takes carbohydrate 140 ± grams, calories 1790 ±, and is practically aglycosuric with 6 units of crystalline and 28 of protamine insulin a day. If Miss P., like Miss M., had been able to have had the advantage of exercise, very likely her insulin dosage could have been halved. These 2 cases suggest that an adult requires between 34 and 80 units of insulin daily. Holm's experiments would substantiate this opinion. Best, transferring his figures for the insulin requirement of the dog, estimates 100 units per day would be about the figure for an adult human. When, therefore, patients claim they require more than 80 or even 50 units, we suspect a complication such as an infection, acidosis, glandular disease, hemochromatosis, or just plain ignorance or carelessness in the quantity and quality of the diet. There are occasional cases, however, who need much more, but they constitute almost a special class by themselves. (See page 379.)

[1] Best: Loc. cit., p. 138.

In a summary of 9 cases of total pancreatectomy, 4 of which were at the Mayo Clinic,[1] the insulin requirements are reported. These did not exceed 40 units in any instance and of those 8 cases surviving over two weeks 26 units were the lowest number of units administered daily.

4. **Efficiency in the Use of Insulin.**—To attain maximum efficiency in the use of insulin its continuous administration would be necessary. But even this would not quite imitate nature unless the supply introduced could be varied according to the carbohydrate demand of the hour, nay, even minute. Protamine zinc insulin meets this need to a greater extent than regular insulin or crystalline insulin because of its longer action, but fails in that it does not automatically adjust itself to the additional load of carbohydrate which a meal demands or the decreased necessity for it induced by exercise; moreover, it presupposes a continuous supply of carbohydrate furnished by food or from body storage. Only under such circumstances would the long effective protamine zinc insulin act at the best advantage. The Toronto workers recognized this situation when regular insulin was introduced and, to meet it, early taught us the advantages of the multiple over the single dose. Holm showed this beautifully with depancreatized dogs. With a constant intravenous injection of insulin Bertram[2] calculates from Holm's experiments that a normal adult, weight 60 kilograms, requires 7.8 units per day when fasting and 48 units when living upon a diet the caloric value of which is derived exclusively from carbohydrate. Martin, Drury and Strouse[3] have described a method for determining the "basal insulin requirement."

5. **Types of Insulin.**—There are two types of insulin, the quick-acting regular insulin or crystalline insulin and the slowly-acting protamine zinc insulin. Experimentally other preparations, such as histone and globin insulin, and many other varieties especially in Germany,[4] have been used. The basic action of the various insulins is the same. All lower the sugar in the blood and in consequence that in the urine. All favor the storage of carbohydrate as glycogen in the skin, liver and muscles and its utilization principally in the last-named. As a result, calories are conserved, not lost, acidosis is prevented and thus the processes of metabolism function normally. Indirectly all insulins are deterrent to the breakdown of protein, and the waste of its carbohydrate fraction and ensuing acidosis. Best[5] states the "action of insulin

[1] Waugh, Dixon, Clagett, Bollman, Sprague and Comfort: Proc. Staff Meetings Mayo Clinic, **21**, 25, 1946.

[2] Bertram: Loc. cit., p. 87.

[3] Martin, Drury and Strouse: Arch. Int. Med., **66**, 78, 1940.

[4] For a review of these consult Die Moderne Insulinbehandlung insbesondere mit Depotpräparaten. Verhandl. d. Gesellsch. f. Verdauungs- u. Stoffwechselkr., **14**, 201–289, 1939. See also page 368 for discussion of histone and globin insulin and insulin mixtures.

[5] Best: Research Defense Soc. Pub., **26**, Nr. 3, 1938.

is to remove all the signs and symptoms of diabetes. To be more specific, insulin accelerates the formation of a complex sugar which is apparently necessary for the proper functioning of the animal organism. It increases slightly the combustion of sugar in the body and it prevents the wasteful formation of excess amounts of sugar from other substances."

The duration of action of a given dose of insulin is influenced by various factors among which is the size of the dose (with larger doses the effect is exerted over a longer period) and by the intake of food. Thus in the fasting diabetic patient a single injection of regular or crystalline insulin causes a fall in blood sugar which reaches its lowest point in six and seven hours respectively. The blood sugar then rises toward the initial value, regaining it after twelve or fourteen hours. With protamine zinc insulin the fall in blood sugar is gradual and prolonged, persisting over twenty-four hours. Best[1] has reported that in fasting diabetic dogs the duration of effect of protamine zinc insulin may be forty-eight to seventy-two hours. In diabetic patients eating meals at the customary hours, the maximal effect of regular or crystalline insulin taken before breakfast is seen three to five hours after the injection. The maximal effect of protamine zinc insulin under similar conditions is seen in twelve to twenty-four hours after the injection and of globin insulin in six to eight hours.

In normal men and animals kept in the fasting state the administration of regular or crystalline insulin causes a prompt fall to the lowest level in one and a half to two hours, with return to the initial value in from five to seven hours. In normal, as in diabetic subjects, the length of action of crystalline insulin appears to be slightly prolonged as compared with that of regular insulin, the difference being a matter of about two hours.

At present we use protamine zinc insulin in practically all patients requiring insulin, supplementing it if necessary with crystalline insulin; both types of insulin are given in the morning before breakfast with usually no more insulin for the rest of the day.

Crystalline insulin is a purer substance than regular insulin, lasts longer and, thanks to the manufacturers, costs no more. Crystalline insulin and protamine zinc insulin are the insulins now used almost exclusively at the George F. Baker Clinic except when other insulins are employed for experimental purposes, as naturally is always the case. The fewer the types of insulin for sale the less confused will patients be in the course of treatment and obviously the less costly will insulin become. The fewer tools a mechanic has, the more skilled he becomes in the use of each one.

See page 368 for a discussion of histone and globin insulin and of various mixtures of insulin.

---

[1] Best: Personal communication.

Protamine Insulin and Protamine Zinc Insulin. — Protamine insulin has constituted the most notable advance in the treatment of diabetes since the discovery of insulin in 1921. It is true the action of regular insulin was dramatic in lowering the blood sugar and promoting the utilization of carbohydrate with all that that implies, but its effect was short-lived and for adequate control of most cases of diabetes two, three and even four injections were required daily. Protamine insulin, and particularly protamine zinc insulin, changed all this, reducing injections to once in twenty-four hours for two-thirds of our hospital, and therefore severe, cases above the age of fifty-five years during 1941 and for nearly one-half (46 per cent) of the entire age groups. (See Table 47.) These results were obtained without very special endeavor to limit insulin to one dose. Manifestly by design and by wider and better distribution of carbohydrate throughout the day the number of diabetics who could be treated by a single dose of protamine zinc insulin might be somewhat increased. More than a generation was filled with the Naunyn, Allen and Banting eras of diabetic therapy and we deem it quite proper that the half century of diabetic achievement ending in protamine insulin which has opened the door into a fourth epoch should be named after its discoverer in Copenhagen — The Hagedorn era.

Soon after insulin became available, it was found that with depancreatized dogs the most favorable effects were produced when it was administered frequently in small doses, because of the excretion of greater amounts of insulin by the kidneys when large rather than small doses were injected and the destruction of insulin by enzymes present in the tissues. As the purity of insulin increased and the evidence of local skin reactions grew less, the duration of the physiological effects which it produced was shortened (Kerr, Best, Campbell and Fletcher[1]). The purification of insulin therefore was not an unmixed blessing.

Hagedorn[2] conceived the idea of producing an insulin compound slowly soluble in tissue fluid by combining it with a basic protein substance. The resulting compound which he produced had an isoelectric zone nearer to the pH of the body than the regular insulin hydrochloride which was definitely acid and therefore more quickly absorbed. For his purpose he resorted to the protamines, described in 1868 by Meischer, and first used by Kossel[3] as protein precipitants about 1890. Of these Hagedorn found the monoprotamines

[1] Kerr, Best, Campbell and Fletcher: Canad. Med. Assn. Jour., 34, 400, 1936; Canad. Pub. Health Jour., 27, 157, 1936. Campbell, Fletcher and Kerr: Am. Jour. Med. Sci., 192, 589, 1936.

[2] Hagedorn, Jensen, Krarup and Wodstrop: Jour. Am. Med. Assn., 106, 177, 1936. Krarup: Clinical Investigations Into the Action of Protamine Insulinate. Copenhagen, G. E. C. Gad., 1935. Hanssen: Jour. Am. Med. Assn., 106, 914, 1936.

[3] Kossel: The Protamine and Histones, Monograph on Biochemistry (Longmans), 1928.

most suitable for his purpose and the best of these proved to be one hitherto undescribed which he obtained from the sperm of *salmo iridius*, the rainbow trout. Alone this maneuver was insufficient to delay absorption, but when the reaction of the solution was adjusted to a hydrogen-ion concentration of pH 7.3, which is similar to that of the body fluids, a precipitate of the protamine insulin took place, necessitating a breakdown of the compound before absorption. This suspension was of practically constant insulin concentration and when deposited in the subcutaneous tissues of the body there was a steady and prolonged absorption of the insulin liberated from the solid particles.

During more than two years Hagedorn and his associates Jensen, Krarup and Wodstrop,[1] at the Steno Memorial Hospital in Copenhagen, studied the action of protamine insulin clinically. As a rule regular insulin was given in the morning and protamine insulin in the evening, but occasionally protamine insulin alone was employed. By these means the peaks and valleys of the blood sugar curve, seen with patients treated with regular insulin, were avoided or greatly minimized. Glycosuria disappeared as did signs of acidosis as measured by the urinary ammonia excretion. Insulin reactions were abolished or came on so much more gradually that there was opportunity to treat them early. In certain cases the total dose of insulin could be reduced. In others in which a single dose of insulin was given in twenty-four hours, it was found advisable to increase it somewhat, because of its slow absorption and the possibility with larger doses of leveling the blood sugar for the entire twenty-four hours yet without risk of hypoglycemia.

Hagedorn recognized that protamine insulin acts too slowly for the treatment of a case of diabetic coma and warned against its use for this purpose, although he might well have added that if properly employed it would prevent it. Likewise, for the same reason, it may not control the hyperglycemia of a heavy carbohydrate meal in a severe diabetic, but will prevent it if the carbohydrate is distributed throughout the day.

Confirmation of Hagedorn's results were reported first by members of the George F. Baker Clinic in Boston,[2] later by the Mayo Clinic[3] and the Toronto groups,[4] and subsequently by many others. All and even more than claimed by Hagedorn in his modest and conservative announcement has proved to be true. The effect of a dose of protamine insulin was demonstrable more than twelve hours

[1] Hagedorn, Jensen, Krarup and Wodstrop: Loc. cit., p. 364. Krarup: Loc. cit., p. 364. Hanssen: Loc. cit., p. 364.

[2] Root, White, Marble and Stotz: Jour. Am. Med. Assn., 106, 180, 1936. Joslin, Root, White, Marble, Joslin and Lynch: New England Jour. Med., 214, 1079, 1936.

[3] Sprague, Blum, Osterberg, Kepler and Wilder: Jour. Am. Med. Assn., 106, 1701, 1936. Wilder: Proc. Mayo Clin. Staff Meet., 11, 257, 1936.

[4] Kerr, Best, Campbell and Fletcher: Loc. cit., p. 364. Campbell, Fletcher and Kerr: Loc. cit., p. 364.

later. Thus it became possible for the diabetic to begin his day with a normal fasting blood sugar. Beecher and Krogh[1] found that regular insulin disappeared from the tissue in about forty-five minutes, whereas protamine insulin required about five hours.

The insertion of zinc into the protamine insulin compound more than doubled its lasting therapeutic quality. It represented the result of research, first, of Abel who crystallized insulin in 1925 and, later, the discovery of Scott and Fisher of the presence of zinc in the insulin molecule. By the addition of zinc the action of the preparation protamine zinc insulin extends for fully forty-eight hours, although with diminishing effect. It is only when protamine zinc insulin has been omitted for this length of time that one is justified in testing the power of a new preparation or modification of insulin. In general when the dose of protamine zinc insulin is increased the duration of effect is prolonged rather than its intensity. However, one must not depend upon this statement too implicitly and be reckless in the prescribing of large doses of protamine zinc insulin.

Remembering that protamine zinc insulin is constantly acting and thus tends to reduce a high diabetic blood sugar toward a normal level and that it acts by night quite as much as by day and with particular effectiveness because the patient is then without food, one must be especially cautious if it is decided to add a dose of quick-acting insulin, crystalline insulin or regular insulin, before breakfast to the treatment of a patient already upon protamine zinc insulin. Certainly the breakfast should not be deferred long after the double injections of crystalline insulin and protamine zinc insulin, because otherwise a reaction might ensue. For this reason some patients find it advantageous to take their breakfast fruit at the same time they make the injections.

On the other hand, if protamine zinc insulin is given alone, it can be given with less attention to time before meals, because its action begins so gradually, and being less violent, it is less necessary to protect the patient with food.

Frequent feedings are always useful for the patient taking protamine zinc insulin and for several reasons. First, as already said, the lowering of the total carbohydrate at a meal by the taking away of a small quantity for lunches, brings the carbohydrate at that meal to a level, which the slowly-acting protamine zinc insulin can control. Second, these feedings also protect against the danger of reactions between meals when the blood sugar is low. Third, it is always advantageous in the administration of carbohydrate to a diabetic to get the benefit which results from the falling tide of a blood-sugar curve, because that decidedly favors the utilization of carbohydrate in contrast to a rising blood-sugar curve which hinders it. Fourth, by promotion of oxidation of carbohydrate between meals the development of acidosis is averted. Fifth, frequent feedings of carbohy-

[1] Beecher and Krogh: Nature, **137**, 458, 1936.

drate favor its utilization.[1] Indeed frequent feedings to an individual supplied with insulin, endogenous or exogenous, constitute a sort of Staub-Traugott[2] phenomenon.

Shifting From Regular or Crystalline Insulin to Protamine Zinc Insulin.—The time required to shift from regular or crystalline insulin to protamine zinc insulin depends upon the severity of the case of diabetes and varies from three to ten days. If one proceeds more rapidly either marked glycosuria is apt to occur or reactions appear. The merit of protamine zinc insulin is that it acts slowly and it simply shows ignorance of this principle in diabetic therapy to expect protamine zinc insulin to show its full effect in a few days, much less in a few hours. Patience, confidence, intelligence and coöperation between doctor and patient are necessary to secure the full benefit of protamine zinc insulin. But don't attempt to paint the lily—in other words, think twice before changing a diabetic to protamine zinc insulin who has done marvelously well for years with regular insulin or crystalline insulin.

The method we now employ in changing from crystalline to protamine zinc insulin is to inject the same number of units of crystalline insulin before breakfast, which the patient has been in the habit of taking, and at the same time a quantity of protamine zinc insulin which is equal to the remainder of the total units of crystalline insulin previously taken by the patient in the twenty-four hours. With children the number of units so injected may need to be increased one-fourth, more or less. Such rearrangements often work out so that one-third of the total insulin for the twenty-four hours will be crystalline insulin and two-thirds will be protamine zinc insulin. Reactions can and do occur with protamine zinc insulin alone, just as they do with regular insulin or crystalline insulin, but they are far more apt to occur if crystalline insulin is given with protamine zinc insulin. The clinician should always remember that when using protamine zinc insulin the patient begins the day with the blood sugar at a much lower level than when upon crystalline or regular insulin alone, because the diabetes has been controlled during the night.

6. **The Number of Doses, Their Distribution and the Average Dose of the Insulins.**—Protamine zinc insulin has simplified these problems greatly and fully as much for the doctor as the patient. Protamine zinc insulin is given once a day and always at our clinic before breakfast. In this way familiarity with its effect is learned, simplicity of treatment attained, and the confusion avoided to which multiple methods would lead. For the general plan of treatment and for specific details of clinical administration of protamine zinc insulin, to avoid duplication the reader is referred to pages 364-367.

If the patient should be compelled to be dependent upon crystal-

---

[1] Grote: Loc. cit., p. 147.
[2] Staub—Traugott phenomenon: See refs. 6 and 7, p. 146.

line insulin or regular insulin, protamine zinc insulin not being available, it is quite possible that in a mild case of diabetes one injection daily would suffice (see page 363 for a discussion of the action of crystalline insulin), and it usually would be best to give that before breakfast; if two doses are necessary, doses before breakfast and supper are given.   If these doses reach the level of 20 to 30 units each and are still inadequate to control glycosuria, then 3 or 4 doses a day may be advisable.   Often, particularly, with young people with severe diabetes, it will be found helpful to give the third dose at bedtime, i. e., 10 P.M. to midnight.   By so doing, one decreases the tendency for the blood sugar to rise in the early morning hours and an adequate dose at bedtime may enable a patient with severe diabetes to awaken with a sugar-free urine. This late evening dose is usually given with little or no food, in contra-distinction to the more liberal lunch when protamine zinc insulin is employed, and must be relatively small, 2, 4 or 6 units, in order not to provoke hypoglycemia.   Some patients require a dose of insulin before each of the three meals plus the bedtime dose.   We have not thought it advisable to give insulin "by the clock," i. e., every six, eight or twelve hours regardless of meals, because of the danger of producing hypoglycemia.

In the presence of complications in addition to a simple holding dose of protamine zinc insulin we often resort to supplementary doses of insulin utilizing the fraction prescription as described on page 334.

The quantity of insulin administered to the average diabetic as well as the percentage of diabetics taking it, is rising in the treatment of diabetes rather than falling, first, because the quantity of carbohydrate in the diabetic diet has been steadily going up throughout the country and, second, because the proportion of severe diabetics living is so much greater, particularly children and young adults, who owe their preservation to insulin, and finally because of the obvious good it does.   See Fig. 10.

7. **Experimental Insulins With Prolonged Actions.**—Since the introduction upon the market of slowly acting protamine zinc insulin in 1937, many attempts have been made to modify and to improve its action.   These investigations have been stimulated primarily by the recognition that one-third to one-half of the patients using protamine zinc insulin need a supplementary injection of a quick-acting insulin, as crystalline or regular insulin, in order to insure a satisfactory blood sugar the earlier part of the day.   This is necessitated by the slow initial effect of protamine zinc insulin.

Globin Insulin.—Globin insulin[1] is prepared by combining insulin with globin, a simple protein obtained from beef erythrocytes.   The market preparation contains 3.8 mg. of globin and 0.3 mg. of zinc per 100 units of insulin.   The first clinical report, published by

---

[1] Reiner, Searle and Lang: Proc. Soc. Exp. Biol. and Med., **40**, 171, 1939.

Bauman in 1939,[1] stressed (1) that owing to its shorter action globin insulin was less apt to produce hypoglycemia during the night than was protamine zinc insulin; (2) the lack of local allergic reactions to this preparation; (3) that whereas mild and moderately severe diabetics were adequately controlled, severe diabetics were only fairly well regulated with globin insulin. Further reports have been made by Bauman,[2][3] Mosenthal,[4] Marks,[5] Andrew and Groat,[6] Paul,[0] Protas[8] Levitt and Schaus,[9] Duncan and Barnes[17] and Trasoff, Borden and Mintz.[11]

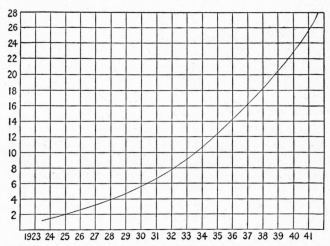

Fig. 10.—The accelerating use of insulin. (Courtesy of C. H. Best.)

Bailey and Marble[12] studied the effect of globin insulin in 12 cases at the New England Deaconess Hospital, 5 of whom remained in the Hospital from seventy-four to one hundred and thirty-two days for the study. The effects of globin insulin, histone zinc insulin and clear protamine zinc insulin were compared with the market protamine zinc and crystalline insulins. They stress the importance of using moderately severe or severe diabetics in testing an insulin, for almost any type of insulin will control a mild diabetic. The patients

[1] Bauman: Am. Jour. Med. Sci., **198**, 475, 1939.
[2] Bauman: Proc. Soc. Exper. Biol. and Med., **40**, 170, 1939.
[3] Bauman: Am. Jour. Med. Sci., **200**, 299, 1940; Bull. New England Med. Center, **5**, 3, 1943.
[4] Mosenthal: Jour. Am. Med. Assn., **125**, 483, 1944.
[5] Marks: Med. Clin. North America, **24**, 649, 1940.
[6] Andrew and Groat: New York State Jour. Med., **40**, 913, 1940.
[7] Paul: Med. World, **61**, 443, 1943.
[8] Protas: Med. Ann. Dist. of Columbia, **13**, 254, 1944.
[9] Levitt and Schaus: Med. Times, **70**, 187, 1942.
[10] Duncan and Barnes: Am. Jour. Med. Sci., **202**, 553, 1941.
[11] Trasoff, Borden and Mintz: Am. Jour. Digest. Dis., **12**, 313, 1945.
[12] Bailey and Marble: Jour. Am. Med. Assn., **118**, 683, 1942.

24

were young, coöperative, free of complications and took from 40 to 80 units of insulin daily. Figure 11 shows the composite insulin curves obtained from the 5 test patients during a period of fasting. Each patient was later regulated in the hospital on each type of experimental insulin for further study.

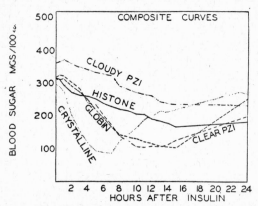

FIG. 11.—Each curve represents the composite effect of a single subcutaneous injection of insulin into a fasting diabetic subject. The curve for globin insulin is a composite of 10 curves, histone zinc insulin 10 curves, turbid PZI 4 curves, clear PZI 10 curves and crystalline insulin 6 curves. Blood sugar determinations were made hourly from 8:00 A.M. until 11:00 P.M. or 12 midnight and then again at 7:00 and 8 00 A.M. the following morning. No food was given throughout the test. In 3 cases, 0.15 unit of insulin per kilogram of body weight was given on separate days, whereas in 2 cases 0.20 unit per kilogram was used. No blood samples were taken between the 15th and 23rd hour.

The following conclusions regarding globin insulin were reached by Bailey and Marble:

(1) Globin insulin has a rate and duration of action between that of crystalline insulin and that of turbid (market) protamine zinc insulin. Its action lasts for eighteen to twenty-four hours and usually permits a normal fasting blood sugar. (2) The initial action is not as great as with crystalline insulin. (3) A moderate rise in blood sugar occurs between 7 and 11 A.M. which may be lessened if the insulin is taken forty-five to sixty minutes before breakfast. (4) There is a tendency for a large, rapid fall in blood sugar between 2 and 5 P.M. with a marked tendency to insulin reactions unless a mid-afternoon lunch is taken. (5) A bedtime lunch is best omitted to avoid hyperglycemia at night. (6) No local cutaneous (allergic) reactions were noted. (Subsequently such were observed, Authors.)

Further experience with globin insulin since the above study confirms the original result that globin insulin may cause a marked fall in the afternoon blood sugar with unpleasant symptoms. Repeatedly we have seen patients miserable with insulin reactions which occur while at work. Despite the recommendation of an afternoon lunch this is not infrequently forgotten with serious results. One patient, Case 20814, had local allergic reactions to globin insulin.

Although globin insulin will control adequately the blood sugars of mild and some moderately severe cases, its action is not satisfactory for severe cases.

Insulin Mixtures.—Much work on insulin mixtures has been carried out by Peck[1] and by Colwell.[2] When crystalline (or amorphous) insulin is mixed with turbid protamine zinc insulin, the result, according to Colwell, is an insulin with a monophasic action which is more prompt and intense and with less prolonged activity than commercial protamine zinc insulin. He determined the amount of soluble insulin in the supernatant fluid of insulin mixtures and found only 0.9 to 2.0 units per 80 units of mixture in the ratios most commonly used (3 : 1, 2 : 1, 1 : 1 parts of insulin to protamine zinc insulin). Colwell believes that fully 85 per cent of diabetic patients requiring protamine zinc insulin supplemented with regular or crystalline insulin can be satisfactorily regulated on a single dose of the 2 : 1 mixture (two parts of crystalline insulin to one part of protamine zinc insulin), and that 97 per cent can be well regulated using some insulin mixture. According to Peck, mixtures made of equal parts insulin and protamine zinc insulin do not show a significantly different action from that obtained when using protamine zinc insulin alone, whereas combinations containing more than three parts of insulin to one part of protamine zinc insulin result in too short a time activity and too great an intensity of effect during the day. From clinical experience he has found mixtures containing 2 : 1 or 3 : 2 parts of insulin to protamine zinc insulin the most useful combination. Ulrich[3] favors the 3 : 2 mixture.

The preparation obtained by mixing protamine zinc insulin with crystalline insulin has a pH between the two. Both Colwell[4] and Peck[5] believe that these mixtures are stable for several months.

The outstanding advantages of insulin mixtures is that only one injection is needed in patients who might otherwise require protamine zinc insulin supplemented with crystalline or regular insulin, and Colwell believes that its waning action during the night lessens the danger of nocturnal hypoglycemia. A disadvantage, however, is the difficulty encountered when the patient attempts to mix the two insulins in a syringe before injection. Although the more intelligent and dexterous patient may do this correctly following the technique outlined by Peck,[6] many will undoubtedly make errors. Our patients are taught to vary their crystalline and prota-

[1] Peck: Ann. Int. Med., **18**, 177, 1943.
[2] Colwell: Arch. Int. Med., **74**, 331, 1944.
[3] Ulrich: Ann. Int. Med., **14**, 1166, 1941.
[4] Colwell: Jour. Am. Med. Assn., **122**, 1231, 1943.
[5] Peck: Proc. Am. Diabetes Assn., **2**, 69, 1942.
[6] Peck: Jour. Indiana Med. Assoc., **36**, 340, 1943.

mine zinc insulin at home when necessary as indicated by their fasting and noon samples of urine. With the insulin mixtures the ratio cannot be changed easily by the patient. Nevertheless, it is apparent that many patients can be well controlled on the insulin mixtures.

Modified Protamine Zinc Insulin.—Since the slow onset of action of turbid protamine zinc insulin often requires a supplementary injection of a rapidly acting insulin, MacBryde[1] favors the use of a single insulin which contains 25 per cent rapid activity and 75 per cent slow activity. This proportion conformed to the ratio needed by the majority of his patients requiring separate injections of insulin and protamine zinc insulin.

Such an insulin has been prepared for experimental study by Eli Lilly and Company and contains one-half the amount of protamine and zinc contained in the market protamine zinc insulin—namely 0.625 mg. of protamine and 0.1 mg. of zinc per 100 units. This turbid preparation has a pH of 7.2.

Using this preparation MacBryde reported that he was able to regulate satisfactorily 90 per cent of 110 diabetic patients. Sixty-four per cent of his well regulated patients required over 40 units daily and some as high as 120 units (average 73 units). In comparison with the 2 : 1 mixture (insulin to protamine zinc insulin) discussed above, MacBryde and Reiss[1] obtained superior diabetic control in each of 10 patients using modified protamine zinc insulin although Peck[2] has claimed the opposite results. Reports by Mac-Bryde and Roberts[3] comparing the results obtained using modified protamine zinc insulin as compared with globin zinc insulin, insulin mixtures, histone zinc insulin and standard protamine zinc insulin, have in each case favored the use of modified protamine zinc insulin.

In a group of 26 patients at the New England Deaconess Hospital with whom we have used this preparation we have obtained satisfactory results although no careful statistical study has been conducted.

Del Fierro and Sevringhaus[4] also report favorable results in 14 of 16 patients and believe that the modified protamine zinc insulin is the best type of protamine zinc insulin for most diabetics who require 40 or more units of insulin daily. Recently, however, the stability of the soluble insulin in this preparation has been questioned which, if true, might make the results with this insulin variable, depending on its age, since fresh lots of insulin would contain a larger amount of soluble insulin than older ones. MacBryde is continuing his efforts to improve this insulin.

[1] MacBryde and Reiss: Jour. Clin. Endocrinology, **4**, 469, 1944.
[2] Peck: Personal communication.
[3] MacBryde and Roberts: Jour. Clin. Invest., **22**, 791, 1943; Jour. Am. Med. Assn., **122**, 1225, 1943.
[4] Del Fierro and Sevringhaus: Ann. Int. Med., **22**, 667, 1945.

Histone Insulin.—Histone (zinc) insulin contains 3.2 mg. of histone, a protein obtained from the thymus gland and 0.2 mg. of zinc per 100 units of insulin and like the standard protamine zinc insulin is turbid with a pH of 7.0±. Composite curves from the study by Bailey and Marble shown in Figure 11 reveal that except for a slight initial action, presumably due to a small amount of soluble insulin present, the action of histone zinc insulin closely parallels the action of standard protamine zinc insulin. Its duration of action, however, seems slightly less prolonged. The general conclusions regarding histone insulin are: (1) Histone zinc insulin is effective for at least twenty-four hours and allows a normal fasting blood sugar. (2) During the first two hours following injection into a fasting diabetic subject there is a definite though moderate fall in blood sugar presumably due to a small amount of soluble insulin in the preparation. (3) The action of histone zinc insulin resembles closely that of turbid protamine zinc insulin except for the initial action and probably for a slightly less prolonged effect. (4) Fewer hypoglycemic reactions occurred than when using the turbid protamine zinc insulin alone or supplemented with crystalline insulin. The few reactions observed were similar to those seen after the administration of turbid protamine zinc insulin. (5) A bedtime lunch is advisable, as with turbid protamine zinc insulin to avoid nocturnal hypoglycemia. (6) No local cutaneous (allergic) reactions were noticed. (7) For patients requiring doses of insulin larger than 30 to 40 units daily, a single injection of histone zinc insulin allows better diabetic control than does a single injection of the turbid protamine zinc insulin variety.

Two definite disadvantages were apparent. Particularly with the U-80 strength, a precipitation frequently occurred around the neck of the vial requiring prolonged mixing before injection. In some vials, clumps of precipitated insulin were found. Possibly because some insulin was lost in this way patients often required a larger dose of histone zinc insulin than was needed with standard protamine zinc insulin supplemented with crystalline insulin.

Further use of histone insulin has borne out these earlier conclusions. In view of these objections and since the amount of free insulin seems unduly small, the use of histone insulin is not advised. MacBryde and Roberts[1] obtained similar results except that no initial rapid action was detected in their patients. Barnes, Cuttle and Duncan[2] report that whereas the onset of action of histone zinc insulin is less abrupt and more prolonged than that of unmodified or crystalline insulin its onset of action is more prompt than that of protamine zinc insulin.

Clear Protamine Zinc Insulin.—In a study of an experimental clear protamine zinc insulin containing 3.8 mg. of protamine and 0.31 mg. of zinc per 100 units of insulin, Bailey and Marble found the preparation similar in its action to globin insulin. It is a clear solution, having a pH of 3.3 to 3.5. Like globin insulin its rate and duration of action is between that of crystalline and that of protamine zinc insulin (see Fig. 11) and the same precaution concerning an afternoon lunch to avoid hypoglycemia is necessary. Despite this apparent similarity, however, it was found that with clear protamine zinc insulin it is more difficult to control the diabetic condition than with the use of globin insulin possibly due to a slightly longer duration of action of the latter.

It is encouraging that attempts are being made to find a better insulin. It would be desirable to have a long acting insulin similar to protamine zinc insulin which in addition provided some rapid action whereby a larger proportion of diabetics could be regulated

[1] MacBryde and Roberts: Loc. cit., p. 372.
[2] Barnes, Cuttle and Duncan: Jour. Pharm. and Exp. Therap., **72**, 331, 1941.

with a single injection. This would seem preferable to the use of extemporaneous insulin mixtures even though the latter secured similar results. The amount of rapid action needed in such a preparation has not been definitely decided although it is probably in the vicinity of 25 per cent. When such an insulin can be prepared which is *stable* and contains the optimum amount of soluble insulin it is probable that it will supplant the present market variety of protamine zinc insulin. In the meantime, good diabetic control can be afforded by the use of protamine zinc insulin supplemented when necessary by an injection of crystalline or amorphous insulin.

8. **An Insulin Reaction.**—Occasionally the action of insulin is so great that the blood sugar is lowered below the normal level and a whole train of phenomena arise, dependent in part upon the low blood sugar *per se*, the lessened glycogen in the tissues or the excess of protective counter-regulatory processes set in motion to raise the blood sugar. The combination of all these processes is known as an insulin reaction or insulin shock. An insulin shock is dependent upon the higher centers of the brain being intact; it does not take place in a spinal animal or in an animal under the influence of a general anesthetic. So often the harmful effects of a low blood sugar are emphasized that we wish to point out first of all how such a condition may be advantageously utilized. When the blood sugar drops the counter-regulatory mechanism of the body, the suprarenals and sympathetic system, through the production of adrenalin relieve it by favoring the discharge of glycogen from the liver. If this counter-regulation goes too far and the liver glycogen is depleted unduly, then the liver acts less well in furthering carbohydrate metabolism. Under such conditions even acidosis is said to occur,[1] just as it does as a result of uncontrolled diabetes when the liver is deprived of glycogen and filled with fat. This state of an approaching depletion of glycogen in the liver can be forestalled by the administration of carbohydrate, and if this is done at such a time, *i. e.*, when the blood sugar is already low and falling, apparently the carbohydrate is very well tolerated, so well in fact that the favorable phenomenon has been noted by patients. They frequently report that if at the first sign of an insulin reaction they take carbohydrate, it is tolerated so well that it counts as a pure addition to the carbohydrate allowance and they need not deduct it from the subsequent meal. That is why patients susceptible to insulin and exposed by occupation to a low blood sugar can advantageously take a minimal dose of carbohydrate hourly on the hour between meals. If the intake of carbohydrate is delayed, much more carbohydrate will be required to offset the hypoglycemia and the harmful effect of the reaction will be prolonged into the next day as shown by the total glucose excreted. The good effects of a low blood sugar often are noted

---

[1] I have seen this in pregnancy.

when a case of diabetic coma is overtreated and the blood sugar is reduced to 0.05 to 0.08 per cent. Under such circumstances often for twenty-four hours carbohydrate is utilized remarkably well with little or no insulin. (See Chapter XI, Hypoglycemia.) This is in line with treatment by Überinsulinierung as recommended by Störring in Umber's clinic.[1]

Why it is that symptoms of an insulin reaction are absent in glycogen storage (von Gierke's) disease when hypoglycemia is extreme, I cannot fathom.

9. **How Many Grams of Carbohydrate Will One Unit of Insulin Metabolize?**—This question no one can answer, although a mathematical attempt has been made by Miller and Allen.[2] There are always adjustments required for exercise and diet. Even if these two factors are constant the improvement of the condition of the patient overthrows one's calculations. Then, too, there are many complications in diabetes which affect the strength of the unit. In diabetic coma several units may be necessary for the utilization of 1 gram carbohydrate, but as acidotic symptoms subside, 1 unit of insulin becomes more efficacious. The crippling effect of infections upon the power of insulin is well known. Other facts are discussed under the section Insulin Resistance, pages 379–386. In general the value of a unit decreases with the number given and follows the law of a diminishing return. The first 10 units are more effective than the second 10, and so on. A given unitage divided in small doses exerts a greater effect than in one large dose. In the latter case the insulin is probably excreted or destroyed. One of our vistors, I regret forgetting his identity, proposed in the administration of the large dose of insulin in diabetic coma to give it in multiple sites rather than in one locality. There is another factor, namely, that insulin cannot act with greatest efficiency unless given an opportunity to display its power. An orator needs an audience to show what he can do, and insulin needs carbohydrate. Thus it has been claimed repeatedly by those advocating the higher carbohydrate diet that the carbohydrate can be doubled with little or no additional requirement for insulin provided total calories are controlled. But we are still somewhat skeptical. All will agree that the whole human machine works better when a substantial amount of carbohydrate is being burned and that carbohydrate and fat metabolism profit by avoidance of either extremely low or extremely high respiratory quotients. Exceptionally there may be no lack of carbohydrate to burn, but it may be in a form which is not combustible. Thus, plenty of carbohydrate may be administered in the diet to a patient with hemochromatosis, but because the glycogen storage facilities of the body are impaired, particularly in liver and skin (perhaps also muscles), insulin may not find any glycogen upon

[1] Störring: Med. Klin., **32**, 1589, 1936.
[2] Miller and Allen: Ann. Int. Med., **13**, 636, 1939.

which it can act. This is only one of the many states in which insulin is not blamable. *In general 1 unit of insulin will metabolize 1 or 2 grams of carbohydrate, and perhaps even 3 to 6 grams, Newburgh[1] says 7, and Holm[2] even 8.75, but it is impossible to state definitely, because we never know how many units the patient's pancreas is producing each day or at the moment.* Therefore it is dangerous to prescribe insulin in arbitrary or schematic fashion; in general the method of trial and error should be adopted, always erring on the side of low and frequent rather than of high and single dosage. Whenever we read that for each gram of glucose lost in the urine or given intravenously 1 unit of insulin should be injected, we shrug our shoulders and exclaim—*Prenez garde!*

Porges[3] points out that children have a low sugar threshold and react with a high glucose equivalent to insulin, but that old people with a high threshold react less well. A similar state is noticeable in cases with a high blood-pressure.

In his Goulstonian Lectures Himsworth[4] elaborates his theory that the height of the blood sugar can be regarded as a "head of pressure" which in health is within normal limits compatible with normal utilization of carbohydrate by the tissues. If, however, the ability of the tissues to use sugar is diminished either by lack of insulin or impairment of insulin action, compensation is made through an appropriate increase in the head of pressure of sugar in the blood. The rate of utilization of sugar by the tissues is thus maintained relatively constant. We cannot reconcile this with the presence of marked glycosuria when the blood sugar rises tenfold, namely 1.0 per cent.

10. **Methods for Administration of Insulin.**—Many methods for the introduction of insulin into the body other than by the needle, subcutaneously or intravenously, have been tried without practical success. Major[5] has mixed insulin with diethylene glycol monoethyl ether and when thus mixed it can be introduced by rubbing into the skin in animals with a resultant fall in blood sugar. He has also shown the absorption in 92 per cent of experiments on diabetic dogs in whom he has inserted pinacol tablets into the intestinal loop. Hermann and Kassowitz,[6] using animals, and Pribram,[7] in a group of 20 diabetics, have demonstrated the percutaneous action of insulin applied in an ointment. All methods of introduction such as the conjunctival, oral, rectal, vaginal and by inunction, have failed to be clinically useful because in general large amounts of insulin are required to produce even variable or slight effects upon the blood sugar[8]. Brahn studied the effect of insulin suppositories (rectal)

[1] Newburgh and Waller: Jour. Clin. Invest., **11**, 995, 1932.
[2] Holm: Arch. f. exp. Path. u. Pharmakol., **121**, 368, 1927.
[3] Porges: Med. Klin., **31**, 10, 1935.
[4] Himsworth: Lancet, **1**, 1, 1939; Proc. Soc. Exp. Biol. and Med., **37**, 338, 1937; Ibid., **38**, 721, 1938.
[5] Major: Am. Jour. Med. Sci., **192**, 257, 1936; Proc. Soc. Exp. Biol. and Med., **34**, 775, 1936; Ibid., **37**, 338, 1937; Ibid , **38**, 721, 1938.
[6] Hermann and Kassowitz: Klin. Wchnschr., **15**, 129, 1935.
[7] Pribram: Idem, p. 1534.
[8] Brahn: Lancet, **1**, 829, 1940.

upon the blood sugar of rabbits and normal persons. He found that the action sets in quickly, attaining its maximum in thirty to forty minutes; the duration of effect was from one to two hours. He quotes Wuhrman[1] as finding that one suppository unit is equivalent to about 10 injection units (!). (See further discussion on page 143.)

Theoretically, the intravenous administration of insulin should be more effective as it is more rapid than the subcutaneous but, aside from the disadvantage of puncturing a vein, it has been discarded because a disproportionate portion of the insulin so introduced is possibly excreted in the urine. Even in coma we give insulin subcutaneously whenever we give it intravenously, as is occasionally necessary in advanced cases.

11. **Site of Injection. Tumefactions. Insulin Atrophies.**—The site of an injection of insulin should be changed so frequently that not more than 1 dose is given in the same spot in a month. Children prefer no alterations in location, partly from their desire for routine, and also partly because frequent injection in the same area destroys the sensibility of the skin and subcutaneous tissue. When so administered the insulin is poorly absorbed and its effect to a greater or less degree nullified. Furthermore, infections at the site of injection may result more easily. Recently an uncontrolled fat diabetic girl showed abscesses in the upper part of the thigh where she claimed no insulin had been injected. Although she very likely spoke the truth, these probably did follow the introduction of insulin, the infection having spread along the lymphatics, an explanation which has been suggested for insulin atrophies occurring at a distance from the point of injection. For convenience it is well for patients to construct an insulin map of the body upon which points of insertion for the needle for a month can be recorded and thus surely one can avoid duplication of site. If insulin is injected often in the same area, as a rule, tumefactions result and, if the injections are long-continued, necrosis of the subcutaneous tissue occurs. Such tissue is more readily susceptible to infections and, in fact, about the only infections one sees as a result of the use of insulin take place under such circumstances. Obviously insulin given in such an area is poorly absorbed and it was pathetic to hear a patient say he always took his insulin in a given area, where as a matter of fact there was a tumefaction, because if he injected it elsewhere he would bring on a reaction. Therefore, impress upon patients that if insulin is scattered, less insulin will be required.

The advantage of injecting insulin into a fresh site was shown strikingly in our insulin resistant Case 14483 who for one and one-half years has taken 300 to 600 units of insulin daily. On January 4, 1936, when 440 units were being given daily into the thighs, the site of injection was changed to the abdominal wall. Severe hypoglycemic reactions occurred. When stabilization was secured several days later, 340 units, or 100 units less than the previous dosage, proved adequate.

Wuhrman: Schweiz. med. Wchnschr., **69**, 35, 787, 1939.

Insulin is generally injected by patients themselves into their thighs. With a little design by moving the line of the sites of injection each week of the month outwards and each day an inch downwards, a repetition of injections in the same area is avoided.

Other localities for insulin injection include the arms, particularly the deltoid and triceps regions, the upper, not the lower portions of the buttocks, and the abdominal wall. In the last-named situation needles shortened to $\frac{3}{8}$ inch can be employed. The needle best liked by the authors' patients is $\frac{1}{2}$ inch long and 26 gauge. It is remarkable that with the widespread use of insulin by hundreds of thousands of diabetics so few accidents occur, perhaps one abscess in half a million to a million injections. It is proof of the intelligence of the average diabetic. The wife of one of my patients placed cleaning fluid in an empty insulin vial for use upon a trip and, forgetting to destroy the bottle upon returning home, the husband injected the contents into his right forearm. The subsequent two weeks, spent in the hospital, afforded him an excellent opportunity to bring his diabetic knowledge up to date.

12. **Administration of Insulin.**—The danger of confusion in measuring the dose of insulin is real. Patients fail to comprehend that a unit is a unit and that, whereas 1 cc. of U-20 insulin contains 20 units, 1 cc. of U-40 insulin contains 40 units, and so on. In order to guard against errors it is well to verify the patient's dosage at each visit. Even a clergyman and a doctor make mistakes, and patients who have taken insulin over a period of years are quite as likely to be wrong in their reports as those just beginning. Partly for this reason, the simplest type of syringe is desirable and this we have found to be a syringe marked only with divisions into tenths of 1 cc. For most patients the U-40 strength is desirable although U-80 strength is employed if more than 40 units are to be injected at one time.

Regular or crystalline insulin will maintain its potency for many months even at room temperature. Protamine zinc insulin is quite stable, but less so than clear varieties. Consequently, it is best to teach patients to keep their reserve supply in the refrigerator, allowing simply the bottle in current use to remain at room temperature. On the other hand, the loss of potency by protamine zinc insulin is slow enough that patients, away from home or living under unusual conditions in which the insulin cannot be kept in a cool place, may be assured that their insulin will maintain practically all of its potency, and any loss may be easily compensated for by slight increases in the number of units taken, depending, of course, upon the day-by-day urine tests for sugar. Insulin should not be used if it has been frozen.

The ideal method of sterilizing the insulin syringe and needle is. by boiling for five minutes. Patients who are away from home may find it difficult or impossible to sterilize their equipment by boiling.

For these, sterilization by alcohol (70 per cent by volume, isopropyl alcohol preferably, is necessary). Various traveling kits are on the market to meet this situation. Because of the time taken in water sterilization many patients use alcohol even at home. If this is done, a dish or strong test-tube or four ounce bottle provided with a cover can be used; this should be sterilized by boiling at least once a week and the alcohol changed. When removing the syringe and needle from the alcohol all traces of alcohol should be blown out by motion of the plunger. This is important because the alcohol may alter the protamine zinc insulin and besides may lead to irritation when introduced beneath the skin. Sterilization by alcohol must always be regarded as second best, and patients should be encouraged to sterilize by boiling when possible.

13. **Lipodystrophy (Insulin Atrophies).**—See page 597.

14. **Improvement of Diabetes to be Assumed in Planning Treatment With Insulin.**—Improvement of the diabetes and along with it of the condition of the patient will take place with almost any kind of intelligent diabetic treatment if faithfully followed. With insulin the possibilities for improvement have been greatly augmented and such gains both doctor and patient must be alert to recognize. Tolerance for carbohydrate may advance so rapidly that insulin reactions occur needlessly and occasionally the need for insulin disappears. In the very young and in the very old, insulin should be begun with small doses. The young, at the onset of their diabetes, and the old respond quickly to insulin, and by the use of small doses one escapes reactions which at the beginning of treatment one desires to avoid especially in these two age groups. Not uncommonly diabetic children respond so well to treatment with diet and insulin that one is puzzled to know whether they really do have diabetes after all. In such cases months may be necessary to clarify the diagnosis. And in elderly people persistence in a suitable dietetic régime with insulin yields such excellent results that it is easy to overdose the patient.

15. **Resistance to Insulin.**—From time to time, since the introduction of insulin, reports have appeared regarding rare individuals with whom extraordinarily large amounts of insulin have been required in order to control the diabetic condition. Thus in the patient of Levi and Friedman[1] in whom diabetes was accompanied by chronic lymphatic leukemia, 76,195 units were administered in forty-seven days; on four successive days, the patient received 4000 units in each twenty-four hours. Such patients have been described as exhibiting "resistance" or perhaps more properly, "insensitiveness," to insulin.[2] In certain of the cases reported in the literature some factor has been apparent to which it seemed reasonable to assign the responsibility for the condition. In others despite extensive study, at times including postmortem examination, no cause

[1] Levi and Friedman: New England Jour. Med., **225**, 975, 1941.
[2] Himsworth: Lancet, Loc. cit., p. 144.

for the high requirement of insulin has been found.[1]   In general, clinicians have not regarded an insulin dosage as extraordinarily high unless it exceeded 100 units daily and cases have not been regarded as "resistant" to insulin unless a daily requirement of 200 or more units of insulin existed over a considerable period of time.   In our own series, 7 such patients have been seen and studied to date.   The case histories of these patients are summarized briefly below.

1. Case 6247, a physician, aged fifty-two years, reported by Root,[2] was observed in Boston in 1927. At this time the urine was not sugar-free with 100 units of insulin daily. A few months later the insulin had to be increased until finally he was taking 1600 units of insulin a day in spite of which he died in coma. At autopsy advanced hemochromatosis involving the pancreas, liver and heart, as well as the skin was found.

2. Case 14483, reported by Marble,[3] was thirty-five years old when first seen. She had been troubled with generalized arthritis since 1926 and at the time of our first observation in 1935 she was already markedly crippled. Since then the arthritic process has continued to progress despite careful treatment directed by arthritic and orthopedic consultants. During a ten months' stay at the Deaconess Hospital in 1935 and 1936 many studies were carried out in an attempt to elucidate the cause of her high requirement for insulin which at one time reached 530 units a day (subsequently at home she took as much as 675 units in one day). No direct evidence was obtained to indicate a pituitary, adrenal, thyroid or gonadal influence as being responsible for the resistance to insulin. In addition to arthritis the patient has exhibited at one time or another marked general glandular enlargement, slight to moderate hepatomegaly and splenomegaly and eosinophilia of striking degree. During her initial stay in the hospital control of her condition was followed by a gratifying gain in weight and strength. In June, 1946, her diabetic condition was under good control with 100 to 125 units of insulin daily. Her arthritis was causing much crippling, discomfort and weakness.

3. Case 17269, male, aged thirty years, was first seen on September 30, 1938. He had had diabetes since January, 1931, and had usually taken a total of 50 units of insulin a day. For the four days prior to his admission to the Deaconess Hospital he had taken from 400 to 800 units of insulin daily and still had much sugar in the urine. In the hospital it was found that his high requirement was genuine; during the first twenty-four hours in the hospital he required 910 units of insulin and in the second twenty-four hours 750 units of insulin. Subsequently his requirement fell so that when last heard from in December 1945, his diabetic condition seemed under good control with 80 units of insulin daily. Detailed studies failed to disclose any cause for the remarkable resistance to insulin.

4. Case 17162, a clergyman, aged thirty-three years, with onset of diabetes in June, 1938, was first seen on September 19, 1938. At that time he spent ten days at the Deaconess Hospital and at discharge was asked to take 26 units of insulin daily. He was not seen again until December 31 when he entered the hospital in diabetic coma with a blood-sugar value of 0.92 per cent and a plasma CO_2 content of 8 volumes per cent. Large doses of insulin were required to bring about recovery from the acidosis and in the subsequent ten days larger doses than usual were necessary to keep the diabetic condition under control. However, he was apparently

[1] Glass, Spingarn and Pollack: Arch. Int. Med., **70**, 221, 1942.
[2] Root: New England Jour. Med., **201**, 201, 1929.
[3] Marble: Arch. Int. Med., **62**, 432, 1938.

in good condition when he left the hospital on January 11, 1939, with the advice to take 112 units of insulin daily. He was again admitted, however, on January 17 in diabetic coma. This time even larger amounts of insulin were required not only during the stage of acute illness but in the week following. Despite the fact, however, that on the preceding day he had received 482 units of insulin, on January 26 the patient was again in diabetic coma and in the next twenty-four-hour period 2312 units of insulin were necessary to overcome the acidosis. His requirement gradually fell in the following days, but even on February 23 he was still taking 1200 or more units daily. Many studies were carried out with this patient but no definite cause of the extraordinary insulin requirement was established. In December 1940 he was taking only 45 units of insulin a day. He died on December 31, 1943 of bronchopneumonia; autopsy disclosed fibrosis and atrophy of the pancreas, pancreatic calculi and fatty cirrhosis of the liver.

5. Case 15761, female, was first seen on June 13, 1937, at the age of forty. The onset of diabetes had been in January, 1935. Her diabetic life had not been extraordinary up until about April 1, 1939. She had spent sixteen days at the Deaconess Hospital in January, 1939; at that time her insulin requirement was 64 units of insulin daily. On or about April 1 she noted that her urine tests for sugar were poor despite increases of insulin dosage ordinarily used. Consequently she had increased the amount so that on the day before her admission on May 8 she had taken 502 units. She spent three months in the hospital in the summer of 1939. The insulin dosage was gradually increased until for a period of three weeks she took from 1700 to 2100 units of insulin daily. Following this her requirement gradually fell so that in August, 1940, her diabetes was under good control on 208 units of insulin daily. By March 1941 she had been able to reduce the daily dosage to 100 units or less and in the five succeeding years the requirement has remained between 50 and 100 units. With this patient as with the two just mentioned no cause for the remarkably high requirement for insulin was found. It is true that this patient exhibited pronounced local skin responses to most varieties of insulin. When last seen on March 29, 1946 her diabetic condition was under good control on a diet of C202, P88, F119, and 60 to 70 units of insulin daily. For about six months she had had considerable discomfort from rheumatoid arthritis affecting chiefly the fingers and wrists, but otherwise was in good general health.

6. Case 18425, male, with onset of diabetes in September, 1937, was first seen on September 11, 1939, at the age of thirty-nine. Since February, 1939 his insulin requirement had gradually increased. He was discharged from the Deaconess Hospital on October 4, 1939 on 226 units of insulin a day only to return two weeks later having found at home that he needed still larger amounts of insulin. During this second admission it was necessary to increase the amount of insulin as high as 690 units in one day. At discharge on November 16 he was advised to take 450 units a day. In July 1940 he was taking from 400 to 500 units of insulin daily and by November 1940 had reduced the amount to 275 units daily. Subsequently he was able to lower the dosage still further and for the last few years his requirement has averaged 125 units a day. When last heard from in April 1946, he was feeling well.

7. Case 22003, a sixty-two-year-old woman with diabetes of twenty years' duration, was admitted to the Deaconess Hospital on August 7, 1942. She had taken insulin intermittently since February 1940. Her dosage in October 1941 was 10 units of unmodified and 20 units of protamine zinc insulin daily. Thereafter her requirement gradually increased until over a period of months a total of 2900 units daily was reached. When admitted to the Deaconess Hospital on August 7, 1942, she was taking 2000 units

a day. When discharged on October 17 on a diet of C172, P104, F89, the diabetic condition was under satisfactory control on 750 units of U-500 unmodified insulin daily. Extensive studies had disclosed no cause for the remarkable insensitiveness to insulin, although delay in absorption from the subcutaneous spaces was suggested by observations using radioactive insulin[1] and by studies of the respiratory quotient[1] following glucose and insulin (the rise was greater after 200 units intravenously than after 400 units subcutaneously). Inelastic, thickened, firm and rather fibrous subcutaneous tissue over certain parts of the body of this patient undoubtedly affected the absorption of insulin. Dr. Francis C. Lowell in studies, results of which he has reported, found that this patient was resistant to both human and market insulin;[2] he found in her blood anti-insulin substances in low concentration.[3] The patient's insulin requirement gradually fell so that in October 1943 she was taking 200 units daily. When last heard from on June 8, 1946, she was taking from 190 to 220 units of insulin daily and was feeling well.

In addition to the 7 patients listed above, our own series includes a small group of patients in whom control of diabetes has necessitated the use of 100 to 150 units of insulin daily for long periods under ordinary circumstances. Still others have required from 100 to 1000 or more units during short periods, chiefly in the presence of acidosis or acute infections with high fever. An extraordinary example of the effect of infection and marked disturbance of liver function with jaundice is given in the following case history.

Case 19110 was 69.9 years old when first seen on June 17, 1940. The onset of symptoms of diabetes had been in January, 1940. Sugar had been found in the urine first in February at the time of a recurrence of jaundice, 6 attacks of which she had suffered in the preceding six years. Insulin was begun in February; in March she was taking 30 units daily. Suddenly in May the insulin requirement rose so that by June 18 she exhibited glycosuria despite 110 units daily. At the time of admission to the New England Deaconess Hospital the urine contained large amounts of sugar together with small amounts of diacetic acid. Larger and larger doses of insulin were given until on the day before cholecystectomy and choledochostomy on June 26, 530 units were administered. At operation cholecystitis and two large stones in the common bile duct were found. In the ten days following operation the amount of insulin given daily varied from 600 to 800 units, reaching a total of 1000 units on July 3. The requirement then gradually fell so that on July 14 the diabetic condition became reasonably well controlled on 92 to 116 units a day. Following operation the jaundice gradually cleared up and the general condition improved. In September 1940, the patient was feeling well, sugar-free and the insulin requirement had fallen to 18 units daily! A month later she was able to give up insulin entirely. When last heard from on April 18, 1946, she was feeling well and had taken no insulin since October 1940.

When the cause of a high requirement for insulin can be found it will fall under one of the following heads:

1. Acidosis.—In the ketosis and coma of uncontrolled diabetes a dose of insulin usually does not exert the same effect upon the blood

[1] Root, Irvine, Evans, Reiner and Carpenter: Loc. cit., p. 143.
[2] Lowell: Jour. Clin. Invest , 23, 225, 1944.
[3] Lowell: Jour. Clin. Invest., 23, 233, 1944.

sugar as can be demonstrated when the acidosis has been overcome; in fact, often the effect seen is only a fraction of that which would be obtained under ordinary conditions. The average case of diabetic coma requires about 200 units of insulin during the first twenty-four hours of treatment in order that recovery may take place and it is not uncommon to find need for 200 to 500 units during this period, particularly if the insulin is not given in large doses during the first three hours. (See page 453.) Doses of from 500 to 1000 units during the first twenty-four hours of treatment of coma are not unusual and occasionally amounts exceeding 1000 units are necessary.

2. Infections.—It is a matter of everyday experience that an acute infection may cause a flare-up in a diabetic condition with increase in blood and urinary sugar and a tendency to ketosis. In general, the more pronounced the infection the greater the effect seen upon the diabetes, although often a relatively mild infection such as a common cold without fever may produce a noticeable effect. Early in treatment patients must be taught to expect this and during infections to test the urine more frequently and to take additional insulin according to needs.

In Wayburn's[1] patient the extraordinarily large requirement of insulin was regarded as due to pulmonary tuberculosis.

In more prolonged or chronic infections, the insulin requirement may decrease as time goes on. Furthermore, as Greene and Keohen[2] have pointed out, the behavior of the insulin requirement in infections is not entirely uniform or predictable. They found that insulin resistance did not develop in all cases of infection or fever (including idiopathic fever, fever due to foreign protein injection and fever produced by the cabinet method) or to administration of histamine or epinephrine. The occurrence of an increased insulin requirement was not related to sex, age, height and duration of the fever or to the apparent toxemia. For some reason insulin resistance appeared to develop more frequently in mild than in severe cases.

3. Destructive processes in the pancreas with marked encroachment upon the insulin producing tissue as in cancer, hemochromatosis, calculi[3] and acute pancreatitis. However, it should be pointed out that the margin of safety as regards the pancreas is great since approximately nine-tenths of the gland must be removed in order to produce diabetes. Furthermore, even with complete removal of the pancreas in human subjects,[4] the insulin requirement appears not to be more than 40 or 50 units daily with individuals on a usual type of diabetic diet. This makes understandable the case reported by Urmy, Jones and Wood,[5] in which despite the fact that at

[1] Wayburn: Am. Jour. Med. Sci., 190, 157, 1935.
[2] Greene and Keohen: Jour. Am. Med. Assn., 121, 173, 1943.
[3] Mason: Jour. Clin. Invest., 9, 31, 1931.
[4] Waugh, Dixon, Clagett, Bollman, Sprague and Comfort: Loc. cit., p. 140.
[5] Urmy, Jones and Wood: Am. Jour. Med. Sci., 182, 662, 1931.

autopsy it was evident that 95 per cent of the islet tissue had been destroyed by the encroachment of an adenocarcinoma, only mild diabetes had developed during the last one and a half years of life. The diabetes was mild in Grafe's[1] case although at autopsy a cancer was found to involve the entire pancreas and on microscopic examination no normal tissue was found. It seems likely that at least part of the high insulin requirement seen occasionally, although by no means invariably, in patients with hemochromatosis[2,3] may be due to a disturbance of liver function incident to the cirrhosis. Mention has already been made of our patient with hemochromatosis whose insulin requirement amounted to 1600 units daily at the time of death. Our patients, Cases 3194 and 11558, whose pancreases weighed 15 and 12 grams, required daily only 80 and 28 units respectively.

4. Disturbance of liver function as a cirrhosis or in the chronic passive congestion of cardiac decompensation:[4] such complicating diseases may disturb the normal function of the liver. This organ is a great transforming agent not only of carbohydrate but also of protein and fat, storing, yielding up or modifying these substances as bodily needs arise. Interference with the function of the liver may well lead to a heightening of a diabetic condition.[5]

Mason and Sly[6] concluded that the insulin resistance of their patient was due to a marked lessening of the liver's ability to convert dextrose to glycogen or an intermediate product in this conversion. Boller and Uberrack[7] showed that enormous doses of insulin are often tolerated by patients with parenchymatous damage of the liver. Case 6533 reported by Root[8] with a severe, acute hepatitis, jaundice, anuria and acidosis required 500 units of insulin in one day, although her usual dose was only 30 units a day.

5. Complicating disease of endocrine glands other than the pancreas, notably the thyroid, the pituitary and the adrenals. It is possible that by excessive action of the secretion of the anterior pituitary gland and the adrenal cortex upon the liver, pancreas and peripheral tissues, an aggravation of the diabetic state may be produced and large amounts of insulin needed for correction of the abnormal processes. At the present time tests are not available to demonstrate disturbances of this type. In the diabetic patient of Pullen and Sodeman[9] insulin resistance was present together with many of the findings characteristic of Cushing's disease. The effect of an excess of a thyroid secretion appears to be clear cut; it seems

[1] Grafe: Metabolic Diseases and Their Treatment, Philadelphia, Lea & Febiger, p. 249, 1933.
[2] Engel: Klin. Wchnschr., 13, 1682, 1934.
[3] Gray: Ann. Int. Med., 19, 501, 1943.
[4] Pollack: Proc. Staff Meet. Mayo Clinic, 8, 453, 1933
[5] Strouse, Rosenbaum, Levy and Soskin: Jour. Clin. Endocrinology, 1, 831, 1941.
[6] Mason and Sly: Jour. Am. Med. Assn., 108, 2016, 1937.
[7] Boller and Uberrack: Klin. Wchnschr., 11, 671, 1932.
[8] Root: New England Jour. Med., 212, 545, 1935.
[9] Pullen and Sodeman: Jour. Clin. Endocrinology, 3, 345, 1943.

fairly well established that action here is upon liver stores causing increased formation of blood sugar.[1] Warvel's[2] patient, a girl, who received large amounts of insulin for ten months, was found at postmortem examination, after death in diabetic coma, to have a tumor of the pineal gland.

6. Resistance to insulin may be accompanied by urticaria and other allergic manifestations, including allergy to insulin itself. However, insulin resistance and allergy to insulin may exist independently.

The remarkable patient of Glassberg, Somogyi and Taussig[3] developed local and urticarial reactions first, and later, insulin resistance, with disappearance of skin reactions. Three hundred units of insulin were required to reduce her blood sugar from 0.30 to 0.08 per cent in three hours. Urticaria in Rudy's[4] patient, a woman aged sixty-five years, was accompanied by insulin resistance to the extent that whereas she had a few days before been sugar-free on a diet containing 100 grams of carbohydrate daily without insulin, during the period of urticaria she required 515 units of insulin in twenty-four hours. Cases of insulin resistance associated with allergy have been reported by Hart and Vicens[5] and Shepardson, Gable and Withrow.[6]

7. Other Causes.—In a high percentage of cases, no complicating condition may be apparent on which to place the blame for insulin resistance. Furthermore, in cases in which it appears likely that a recognized complication may be responsible for a high insulin requirement, it is difficult to be certain that such a connection exists. As a consequence, workers have attempted to uncover causes for insulin resistance not apparent on the surface and not represented by manifest disease. Thus, acting upon the knowledge that extracts of the anterior pituitary and adrenal cortex possess diabetogenic properties, attempts have been made to demonstrate an anti-insulin effect of the blood plasma of insulin resistant patients. Glen and Eaton,[7] Wayburn and Beckh[8] and Marble, Fernald and Smith[9] reported that the serum of certain insulin resistant patients had an insulin-antagonizing effect as shown by protection tests in mice or rabbits.

A second approach led Lowell[10] to conclude that insulin resistance may occur on an immunologic basis. He found in sera from two insulin resistant patients neutralizing antibodies for crystalline insulin which under certain circumstances exhibited species speci-

[1] Hills, Sharpe and Gray: Bull. Johns Hopkins Hosp., **55**, 193, 1934.
[2] Warvel: Personal communication to the authors.
[3] Glassberg, Somogyi and Taussig: Arch. Int. Med., **40**, 676, 1927.
[4] Rudy: New England Jour. Med., **204**, 791, 1931.
[5] Hart and Vicens: Jour. Clin. Endocrinology, **1**, 399, 1941.
[6] Shepardson, Gable and Withrow: Calif. and West. Med., **60**, 201, 1944.
[7] Glen and Eaton: Loc. cit., p. 128.
[8] Wayburn and Beckh: Jour. Clin. Endocrinology, **2**, 511, 1942.
[9] Marble, Fernald and Smith: Loc. cit., p. 128.
[10] Lowell: Proc. Soc. Exper. Biol. and Med., **50**, 167, 1942; loc. cit., p. 382.

25

ficity. Lowell regarded insulin-neutralizing and skin-sensitizing (allergic) antibodies as distinct. Lerman[1] likewise found antibodies (precipitins and passive-transfer antibodies) in the serum of patients with insulin resistance but concluded that they were antiharmonic. Lerman believed insulin resistance to be dependent upon the appearance and concentration in the body of antibodies to insulin. Lerman made the practical suggestion that repeated administration of insulin rather than its omission offers a means for overcoming insulin resistance.

For further discussion regarding insensitiveness to insulin (see p. 143); regarding allergy to insulin (see p. 464); and for articles regarding insulin resistance see the papers by Martin *et al.*,[2] Eichbaum,[3] Lozinski and Frohlich[4] and Schloss.[5]

16. **Insulin in Non-diabetic States.**—Although little is known concerning the effect of insulin upon the carbohydrate metabolism in non-diabetic persons it has been used in a variety of conditions including pregnancy, cardiac, thyroid and liver disease, peptic ulcers, acute infections and various skin affections. It may be useful, particularly when under nutrition is a problem. A temporary loss of carbohydrate tolerance during the administration of insulin under such circumstances has been noted in certain patients and also in experimental animals. However, in Blotner's studies the tolerance always returned to normal.

Thin undernourished individuals whose emaciation is due to poor appetite can be helped to take more food. The practice of using insulin in non-diabetic patients to increase weight began in 1923 and was soon adopted for non-diabetic tuberculous cases. The mode of its action is not entirely clear. Insulin is only one of many factors influencing appetite and nutrition and not all patients with tuberculosis react to its use in the same way. F. M. Allen advised beginning with 5 units three times a day and increasing to 40 units three times a day. The protection against shock depends not so much on large quantities of carbohydrate as the repeated administration of such small amounts as 10 grams. Occasionally much larger doses of insulin were given. Individualization of the dose should be emphasized and especially in cases where tuberculosis of the adrenals or liver is present. In such cases dangerous hypoglycemia may occur.

In general less is heard today than formerly of the therapeutic use of insulin to combat undernutrition.

See Blotner's article[6] for his own investigations and the articles of F. M. Allen[7] for a review of the literature.

[1] Lerman: Am. Jour. Med. Sci., **207**, 354, 1944.

[2] Martin, Martin, Lyster and Strouse: Jcur. Clin. Endocrinology, **1**, 387, 1941.

[3] Eichbaum: Folia Clinica et Biol. (São Paulo), **14**, 9, 1942.

[4] Lozinski and Frohlich: Canad. Med. Assn. Jour., **46**, 62, 1942.

[5] Schloss: Ann. Int. Med., **19**, 533, 1943.

[6] Blotner: Jour. Am. Med. Assn., **100**, 88, 1933.

[7] Allen: Am. Rev. Tuberc., **33**, 230, 1936. Allen, Douglass, Warren and Pottinger: Am. Rev. Tuberc., **33**, 257, 1936.

CHAPTER XI

HYPOGLYCEMIA DUE TO INSULIN.

REVISED BY ALEXANDER MARBLE, M.D. AND PRISCILLA WHITE, M.D.

A. Introduction.—Insulin reactions constitute one of the major problems in the treatment of diabetes. It is not an indifferent matter for a clergyman, a girl or a boy to be sent to jail upon the supposition that he or she is drunk or to a hospital as an epileptic; for students to fail in a long written or oral examination upon which a rating for the year depends; or for directors of large corporations to develop irritability, garrulousness, tremor or somnolence at an annual meeting of their boards. The fear of a reaction is almost worse than the actuality. Moreover, the dangers of a reaction to limb and life, the diabetic's and his companion's, apart from those which injure the reputation, are by no means trifling. The fatalities are few, although probably the unrecorded instances exceed in number those which have appeared in the literature.

Adlersberg and Dolger[1] bring out the fact that, because of mental and physical changes present during hypoglycemia, actions may be committed which are against law and accepted conventions and urge that some uniform legislative procedure be established to deal with such incidents. However, these considerations should not receive undue emphasis and one would agree whole-heartedly with the authors in concluding that: "The difficulties described should not stigmatize the diabetic patient as an inferior in our highly competitive society. It should be stated that the overwhelming majority of diabetics are capable of becoming an integral part of society, suffering no appreciable handicap, but on the contrary successfully fulfilling their obligations in all fields of human endeavor."

It is imperative that diabetic patients avoid frequent insulin reactions. Not only are they inconveniencing and embarrassing to the patient but their occurrence reflects upon the ability of diabetic individuals as a whole to take a normal part in everyday life. Among the disadvantages to the patient is the fact that, as brought out by Somogyi,[2] hypoglycemia induced by insulin leads to hyperglycemia because the process of hepatic glycogenolysis set in motion to correct the hypoglycemia overshoots the mark with the result that hyperglycemia results.

Even before the introduction of insulin, hypoglycemia had begun

[1] Adlersberg and Dolger: Loc. cit., p. 89.
[2] Somogyi: Proc. Soc. Exp. Biol. and Med., **38**, 51, 1938. See also Somogyi, Weichselbaum and Neinbrecker: Ibid., **37**, 62, 1937.

to appear as a serious factor in the treatment of diabetes. In 1921, 3 cases were reported under the title, "The Critical Period of Hypoglycemia in Undernutrition,"[1] and subsequently a fourth was rescued by Root from impending death by the giving of orange juice. Four similar cases occurred in neighboring clinics. See page 415.

B. **Symptoms.**—When, following an injection of insulin, an individual develops several symptoms of a group characterized by hunger, nervous instability, sweating, numbness or tingling of the tongue or lips, double vision, headache, faintness, tremor, unsteady gait, rapid heart action, somnolence or unconsciousness and convulsions, he is said to be having an insulin reaction. Such reactions appear most commonly three or four hours after a meal before which unmodified insulin has been given, but may occur in the interval between the administration of the insulin and the taking of food if that interval is unduly prolonged. They occur six to eight hours after the administration of globin insulin and nearer twenty-four hours after the administration of protamine zinc insulin. Lack of an adequate food supply, particularly carbohydrate, either in the diet or as a reserve stored in the body, favors an insulin reaction and the same effect would occur if the food were unutilized, remaining unabsorbed in the stomach or lost by diarrhea. Consequently a meager diet and emaciation make one susceptible. Likewise unusual or strenuous exercise by its demand for sources of energy may precipitate hypoglycemia. This is especially apparent if carbohydrate is deficient in the diet or if the amount of glycogen in the liver and muscles is low. In fact, anything which depletes glycogen stores, such as overaction of the endocrine glands —adrenals, thyroid, pituitary—or a drug like phloridzin, or anything which curtails the capacity for glycogen storage either in the liver, by its extirpation or disease, or in the muscles, as in progressive muscular dystrophy, will accomplish the same result. That ketonuria may occur in hypoglycemia has been emphasized by Somogyi[2] and Drey.[3]

The symptoms of an insulin reaction often are said to develop when the blood sugar is at a normal level or even above. Such instances have not come to the personal attention of the authors. It is true that sudden falls of the blood sugar from high levels to levels only slightly below 100 mg. per cent may give rise to symptoms of a reaction which would never be felt under ordinary conditions, and we are willing to concede that a temporary reaction hardly severe enough to demand treatment may then appear, but none of us recall even a situation of this type unless the blood sugar has fallen to at least 80 mg. per cent. From the very inauguration of

[1] Joslin: Med. Clin. North America, **4**, 1723, 1921.
[2] Somogyi: Jour. Biol. Chem., **141**, 219, 1941. Somogyi and Weichselbaum: Ibid., **145**, 567, 1942.
[3] Drey: Ann. Int. Med., **22**, 811, 1945.

treatment with insulin in 1922 we have endeavored to secure the blood for determination of sugar before administering carbohydrate for a supposed reaction. This policy has certainly lowered the number of supposed or feigned reactions in children. We are as insistent upon this rule today as we were twenty-four years ago.

The correctness of the above view is supported by the diminishing number of reports of alleged insulin reactions in the presence of hyperglycemia or even of a normal blood sugar. Falta[1] shared this belief.

Furthermore, patients often attribute symptoms, such as nervousness and sweating, directly due to intercurrent disease or complications, to insulin. Again confusion occurs in patients' minds regarding an insulin reaction when they note the characteristic symptoms and yet find that the urine contains sugar. They do not realize that the glycosuria demonstrated by their Benedict test may represent sugar which passed through the kidneys minutes or hours previously and then was retained with the urine in the bladder. In a true reaction a second freshly passed specimen of urine will be found to be sugar-free provided the bladder was thoroughly emptied at the previous micturition. At such times a therapeutic test of the genuineness of a reaction is the recovery following the giving of 5 to 20 grams of carbohydrate.

The severity of an insulin reaction is by no means definitely commensurate with the extent of the hypoglycemia. Sigwald[2] emphasized this point repeatedly. Particularly in children blood-sugar levels of 40 mg. per cent may be present without recognizable symptoms. Rabbits kept quietly at rest may exhibit low blood-sugar values without symptoms, only to have them appear at the clap of the hand. A diabetic in seemingly good condition jumped off a haymow in company with 30 other diabetics and instantly went into a reaction. However, this happened to none of the others. With necrosis of the mid-brain Högler and Zell[3] showed a lowering of the blood sugar in rabbits might be extreme without bringing on convulsions. Phenobarbital acts similarly. During a severe insulin reaction there may be actually no "true" sugar in the blood;[4] any blood-sugar value of 15 to 25 milligrams per cent obtained by methods currently used must be regarded as representing almost entirely, if not entirely, non-glucose reducing substances.

Rabinowitch and Peters[5] reported in 1929 the case of a young diabetic who had for six hours a "true" blood sugar of zero without symptoms! Maddock and Trimble[6] examined the blood of several

[1] Falta: P. 95, loc. cit., p. 85.
[2] Sigwald: L'Hypoglycemie, Paris, G. Doin et Cie, 1932.
[3] Högler and Zell: Ztschr. f. d. ges. exp. Med., **86**, 158, 1933.
[4] Dotti and Hrubetz: Jour. Biol. Chem., **113**, 141, 1936.
[5] Rabinowitch and Peters: Am. Jour. Med. Sci., **178**, 29, 1929.
[6] Maddock and Trimble: Jour. Am. Med. Assn., **91**, 616, 1928.

patients at hourly intervals for the content of sugar. They were astonished to find how frequently values as low as 50 milligrams per cent occurred with or without symptoms. Smith's[1] case had aglycemia but hypoglycemic symptoms were present. We have at times observed patients with "true" blood-sugar levels of zero or nearly so, but almost invariably with symptoms of hypoglycemia.

When a diabetic child becomes quiet, lacks interest and is unnaturally good; when an adult diabetic acts ambitionless, depressed and morose, or an elderly man or woman weak and faint, one should suspect that the blood sugar has fallen below normal. If the occasion is some hours after meals, particularly if the patient has had an active period of exercise, and if one learns that he took his usual dose of insulin and in haste ate less than usual, one feels reasonably sure that the suspected diagnosis is correct. The surmise changes to certainty if one finds a tremor of the hands with moisture in the palms and a few beads of sweat on the forehead. Diabetics in such a condition respond to questions like an automaton and give the impression that soon they may become unconscious or, quite the reverse, become emotionally unstable.

The question is often raised as to whether prolonged and frequent attacks of hypoglycemia lower the mentality permanently. We have no evidence that this is the case if the attacks are of brief duration. It is true that Case 18919, a woman aged forty-two years when seen in 1940, with diabetes of fifteen years' duration, showed such definite evidences of personality changes, loss of memory and inability to cerebrate normally six months after an attack of hypoglycemia with unconsciousness which lasted two weeks, that she required the constant supervision of a nurse. However, she was a chronic alcoholic and mentally unstable before the attack. (See reference to Störring, page 394.) Writing of prolonged attacks of hypoglycemia, Aitken[2] stated, "Although the intelligence quotient has been reported as dramatically improved[3] by the total relief of hyperinsulinism, some cases show marked residual deterioration." The persistence of serious mental changes is to be feared if hypoglycemia is prolonged by reason of the giving of insulin during a reaction mistakenly thought to be due to diabetic coma, as in the twenty-two-year old man described by Klein and Ligterink.[4]

In 40 healthy students aged seventeen to twenty-three years Davis[5] found that insulin in doses of 0.05 units per kilogram of body weight produced the most dysrhythmia in electroencephalograms in those subjects in whom preinsulin records indicated slow dysrhythmic activity. The incidence of epilepsy with abnormal

[1] Smith: Boston Med. and Surg. Jour., **195**, 663. 1926.
[2] Aitken: Med. Clin. North America, **20**, 393, 1936.
[3] Powell: Am. Med., **40**, 172, 1934.
[4] Klein and Ligterink: Arch. Int. Med., **65**, 1085, 1940.
[5] Davis: Arch. Neurol. and Psychiat., **49**, 186, 1943.

electroencephalographic tracings in insulin-treated diabetic children in our series amounted to 2.3 per cent. (See pp. 568 and 759.) Of 35 of our diabetic patients who had had frequent severe insulin reactions, 18 had abnormal electroencephalograms.[1]

C. **Symptoms Characteristic of Reactions Due to Protamine Zinc Insulin.**—The onset of symptoms following overdosage with protamine zinc insulin is usually slower and more gradual than that following regular or crystalline insulin. Whereas reactions due to the latter varieties occur usually within three or four hours after a given dose has been injected, those following protamine zinc insulin do not appear until within twelve to twenty-four hours after the injection. Since protamine zinc insulin is usually prescribed before breakfast this means that hypoglycemic attacks due to this type of insulin occur usually during the night time and particularly during the hours from midnight to morning. A patient who has received too large amounts of protamine zinc insulin may be awakened by symptoms of a reaction at from 2 to 6 A.M. or may be found in a stupor or unconscious state by his family in the morning when he does not arise at the usual hour. Another important feature is that treatment of reactions due to protamine zinc insulin may often require repetition at hourly or half-hourly intervals because of the persistence of the tendency to hypoglycemia.

Our continued experience with protamine zinc insulin has been that reactions are less common with this type of insulin than with the use of regular insulin alone. Lowrie and Foster[2] likewise reported that not only did reactions occur less frequently with protamine zinc insulin than with regular insulin, but they were in general less severe. The symptoms of reactions due to protamine zinc insulin occurred in the following order: nervousness and trembling, weakness, hunger, sweating, blurring of vision, headache, faintness, somnolence, dizziness, nausea, paresthesia, disorientation and coma. One patient had two attacks of transitory hemiplegia.

Symptoms following protamine zinc insulin often consist of headache, usually occipital, and mild nausea, rather than trembling, sweating, tachycardia, and the other symptoms of a more acute nature occurring with hypoglycemia following unmodified insulin. Occasionally the nausea may be marked and vomiting may occur. The family of Case 16333, a thirteen-year-old boy, were awakened at 3 A.M. by shrieks from the boy's room. Hurrying there, they found the patient in convulsions and vomiting. With much effort orange juice was administered but soon vomited. Other attempts were made to give carbohydrate but vomiting continued until the patient was admitted to the New England Deaconess Hospital at 8 A.M. Apparently enough carbohydrate had been absorbed to overcome stupor and convulsions. Following the giving of food

[1] Greenblatt, Murray and Root: New England Jour. Med., **234**, 119, 1946.
[2] Lowrie and Foster: Am. Jour. Digest. Dis., **7**, 101, 1940.

at the hospital his vomiting ceased, the nausea cleared up, and his further course was uneventful.

The difference in the clinical picture of reactions due to insulin and protamine insulin are what one would expect. With protamine insulin the symptoms as a rule come on more slowly, are more easily recognized by the patient, are less severe, and treatment must be repeated hourly. However, it is because of the seemingly innocuousness of the symptoms that danger exists. The patient may drift into unconsciousness and one can conceive of a fatal issue. Fortunately, this did not occur with Mary Q., Case 4715, aged sixteen years, diabetes of eleven years' duration in 1936. Following two days of mountain climbing during which her father expertly averted trouble by adjustments of diet and regular and protamine insulin, she returned home and the next day took a nap after a noon luncheon. She was later discovered unconscious and six hours passed before recovery supervened. In this instance the diabetes as a whole had improved so much from exercise, plus diet and insulin, that the favorable effect of all three was prolonged. Perhaps with regular insulin alone, the distressing incident would not have taken place. When last heard from in April, 1946, the patient, now almost twenty-six years of age, was in good condition, taking 67 units of insulin daily.

A clever diabetic college graduate, Case 7736, undergoing an exercise test following transfer to protamine insulin, slipped into an insulin reaction and later was discovered as "an unknown male" admission at the Boston City Hospital, promptly diagnosed and quickly relieved. If so intelligent a patient as he was caught unawares, how easily this might happen with others.

D. **Classification of Symptoms.**—The symptoms of hypoglycemia, particularly relating to the nervous system, were thoroughly studied and classified by J. Wilder[1] and amplified by Falta.[2] They can be grouped in three types according as to whether they concern the (a) vegetative (sympathetic) nervous system, (b) the central nervous system, or (c) are psychical.

(a) **Sympathetic Nervous System.**—Belonging in this group are: (1) Hunger and faintness. (2) Muscular weakness. Motion of arms and legs, speech and even standing may be difficult. The extremities are as "heavy as lead." Tremor may be pronounced. A little three-year-old's hand trembled as he tried to raise his baby spoon to his mouth. Taubenhaus and Schwarz[3] measured the tone of the biceps muscle in fasting healthy persons following the injection of insulin and found that this fell along with the blood sugar, independent of accompanying hypoglycemic symptoms. After the giving

---

[1] Wilder, J.: Deutsch. Ztschr. f. Nervenh., **112**, 192, 1929; Klinik und Therapie der Zuckermangelkrankheit, Leipzig, Weidman & Co., 1936.

[2] Falta: P. 118, loc. cit., p. 85.

[3] Taubenhaus and Schwarz: Wien. Arch. f. inn. Med., **30**, 271, 1937.

of sugar the muscle tone rose to its original value. It appears that the decrease in tone occurs before any other hypoglycemic symptom. (3) Sweating. Beads of sweat may appear on the forehead and the palms, soles and axillæ often become moist. The night clothes may be drenched, and if this occurs after an operation, leads to confusion with surgical shock. Sweating is a valuable differential diagnostic sign between an insulin reaction and diabetic coma. (4) The pulse and blood-pressure vary with the stage of the reaction and the epinephrin response. There may be definite, though almost invariably temporary, changes in the electrocardiogram. (See pages 516 and 519.) (5) A leukocytosis is not infrequent although one does not see values as high as in diabetic coma. (6) Vomiting, representing, according to Falta,[1] a lowered tone in the splanchnic area and pains in the lower abdomen are uncommon (except that nausea and vomiting may occur in association with hypoglycemia due to protamine zinc insulin), whereas (7) paresthesiæ, such as numbness of the lips, are common. Falta adds, as less common symptoms and signs, salivation, lacrimation, and desire to urinate.

(b) **Central Nervous System.**—(1) Those of bulbo-pontine character include chiefly disturbances of speech, inability to formulate words but ability to understand, mask-like facies, and slowness to react or lack of reaction of, or dilatation of, the pupils. (2) Symptoms of corticospinal origin include: Jacksonian twitchings, double vision, mono- and hemiplegias, loss of reflexes, positive Babinski, involuntary micturition or defecation, severe tonic or clonic cramps (at times epileptiform), aphasia, amnesia, apraxia, and occasionally hallucinations. (3) Striothalamic symptoms may be akinetic or hyperkinetic. The patient knows he should take his sugar, but cannot take it out of his pocket and put it into his mouth. He may exhibit a fixed gaze and glassy eyes. Hyperkinetic symptoms include: athetotic or choreiform motions, grimaces, loud speaking, a compulsion to cry, laugh, or be ridiculous. (4) Central vegetative signs include: variations in regulation of temperature, somnolence, faintness, collapse, and temporary blindness.

(c) **Psychical Manifestations.**—These include loss of consciousness and may be followed by prolonged stupor. A patient may be stuporous rather than comatose; although he understands what is said to him, he cannot bring himself to expression. Other signs include catatonia and a state of excitement which may merge into actual dementia. Confusion with alcoholism is easy and therefore diabetics should leave alcohol alone. Psychoses, periods of hysteria, anxiety and depression, and attacks of violence, or attempts at suicide may occur.

Himwich's[2] classification, based on Frostig's[3] observations in

---

[1] Falta: P. 91, loc. cit., p. 85.
[2] Himwich: Am. Jour. Digest. Dis., **11**, 1, 1944.
[3] Frostig: Am. Jour. Psychiat., **96**, 1167, 1940.

insulin-treated schizophrenics, divides hypoglycemic symptoms in 5 groups whose unvaried order of appearance is explained on the basis of the metabolic rate of each region in the brain.[1] According to Himwich, first to suffer from sugar deprivation are, phylogenetically speaking, the newest portions of the brain, the cerebral hemispheres and parts of the cerebellum, which metabolize at the highest rate. Then, in turn, each succeeding lower portion of the brain becomes involved. The medulla oblongata, the oldest part of the brain and the portion with the lowest metabolic rate, functions long after higher centers are able to do so. The 5 phases described by Himwich are: (*a*) cortical, (*b*) subcorticodiencephalic, (*c*) mesencephalic, (*d*) premyelencephalic and (*e*) myelencephalic. Naturally the fifth stage is the most dangerous and is recognized by deep coma and the predominance of parasympathetic signs. The patient's respiration is shallow, the heart rate is slow, the skin is pale and the pupils are contracted, no longer reacting to light. Perspiration and a subnormal temperature are present. The muscles are relaxed, the tendon jerks depressed and the corneal reflex entirely lost. Prompt treatment is imperative.

Störring,[2] in an analysis of 1200 insulin-treated diabetics, found that neurovegetative symptoms were common in hypoglycemia, whereas purely psychotic symptoms were rare. He concluded that psychotic symptoms occur only in patients with an hereditary background of psychosis.

Weber and Blum[3] in reporting a case of acute pulmonary edema combined with hypoglycemic coma, discuss the physical signs of hypoglycemia. Harrison and Finks[4] emphasize that hypoglycemia may be the trigger factor producing arrhythmias, angina, hypertensive encephalopathies, carotid sinus syncope and circulatory disturbances of the menopause.

E. **Fatal Cases During Insulin Reaction.**—No patient has died at the Deaconess Hospital of hypoglycemia due to insulin. However, Case 6884, a young woman aged 29.9 years, with diabetes of 16.6 years' duration, developed a reaction at the Deaconess Hospital while undergoing treatment for diabetic neuritis which, eventually, proved fatal. Her death occurred in the nearby Psychopathic Hospital on October 5, 1944, where she was transferred after several weeks of a vegetative existence at the Deaconess. Senile plaques were found in the brain in addition to diffuse vascular disease and intercapillary glomerulosclerosis. Three of our patients, living many miles away and not under our direct care, have died following an overdose of insulin. In addition 4 others seen in consultations have succumbed—one, a young girl, in the course of thirty-six

[1] Himwich and Fazekas: Am. Jour. Physiol,, **132**, 454, 1941.
[2] Störring: Deutsch. med. Wchnschr., **1**, 10, 1937.
[3] Weber and Blum: Jour. Neurol. and Psychiat., **5**, 37, 1942.
[4] Harrison and Finks: Am. Heart Jour., **26**, 147, 1943.

hours, never recovered from unconsciousness after being given 200 units of insulin when found unconscious as the result of a reaction which the attending physician mistook for diabetic coma; another, a young man, similarly after 60 units; and the third, a child, after an exhausting illness when the apathy, extreme weakness and unconsciousness were ascribed to the illness and left untreated. The diagnosis in this last case was missed in an excellent clinic partly because sympathy for the child delayed a venous blood-sugar test and partly because at that time a method for a capillary blood test was not available.

A fourth patient, a school teacher, returned to her home at 6:30 P.M. and behaved queerly. When a physician arrived thirty minutes later she was unconscious and having convulsions. Unable to obtain a urine test, he diagnosed coma and gave 200 units of insulin during the night. The next day the hypoglycemia was recognized and treated with intravenous glucose until the blood sugar was well above normal, but she died.[1]

A fifth[2] case developed hypoglycemia every afternoon, unrecognized, because the blood sugar was tested only before breakfast, and the dose of insulin increased each day because the fasting blood sugar was high. She recovered consciousness with 10 grams glucose given intravenously, lapsed one hour later but again recovered with a second such injection. One hour later she again lapsed into unconsciousness and died when glucose injection was delayed.

The sixth case was a man of 76.3 years, duration of diabetes 5.2 years, who had taken insulin 4.5 years and protamine or protamine zinc insulin for the preceding 3.7 years. Arriving at a friend's house after a long railroad journey in the late morning he drove about the country, sight-seeing and probably was without food several hours longer than usual. He acted queerly just before lunch, became violent, and then lapsed into unconsciousness; when he did not recover with 10 to 25 grams glucose intravenously and failed to swallow, the physician, thinking he was in diabetic coma, gave a "good shot" of insulin. Death occurred five days later, despite large quantities of glucose subcutaneously, and the autopsy revealed nothing definite except possible capillary hemorrhages in the brain. The seventh case, age sixteen years, became unconscious suddenly. When the blood sugar was found to be 39 mg. per cent, 450 grams glucose were given in divided doses in twelve hours. She was seen by one of us in consultation on the fifth day, but death occurred on the sixth day of unconsciousness, July 7, 1940.

The experience of workers using insulin shock treatment for schizophrenia has been that occasionally patients remain comatose even after sufficient glucose has been given by gavage and

---

[1] Root: Compt. rend. de Cong. franc. de méd., XXIIIe Session, Quebec, 1934, Paris, Masson et Cie, p. 136, 1935.
[2] Root: Lancet, ii, 544, 1926.

intravenously to raise the blood sugar to abnormally high levels. This condition of protracted coma is a dangerous complication. In patients recovering, the coma may persist for hours, days, or weeks, gradually merging into a state of catatonic stupor before awakening. In certain patients fever, rapid pulse and respiration, convulsions, vomiting, and diarrhea may occur. Death or permanent brain damage may result. An interesting observation which has been made in this connection is that not infrequently following recovery from protracted coma dramatic psychiatric improvement takes place.[1]

It is rare indeed for a single dose of insulin even though quite large to have serious consequences. Almost invariably if the patient is kept warm and no more insulin is given recovery will take place in time. This does not apply, of course, to the enormous doses given in the insulin shock treatment for schizophrenia. Case 1542, a woman, aged sixty years, the first patient in New England to receive insulin, in August, 1922, repeated by mistake her morning dose of insulin which consisted of 6 units of crystalline and 36 units of protamine zinc insulin. She was alone in the house. Unconsciousness resulted and continued from 11 A.M. to 4 P.M. when spontaneous recovery took place. There were no unpleasant sequelæ. Dr. F. B. Peck of Eli Lilly & Co. told us of a patient who was given 200 units of protamine zinc insulin in one dose. She was treated in a hospital and given frequent feedings. No ill effects were observed but no insulin was necessary for the following three days. The real hazard in such patients is that the unconsciousness of the insulin reaction be confused with that of diabetic coma and more insulin given.

Bowen and Beck[2] collected 19 fatal cases of insulin reactions in the literature, and Sigwald enumerated 24 cases.[3] Falta[4] referred to an instance of drowning during an attack of hypoglycemia. Lawrence, Meger and Nevin[5] report 6 fatal cases and Roche[6] 2 fatal cases. Mann considers deaths due to lack of glucose in the nervous system.

The prognosis of an insulin reaction is almost invariably good if it is diagnosed reasonably early. Early recognition is vital as the foregoing cases show. For this reason Table 51 (see page 444) is inserted, because it contains the salient points of differential diagnosis between an insulin reaction and diabetic coma. The prognosis, however, is by no means that of the disease *per se* but rather is de-

[1] Wortis and Lambert: Am. Jour. Psych., **96**, 335, 1939.
[2] Bowen and Beck: Ann. Int. Med., **6**, 1412, 1933.
[3] Sigwald: Loc. cit., p. 389.
[4] Falta: Klin. Wchnschr., **14**, 697, 1935.
[5] Lawrence, Meger and Nevin: Quart. Jour. Med., **11**, 181, 1942.
[6] Roche: Brit. Med. Jour., **2**, 35, 1942.
[7] Mann: Jour. Am. Med. Assn., **126**, 467, 1944.

pendent upon the doctor who treats it and the physical injury to which the reaction may expose the patient.

If a patient has a convulsion, one worries, fearing organic damage to the central nervous system. Residual signs, local paralysis, hemiplegia are alarming, although they may disappear within twenty-four hours. Allan and Crommelin[1] and Murphy and Purtell[2] each reported a child with evidence of residual cerebral damage. In certain cases a fall during a reaction or a supposed reaction complicates the picture because it may have nothing to do with a reaction, but prove to be a cerebral hemorrhage to which prolonged diabetes made the diabetic susceptible. The differential diagnosis here includes traumatic hemorrhage.

Any clinic in which large numbers of diabetic patients are treated is confronted often with insulin reactions, not only in patients in the hospital, but in those previously, often quite recently, discharged. It is for this reason we ask our patients to carry an identification card in their pocket. This reads as follows:

> I am a Diabetic.
> Am I in insulin shock or diabetic coma?
>
> If sugar, orange juice or sweetened fluids do not cause definite improvement in fifteen minutes, please call a doctor or send me *immediately* to a hospital.

It is much better to prevent than to be obliged to treat an insulin reaction. Insistence upon 5 grams of carbohydrate between meals and upon retiring with an extra dose within two hours after a meal if an automobile is to be driven is good prophylaxis. Diabetics taking insulin should avoid alcohol.

Never blame insulin for a death unless to good clinical evidence is added the corroboration of a skilful and complete postmortem examination! Case 2528, a twenty-six-year-old woman with diabetes of over fifteen years' duration, died suddenly eleven days after an appendectomy just as she was about to be discharged from the hospital. Although at the time it was suggested that an insulin reaction might have been the cause of sudden death, autopsy disclosed a pulmonary embolism. Another example was afforded in the experience with Case 1500 whose wife telegraphed as follows: "P. B. died early today from bad insulin reaction." We all doubted the accuracy of the diagnosis and although a partial autopsy had been performed to carry out our patient's desire to give us his pancreas, a second postmortem examination was carried out the next day although it necessitated a trip of over 400 miles. It proved well worth while because it revealed a typical acute coronary occlusion. The frothing at his lips, noted when he was found dying in the

[1] Allan and Crommelin: Jour. Am. Med. Assn., **118**, 373, 1942.
[2] Murphy and Purtell: Am. Jour. Digest. Dis., **10**, 103, 1943.

middle of the night, was due to pulmonary edema, rather than to a convulsion. Deaths from insulin reactions have, in our experience occurred only after symptoms lasting for some hours rather than suddenly. This patient had taken regular insulin for fourteen years; the onset of diabetes had been at the age of forty-one and death at sixty-three years.

At times it may be most difficult to decide whether or not hypoglycemia was responsible for death. An instance in point is Case 5896, aged twenty years, with onset of diabetes at the age of eight and eight-tenths years, who was found dead on the floor of her apartment in a Southern city. She had apparently been dead for three days and the possibility arose that she had died from an overdose of insulin. However, there were no data either in a clinical or a laboratory way to support this diagnosis. No autopsy was done. The patient had been married for about a year and was about four months pregnant at the time of her death. She was taking 58 units of unmodified insulin a day. She was seen by a prominent physician five days before she was found dead, at which time the urine was free from sugar, although it did contain a faint trace of ketone bodies. Apparently she was doing well diabetically, was feeling fine, and was happy.

Likewise doubt must exist as to the cause of death of Case 13859 who died at the age of forty-seven and seven-tenths years after five years of diabetes. This man was given in a hospital 40 units of insulin at about 11 A.M. because of the finding of a large amount of sugar in the urine. It was not known at this time that the fasting blood sugar was 128 mg. per cent. The patient died at 2 P.M., three hours after the insulin had been given. No autopsy was performed.

The widespread use of the insulin shock treatment for schizophrenia introduced by Sakel in 1928 has afforded much opportunity for studies of the changes taking place in the body as the result of the administration of large doses of insulin. To summarize adequately all of the contributions would require much space. In a supplement to the May, 1938, number of the *American Journal of Psychiatry* were published the Proceedings of the 89th Meeting of the Swiss Psychiatric Association a year before. This meeting was given over to the discussion of the treatment of schizophrenia with insulin and cardiazol. Sixty-eight different communications on all phases of the subject are included in the supplement.[1]

Allen[2] states that no animal ever succumbs to insulin hypoglycemia while eating up to the capacity of a normal hungry individual of the species, since loss of appetite always precedes any dangerous symptoms. The insulin dosage which can be tolerated without intoxication varies according to the species; for a strong man it

---

[1] Am. Jour. Psych., vol. **94**, Suppl., 1938.
[2] Allen: New England Jour. Med., **219**, 77, 1938.

is probably 15 units per kilogram and somewhat less for the dog and cat. For the rabbit it is 35 to 40 units per kg., for the mouse 1000, and for the rat 2000 to 4000 units, and for birds still higher. Tietz[1] and co-workers found a consistent rise in blood adrenalin during the deep stages of insulin coma with a drop after termination. In one patient who failed to arouse when sugar was given by gavage, the blood adrenalin continued high but fell following the administration of glucose intravenously. The latter procedure immediately aroused the patient. Keyes[2] studied the changes in the components of the blood serum in otherwise normal male schizophrenic patients undergoing insulin shock treatment. At the height of the reaction the following changes were noted: (1) a moderate increase of protein, (2) a marked increase in potassium, (3) in all but one case a significant decrease in non-protein nitrogen, and (4) in all but one case a slight rise in the sodium. Studies in dogs give similar results. The changes in the serum potassium were ascribed in large part to adrenal hyperactivity in response to hypoglycemia. Haid[3] reported a fall in blood calcium.

Various workers have studied the anatomical changes brought about by prolonged hypoglycemia. These consist almost entirely of abnormalities in the central nervous system seen only on microscopic examination. Weil, Liebert and Heilbrunn[4] found that rabbits dying in insulin convulsions showed marked disintegration of ganglion cells with liquefaction, vacuolization, and homogenization. Weeks or months after repeated insulin shocks there was evidence of marked shrinkage of the cytoplasm and nuclei. Zimmerman[5] studied the lesions of the nervous system in cats following large doses of insulin. The anatomical lesions included widespread cortical necrosis affecting the ganglion cells. When the hypoglycemia was of short duration the changes were apparently reversible and the animals recovered functionally and anatomically. Yannet[6] also studied the effect of insulin hypoglycemia on cats. In the muscles he found no significant changes in the distribution of water or potassium during or after severe hypoglycemia. In the brain, however, there was a shift of water from the extracellular spaces into the cells. Of the animals surviving the hypoglycemia, about one-half showed no central nervous system lesions. Chemically a significant loss of intracellular potassium could be demonstrated. The other half of the surviving animals showed evidence of widespread cerebral damage with marked loss of cellular water leading to shrinkage of the cells and decrease in the concentration of intracellular potassium. The total water content of the brain remained the same.

[1] Tietz, Dornheggen and Goldman: Endocrinology, **26**, 641, 1940.
[2] Keyes: Am. Jour. Physiol., **123**, 608, 1938.
[3] Haid: Ztschr. f. klin. Med., **139**, 485, 1941.
[4] Weil, Liebert and Heilbrunn: Arch. Neurol. and Psychiat., **39**, 467, 1938.
[5] Zimmerman: Arch. Path., **28**, 276, 1939.
[6] Yannet: Arch. Neurol. and Psychiat., **42**, 237, 395, 1939.

Moersch and Kernohan[1] found at autopsy in 2 cases of islet-cell tumor of the pancreas multiple petechial hemorrhages and degeneration of some of the nerve cells. Layne and Baker[2] point out that any associated chronic disease that might affect the brain, such as alcoholism, arteriosclerosis, or prolonged chronic infection, will tend to make the patient much more susceptible to irreversible cerebral changes when marked hypoglycemia develops.

Sahs and Alexander[3] reviewed twenty-five articles describing changes in the brain brought about by hypoglycemia. They summarize these changes as follows: "irregular dilatation of intracerebral vessels, indicating varying degrees of sluggish flow; multiple thrombi and perivascular extravasations, notably in the basal ganglia and medulla oblongata, but involving other areas as well; foci of blanching in the central and upper parietal regions of the cortex, and interstitial edema, with swelling of oligodendroglia cells in the cerebral white matter. . . . Evidence is present to support the anoxic theory of hypoglycemic shock." Himwich, Bowman, Wortis and Fazekas[4] studied the metabolism of the brain by determining the glucose and oxygen content of the blood collected simultaneously from the internal jugular vein and the femoral artery. They found that the oxygen utilization of the brain, and, therefore, its metabolic rate were decreased during severe hypoglycemia. Soskin[5] points out that marked hypoglycemia drives the available supply of sugar from the blood, below the minimal requirements of the tissues. Under such conditions the *muscle* may have recourse to its stored glycogen, or may perhaps turn to protein and fat as a source of energy, but *nerve tissue* has little stored carbohydrate and cannot utilize protein or fat. Therefore nerve tissue during marked hypoglycemia is unable to maintain even the minimal rate of metabolism compatible with well-being. Thus prolonged insulin hypoglycemia may lead to irreversible damage to the central nervous system.

F. **Treatment of Insulin Reactions.**—Treatment of an insulin reaction is simple and 5 or 10 grams of glucose orally usually relieve the patient in a few minutes. Lower concentrations (5 per cent) of glucose orally produced more rapid recoveries than high concentrations (30 per cent) in the experience of Golden and Goldfarb.[6] Occasionally three times as much is required, and sometimes it is necessary to inject the glucose intravenously in which case, as a rule, the response is so prompt that before 10 cc. of a 50 per cent solution are introduced recovery has occurred. Indeed, the effect is sometimes so prompt and startling as to lead one to wonder how

[1] Moersch and Kernohan: Arch. Neurol. and Psychiat., **39**, 242, 1938.
[2] Layne and Baker: Minnesota Med., **22**, 771, 1939.
[3] Sahs and Alexander: Arch. Neurol. and Psychiat., **42**, 286, 1939.
[4] Himwich, Bowman, Wortis and Fazekas: Science, **86**, 271, 1937. Himwich Frostig, Fazekas and Hadidian: Am. Jour. Psych., **96**, 371, 1939.
[5] Soskin: Arch. Neurol. and Psychiat., **42**, 563, 1939.
[6] Golden and Goldfarb: Proc. Soc. Exper. Biol. and Med., **51**, 134. 1942.

so little carbohydrate could accomplish so great a miracle. The longer the period of an insulin reaction and the unconsciousness, the more carbohydrate is required, and in one of the fatal cases seen in consultation 200 grams of glucose were given intravenously and subcutaneously before the blood sugar began to rise. Even then the damage may be done and the condition irremediable.

If the patient will not swallow, glucose can be introduced by catheter through the nose. We have known no harm to result, but we have been told of liquids forced upon patients during a reaction and entering the lungs. Glucose, corn syrup, molasses, and honey have all been used. Corn syrup can be given diluted with twice its volume of water by rectum, but its efficacy is questionable. Warm liquids are preferable to cold.

Various substitutes for glucose, such as levulose and cane sugar, have been tried, but none are quite as good. Of course, for the mild group of symptoms, which accompanies a slight lowering of the blood sugar, carbohydrate in any form, and even protein, might suffice. Food requiring time for digestion and absorption is preferable in the *prophylaxis* of insulin shock.

Adrenalin will mobilize glucose in the blood provided glycogen is available in the body. Consequently one can give to an adult, in a reaction which has occurred not too many hours after a meal, 1 cc. of 1 to 1000 solution of adrenalin or one-half this dose for a child. Pituitary extract (solution of posterior pituitary, surgical, U.S.P.) in dosage of 0.3 to 0.5 cc. subcutaneously is likewise helpful. Even if the injection of adrenalin or pituitrin is effective, it should be followed by carbohydrate, because otherwise the recovery might be temporary.

The injection of potassium salts to alleviate the symptoms of hypoglycemia has been suggested.[1] The basis of this type of therapy is the fact that when insulin is given to either normal or diabetic individuals the serum potassium falls along with the blood sugar.[2] As Talbott and Schwab[3] remark, potassium appears to have a biological action antagonistic to that of insulin. Incidentally, according to McQuarrie, sodium (as chloride) exerts a favorable, although perhaps temporary, influence on the carbohydrate metabolism of diabetic children taking simplified diets low in potassium.

Cases of extreme hypoglycemia with convulsions are treated with glucose, but if the low blood sugar has been present for a long time, in addition we insert a cannula into a vein and give 5 per cent glucose constantly along with 4 cc. of 1 to 1000 adrenalin per 1000 cc. of glucose solution. Indeed, if consciousness does not return promptly (or within one hour) we employ constant intravenous administration of 10 per cent glucose solution to maintain the blood sugar at a level

[1] McQuarrie, Thompson and Anderson: Jour. Nutrition, 11, 77, 1936.
[2] Kerr: Jour. Biol. Chem., 78, 35, 1938.
[3] Talbott and Schwab: New England Jour. Med., 222, 585, 1940.

of approximately 200 mg. per cent.   The use of hypertonic solutions of sodium chloride, sucrose, or sorbitol may be tried to combat cerebral edema, if lumbar puncture indicates its presence.   Oxygen under positive pressure is indicated if the patient has cyanosis. Suction may be necessary to aspirate fluid in bronchi resulting from pulmonary edema.   Fresh whole blood, 500 cc., may be used to supply respiratory enzymes since a toxic action of hypoglycemia on the respiratory enzymes of the brain has been shown by Komesarenko and Maevskajo.[1]   Sodium phenobarbital or other barbiturates are valuable as anticonvulsants.

One should not hesitate to seek aid in the treatment of patients with profound and prolonged hypoglycemia.   Our severest case to recover did so with the help of consultants with special training in anesthesia, laryngology and neurology.

[1] Komesarenko and Maevskajo: Jour. Med. Ukraine, **10**, 1145, 1940.

CHAPTER XII.

HYPERINSULINISM.

By Alexander Marble, M.D.

A. INTRODUCTION.

Hyperinsulinism is a condition in which, because of excessive secretion by the islands of Langerhans of the pancreas, spontaneous hypoglycemia is present; this develops upon fasting, and with physical activity the tendency is greater. It is relieved by food and, in the well-nourished individual, slightly and transiently by the injection of adrenalin or pituitary extract. The symptoms are much the same as those caused by an overdose of injected insulin and vary quite as much from person to person and from attack to attack as is true in hypoglycemia artificially produced. Characteristically the patient with hyperinsulinism suffers periods of nervousness, trembling, sweating, weakness, unsteadiness of gait, emotional instability, inability to concentrate, bizarre behavior, mental confusion, and often increasing drowsiness leading up to total unconsciousness with or without convulsions. The condition is seen in its most definite form in those patients possessing an islet-cell tumor of the pancreas. Hyperinsulinism without tumor is said to exist and is considered to be due to general hypertrophy or hyperplasia of islet tissue. However, the diagnosis of functional hyperinsulinism is by no means as satisfying as that of hyperinsulinism with tumor. At any rate, the term "hyperinsulinism" should be reserved for that state in which excessive secretion of insulin occurs due to overactivity of islet tissue.[1] In the differential diagnosis between hyperinsulinism and other forms of chronic hypoglycemia, one must consider particularly diseases of the liver affecting glycogen storage and conditions associated with hypofunctioning of the adrenal cortex, the anterior lobe of the pituitary and the thyroid.

B. TUMORS OF ISLANDS OF LANGERHANS.

1. **Incidence.**—Although, in 1926, Warren[2] was able to collect 20 instances of adenoma of the islands of Langerhans, the clinical significance of the finding was not appreciated at that time. It is true that, in 1924, Harris[3] had described a syndrome which was termed "hyperinsulinism," but it was not until 1927 that the first case of hypoglycemia (with recurring attacks of convulsions and

[1] Gorsuch and Rynearson: Med. Clin. North America, **28**, 985, 1944.
[2] Warren: Loc. cit., p. 197, ref. 5.
[3] Harris: Jour. Am. Med. Assn., **83**, 729, 1924.

unconsciousness and fatal issue in hypoglycemia), due to a tumor (carcinoma) of the islands of Langerhans, was reported with operative and necropsy findings by Wilder and associates from the Mayo Clinic.[1] During the last few weeks of the patient's life the hypoglycemia was so severe as to necessitate the taking of 1000 grams of cane sugar daily. Metastases in the liver developed, and potent insulin was obtained subsequently from these. This finding, incidentally, was conclusive proof that insulin is the product of the beta cells of the islands of Langerhans. The first report of the cure of a patient by surgical removal of a tumor (carcinoma) of the island cells of the pancreas was made in 1929 by Howland, Campbell, Maltby and Robinson.[2]

Since these early reports, the literature on the subject has become voluminous, partly because of repetitions in the publication of cases. Whipple and Frantz[3-8] have kept a register of reported cases and have published from time to time critical summaries of the accumulated experience. In reviewing the literature for a paper submitted for publication March 16, 1944, Frantz[7] found a total of 149 cases of islet cell tumor with hypoglycemia. Of the 149, 106 were shown to be benign, 28 were questionably malignant and 15 were proven malignant since there were metastases in adjacent organs. It should be noted that the cases referred to represent those with hypoglycemia; pancreatic tumors, having all the morphological characteristics of islet-cell growths, are found at operation and autopsy, in patients without clinical or laboratory evidence of hypoglycemia.

2. **Pathology.**—Although islet-cell tumors occur most commonly in the tail of the pancreas, it must be borne in mind, as noted by Duff,[9] in an analysis of reported cases, that 25 per cent are located either in the head or at the junction of the tail and body of the organ. Duff found that multiple adenomata had been encountered in about 12 per cent of cases. In Maxeiner's[10] case, clinical recovery from attacks of hypoglycemic seizures followed the removal of 75 per cent of the pancreas which on examination was found to contain 8 small islet-cell tumors.

Most of the reported adenomata have varied from 1 to 2 cm. in diameter although some have been quite large. In Brunschwig's[11] case the tumor was 13 x 10 cm. and in its greatest diameter, 15 cm.;

1 Wilder, Allan, Power and Robertson: Loc. cit., p. 197.
2 Howland, Campbell, Maltby and Robinson: Jour. Am. Med. Assn., **93**, 674, 1929.
3 Whipple and Frantz: Loc. cit., p. 197.
4 Frantz: Ann. Surg., **112**, 161, 1940.
5 Frantz: New York State Jour. Med., **41**, 881, 1941.
6 Whipple, Bauman and Hamlin: Am. Jour. Med. Sci., **201**, 629, 1941.
7 Frantz: Ann. Surg., **119**, 824, 1944.
8 Whipple: Surgery, **16**, 289, 1944.
9 Duff: Am. Jour. Med. Sci., **203**, 437, 1942.
10 Maxeiner: Journal-Lancet, **65**, 256, 1945.
11 Brunschwig: Surgery, **9**, 554, 1941.

it weighed 673 grams. In the case reported by O'Leary and Womack[1] the growth was likewise large, measuring 11 x 9 x 9 cm. and weighing 500 grams. In his article published in 1942, Duff[2] stated that hyperinsulinism had not been observed in association with adenomata less than 1 cm. in diameter. However, in 1944 Priestley, Comfort and Radcliffe[3] reported that in a case of hyperinsulinism in which total pancreatectomy had been carried out, prolonged search throughout the pancreas finally revealed in the head of the organ a cellular adenoma of the islands of Langerhans, measuring 8 x 5 x 5 mm. Islet-cell tumors usually appear grossly as pink or purplish nodules which are somewhat firmer than surrounding pancreatic tissue.

The histological pattern of islet-cell adenomata was carefully studied in 9 tumors by Laidlaw[4] who found them structurally to resemble gigantic islets of Langerhans. As in normal islet tissue, the adenomata contain rich capillary networks bordered by rows of columnar and cuboidal cells. Laidlaw found no hydropic degeneration and no increased mitosis. With differential stains he found that most of the cells take the granule stain of the beta cell with here and there an alpha cell. Frequently portions of pancreatic ducts and ductules have been seen.

Frantz[5] has stressed that one often has much difficulty histologically in differentiating between malignant and benign islet-cell tumors. Usually the tumors show encapsulation; the capsule may be complete or incomplete. In certain others belonging in the questionable group, there is no capsule and tumor cells are found in the blood vessels.

Microscopic examination of tumor tissue from our own 4 patients with adenomata showed the capsule of the tumor to be incomplete in each of 3 cases in which there was enough tissue available for satisfactory examination. In 2 of the 4 cases, blood vessel invasion was noted. However, patients from whom tumors of this sort were removed have remained alive, as in the case of our patients, many months or years after operation. Frantz[6] states that "in the group of suspicious tumors, the suspicion of the pathologist, not the surgeon, has yet to be confirmed in a single case by follow-up data." The suggestion is made that these tumors may be analogous to the "adenoma malignum" type of carcinoma of the thyroid, which is slow growing and late to metastasize. This affords sufficient basis for urging surgical exploration in any patient in whom the diagnosis of probable islet-cell tumor has been made.

[1] O'Leary and Womack: Arch. Path., 17, 291, 1934.
[2] Duff: Loc. cit., p. 404.
[3] Priestley, Comfort and Radcliffe: Ann. Surg., 119, 211, 1944.
[4] Laidlaw: Am. J. Path., 14, 125, 1938.
[5] Frantz: Loc. cit., p. 404, ref. 4.
[6] Frantz: Loc. cit., p. 404, ref. 7.

3. **Diagnosis.**—Whenever marked hypoglycemia with values below 60 mg. and most certainly below 50 mg. per 100 cc., regularly develops upon fasting, the presence of an islet-cell tumor must be assumed until proven otherwise, provided that by careful study extra-pancreatic causes for hypoglycemia have been excluded. These include diseases of the liver affecting glycogen storage and conditions associated with hypofunctioning of the adrenal cortex, the anterior lobe of the pituitary gland and the thyroid gland. Since conclusive evidence is lacking to indicate that the postprandial hypoglycemia described by some[1] in patients suffering from chronic fatigue is due to excessive nervous stimulation of islet tissue, the term "hypoglycemia" rather than "hyperinsulinism" is to be preferred in this connection and the condition regarded as not proved to be of pancreatic origin.[2]

No elaborate diagnostic procedures are necessary. The characteristic symptoms associated with well-marked hypoglycemia brought on by fasting, increased by physical exertion and relieved by food, are the important features. As an aid in the diagnosis, the glucose tolerance test is of value only if carried out for a sufficient length of time, i. e., four, five or six hours. Characteristically, the blood sugar (fasting) starts at a low level, below 60 mg. and usually approximately 40 mg. per 100 cc. Following the giving of glucose, the rise in blood sugar may be within normal limits or the curve may be diabetic in type.[3] Conn and Conn[4] have suggested that the type of curve depends upon the amount of carbohydrate in the diet of the preceding few days; diets high in carbohydrate increase sugar tolerance and those low in carbohydrate lower it. The glucose tolerance curve up to the third hour may, therefore, be essentially normal or mildly diabetic in type except for the initial value. After three hours, however, the blood sugar usually falls rather sharply to a low level (in our cases to approximately 40 mg. per cent) and in the fourth, fifth and sixth hours shows *no tendency to rise spontaneously* toward normal. This last fact is of importance: in the normal individual one often obtains a hypoglycemic phase in the glucose tolerance test but, presumably due to the compensatory secretion of epinephrine, there is a spontaneous return to normal values. Such does not occur in hyperinsulinism probably because of the continuous secretion of insulin by the islet-cell tumor.

The glucose tolerance curve in patients with hyperinsulinism differs from that described by Portis[1] in patients with postprandial hypoglycemia associated with "vagotonia" and fatigue in the following particulars: (1) in the latter condition, the fasting blood sugar, although perhaps lower than the average normal, is not

[1] Portis: Jour. Am. Med. Assn., **126**, 413, 1944.
[2] Keating and Wilder: Southern Med. and Surg., **103**, 125, 1941.
[3] Whipple, Bauman and Hamlin: Loc. cit., p. 404.
[4] Conn and Conn: Arch. Int. Med., **68**, 876, 1941.

depressed to the extent seen in hyperinsulinism; (2) the curve tends to be flat; (3) the lowest blood sugar usually occurs two, three or four hours after the administration of glucose; and (4) there is a tendency for the blood sugar to return to normal without the administration of food or glucose.

Various secondary tests may be carried out, including blood sugar studies following the giving of epinephrine, pituitary extract, ergotamine and insulin. One would anticipate that the blood sugar raising effect of epinephrine and pituitary extract would be less, and the blood sugar lowering effect of insulin would be greater, than in normal individuals studied under the same conditions. This is in general true but our experience has been the same as that of other workers, namely, that although the results obtained are interesting, they are apt to be variable and do not contribute significantly to the diagnosis.

4. **Surgical Treatment.**—Once the diagnosis of a probable islet-cell tumor has been made, exploration should be urged not only for symptomatic relief but also because of the possible danger of damage to the central nervous system produced by repeated attacks of prolonged hypoglycemia and, thirdly, because of the possibility of malignant degeneration of a tumor originally benign.

The approach to the pancreas through a long curved transverse incision above the umbilicus and through both recti, as advocated by Whipple,[1] has proved to be satisfactory. In the exploration one cannot overemphasize the importance of freeing the pancreas thoroughly so that it may be palpated throughout its extent from the tip of the tail to the head, and so that it may be visualized over as large a part of its course as possible. This means that infinite pains and patience are required and that at times the operation will be a long one. Of our five patients, two had been operated on previously by good surgeons and yet the tumor was overlooked. Palpation must be sufficiently thorough and delicate that a tiny nodule embedded within the substance of the pancreas and not visible from either surface may be located.[2] If one has felt sure of the diagnosis prior to operation, then one should carry the exploration to the limit in an attempt to demonstrate a tumor. Even though one nodule has been found, the exploration should be continued because of the relatively high incidence of multiple tumors.[3]

It is surprising how well patients withstand the manipulation of the pancreas and the removal of the tumors. With the exception of our one patient who had a carcinoma with metastases, all did well postoperatively. One patient suffered from bronchopneumonia transiently, but left the hospital in good condition one month after operation.

[1] Whipple and Frantz: Loc. cit., p. 197.
[2] Isaacs: Jour. Am. Med. Assn., **130**, 404, 1946.
[3] Duff: Loc. cit., p. 404.

5. **Authors' Cases of Hyperinsulinism.**—Between 1939 and 1942 we encountered 5 proved cases of hyperinsulinism due to islet-cell tumors. In 4 of the 5 cases, removal of a single adenoma resulted in the relief of symptoms which has persisted to date (four to seven years after operation). In 1 case (Case 3), death followed seven weeks after operation which disclosed an islet-cell carcinoma with multiple metastases in the liver. All operations were performed by Dr. L. S. McKittrick and Dr. T. C. Pratt. Three of the patients were females and two were males. The ages at the time of operation ranged from sixteen to fifty-nine years. The period from the onset of symptoms to the time of operation varied from two to eight years. In 3 cases the tumor was in the head, in one in the body and in one in the tail of the pancreas. Two of the patients had been operated upon previously without the finding of a tumor. The case histories, reported in detail elsewhere,[1] are summarized briefly below.

Case 1, Miss P. F., a high school student aged sixteen years, was first seen on November 23, 1938. She had been well up until the summer of 1933 at which time she began to have occasional spells of stupor, passing into definite unconsciousness. Following one such attack she was admitted to a hospital where she spent four weeks; the diagnosis of hyperinsulinism was made and the patient discharged with instructions as to diet. She was readmitted in January, 1934 and, following a period of study, was operated upon in February. At the laparotomy no tumor of the pancreas could be seen or felt and only a small piece of the tail of the pancreas was removed for study. Histological examination showed this to be normal pancreas. Her case was reported by Boone in 1934.[2]

Following the operation, strangely enough, the patient was free from significant attacks until August, 1938. At this time they recurred, and in one week she had three spells. On November 8, 1938, a bad attack occurred at school and she was admitted to another hospital where she remained until November 23.

At our first examination on November 28 the blood sugar was 50 mg. per cent at five hours after lunch. The physical examination was essentially negative except for undernutrition and carious teeth. Laboratory tests other than that for blood sugar were normal. The patient continued to have spells of unconsciousness, particularly in the early morning after an overnight fast. Consequently arrangements were made for her to enter the Deaconess Hospital, which she did on January 3, 1939. Following studies which confirmed the diagnosis of recurring hypoglycemia, exploratory operation was carried out on January 16, 1939. Although careful examination of the body and tail of the pancreas failed to reveal a tumor, a definite area of thickening was felt in the head of the organ. Exploratory incision was made directly over this point and a somewhat lobulated, reddish-purple, seemingly encapsulated nodule was exposed and removed. Microscopic examination showed the tumor to be an islet cell adenoma. Assay of the tissue for insulin, kindly carried out by Mr. George B. Walden in the Lilly Research Laboratories, yielded a value of 7 units per gram, or two to three times the normal.

The patient has been seen or heard from at intervals since operation and has continued in good condition. There have been no attacks suggest-

[1] Marble and McKittrick: New England Jour. Med., accepted for publication.
[2] Boone: New England Jour. Med., **211**, 49, 1934.

ing hypoglycemia, random blood sugar values have been normal and glucose tolerance tests have shown a normal response. A fasting blood-sugar on May 18, 1946, was 84 mg. per 100 cc. When last heard from in August 1946, over seven and a half years after operation, she had continued to be free from attacks suggesting hypoglycemia.

Case 2. Mrs. L. H., aged forty-nine years, admitted to the New England Deaconess Hospital on June 20, 1939, had been well up until about January 1931, at which time she began to experience attacks of weakness and drowsiness which were relieved by the taking of orange juice. Over the next three years she took much extra food so that her weight increased to over 200 pounds. There were frequent attacks of the sort described. Some of these were severe enough to precipitate total unconsciousness, for which she had been treated during admissions to her local hospital.

On admission to the New England Deaconess Hospital physical examination was essentially negative except for obesity and for the fact that mental reactions often were very slow. Despite additional feedings, periods of drowsiness were frequent. Fasting blood sugar values varied from 31 to 46 mg. per cent. The glucose tolerance curve was characterized by an extremely low initial value, a normal course for the first three hours after the giving of glucose, and then a gradual fall to 38 mg. per cent five hours after the giving of glucose.

On June 28 at exploratory laparotomy a solitary tumor was found in the body of the pancreas and removed without incident. Following operation the postoperative course was uneventful and blood sugar values remained well within a normal range.

Histological examination of the tissue from the tumor showed a typical islet-cell adenoma. Assay of the adenoma by Mr. Walden showed it to contain over 100 units of insulin per gram of tissue in contrast to the normal of 2 to 3 units per gram.

A glucose tolerance test carried out on July 18 gave normal results. Glucose tolerance tests performed in October 1939 and May 1942 were also entirely normal. The patient was last heard from on August 4, 1946. She considers herself in very good health and has had no further hypoglycemic attacks.

Case 3, Mrs. F. H., was first seen on September 15, 1938, at which time she was fifty-eight years old. She had been well up until June, 1935; at this time she began to suffer occasional fainting spells and attacks of coma during which she would remain in a dazed and drowsy condition for twelve to forty-eight hours. During minor episodes, mental confusion, speech disturbances and blankness of vision were common. As time went on, her fainting spells became more common until in 1937 she was having one or two a day. Attacks at 5 A.M. were common unless food was taken at bedtime. During a hospital stay in June, 1938, the fasting blood sugar was as low as 27 mg. per cent. A diet high in fat and low in protein and carbohydrate was advised and on this the patient did fairly well for a while. Then the symptoms recurred and feedings had to be increased to every two or three hours in order to prevent attacks.

At the time of admission to the New England Deaconess Hospital on September 15, 1938 she was obese. The fasting blood sugar varied from 30 to 50 mg. per cent. At one time during the course of a day a value as low as 20 mg. per cent was obtained after exercise. The glucose tolerance curve was characterized by a subnormal initial value, a normal course up to three and a half hours after the giving of glucose with a sharp falling away of values until that of 35 mg. per cent was reached at the end of five hours. The diagnosis of islet-cell tumor of the pancreas was made and operation advised. For personal reasons the patient preferred to go home to consider the matter but promised to return for operation.

Shortly after her return home the patient slipped and fell, suffering injuries which kept her in bed for twenty weeks. During this time, but to a much greater extent when she resumed her activity, the attacks incident to hypoglycemia took place at frequent intervals. She was delayed by one thing and another and did not reënter the Deaconess Hospital until September 12, 1939, a year after her first admission. She now found that she required food about every three hours; otherwise her vision would become blurred and then would follow mental dullness, stupor, and unconsciousness, at times with convulsions. The attacks were definitely hastened by exercise and relieved by food. Physical examination at this second admission showed her to be even more obese than a year before. The blood sugar on the morning after admission was 29 mg. per cent despite the fact that orange juice had been given within an hour of the time of drawing the blood. All blood sugar values during the four days after admission were subnormal, in fact it was so difficult to keep the patient out of hypoglycemia with the resulting stupor, that it was decided to proceed at once with exploratory operation.

Laparotomy on September 16 disclosed a tumor in the tail of the pancreas with multiple nodules in the liver. The pancreatic tumor .was excised and material was removed from one of the nodules for histological examination. Microscopic study showed the tissue of the primary tumor and of the metastatic nodule to be composed of an island-cell carcinoma (mixed cell type) with marked hyalinization.

The postoperative course was complicated first by bronchopneumonia, persistent purulent discharge from the pancreatic wound, an abscess of the right arm, marked anorexia, and particularly by extraordinary and persistent shortness of breath and rapid respiration. Physical examination and roentgen-rays of the chest yielded no findings which entirely explained the shortness of breath at bed-rest. Finally, however, about six weeks after the operation she seemed somewhat better and was allowed to sit in a chair for short periods. Suddenly, on November 3 she collapsed and died within a few minutes.

The behavior of the blood sugar in the postoperative period was extraordinary. During the first week the values were at a high normal level; then they gradually increased so that fasting values as high as 250 mg. per cent were obtained, at which time glycosuria to the extent of 35 grams per twenty-four hours was present. It became necessary, therefore, to begin insulin, which was then continued for a full month in dosage of 12 to 16 units of the protamine zinc variety daily in the morning before breakfast. With such treatment the glycosuria cleared up, blood sugar values were maintained at a satisfactory level and finally insulin was discontinued. During the last ten days of the patient's life no insulin was given. The fasting blood sugar on the day before death was 150 mg. per cent. No similar instance of the development of transitory diabetes following removal of a pancreatic tumor has come to our attention, although various observers have noted transient hyperglycemia after removal of an adenoma.

At postmortem examination the pancreatic wound was well healed and there was no evidence of diffuse pancreatitis. Many nodules of varying size were found in the liver. The immediate cause of death was acute pulmonary embolism with a large antemortem clot in the right pulmonary artery. The origin of the embolus was in an extraordinarily long thrombus in the superior vena cava. There was in addition thrombophlebitis of marked degree in the right brachial vein. The autopsy findings have been reported in detail by Gray.[1]

Case 4, Mr. E. R., a thirty-two-year-old bartender and taxi driver, was first seen on October 23, 1941. He had been admitted to a hospital on

---

[1] Gray: Am. Jour. Path., **18**, 633, 1942.

October 1, 1940, with the complaint that for one year he had experienced attacks of twitching of the face and neck, some staggering in gait, weakness, dizziness and sleepiness, all relieved by food. Blood-sugar studies had shown extremely low values and the diagnosis of probable islet-cell tumor was made. On October 15, 1940 he was operated upon but no tumor could be felt in the pancreas. Blood-sugar values continued to be low and attacks persisted despite a high protein, low carbohydrate diet and phenobarbital daily.

Questioning upon admission to the New England Deaconess Hospital revealed that symptoms had included the following: drowsiness leading to unconsciousness, weakness, sweating, rapid heart action, trembling and nervousness, numbness especially about the lips, inability to concentrate or to think clearly, staggering gait as that of a drunken man, twitching of the hands and face, pugnaciousness, aggressiveness and blurring of vision. The first symptom noted was usually drowsiness. Attacks were definitely brought on more easily by exercise and by prolonged abstinence from food. Food gave relief almost immediately. The patient first noticed his trouble because of difficulty at times in tying his tie. As a bartender he got along fairly well, because he could usually forestall attacks by taking food, but even so, at times he would get orders mixed up. Once while a taxi driver, he pulled his car up to the curb, got out and walked aimlessly five blocks before a friend saw that something was wrong and took care of him; afterward, the patient did not recall having walked the five blocks.

Physical examination and laboratory studies showed no abnormalities except for low blood-sugar values. At exploratory laparotomy carried out on October 30 an encapsulated, soft, mottled red-gray tumor measuring 1.5 x 1.5 x 1.7 cm. was removed from the pancreas. On microscopic examination it proved to be an "adenoma of insular origin, chiefly beta cells; scattered foci of ductal epithelium." Dr. J. H. Waite transplanted under sterile conditions a small bit of the tumor into the anterior chamber of the eye of a normal rabbit; however, the tumor failed to develop and no signs of excessive insulin activity were evident from periodic tests of the rabbit's blood sugar. (In this connection the report of Lups[1] is of interest. It is stated that a tissue culture extract from an islet-cell adenoma was active in lowering the blood sugar level of rats.)

Following operation the patient developed bronchopneumonia and was uncomfortable during the first several days after operation, but gradually improved and left the hospital on December 1 in good condition. From his home physician it was learned that up to the time of last observation in May, 1946, he had continued to feel well and had had no attacks suggesting hypoglycemia.

Case 5, Mr. S. F., a forty-five-year-old farmer, was admitted to the New England Deaconess Hospital on November 8, 1941. He had felt well up until three years before, when he began to notice dizziness brought on particularly by exercise and relieved by eating. Symptoms gradually increased to include weakness, fatigue and at times a change in temperament, irritability and a feeling of mental confusion. Various types of medical treatment had proved ineffective.

The first indication of difficulty came one day in the spring of 1938 while plowing corn. He noticed increasing difficulty and finally, when he stopped and let go of the reins which had been partly supporting him, he felt dizzy and sank to the ground. When he finally got to the house and obtained food, he felt relieved at once. This episode was the beginning of a long series of similar experiences. He soon adopted a schedule of taking orange juice or other food as soon as he arose in the morning, before starting work. During the last several months he had to give up most of the

---

[1] Lups: Acta Med. Scandin., 117, 261, 1944.

work about the farm because of the danger of hypoglycemic attacks. He ate regularly between meals and carried sugar in his pocket at all times. When attempts were made to arouse him from a hypoglycemic stupor, at times he would be simply confused and coöperate with difficulty, and at other times he would be pugnacious.

Physical examination and laboratory studies gave essentially normal findings except for abnormally low blood sugar values. The blood sugar on November 10 was 41 mg. per 100 cc. and subsequent values were uniformly at a low level, usually below 50 mg. per 100 cc.

Operation was carried out on November 18 under gas-oxygen and ether anesthesia. Following difficult exposure of the pancreas, painstaking exploration finally revealed a small, firm area within the pancreatic tissue at the free margin of the head in the duodenal loop. Further investigation proved difficult, because of the extreme vascularity of the region, but by blunt dissection a deep purplish encapsulated tumor about 1 cm. in its greatest diameter was removed in one piece. Histological examination of the tumor showed an adenoma of the islet cells with hyalinized stroma.

The postoperative course was uneventful. No further hypoglycemic attacks were experienced and blood-sugar values were within the normal range. He has continued well to date. Almost five years after operation, he wrote on August 4, 1946, that he had been in excellent health and had had no further difficulty of the sort which he had experienced prior to the operation.

C. HYPERINSULINISM WITHOUT ISLET-CELL TUMOR.

As has been previously mentioned, certain patients in whom the diagnosis of a pancreatic tumor seemed likely from the clinical findings have been found at operation to have no tumor. Some surgeons, first of whom were the Finneys,[1] encountering such a situation, have carried out resections of the pancreas following the principle of subtotal thyroidectomy for hyperthyroidism. Such a procedure definitely assumes that the hypoglycemia is due to an excessive secretion of insulin. This point of view has been upheld, particularly by Harris,[2] who believes that hyperinsulinism occurs more frequently than is commonly believed.

One should certainly be most cautious in making the diagnosis of hyperinsulinism without islet-cell tumor. In making such a diagnosis in the patient who has not been surgically explored, one takes for granted, first, that there is no islet-cell tumor present and, second, that the hypoglycemic attacks are not due to disturbances outside the pancreas. Even in those patients in whom no tumor can be found at operation, the possibility always exists that the growth is so small or so well hidden that it has been overlooked. That this is a real possibility has been amply shown by the experience of surgeons who more than once at second operations have found tumors overlooked at the first exploration.[3] Two of our patients (Cases 1 and 4) are cases in point. The possibility of the presence

[1] Finney and Finney: Ann. Surg., 88, 584, 1928.
[2] Harris: Cyclopedia of Med. (Piersol), 13, 184, 1936.
[3] Whipple: Loc. cit., p. 404.

of an adenoma in aberrant pancreatic tissue must likewise be considered.[1]

On the other hand, the literature contains enough reports of partial or complete relief of symptoms following subtotal resection of the pancreas that the procedure is justifiable if no tumor can be found. Experience has shown that to be successful, resection must be radical.[2] Not infrequently in cases of resection, minute examination of the portion of the pancreas removed at operation has revealed one or more tiny adenomata which were not identified by the surgeon.

D. NON-SURGICAL TREATMENT OF HYPERINSULINISM.

It cannot be emphasized too strongly that if the history, symptoms and laboratory findings suggest the probable diagnosis of an islet cell tumor, abdominal exploration should be advised for the following reasons: (1) surgical removal of an adenoma effects a complete cure; (2) "medical" treatment is often unsatisfactory; (3) there is a real danger of the presence or development of malignancy in an islet cell tumor, if present; (4) irreparable damage to the body, especially to the central nervous system, may result from repeated attacks of hypoglycemia over a long period of time.

However, in certain instances the clinical findings may be far from clear-cut and blood-sugar values only slightly and inconstantly below the lower limit of normal. With such patients and with those in whom exploration fails to reveal a tumor, non-surgical treatment must be resorted to. This consists of therapy demanded by acute attacks of hypoglycemia and that made desirable to prevent their frequent occurrence.

In acute attacks relief is best secured by the administration of carbohydrate in a form easily available to the body. If the patient is able to coöperate, orange or other fruit juices, ginger ale, sugar, candy, milk, etc., may be given by mouth. Wilder[3] prefers milk and bread to fruit juice or sugar. In unconscious patients, the injection of glucose (10 to 20 cc. 50 per cent solution) intravenously usually gives prompt relief. The administration of 0.5 to 1.0 cc. of epinephrine or pituitary extract subcutaneously may be of assistance just as in patients experiencing hypoglycemia due to injected insulin.

In the prevention of attacks, a diet low in carbohydrate and high in protein[4,5] has been found most helpful. A high-fat diet is likewise advantageous but care must be taken not to produce obesity by a too-liberal use of fat. The total food supplied for the day is best

[1] Holman, Wood & Stockton: Arch. Surg., **47**, 165, 1943.
[2] Brush and McClure: Ann. Surg., **120**, 750, 1944.
[3] Wilder: P. 400, loc. cit., p. 55.
[4] Conn: Jour. Clin. Invest., **15**, 673, 1936.
[5] Conn and Conn: Arch. Int. Med., **68**, 876, 1941.

divided into 3 main meals and 3 lunches; the lunches, given in the forenoon, afternoon and at bedtime, should be made up not of pure carbohydrate as fruit juice or ginger ale but of food containing protein and fat as well in order to take advantage of the more prolonged effect of these dietary components on the blood sugar. We have had no experience in the use of insulin with patients with hyperinsulinism; this was suggested by John[1] with the idea that a dose given regularly one-half hour after meals would depress insular activity. Certainly one would hesitate to employ this method with patients possessing a strong tendency to hypoglycemic attacks.

Drugs are not of striking value in the prevention of hypoglycemic attacks. Although one usually regards the effect of epinephrine as quite transient, Conn and Conn[2] regard the daily administration of this drug as an useful adjunct in treatment. Epinephrine in oil with its prolonged action would seem to be a desirable preparation. Phenobarbital and related sedatives may help in preventing convulsions and lesser physical manifestations although it is doubtful that hypoglycemia is appreciably altered. Thyroid extract, extracts of posterior pituitary, ephedrine, bromides, atropine or belladonna and caffeine have also been suggested but their use either does not give relief or produces other effects in the body which makes their continued administration undesirable.[3]

Theoretically, at least, alloxan might be of value in the treatment of hyperinsulinism. Brunschwig and his associates[4] injected alloxan into a thirty-two year old man with an islet-cell carcinoma of the pancreas with metastases to the liver. Temporary improvement lasting several days and in one instance twenty-one days during which no hypoglycemic reaction occurred, followed each series of injections. The great danger in using this drug is emphasized, however, in another case reported at the same time in which a man with recurrent carcinoma of the rectum was given alloxan and died six hours later. See also report of case on page 181.

Since physical activity accentuates the tendency to hypoglycemia, exercise must be taken in moderation. Before periods of unusual exertion, additional food, preferably of a type requiring some digestion, should be taken prophylactically.

In the treatment of hypoglycemia not due to injected insulin or to hyperinsulinism (see Section E which follows), therapy must be directed toward the underlying cause.

E. CHRONIC SPONTANEOUS HYPOGLYCEMIA ARISING OUTSIDE THE PANCREAS.

Apart from true hyperinsulinism, hypoglycemia may occur: (1) in long-continued undernutrition; (2) following prolonged exercise;

[1] John: Endocrinology, **17**, 583, 1933.
[2] Conn and Conn: Arch. Int. Med., **68**, 1105, 1941.
[3] Wilder: P. 400, loc. cit., p. 55.
[4] Brunschwig, Allen, Owens and Thornton: Loc. cit., p. 180.

(3) as a result of an overdose of insulin (see Chapter XI); (4) in "neurogenic" hypoglycemia; (5) in Addison's disease or in other conditions affecting the suprarenal glands; (6) in hypothyroidism; (7) in hypopituitarism; (8) following extirpation of the liver in animals or in markedly destructive liver disease in man; (9) in miscellaneous conditions.

1. **Undernutrition.**—The low diet of the Allen undernutrition era predisposed to hypoglycemia, and not long after it had begun instances of this occurred among the authors' patients.[1] The first deaths were startling and at the time unexplained. Space here permits mention of one case only. A man, Case 1831, with onset of diabetes, in April, 1917, at the age of thirty-eight years, entered the hospital, May 5, 1920. Acidosis was present, glycosuria 2.4 per cent, and the blood sugar 0.36 per cent. After four days of under-nutrition, during which the total calories consumed amounted to less than 900, followed by two days of fasting, the patient failed to become sugar-free and the blood sugar remained 0.27 per cent. Upon resumption of 14 to 35 grams of protein per day and 3 to 8 grams of fat, the blood sugar dropped to 0.11 per cent and on the next day to 0.05 per cent. This unusually low value was assumed in the laboratory to be erroneous and, unfortunately, not reported. Upon the following morning the patient became irrational, dis-oriented, but an hour afterward was again apparently normal, and was able to sit up and even walked around. Physical examination was negative. The next morning he could not be roused, coma gradually deepened, though unassociated with acidosis, and death occurred in a few hours. The blood sugar was 0.04 per cent. No marked loss of weight during hospital stay was observed, though he had lost 72 pounds in the three years before admission. Quantitative examinations of the nitrogen in the urine were made and showed an average excretion of 16.9 grams from the tenth to the sixth day before death and an average excretion of 19.6 grams on four of the five days preceding death. No autopsy was allowed.

Marked loss of weight characterized all cases for whom the data were recorded. In 2 of the cases, sudden decline in weight, although already low, took place shortly prior to the hypoglycemia. In 2 instances the excretion of urinary nitrogen per kilogram body weight was high. The metabolism in Case 1085, who presumably died of hypoglycemia a few days later, was −40 per cent.

In any discussion of hypoglycemia due to undernutrition properly must be placed the hypoglycemia which occurs during the end-stages of a chronic and wasting disease. Case 11419 with advanced tuber-culosis died in hypoglycemia, although no insulin had been given for several days prior to death and large amounts of carbohydrate were administered frequently. Hypoglycemia undoubtedly occurs

---

[1] Joslin: Loc. cit., p. 388.

in afebrile cachexia; certainly some of the symptoms of cachectic patients are explainable on this basis.

Hypoglycemia is well known in the new-born infant and during lactation, in the course of diarrhea and even of a slowly absorbed meal from whatever cause. Sigwald[1] cites its occurrence as a result of cold or dehydration. Consider its possible wholesale occurrence in famine and in voluntary starvation, as practiced by religious fanatics in olden times, and how comparatively easy it would be for ascetic monks or magicians to go into a trance, see visions and dream dreams at the conclusion of a physical orgy of ecstatic fury. What a field for physiological interpretation of the past. And there is a quasi humorous or practical side universally recognized in never trying to make a bargain or to seek a contribution for research or the hospital when the prospect's stomach is empty.

That hyperglycemia of severe grade with blood-sugar values below 40 mg. per cent and coma can, and does, occur in persons subjected to prolonged undernourishment has been shown by Gounelle and Marche.[2] Their observations were made on individuals who were on inadequate diets in France in 1941 and 1942. Of particular interest was the occurrence of spontaneous hypoglycemia in persons whose diets were deficient in protein and fat and not in carbohydrate.

2. **Exercise.**—Levine and his associates[3] found the blood sugar to be moderately diminished in 2, and markedly diminished in 4, of 11 marathon runners studied. A close correlation existed between the physical condition of the runners at the finish of the race and the level of the blood sugar. Those competitors who had extremely low blood-sugar values presented a picture of shock, not unlike that produced by an overdose of insulin. Blood-sugar figures as low as 49 and 50 mg. per cent were obtained, but when these same individuals ate candy during the run the percentages were 92 and 114 mg. per cent and they finished in good condition.

Soon after the beginning of exercise there is an initial rise in blood sugar, as Levine and his co-workers, as well as Rakestraw[4] previously, showed. This rise persists in the severe diabetic, untreated with insulin (see page 357), but if the diabetic is given insulin, his blood sugar will fall after exercise in the same manner as that of a normal individual or mild diabetic who can manufacture enough of his own.

3. **Hypoglycemia Due to Insulin** (See Chapter XI).

4. **"Neurogenic" Hypoglycemia.**—The recurring hypoglycemia described by Portis[5] and other workers[6] in association with "vago-

[1] Sigwald: Loc. cit., p. 389.
[2] Gounelle and Marche: Occupational Med., 1, 48, 1946.
[3] Levine, Gordon and Derick: Jour. Am. Med. Assn., 82, 1778, 1924. Gordon, Kohn, Levine, Matton, Scriver and Whiting: Jour. Am. Med. Assn., 85, 508, 1925.
[4] Rakestraw: Jour. Biol. Chem., 56, 121, 1923.
[5] Portis: Loc. cit., p. 406.
[6] Donnelly and Palmer: South. Med. & Surg., 106, 363, 1944.

tonia" and fatigue has been discussed previously. Relief is said to follow the use of between-meal feedings and atropine. Wilder[1] suggests that "neurogenic" hypoglycemia may be the result of the direct nervous influence on the glycogen mechanism of the liver.

5. Conditions Affecting the Suprarenal Glands.—A low blood sugar is often found in Addison's disease and has been referred to by Wadi[2] and Porges.[3] A case of Rabinovitch and Barden[4] who died in hypoglycemia was found at autopsy to have the adrenal medulla entirely replaced by lymphoid tissue. Anderson's case[5] of fatal hypoglycemia had an adrenal tumor. See page 737.

6. Hypothyroidism.—Hypoglycemia of mild degree may occur in cases of thyroid insufficiency. Such has been reported by Campbell,[6] Gardiner-Hill,[7] Zubiram[8] and Holman.[9] Goldzieher,[10] in studying 112 cases of hypoglycemia, stresses the importance of pituitary and thyroid lesions. Such hypoglycemia is usually of little clinical importance, however.

7. Hypopituitarism.—The increased carbohydrate tolerance found in states of diminished pituitary secretion is discussed in Chapter XXVII (page 724). Pituitary extract is an insulin antagonist and decrease in its effectiveness may well render an individual insulin-sensitive, just as Houssay has shown to be the case with hypophysectomized animals. Wilder[11] has described a condition of "hypophysäre-spontanhypoglykämie," characterized by symptoms of hypoglycemia in association with pituitary disturbances. The woman, aged forty-eight years, with Simmonds' disease reported by Mogensen[12] had blood-sugar values as low as 38 mg. per cent. Lloyd's[13] patient who died in convulsions had a pituitary tumor and hypertrophy of the islands of Langerhans and of the parathyroid glands. Farquharson, Belt and Duff[14] found blood-sugar values as low as 28 mg. per cent in 3 patients with Simmonds' disease. Following the giving of glucose in a tolerance test, relatively slight increases in blood-sugar values were observed.

8. Disease or Removal of the Liver.—The sugar in the circulating blood has for its source the glycogen in the liver. When this glycogen reserve is depleted, hypoglycemia, unrelieved by the administration of epinephrine, pituitrin or thyroid extract, may result. The factor

[1] Wilder: P. 357; loc. cit., p. 55.
[2] Wadi: Klin. Wchnschr., **7**, 2107, 1928.
[3] Porges: Ztschr. f. klin. Med., **69**, 341, 1910.
[4] Rabinovitch and Barden: Am. Jour. Med. Sci., **184**, 494, 1932.
[5] Anderson: Am. Jour. Med. Sci., **180**, 71, 1930.
[6] Campbell: Jour. Kansas Med. Soc., **30**, 365, 1929.
[7] Gardiner-Hill, Brett and Smith: Quart. Jour. Med., **18**, 327, 1925.
[8] Zubiram: Med. Mexico, **9**, 306, 1929. Cited by Harris: Ann. Int. Med., **7**, 1084, 1934.
[9] Holman: Bull. Johns Hopkins Hosp., **34**, 69, 1923.
[10] Goldzieher: Endocrinology, **20**, 86, 1936.
[11] Wilder: Deutsch. Ztschr. f. Nervenh., **112**, 192, 1930.
[12] Mogensen: Endocrinology, **27**, 194, 1940.
[13] Lloyd: Bull. Johns Hopkins Hosp., **45**, 1, 1929.
[14] Farquharson, Belt and Duff: Trans. Am. Clin. and Clim. Assn., **54**, 106, 1938.

of safety is large, however, and Mann[1] has shown that permanent reduction of hepatic tissue to less than 15 per cent results in only slight changes in the blood-sugar level. This is undoubtedly the reason why it is so difficult to devise a test which will indicate the function of the liver. It is significant that in depancreatized dogs a fall in blood sugar occurs steadily following hepatectomy, as in the normal animal. Briggs[2] cites 7 references concerning hypoglycemia in connection with destructive disease of the liver. Hypoglycemia is known to occur following toxic damage to the liver from chloroform, carbon tetrachloride and guanidine,[3] from phosphorus,[4] from hydrazine,[5] and following infections of the liver itself.[6] Whenever carbohydrate fails to be stored as a reserve in the liver, then the train of hypoglycemic symptoms appears and it would appear to be in some way because of the liver that the blood sugar fluctuates to extremes in brief periods. It is in the hepatic vein that one finds the highest blood-sugar.

Chronic hypoglycemia occurs characteristically in von Gierke's disease (glycogen-storage disease; glycogenosis). In this condition the liver is enlarged and filled with glycogen. Yet despite this superabundance of carbohydrate stores in the body the individual suffers from want of usable sugar due presumably to diminution or lack in the amount of glycogenolytic enzyme or glycogenase in the liver. The fasting blood sugar is consistently low and fasting acetonuria, lipemia and hypercholesterolemia are not uncommon.[7] Erbon[8] and Sackel[9] have brought forth evidence to indicate that von Gierke's disease is a condition apart from hyperinsulinism. The latter investigator found an approximately normal or only slightly decreased rate of postmortem glycogenolysis in samples of liver from 2 cases of hyperinsulinism. Interestingly enough in von Gierke's disease the patient experiences no symptoms as a result of the hypoglycemia, even though the blood sugar may be extremely low. Wagner's monograph[10] on "Die Speicherkrankheiten" is a classic in this field.

Coller and Jackson[11] describe 3 patients with hypoglycemia which they regard as due to liver damage arising from gall-bladder disease. Following operation, at which, incidentally, no abnormalities were noted in the pancreas, a return toward normal dextrose tolerance

[1] Mann: Medicine, **6**, 419, 1927.

[2] Briggs: Minnesota Med., **17**, 527, 1934.

[3] Minot and Cutler: Jour. Clin. Invest., **6**, 369, 1928. Minot: Jour Pharm. and Exp. Therap., **43**, 295, 1931.

[4] Frank and Isaac: Arch. f. exp. Path. u. Pharmakol., **64**, 274, 1911.

[5] Underhill: Jour. Biol. Chem., **10**, 159, 1911. Bodansky: Am. Jour. Physiol., **66**, 375, 1923.

[6] Lyon: Acta med. Orient., **4**, 401, 1945.

[7] Schneider: Cleveland Clinic Quart., **13**, 34, 1946.

[8] Erbon: Ztschr. f. klin. Med., **134**, 31, 1938.

[9] Sackel: Jour. Clin. Invest., **18**, 723, 1939.

[10] Wagner: Ergebn. d. inn. Med. u. Kinderheilk., **53**, 586, 1937.

[11] Coller and Jackson: Jour. Am. Med. Assn., **112**, 128, 1939.

was obtained. Coller and Jackson believe that long-standing gall-bladder disease may bring about important disturbances in carbohydrate metabolism and on this basis urge early operation. It is interesting that in these 3 patients following removal of the gall-bladder, improvement was gradual, rather than dramatic, as when pancreatic adenomata are removed.

9. **Other Conditions.**—McCrudden and Sargent,[1] Sendrail and Planques,[2] and Scheimann[3] have reported low blood-sugar values in progressive muscular dystrophy. MacLean and Sullivan[4] noted hypoglycemia in patients with status thymolymphaticus, although seldom, if ever, were blood-sugar values low enough to provoke symptoms.

Herrmann and Gius[5] found at operation in their patient with hypoglycemia not an adenoma but only a calcareous mass in which no pancreatic tissue could be found. Surprisingly enough, the removal of the mass apparently overcame the hypoglycemia and dextrose tolerance tests became normal. The man, aged forty-nine years, reported by Brinck and Sponholz[6] likewise was found to have pancreatic stones. In this patient the tendency to hypoglycemia seemed not to have been as marked as in cases of islet-cell adenomata, since the lowest blood sugar recorded was one of 59 mg. per cent. In addition to the calculi in the pancreas there was a marked degree of lipomatosis of the entire pancreas and histologically there appeared to be an almost complete disappearance of the acinar tissue. There was in addition atrophy of the liver with fatty infiltration.

[1] McCrudden and Sargent: Arch. Int. Med., **17**, 465, 1916.

[2] Sendrail and Planques: Gaz. d. hôp., **100**, 1105, 1137, 1927. Cited by Moore *et al.*: Brit. Med. Jour., **2**, 837, 1931.

[3] Scheimann: Arch. f. Psychiat., **87**, 665, 1929.

[4] MacLean and Sullivan: Proc. Soc. Exp. Biol. and Med., **23**, 425, 1926.

[5] Herrmann and Gius: Jour. Am. Med. Assn., **108**, 1402, 1937.

[6] Brinck and Sponholz: Deutsch. Ztschr. f. Verdauungs- und Stoffwechselkrankh. **1**, 1, 1938.

CHAPTER XIII.

DIABETIC COMA.

REVISED BY HOWARD F. ROOT, M.D., AND ALEXANDER MARBLE, M.D.

A. DEFINITION.

DIABETIC coma is the unique complication of diabetes; it is the end result of the disease when uncontrolled. Strictly speaking, it is the condition of unconsciousness accompanying the more severe grades of diabetic acidosis. Actually, the term is often more loosely applied and, in the authors' opinion, advantageously so. If one limits the diagnosis of diabetic coma to unconsciousness so profound that no stimulus, however great, will produce a response, then relatively little material will be available for profitable consideration and for the evaluation of features of treatment.

Since acidosis varies widely in severity without sharp transitions from one stage to another, arbitrary standards of classification must be set up. For some years it has been our custom to classify any case of diabetic acidosis as one of diabetic coma when the carbon dioxide combining power (or more recently, the carbon dioxide content) of the blood plasma is 20 volumes per cent (9 milliequivalents per liter) or less. This arbitrary division of cases is at times unsatisfactory, but it has the advantage of affording an accurate way of putting into one group a series of cases for future study and comparison. The figure of 20 volumes per cent has the following basis to commend it; in the pre-insulin days most cases of diabetic acidosis with a CO_2 of above 20 volumes per cent recovered; most, though not all,[1] of those with values below this, died. Hence, our series include, in a rough sense, those patients who without the aid of insulin would have died.

Comparison of the mortality from coma in different clinics is of uncertain value, but we do believe that improvement in the treatment of coma year by year in one's own hospital should be the common aim.

B. INCIDENCE.

At one time diabetic coma was regarded as the almost inevitable culmination of a diabetic history. Before insulin it was the exceedingly rare diabetic child who lived for more than two years. With few exceptions, every child with diabetes died in coma within a matter of months from the time of the onset of the condition. In the experience of the senior author, 63.8 per cent of all patients

---

[1] Joslin: Bull. Johns Hopkins Hosp., **29**, 82, 1918; Med. Clin. North America, **1**, 895, 1918.

dying in the Naunyn era from 1898 to 1914, died in coma; with treatment by undernutrition the figure fell during the years 1914 to 1922 to 41.5 per cent. With the introduction of insulin in 1922 and the beginning of a new era in diabetes, diabetic coma became much less frequent and when once acquired could be much more successfully treated. Thus, in the years 1936 to 1946 only 4.4 per cent of deaths among the authors' diabetic patients, no matter where in the world they died, were in coma. (See Fig. 12.) Despite this markedly lowered incidence and mortality, diabetic coma still occurs all too frequently. Among 2112 admissions for diabetes (including a few for non-diabetic glycosuria) to the New England Deaconess Hospital in 1945 there were 32 cases of coma, representing 1.5 per cent of the total. From May, 1923 to January, 1946 we have seen in all 651 cases (in 495 patients) of diabetic acidosis in which the CO_2 combining power, or content, of the blood plasma was 20 volumes per cent (9 milliequivalents per liter) or below.

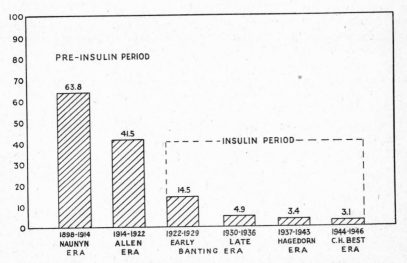

Fig. 12.—Coma as a cause of death. Percentage of all deaths due to diabetic coma. Patients of all ages. Prepared by the Statistical Department of the Metropolitan Life Insurance Company. Values given above for years since 1922 differ slightly in arrangement from those in Table 26.

Baker[1] summarized the clinical findings and outcome of 108 consecutive cases treated at the Mayo Clinic among patients seen from October, 1923, to January, 1934. With three exceptions the cases all had an initial plasma CO_2 combining power of less than 25 volumes per cent. Seventeen, or 15.7 per cent, of the patients died.

Dillon and Dyer[2] stated that among 3009 admissions of diabetic

[1] Baker: Arch. Int. Med., **58**, 373, 1936.
[2] Dillon and Dyer: Ann. Int. Med., **11**, 602, 1937.

patients to the wards of the Metabolic Division of the Philadelphia General Hospital in the six years from 1931 to 1936, there were 268 admissions of patients in severe acidosis. Of these, 167, or 43.7 per cent, resulted in death. It is obvious from an examination of the data of Dillon and Dyer that a large proportion of their patients reached the hospital in extremely poor condition.

From the Montreal General Hospital, Rabinowitch, Fowler and Bensley[1] reported 125 cases of severe acidosis; excluded from this group were other patients in acidosis who were not definitely drowsy. Among the 125 patients there were 33 deaths, a case mortality of 26.4 per cent. In statistics quoted by Rabinowitch and associates the statement is made that in New York City in 1933 coma accounted for about 35 per cent of all deaths among diabetic individuals; in 1937, however, coma caused only 179 fatalities among a total of 2669 deaths, an incidence of 6.7 per cent.

Owens and Rockwern[2] analyzed the records of all diabetic patients admitted in ketosis to the Cincinnati General Hospital for the fifteen years from 1923 to 1936. They found 92 cases which satisfied clinical and laboratory requirements for impending or actual coma. Patients with mild acidosis without significant mental symptoms were not included. Of the 92 patients there were 47 deaths, a mortality of 51.1 per cent.

Between the years of 1933 and 1938 there were approximately 1100 admissions for diabetes to the Toronto General Hospital.[3] Of these, 114 died, 14 in coma and 100 without coma. Among the coma deaths 9 were in females and 5 in males. The average age at the time of death was forty-five and two-tenths years in contrast to that of sixty-one and eight-tenths years in those patients dying without coma. In 6 of the 14 cases the event precipitating coma was infection; in the remaining 8 the cause was thought to be neglect of treatment.

Among the last 1865 patients admitted to the metabolic services at four Philadelphia hospitals, 220 had diabetic acidosis, of whom 52, or 23.6 per cent, died. Excluding those patients with complications, the mortality rate was 5 per cent.[4]

Danowski, Winkler and Peters[5] report that in 188 cases of diabetic acidosis treated at the New Haven Hospital between 1924 and 1944, 34 cases died. Of the 34, 26 had peripheral vascular collapse. The fatal cases received on an average 246 units and the recovered cases received on an average 205 units of insulin in twenty hours. In 19 of the 34 fatal cases and in 19 of the recovered cases, the blood sugar had risen instead of fallen at the end of the first four to seven

[1] Rabinowitch, Fowler and Bensley: Ann. Int. Med., **12**, 1403, 1939.
[2] Owens and Rockwern: Am. Jour. Med. Sci., **198**, 252, 1939.
[3] Fletcher and Graham: Canad. Med. Assn. Jour., **41**, 566, 1939.
[4] Beardwood: Jour. Am. Med. Assn., **117**, 1701, 1942.
[5] Danowski, Winkler and Peters: Yale Jour. Biol. and Med., **18**, 405, 1946.

hours of treatment. One of their conclusions is that glucose solution may aggravate the salt deficit of diabetic coma if given subcutaneously.

These reports force upon us the realization that diabetic coma is still an important problem. Since most cases are needless, efforts must be redoubled in order to educate the public and medical profession alike so that diabetic coma may be avoided. Furthermore, one must constantly reëmphasize the importance of prompt recognition of the condition and early institution of energetic treatment. That knowledge on the part of the patient is of great value is shown by the causes of death among 225 diabetic doctors. In the period of 1897 to 1914, 4 in 8 (50 per cent) of the deaths were in coma, in 1914 to 1922, 32 per cent, and from 1937 to 1946, only 1 per cent of the deaths were in coma. Contrast these figures with those for the diabetic patients generally, as shown in Figure 12. (See also pages 229 and 323.)

C. THE PATHOLOGICAL PHYSIOLOGY OF DIABETIC COMA.

Continued study of the chemical processes by which ketone bodies ("acetone bodies") are formed from fatty acids has led to modifications of former concepts.[1,2] Improved methods for estimation of ketones, which make possible the determination of very small amounts, have shown their presence in the blood of normal individuals. It has been demonstrated that fatty acids with an odd, as well as those with an even, number of carbon atoms give rise to ketone bodies.

According to the Knoop theory, of *successive beta oxidation*, formerly widely accepted but now discredited by most workers, the breakdown of fatty acids takes place in regular sequence by oxidation at the β carbon atom with the production of a new fatty acid containing two less carbon atoms. Normally this process is carried to completion, but in the diabetic individual, due to inadequate oxidation of carbohydrate, the process stops short at the stage of butyric acid, when the fatty acid chain has been reduced to 4 carbon atoms. Without control of the diabetic condition and the regaining of the ability to oxidize carbohydrate, abnormal products of the decomposition of butyric acid accumulate in the body. Aceto-acetic ("diacetic") acid and β-hydroxybutyric acid are probably formed first and from these acetone results. These "acetone bodies" accumulate in great excess in the blood and body tissues generally, overflowing then into the urine.

The structural formulæ of butyric acid, beta-hydroxybutyric acid, aceto-acetic acid, and acetone are shown on p. 424.

[1] Soskin and Levine: Am. Jour. Digest. Dis., **11**, 305, 1944; Arch. Int. Med., **68**, 674, 1941.
[2] Stadie: Loc. cit., p. 114.

Aceto-acetic acid occurs in two forms, the keto- and the enol-form. The former is the more stable of the two and it appears that it and beta-hydroxybutyric acid are relatively non-toxic, as contrasted with the labile enolform. By loss of carbon dioxide aceto-acetic acid is converted into acetone.

Butyric acid.	Beta-hydroxybutyric acid.	Aceto-acetic acid (diacetic acid).		Acetone.
		Ketoform.	Enolform.	
CH_3	CH_3	CH_3	CH_3	CH_3
CH_2	$CHOH$	CO	CHO	CO
CH_2	CH_2	CH_2	CH	CH_3
$COOH$	$COOH$	$COOH$	$COOH$	

The failure to find butyric and acetic acids in ketone-producing liver led Hurtley[1] to propose the theory of *multiple alternate oxidation*. According to this concept, the intact fatty acid chain is first oxidized at alternate carbon atoms and then split into blocks of four carbon atoms each. This explanation accounted for the greater than 1:1 ratio of ketogenesis from the higher fatty acids as well as other chemical observations, and was accepted by Deuel,[2,3] Jowett and Quastel,[4] and Stadie, Zapp and Lukens.[5] Stadie and associates have given additional support to those[6] who have attacked the validity of the Knoop theory.

Studies of the ketogenic properties of other fatty acids by Jowett and Quastel and MacKay and co-workers[7,8] showed a greater production of ketone from certain acids containing fewer carbon atoms and led to a new theory which they term the *"beta-oxidation-acetic acid condensation hypothesis."* MacKay holds that all fatty acid chains, whether odd or even, may be subject to oxidation at each alternate carbon atom. Ketones are formed by the condensation of two acetic acid molecules. Subsequently Swendseid *et al.*,[9] using acetic acid containing heavy carbon demonstrated the chemical reaction in experiments *in vitro*.

It is generally believed that diabetic muscle can oxidize the acetone bodies as well as normal muscle and that their accumulation in the patient with uncontrolled diabetes is due simply to a rate of formation which exceeds the capacity of the tissues for utilization.

The oxidation of excess ketone bodies in the peripheral tissues, although usually readily carried out may still have definite limits.

[1] Hurtley: Loc. cit., p. 114.
[2] Butts, Cutler, Hallman and Deuel: Jour. Boil. Chem., 109, 597, 1935.
[3] Deuel, Hallman, Butts and Murray: Jour. Biol. Chem., 116, 621, 1936.
[4] Jowett and Quastel: Biochem. Jour., 29, 2181, 1935.
[5] Stadie, Zapp and Lukens: Jour. Biol. Chem., 132, 423, 1940.
[6] Poczka: Deutsch. Arch. klin. Med., 183, 170, 1938-39.
[7] MacKay, Wick and Barnum: Loc. cit., p. 114.
[8] MacKay, Barnes, Carne and Wick: Loc. cit., p. 114.
[9] Swendseid, Barnes, Hemingway and Nier: Jour. Biol. Chem., 142, 47, 1942.

When glycogen stores are depleted by excessive work, as described by Barach,[1] by starvation or by phloridzin as described by Mirsky and Nelson,[2] increased oxidation of protein and fat may result in ketonuria. It is in diabetes, however, where the depletion of glycogen stores is combined with the limitation of the power of oxidizing carbohydrate, *even if available*, that severe degrees of ketosis have had the greatest clinical significance.

The body is capable of withstanding a certain amount of increase in the content of acetone bodies. Thus, a certain portion of the ketone acids, because of their weak acid character, can be excreted as free acid in highly acid urine and another fraction is neutralized by ammonia and excreted. Furthermore, carbon dioxide is displaced from bicarbonate of the plasma by the ketone acids and by means of this buffer action and that of the blood proteins, considerable amounts of acid can be taken up without appreciable change in the hydrogen-ion concentration of the blood. This bodily defence is not perfect, however. When excessive amounts of ketone acids accumulate, a certain portion is excreted in the urine along with fixed base, chiefly sodium. This process withdraws elements from the body which can be replaced only from extraneous sources. The reduction in the fixed base of the blood means a reduction in the total salt or electrolyte concentration of the body fluids. To meet this, fluid is excreted with consequent dehydration. The result is lowered body fluid volume with a diminished concentration of base. The volume of circulating blood is further decreased by stasis of fluid in the peripheral tissues.

A peculiarly important place may be assigned to potassium[3] although the loss of sodium in acidosis is known to be excessive. Guest[4] states that the rapid development of severe acidosis is accompanied by excessive phosphaturia which results mainly from the decomposition of labile organic phosphate in the blood and tissue cells. In the blood, all decreases in concentration of the organic phosphate are associated with decreases in the concentration of potassium. During recovery from acidosis, the restoration of normal chemical structure of the blood involves the replacement of potassium concomitantly with resynthesis of the organic phosphates of the blood cells. The glycolytic enzyme system by which the organic phosphates are formed and decomposed may be regarded as the principal mechanism in maintaining the acid-base equilibrium of the blood. In reporting 5 cases of severe diabetic acidosis in children, Guest records an excretion of phosphorus at the rate of 164 milligrams per hour during the first few hours of treatment and rapid decline at the end of eighteen hours to only 2 milligrams

[1] Barach: Am. Jour. Digest. Dis., **10**, 134, 1943.
[2] Mirsky and Nelson: Am. Jour. Dis. Child., **67**, 100, 1944.
[3] Darrow: New England Jour. Med., **233**, 91, 1945.
[4] Guest: Am. Jour. Dis. Child., **64**, 401, 1942.

per hour. This rapid loss of phosphate in the acute stage means an excessive excretion of potassium as well as phosphorus due to a breakdown of intracellular constituents. During the period of recovery, organic phosphates are reformed in the tissues and with normal concentration restored the normal excretion of potassium occurs in the urine. Kaplan, Franks and Friedgood[1] found that in coma in rats with alloxan diabetes, the same rise in inorganic phosphate of the blood and change in liver phosphate and glycogen occurred as they found in human cases of diabetic coma. In the past, the knowledge that an elevation of the blood potassium from 5 milliequivalents to 10 milliequivalents per liter might cause heart block and that an elevation to 12 or 15 milliequivalents might be fatal has prevented attempts to administer potassium solutions intravenously. However, the fact that the tissue cells have lost much potassium and that the danger of an excessive increase may be checked by watching changes in the blood phosphate has led to trial administration of solutions containing potassium.

A deficiency of serum potassium may result in paralysis of the voluntary muscles as in the case reported by Holler.[2] A girl aged eighteen years, with diabetes for three years, had been irregularly treated and had omitted insulin for five days prior to her admission in profound diabetic coma. The blood sugar was 400 mg. per 100 cc. She was given during the next nineteen hours 500 to 750 cc. of 5 per cent glucose in isotonic solution of three chlorides each hour intravenously and 25 units of crystalline insulin given subcutaneously each half hour. The acidosis lessened and she was improving until, after twelve hours of treatment, she began to have respiratory distress. At the end of twenty-one hours the distress was extreme and soon it appeared that she was at the point of death from paralysis of the muscles of respiration. She was placed in a Drinker respirator. At this time the blood CO_2 combining power was 50 volumes per cent and the blood sugar 221 mg. per 100 cc. After three hours it was discovered that the potassium of the serum was markedly lowered: 2.5 milliequivalents per liter (9.8 mg. per 100 cc.). She was given 1.5 gm. of potassium chloride in a 2 per cent solution in distilled water intravenously slowly and at the end of twenty minutes her breathing became normal. Later a second infusion of 200 cc. of a 2 per cent solution of potassium chloride mixed with isotonic sodium chloride solution was given, with complete and permanent relief. The author suggested various possible explanations for the potassium deficiency. Dehydration or diuresis may cause a loss of potassium in the urine, and this loss occurred particularly in 2 cases studied by Atchley and associates,[3] when insulin

[1] Kaplan, Franks and Friedgood: Science, **102**, 447, 1945.
[2] Holler: Jour. Am. Med. Assn., **131**, 1186, 1946.
[3] Atchley, Loeb, Richards, Benedict and Driscoll: Jour. Clin. Invest., **12**, 297, 1933.

was withdrawn from treatment of the patient. With the restoration of insulin and fluid, an abrupt retention of potassium as well as sodium and water occurred. In depancreatized dogs receiving anterior pituitary extract, Foglia[1] found a decrease in the serum potassium to 11.3 mg. from normal levels of 18.9 mg. per 100 cc. The deposition of glycogen in the rat liver is accompanied by the deposition of potassium and reduction in serum potassium according to Fenn.[2]

Holler's patient received a total of 17,750 cc. of fluid and excreted 15,325 cc. of urine in twenty-four hours. She received 9000 cc. of a 5 per cent glucose solution in isotonic solution of three chlorides, an amount certainly adequate to explain the diuresis. He refers also to a record from the Massachusetts General Hospital[3] of a death occurring in diabetic coma treated with glucose. The period before death was characterized by "peculiar, gasping respirations," possibly due to "low serum potassium." As suggested by Holler, the possibility of producing potassium deficiency when diabetic acidosis is treated by large amounts of glucose solution in addition to insulin must be borne in mind. This clinical trial of excessive glucose administration in coma scarcely needs or justifies repetition.

A specific depletion of intracellular potassium which accompanies diabetic coma may be grossly magnified by a diuresis artificially induced.

Not only are the fixed bases lost in the urine but also there is a depletion of body chloride. This is due in part to the vomiting which is the almost invariable accompaniment of diabetic acidosis, to the marked diuresis which is so characteristic and which is due probably to the effect of the ketone acids, and possibly in part to the replacement of the chloride ion by the oxybutyric anion and the subsequent excretion of chloride as ammonium chloride.

The end-results of the above processes are (1) hemo-concentration and dehydration; (2) depletion of both fixed base and chloride of the body; (3) lowering of the plasma CO_2 combining power; (4) shift in the pH of the blood toward the acid side; (5) depletion of glycogen stores in liver and muscles.

The clinical picture of diabetic coma—the Kussmaul respiration, the gastro-intestinal symptoms, the circulatory failure, dehydration, and the stupor—are attributable in large part to the toxic effects of the ketone bodies (and possibly certain other as yet unidentified acids) particularly on the central nervous system and its regulatory centers. The dehydration and disturbances in intra-cellular electrolyte economy may be important factors in causing death, as is

[1] Foglia, Gerschman, Marenzi, Munoz and Rietti: Compt. rend. Soc. de biol., **126,** 152, 1937.

[2] Fenn: Jour. Biol. Chem., **128,** 297, 1939.

[3] Cabot Case 30451, New England Jour. Med., **231,** 657, 1944.

emphasized by Gamble[1] and by Sprague,[2] as well as by most recent students of coma.

It has long been held that the utilization of carbohydrate exerts an antiketogenic effect and the primary aim in treatment of diabetic coma is to improve the oxidation of glucose. Woodyatt[3] held that the oxidation of sugar not only spared the oxidation of fatty acids but had an additional antiketogenic effect. Stadie emphasizes total magnitude of the fat metabolism and regards the metabolism of 2.5 grams fat per kilogram as the upper limit, beyond which ketosis will occur. Mirsky and Soskin regard the presence of glycogen in the liver as the essential condition to avoid ketosis. It should be noted that coma patients can die with livers well supplied with glycogen.[4] Probably in the well treated coma case both an increase in glucose oxidation and an increase in glycogen storage occur.

D. CLINICAL MATERIAL IN DIABETIC COMA.

The entire series treated by the authors at the New England Deaconess Hospital from May 1923 to January 1946 includes, as stated above, 651 instances of coma in 495 patients. From time to time reports have been published describing successive groups of these cases.[5] In Table 48 are summarized the datag iven in nine articles published to date, together with those of a tenth group representing cases which have occurred since the writing of the last report in January 1942.

The average age of patients varied in the different series only from 26.1 to 31.6 years. Extremes of age are seen. Case 19034 was only eleven months while Case 7210 was 77.5 years of age at the time of coma. For Case 7210 this was a third attack. Both the baby and the elderly woman recovered and, as far as we have been able to discover, the latter is the oldest patient on record to have recovered from an attack of diabetic coma. Case 6960 was 77.3 years of age when she recovered from coma in May 1943. In Dillon and Dyer's[6] series there was one woman aged eighty-three years who entered the hospital with a blood sugar of 896 milligrams, and a CO_2 combining power of 18 volumes, per cent; she died, however, eleven hours after admission and postmortem examination showed abscesses of the kidneys and lungs. Our Case 7210 had had two other attacks of coma and one of very severe acidosis which had been brought on by omission of insulin, but it was felt that,

[1] Gamble: Extracellular Fluid, Harvard Dept. of Pediatrics, Chart 40, 1942.
[2] Sprague: P. 117; loc. cit., p. 314.
[3] Woodyatt: In Cecil's Textbook of Medicine, 6th ed., Philadelphia, W. B. Saunders Company, p. 610, 1943.
[4] Root: Med. Clin, North America, in press.
[5] Joslin and others: Med. Clin. North America, **8**, 1873, 1925; **10**, 1281, 1927; **13**, 11, 1929; **15**, 829, 1932; **16**, 793, 1933; New England Jour. Med., **212**, 288, 1935; Arch. Int. Med., **59**, 175, 1937; Jour. Am. Med. Assn., **119**, 1160, 1942.
[6] Dillon and Dyer: Loc. cit., p. 421.

TABLE 48.—651 CASES OF DIABETIC COMA.

Summary Table—Comparative Study, by Averages, of the Ten Series.

Series and number of cases	Age at coma, years.	Duration of D.M., years.	Date.	Blood. Sugar, per cent. 1st day.	Sugar, per cent. 2d day.	Plasma CO_2 combining power, vol. %. 1st day.	2d day.	3d day.	Non-protein nitrogen, mg. per 100 cc. 1st day.	Urine at entrance. Diacetic acid.	Sugar, per cent.	Insulin units. 1st day.	2d day.	3d day.	Fatal cases. No.	Per cent.
I 24 Cases	31.5$_{24}$	2.4$_{24}$	May, 1923, to Mar., 1925	0.47$_{23}$	0.20$_{20}$	15$_{24}$	33$_{20}$	31$_{10}$	47$_{16}$	+++++$_{24}$	3.3$_{24}$	154$_{24}$	63$_{12}$	58$_{11}$	5	21
II 28 Cases	31.6$_{28}$	2.8$_{28}$	Apr., 1925, to Feb., 1927	0.49$_{28}$	0.20$_{20}$	14$_{28}$	29$_{20}$	30$_{10}$	46$_{11}$	+++$_{28}$	3.4$_{28}$	166$_{28}$	59$_{26}$	49$_{26}$	4	14
III 53 Cases	29.1$_{53}$	4.0$_{53}$	Mar., 1927, to Feb., 1929	0.53$_{52}$	0.21$_{46}$	13$_{53}$	28$_{37}$	38$_{11}$	60$_{33}$	+++$_{51}$	3.1$_{53}$	183$_{53}$	40$_{00}$	39$_{40}$	5	9
IV 74 Cases	31.3$_{74}$	3.5$_{74}$	Feb., 1929, to Aug., 1931	0.49$_{74}$	0.20$_{51}$	11$_{73}$	29$_{42}$	35$_{11}$	48$_{52}$	++$_{74}$	3.7$_{74}$	257$_{74}$	49$_{65}$	41$_{63}$	13	18
V 42 Cases	26.1$_{42}$	3.5$_{42}$	Aug., 1931, to Oct., 1932	0.47$_{43}$	0.15$_{37}$	12$_{42}$	28$_{38}$	33$_{5}$	37$_{17}$	++$_{43}$	3.9$_{40}$	201$_{43}$	51$_{41}$	45$_{39}$	2	5
VI 55 Cases	28.5$_{55}$	4.3$_{55}$	Oct., 1932, to Oct., 1934	0.51$_{55}$	0.17$_{46}$	12$_{55}$	29$_{31}$	34$_{9}$	49$_{28}$	++$_{54}$	3.6$_{54}$	196$_{55}$	52$_{51}$	44$_{40}$	6	11
VII 42 Cases	28.2$_{42}$	5.6$_{42}$	Oct., 1934, to Jan., 1936	0.54$_{42}$	0.20$_{39}$	11$_{42}$	30$_{94}$	41$_{5}$	49$_{18}$	++$_{43}$	3.7$_{42}$	210$_{41}$	66$_{41}$	61$_{41}$	3	7
VIII 145 Cases	29.7$_{145}$	5.2$_{145}$	Jan., 1936, to Jan., 1940	0.50$_{144}$	0.17$_{127}$	10$_{144}$	30$_{112}$	46$_{98}$	37$_{84}$	++$_{141}$	3.6$_{144}$	192*$_{141}$ 35†$_{63}$	43*$_{33}$ 36†$_{96}$	41*$_{27}$ 38†$_{106}$	17	12
IX 62 Cases	27.6$_{62}$	5.3$_{62}$	Jan., 1940, to Jan., 1942	0.44$_{62}$	0.15$_{60}$	12$_{62}$	36$_{47}$	47$_{34}$	41$_{11}$	++$_{14}$	3.2$_{45}$	207*$_{63}$ 37†$_{51}$	43*$_{60}$ 42†$_{51}$	30*$_{60}$ 42†$_{61}$	3	5
X 126 Cases	28.1$_{126}$	6.7$_{126}$	Jan., 1942, to Jan., 1946	0.52$_{125}$	0.15$_{133}$	14$_{125}$	37	33$_{11}$	55$_{39}$	+++$_{111}$	3.3$_{117}$	254*$_{124}$ 28†$_{108}$	30*$_{120}$ 39†$_{122}$	29* 39†	3	2.4
Total and averages 651 cases	29.3	5.5	.....	0.51	..	13	33	38	50	+++	3.4	225	64	62	61	9.4

*Unmodified insulin. †Protamine zinc insulin. The subfigures indicate the number of determinations upon which the average is computed in each series.

although for some months she had been poorly regulated, this last attack was precipitated by a urinary tract infection. She responded well to treatment but died at the age of 78.8 years of cerebral hemorrhage. In all of our series there have been 8 recoveries among 10 instances of coma in 7 patients seventy years of age and over at the time of the attack of coma.

Among the 495 patients there were 182 males and 313 females. The preponderance of females is all the more striking when one considers that in the age group chiefly concerned (153 of our cases were under fifteen years of age) diabetes is fully as common in males as in females.

The duration of diabetes prior to the onset of coma varied from 2.4 years in Series I, which ran from May, 1923 to March, 1925, to 6.7 years in Series X, which ran from January, 1942 to January, 1946. These figures and others in the same column of Table 48 are influenced by various factors. Thus the figure is increased appreciably in some series by the inclusion of a great number of cases of long-standing who are chronic offenders. Then, too, in the period from May, 1923, to March, 1925, the patients had scarcely had time to live longer than 2.4 years with their diabetes because it was not until August 7, 1922 that the first dose of insulin was given at the New England Deaconess Hospital.

E. ETIOLOGY.

The usual causes of coma are preventable. We teach patients that coma occurs because of (1) too much food, (2) too little insulin, or (3) an infection. Too much food may mean the deliberate breaking of diet, or the consumption of body tissue as in undiagnosed diabetes, fever or hyperthyroidism. Too little insulin often means no insulin, due to its omission from carelessness or ignorance, or the discovery of diabetes with the onset of coma. The influence of infections is real. Patients may be progressing serenely, with diet, insulin and exercise well balanced, when, with the development of a carbuncle, pneumonia, upper respiratory infection or other acute febrile illness, acidosis may be precipitated.

An insulin-treated diabetic should be taught that if he omits his insulin, he is in danger of coma. When sugar appears in the urine, even though he curtails or omits his diet, he must be made to realize that he can consume his own tissues and that he always requires insulin as long as sugar shows.

Irregularities of diet exceed by far any other cause of coma. In 145 consecutive cases of coma it seemed definite that in 72 the cause was breaking of diet, too little or no insulin, or both. There were 18 other cases in which the cause was not apparent, but we suspect that in most of them it was diet-breaking or inadequate insulin dosage In general associated with overeating, there is almost invariably a deficiency in insulin.

In the same series of 145 cases there were 24 in which infections probably played a large part in causing the acidosis. Among these there were 6 instances of upper respiratory infection, 3 of carbuncles, 3 of pneumonia, 2 of labial abscesses, and 1 each of infection and gangrene of the foot, epididymitis, pulmonary tuberculosis, hepatitis, sinusitis, acute rheumatic fever, urinary tract infection, appendicitis, cellulitis of the neck and meningococcic meningitis. In only one case (15656) did it seem at all likely that hyperthyroidism may have been a precipitating factor. However, at times acute thyrotoxicosis ("thyroid storm") and diabetic coma may occur together to produce a most unusual and alarming clinical picture. Two such instances, occurring in Cases 4289 and 13172, were reported by Root.[1]

In this series of 145 cases, toxemia of pregnancy and cardiac decompensation seemed in one case each to be associated with the precipitation of acidosis. In 4 instances coma occurred in periods of marked insensitiveness to insulin; Case 17162 developed diabetic coma with a blood sugar of 0.43 per cent and a CO_2 of 5 volumes per cent despite the fact that in the few days just prior to this his insulin dosage had ranged from 300 to 480 units daily. During this attack of coma 2312 units of insulin were required during the first twenty-four hours of treatment. Recovery ensued. (See page 380.)

In 50 recent cases the omission of insulin was an important factor in 27 instances, although dietary error was also present. In 6 instances overeating and in 9 cases infections, chiefly respiratory, seemed from the history to be of major importance. Mirsky[2] fed diabetic patients in the hospital ward large amounts of carbohydrate without producing acidosis and concluded that excessive carbohydrate ingestion is less important than the omission of insulin in causing coma. He states, "Needless to say, excessive amounts of carbohydrate, such as we used, are contra-indicated as a therapeutic procedure, because of the polyuria and resultant loss of weight on the one hand and the possible danger of pancreatic exhaustion on the other."

In 4 patients the onset of coma coincided with that of menstruation. Others, as Harrop and Mosenthal[3] and Bertram,[4] commented upon the influence of menstruation in increasing or precipitating acidosis. Bertram mentioned one patient who in 8 of her 17 attacks of coma suffered the illness at the onset of the menses.

The diabetic is not immune to conditions other than acidosis which cause nausea and vomiting, such as acute gastro-intestinal upsets, acute appendicitis and acute infectious diseases. Any one of these conditions can and will precipitate coma. One state passes

[1] Root: Medical Papers dedicated to Henry A. Christian, Baltimore, Waverly Press, Inc., p. 434, 1936.

[2] Mirsky: Jour. Am. Med. Assn., **118**, 690, 1942.

[3] Harrop and Mosenthal: Bull. Johns Hopkins Hosp., **29**, 161, 1918.

[4] Bertram: P. 36; loc. cit., p. 87.

quickly into the other, each masking the other and making the end-result more serious. Unable to take food, the uneducated, unprepared diabetic patient omits his insulin and coma follows. We have been forced to conclude that in diabetes vomiting is an evil omen, and unless heeded may lead to death. We have heard the story over and over from patients that because they felt sick, perhaps vomited and so could not take food, they reasoned that, therefore, they did not need to take their insulin, and we regret to state that sometimes the discontinuance of insulin was carried out on their physicians' advice.

Because an infection may frequently be the precipitating cause of acidosis, it is imperative that at the outset of treatment of a case of coma, a complete physical examination be done. It must always be borne in mind that fever is not present in uncomplicated diabetic coma; in extremely severe acidosis the temperature is normal or below. Consequently, if after partial recovery fever is found to be present, or if in any way the case does not respond in a straightforward manner, a complication should be suspected and an even more thorough physical examination often in association with a surgeon, and including an otoscopic and a pelvic and rectal examination be done in order to ascertain the underlying difficulty.

The important influence of infection on the precipitation and course of diabetic coma is illustrated by the following case reports.

Case 23974, engineer, age thirty-one years, diabetes nine years in duration, was admitted November 30, 1943 in profound diabetic coma. He had broken diet on Thanksgiving Day. Nausea and vomiting began the next day, became worse on the second day and therefore insulin was omitted. On the third day without insulin he became entirely unconscious with labored breathing. Upon admission the blood-pressure could not be obtained and the pulse was hardly perceptible. After treatment was begun the blood-pressure rose to systolic 50 and diastolic 30. The eyeballs were extremely soft, Kussmaul respiration was extreme and he was completely unconscious. The blood sugar 1540 milligrams per cent, the blood CO_2 9 volumes per cent, blood acetone 130 milligrams per cent and the non-protein nitrogen was 91 milligrams per 100 cc. Dehydration was extreme. Examination of the lungs showed no râles but there was an amphoric quality to the respiratory murmur. In the first few minutes after admission he received 200 units of insulin subcutaneously and 100 units intravenously; during the first five hours in the hospital he received a total of 700 units of insulin intravenously and 600 units subcutaneously. During these five hours the blood sugar fell to 1080 milligrams and the CO_2 rose to 20 volumes per cent. At the end of eighteen hours the blood sugar had fallen to 222 milligrams. The catheterized urine upon admission showed 5.3 per cent sugar but only a slightly positive test for diacetic acid. From that time on, no urine was obtained although he received 6000 cc. of salt solution intravenously in the first ten hours. An x-ray showed bilateral bronchial pneumonia; continuous intravenous administration of penicillin was begun and continued for three days until the pneumonia cleared. The secretion of urine began at the end of twelve hours and continued in normal quantity. However, the non-protein nitrogen of the blood rose to 130 milligrams and remained elevated for two weeks. During this time anorexia and vomiting were so frequent that during the first few days he was fed by intravenous administration of 5 per cent glucose solution in normal salt solution, usually with the addition of ⅙ molar sodium lactate solution in an attempt to raise the blood CO_2 values which persisted at a level of 30 to 40 volumes per cent during this period of nitrogen retention. The urine showed a moderate amount of albumin upon admission but only a few white blood cells. At the end of two weeks the non-protein nitrogen of the blood fell to normal. At this time it was supposed that he might have an underlying chronic pyelonephritis. After his recovery intravenous pyelograms revealed normal kidney outlines and apparently normal kidney function. His recovery was complete and on November 16, 1945 he was taking 6 units of crystalline and 42 units of protamine zinc insulin daily. He weighed 154 pounds and his diet was carbohydrate 173 grams, protein 97 grams and fat 118 grams. He illustrates the serious but temporary impairment in renal function brought about in diabetic coma when complicated by severe infection.

Case 22682, clerk, aged nineteen years with diabetes of four months' duration untreated and unrecognized until she developed serious acidosis, entered April 10, 1943, profoundly unconscious and anuric. A respiratory infection began four days previously, glycosuria was discovered two days previously and she had become unconscious twenty-four hours before admission. She was transferred from another hospital because of her anuria. Upon admission the blood sugar was 534 milligrams per cent, the blood CO_2 was 12 volumes per cent and non-protein nitrogen was 55 milligrams per 100 cc. Following the administration of 200 units of insulin the blood sugar fell to 165 milligrams and the CO_2 rose to 21 volumes per cent. On admission the eyeballs were soft and gastric lavage yielded 800 cc. of black tarry material. She died six hours after admission. Postmortem examination showed extreme streptococcus infection of the throat with membrane formation in the pharynx, palate and nose. There was pus in the sphenoid and ethmoid sinuses and early invasion of the pituitary fossa was present. In addition there were early cholesterosis of the gall-bladder and early atheromatosis of the aorta.

Case 13274, a mechanic, aged thirty-four and four-tenths years, was admitted in acidosis on April 10, 1937, having been ill at home for about a week; prior to this he had lost weight for two to four months. On the day before admission he had had nausea, vomiting, labored breathing, and become drowsy. On physical examination our colleague, Dr. W. J. Clauser, noted fever, stiffness of the neck and a positive Kernig sign and suspected meningitis. Lumbar puncture yielded cloudy, slightly purulent fluid containing meningococci. With repeated lumbar taps and administration of antimeningococcus serum, he made a gradual recovery. He was alive in February, 1946.

A study of 126 cases, as summarized in Table 49, shows no striking correlation between the incidence of coma and the duration of diabetes. The relatively large number of cases occurring within the first year of diabetes includes chiefly patients with hitherto unrecognized diabetes. The continued occurrence of coma in patients who have had diabetes more than one year demands that the education of a patient not stop with the initial contact but that it be a continuous process. The diabetic patient must be made to realize the value of careful treatment and be made to assume responsibility for himself.

28

TABLE 49.—DURATION OF DIABETES PRIOR TO COMA IN 126 CONSECUTIVE CASES.
(Series X, Table 48.)

Duration of diabetes, years.	No. of cases of coma.	Duration of diabetes, years.	No. of cases of coma.
0–1	17*	11–12	2
1–2	6	12–13	4
2–3	13	13–14	7
3–4	11	14–15	4
4–5	9	15–16	2
5–6	4	16–17	0
6–7	18	17–18	2
7–8	11	18–19	2
8–9	2	19–20	0
9–10	5	Over 20	3
10–11	4		

* In 9 of the 17 cases the duration of diabetes was one-half year or less.

We share Woodyatt's[1] belief that it is not enough for a patient to be familiar with the technical details of testing the urine, calculating the diet and giving insulin. He must know the conditions which may bring on acidosis so that he may thus prevent or check it. He must know the rules of treatment so well that in an emergency he will act reflexly in accordance with them.

In our cases of diabetic coma there has been a relatively large number of patients in whom the disease had not been recognized until the onset of acidosis. In 145 cases there were 19 instances of coma in patients with unrecognized diabetes or untreated diabetes of recent onset. Even more striking was the experience of Dillon and Dyer[2] in this respect; of their 224 patients with diabetic coma, 82 did not know that they had diabetes at the onset of acidosis which caused them to be admitted to the Philadelphia General Hospital. These cases present a difficult problem, and it is only by education and stimulation of the interest of physicians and laity alike regarding the importance of early recognition of the disease that progress can be made.

F. THE SYMPTOMS AND SIGNS OF DIABETIC COMA.

1. **Warning Signs and Directions to Patients.**—The symptoms of diabetic coma are notoriously vague and even to a doctor the diagnosis often proves elusive. The spectre of threatening diabetic coma should always haunt the physician, particularly when the patient is first seen. It is astonishing how insidiously coma steals over a patient, and we have given up expecting nurses, unless they have had great experience with diabetic patients, to recognize its approach. It is better to treat any symptom out of the ordinary as premonitory of coma and better for patients when they feel sick to begin coma precautions than to run the risk of beginning treatment too late. Despite the only too large number of cases of diabetic

[1] Woodyatt: Med. Clin. North America, **21**, 11, 1937.
[2] Dillon and Dyer: Loc. cit., p. 421.

coma which we have seen, more than once we have been chagrined at having failed to realize its presence. Anything unusual should arouse suspicion, and one should instantly investigate any of the following symptoms: headache, anorexia, restlessness, weakness, listlessness, nausea, vomiting, drowsiness, and painful, rapid or deep breathing. In the presence of fever always be on the alert for coma.

Rules for the prevention of coma are taught to all patients and they are instructed to follow them whenever they feel indisposed from any cause whatsoever. These measures can do no harm in any condition and by their adoption in the early stages of acidosis will avert it in all but the most desperate cases. They are as follows: (1) Go to bed whenever indisposed; (2) keep warm; (3) call the doctor after first having examined the urine for sugar; (4) secure a nurse or at least someone to wait upon you and save your strength; (5) drink a glass of liquid each hour—such as coffee, tea, broths, diluted orange juice, water, oatmeal gruel; (6) move the bowels by enema, and, if liquids have not been retained by mouth, follow the enema by an injection of 1 pint of lukewarm water containing a teaspoonful of salt; (7) on the advice of your doctor take appropriate doses of rapidly-acting insulin as long as the urine contains sugar.

2. **Symptoms.**—As stated above, there are no symptoms which are invariably found but usually the onset of definite acidosis is attended by headache, malaise, nausea, vomiting, abdominal pain and pains variously over the body including the extremities. Often these symptoms have been preceded by thirst, polyuria and other classical symptoms of uncontrolled diabetes. Useful in diagnosis is the history of irregularity in treatment with diet or insulin, of an infection or of a state in which there is increased metabolism. If proper treatment is not instituted, the vomiting and abdominal pain continue and the breathing becomes labored.

The saturation of the body with "acetone bodies" is reflected in the fruity odor of the breath which sometimes is so marked that the peculiar smell in the sick room is apparent to those entering. Drowsiness comes, proceeds to stupor and passes finally into coma. Complete unconsciousness truly represents an advanced stage; fortunately most patients when brought to the hospital for treatment can be aroused if sufficient stimulus be applied. It is striking how much acidosis may be present without unconsciousness. Case 9783 *walked* into the hospital at 8 A.M. January 9, 1931. A determination of the plasma CO_2 combining power shortly after entrance gave a value of 4 volumes per cent(!). Energetic treatment with supportive measures and 430 units of insulin were of no avail and he died seven hours after admission. In the pre-insulin days Case 1870 *walked* into the hospital at 9 A.M. February 11, 1921. Although marked Kussmaul respiration was present, the mental state was affected only to the point of drowsiness. However, this patient was dead by 10 P.M., thirteen hours after admission.

3. **Signs.**—When first seen, the patient in full-blown diabetic coma presents a distressing picture. He lies in bed, unconscious or semiconscious, often moaning as with pain, with a dry, cold skin, flushed drawn face, and obviously dehydrated tissues. One evidence of the dehydration may be a pleural friction rub, which may disappear rapidly with the administration of fluids, as was described by Armanino and Pry[1] in 5 cases. Respirations are of the long, deep rapid Kussmaul ("air-hunger") type. The air-hunger may be replaced by shallow respiration when death approaches. The eyeballs are soft, the mouth and tongue are dry and present a dirty coating. At intervals the patient vomits dark brown material, obviously changed blood. On being turned or examined, cries as of pain may be occasioned. The abdominal findings may closely simulate those of acute appendicitis. The extremities are cold and the body temperature, in the absence of accompanying infection, is often below normal. The pulse is rapid and weak and the blood-pressure low. Often the muscles are flaccid, the tendon reflexes diminished or absent and the pupils dilated. Falta[2] states that the Loewi reaction (dilation of the pupil when a drop of epinephrine is applied to the eye) is often strongly positive.

As regards the respiration Knipping and Armiejevic[3] have shown that the minute volume and the respiratory equivalent (relationship between the respiratory volume and the O_2 consumption) are increased. The pulse is rapid and of poor quality. There may occur a decrease in the amount of circulating blood so that the blood collects in the periphery of the body[4,5] and, as Falta[2] puts it, "das Herz läuft leer." According to him the disturbance of circulation is therefore chiefly peripheral and the resulting fall in blood-pressure is refractory to digitalis.

G. LABORATORY FINDINGS IN DIABETIC COMA.

In the following discussion reference is made again to the summary Table 48 which gives the average results in the ten series of coma cases treated thus far.

1. **Blood Sugar.**—The average initial blood sugar varied surprisingly little from series to series being between 0.44 and 0.54 per cent. This had, on the average, fallen on the second day after admission to a satisfactory (diabetic) level. A high blood sugar does not necessarily imply a poor prognosis. Among 651 cases of coma we have seen in all 24 cases in which the initial blood sugar was 1 per cent (1000 milligrams per 100 cc.) or above. Of these 19 re-

[1] Armanino and Ory: Am. Jour. Med. Sci., **211**, 597, 1946.

[2] Falta: Die Zuckerkrankheit, Berlin and Vienna, Urban & Schwarzenberg, 1936.

[3] Knipping and Armiejevic: Ztschr. f. exp. Med., **74**, 787, 1930.

[4] Eppinger, Kisch and Schwartz: Das Versagen des Kreislaufes, Berlin, Julius Springer, 1927.

[5] Lauter and Baumaun: Arch. f. klin. Med., **159**, H. 1–2, 1928.

covered and 5 died. In our series the highest blood sugar with recovery of the patient was 1.68[1] per cent. (See page 169.)

If it is true that in diabetic coma the level of the blood sugar depends not merely upon food ingestion but upon the degree of excessive glucose formation from protein and fat as well as from glycogen, then a relation exists between the severity of the metabolic disorder and the blood-sugar level. In Table 50 the correlation of blood-sugar levels and the insulin requirement in 173 coma cases indicates that this relationship should not be neglected.

TABLE 50.—BLOOD-SUGAR LEVEL CORRELATED WITH INSULIN DOSE IN 173 COMA CASES.

October 21, 1940, to January 1, 1946.

Blood sugar on admission, mg. per 100 cc.	Cases.	Average insulin in first 24 hours, units.
1300–1600	2	1219
1000–1300	5	815
600–1000	39	368
400–600	60	247
200–400	67	161

Two adults whose blood-sugar values were 1380 and 1540 milligrams per cent with recovery required an average of 1219 units in the first twenty-four hours. The decline in insulin requirement parallels the initial blood-sugar level. In 67 cases in whom the blood-sugar level was between 200 and 400 milligrams, the average insulin dose was only 161 units. It is true that in some of these patients insulin had been given prior to admission by the house physician, often in liberal amount upon our recommendation by telephone.

Dillon and Dyer[2] reported 25 cases of diabetic coma in which the blood sugar was 1000 milligrams per cent or more on admission to the Philadelphia General Hospital. Of these 9 recovered and 16 died. Sixteen were women and 9 were men. The ages varied between twenty-one and fifty-nine years. Fourteen of the 25 patients were negroes. Recovery took place in a colored woman, aged twenty-one years, who entered with a blood sugar of 1850 milligrams per cent, a plasma CO_2 combining power of 13 volumes per cent, and blood urea nitrogen of 95 milligrams per cent.

2. **Blood CO_2.**—The average CO_2 combining power of the blood plasma on admission was also surprisingly constant, varying in the different groups of patients from 10 to 15 volumes per cent. This rose on succeeding days so that on the second day (usually twelve to eighteen hours after admission) the average values varied from 28 to 37 per cent. In Series VIII by the third day it had reached a higher level than in any of the preceding series although in that particular series it was the lowest at entrance. In Fig. 13 variations in CO_2 content of the plasma, expressed in milliequivalents per liter, are shown in relation to the acid-base composition of the blood plasma.

[1] Curtis and Dixon: Loc. cit., p. 169.
[2] Dillon and Dyer: Loc. cit., p. 421.

3. **Blood Acetone.**—An abnormal concentration of acetone bodies in the blood is an essential feature of diabetic coma (Root[1]). It is usually proportional to the severity of coma and the amount of treatment required for recovery; this is especially so if due allowance is made for the fact that the susceptibility of the brain to acidosis will

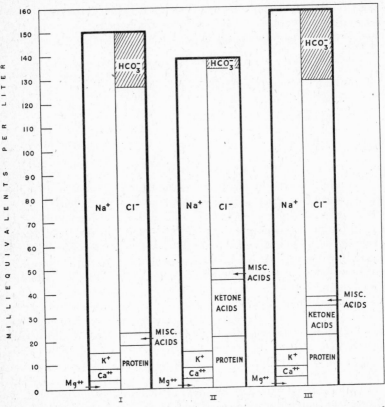

Fig. 13.—Acid-base composition of the blood plasma in a normal, *I*, compared with a case of diabetic coma, *II*, diabetic ketosis with alkalosis resulting from alkaline therapy, *III*. The data are charted after the method of Gamble. *II*, Diabetic coma with vomiting for several days. Dehydration was marked. Blood CO_2 content 4 milliequivalents, total base 139 milliequivalents. *III*, Diabetes of long duration, man twenty-six years of age. Vomiting for seven days with mild grippe. He took soda bicarbonate and Amphojel in large quantities. Blood CO_2 content 33.6 milliequivalents. Blood ketones 73 mg. per 100 cc. Blood chloride 89 miliequivalents per liter.

be affected by the age of the patient, by the duration of the diabetes, by the presence or absence of acute infection and especially by such other factors as coexisting arteriosclerosis and nephritic lesions. In a summary of determinations of total acetone bodies in the

[1] Root: Jour. Am., Med. Assn. **127**, 557, 1945.

whole blood of 31 cases of diabetic coma in which the blood carbon dioxide content was 20 volumes or less and 10 cases of ketosis in which the acidosis was not so severe as given by Root, 2 patients who recovered showed values of 195 milligrams total acetone bodies per 100 cc. No patient actually in coma had less than 60 milligrams of acetone, diacetic acid and beta-oxybutyric acid in 100 cc. of blood. Indeed, complete unconsciousness did not occur with acetone values under 100 milligrams with a single exception. This girl, aged nineteen years, was anuric and death occurred as a result of a purulent involvement of the sinuses and beginning meningitis. This low concentration of acetone bodies is consistent with the disappearance of acetone bodies in the urine during the last few hours of life in severe acidosis and is in some way related to the terminal cachexia of diabetes and severe infection. Twenty-one patients had blood acetone values of over 100 milligrams. Of these, 10 were female, 11 male and only 2 were over the age of forty years. The highest blood-sugar values and the highest insulin doses were required in the groups with the highest blood acetone values. Thus the average blood sugar for the patients with blood acetone values above 140 milligrams was 748 milligrams and the insulin requirement during the first twenty-four hours for this group of patients was 553 units. The effect of impaired renal function in causing retention of acetone bodies was shown in a woman of seventy-six years who entered with gangrene and auricular fibrillation. The blood acetone value was 133 milligrams, yet the blood carbon dioxide content was 38 volumes per cent. She made a good recovery after thigh amputation. The rapidity with which the concentration of total acetone bodies in the blood of patients declines under treatment for diabetic coma seems roughly to parallel that of the decline in the blood sugar.

Poulsen[1] has devised a method for determining total acetone bodies in capillary blood which requires only 0.2 cc. of blood. He found that brief intense muscular exertion did not cause an increase in ketone bodies in the blood, whereas more prolonged work performance led to a definite increase in ketone bodies in the blood. He records blood acetone values up to 120 milligrams per 100 cc. in cases of severe ketosis.

Bertram[2] records values for total acetone (acetone and diacetic acid, but not including β-oxybutyric acid) as high as 135 milligrams per cent and for β-oxybutyric acid as high as 213 milligrams per cent. He believes the greatest toxic effect to be due to the acetone and diacetic acid content of the blood exceeds 70 milligrams per cent. The highest value that we have found so far in diabetic coma

[1] Poulsen: Studies on the Ketosis in Diabetes Mellitus, Copenhagen, Steno Memorial Hospital, 1941.
[2] Bertram: P. 51; loc. cit., p. 87.

has been 195 milligrams per cent for acetone bodies including acetone, diacetic acid and β-oxybutyric acid.

4. **Blood Non-protein Nitrogen.**—An elevation in the non-protein nitrogen content of the blood occurs frequently. Average values in the different groups have varied from 37 to 60 milligrams per cent in the initial blood samples. Among the 145 cases in Series VIII, 47, or 32.4 per cent, had on admission a non-protein nitrogen value of 45 milligrams per cent or over. Of these, 6 died, but none of the deaths was among the 5 patients in whom the non-protein nitrogen values were highest, 89 milligrams to 140 milligrams per cent.

5. **Urine Findings.**—The urine almost invariably contained on admission a large quantity of diacetic acid as shown by a definitely positive ferric chloride (Gerhardt) reaction. Only in cases in which there is associated renal block does one see a negative test for acetone bodies, and in these cases the blood plasma will invariably be found to give a positive test for acetone. Rare exceptions to this rule have been reported but it is doubtful if these were cases of true diabetic coma. In Case 25957 the urine gave no test for diacetic acid or acetone but the blood acetone content was 70 milligrams per 100 cc. and the blood non-protein nitrogen was 63 milligrams. Briggs[1] regarded it impossible that acetone should be present in the blood and absent in the urine because acetone diffuses so rapidly and furthermore it is not even necessary for acetone to pass the kidneys to get into the bladder urine. Incidentally, Briggs described an ingenious method for detecting ketosis. In his procedure the patient blows rapidly through a bent glass drinking tube into about 3 cc. of Nessler's reagent in a large test-tube until a white opalescence appears. The number of blows required to give the test depends upon the concentration of the acetone in the breath and the volume of expirations. If the patient is comatose the test-tube containing the Nessler's reagent is fitted with a two-holed stopper thereby providing for both inlet and outlet tubes of glass; these are connected with short pieces of rubber tubing. The free end of the inlet tubing is placed in the patient's mouth and suction is applied by an operator on the outlet tubing. A few bubbles drawn through the rubber at the end of the 3 successive expirations gives an intense white cloud in the presence of severe ketosis.

Hyperglycemic stupor with hyperpyrexia described the condition of Case 23935, age nineteen years, reported by Root.[2] The patient had entered another hospital twenty-four hours before in early coma, where he had received 400 grams glucose as orange juice and by intravenous injection. Insulin was delayed until he was unconscious. Then insulin in large amounts was given. Upon transfer to the Deaconess Hospital the blood and urine contained no acetone

[1] Briggs: Jour. Lab. and Clin. Med., **25**, 603, 1940.
[2] Root: Loc. cit., p. 428.

bodies but the blood sugar was 678 milligrams. Autopsy was negative.

Richardson[1] described a case of diabetic coma with a CO_2 of 7 volumes per cent who nevertheless had no diacetic acid or acetone in the urine. He discusses as possible causes for such a condition (a) dehydration with accompanying decrease in the total base of the body, (b) the excretion of all the ketones as β-hydroxybutyric acid rather than as diacetic acid or acetone and (c) pathological changes in the kidney which may impair the excretion of ketones. Labbé and Boulin[2] likewise have called attention to the possibility of diabetic coma with a negative test for diacetic acid in the urine. Usually, however, the demonstration of acetone or of diacetic acid in the urine is a requisite for diagnosis.

The amount of sugar in the urine varied on the average between 3 and 4 per cent; strikingly high values are rarely seen. The urine usually gives a positive test for albumin and the astonishing showers of granular casts seen in the sediment are a classical and frequent finding.

6. **Blood Chloride and Anuria.**—The fact that the chloride of the blood plasma is frequently lowered has already been mentioned. It is noteworthy that subsequent to this, urinary secretion may cease and retention of non-protein nitrogen elements follow. In 3 cases reported by Root[3] injections of 50 cc. to 130 cc. of 10 per cent salt solution intravenously induced urination and relieved dangerous nitrogen retention. This measure may succeed after patients have been given, without benefit, large amounts of physiological salt solution parenterally as well as hypertonic glucose solution intravenously, but the indication for such treatment is a low percentage of salt in the blood; it is possible that a diminution in the sodium rather than the chloride content of the blood is the responsible factor, but data are not complete on this point. Recently Krarup[4] has reported upon the successful use of 1 liter of 1.3 per cent sodium bicarbonate solution intravenously daily for three days in a patient who developed anuria and an elevated blood urea following diabetic coma. In Krarup's patient the plasma chloride was normal but the alkali reserve was still low. His case was therefore not comparable to those reported by Root.

7. **Hematologic Changes.**—Leucocytosis is the rule in coma and values from 15,000 to 50,000 white blood corpuscles per cubic millimeter are commonly found even though there be no accompanying infection. The highest count in our series was 92,000, in Case 13074. Lawrence[5] has called attention to the increase in formed elements of the blood with a color index over 1, due to dehydration

[1] Richardson: Med. Clin. North America, **16**, 257, 1932.
[2] Labbé and Boulin: Bull. et mém. Soc. méd. de hôp. de Paris, **49**, 313, 1933.
[3] Root: Loc. cit., p. 254.
[4] Krarup: Jour. Am. Med. Assn., **114**, 1604, 1940.
[5] Lawrence: Brit. Med. Jour., **2**, 145, 1932.

and hemo concentration. Heck and Hall[1] state that along with leucocytosis, diabetic coma is commonly associated with a leukemoid reaction. The myeloid immaturity disappears promptly upon control of the acidosis. They cite the case of one patient treated at the Mayo Clinic in whom the white blood count was 25,000 and the differential count showed 2.3 per cent metamyelocytes, 0.7 per cent myelocytes, and 0.3 per cent promyelocytes.

H. THE DIFFERENTIAL DIAGNOSIS IN DIABETIC COMA.

An unconscious patient always presents a problem in diagnosis. When the patient is a known diabetic the possibility of diabetic coma comes quickly to mind. One should not, however, forget that coma may be the first striking evidence of diabetes and that the patient may be brought to the physician without any knowledge on the part of the family that diabetes is present. The past history and events leading up to the present illness are, nevertheless, of great value in calling attention to the correct diagnosis. In differential diagnosis one must consider the following: severe hypoglycemia, cerebral hemorrhage, uremia, meningitis, poisoning as by barbital, and toxicity from overwhelming infections. The history, physical findings, examination of the urine, and determination of the blood sugar will allow ready diagnosis in almost every instance.

Bowen, Roufa and Clinger[2] have called attention to the confusion which may arise between marked salicylate poisoning and diabetic acidosis because of the close similarity of the clinical picture. Their patient, a boy, aged eighteen months, exhibited stupor, Kussmaul respiration and dehydration, and the urine gave a 3+ reduction with Benedict's solution. A strongly positive ferric chloride test was reported (violet color due to salicylates). The blood sugar was 87 mg. per 100 cc. and the CO_2 capacity of the blood plasma, 50 volumes per cent. The child was discharged clinically well three days after admission. The authors believe that the dyspnea of salicylate poisoning can be more reasonably explained on the basis of an irritative action on the respiratory center than an acidosis. In Labbé's[3] case, however, a definite acidosis existed with a lowering of the CO_2 combining power of the plasma to 18 volumes per cent. His patient was a woman, aged twenty-five years, who had been receiving 12 grams of sodium salicylate a day (with sodium bicarbonate) because of acute articular rheumatism.

In patients receiving insulin the differentiation between diabetic coma and an insulin reaction (hypoglycemia) may at times be confusing to the family of the patient and even to the doctor. The necessity of immediate action designed to obtain urine and blood

[1] Heck and Hall: Jour. Am. Med. Assn., **112**, 95, 1939.
[2] Bowen, Roufa and Clinger: Jour. Am. Med. Assn., **107**, 276, 1936.
[3] Labbé: Jour. Am. Med. Assn. (Paris letter), **106**, 55, 1936.

tests and settle the diagnosis cannot be exaggerated. The giving of more insulin to a patient already in hypoglycemia, or the withholding of insulin when the patient is in coma may lead to a fatal outcome. Diabetic coma comes on gradually over a period of hours or days, whereas an insulin reaction is manifest in a much shorter interval, even minutes. It is true that in reactions due to protamine zinc insulin the onset of symptoms is usually gradual, as would be anticipated with the use of a preparation which acts so slowly. The symptoms of the usual reaction due to regular or crystalline insulin are: nervousness, sweating, faintness, headache, hunger, and double vision. Only rarely does the condition progress to unconsciousness with or without convulsions. Reactions due to protamine zinc insulin are often accompanied by headache, particularly occipital, and occasionally by nausea and at times even vomiting. Although at the time of an insulin reaction the first specimen of urine may contain sugar, a second specimen obtained fifteen or twenty minutes later will invariably be sugar-free. Treatment, which consists in supplying readily available carbohydrate by mouth, under the skin, or by vein, usually gives prompt relief. More than one administration of carbohydrate may be necessary to bring about complete recovery from a reaction due to protamine zinc insulin.

When faced with the problem of unconsciousness of a diabetic patient at home or under conditions in which laboratory studies are difficult to carry out, it is justifiable to give a small amount of concentrated sterile glucose solution intravenously. If prompt and complete recovery takes place, an insulin reaction was probably the presenting condition; if no improvement is noted in a very few minutes, the condition is possibly that of diabetic coma and more exact study, usually with immediate hospitalization, is indicated.

It should be emphasized that recovery following the giving of glucose intravenously should be prompt and definite if one is to assume that the condition is one of hypoglycemia. Otherwise laboratory confirmation is imperative. In our own Case 2967, reported in detail elsewhere,[1] enough improvement followed intravenous injections of glucose that doctors and nurses felt that their original diagnosis of hypoglycemic coma was verified and yet the patient died two hours after admission to the hospital. Information from the laboratory, obtained too late to be of help, showed that the unconsciousness was that of profound diabetic coma in that end-stage in which Kussmaul respiration had given way to the pre-terminal breathing of the moribund.

Exercise extraordinary care before giving insulin if there is a possibility of insulin shock. Likewise, remember death lurks also if diabetic coma continues without insulin. Be forehanded. Always plan ahead as to how laboratory aids can be promptly secured.

[1] Joslin and others: Arch. Int. Med., 59, 175, 1937.

TABLE 51.—DIABETIC COMA AND INSULIN REACTION. DIFFERENTIAL DIAGNOSIS.

	Diabetic coma.	Insulin reaction.*
1. Onset	Slow—days	Sudden—minutes.
2. Food	Too much	Too little.
3. Insulin	Too little	Too much.
4. Presence of infection	Frequent	None.
5. Thirst	Extreme	Absent.
6. Hunger	Absent	Frequent.
7. Vomiting	Common	Seldom.
8. Pain in abdomen	Frequent	Absent.
9. Fever	Absent except with infection	Absent.
10. Skin	Dry	Moist.
11. Tremor	Absent	Frequent.
12. Vision	Dim	Double.
13. Eyeballs	Soft	Normal.
14. Appearance	Florid—extremely ill	Pale—weak—faint.
15. Respiration	Air-hunger	Normal.
16. Blood-pressure	Tends to fall	Tends to rise.
17. Mental state	Restless—distressed	Apathetic—irritable —hysterical.
18. Unconsciousness	Gradually approaches	May intervene suddenly.
19. Urine: sugar	Present	Absent (always in 2d specimen).
20. Urine: diacetic acid and acetone	Present	Absent.
21. Blood sugar	High	Low.
22. Specific treatment	Insulin—fluid—salt	Carbohydrate.
23 Response to treatment	Gradual—hours	Quick—minutes.

* The features of an insulin reaction listed in this table are those observed after rapidly-acting insulin, regular or crystalline. In certain respects reactions due to the slowly-acting protamine zinc insulin may differ. Headache, particularly occipital, nausea, and even vomiting may occur. These symptoms make the differential diagnosis between reactions from protamine zinc insulin and coma more difficult than that between regular or crystalline insulin and coma.

Dr. L. S. McKittrick,[1] our surgical colleague, who sees in consultation many of our coma cases, has discussed from the surgical viewpoint the differential diagnosis and treatment of a diabetic patient with nausea, vomiting and abdominal pain. He states that in a diabetic, malaise, drowsiness, vomiting and diffuse abdominal pain associated with widespread tenderness and spasm are so suggestive of acidosis, without demonstrable intra-abdominal pathological changes, that operation should not be done unless the abdominal symptoms persist after three or four hours of adequate treatment with insulin. Conversely, a history of abdominal pain with or without vomiting, when associated with localized and definite abdominal tenderness, usually with spasm, is suggestive of a surgical lesion within the abdomen in the patient with diabetic acidosis, just as is the case in the non-diabetic patient, and may be an indication for immediate operation. In that rare case, in which definite differentiation is impossible and yet imperative, it may be safer to open the abdomen under local anesthesia than to suffer further delay.

[1] McKittrick: New England Jour. Med., **209**, 1033, 1933.

Beardwood[1] has discussed in detail the abdominal symptomatology of diabetic acidosis recording his observations in 114 cases. Among these the onset of acidosis was accompanied in the majority of cases by symptoms referable to the gastro-intestinal tract. He lists the theories which have been advanced to explain the occurrence of such symptoms, namely, that they are due to (1) acute pancreatitis, (2) to intense spasm of the gastro-intestinal tract or that (3) they represent a defense mechanism set up to rid the body of the acid ions of the gastric juice. Admittedly none of these explanations is adequate. For further discussion see the paper by Walker.[2]

I. THE MORTALITY AND CAUSES OF DEATH IN DIABETIC COMA.

In the right-most column of Table 52 is given the mortality of the 10 groups of cases previously discussed. It has varied from 2.4 per cent in Series X to 21 per cent in Series I. Among the 651 coma admissions in 495 patients in the entire series there have been a total of 61 fatal cases, a case mortality of 9.4 per cent.

TABLE 52.—DEATHS IN COMA COMPARED WITH TOTAL DIABETIC DEATHS.

New England Deaconess Hospital, May, 1923, to January 1, 1946.
(Authors' patients only.)

	Total diabetic deaths.	Deaths from diabetic coma.	
		No.	Per cent of total.
1923 (from May)	7	2	28.6
1924	19	3	15.8
1925	20	2	10.0
1926	18	1	5.5
1927	19	3	15.7
1928	24	3	12.5
1929	33	3	9.1
1930	39	4	10.3
1931	28	7	25.0
1932	41	2	4.9
1933	31	4	12.9
1934	37	1	2.7
1935	26	3	11.6
1936	43	4	9.3
1937	45	4	8.9
1938	38	2	5.3
1939	44	7	16.0
1940	33	3	9.1
1941	27	0	0.0
1942	37	0	0.0
1943	30	1	3.3
1944	24	1	4.1
1945	52	1	1.9
	715	61	8.5

From May, 1923, to January 1, 1946, there have been 715 deaths among diabetic patients under our care at the New England Deacon-

[1] Beardwood: Jour. Am. Med. Assn., **105**, 1168, 1935.
[2] Walker: Ann. Int. Med., **9**, 1178, 1936.

ess Hospital; 61 of these patients, or 8.5 per cent entered in diabetic coma. In Table 52 the fatal cases are listed by years. The causes of death in these cases are discussed in the following paragraph:

1. Causes of Death During Coma and After Discharge From the Hospital.—As stated above there have been 61 deaths in the entire series of 651 attacks of coma in 495 patients. Of the 434 patients who left the hospital after recovery from coma, 67 have since died, and the remaining 367 were known to be alive on January 1, 1946.

In Table 53 are listed the causes of death of the 128 cases. Noteworthy is the fact that of the 67 cases dying after leaving the hospital following recovery from coma, 12 subsequently died elsewhere in another attack of diabetic coma and 15, or 22.4 per cent, died of tuberculosis.

TABLE 53.—CAUSES OF DEATH IN 128 CASES DURING OR FOLLOWING COMA. (1923–1946.)

Causes of death.	Fatal coma cases, New England Deaconess Hospital.	Cases dying after discharge following recovery from coma
Uncomplicated coma	22	12
Sepsis and metastatic infection	18	4
Pneumonia (1 with positive blood culture)	9	5
Pancreatitis	3	0
Cardiac	3	13
Pulmonary embolism	1	0
Pulmonary infarct with empyema	1	0
Hemorrhage from duodenal ulcer	1	0
Cerebral softening	1	0
? Alkalosis	1	0
Infected burn	1	0
Tuberculosis	0	15
Cancer	0	4
Meningitis	0	2
Gangrene	0	1
Hypoglycemia	0	2
Trauma	0	2
Alcoholism	0	1
Intestinal obstruction	0	1
Nephritis	0	3
Suicide	0	1
Found dead	0	1
Total	61	67

The average duration of diabetes among the 61 fatal (in the hospital) coma cases was 4.0 years and among the 67 cases dying after recovery from coma, 9.2 years. The latter figure is high enough to show that despite one or more attacks of coma the life expectancy of the diabetic is now steadily increasing. The still more encouraging fact is that the average duration of diabetes to January 1, 1945 of the living 246 coma cases who developed diabetes prior to January 1, 1940 was already 15.5 years.

In 166 diabetic autopsies studied by Vartiainen[1] coma was present

[1] Vartiainen: Acta med. Scand., **118**, 575, 1944.

in 63 cases of whom 39 were in the pre-insulin era and 24 in the insulin era. Of these 32 had no complications.

Root and Bloor[1] found among patients who had had diabetic coma, 17.8 per cent developed pulmonary tuberculosis within five years after recovery from coma. Of the 128 coma cases who died either within or outside of the hospital, tuberculosis caused 15 deaths. The effect of the metabolic disturbance in coma upon a chronic infection and the susceptibility to tuberculosis again emphasize the tragic character of this complication.

2. **Autopsy Findings.**—Of our 61 fatal (hospital) cases, permission for a postmortem examination was secured in 42 instances. In Table 54 are listed the chief causes of death in these cases.

TABLE 54.—DIABETIC COMA. CAUSES OF DEATH IN 42 AUTOPSIED CASES DYING BEFORE HOSPITAL DISCHARGE (ONE HOUR TO SIXTY-THREE DAYS AFTER ADMISSION).

	Cases.
Coma uncomplicated	11
Septicemia following local infections (neck, 4; labium, 3; kidney, 2; appendix, 1; foot, 1; mastoid, 1; prostate, 1; sinuses, 1)	14
Multiple renal abscesses (septicemia not proved)	1
Acute pancreatitis	3
Pneumonia	6
Other causes (1 case each with pulmonary embolism, infarct of lung with empyema, hemorrhage from duodenal ulcer, cerebral softening, and unexplained—? alkalosis, and 2 from coronary occlusion)	7
	42

Study of Table 54 shows that 24 of the 42 patients had infections of serious degree, in most instances in themselves carrying a fatal prognosis. However, there were 11 patients—more than one-fourth of the total—in whom autopsy disclosed no complication. These were the needless deaths, the deaths due to neglect on someone's part.

The serious character of the complications present in fatal cases of diabetic coma is well brought out in Table 54. In 14 patients there was septicemia and in another multiple renal abscesses. Three of the patients (Cases 3267, 9987 and 10115) were found on postmortem examination to have acute pancreatitis; these and a fourth case (14370), seen in another hospital, have been reported by Root.[2] In this series of 4 cases the diagnosis of acute pancreatitis was not made during life; this experience illustrates strikingly the value of autopsies in patients dying in diabetic coma. In the differential diagnosis of acute pancreatitis one should consider acute hepatitis, perforated ulcer, and acute cholecystitis. In Root's 4 cases fatty infiltration and enlargement of the liver were found.

Dillon, Riggs and Dyer[3] found that in 8 patients (ages fourteen

---

[1] Root and Bloor: Am. Rev. Tuberc., **39**, 714, 1939.
[2] Root: Loc. cit., p. 207.
[3] Dillon, Riggs and Dyer: Am. Jour. Med. Sci., **192**, 360, 1936.

to forty-five years) dying with uncomplicated diabetic acidosis, brain lesions similar to those seen in acute asphyxia were present with the primary pathological changes occurring in the cerebral capillary bed. They report that the capillaries were dilated and that the endothelial cells showed degenerative changes with increased permeability of the walls, as evidenced by the presence of perivascular and pericellular edema. There was proliferation of neuroglia, especially in the subependymal and marginal areas; acute degenerative changes in the ganglion cells were seen. The capillary changes were identical throughout the brain, but the degree of cellular destruction varied in different localities. The degeneration of the ganglion cells was greatest in the third and fourth cortical layers, in the extra-pyramidal system, in the cerebral vegetative centers of the diencephalon and of the medulla, in the olivocerebellar system and in Sommer's sector of Ammon's horn. The choroid plexus was severely damaged.

J. THE PROGNOSIS IN DIABETIC COMA.

Important factors in the prognosis of diabetic coma are (1) the severity of the acidosis; (2) the duration and degree of unconsciousness before the institution of treatment; (3) the age of the patient; (4) the cardio-vascular-renal status of the patient; (5) complicating conditions, which are often responsible for the precipitation of the acidosis; (6) grossly abnormal laboratory findings.

1. **Severity of Acidosis.**—Naturally those cases in which acidosis is most severe warrant a less favorable prognosis. This in itself is by no means a safe guide, however. Among our 651 cases there have been 85 with a plasma CO_2 combining power, or content, of 5 volumes per cent or less, and of these 73 recovered. There were 18 cases with a value of 2 volumes per cent and even of these 14 recovered. Furthermore, 18 of our 61 fatal cases had a plasma CO_2 value of 15 volumes per cent or more on admission. A more important point is the character of the response to energetic treatment with insulin, fluids and salt.

Rabinowitch[1] has criticized the use of plasma CO_2 values as an index to severity of coma. All would concede that, as pointed out above, the plasma CO_2 is by no means invariably a safe guide, either as to the severity of acidosis or as to prognosis in any individual case. However, it is instructive to note that in our own series of cases there has been some correlation between the CO_2 value and mortality, especially in the series up to 1940. This is shown in Table 55. Thirty-two, or 13.3 per cent, of 240 patients with a CO_2 of 10 volumes per cent or lower died, whereas among 397 patients with a CO_2 of from 11 to 20 volumes per cent, there were 26 deaths, or only 6.5 per cent mortality. It is true that among the unconscious

[1] Rabinowitch, Fowler and Bensley: Loc. cit., p. 422.

patients the percentage of deaths was essentially the same in the group with a CO_2 value above 10 volumes per cent as in the group with low values. In the latter series the number of deaths is too low for statistical comparison.

TABLE 55.—MENTAL CONDITION AND PLASMA CO_2 VS. MORTALITY IN DIABETIC COMA.

1923–1939.*

Mental condition.	Plasma CO_2, 10 vols. per cent or below.		Plasma CO_2, 11 to 20 vols. per cent.		Total cases.	
	No. of cases.	Mortality, per cent.	No. of cases.	Mortality, per cent.	No. of cases.	Mortality, per cent.
Conscious	53	5.7	134	2.2	187	3.2
Drowsy or semiconscious	76	11.8	106	6.6	182	8.8
Unconscious	55	34.5	28	35.7	83	35.0
Totals and averages	184	16.8	268	7.1	452	11.2

* Eleven cases with incomplete data have been excluded.

1940–1945.*

Conscious	5	0.0	33	3.0	38	2.6
Drowsy or semiconscious	32	0.0	76	1.3	108	0.9
Unconscious	19	5.3	20	15.0	39	10.3
Totals and averages	56	1.8	129	3.9	185	3.2

* Three cases with incomplete data have been excluded.

It cannot be too strongly emphasized that no single factor is all-important in prognosis. Patients with extreme acidosis, patients with marked hyperglycemia, elderly patients, patients unconscious for hours, and patients in circulatory collapse—all *may* get well with proper treatment. It is usually a combination of adverse influences which is disastrous. It is the complete situation in any individual case which is important in prognosis.

2. **Duration and Degree of Unconsciousness.**—The duration of unconsciousness before treatment is begun is of much importance in prognosis. It has been said by some that if a patient is unconscious for eight hours, by others twelve hours, that the outlook is very grave. It is difficult to speak in such exact terms, and no case should be regarded as hopeless, but the general implication is correct. Very unfavorable is the disappearance of Kussmaul respiration and onset of feeble, gasping respiration due to effect upon the respiratory center.

The determination of unconsciousness is not as easy as it would appear at first glance. A patient may be so stuporous and his mentality so clouded that he be difficult to arouse and later, after recovery, not recall important incidents and yet at the time may respond to questions or to painful stimuli. Accordingly, certain arbitrary standards must be set up. Dillon and Dyer[1] term a patient uncon-

[1] Dillon and Dyer: Loc. cit., p. 421.

29

scious if he is unable to be aroused sufficiently to answer "yes" or "no" to some simple question. Rabinowitch, Fowler and Bensley[1] divide acidotic patients into those with threatening coma who exhibit no drowsiness at all, and those with coma. In the latter group they recognize four stages; patients are classified as drowsy, semiconscious, unconscious but respond to pain, and completely unconscious. Pain is elicited by touching the conjunctivæ.

The degree of unconsciousness is certainly an important factor in the prognosis. However, our experience is not in agreement with that of Rabinowitch and associates or of Owens and Rockwern,[2] who regard total unconsciousness as almost precluding recovery. In the series at the Montreal General Hospital, all of 11 patients who were completely unconscious on admission to the hospital died. Of 40 unconscious patients at the Cincinnati General Hospital, 27 died. Our own experience, shown in Table 55, emphasizes the decline in the mortality of the totally unconscious patients in the period between 1940 and 1946 as compared with the period between 1923 and 1939. We believe that the fact that only four, or 10.3 per cent, out of 39 totally unconscious patients died in the later period is due largely to the use of larger doses of insulin during the first two or three hours of treatment. Thus the average patient with coma received 212 units in the first three hours of treatment in this later period, and these unconscious patients often received from 300 to 700 units of insulin in the first three hours of treatment. The advantage of this rapid and aggressive treatment is double. First, it checks the downward progress of the acidosis. Second, the rapid improvement brought about in the patient's condition makes possible the diagnosis of complications and more important still, control of the acidosis is of utmost importance in aiding the treatment of complications particularly of an infectious nature. This is well illustrated in Case 23974 described on page 432 in whom recovery from unconsciousness occurred despite bilateral progressive pneumonia, anuria, and marked nitrogen retention. He received 1300 units during the first five hours of treatment.

3. **Age of Patient.**—The age of the patient is a third important factor in prognosis. Youth carries with it a great advantage. Among 651 instances of coma in our entire series 153 were patients under fifteen years of age at the time of the attack of coma. Of these, there has been only one death and that was in a girl (Case 9162) fourteen years of age with diabetes of 3.8 years' duration who entered the hospital in a moribund state after three days of nausea, vomiting and abdominal pain at home and died in less than one hour. Even if one enlarges the group of coma cases among juvenile patients to include all instances occurring in patients under twenty years of age at the time of coma, one finds that there

[1] Rabinowitch, Fowler and Bensley: Loc. cit., p. 422.
[2] Owens and Rockwern: Loc. cit., p. 422.

have been but 8 deaths among 305 instances of coma. This case mortality of 2.6 per cent contrasts sharply with that of 15.3 per cent among patients twenty years of age or older (53 deaths in 346 cases). Table 56 shows the mortality in 651 cases by decades. The benefit conferred by youth is clearly demonstrated.

TABLE 56.—INCREASING DANGER OF COMA WITH ADVANCING AGE.

Age at coma, by decades.	Total cases.	Deaths.	
		No.	Per cent.
First	39	0	0
Second	266	8	3.0
Third	83	5	6.0
Fourth	88	8	9.0
Fifth	70	11	15.5
Sixth	65	22	33.8
Seventh	29	5	17.2
Eighth	11	2	18.1
Totals and averages	651	61	9.4

4. **Cardiovascular Status.**—A fourth factor in prognosis which is in large measure influenced by each of the preceding two points, is the state of the cardiovascular system. Circulatory collapse which fails to respond to supportive treatment is seen almost exclusively in adult patients, because gross neglect is required to produce such a situation in a child. With adult patients a blood-pressure which is subnormal (below 90 millimeters mercury) and with treatment fails to rise or continues to fall, signifies a grave prognosis. In patients with previously normal cardiac function, irregularities of the pulse may be a bad sign. With circulatory collapse which does not respond to treatment, oliguria and eventual anuria are the rule, and exitus often takes place within a few hours. One may with enormous doses of insulin in such cases control the blood sugar and cause some rise in the carbon dioxide combining power of the blood plasma, but the blood non-protein nitrogen rises and the patient's clinical condition grows progressively worse.

5. **Complications.**—When diabetic coma is complicated by some other acute condition, the prognosis is, of course, determined by the nature and severity of the complication. It is significant and indeed encouraging that as years go by, deaths from diabetic coma occur more and more in patients with serious complications, in themselves carrying a high mortality, apart from the diabetic acidosis. This is as it should be, and one should strive to eliminate deaths from diabetic coma on any other basis. Even in the presence of complications, the diabetic condition can almost invariably be brought under control and all efforts should be exerted toward this end, even though "chemical" improvement may not be accompanied by clinical recovery. Needless to add, the treatment of complications, particularly infections, including pneumonia, should be modern and energetic; full use of the newer chemotherapeutic agents should be made.

6. **Laboratory Data.**—In estimating the prognosis in any given case the clinical condition of the patient and his response to treatment must be accorded greater weight than abnormal values obtained in laboratory studies. Grossly abnormal blood values, although indicating a severe condition, do not by any means point to a bad outcome. Reference has already been made to the fact that of our 24 patients who on admission had a blood sugar of 1000 milligrams per cent or above, 19, or 79.1 per cent, recovered. Likewise, extreme reduction in plasma CO_2 values does not imply a fatal outcome; 208, or 86.7 per cent, of our 240 cases with an initial CO_2 of 10 volumes per cent or less recovered. Even high values for the blood non-protein nitrogen do not necessarily imply poor prognosis. Among 651 cases of coma 27 had a non-protein nitrogen value of 80 milligrams per cent or more on admission; of these 17, or 63.0 per cent recovered. Patients with preëxisting nephritis, however, have a definite handicap. In most patients the elevation of the non-protein nitrogen, together with the albuminuria and cylindruria are indications simply of temporary renal impairment, reversible in nature. Bertram[1] believes the outlook to be bad when the total acetone content of the blood (acetone $+$ diacetic acid, but not including β-oxybutyric acid) is greater than 70 milligrams per cent. He regards the level of β-oxybutyric acid alone as of no significance, a point consistent with the fact as mentioned by Best and Taylor[2] that β-oxybutyric acid is a relatively non-toxic product as contrasted with diacetic (aceto-acetic) acid which probably derives toxicity from the enolic form, $CH_3COHCHCOOH$. The amount of β-oxybutyric acid formed by a diabetic in acidosis during twenty-four hours is far more than is realized. Thirty to 40 grams of total ketone bodies per day are not uncommon in precomatose stages.[3] Case 4 once held a world's record for acid production.[4] This patient excreted during three successive days of coma a total of 437 grams of β-oxybutyric acid as calculated from the β-oxybutyric acid and diacetic acid in the urine or the equivalent of 1 gram hydrochloric acid per kilogram body weight.

We have had no experience with determinations of the freezing-point of the serum, but Bertram regards a depression to 0.68° or below as indicative of marked retention of ketone bodies and therefore of doubtful prognosis.

The leucocytosis which is so characteristic of diabetic coma is of no value in prognosis. Bertram has carried out determinations of the blood sedimentation rate and finds this value of no practical meaning.

[1] Bertram: Loc. cit., page 87.
[2] Best and Taylor: Page 574, loc. cit., p. 116.
[3] Falta: P. 101; Loc. cit., p. 85.
[4] Joslin: Jour. Med. Res., **6**, 306, 1901.

K. THE TREATMENT OF DIABETIC COMA.

1. **Preparation Prior to Hospital Admission.**—A patient in diabetic coma deserves to be in a hospital. By this means every facility is afforded for constant observation with uninterrupted treatment, including the administration of parenteral fluids, and as frequent analyses of the blood and urine as may be necessary. If one learns by telephone that a patient at home is to be brought to the hospital, a preliminary dose of 20 to 40 units of insulin given by the home physician or the family may be advised provided the diagnosis seems certain. A bed at the hospital should be prepared and necessary equipment as blankets, hot-water bottles, stomach and rectal tubes, salt and glucose solutions, insulin, and stimulants assembled so that when the patient arrives, treatment begins. A laboratory technician should be instantly available and continuously so until the patient is out of danger so that no time is lost in getting reports.

2. **Insulin.**—On admission, after the diagnosis has been verified by history, physical examination and examination of the urine, a preliminary subcutaneous dose of insulin usually of 20 to 100 units is given. This dose must be varied to suit the age of the patient, the degree of acidosis, and previous insulin administration. The insulin should be of the unmodified, "regular" or crystalline type; protamine zinc insulin acts so slowly that it should not be used except as an adjunct to treatment with the other varieties.

The chief objective in this first few hours of treatment is to give as much insulin as is needed. In 478 cases[1] treated between 1923 and August 1940, the average amount of insulin given in the first three hours was 83 units. Deaths numbered 58, or 12 per cent. In 123 cases from August, 1940 to May 1, 1944, the average dose of insulin in the first three hours was 216 units and only 2 deaths occurred, or 1.2 per cent. Insulin resistance increases as acidosis advances. It is the insulin given in the first few hours which counts most heavily. Since May, 1944 in 50 cases the average insulin given in the first three hours was 210 units, and of these cases 2 per cent died.

Provided acidosis is marked enough and the blood sugar high enough, a dose of insulin similar in size to the initial dose may be given every half-hour until there is clinical and chemical evidence of improvement. Then urine specimens are secured at intervals of one or two hours with instructions to give insulin according to the Benedict's test, for example, 20 units for a red or orange test, 15 for a yellow, and 10 for a yellow-green test. This dosage, too, must be varied depending on the severity of the acidosis, the age of the patient, and the response to treatment. Unless forced to do so, we prefer not to catheterize patients, for fear of resulting infection. Instead we make frequent blood-sugar estimations (capillary blood

[1] Root: Loc. cit., p. 438.

may be conveniently used) as a guide to treatment if urine specimens cannot be secured.

As indicated above, our custom has been to give insulin in divided doses at frequent intervals, regulating the amount according to the severity of the acidosis and the response to treatment. This method has been successful in our hands and is the one used by most clinicians.[1] Fowler, Bensley and Rabinowitch[2] proposed the more or less routine administration of a definitely large amount, such as 400 units at the outset of treatment, dividing this amount between insulin of rapidly-acting and protamine zinc types. These workers at the Montreal General Hospital advise the immediate and simultaneous injection of 100 units of unmodified insulin intravenously, 100 units of unmodified insulin and 200 units of protamine zinc insulin subcutaneously, along with larger amounts of carbohydrate. Of 26 patients treated by this new method, 6 died. It seems to the authors more logical to adjust the size of the dose to the severity of the acidosis and the response to treatment; this implies constant and personal supervision by the physician during the all-important first six to twenty-four hours of treatment but a coma case deserves no less than this.

The average amount of insulin used in our cases (see Table 48) in the first twenty-four hours varied from 154 units for Series I, in the early days of insulin experience, to 252 units in Series IV, from February, 1929 to September, 1931. This latter group included several severe cases and the mortality for this period was 18 per cent. In Series X the average amount in the first twenty-four hours was 254 units of unmodified, and 28 units of protamine zinc insulin, with an average total of 282 units for the 126 patients.

At times extraordinary amounts of insulin are necessary. There should be no hesitancy in using enough to obtain results, remembering that in the presence of acidosis a unit of insulin cannot be taken at face value. In addition to close observation of the clinical condition of the patient, tests of blood and urine must be frequent. Of the 651 cases of coma 40 were given 500 units of insulin or more during the first twenty-four hours after admission. In 2 cases which have been reported in detail elsewhere, Root and Riseman[3] used 1280 and 850 units respectively during the first twenty-four hours of treatment. In each instance during the first few hours of treatment the patient had failed to respond to the usual energetic treatment with the development of anuria, but recovery took place when still larger amounts of insulin were given.

Wiener[4] has reported a case of a man aged fifty-eight years with extreme insensitiveness to insulin who, in one twenty-four hour

[1] Duncan and Jewesbury: Med. Clin. North America, **23**, 1533, 1939.
[2] Fowler, Bensley and Rabinowitch: Canad. Med. Assn. Jour., **42**, 336, 1940.
[3] Root and Riseman: Jour. Am. Med. Assn., **110**, 1730, 1938.
[4] Wiener: Am. Jour. Med. Sci., **196**, 211, 1938.

period, was given 3250 units of unmodified insulin in order to bring about recovery from acidosis.

Grafe's[1] patient, admitted to the hospital with a blood sugar of 1365 milligrams per cent, was given 1940 units of insulin in the first and 1300 units in the second twenty-four hours of treatment. Grafe speculates as to whether this remarkable insensitiveness to insulin was associated with the chronic pulmonary tuberculosis and acute gastro-enteritis which complicated the diabetic acidosis in this fifty-five-year-old man.

A case of severe coma complicated by chronic laryngeal obstruction reported by Gorman, Harwood and White[2] required for recovery 3620 units of insulin in twenty hours. The patient entered with a blood sugar of 1240 milligrams. The blood CO_2 was 3.8 m. eq. per liter and the non-protein nitrogen value was 108 milligrams per 100 cc. No glucose was given during the first twenty hours. The patient developed auricular fibrillation and received cedilanid.

If the patient is in circulatory collapse, so that doubt exists about the absorption of insulin, it is well to give it intravenously as well as subcutaneously. In addition to insuring absorption, intravenous administration, as Penson and Wohl[3] have pointed out, brings about an earlier and more pronounced, though less prolonged, hypoglycemic effect than subcutaneous injection.

A patient may rarely pass from diabetic coma into the unconsciousness which attends hypoglycemia without striking warning signs and such a possibility one should always remember. This is explainable on the assumption that the signs of marked hypoglycemia are dependent upon the integrity of higher nerve centers as evidenced by the fact that there are no physical signs of hypoglycemia in the spinal or anesthetized animal.[4] Therefore, orders should be so written that no insulin is given if the Benedict's test is green or blue and as a further precaution, frequent determinations of the blood sugar are advisable at this stage of treatment.

3. **Fluids.**—Dehydration is one of the striking clinical features of diabetic coma. The skin is dry and inelastic, the tongue and mucous membranes of the mouth are parched, the eyeballs are soft, and the subcutaneous tissues are obviously depleted of fluid. Atchley[5] and co-workers in a study of 2 diabetic patients with experimental acidosis demonstrated this loss of intra- and extracellular body water and electrolytes following the withdrawal of insulin therapy and the reversal of the process when insulin is resumed.

Sunderman and Dohan[6] compared the extracellular water of

[1] Grafe: Verhandl. deutsch. Gesellsch. f. inn. Med., p. 78, 1937.

[2] Gorman, Harwood and White: New England Jour. Med., **234**, 500, 1946.

[3] Penson and Wohl: Presse méd., **43**, 63, 1935.

[4] Best: Loc. cit., p. 136.

[5] Atchley, Loeb, Richards, Benedict and Driscoll: Jour. Clin. Invest., **12**, 297, 1933.

[6] Sunderman and Dohan: Am. Jour. Physiol., **132**, 418, 1941.

dogs in which diabetic ketosis was produced with that of normal controls. Although the total volume of serum in the circulation was decreased, when compared with a healthy state, actually the serum volume per kilogram of body weight was consistently increased. Also the extracellular water per unit of body weight was increased. These measurements were consistent with dehydration of the body as a whole, and yet with such alteration in the intracellular fluids as to increase the water outside the cells. Insulin had a marked effect in readjusting the partition of water and electrolytes between cells and serum.

Anuria in a diabetic woman apparently due to dehydration but associated with blood non-protein nitrogen of 100 milligrams per cent was described by Styron and Leadbetter[1] as an example of anuria due to extrarenal azotemia. Relief followed the administration of saline together with the use of insulin.

Treatment must have, then, as one of the primary aims, the restoration of fluid and electrolytes to the body. This is best done by the prompt intravenous administration of 1500 to 2000 cc. of physiologic solution of sodium chloride which may be repeated if the condition of the patient so indicates. In selected cases a subcutaneous infusion of 1000 to 1500 cc. of salt solution may be given. When the need is urgent, fluid may be administered both intravenously and subcutaneously at the outset. We have never observed embarrassment of the heart to follow even such liberal quantities of fluid. Campbell, Reeser and Kepler[2] gave their patient 9875 cc. of fluid, in the first 12 hours of treatment; they emphasize the importance of supplying adequate amounts.

In the 2 patients reported by Root and Riseman, already cited, not only were large quantities of insulin necessary, but in addition extraordinarily large amounts of fluid were given. In one patient 13,800 cc. and in the other 11,600 cc. of total fluid were given during the first twenty-nine hours of treatment. No sign of cardiac failure was seen in either case, although it must be admitted that both were fundamentally normal as regards the cardio-vascular-renal system. Stephens and Burtness[3] record a patient with coma who entered the hospital with a blood-sugar level of 1550 milligrams and who received 11,500 cc. of intravenous fluid in twenty-four hours without evidence of circulatory overloading. During this time 495 units of insulin were given and the total of the urinary output was only a few hundred cubic centimeters. In elderly patients, particularly in the presence of heart and kidney disease, one must proceed somewhat more cautiously in the giving of very large amounts of fluid parenterally. Obviously so much fluid would be contraindicated if the patient were not dehydrated.

[1] Styron and Leadbetter: New England Jour. Med., **230**, 731, 1944.
[2] Campbell, Reeser and Kepler: Proc. Staff Meet., Mayo Clinic, **15**, 520, 1940.
[3] Stephens and Burtness: California and West. Med., **61**, 66, 1944.

All solutions should be slightly above body temperature, should be given slowly, and with great caution to avoid infection or unnecessary trauma. Following a cleansing enema, salt solution may at times be given rectally with success. This must be done with care; Bertram[1] mentions a patient in whom sepsis developed following intestinal necrosis at the site of insertion of a rectal tube. Avoid pressure from hot water bottles since slight pressure during coma may result in gangrene as occurred in two adolescent diabetic patients reported by Whittaker.[2] After gastric lavage, fluids as broths, orange juice or ginger ale may be given cautiously by mouth. Usually it is preferable to wait perhaps an hour after gastric lavage and then begin by limiting such fluids to 100 cc. per hour. Although the treatment of dehydration and shock is of great importance, remember that uncontrolled diabetes is at the basis of coma. Give enough insulin early!

4. **Gastric Lavage.**—Gastric lavage should be carried out routinely unless the patient is *in extremis* or in such condition that the procedure involved would be dangerous. Usually one's efforts will be rewarded by finding the stomach filled with sizable quantities of fluid, food remains and old blood. Removal of such contents and gentle lavage with warm water or normal salt solution relieves the abdominal distress, stops vomiting, and prepares the way for the early administration of fluids by mouth. The importance of gastric lavage is suggested in the work of Burgess, Scott and Ivy[3] who found that in dogs prolonged distention of the stomach with water introduced into a balloon caused marked changes in the wall of the stomach and resulted in death within a period of from twenty-six to ninety hours even though there was no significant fall in blood chlorides or dehydration. Definite abnormalities in the electrocardiogram were also noted.

John[4] regards the washing out of the stomach as an important procedure and cites 1 case in which death occurred because this was not done. The patient was brought out of coma chemically, but suddenly became cyanotic and the respirations ceased although the heart continued to beat. At autopsy it was found that stomach contents had been regurgitated, had trickled down the trachea and choked the patient to death.

5. **Circulatory Stimulants.**—Circulatory stimulants are practically never needed with children and in adults rarely produce startling or lasting results. Epinephrine in doses of 0.3 to 1 cc. may be given subcutaneously for extreme collapse. Ephedrine sulphate gives a more prolonged effect in raising blood-pressure and may be given subcutaneously in doses of 0.5 to 1 cc. (25 to 50 mg.). Either epinephrine or ephedrine may be given intravenously in emergencies

---

[1] Bertram: P. 39, loc. cit., p. 87.
[2] Whittaker: Brit. Med. Jour., 2, 469, 1944.
[3] Burgess, Scott and Ivy: Arch. Int. Med., 49, 439, 1932.
[4] John: Jour. Am. Med. Assn., 105, 587, 1935.

but usually if the situation is grave enough to warrant such medication, the prognosis is bad.

The previous statement has been questioned by Bertram, who believes that energetic support of the circulation is necessary in order to counteract the development of cardio-vascular collapse. Accordingly, early in treatment he gives 0.3–0.4 milligrams of strophanthin intravenously. In extreme failure of the circulation he recommends the addition of sympatol or adrenalin to a constant intravenous drip in amount of 1 to 2.5 cc. of a 1 to 1000 solution hourly, following the blood-pressure all the while. While by no means deprecating the use of drugs, we must reiterate that we have encountered no case in which such medication has appeared to be life-saving.

6. **Blood Transfusion.**—Blood transfusion has been carried out with relatively few of our patients. There have been occasional transfusions in selected cases but it has always been extremely difficult to evaluate the effect, and to know whether the benefits obtained were due to the transfusion or to other factors. The chief use of blood transfusions is, of course, upon the theory of combating circulatory collapse; if one could anticipate in advance which patients would not respond favorably to treatment in this regard, blood transfusions could be performed earlier and better opportunity for judging their value be had. So often the need for unusual measures is not, or cannot be, appreciated until the patient has been in the hospital a few hours and the lack of satisfactory response to treatment noted. By the time a donor has been secured and the transfusion of blood given, still further time is lost during which the patient's condition may have become steadily worse.

Our recent experience leads us to believe that the intravenous infusion of simple physiologic solution of sodium chloride is a proper and satisfactory way of treating circulatory collapse, and we shall use it in the future in those patients who enter with a weak, rapid pulse and low blood pressure or develop such despite energetic treatment.

7. **Glucose and Food.**—It is our practice almost never to add glucose to the subcutaneous and intravenous infusions used at the outset of treatment. Our reasons are as follows: (1) Glucose is already flooding the blood and body tissues generally in the patient with diabetic coma and can be utilized just as satisfactorily as injected glucose if adequate amounts of insulin are supplied. Actually when glucose solution was administered intravenously to patients in diabetic coma Root and Carpenter[1] found no evidence from the respiratory quotient that such glucose was oxidized. (2) Under certain conditions added glucose may precipitate renal

---

[1] Root and Carpenter: Am. Jour. Med. Sci., **206**, 234, 1943.

block. From experiments on animals, Allen[1] reports that large injections of glucose subcutaneously may result in oliguria.

Helmholz and Bollman[2] found that the kidney can produce a marked diuresis in response to high concentrations of glucose brought about by injection. As a result of this process marked hydropic degeneration of the convoluted tubules occurred and a temporary anuria developed. In experimental animals these changes were reversible. In the cases reported by Root and Riseman[3] the condition of the patients became worse rather than better following the parenteral administration of glucose; recovery took place with the use of large amounts of a physiologic solution of sodium chloride intravenously together with extraordinarily large amounts of insulin. (3) Serial determinations of the blood sugar afford an excellent guide to treatment during the first several hours in the hospital. Obviously such values are robbed of their significance if a constant infusion of glucose is being carried out. (4) When glucose is given at a rate exceeding caloric needs, such as 100–400 grams within a few hours, a considerable portion of this glucose may be converted to fat, as suggested by Drury.[4] When diabetic rats received large quantities of sugar and insulin, only a small part was oxidized and most of the carbohydrate was stored as fat, according to Pauls and Drury.[5] (5) A deficiency of serum potassium with resulting paralysis of voluntary muscles has followed the use of large amounts of glucose in coma. (See page 426.)

The administration of food should be begun as soon as a marked decline in the blood sugar and the clinical improvement of the patient indicates that sufficient insulin has been given to make possible the utilization of carbohydrate given. In some instances orange juice or oatmeal gruel may be given in amounts furnishing 10 grams carbohydrate per hour beginning as early as the sixth or eighth hour after admission. In others intravenous administration of glucose is necessary for the first few days as in Case 23974 (see page 432). It is important to remember the tremendous disturbance in protein metabolism during serious acidosis and that protein is needed as well as carbohydrate. In Case 20945, a boy aged fifteen years, admitted in coma, Root and Carpenter[6] recorded nitrogen elimination of 1109 milligrams per hour during the first three hours after treatment which fell to a rate of 339 milligrams per hour as improvement took place with insulin treatment. This case illustrated the marked degree of protein break-down and probable glucose formation therefrom and the rapid change in protein metabolism brought about by treatment with insulin.

[1] Allen: Trans. Assn. Am. Physiol., 53, 320, 1938.
[2] Helmholz and Bollman: Jour. Lab. and Clin. Med., 25, 1180, 1940.
[3] Root and Riseman: Loc. cit., p. 454.
[4] Drury: Am. Jour. Physiol., 131, 536, 1940.
[5] Pauls and Drury: Jour. Biol. Chem., 145, 481, 1942.
[6] Root and Carpenter: Loc. cit., p. 458.

In this regard we disagree with Bertram,[1] Himsworth,[2] Peters,[3] Conn[4] and others who give insulin and glucose simultaneously. Of 651 instances of coma we have had 61 deaths and of these only 22 have been such that death could be ascribed to diabetes alone. Among this number there are no cases which, in our opinion, might have been saved by the administration of glucose. When it is evident by the improvement of the patient and by the decline in blood sugar, which indicates that sufficient insulin has been given so that excessive glucose in the body fluid is being utilized, the administration of food is begun. Ten grams of carbohydrate per hour either as orange juice or gruel by mouth or glucose by injection may be given. Our aim is to provide for the patient receiving and utilizing 100 to 200 grams of carbohydrate in the first twenty-four hours. Except in profoundly unconscious patients carbohydrate administration is usually begun from eight to twelve hours after admission.

8. **Cleansing Enema.**—A cleansing enema is routinely given to relieve abdominal distention and promote intestinal tone.

9. **Alkalies.**—Experience has amply shown that alkalies are needless and if given in quantities necessary for effectiveness in a purely chemical sense may be actually harmful. The danger of the use of soda has been fully discussed in previous publications. Kydd[5] has lent support to the opinion that without alkalies, treatment with insulin, fluids, sodium chloride, and carbohydrate suffices to provide for recovery from diabetic acidosis and eventual restoration of the body electrolytes. Falta[6] states that in recent years he has almost always carried out treatment without alkalies. He mentions that alkaline solutions given intravenously may check diuresis and lead to insulin edema.

Hartmann[7] recommends the use of racemic sodium lactate in diabetic coma to hasten recovery from acidosis. However, the mortality among his series of children was rather high. Unfortunately Hartmann's results are a little difficult to interpret as to the merits of sodium lactate alone because he recommends methods in the use and dosage of insulin which in our belief do not allow maximal success. It is possible that sodium lactate may prove helpful in selected patients in whom acidosis persists for an unusually long period despite control of hyperglycemia.

Kepler[8] of the Mayo Clinic regards large amounts of sodium bicarbonate as definitely contraindicated. He does advise its use in

[1] Bertram: Klin. Wchnschr., **11**, 1998, 1932.
[2] Himsworth: Lancet, **2**, 165, 1932.
[3] Peters: Yale Jour. Biol. and Med., **17**, 685, 1943.
[4] Conn: Univ. Hosp. Bull., Ann Arbor, **11**, 50, 1945.
[5] Kydd: Jour. Clin. Invest., **12**, 1169, 1933.
[6] Falta: P. 279, loc. cit., p. 85.
[7] Hartmann: Arch. Int. Med., **56**, 413, 1935.
[8] Kepler: Med. Clin. North America. **22**, 979, 1938. See also Campbell, **Reeser** and Kepler. Loc. cit., p. 456.

certain patients in whom there is an unusual lag in the recovery of the carbon dioxide combining power of the blood plasma; in such cases he gives 250 to 500 cc. of a solution of 5 per cent sodium bicarbonate intravenously. Bertram's[1] custom is apparently about the same. However, it is extremely doubtful that a mild acidosis characterized by a plasma CO_2 of 20 to 50 volumes per cent is of any great harm to the patient on the day following admission for coma, provided the clinical condition seems good and ketonuria has ceased.

Erickson and Kepler[2] reported the case of a diabetic patient in whom alkalosis occurred from overdosage with soda. This patient, a man aged forty-two years, upon developing the signs of ketosis took at home in all about 250 grams of soda on the day prior to admission to the Mayo Clinic. Upon arrival he presented most of the clinical signs of severe diabetic acidosis with the exception that his respirations were shallow rather than labored. The urine contained much sugar and diacetic acid. The CO_2 combining power of the plasma was 80.6 volumes per cent. This patient, with appropriate treatment, made a good recovery and left the hospital in ten days in good condition.

Kirk[3] reports 2 cases of diabetic coma relieved by solutions of bicarbonate of soda, administered intravenously. However, it would appear that his patients entered the hospital in only moderately severe acidosis and one wonders if they would not have benefited from larger doses of insulin given earlier. One patient was a man, aged fifty-six years, scarcely more than drowsy, whose blood sugar was 490 milligrams per cent. Since following 120 units of insulin the blood sugar did not fall satisfactorily, the soda was given. The second patient, a woman whose blood sugar was only 200 milligrams per cent on admission, was given soda because she did not become conscious during the first few hours of her stay. Both patients recovered.

As previously stated, among our entire series of coma cases there have been 22 deaths which could be ascribed to diabetes alone. Examination of their records in retrospect fails to convince us that the use of alkalis would have altered the outcome in a single instance.

10. **Treatment in Convalescence.**—Following recovery from acute acidosis, return to normal is usually steady and rapid except in patients long unconscious and in severe shock. Even on the day after admission the average patient is able to take a soft-solid diet and within two or three days is well on the way toward a regular maintenance diet. Indeed, improvement in general condition is often so rapid that one is apt to forget that the patient has suffered a terrific bodily insult from which prompt restitution to normal physiology and chemistry must be more apparent than real. Activity for a few days should be limited and a gradual return to a normal

[1] Bertram: P. 102, loc. cit., p. 87.
[2] Erickson and Kepler: Proc. Staff Meet. Mayo Clin., 14, 28, 1939.
[3] Kirk: Lancet, 1, 505, 1939.

life insisted upon. An occasional complication is the appearance of edema of the extremities due to over-compensation in the matter of fluid retention.

L. COMPLICATIONS OF DIABETIC COMA.

Any complicating condition may alter materially the prognosis in a given case of coma. Space does not permit mention of many interesting and instructive cases in this regard. However, it seems worth while to discuss briefly certain incidents which may occur in the course of the treatment.

1. **Hypoglycemia.**—Occasionally treatment may be so energetic that the blood sugar may be forced to hypoglycemic levels. It has already been mentioned that the patient can pass from diabetic coma to insulin shock without any striking sign of such an occurrence. Hence fairly frequent blood-sugar estimations are a valuable aid in treatment. Possibly because it is our invariable rule to begin to give frequent and small amounts of carbohydrate by mouth as soon as tolerated by the patient, we have never seen hypoglycemia following recovery from diabetic coma which gave rise to or resulted in any serious difficulty.

2. **The Return to a Condition of Coma After Apparent Recovery.**— Such a complication is uncommon in a well-regulated hospital, but it does occur. Without adequate laboratory facilities it is sure to be met with more frequently. The secret of its avoidance is constant careful observation of the patient and as frequent laboratory tests as are necessary.

3. **Circulatory Collapse.**—Because of its importance, a further word may well be said regarding the treatment of profound shock characterized by a blood-pressure below 90 mm. of mercury (at other times too low to measure), rapid pulse, and eventual anuria. This state is not limited to older patients and may be seen in advanced coma at any age. One must agree with Lande[1] regarding the poor prognosis which attends such a case. On the other hand, we have seen unexpected recovery in a pulseless patient, aged seventy years, treated with the methods outlined above. Cases 6803, 7047 and 10970 had blood-pressures from 0 to 80 mm. Hg, but made good recoveries. Lawrence[2] has reported the use intravenously of gum acacia solutions and large amounts (4 to over 5 liters) of salt solution, both isotonic and hypertonic, to raise the blood-pressure and counteract dehydration. Ralli and Waterhouse[3] stress the importance of large amounts of fluid. Labbé and Boulin[4] hold that the use intravenously of adrenalin 1 milligram in 1500 cc. of normal salt solution is of great value. Bertram[1] and Falta[2] use various circulatory stimulants including strophanthin, cardiazol, hexeton, coramin,

---

[1] Lande: Jour. Am. Med. Assn., **101**, 9, 1933.
[2] Lawrence: Brit. Med. Jour., **1**, 690, 1930.
[3] Ralli and Waterhouse: Am. Jour. Med. Sci., **187**, 607, 1934.
[4] Labbé and Boulin: Presse méd., **41**, 1705, 1933. Labbé: Leçons Cliniques, Paris, Masson et Cie, p. 160, 1932.

strychnine, caffein, camphor preparations, and sympatol. In marked collapse Bertram recommends the careful use of a constant intravenous infusion containing sympatol ,or adrenalin. Bopp[3] believes that coramin given intravenously is of great value in treating circulatory collapse occurring in diabetic coma. We shall continue to use normal salt solution in amounts from 3 to 5 or more liters administered subcutaneously and intravenously in addition to fluids by mouth and rectum. When indicated this will be supplemented by adrenalin or ephedrine subcutaneously or intravenously. For anuria accompanied by a subnormal blood salt we shall use 10 per cent salt solution in 60 cc. quantities as described on pages 254 and 441. The use of transfusion of whole blood will also be given further trial in cases with low blood-pressure under 70 mm. of mercury.

Distribution of Population by Age.—The chart below became available too late for inclusion in the text at the proper place but is so valuable that it is inserted here. It shows the growing proportion of older individuals in the United States with the bringing of more persons into the age zones in which diabetes is most common, thereby increasing the number of those requiring insulin.

PER CENT DISTRIBUTION OF TOTAL POPULATION BY AGE
UNITED STATES, 1900 to 2000 *

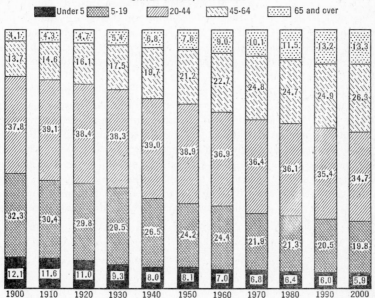

Under 5   5-19   20-44   45-64   65 and over

* Prepared by the Statistical Bureau of the Metropolitan Life Insurance Company. Figures up to and including those for 1940 are based on census data; the others are estimates.

    1 Bertram: Loc. cit., p. 87.
    2 Falta: P. 279, loc. cit., p. 85.
    3 Bopp: Deutsch. med. Wchnschr., 61, 218, 1935.

CHAPTER XIV.

ALLERGY AND DIABETES.

REVISED BY C. CABELL BAILEY, M. D.

Introduction.—Allergic conditions may exist in diabetic patients, just as in non-diabetics, and when present may complicate diabetic treatment. In addition the diabetic may exhibit hypersensitiveness to insulin, which may be not only troublesome but also at times serious. The lipodystrophies observed in diabetics, consisting chiefly of insulin atrophies, insulin lumps and perhaps necrobiosis lipoidica diabeticorum, may represent local allergic manifestations, but the etiology of these conditions is unknown and they are discussed elsewhere.

A. ALLERGIC STATES PECULIAR TO DIABETES.

Hypersensitiveness to Insulin

Shortly after the discovery of insulin, reports began to appear of allergic phenomena developing after its use. One of the earliest papers[1] described 4 cases of urticaria developing among the first 83 patients treated with insulin. Fundamental articles and reviews are those of Tuft,[2] Allan and Scherer,[3] Davidson,[4] Lewis,[5] Abrahamson,[6] and Herzstein and Pollack.[7] Sensitiveness to insulin has also been known to occur in non-diabetics and at least 3 such cases have been reported.[8,9,10]

1. **Types of Allergic Manifestations.**—The most common allergic reactions following the injection of insulin are local responses; these vary greatly in severity and duration and apparently are more common since the introduction of protamine zinc insulin. Patients usually describe a stinging, burning, or itching sensation at the site of the injection, and in from one-half to several hours the affected tissues become indurated. The indurations may vary from one to several centimeters in diameter, may be warm to touch, and may be surrounded by a small or large area of erythema. Pain or soreness is present in almost all cases. In some patients the indurations

---

[1] Joslin, Gray and Root: Jour. Metab. Res., **2**, 651, 1922.
[2] Tuft: Am. Jour. Med. Sci., **176**, 707, 1928.
[3] Allan and Scherer: Endocrinology, **16**, 417, 1932.
[4] Davidson: Jour. Allergy, **6**, 71, 1934.
[5] Lewis: Jour. Am. Med. Assn., **108**, 1336, 1937.
[6] Abrahamson: Jour. Clin. Endocrin., **1**, 402, 1941.
[7] Herzstein and Pollack: Jour. Mt. Sinai Hosp., **6**, 3, 1939.
[8] Sammis: Jour. Allergy, **6**, 387, 1935.
[9] Cohen and Simon: Jour. Allergy, **9**, 503, 1938.
[10] Ulrich, Hooker and Smith: New England Jour. Med., **221**, 522, 1939.

disappear in from six to twenty-four hours while in others each area may last several days.

Far more spectacular, and fortunately much less common, are the generalized allergic reactions. Chief among these are the urticarial responses which are annoying mainly because of the associated itching.

Frequently the generalized reactions are accompanied by angioneurotic edema involving especially the loose tissues of the eyelids and lips. When most severe, such reactions may in rare instances be accompanied by laryngeal edema and produce interference with respiration. This type of generalized reaction usually appears within one-half hour after the insulin injection and may disappear spontaneously within one to several hours. Occasionally patients have first a period of only local reaction at the injection site followed in a few days or weeks by a general reaction, while still others as described by Watson[1] may have no reaction for several days followed by local reactions which increase in intensity until finally a generalized allergic response develops. The use of ephedrine usually gives very prompt relief but may need to be repeated frequently. Less frequent allergic responses have been those of gastro-intestinal symptoms,[2] non-thrombocytopenic purpura,[3] and various combinations of untoward effects.

The most serious allergic response to insulin is anaphylactic shock. Such reactions usually follow a period when insulin was omitted for a time and then resumed. Unconsciousness, dyspnea, fall in blood pressure, and cyanosis, in addition to edema and urticaria may develop and the patient may appear moribund. Fortunately no fatal cases have been reported, although one patient discontinued insulin because of severe allergy and died in diabetic coma.[4] Case 26598 developed anaphylactic shock at the George F. Baker Clinic following the first injection of insulin she ever received but fortunately recovered, was desensitized and later received insulin without difficulty. Wechsler *et al.*[5] describe a sixty-five year old female who had three such reactions, the first of which simulated a coronary occlusion.

2. **Incidence.**—Small localized reactions at the site of insulin injection at the beginning of therapy are common. They are observed after the use of unmodified (regular or crystalline) insulin and probably more frequently after the injection of modified (protamine zinc) insulin. In most cases such reactions are mild, of short duration, and cause little discomfort to the patient. Perhaps 15 to 30 per cent of the cases have some local reaction at the beginning of insulin therapy.

[1] Watson: Canadian Med. Assoc. Jour., **47**, 336, 1942.
[2] Bayer: Jour. Am. Med. Assn., **102**, 1934, 1934.
[3] Kern and Langner: Jour. Am. Med. Assn., **113**, 198, 1939.
[4] Strauss: Klin. Wchnschr., **4**, 491, 1925.
[5] Wechsler, Farmer and Urban: Jour. Lab. and Clin. Med., **26**, 1090, 1941.

The first insulin preparations were less pure than those commercially available today and undoubtedly some of the untoward effects were not due to insulin. With improved methods of production, these reactions became less frequent. Allan and Scherer pointed out an increase in the incidence of true insulin allergy as the years passed and suggested as a possible cause in some cases that sensitization to insulin given in previous years had occurred, with such cases becoming more numerous as the general diabetic population increased. As will be shown, the histories of many reported allergic cases bear out this idea. Allan and Scherer reported 161 cases with allergic reactions in a total of 1907 cases, an incidence of 8.4 per cent. Collens, Lerner and Fialka[1] had 30 patients with local allergic reactions in a group of 407 cases, an incidence of 7.3 per cent. In 108 cases of diabetic coma, Baker[2] mentioned 3 cases of insulin allergy which complicated the treatment of coma. Kern and Langner reported that 17, or 16.3 per cent, of 104 diabetics given protamine zinc insulin had local reactions.

In contrast to the local manifestations of allergy, generalized reactions are exceedingly rare. Based on an estimate of 700,000 diabetics in the United States and of 350,000 using insulin and considering the various ways in which the varieties of insulin are given, it seems likely that at least 500,000 insulin injections are given daily. In proportion to this number, how few cases of severe allergy are reported! At the New England Deaconess Hospital about 60,000 insulin injections are given each year. In the calendar year 1939 there were 1823 admissions of diabetic patients to the George F. Baker Clinic. Of this number about 90 per cent took insulin and only 2 patients had a generalized reaction. In a group of 20,000 true diabetics, not all of whom have required insulin, there are only 21 who are known to have had insulin hypersensitiveness with generalized reactions. Rathery *et al.*[3] mention that in diabetics, as with any patient demonstrating allergy, the *terrain* plays a preponderant rôle, because the same insulin used with other diabetic patients does not produce any trouble.

3. **Theories of Causes of Allergy With Insulin Administration.** — As Cohen and Simon have stated, hypersensitivity to insulin has been ascribed to (1) the insulin protein itself, (2) the protein characteristic of the animal from which it was obtained, (3) some extraneous substance of the pancreas not removed in the isolation of insulin, or (4) to substances added to the insulin, of chemical nature, or of protein character such as protamine. Cases illustrating each condition have been reported. In the few cases where allergic manifestations followed the initial injection of insulin the presence

---

[1] Collens, Lerner and Fialka: Am. Jour. Med. Sci., **188**, 528, 1934.

[2] Baker: Arch. Int. Med., **58**, 373, 1936.

[3] Rathery, Bargeton, Maschas and Turiaf: Bull. et mém. Soc. méd. d. hôp. de Paris, **55**, 580, 1939.

of an inherited allergy or atopy to insulin protein was suggested, in contrast to the cases and animal experiments in which the sensitizing power of insulin as a protein had been shown to indicate the presence of true anaphylaxis after repeated administrations.

In the early years of insulin therapy the untoward local reactions were occasionally produced by preservatives, such as tricresol, used in the insulin, or by the injection of alcohol sometimes used to sterilize the needle and syringe, and in a few cases by formalin which had been added to the alcohol, employed for sterilization of the skin. These reactions are less likely to occur if the insulin is given subcutaneously as is proper, instead of being given partly in the intra-dermal layers of the skin, as is sometimes done by error.[1,2]

Besides these local reactions various studies have shown that humans and animals may be sensitized to the insulin molecule itself and show true allergy or anaphylaxis. Such sensitiveness has been demonstrated with insulins from all companies and laboratories, and with insulin of all types derived from all sources, including crystalline insulin and even human insulin.[3] A hypersensitive response has been demonstrated with as little as 1/2,000,000 unit of insulin.[4] Insulin would certainly be expected to possess antigenic properties because "crystalline insulin exhibits all the properties of a typical protein. . . . All evidence points to the fact that the crystalline insulin protein is chemically a homogeneous substance and represents the hormone itself."[5] There is evidence that insulin contains two kinds of protein, one characteristic of the hormone, and the other characteristic of the pancreatic protein of the species from which the insulin was obtained, though usually not characteristic of other proteins of the same animal. Sensitivity to the hormone protein is illustrated by patients who react to insulin from all sources including crystalline insulin. Examples of sensitivity to the organ protein of a certain species are patients sensitive only to the insulin derived from that certain species, but who are not sensitive to other proteins of the same species. Further support of this theory was given by Abel, quoted by Davidson, . . . "The best theory that can be offered at present for the insulins of different species of animals is this: That while these insulins all have the same composition and crystalline form, they differ in respect to the interior arrangement of the component amino acids, and it is on this, just as in the case with various proteins from different animals, that the difference in allergic response rests."

Page and Bauman injected 81 diabetic non-allergic pat'ents intra-

[1] Bryce: Med. Jour. Australia, **1**, 371, 1933.

[2] Kern and Langner: Loc. cit., p. 465.

[3] Campbell, Gardiner and Scott: Jour. Clin. Invest., **9**, 28, 1930.

[4] Esten and Dumm: Internat. M. Digest, **40**, 16, 1942.

[5] Jensen: Insulin: Its Chemistry and Physiology, New York, Oxford University Press, 1938.

dermally with various insulins and insulin modifiers,[1] and found the following percentage of positive local reactions: protamine 18.5, native globin (beef) 2.4, acid control 1.2, zinc chloride control 41.9, insulin (beef) 24.6, and crystalline insulin (recrystallized, zinc free) 4.8. They stress the low incidence of allergic reaction following the use of globin insulin.

The earliest investigators[2,3] of the protamines were unsuccessful in demonstrating antigenic properties although the increased incidence of local reactions with protamine zinc insulin would seem to incriminate the protamine added to the insulin. However, Kern and Langner,[4] using a suitable protamine test solution, performed skin tests on 104 diabetic patients using protamine zinc insulin and of whom there were 17 patients experiencing local reactions with its use, on 100 non-diabetics as controls, and on 8 allergic non-diabetic patients who were sensitive by skin tests to salmon muscle protein. In all cases the results were negative. To explain the frequent reactions with protamine insulins, where the addition of protamine to insulin seemed to increase the sensitivity to insulin, these authors made the interesting speculation that there was evidence that the addition to a true antigen of a substance possessing in itself no antigenic properties made sensitization to that antigen in an animal easier than the injection of the antigen alone.

Allan and Scherer remarked that it is presumably impossible for man to become hypersensitive to a material which is produced in his own body. Since crystalline insulin is supposedly the pure hormone, allergic reactions with it indicate that the hormone molecule differs in the different species, or that there is a protein attached to it. Bryce found it difficult to conceive of sensitiveness to insulin being acquired if the human hormone does not differ in chemical composition from that derived from other species, and suggested that it was possible that fresh antigenic properties were conferred upon the insulin during the course of its preparation *in vitro*. Sensitiveness to human insulin has already been mentioned. Of related interest is the observation of sensitiveness to human pituitrin.[5] Sensitiveness to posterior pituitary extract is not uncommon.[6]

4. **Experimental Studies.**—Barral and Roux[7] produced hypersensitiveness to insulin in guinea pigs. Animals sensitized in this way did not go into shock when injected with pancreas extracts, and *vice versa*, animals sensitized with pancreas extracts did not go into shock when injected with insulin. Lewis[8] used the Schultz-Dale

[1] Page and Bauman: Jour. Am. Med. Assn., **124**, 704, 1944.
[2] Taylor: Jour. Biol. Chem., **5**, 311, 1908.
[3] Wells: The Chemical Aspects of Immunity, 2d ed., New York, The Chemical Catalogue Company, 1929.
[4] Kern and Langner: Loc. cit., p. 465.
[5] Simon and Ryder: Jour. Am. Med. Assn., **106**, 512, 1936.
[6] McMann: Jour. Am. Med. Assn., **113**, 1488, 1939.
[7] Barral and Roux: Compt. rend. Soc. de Biol., **106**, 292, 1931.
[8] Lewis: Loc. cit., p. 464.

technique to study the antigenic properties of insulin. Uteri of virgin guinea pigs which had been sensitized to beef insulin reacted when exposed to beef insulin, but not when exposed to beef pancreas protein or beef serum. This experiment showed that the insulin protein was distinct from most of the protein of the pancreas. Lewis believed that the absence of reaction with beef serum, which is a strongly species specific antigen, indicated that insulin is not species specific. Uteri sensitized with either beef or pork insulin reacted when a strip of uterus was exposed to the insulin not used for the sensitization. He concluded from his various experiments that insulin proteins from different animal sources were immunologically closely related but not completely identical. Bernstein, Kirsner and Turner[1] also produced anaphylaxis in guinea pigs by sensitization with insulin. They were better able to demonstrate anaphylaxis with insulin after a preliminary sensitization with a combination of insulin and horse serum. The theories of Kern and Langner concerning the sensitizing properties of a combination of insulin and protamine have already been mentioned. Using protamine solutions only, and in amounts much larger than a diabetic patient would receive in therapeutic doses of protamine zinc insulin, Kern and Langner were unable to demonstrate anaphylaxis to protamine in guinea pigs.

5. **Proof of Insulin Sensitivity in Man.**—Various techniques have been used to prove that hypersensitiveness to insulin may occur in man. Practically all authors have used skin tests as the simplest method of proof. Tuft[2] was about the first investigator to try a passive transfer test, according to the Prausnitz-Küstner technique, and in obtaining positive tests he demonstrated the presence of specific reacting antibodies or reagins. He was able to show the presence of precipitins, but attempts to demonstrate complement-fixing antibodies and anaphylactic antibodies in the patient's serum were unsuccessful. His patient's serum was tested at intervals; the precipitins disappeared in a few weeks, but the reagins persisted for two or three months. Positive passive transfer tests were reported by Campbell, Gardiner and Scott, Bryce, and Sammis; such tests were unsuccessful in the cases reported by Murphy, Beardwood and Miller,[3] and Ulrich, Hooker and Smith.

6. **Antibodies for Crystalline Insulin.**—The existence of two antibodies for crystalline insulin has been demonstrated by Lowell[4,5,6] in two patients who had both insulin resistance requiring large doses of insulin and also sensitivity to injected insulin. The first antibody was thermostabile and insulin neutralizing capable of destroying the physiological effect of crystalline insulin. Mice injected

---

1 Bernstein, Kirsner and Turner: Jour. Lab. and Clin. Med., **23**, 938, 1938.
2 Tuft: Loc. cit., p. 464.
3 Murphy, Beardwood and Miller: J. Allergy, **5**, 606, 1934.
4 Lowell: Proc. Soc. Exp. Biol. and Med., **50**, 167, 1942.
5 Lowell: Loc. cit., p. 382, ref. 2.
6 Lowell: Loc. cit., p. 382, ref. 3.

with 0.5 cc. of such a patient's serum to which was added 0.02 units of crystalline insulin failed to develop hypoglycemia. When normal serum was substituted, this amount of insulin regularly produced hypoglycemic convulsions. In one human subject, the patient obtained a marked insulin effect from 30 units of human insulin intravenously yet had little or no effect from 30 units of crystalline insulin. It was suggested that this insulin-neutralizing antibody accounted for the patient's resistance to crystalline insulin. Since the patient responded well to human insulin Lowell suggested that the part of the molecule which served as antigen for the neutralizing antibody was characteristic for insulin derived from beef and pork pancreas and was not the part of the molecule which acted physiologically as insulin. The second antibody was heat-labile and conferred sensitivity on normal skin as evidenced by passive transfer tests. The generalized urticaria which followed the injection of insulin was attributed to this antibody.

Loveless[1] demonstrated the presence of reagins which are thermolabile sensitizing antibodies in the blood of a diabetic woman highly allergic to insulin as measured by passive sensitization studies done with serum dilutions. During desensitization treatment the serum acquire a second antibody which was thermostable and adequate to neutralize 0.1 unit of crystalline insulin per ml. as revealed by testing serum-insulin mixtures in sensitized skin. The thermostable antibody was capable of inactivating the hormonal function of insulin when injected into mice with lethal doses of crystalline insulin.

7. **Nature of the Allergic Response.**—Characteristic of the majority of the reported cases of hypersensitiveness to insulin having generalized reactions is the fact that these patients have received insulin in the past and it has been *omitted for a period* of months or years. With *resumption* of insulin therapy, after a period of days which might be considered to be an incubation period such as is observed in serum disease, then local or generalized allergic responses appear.[2] Bernstein *et al.* point out that this evidence of the sensitizing property of insulin is shown after "a period of insulin freedom which permits the sensitization to manifest itself, whereas such sensitization had been previously obscured by the frequent therapeutic (an incidentally desensitizing) injections." The appearance of allergic phenomena after resumption of insulin therapy has been variously reported as coming after a period of five to fifteen days, but usually occurs in from six to ten days. The similarity of these acquired responses to serum disease and to drug hypersensitiveness, has been mentioned by several authors. Tuft stated that insulin hypersensitiveness with generalized responses closely resembles serum disease, because "both are acquired or induced forms of hypersensitiveness, in both conditions the reaction does not occur

---

[1] Loveless: Fed. Proc., **5**, 250, 1946.
[2] Root: Jour. Amer. Med. Assn., **131**, 822, 1946.

following the initial or sensitizing injection but rather after a variable latent period, and urticaria is present in both as part of the reaction. Also, in both instances following the reaction, positive skin tests to the offending antigen are obtained and antibodies are detectable in the patient's serum: precipitins and antiphylactins in the case of serum disease and precipitins and reagins in insulin hypersensitiveness. These antibodies persist in both conditions for only a short period after the occurrence of the reaction . . . but cutaneous sensitivity persists apparently for a considerable period of time." Tuft also observed that with insulin there was evidence indicative of immunological specificity, because, as with lens protein, insulin protein derived from various species of animals is immunologically and probably chemically similar to the insulin protein of all other species of animals but different from the proteins of other tissues of the same animal. Since patients were not sensitive to the proteins of the other tissues of the animal, Campbell *et al.* thought that there was sensitization to organ protein as well as to the insulin protein.

8. **Eosinophilia.**—The association of eosinophilia with clinical allergic conditions and in experimental anaphylaxis has been known for decades, though the reasons for this are not understood.[1] The administration of insulin apparently has something to do with the production of eosinophiles. When the routine admission blood smears of 293 consecutive admissions to the George F. Baker Clinic were classified, it was found that eosinophilia of 3 per cent or more was present in 15.6 per cent of 83 patients not taking insulin, as compared with 28.6 per cent of 210 patients receiving insulin. The type of insulin seemed less important since eosinophilia was demonstrated in 22.4 per cent of those taking only regular insulin and in 29.1 per cent of those using only protamine zinc insulin. Except for 1 case with asthma and 1 case with eczema, no patient with an elevated eosinophile count was diagnosed as having any allergic condition. There were several cases having an allergic condition but who did not have an eosinophilia.

9. **Treatment of Insulin Hypersensitiveness.**—Depending upon the degree of sensitivity, the severity of the diabetes and the demands of the occasion, a patient who has hypersensitiveness to insulin can be treated in several ways.

(*a*) **Spontaneous Desensitization.**—Fortunately, the great majority of patients allergic to insulin have only local allergic reactions. Almost all will spontaneously overcome their hypersensitivity by continuing the insulin providing the reactions are not too severe, and they can tolerate the local discomfort for a few days or weeks. If a patient needs insulin and the allergic response is not too unbearable, then the patient should certainly be encouraged to take

[1] Ringoen: Eosinophile Leucocytes and Eosinophilia, in Handbook of Hematology, H. Downey, editor, New York, Paul B. Hoeber, Inc., pp. 180–229, 1938.

insulin for several weeks in the hope that spontaneous desensitization will occur.

(*b*) **Change Brand of Insulin.**—A few hypersensitive patients have been reported to be sensitive to insulin derived from only one species of animal, or from one manufacturer.[1,2] Collens *et al.* reported that 25 of 30 cases with protein reactions responded by merely changing the type of commercial insulin used. In our experience only a very small per cent of the cases have responded in this way. This is understandable when one considers that of the four American companies making insulin, Squibb, Sharpe & Dohme (Mulford) and Burroughs-Wellcome use beef pancreas exclusively whereas Eli Lilly Company uses a mixture of beef and pork pancreases. Certain manufacturers have on hand or will prepare upon request insulin from either beef or pork pancreases alone.

(*c*) **Low Carbohydrate Diets.**—The use of diets low in carbohydrate to avoid the use of insulin in patients with insulin sensitivity is rarely justified. The advantages of treating a diabetic with an adequate diet, protected if necessary with the addition of sufficient insulin, are so well known that one should hesitate before reducing the carbohydrate below 150 grams a day to avoid the use of insulin. Only in rare cases where desensitization cannot be accomplished or in mild diabetics, especially elderly ones, does the adoption of the low carbohydrate diet seem reasonable. Infection in the diabetic patient may suddenly and markedly increase the insulin requirement even in the mild case. In such cases of insulin allergy treated by diet alone, the use of emergency desensitization methods might be necessary to prevent acidosis.

(*d*) **Desensitization.**—Patients who require desensitization are those sensitive to all types of insulin and those who develop generalized allergic responses. Descriptions of programs for rapid desensitization[3,4,5,6] requiring less than a day, and for slow desensitization,[7,8] using the ordinary method of intradermal desensitization, are easily obtainable. The usual method is to begin with a very small dose of diluted insulin and to increase rapidly the amount injected at frequent intervals as long as there is no significant local or general response. Should the latter occur one starts again from the last non-reacting dose. A wise procedure is to use crystalline or regular insulin as the desensitizing agent.

The program of desensitization usually followed at the George F. Baker Clinic calls for an initial dose of 1/1000 unit of insulin sub-

[1] Collens, Lerner and Fialka: Loc. cit., p. 466.
[2] Grishaw: Jour. Am. Med. Assn., **97**, 1885, 1931.
[3] Allan and Scherer: Loc. cit., p. 464.
[4] Bayer: Loc. cit., p. 465.
[5] Corcoran: Am. Jour. Med. Sci., **196**, 359, 1938.
[6] Ulrich, Hooker and Smith: Loc. cit., p. 464.
[7] Bryce: Loc. cit., p. 467.
[8] Herold: New Orleans Med. and Surg. Jour., **91**, 163, 1938.

cutaneously. If no significant local reaction occurs the dose is approximately doubled with each succeeding dose. When no emergency exists 4 daily doses are ordinarily given; thus the insulin dose in units the first day would be 1/1000—1/500—1/250—1/125, the second day 1/100—1/50—1/25—1/12—and the third day 1/5— 1/2—1—2. The first day's solution is prepared by placing 4 units of crystalline insulin under aseptic conditions in 40 cc. of normal saline and then further dilution by mixing 1 cc. of the resulting solution with 9 cc. of normal saline. The final preparation contains 1/1000 unit of insulin in 1/10 cc. of solution. Desensitization as a life-saving measure in cases of hypersensitive diabetic coma cases has been reported.[1,2]

Case 11934 was admitted to the Deaconess Hospital in acidosis with a blood sugar of 303 mg. per cent, blood CO_2 combining power of 37 vol. per cent and with 4+ diacetic acid in the urine. She had an infected foot and had vomited ten times during the day. Insulin begun two days earlier had resulted in generalized urticaria and was therefore discontinued. Rapid desensitization was instigated beginning with 1/1000 unit of insulin and the dose doubled every 20 minutes. In this way desensitization was accomplished within five hours. In this case the blood precipitin test for antibodies was negative but the passive transfer test was positive. '

Following desensitization there are sometimes unexpected findings. Campbell *et al.* reported that one patient developed local desensitization for only crystalline insulin on a part of only one thigh. Allan and Scherer reported a case where allergic responses did not occur on the thighs where insulin was ordinarily given but did appear after injections in the arms. Some patients may subsequently be able to tolerate therapeutic doses of insulin easily, but may still have positive skin tests,[3] or occasionally still have local reactions.[4,5] Desensitization may not be permanent, for after a period of regularly using insulin satisfactorily allergic symptoms have been reported as recurring.[6] Bayer advised that after desensitization had been brought about a patient should continue the use of insulin without interruption unless there is good evidence that the insulin may be discontinued permanently.

(*e*) **Non-specific Desensitization With Histamine.**—Following the evidence that allergic symptoms may be brought about by the release of histamine or a histamine-like substance as a result of the allergic reaction, attempts were made to desensitize with histamine itself. Collens *et al.* were the first to apply this treatment to a diabetic hypersensitive to insulin of all kinds. After a program of injections of histamine phosphate there was progressive decrease in

[1] Allan and Scherer: Loc. cit., p. 464.
[2] Baker: Loc. cit., p. 466.
[3] Herold: Loc. cit., p. 472.
[4] Bayer: Loc. cit., p. 465.
[5] Collens, Lerner and Fialka: Loc. cit., p. 466.
[6] Ulrich, Hooker and Smith: Loc. cit., p. 464.

the severity of the insulin sensitivity reactions until there were no local reactions. This was probably not a case of spontaneous desensitization because the patient had been having local reactions for a year before the histamine treatment was started. Herzstein and Pollack[1] reported a case where an attempt at desensitization with histamine phosphate was not successful, and the patient was finally desensitized to protamine zinc insulin. Roth and Rynearson[2] reported a case where desensitization with histamine was successful.

(f) **Benadryl.**—Only one report[3] is available on the use of the new synthetic antihistamine drug Benadryl in cases of insulin allergy. Horton and his associates[4] at the Mayo Clinic have obtained encouraging results with other forms of allergy and it appears quite possible that the use of this drug may prove helpful in insulin hypersensitiveness as well.

(g) **Histaminase.**—Although earlier reports[2] suggested that histaminase might be of some value in occasional cases of insulin allergy Best and McHenry[5] believe there is no physiological basis on which to base its clinical use. It is no longer used to any extent for this purpose.

(h) **"Immunological" Desensitization.**—A final type of treatment might possibly be called "immunological" desensitization and will be discussed in a following section. (See page 476.)

10. **Cases of Hypersensitiveness to Insulin.**—Only a few illustrative cases will be described.

Case 21137, a man aged forty-three years at onset of diabetes in 1939 was first seen in February 1945. He had taken insulin without difficulty for five weeks in 1939 during the time he was treated for an infected toe. On March 6, 1945 he was again started on insulin—8 units of protamine zinc insulin—because his blood sugar was 232 mg. per cent and urine showed 3.2 per cent glycosuria. Ten days later he suddenly developed generalized urticaria, with marked angioneurotic edema of his face, hands and lower extremities. A few days later he was desensitized to insulin beginning with 1/1000 unit of crystalline insulin and the dose doubled with each subsequent injection. He was given 5 doses the first and second day and received undiluted insulin 1 and 2 units on the third day. Thereafter he was changed to protamine zinc insulin which he has continued to take without evidence of local or general allergic reactions.

Case 27012, a woman aged forty-five years at the onset of her diabetes in 1939, was first admitted to the New England Deaconess Hospital in June 1945. She had taken insulin for a few weeks in 1943, two years previously, but had discontinued it because of local allergic reactions at the site of injections. Insulin was resumed on admission to the hospital since her blood sugar was 338 mg. per cent and the urine revealed 3.2 per cent sugar. About four hours later the patient developed marked generalized urticaria. Two days later she was desensitized in the usual manner beginning with 1/1000 unit of crystalline insulin and rapidly increasing the dose

[1] Herzstein and Pollack: Loc. cit., p. 464.
[2] Roth and Rynearson: Proc. Staff Meet. Mayo Clin., 14, 353, 1939.
[3] Gastineau and Leavitt: Proc. Staff Meet., Mayo Clinic, 21, 316, 1946.
[4] McElin and Horton: Proc. Staff Meet. Mayo Clin., 20, 417, 1945.
[5] Best and McHenry: Jour. Am. Med. Assn., 115, 235, 1940.

4 times a day. On the third day concentrated insulin was taken without evidence of allergic manifestations. She was then changed to protamine zinc insulin without difficulty and was discharged well controlled with 12 units on July 18, 1945.

Case 3124, a woman aged thirty-seven years at onset of diabetes in October, 1921, was first observed in 1923. Her local physician reported that she had been given insulin when it had first become available and that she responded satisfactorily. The insulin supply temporarily failed and when it was resumed she was found to be sensitive. The sensitiveness had been so marked that on two occasions she had almost succumbed to anaphylactic shock; attempts at desensitization had been unsuccessful. When she came to the New England Deaconess Hospital she had not had insulin for several months and was on a diet of carbohydrate 40 grams, protein 70 grams and fat 130 grams with which she had much glycosuria and some ketosis. She was given insulin 1/100 unit one day, 1/50 unit the next day, and in increasing amounts until once with 3 units there was a local swelling. Subsequently she took 10 units three times a day without difficulty, and when last heard from in December 1944 she was still taking insulin.

Case 26598, a woman aged seventy-three years with diabetes of three months' duration was admitted March 28, 1945 with diabetic neuritis and left peroneal paralysis. She had never received insulin previously but gave a history of hay fever in the spring and fall for fifteen years. Two days later because of an elevated blood sugar and 1.2 per cent glycosuria she was given 8 units of protamine zinc insulin. Within thirty minutes the patient developed itching of the hands, thick speech and slight dyspnea. Following temporary improvement she rapidly became unconscious and pale two hours later with a fall in blood pressure and the development of urticaria and angioneurotic edema. She made an uneventful recovery. An intradermal test with 1/100 unit of insulin 3 days later was markedly positive hence desensitization was begun with an injection of 1/1000 unit of insulin. Within three days she was able to take concentrated insulin but still had small local reactions at the site of injection on discharge April 15, 1945.

Case 17757, a woman aged forty-eight years at onset of diabetes in 1938, was first observed in January, 1939. For two months previously at another hospital she had been given insulin, but for the three months' stay at the New England Deaconess Hospital for coronary thrombosis the blood sugars remained remarkably low and she was given no insulin. She was readmitted in December, 1939, with a blood sugar of 0.42 per cent and was started on both crystalline insulin and protamine zinc insulin. As much as 24 units of crystalline insulin and 60 units of protamine zinc insulin were required to bring the fasting blood sugar as low as 0.20 per cent. Six days later she developed generalized urticaria. Intradermal skin tests were markedly positive with every variety of insulin, but not with solutions of sodium chloride, zinc sulfate or protamine. An attempt at intradermal desensitization was tried but she continued to have wheals and pseudopods with as little as 1/500 unit. The patient was then started on histaminase ("Torantil") orally in a dosage of 30 to 40 units per day. Slow decrease in the amount of urticaria followed. She was finally given only crystalline insulin and the blood sugars became more normal. At discharge in January, 1940 the patient was taking 36 units of crystalline insulin, occasionally had hives, and an intradermal skin test with crystalline insulin was still markedly positive. When last seen in March, 1946 her diabetic condition was still well controlled with a single injection of 10 units of crystalline insulin.

11. **Insulin Resistance.**—Allergy to insulin and so-called insulin resistance may exist simultaneously.[1,2,3] The latter subject is dealt with at length on page 385. That the two may coexist is well illustrated by the case of Hart and Vicens.[4] A sixty year old man was admitted to the hospital in acidosis and received regular insulin with the development of a general as well as a local allergic reaction. Within the next three days his daily insulin dose rose to 920 units. Seven weeks later, however, his insulin requirement had reduced to such an extent that hypoglycemic reactions occurred with only 10 units daily; whereby insulin was discontinued.

Lowell[5] has shown that allergic antibodies and insulin neutralizing antibodies may exist in a patient's serum together, but need not vary in a parallel fashion.

Karr and his collaborators[6,7] reported the case of a woman who developed local reactions to insulin injections and in addition became resistant to insulin, requiring at one time over 600 units daily, and even then the fasting blood sugar values were over 200 mg. per cent. Precipitins were demonstrated in the blood serum. The treatment she received might be called "immunological" desensitization. After a rabbit was sensitized with the patient's serum, the animal's serum showed allergic antibodies by the precipitin test using insulin as the antigen. The patient was found to be sensitive to this rabbit serum. She was desensitized with it and then given 5 cc. intramuscularly. About a week later the patient had insulin shocks, the insulin requirement steadily decreased, and after about a month insulin was discontinued while the patient was using a liberal carbohydrate diet. However, a glucose tolerance test was still characteristic of diabetes.

B. ALLERGIC STATES NOT PECULIAR TO DIABETES.

A. Incidence of Allergic Conditions in Diabetics.

It is generally believed that the ordinary allergic states are not frequently found in diabetic patients. Swern[8] found only 6 diabetics in a group of 4000 allergic patients, chiefly asthmatic, studied in a period of ten years. On 61 allergic cases who were over thirty years of age, overweight and not fasting, blood-sugar determinations were made. Most values ranged from 80 to 130 mg. per cent and none were over 160 mg. per cent. Wilmer, Miller and Beardwood[9] had

[1] Glassberg, Somogyi and Taussig: Loc. cit., p. 385.
[2] Rudy: Loc. cit., p. 385.
[3] Goldner and Ricketts: Jour. Clin. Endocrin., 2, 595, 1942.
[4] Hart and Vicens: Jour. Clin. Endocrin., 1, 399, 1941.
[5] Lowell: Loc. cit., p. 382, ref. 3.
[6] Karr, Kreidler, Scull and Petty: Am. Jour. Med. Sci., 181, 293, 1931.
[7] Karr, Scull and Petty: Jour. Lab. and Clin. Med., 18, 1203, 1933.
[8] Swern: Jour. Allergy, 2, 375, 1931.
[9] Wilmer, Miller and Beardwood: Southern Med. Jour., 29, 197, 1936.

only 2 diabetic patients in a group of 4762 allergic cases, both of whom had bacterial (intrinsic) asthma. In a group of 1870 diabetics, only 2 cases were proven definitely to be allergic. However, these authors believed that in allergic persons some disturbance of carbohydrate metabolism occurs which might result from a glandular dysfunction and might accompany or form the background of the allergic disease. One hundred patients with various sorts of allergy were examined by means of glucose tolerance tests. According to their tests, normal patients and allergic patients with intrinsic allergy had similar glucose tolerance curves, whereas hay-fever cases and allergic cases in general in whom there was demonstrable sensitivity apparently had a greater tolerance for glucose since the blood-sugar curve did not rise so high during the standard three hour test. Abrahamson[1] reports 12 non-diabetic asthmatic patients in which asthma was associated with low blood sugars. By giving 100 grams of glucose he was able to reproduce the attacks for when blood-sugar values reaches 48 to 64 mg. per cent after four to seven hours, asthma occurred. Marked improvement followed the use of low carbohydrate, high fat diets with frequent small in between meals. Goltman[2] also believes that a great many allergic individuals have a low fasting blood sugar and very definitely increased sugar tolerance.

In contrast to this view, Wagner and Rackemann[3] studied glucose tolerance tests in asthmatics and concluded that the tests were normal for allergic cases and that whatever the fundamental nature of allergy might be, it is not concerned with the blood-sugar level.

Allergy or at least an allergic history is not rare in diabetes. Kern's[4] studies confirmed the usual belief that diabetes and allergy seldom occur in the same patient only if the phrase, "at the same time," was added. His statistics demonstrated that the past medical histories of diabetics showed an even higher incidence of allergy than those of persons in the community at large. Table 57 is reproduced from Kern's article:

TABLE 57.—PERCENTAGE OF FAMILY INCIDENCE OF DIABETES AND ALLERGY IN CONTROLS, ALLERGICS AND DIABETICS. (AFTER KERN.[4])

No. of cases.	Group.	Family history positive.	
		For diabetes, per cent.	For allergy, per cent.
500	Controls	6.2	11.2
500	Asthma or hay-fever . . .	21.0	80.4
100	Chiefly food allergy	35.0	85.0
300	Diabetics	25.3	29.3

Other studies by the same author showed that diabetic parents tended to have allergic children but that allergic patients only

---

[1] Abrahamson: Jour. Clin. Endocrin., **1**, 402, 1941.
[2] Goltman: Southern Med. Jour., **38**, 854, 1942.
[3] Wagner and Rackemann: Jour. Allergy, **8**, 353, 1937.
[4] Kern: Trans. Assn. Am. Phys., **49**, 23, 1934.

infrequently had diabetic children. Kern commented that this is what one would expect since diabetes is a recessive and allergy a dominant characteristic. In 300 diabetic patients a personal allergy history was positive in 20.3 per cent (61 patients). In 46 of these 61 patients allergic reactions had ceased before the diabetes began. It might be added that it is not strange for diabetics to have children who have allergy because allergy often develops in early life. Furthermore, diabetes does not usually appear in children of allergics because the disease usually appears in middle life.

The alleged infrequency of allergic conditions in association with diabetes is probably more apparent than real. Our experience suggests that with a more careful history and search for allergic symptoms the diabetics may have just as much allergy as nondiabetics. The diabetic cases have had allergy of varied types, and this applies to patients with non-diabetic glycosuria as well.

B. Asthma.

In a group of 16,016 true diabetics, only 30 cases with bronchial asthma were recognized, 22 of whom were adults. Among approximately 10,000 diabetic admissions to the New England Deaconess Hospital during the past six years, only 21 cases of asthma have been detected. It seems probable that some mild cases were overlooked owing to failure to question the patient regarding allergic disease. Both intrinsic and extrinsic asthma have been observed. In some cases the asthma began years before the onset of the diabetes, and in others the reverse was true. Case 5079, a woman aged thirty-eight years in 1924 when she developed asthma, was first found to have glucosuria when she was examined because of the asthma six months later. There were no symptoms of diabetes at that time. She was alive and active April 1946, taking 42 units of insulin, but still has occasional severe asthma believed by Dr. Francis Rackemann to represent primarily a bacterial allergy. Case 16705, a man who had been asthmatic for years, developed hives at the age of forty-two years in 1935, and on check-up for this condition glycosuria was found. Case 17701, a man aged seventy-one years in 1939 at the onset of diabetes, had had asthma for five years. The diabetes had never been severe enough to require insulin but he reported a curious relief of asthmatic symptoms after the onset of diabetes.

In 1400 juvenile diabetics there have been at least 11 with asthma. In 6 cases the asthma began before the diabetes, in 2 after the diabetes, and in 3 cases the onset date of the asthma was not stated. As with adults, the asthma was of both intrinsic and extrinsic types.

Several cases of asthma in the entire group have had to use epinephrine at various times, but except in one case, no significant effect on the blood-sugar level and diabetic control has been noted. Case 3717, a boy, aged fifteen years in 1923 when the diabetes began, had had bronchial asthma since infancy. The asthma has always been severe and he is sensitive to the inhalants, eggs, milk, and other antigens. Attacks have been almost of daily occurrence and he has taken from 4 to 24 injections of epinephrine (up to 0.8 cc. of 1 to 1000 solution) a day.

Despite the fact that epinephrine temporarily raises the blood sugar, the diabetic with asthma soon learns to adjust his insulin accordingly. Case 5079 frequently needs to double her usual insulin dose of approximately 36 units during a siege of asthma.

C. Miscellaneous Allergic States.

Hay-fever has been observed as an incidental finding in many diabetic patients. Hives, not due to hypersensitiveness to insulin, has been noted, and has usually been due to sensitivity to certain foods. Diabetic patients have been observed with urticaria of serum disease, with eczema, and with migraine of the common and the abdominal types. Two cases of drug sensitivity have recently been observed, one who develops a marked dermatitis and eczema to applications of hexylresorcinol solution, and the other to applications of tincture of metaphen. Case 18773 develops a localized dermatitis to any application of a metal to or near the skin. Dermatitis occurs if he has coins or keys in the trouser pockets, uses uncovered garters, or wears a wrist watch or gold frame glasses. He has no personal or family history of allergy.

D. Relationships of Ordinary Allergy, Anaphylaxis, and Insulin.

Certain aspects in the relationship of administration of insulin to allergy are worthy of mention. Lee[1] summarized findings of other workers in which it was shown that drugs which stimulate the sympathetic nervous system inhibit anaphylaxis, that sympatheticotonia during anaphylaxis should inhibit anaphylaxis, and that the amount of epinephrine in the blood increases after the injection of insulin. In his own experiments, using guinea pigs sensitized to horse serum, he found that hypoglycemia after insulin injection was relatively less during anaphylactic shock. He also found that both unilateral and bilateral vagotomy augmented anaphylactic symptoms, and that insulin inhibited this augmenting action, thereby showing some correlation between insulin, anaphylaxis and the vagus.

Bartelheimer and Afendulis[2] observed that repeated insulin reactions in guinea pigs seemed to reduce the severity of anaphylaxis in the animals when sensitized to horse serum. If insulin was inac-

---

[1] Lee: Jour. Chosen Med. Assn., (Abstract Section), **24**, 97, 1934.
[2] Bartelheimer and Afendulis: Ztschr. f. d. ges. exper. Med., **104**, 31, 1938.

tivated with cystine hydrochloride before injection there was no modification of a typical anaphylactic shock. They reported that the blood of animals in insulin shock, when tested by physiological methods based on a fall of blood-pressure, resulted in the same drop as produced by injection of 0.001 milligram of histamine. Therefore they concluded that in insulin shock, histamine or histamine-like substances were set free in the blood, and that after repeated insulin injections the organism loses its sensitivity to the histamine-like substance, to result in decreased response to anaphylactic shock where the etiological agent is histamine.

These findings have been applied to humans. Wegierko[1] observed that asthmatics got relief with the first signs of insulin shock. Consequently, he treated asthmatics with a series of insulin shocks, not as severe as those used for schizophrenic patients, and the asthma was relieved for eighteen to twenty-four hours. After a course of ten to fifteen shocks he believed that the asthmatics were definitely improved. Swern[2] believed that skin reactions of asthmatics apparently decreased with the onset of diabetic symptoms and that asthma improved with treatment of the diabetes but he did not mention the use of insulin. Joseph[3] reported that he treated 104 cases of hay-fever and asthma with 8 units of insulin arbitrarily given every other day and that most patients had marked benefit from the insulin treatment, usually after the fourth injection. One might theorize that this resulted from a secondary increase of secretion of epinephrine following the injection of insulin.

[1] Wegierko: Presse méd., **44**, 731, 1936.
[2] Swern: Loc. cit., p. 476.
[3] Joseph: Med. Rec., **149**, 16, 1939.

CHAPTER XV.

CARDIO–RENAL–VASCULAR DISEASE.

Revised by Howard F. Root, M.D.

A. INCIDENCE OF CARDIO–RENAL–VASCULAR DISEASE.

Arteriosclerotic changes in early stages and of mild degree are easily discernible by careful pathological study in many individuals as early as the third decade, whether the population studied is composed of diabetics or non-diabetics. It is the unusual frequency of advanced lesions of occlusive vascular disease, involving chiefly the coronary vessels and the leg arteries, which provides the outstanding features of diabetic morbidity- and mortality-rates. In recent years chronic renal disease associated with diabetic retinopathy has assumed an important position, especially in young patients with diabetes of long duration. In 84 cases of childhood diabetes dying after more than ten years' duration, 31 died of nephritis. (See page 768.) An elucidation of the relative importance of the various causative factors, together with improvements in our methods of preventing and of treating these complications when they arise, represent without doubt the most urgent need in diabetic treatment today.

The diabetic lives and dies in the arteriosclerotic zone; lives in it, because two-thirds of the 25,148 true diabetics in the present series originated after thirty-nine years of age; died in it, because although the average age at death of 326 cases in the Naunyn period was 44.5 years, the average age at death of the 651 fatal cases in the Charles H. Best era was 64.5 years.

Exposure of the patient to the influence of diabetes was not long enough in Naunyn's time to show whether it would result in arteriosclerosis. The average duration of the disease was then only 4.9 years and the few diabetics who exceeded this limit were the mild old cases who already presented at the onset of diabetes the vascular changes consistent with their age. (See Table 59 and page 483.)

The length of exposure was greater in the Allen period, but has become still more evident in the Charles H. Best epoch. Seven hundred and forty-nine children who have had diabetes for more than fifteen years attest this, as well as the average duration of the disease in 651 recently fatal cases of all ages which has become 14.1 years.

As a cause of death of the diabetic, arteriosclerosis has risen three-fold (333 per cent) in importance, and coma has dropped to one-twentieth of its former incidence. (See Table 59.) Yet the pre-

31

mature development of arteriosclerosis is already yielding to better dietary and insulin treatment.

1. **Criteria for the Incidence of Arteriosclerosis.**—The best criteria are furnished by autopsies, next by the causes of death found on the death certificates of diabetics, although here certain instances would escape detection. The third source is the evidence obtained from clinical and physical examination plus the help of the roentgen ray. The living cases have been investigated with increasing care in recent years for signs of arteriosclerosis. Attention has been paid to the peripheral arteries by means of roentgenograms of the lower extremities and classification of the sclerosis of the radial arteries in four grades: (1) palpable; (2) roll under finger; (3) tortuous; (4) beaded or pipe-stem.

TABLE 58.—AORTIC ATHEROSCLEROSIS IN 23 DIABETICS AND 170 NON-DIABETICS OF SIMILAR AGE AT AUTOPSY.

Grade of sclerosis.	Diabetes less than one year in duration.		Non-diabetics.	
	Number.	Per cent.	Number.	Per cent.
Slight	14	61	94	55
Moderate and advanced	9	39	76	46

TABLE 59.—INFLUENCE OF DURATION OF DIABETES UPON PERCENTAGE OF TOTAL DEATHS IN DIABETICS DUE TO ARTERIOSCLEROSIS AND DIABETIC COMA.

Epoch.	Average duration of diabetes yrs.*	Deaths, total.	Coma per cent.	Arteriosclerosis, per cent.	Average age at death, yrs.
Naunyn:					
1898 to June, 1914	4.9	326	64	17	44.5
Allen:					
June, 1914, to Aug., 1922 . . .	6.1	836	42	24	46.7
Banting:					
Aug., 1922, to Dec. 31, 1925 . . .	7.5	537	21	41	54.3
Jan., 1926, to Dec. 31, 1929 . . .	8.4	918	11	49	60.0
Jan., 1930, to Dec. 31, 1934 . . .	10.0	1741	5	58	62.7
Jan., 1935, to Dec. 31, 1936 . . .	11.6	793	4	59	63.9
Hagedorn:					
Jan., 1937, to Dec. 31, 1939 . . .	12.4	1229	4	62	64.8
Jan., 1940, to Dec. 31, 1943 . . .	13.3	1354	3	66	65.0
Charles H. Best:					
Jan., 1944, to date†	14.1	651	3	67	64.5

* Based on cases of known duration.
† Deaths reported through May 15, 1946.

Clinical data which allow inferences to be drawn upon the existence of arteriosclerosis in the brain, heart, eyes and kidneys must be utilized. Conclusions upon the presence of arteriosclerosis in the living cases of this series, however, will err on the side of too low a percentage as is emphasized by Rabinowitch.[1]

(a) **Evidence From Autopsies.**—Autopsy examinations of 484 diabetics described by Warren[2] showed arteriosclerosis present in all

[1] Rabinowitch: Ann. Int. Med., **8**, 1436, 1935. Rabinowitch, Ritchie and McKee: Ann. Int. Med., **7**, 1478, 1934.
[2] Warren: P. 128; loc. cit., p. 196.

but 50 cases, of whom 36 were under thirty years of age. Arteriosclerosis caused the death of 143 cases, 30 per cent, of whom 1 died of acute coronary thrombosis at thirty-three years. The decade of onset in which arteriosclerosis did not present gross manifestations at autopsy was the first, thus making it the only decade in diabetes immune to arteriosclerosis. In the second decade among 29 cases arteriosclerosis was present in 12, or 41 per cent.

(*b*) **Evidence From Fatal Cases.**—Of our true diabetics, 8384 have died. These have been classified in five groups, the Naunyn, 1898 to 1914, the Allen, 1914 to 1922, the early and later Banting, 1922 to 1929 and 1930 to 1937, the Hagedorn to December 31, 1943 and the Charles H. Best to May 15, 1946. (See page 482.) Analysis of the causes of death of these patients in order to determine the part played by arteriosclerosis has been made upon the following basis: The term arteriosclerosis has been taken to include all deaths under the headings (*a*) arteriosclerosis and gangrene, (*b*) apoplexy or its synonyms. Acute disease of the heart and kidney are for all practical purposes in such a compilation absent and consequently all (*c*) cardiac and (*d*) nephritic deaths are included in the arteriosclerotic group. Table 59 is compiled in this manner and indicates the increasing frequency of arteriosclerosis on the death certificate, rising as it does from 17 per cent in the Naunyn era to 67 per cent in the Charles H. Best era. The table also shows the increasing duration of the disease from 4.9 to 14.1 years and that diabetics are growing old because the average age at death in the Naunyn era was 44.5 years, and in the Charles H. Best era 64.5 years.

That the development of arteriosclerosis is excessive and has become the major cause of death among diabetics generally, just as it has at the Deaconess Hospital, is amply confirmed by many writers, including Nathanson,[1] Blotner,[2] Rabinowitch,[3] Wilder.[4] Enklewitz[5] and Sprague.[6] Root and Sharkey[7] for the first time demonstrated that its excessive development followed the onset of diabetes.

Coronary occlusion was the cause of death in 11 per cent of 139 cases reported by Dry and Tessmer.[8] The excessive frequency and the early development of arteriosclerosis in diabetic patients is brought out by a comparison of the autopsy findings in 193 diabetic and 2250 non-diabetic patients by Lisa, Magiday, Galloway, and Hart.[9] Their patients were classified by age and analysis showed

[1] Nathanson: Am. Jour. Med. Sci., **183**, 495, 1932.
[2] Blotner: New England Jour. Med., **203**, 709, 1930.
[3] Rabinowitch: Loc. cit., p. 480.
[4] Wilder: South. Med. Jour., **19**, 241, 1926.
[5] Enklewitz: Am. Heart Jour., **9**, 386, 1934.
[6] Sprague: P. 122; loc. cit., p. 314.
[7] Root and Sharkey: Ann. Int. Med., **9**, 873, 1936.
[8] Dry and Tessmer: Minnesota Med., **24**, 96, 1941.
[9] Lisa, Magiday, Galloway and Hart: Jour. Am. Med. Assn., **120**, 192, 1942.

that arteriosclerosis, especially in the severest form, appears more often in a diabetic patient at practically all ages. This was true not only in the coronary arteries and the aorta, but also in the kidneys.

In Table 58 are shown a comparison of the degree of atherosclerosis in the aorta of 23 diabetics whose diabetes was of less than one year in duration with 170 non-diabetics of similar age at autopsy. It will be seen that slight degrees of atherosclerosis were observed in 61 per cent of the diabetics and in 55 per cent of the non-diabetics, whereas moderate and advanced changes occurred in 39 per cent of the diabetics and in 46 per cent of the non-diabetics. Certainly it is clear from this that the amount of aortic change in diabetics in the early stage of the disease is very nearly the same as with non-diabetics. No such difference appears as is evidenced in the series of diabetics of long duration as compared with non-diabetics. Clearly the excessive degrees of atherosclerosis are in some manner related to diabetes of long duration.

The influence of the duration of diabetes upon the percentage of total deaths of diabetics due to arteriosclerosis has been studied. When the duration was five to nine years, the percentage of total deaths from arteriosclerosis was 36 per cent, when ten to fourteen years it was 49 per cent, when fifteen to nineteen years it was 67 per cent and from twenty years onward, 58 per cent (the decrease in the last period possibly being due to the unusually large number of death certificates in this period bearing the term "diabetes" only). It is true that the long cases formerly were toward middle life and so an increasing duration brought all these patients into the realm of arteriosclerosis, but this could hardly account for the steady increase shown.

(c) **Clinical Evidence of Arteriosclerosis.**—The living cases of diabetes of ten or more years' duration are considerably behind the dead in their percentage of arteriosclerosis. The first two decades can almost be disregarded because with better treatment almost no calcification in the arteries is found now. From the third decade onward its frequency and severity increase with the age and the duration of diabetes.

The roentgen-ray has been an increasing help in the clinical study of arteriosclerosis since 324 of our diabetics were studied in this manner by Dr. L. B. Morrison and Dr. I. K. Bogan.[1] Of course uncalcified arteries do not show by roentgenogram and consequently a considerable number of atheromatous cases are overlooked. This makes their positive findings all the more impressive.

Four reports from the University Hospital, Philadelphia,[2] present

---

[1] Morrison and Bogan: Am. Jour. Med. Sci., **174**, 313, 1927.
[2] Diabetes Mellitus as Observed in 100 Cases for Ten or More Years: I. General Observations, Richardson and Bowie, p. 1; II. Cardiac Studies, Edeiken, p. 8; III. Ocular Findings, Leopold, p. 16; IV. Peripheral Vascular Findings in, 89 of These Cases, Naide, p. 23. Am. Jour. Med. Sci., **209**, 1, 1945.

a study of 100 patients who had had diabetes for ten years or more. The diabetes did not always progress to greater severity. Comparison of the diet and insulin at the beginning and at the end of a five year period revealed that the diabetes of 45 per cent of the patients had not advanced. Ten patients required less insulin at the end than at the beginning of the period. Of the 55 who required more insulin, a number had also received increases in diet. Acidosis occurred in 3 of the group. Anemia of a mild degree was present in 26 patients. Chronic or repeated acute infections occurred in 39 patients. Hypertension (systolic blood pressure 160 mm.) was present in 38 per cent, all past fifty years of age; the incidence increased with each decade. The incidence of hypertension apparently was not dependent on duration, control or severity of the diabetes. Only 3 patients under 50 had abnormalities of the heart which could be attributed to their diabetic state. The 3 patients were twenty-four, thirty and forty-seven years of age and had had diabetes for fifteen or sixteen years. The low incidence of cardiovascular abnormalities in this younger group receiving a high carbohydrate-low fat diet compared to reports in the literature regarding patients on a high fat-low carbohydrate diet is suggestive of the value of the high carbohydrate-low fat diet in reducing the incidence of premature cardiovascular abnormalities. Complicated cataracts were fewer in diabetic patients treated for ten years than in the untreated. Subcapsular "snow flake" cataracts were still found in the diabetic patients treated for ten years. The diabetic patients treated for ten years showed an incidence of sclerosis similar to that of the non-diabetic and to the diabetic of varying duration and therapy. Deep retinal hemorrhages and exudates increased with the duration of diabetes and might be slightly decreased by closely observed therapy. Of the 89 patients who were studied from the standpoint of arteriosclerotic occlusive disease in the legs, 3 patients of those under fifty years of age and 30 of those over fifty had evidence of peripheral arteriosclerosis. Premature arteriosclerosis (below fifty) was therefore not common in this group. The severity of the diabetes did not affect the incidence of arteriosclerosis, but the adequately controlled patients had a low incidence of arterial disease. The females had a much higher incidence of arteriosclerotic occlusive disease than males. There were no amputations in the entire group. Neuritis in the extremities was present in 31 of the 89 patients, chiefly in those with arteriosclerosis.

B. THE ETIOLOGY OF THE ARTERIOSCLEROSIS IN DIABETES.

1. **Introduction.**—The problem of the cause of arteriosclerosis is inevitably concerned with the processes of aging and degeneration, since the development of arteriosclerosis is obviously so much more

frequent in later adult life than in early life.   However, it seems clear that other causes than senescence must be accepted if an explanation is to be found for the varying degrees of change in different ages and different races and in different diseases and the obvious connection of vascular changes to definite endogenous and exogenous factors in an appreciable number of cases.   Hueper[1] reviewed the clinical and experimental literature upon arteriosclerosis, presenting the evidence for the senescence theory, the toxin theory and the theories of mechanical trauma and anoxemia.

Four types of arteriosclerosis are commonly recognized.   (1) Atheromatosis is a patchy lesion observed chiefly in the intima of the larger elastic arteries in contrast to the muscular arteries.   (2) Arteriolar sclerosis is a diffuse lesion involving the arterioles and finer branches of the arterial tree frequently observed in patients with hypertension.   Hyaline intimal lesions, hypertrophy and degeneration of the media and thickening of the subendothelial layer of the intima are characteristic.   A close relation exists between hypertension and atherosclerosis, particularly with reference to the coronary arteries (Leary).[2]   (3) Monckeberg's sclerosis represents primary necrosis and calcification of the media of the muscular arteries.   (4) Senile loss of elasticity, and degeneration of the aging process.

Atheromatosis presents nodular patchy lesions of the aorta as well as of the larger, middle-size and even smaller arteries chiefly of the elastic type, although also found in arteries of the muscular type.   The intima first is affected, becomes thickened and the cells often are filled with lipoids.   All active human lesions contain cholesterol in excess.   Only healed or calcified lesions are free from this excess.   Calcification of the plaques with fibrosis of the media develops and gradually the lumen is reduced.   That atherosclerosis is not merely a disease of age is indicated by Leary's series in which advanced coronary sclerosis occurred at twelve and fifteen years of age with numerous coronary deaths in the twenties and thirties. The chief characteristics of arteriolar sclerosis are hypertrophy of the media of the arterioles and small arteries, proliferation of the intima and reduction in the ratio of the thickness of the walls to the diameter of their lumina.

Monckeberg's sclerosis is a patchy involvement of the media without the accumulation of lipoid.   It is not limited to the aged, but is easily demonstrated by roentgenogram in the calcified leg arteries of many patients in the third decade of life, whose diabetes began in childhood.   LaMont's[3] patient was twenty-nine years of age with diabetes of fifteen years' duration when calcified arteries were demonstrable by x-ray throughout the peripheral arterial

[1] Hueper: Arch. Path., **38**, 162, 245, 350, 1944; **39**, 51, 1945.
[2] Leary: Bull. New York Acad. Med., **17**, 887, 1941.
[3] LaMont: Ohio State Med. Jour., **37**, 30, 1941.

system. Thrombosis occurs when by reason of the extension of the lesion from the media to the intimal surface its nutrition is involved and clot formation occurs at the site. The fact that nicotin, irradiated ergosterol as well as adrenalin injections in animals have been shown to cause medial sclerosis rather than atheroma suggests a different etiology from that of atherosclerosis. However, bearing in mind that the two lesions occur together in the same person and in such close relation to one another suggests very strongly that they really are part of the same process. Any or all of these lesions may be associated with senile arteriosclerosis.

Wilder,[1] although recognizing the great incidence of atherosclerosis in diabetes and the importance of its treatment as a complication of diabetes, doubts that the vascular lesions are due solely to diabetes. He stresses the observation that arteriolar sclerosis as judged by hypertension, sclerosis of the retinal artery, and the incidence of nephritis is no more common among diabetic patients than among others. The incidence of visible sclerosis of the retinal arteries seems to be no greater in diabetics than in non-diabetics. On the other hand, the incidence of deep retinal hemorrhages certainly is greater and the conviction is growing that these lesions are fundamentally due to some injury to the walls of the small arterioles and venules, even though it cannot be recognized clinically nor its nature defined. More important still is the emergence of an unusual nephropathy ("intercapillary glomerulosclerosis") with associated retinopathy as a frequent complication in young diabetics of long duration. However, Root and Sharkey,[2] in a study of 175 diabetic autopsies, noted the frequency of changes in the small arterioles in diabetic patients at autopsy and the great frequency of arteriosclerotic nephritis of mild degree.

In discussing glomerulosclerosis, Spuehler and Vollinger[3] considered that the association of diabetes with arteriosclerosis and arteriolosclerosis is generally accepted. They believe that the characteristic changes in diabetic glomerulosclerosis involving the capsular membrane, capillary and basement membrane of the tubules, obtain also in the eye, and explain the frequent development of retinitis. It is true that although mild degrees of nephritis are found in older diabetic patients, death from uremia and vascular nephritis as a chief cause is less common but increasing. Such patients in our experience usually have developed some lesion of the extremities or infection from which they died before nephritis itself was fatal. It is the arteries of the heart (see page 509) and the legs which show the most extensive changes. Herzstein and Weinroth[4] found peripheral arteriosclerosis in 51 per cent of 249 male

[1] Wilder: New Internat. Clin. II, Ser. 2, p. 13, 1939.
[2] Root and Sharkey: Loc. cit., p. 483.
[3] Spuehler and Vollinger: Deutsch. Arch. f. klin. Med., **190**, 321, 1943.
[4] Herzstein and Weinroth: Arch. Int. Med., **76**, 34, 1945.

diabetics. Actually, Dry and Hines[1] found at the Mayo Clinic, arterial insufficiency in the legs of diabetics to be eleven times as frequent as in non-diabetics, and among women arteriosclerosis obliterans was eighty times as frequent in diabetics as in non-diabetics.

Among the factors influencing the arterial system, the vegetative nervous system must be considered because of its control of vascular tone. The influence of heredity in producing arteriosclerosis is best indicated by the frequency of hypertension and arteriosclerosis among the relatives of patients with essential hypertension. Weitz[2] regarded the predisposition to hypertension as a Mendelian dominant character in contrast to many investigators who assign to heredity a definite but a·subordinate influence.

If one is to assume that the development of occlusive vascular disease in the diabetic patient depends not upon the existence of diabetes but upon the coexistence of a hereditary abiotrophy, then first one should expect to be able to show such a frequency of arteriosclerotic lesions in the members of the family of diabetic patients as would indicate a greater hereditary tendency than is present in the general population. If this hereditary abiotrophy accompanies every case of diabetes or hereditary defect in the insulin-manufacturing apparatus then all diabetic patients at certain ages should show the same excessive vascular disease. It is well-known that certain diabetic patients have occlusive vascular disease of such a type as to cause progressive diminution of the arterial lumina so that gangrene in one leg is followed a few years later by gangrene in the other. On the other hand, there are certain diabetic patients who have infected lesions of the feet, requiring amputation of the toe or leg, who go on for years thereafter without developing truly occlusive vascular disease. On this basis one may state, therefore, that if there is a hereditary abiotrophy for arterial disease, it is present in only a limited percentage of diabetic patients since gangrene involves only a small percentage of all diabetic patients.

Two series of 100 diabetic patients each were studied with respect to familial vascular disease. One series consisted of 100 adult diabetics who had had coma. The other 100 cases consisted of diabetic patients who had had surgical lesions of the feet, dependent upon arteriosclerosis. In the coma series, 75 were female and 25 were male, whereas in the series made up of foot cases, 59 were female and 41 were male. Three vascular conditions were sought for in the family: high blood-pressure, cerebral hemorrhage and heart trouble. In the coma series, 53 out of 100 had known of the existence of one or more of these three conditions in a father, mother, brother or sister and sometimes in two or three members of the family. In the foot series, which was made up of older people, 69 patients simi-

[1] Dry and Hines: Ann. Int. Med., **14**, 1893, 1941.
[2] Weitz: Ztschr. f. klin. Med., **96**, 151, 1923.

larly reported one or more of these three conditions in one or more of their relatives.

Although the morphologic and chemical peculiarities of the arteriosclerotic artery wall have been studied carefully, the underlying causal factors are still under debate. The old question whether the injury fundamentally begins in the intima or in the media is of less importance than the fact that different processes or changes appear in the intima and the media, which, indeed, together make up the picture of arteriosclerosis but which can begin independently of each other. The sclerosis of the intima begins as a gradual thickening of the ground substance with later lipoid infiltration and eventually calcification. In the muscles of the media appear necrosis, changes in structure of the elastic tissue and calcium deposition. We can no longer accept the old Virchow idea of an inflammatory process. We know that in addition to the inevitable constitutional and hereditary predisposition, nutritional, toxic and mechanical causes play a rôle.

In a recent study by Lisa, Magiday and Hart[1] the vascular supply in amputated legs was studied in a group of 55 diabetics and 51 non-diabetics. The patients came from the New York City Hospital on Welfare Island. The study emphasizes the extensive character of arteriosclerosis in both diabetics and non-diabetics. They were unable to distinguish types of arteriosclerosis characteristic of diabetes. The most important point in such a study is hinted at by the authors' comment that peripheral occlusive disease is many times more frequent in the diabetic. Actually, at the age mentioned, probably not more than one in fifty individuals have diabetes so that in such a hospital where old age cases are so prominent, the fact that an equal number occurred indicates that diabetes was associated with extensive arteriosclerosis fifty times as frequently as in the non-diabetic. More important still is the effect of diabetes in altering the relation of occlusive vascular disease and sex. These authors had among the women of the series, twenty-eight diabetic cases and eight non-diabetic. These figures would suggest that in women peripheral arteriosclerosis leading to amputation of the leg for gangrene occurred more than 150 times as frequently as it does in non-diabetic women. These figures are in agreement with all previous observations emphasizing the extraordinary influence of diabetes in accelerating the development of vascular disease in the extremities.

The atheromatous intimal thickenings and calcareous deposits characteristic of arteriosclerosis occur in mammals other than man, as well as in birds. The histological changes are similar to those in man but less pronounced in degree, according to Fox.[2] Wild animals showed atherosclerosis as well as animals in captivity. Mammals

---

[1] Lisa, Magiday and Hart: Jour. Am. Med. Assn., **118**, 1353, 1942.
[2] Fox: in Cowdry, Arteriosclerosis, New York, Macmillan Company, p. 153, 1933.

and birds showed the most typical lesions, whereas certain animal families failed to show arteriosclerosis, according to Fox.[1]

The influence of the endocrine glands is well reviewed by Raab.[2] He gives first place to the adrenals because of the presence of the hemodynamic effects of adrenalin, its selective action upon the media, the intimate relationship between the adrenal cortex and the lipoid metabolism (the capacity of the cortical hormone for "fixing" cholesterol in the tissues) and the pathological records of arteriosclerosis in young patients with adrenal tumors. He also stresses the production of medial necrosis and calcification by means of injections of a lipoid extract obtained from the blood of arteriosclerotic and hypertensive patients. Adrenalin-free cortical extracts do not produce changes in the arteries. The presence of vaso-active adrenalin-lipoid combinations in the serum and the sensitization of the arterial wall to adrenalin by cholesterol and cortical lipoids are stressed.

The influence of the thyroid is definite since it is shown that in animals from whom the thyroid has been removed that cholesterin sclerosis is developed most easily. Indeed, even in children with lack of development of the thyroid gland arteriosclerosis has been found. Cases of hyperthyroidism conversely show relatively little arteriosclerosis. A clear relationship exists with the parathyroid glands since there is a special tendency to calcification of the vessels in von Recklinghausen's disease. Also in arteriosclerotic men the oxyphilic cells of the parathyroids are increased.

The influence of the sex glands upon arteriosclerosis is indicated by the rapid advance of arteriosclerotic changes in the period of life when sexual activity ends. Also the loss of the sex glands through castration advances experimental cholesterin atherosclerosis as well as the vitamin D sclerosis of the media.

The effectiveness of prolonged oral administration of vitamin C and the B-complex on the increased capillary fragility in 4 diabetic patients without retinitis or any other complication, even hypertension and in 6 diabetic patients with retinitis, has been tested, with negative results, by Rudy, Beaser and Seligman.[3] The effectiveness of both orally and parenterally administered vitamin P in some patients of this group was studied. Both the hesperidin and the eriodictyol fractions of vitamin P were tested intravenously, separately and combined, with negative results. A similar study of the effect of vitamin P therapy on the increased capillary fragility of thrombopenic purpura (2 cases) and rheumatoid arthritis (1 case) was made, with negative results.

There is little evidence in favor of the belief that infections either

[1] Fox: Bull. New York Acad. Med., 15, 748, 1939.
[2] Raab: Klin. Wchnschr., 18, 611, 1939.
[3] Rudy, Beaser and Seligman: Arch. Int. Med., 73, 18 and 23, 1944.

acute or chronic have much to do with the production of arterio-sclerosis.

Winternitz, Thomas and LeCompte[1] have explained the formation of the plaques which characterize human arteriosclerosis on the assumption that blood extravasated within the wall, especially in the intima, of the aorta and large arteries might be a source of the lipoidal deposits. The authors support their beliefs that the lipoid followed the hemorrhage by showing that there is an extensive vascular network in the intima of normal blood vessels of animals other than man.

Leary,[2] in contrast to Winternitz, questions the etiological rôle of intimal hemorrhage in arteriosclerosis. He holds that the normal intima is not vascularized and that vascularization occurred only in connection with vascular lesions in which repair had taken place. He reasons that since the vessels arose only as a result of a repair process and were of advanced atherosclerotic type the hemorrhages from such vessels must be a late phenomenon and therefore not of etiological importance.

2. **Diet.**—Important components of the diet favoring the development of arteriosclerosis are the lipoids, first of all the cholesterin and the light active ergosterin (vitamin D). The first when present in large amounts favors pure intimal lipoidosis, the second pure medial sclerosis. The best imitation of human arteriosclerosis in experimental animals is obtained by combining the use of cholesterin and vitamin D.

Nicotin is an important poison, because it not only produces acute mobilization of adrenalin but in chronic usage in animal experiments often produces adenoma formation in the adrenal cortex. The iodine content of the diet is important since experimentally iodine in either organic or inorganic form counteracts experimental cholesterin sclerosis. Except for calcification following hypervitaminosis with vitamin D experimentally produced, little is known about the effect of vitamins upon arteriosclerosis. Nevertheless, the long-continued use of diets deficient in vitamins may yet be proved a causative factor in arteriosclerosis. Undernutrition, so far as caloric intake is concerned, has not been proved beyond doubt to influence the degree of arteriosclerosis.

The effect of meat in producing arteriosclerosis is still not established. Stefansson lived for months on a pure meat diet without ill effects upon blood-pressure or kidney function. No one today, so far as we are aware, approves of increasing the protein above the usual standard of a gram per kilogram body weight in the diet of an individual who is developing arteriosclerosis. Does carbohydrate cause arteriosclerosis? If taken in such excess as to produce obesity,

[1] Winternitz, Thomas and LeCompte: Arteriosclerosis, Charles C Thomas, Springfield, 1938.
[2] Leary: Am. Heart Jour., **16**, 549, 1938.

arteriolar sclerosis and hypertension may result, but except in this manner no one would attribute any such function to it. To a non-diabetic carbohydrate is benign. But with the diabetic to use carbohydrate introduces the problem of hyperglycemia which develops when the carbohydrate is not burned. Is a persistent hyperglycemia a cause of arteriosclerosis in diabetes? It is an abnormal condition and any abnormal state would tend to wear out the machine.

Our diabetic children of today constitute an experiment with hyperglycemia. (See Chapter XXVIII.) Briefly it may be said that in the 749 cases with duration fifteen years or more with onset in childhood, nearly 50 per cent of those studied have shown calcified arteries in the legs by roentgen-ray. Abnormalities of fat metabolism appeared to be more injurious than abnormalities of carbohydrate metabolism. We do not believe that a hyperglycemia up to 0.20 per cent is particularly harmful to a diabetic provided the urine is sugar-free, because this is proof that he is not eating carbohydrate uselessly. Acidosis with dehydration may well be an etiological factor in the arteriosclerosis of diabetics, if its action extends over a long period. Prior to insulin the patient with acidosis died too soon to disclose the effect acidosis would produce, but now we are forced to look elsewhere than in diabetes for information.

The acidosis in diabetes may not be exclusively of the ketogenic type, but may in part be related to the diet. Such a disturbance of the acid-base balance, as occurs with heavy protein and other diets, may lead to the development of arteriosclerosis as has been emphasized by workers in the Potter Memorial Clinic in Santa Barbara.[1] Does an excess of fat in the diet lead to arteriosclerosis? The imbibition theory of arteriosclerosis enunciated by Virchow and reaffirmed and amplified by Aschoff[2] and others fits the diabetic situation. Virchow found fat in the intima of the larger arteries and concluded that the fat in the form of cholesterol esters was deposited there by imbibition from the blood stream and that the more fat in the blood the more readily it would be deposited. In the later stages calcium salts would be linked with the cholesterol[3] in the lower layers of the intima and calcified arteries would result. We believe the chief cause of premature development of arteriosclerosis in diabetes, save for advancing age, is an excess of fat in the body (obesity), in the diet, and in the blood due to lack of control of the diabetes. With an excess of fat diabetes often begins and from an excess of fat diabetics die, formerly of coma, recently of arteriosclerosis.

[1] Nuzum, Osborne and Sansum: Arch. Int. Med., 35, 492, 1925. Sansum, Blatherwick and Bowden: Jour. Am. Med. Assn., 86, 178, 1926. Nuzum, Segal, Garland and Osborne: Arch. Int. Med., 37, 733, 1926.
[2] Aschoff: Lectures on Pathology, New York, Paul B. Hoeber. Inc.. 1924.
[3] Westphal and Blum: Deutsch. Arch. f. klin. Med., 152, 331, 1926.

3. **Blood Fat and Cholesterol.**—The fat in the blood tends to be above normal when the diabetes is not under good control. The percentage of fat rises with the severity of the disease,[1] varies particularly, although less than formerly supposed, with the extent of the acidosis and is especially related to the quantity of carbohydrate which is being oxidized, rather than to the fat administered. The larger amount of carbohydrate prescribed of late, together with its better utilization and also quite probably the influence of insulin on the fat metabolism would appear to explain the recent reports upon our cases. For a discussion of fat in blood, see page 170.

Cholesterol, one of the substances always associated with blood fat, is also generally increased in the blood when the diabetes is uncontrolled. Labbé and Heitz[2] found the cholesterol increased in the blood of 18 diabetics and 27 patients with endarteritis obliterans, and attributed a close connection between the cholesterol and the arterial disease. Analyses of aortæ of 25 diabetics and 25 non-diabetics at the Deaconess Hospital by Lehnherr[3] showed greater deposits of cholesterol, total lipid and calcium in the diabetics than in non-diabetics of comparable ages.

When Himsworth[4] produced fatty deposits in the aortæ of rabbits by feeding cholesterol, he tried the effect of choline in preventing the changes. Fat deposits in the liver were reduced, but the arteries were unaffected. In this connection the occurrence of angina pectoris in hereditary xanthomatosis is important. Müller[5] states that as early as 1873 Fagge described a case of xanthomatosis with cardiovascular symptoms. His own experience concerns 17 families, including the histories of 76 persons, 32 men and 44 women. He examined 33 of these persons, ages varying from thirty-one to eighty-five years. They were office workers for the most part. Sixty-eight of the 76 appeared to have had heart disease while 8 had had xanthelasma. In the 68 persons angina pectoris was diagnosed in 59 of whom 38 had died, 14 dying suddenly. In 11 cases signs of cardiac infarction were found. In the 17 families xanthoma tuberosum was noted alone or combined with xanthelasma in 8 families. In 6 families there were records of xanthelasma only. In 37 patients the cholesterol of the blood was estimated and the amount varied from 129 to 560 mg. per 100 cc. In all except 2 cases hypercholesteremia was found. He concludes that these cases confirm the observation on xanthomatosis as a cause of hereditary heart disease. They reveal further that the syndrome of xan-

[1] Gray: Am. Jour. Med. Sci., **168**, 35, 1924. Blix: Studies on Diabetic Lipemia, Lund, p. 125, 1925. Rabinowitch: Ann. Int. Med., **8**, 1436, 1935. Muller: Am. J. Digest. Dis., **12**, 355, 1945.
[2] Labbé and Heitz: Ann. d. med., **18**, 108, 1925.
[3] Lehnherr: New England Jour. Med., **208**, 1307, 1933.
[4] Himsworth: Acta med. Scandin. Supp. 90, p. 158, 1939.
[5] Müller: Arch. Int. Med., **64**, 675, 1939.

thomatosis, hypercholesteremia and angina pectoris presents itself as a definite clinical disease in the 1st, 2d, 3d and 4th generations; that it is a dominant, hereditary disease. In his group not all the cases were due to this condition of xanthomatosis, but it is remarkable how rare were the usual causes of heart disease, rheumatic fever, syphilis and high blood-pressure. Actually in this series only one case had cerebral hemorrhage.

Leary[1] has produced typical coronary atherosclerosis in rabbits by feeding cholesterol and regards it as a specific disorder of the cholesterol metabolism. Page and Bernhard[2] found that this could be prevented if the rabbits were given an organic iodine compound at the same time. Lipemia developed in both groups of rabbits, but lipemia was more marked in the cases that received the iodine. It is evident, therefore, that in addition to lipemia and blood-pressure a third factor must influence the receptivity of tissues to the deposition of fat in their walls. Thus, this individual factor in the tissues of the arterial walls themselves may account for the fact that atherosclerosis develops under some circumstances with very little excessive lipemia whereas in other individuals marked lipemia may lead to comparatively little change.[3]

Gibbs, Buckner, and Bloor[4] studied the cholesterol and the cholesterol-cholesterol-ester ratio in the plasma of diabetics with advanced arteriosclerosis. In normal persons they found the cholesterol ester to be on the average 60 to 65 per cent of the total. In diabetic patients with arteriosclerosis, on the other hand, percentages were 72 in one group and 75 in another. In their group the total amount of cholesterol was about normal in the arteriosclerotic diabetics. They comment on the work of Schönheimer[5] who found that the ester content of calcified arteries was as high as in the uncalcified and therefore denied that esters change to calcium salts. Warren[6] suggested that fluctuation of the sugar concentration, which occurs rapidly in the blood of diabetic patients, might disturb the osmotic pressure relationship and tend to increase the permeability of the lining of the artery. Rabinowitch points to the changes in colloidal pressure due to diabetic glycemia. This would result in an increased hydrostatic pressure which in a long period of time might affect the intima of the artery. We have, therefore, in the metabolism of the diabetic many facts consistent with Virchow's theory and Aschoff's elucidation of it.

[1] Leary: Loc. cit., p. 218.
[2] Page and Bernhard: Arch. Path., **19**, 530, 1935.
[3] See also: Fenz and Zell: Klin. Woch., ii, 1133–1143, 1936; Lande and Sperry. Arch. Path., **22**, 301, 1936; Jobling and Meeker: Arch. Path., **22**, 293, 1936; Keston, Meeker and Jobling: Proc. Soc. Exp. Biol. Med., **34**, 818 1936; Duff: Arch. Path., **22**, 161, 1936.
[4] Gibbs, Buckner and Bloor: New England Jour. Med., **209**, 384, 1933.
[5] Schönheimer: Ztschr. f. phys. Chem., **160**, 61, 1926.
[6] Warren: P. 140: loc. cit., p. 196.

Rabinowitch,[1] and later Gordonoff[2] emphasize the relation of irradiated ergosterol and arteriosclerosis and Rabinowitch[3] holds that dietary treatment with diabetic control are already preventing arteriosclerosis.

C. THE PATHOLOGY OF ARTERIOSCLEROSIS.

Provided he has diabetes long enough every diabetic will die of or with arteriosclerosis, just as will any other individual. One must never forget that the most frequent years for the development of diabetes are around fifty years, a period when susceptibility to arteriosclerosis is greatest.

The first question, therefore, we as clinicians wish to ask the pathologist is: "Does this diabetic patient show more arteriosclerosis than is normal for age, sex, and weight?" This has already been answered in the affirmative. And the second question we would propose is: "Provided this diabetic shows more arteriosclerosis than is normal for his age, is it the same type of arteriosclerosis which is characteristic for his age?" In other words, is the diabetic simply prematurely old or is there anything specific about the type of arteriosclerosis which he presents? Surgically there appears to be a difference between gangrene in the diabetic and non-diabetic, and this implies a difference in the arteriosclerosis or in the tissues in which arteriosclerosis develops. It is true that advanced changes occur both in the media and intima but their occlusive character depends upon the relatively precocious and more advanced intimal atherosclerosis.

Clinically, arteriosclerosis in diabetes attacks the arteries of the heart and legs in preference to the arteries of the brain.

In 175 diabetic autopsies studied by Root and Sharkey[4] cerebral arteriosclerosis was no more frequently a cause of death than in non-diabetics, nor was sclerosis of retinal vessels more frequent in diabetics than in non-diabetics according to Waite and Beetham.[5] Apparently it is the muscular type of arteries in the heart where the effect of diabetes upon the intima is most manifest. In Table 60 an attempt is made to show the changing tendencies in the localization of arteriosclerosis causing death in 4495 diabetics. Evidently the proportion of deaths from arteriosclerosis of the kidneys and extremities is decreasing while that from the brain is stationary and from the heart is increasing. This decrease in the percentage of deaths from arteriosclerosis in the legs is the first hopeful sign in the whole diabetic arteriosclerotic situation.

[1] Rabinowitch: Canad. Med. Assn. Jour., **28**, 162, 1933.
[2] Gordonoff: Progresos Clin., **42**, 721, 1934.
[3] Rabinowitch: Canad. Med. Assn. Jour., **51**, 300, 1944.
[4] Root and Sharkey: New England Jour. Med., **215**, 605, 1936.
[5] Waite and Beetham: New England Jour. Med., **212**, 367, 1935.

TABLE 60.—LOCALIZATION OF TERMINAL LESION IN 4495 DIABETIC DEATHS
DUE TO ARTERIOSCLEROSIS.[1]

Per cent of all deaths.

Site of terminal lesion.	Naunyn era.	Allen era.	Early Banting era.	Late Banting era.	Hagedorn era.	Charles H. Best era.
Brain	18	22	20	18	22	22
Kidneys	18	15	9	8	6	7
Heart	35	40	49	57	60	64
Peripheral gangrene	21	17	19	13	8	4
Unassigned site	9	6	3	4	4	3
Number of deaths	57	203	672	1474	1655	434

D. THE PREVENTION OF ARTERIOSCLEROSIS IN DIABETES.

With physiological overstrain as a cause of arteriosclerosis the diabetic at present is not concerned. He has too little rather than too much physiological strain save that which may result from obesity and hypertension.

But with the second factor, an excess of cholesterol in the blood due to imperfect control of his diabetes, he has the greatest concern. Yet the diabetic must use fat. How much is it safe for him to take to prevent arteriosclerosis? First of all, the quantity must be so low that body weight eventually will be kept normal or a trifle below normal.

As yet we do not favor complete exclusion of foods rich in cholesterol from the diet of the diabetic, although we do limit eggs to 1 daily in patients over fifty years of age. Cholesterol is too valuable a compound of the body to be treated in this cavalier fashion. Cholesterol exists in nearly every cell of the body and this cannot be without cause. It appears to protect against infections. We are going far enough in our present imperfect knowledge of the subject if we provide for the complete oxidation of fat.

E. THE TREATMENT OF ARTERIOSCLEROSIS AND DIABETES.

If a diabetic has known enough to live ten years, be sure you know enough to make him live another ten years before you tamper with his diet. The arteries of the young diabetic are elastic and his diabetes is so pliable and amenable to all types of treatment that you can toss him about in your diabetic salon like a rubber doll. Not so the old diabetic. His arteries are thickened and sometimes hard and his status must be changed as delicately as you would move a choice piece of bric-a-brac. A sudden lowering of the blood-sugar level even to values still above normal might work disastrously to a heart accustomed for years to work on a much higher blood-sugar plane. Therefore, with diabetic patients having angina pectoris be extremely cautious.

[1] Deaths recorded up to May 15, 1946, and tabulated by the Statistical Bureau of the Metropolitan Life Insurance Company.

If the blood sugar is increased as a compensatory phenomenon in arteriosclerosis, it would be important, because in the arteriosclerosis of the legs and in other parts of the body it would hold as well as for the heart. We are not at all sure about this but we are positive that a high blood sugar in a chronic sclerotic should not be lowered suddenly. One must not think of hyperglycemia merely from the diabetic standpoint, but from that of the needs of the entire body. Grote and Umber both doubt that harm can be done to the arteriosclerotic with insulin, and we hold the same opinion provided it is conservatively administered.

F. THE BLOOD PRESSURE.

Surgical treatment of hypertension by lumbodorsal sympathectomy has been employed in a few diabetic patients when other methods of treatment have clearly failed to give relief from symptoms, or to stay a malignant progression. Case 23153, aged forty-five, with diabetes of eight years' duration, had persistent severe headaches unrelieved by medication or diet. Her blood pressure was systolic 210, diastolic 120. She was prepared for operation by a diet providing 600 calories daily which enabled her to lose 50 pounds, and bilateral sympathectomy was carried out by Dr. James Poppen. Relief from the headaches was prompt and has persisted. Her diabetes improved remarkably so that her insulin requirement which had formerly been 70 to 90 units a day, was only 10 units daily at discharge. If the operation is to be carried out on young diabetic patients, it must be done before serious degenerative changes have occurred. Case 6346 entered at the age of twenty-eight years with diabetes of sixteen years' duration, with hypertension and albuminuria, and diabetic retinitis which had been observed to increase during the last three years. His condition seemed doomed to deteriorate. Following sympathectomy he did not regain consciousness and during the next few days developed gangrene of one foot, and died with coronary occlusion. Another of our juvenile patients, Case 5000, was operated upon at another hospital and similarly failed to recover. A third young man, Case 8405, died of shock following splanchnicectomy.

These patients taught us that if sympathectomy is to have benefit in the young group of diabetic patients, it must be performed at an earlier stage. Probably it should be performed before elevation of the diastolic and systolic pressure is constant throughout the twenty-four hours, when a good fall of blood-pressure is obtained after the administration of three hourly doses of sodium amytal and not many months after albuminuria develops and retinal hemorrhages begin. Certainly impairment of renal function indicated by nitrogen retention, congestive heart failure, or angina pectoris should be a contraindication in diabetics. Probably the operation should not

32

be attempted in diabetics past the age of forty-five years who have had diabetes more than five years. Nevertheless, in patients selected carefully, the operation may relieve the symptoms. Lumbar sympathectomy carried out for the relief of vascular spasm in the lower extremities as in the case of Case 17451 was successful.

The importance of the blood-pressure in diabetes lies in its prognostic significance with respect to complications, and the possibility that hypertension is due to a pituitary, adrenal or pluriglandular syndrome. The valuable study of 10,883 persons by Robinson and Brucer[1] indicated that the normal range for systolic blood-pressure is from 90 to 120 millimeters of mercury. The pressure should not rise with age normally. All the cardiovascular complications multiply in the diabetics with hypertension. Among 175 diabetics examined at autopsy a systolic blood-pressure from 150 millimeters to 230 millimeters had been present in 54 per cent. Both gangrene and coronary thrombosis were three times as frequent among patients with hypertension as among those with normal blood-pressure. Major,[2] in an important comparison of the blood-pressure in diabetics with non-diabetics, brings out the point that the systolic blood-pressure was slightly higher in every diabetic patient than in patients in a dispensary hospital series and considerably higher than the blood-pressure in normal persons in the same age group. The blood-pressure in diabetes is slightly below normal until the age of thirty-five years is reached; it then changes to slightly above normal and the interval between diabetic and normal widens as age advances. The above statements are based upon data secured from diabetics since April 1, 1919. Previously, the blood-pressure of diabetics was a trifle higher.

In autopsies at the Deaconess Hospital not only were the larger arteries involved but the arterioles were sclerotic, chiefly in cases with hypertension but also in cases without hypertension. In general, the impression gained from 175 autopsies was that the hypertension was usually secondary to tissue changes involving arterioles as well as arteries. Grote,[3] in discussing Kylin's suggestion that hypertension in diabetes is really due to overfunction of the anterior lobe of the pituitary and, therefore, often associated with insulin resistance, opposes Kylin on the ground that diabetics with hypertension do not show any consistent resistance to insulin. Furthermore, the most resistant cases do not have hypertension.

An adrenal effect upon the blood-pressure is shown by Pijoan,[4] who gave 15 units of insulin intravenously and read the blood sugars and blood-pressures thereafter for ninety minutes in both animals and human beings. In 25 individuals the blood sugar dropped 30 mg. without any change in blood-pressure. Then there occurred

[1] Robinson and Brucer: Arch. Int. Med., **64**, 409, 1939.
[2] Major: Arch. Int. Med., **44**, 797, 1929.
[3] Grote: Deutsch. med. Wchnschr., **61**, 41, 84, 1935.
[4] Pijoan: Proc. Soc. Exp. Biol. and Med., **34**, 37, 1936.

a sharp rise in blood-pressure averaging 40 millimeters of mercury systolic and 10 millimeters diastolic. At this time the blood sugar also rose 30 and 46 mg. In 20 cases of hypertension the same thing occurred only in more striking fashion. Animals from whom the adrenal glands had been removed did not show any changes in blood-pressure. In the Cushing syndrome, mild diabetes, obesity, amenorrhea, osteoporosis, and susceptibility to infection are associated with hypertension. Raab[1] draws an analogy between these symptoms and those characteristic of old age and diabetes. Case 27509, age seventy-six years, presented hirsutism, obesity, hypertension, diabetes and coronary infarction which caused her death. At autopsy the kidneys were granular and contracted, but she also had a cortical adenoma in one adrenal.

Explanations of high blood-pressure in diabetes mellitus on the grounds of disturbances in the relations between cholesterol and the hydrophilic colloids of the plasma are offered by Rabinowitch[2] and by Alvarez and Neuschlosz.[3] The ability to keep cholesterol in solution is dependent upon the presence in the plasma of a sufficient concentration of a hydrophilic albumin and lecithin colloid. A plasma may be supersaturated with cholesterol when the cholesterol amount is not increased, depending on changes in the amount of albumin in the serum. Alvarez and Neuschlosz found in nearly all cases with hypertension that supersaturation exists.

A chronic and slowly progressive pyelonephritis was found commonly in the women studied thoroughly by Bowen and Kutzman.[4] Bacteria isolated from the urine included streptococcus hemolyticus, colon bacillus, staphylococcus and other organisms. It must be sought not only in women but in male diabetic patients when hypertension and albuminuria are found, particularly if associated with retinal changes.

Changes in blood pressure in 482 diabetics under observation for ten years were slight in 220 cases. The systolic pressure rose more than 10 mm. Hg. in 244 cases. In this series, cases of hypertension of severe type and short duration of life were excluded. Three hundred and fifty-eight cases in this series were over forty years of age. The mere fact that so many diabetics were alive at the end of ten years indicates mildness both of diabetes and hypertension. At each decade the group with hypertension increased. The blood-pressure often falls below 90 mm. Hg systolic in coma and conversely rises during an insulin reastion. (See pp. 393, 436, 451 and 462.)

A series of 100 diabetics followed for ten years received in 1939 an average diet of carbohydrate 162 grams, protein 73 grams and

1 Raab: Wien. Klin. Wchnschr., 49, 112, 1936.
2 Rabinowitch: Arch. Int. Med., 46, 752, 1930.
3 Alvarez and Neuschlosz: Klin. Wchnschr., 10, 244, 1931.
4 Bowen and Kutzman: Ann. Int. Med., 17, 3, 1942.

fat 82 grams. Richardson, Bowie, Edeiken, Leopold and Naide[1] report that in 45 of these patients the diabetes did not increase in severity nor did the diabetes appear to influence the development of hypertension. Cardiac enlargement in the hypertensive group occurred only half as frequently as in a non-diabetic hypertensive group.

G. NEPHRITIS AND DIABETES.

Intercapillary Glomerulosclerosis.—For years occasional young diabetic patients have been observed with albuminuria, nephrotic edema, hypertension, renal insufficiency and retinopathy. They were usually regarded as suffering from an independent renal or vascular disease. In 1936, Kimmelstiehl and Wilson[2] described lesions of the glomeruli of the kidneys of diabetic patients who had presented symptoms just mentioned and applied the term intercapillary glomerulosclerosis to these patients. The condition is illustrated in Case 10578, a schoolgirl, aged nineteen years at the onset of diabetes in September, 1928. She had scarlet fever at the age of five years and albuminuria had been present off and on in frequent tests ever since. On October 30, 1931 the urine contained a large trace of albumin. The blood-pressure was 148/84. She was then taking 35 units of insulin a day, the phthalein excretion was 40 per cent in two hours, and the specific gravity of the urine varied between 1.015 and 1.029. The plasma cholesterol was 238 mg. In November, 1932 edema was noted. At this time the plasma cholesterol was 490 mg. and the serum protein 4.7 per cent. The basal metabolism was minus 8 per cent on one occasion and minus 1 per cent on another after a period during which she had received thyroid extract in small amounts. Her weight, which had been 122 pounds, increased to 140 pounds with edema, but it was possible to reduce it 8 pounds by using a diet containing 95 grams of protein daily. The highest plasma cholesterol values varied between 510 and 538 mg. in May, 1933. Death occurred from uremia October 16, 1933. At autopsy the anatomical diagnoses included nephrosis, lipoid histiocytosis of spleen, liver and bone marrow, atheromatous and hyaline arteriosclerosis. Glomeruli of the kidney showed deposits of hyaline material particularly in the central portion, and no normal glomeruli were seen. Some proliferation of the capsular epithelium was present, at times showing definite crescents. Since 1939 the lesion has frequently been noted in our cases. In 40 cases under forty years of age, the typical lesions occurred in 13 cases. (See page 217.) In 50 cases from forty to seventy-five years the typical advanced renal lesions occurred in 8 cases, and in 20 cases slight increase in the axial connective tissue of the glomerular tuft was seen. This change corresponds to Laipply's Grade I lesion.[3]

[1] Richardson, Bowie, Edeiken, Leopold and Naide: Loc. cit., p. 484.
[2] Kimmelstiehl and Wilson: Am. Jour. Path., 12, 83–98, 1936.
[3] Laipply, Eitzen and Dutra: Loc. cit., p. 217.

In the 8 cases reported by Kimmelstiehl and Wilson[1] the striking pathological features were the completely hyalinized condition of many glomeruli and the limitation of the hyalin to the centers of glomeruli or individual lobules in others. Spherical or diffuse hyalin masses lie apparently between the capillaries of the glomerular tufts. A high degree of arteriosclerosis with fatty degeneration of the arterioles was present. In the capsules deposits of hyaline material and lipoid occurred beneath the epithelium. Newburger and Peters[2] report 4 similar cases studied at autopsy with 5 additional cases in which the clinical features were characteristic but no autopsy was done. Their patients presented many of the features of malignant hypertension with marked eye-ground changes. In our case, 10578, in addition to an arcus juvenilis, Dr. W. P. Beetham found marked retinitis with large areas of cotton-wool exudate and many hemorrhages but no choking of the discs. In general the diabetes in the patients of Newburger and Peters was quite mild, whereas in our case the diabetes was of the typical juvenile type. Anson[3] studied the kidneys in 900 autopsies at the Hospital of the Medical College of Virginia and found 6 cases which satisfied the criteria proposed by Kimmelstiehl and Wilson. Horn and Smetana[4] reviewed all cases of diabetes and arteriolar nephrosclerosis in the files of the Presbyterian Hospital. Of 144 patients with diabetes, 22.0 per cent showed intercapillary glomerulosclerosis. Of 126 instances of arteriolar nephrosclerosis without diabetes, 25.4 per cent showed the glomerular lesion. They stated the advanced glomerular lesions occurred only in the diabetics. Goodof,[5] in a review of 214 diabetic autopsies found the lesion in 44 per cent of cases with the condition present rather more frequently in women than in men. Thirty per cent of non-diabetic individuals over seventy years of age have mild lesions of intercapillary glomerulosclerosis. He found advanced lesions only in diabetics.

Henderson[6] studied the renal sections from 313 patients at the Mayo Clinic and found glomerular lesions of intercapillary glomerulosclerosis in 30 cases, an incidence of 9.6 per cent. In an additional 31 cases, diffuse lesions were found which probably represented the early lesion. In 2022 routine autopsies, they found 81 cases of glomerulonephritis in which the lesion occurred in 3.6 per cent. Derow, Altschule and Schlesinger[7] describe a forty-six year old male, diabetic, showing also not only the sclerosis and deposition of hyalin in the central portion of the glomeruli, but also doubly refractile bodies in the renal tubular epithelium. Clinical criteria

[1] Kimmelstiehl and Wilson:: Loc. cit., p. 500.
[2] Newburger and Peters: Arch. Int. Med., **64**, 1252, 1939.
[3] Anson: South. Med. Jour., **31**, 1272, 1938.
[4] Horn and Smetanna: Loc. cit., p. 218.
[5] Goodof: Ann. Int. Med., **22**, 373, 1945.
[6] Henderson: Thesis, Graduate School, Univ. of Minnesota, Marcy, 1944.
[7] Derow, Altschule and Schlesinger: New England Jour. Med., **221**, 1012, 1939.

for recognizing the condition during life are not as yet definite. Evidently the lesion is not peculiar to diabetes. It has been found in subacute bacterial endocarditis. Sclerosis in the pre-glomerular arterioles may be an important feature in the lesion. It may be ranked with retinopathy and neuropathy as more or less specific degenerative complications of diabetes.

Chronic Nephritis.—At autopsy vascular nephritis in early stages is common among diabetics. Warren[1] records in 454 diabetic autopsies, 69 with slight, 51 with moderate and 13 with severe arteriosclerotic lesions in the kidneys. In a comparison of 193 diabetic and 2250 non-diabetic autopsies, Lisa, Magiday, Galloway and Hart[2] found the incidence of renal arteriosclerosis compatible with hypertension more frequent in the diabetics in each decade. In the past the lesions in other arteries have seemed to progress to an advanced stage more rapidly and death has been ascribed to coronary disease, gangrene or cerebral hemorrhage. In recent years, as the number of patients with diabetes of long duration has increased, the frequency of albuminuria, hypertension and chronic nephritis has forced itself upon us, especially in the young. Four cases[3] in young patients with retinal changes producing severe loss of vision impressed upon us all the fact that these patients have not followed diabetic dietary instructions. This is even more striking in the series of 110 patients with retinitis proliferans, (see page 614) in whom chronic nephritis and coronary disease have taken a heavy toll.

Various forms of nephritis are seen in diabetes. Acute glomerulonephritis has been uncommon, although Case 20187 with diabetes of six years' duration, developed at the age of thirty-one years, acute glomerulonephritis with an elevation of blood-pressure, bilateral choked discs, and almost complete blindness from which he made an excellent recovery in June, 1944. He has been well with freedom from albuminuria and with normal blood-pressure and normal eye grounds until August, 1946, with the exception of one period when, during acute grippe he had albuminuria, and hematuria for a period of ten days. Chronic glomerulonephritis is most commonly seen among diabetic patients with edema and often in a nephrotic phase. Hypertension may or may not be present. Albuminuria is marked, often the concentrating power of the kidneys is not greatly reduced, and the phenolphthalein excretion may not be greatly reduced. In addition to bed rest and moderate restriction of fluids and salt intake, injection of acacia solution has been employed in those patients where a great reduction in plasma protein and a reversal of the albumin globulin ratio is present. In Case 7795, age thirty

---

[1] Warren: P. 130, loc. cit., p. 196.
[2] Lisa, Magiday, Galloway and Hart: Loc. cit., p. 483.
[3] Joslin: Med. Clin. North America, 28, 1054, 1944.

years, with diabetes of fifteen years' duration, a loss of 16 pounds, of edema, was accomplished by means of intravenous injections of acacia solution which has persisted for a year and a half, although it is true that in January, 1946 the control of her edema required spending much time off her feet. Digitalis has seemed at times to be helpful and potassium nitrate, 8 grams, daily, has been continued in her case as with others. In Case 21916, age forty-one years, with chronic glomerulonephritis, and the nephrotic syndrome, the administration of 30 grams of acacia in 400 cc. of distilled water was followed some hours later by a severe attack of asthma. The edema was relieved, but no more acacia could be given. A similar reaction occurred in Case 9822, age twenty-six years, with diabetes of sixteen years' duration, although her edema was improved in spite of the severe reaction with acacia. Subsequently she was given an intravenous injection of human albumin solution in salt-free form, and had remained free from edema since November, 1945, until February, 1946. Unfortunately the nephrotic state in the young diabetic of long duration is frequently followed within a period of months or years by the terminal phase with hypertension, nitrogen retention and uremia. Case 7695, with diabetes since the age of sixteen years, had had repeated acidosis. Albuminuria appeared at the age of twenty-six years. During the nephrotic phase with edema and low serum protein, transfusions were used. During the last few months of her life, uremia was established and she finally died on July 11, 1943, age thirty-two years, with a terminal coronary occlusion. At autopsy generalized arteriosclerosis as well as chronic glomerulonephritis combined with vascular nephritis were found. Pure nephrosis with complete recovery has not been seen in our diabetic patients.

Plasma transfusions and intravenous injection of salt-poor albumin solution have been used in the nephrotic stage. Pulmonary edema must be avoided by caution to limit the frequency and speed of injections.

Typical nephrosclerosis associated with hypertension occurs in diabetic patients somewhat less frequently but is not uncommon. Case 26007, age fifty-nine, with diabetes of twenty years' duration, came for her first examination because of severe dyspnea. Although the dyspnea was extreme, she was not drowsy. The urine contained no acetone. The blood sugar was 1000 mg. and the blood CO_2 was 15 volumes per cent, a typical illustration of nephritic acidosis. The non-protein nitrogen was 113 mg. At death on February 16, 1945, the autopsy showed markedly contracted kidneys with extreme arteriolar nephrosclerosis.

H. HEART DISEASE AND DIABETES.

Arteriosclerotic heart disease has become the captain of the men of death among diabetic patients. The change is comparable to the changing death-rate from heart disease in the general population. Thus the death-rate for diseases of the heart in the Registration Area of continental United States rose from 159.1 in 1920 to 318.3 in 1943.[1] The proportion of cardiac deaths to total deaths among diabetics in the Charles H. Best era (44.5 per cent) was seven times that of the Naunyn era (6.1 per cent), indicating the greater age at death due to prolongation of life. (See Table 26.) In 1931 Root and Graybiel[2] were able to collect 210 cases of angina pectoris in 7000 cases of diabetes, but the frequency of coronary arteriosclerosis has greatly increased as other causes of death have diminished. In a comparison of atherosclerotic lesions in the coronary arteries of 349 diabetic patients and 3400 non-diabetic patients at autopsy by sex and decade of age, Root, Bland, Gordon and White[3] found coronary occlusion five times as frequent in the diabetic group. In 110 autopsies at the Deaconess Hospital between 1940 and 1946, coronary arteriosclerosis was noted in 108 cases by Millard and Root.[4] Granting the increasing longevity of diabetic patients, the increase in cardiac disease is greater than can be explained by age alone.

The influence of hypertension is definite since the frequency of both coronary disease and gangrene is more than twice as great among diabetics with hypertension than with normal blood-pressure. In contrast to arteriosclerosis other types of cardiac disease are rare. Congenital heart lesions have occurred in babies of diabetic mothers (see page 774). Dextrocardia with complete situs inversus and angina pectoris radiating to the right arm were observed in Case 13976. Patent interventricular septum was present in Case 19323. The coincidence of hyperthyroidism has accounted for occasional cases of auricular fibrillation in diabetics. Degenerative changes in the myocardium not dependent on coronary disease have been noted by a number of writers. Nathanson[5] described the pale, swollen and cloudy heart muscle as present in nearly every case of acidosis and coma. These changes may well be merely accompaniments of dehydration. Certainly young coma patients without vascular disease show no clinical evidence of myocardial weakness.

1. **Physiology.**—The metabolism of the mammalian heart has been the object of many experimental studies. Blood pyruvate studies, already reported by Yanof[6] in non-diabetic subjects, would be of especial value in diabetics, because this intermediate in carbohydrate metabolism is so greatly influenced by insulin (see page 118). Cruickshank and Stratup[7] found that the normal isolated heart has a respiratory quotient of unity with an adequate supply of

[1] Vital Statistics—Special Reports, Department of Commerce, Washington, D. C.. **21**, No. 8, 149, 1945.
[2] Root and Graybiel: Jour. Am. Med. Assn., **96**, 925, 1931.
[3] Root, Bland, Gordon and White: Jour. Am. Med. Assn., **113**, 27, 1939.
[4] Millard and Root: To be published.
[5] Nathanson: Loc. cit., p. 483.
[6] Yanof: Arch. Int. Med., **69**, 1005, 1942.
[7] Cruickshank and Stratup: Jour. Phys., **77**, 365, 1933.

blood sugar. Upon adding sugar the oxygen consumption rises and the administration of insulin causes a further, increase. When the blood sugar falls to 0.05 per cent, a certain amount of glycogen is used. If insulin is added in hypoglycemia, a synthesis of glycogen results. If hypoglycemia is prolonged and extreme, the respiratory quotient falls, indicating the utilization of non-carbohydrate sources of energy. The characteristic action of insulin, therefore, is to stimulate synthesis of glycogen in the heart. Actually the heart can function when the blood supplied is free from sugar according to Griffith and Waters (personal communication of unpublished results). Working in the Laboratory of Physiology of Toronto University they found that under these circumstances, the lactic acid removed from the blood was negligible if the concentration of lactic acid was about 10 mg. per 100 cc. of blood. No fat was removed from the blood.

Waters, Fletcher and Mirsky[1] studied the utilization of ketone bodies by the heart-lung preparation in order to determine whether there is a fixed ketolytic ratio. They found when the heart-lung preparation was perfused with blood containing various concentrations of glucose and ketone bodies that there was no reason to support the hypothesis that oxidation of ketones depends upon the simultaneous oxidation of carbohydrate, that is, there was no positive correlation between the sugar and ketone body utilization. The heart therefore was dependent upon its own stores. Cruickshank[2] states that diabetic heart muscle invariably shows an increase in glycogen content. Starvation makes little change in cardiac glycogen. As the blood sugar falls the heart quickly resorts to other sources for its energy. In the depancreatized dog, the addition of insulin causes a rapid rise in the respiratory quotient of the heart toward unity. In diabetic animals, less glucose is utilized than by the normal heart, according to von Pomothy[3] and Evans, Grande, Hsu, Lee and Mulder.[4] However, the almost unimpaired utilization of lactate by the hearts of diabetic dogs demonstrated by Evans et al. compensates for this deficiency. Insulin greatly increased the glucose utilization. The fact that the diabetic heart can remove glucose from the blood was also demonstrated by Himwich, Goldfarb and Fazikas.[5] Pollock et al.[6] found that the avoidance of anoxemia and the giving of glucose increased the content of creatin phosphate in the dog's heart, thus affording an explanation of the therapeutic value of glucose and oxygen in cardiac disease. Geiger and Hambourger[7] in experimental studies found the rabbit heart unimproved by using glucose solution of greater concentration than 0.1 per cent.

[1] Waters, Fletcher and Mirsky: Am. Jour. Physiol., 122, 542, 1938.
[2] Cruickshank: Phys. Rev., 16, 597, 1936.
[3] von Pomothy: Biochem. Ztschr., 275, 448, 1935.
[4] Evans, Grande, Hsu, Lee, and Mulder: Quart. Jour. Exp. Phys., 24, 365, 1935.
[5] Himwich, Goldfarb. and Fazikas: Am. Jour. Phys., 114, 273, 1936.
[6] Pollock, Flock, Essex, and Bollman: Proc. Staff Meet. Mayo Clinic, 8, 521, 1933.
[7] Geiger and Hambourger: Am. Heart Jour., 16, 261, 1938.

Liebig[1] found in animals marked increase in glycogen of the heart muscle following a single injection of insulin. Intravenous dextrose injections caused mobilization of glycogen in heart, liver and skeletal muscle with diminution of total carbohydrate in all three. Ellis and Faulkner[2] concluded that an injection of a liter of 5 per cent dextrose solution given slowly would produce less train on the cardiovascular circulation than intravenous injection of 100 cc. of 50 per cent dextrose solution at the rate of 10 cc. per minute.

In experimental coronary occlusion, Himwich, Goldfarb and Nahum[3] noted a loss of glycogen from infarcted areas and an outpouring of lactic acid into the blood stream. Their data indicate also that in diabetic patients with coronary occlusion the use of insulin and glucose may be of great value. It is an incontrovertible fact in our experience that patients with incompetent hearts have been benefited with the use of insulin. Never have we seen any reason to withhold it in reasonable doses. Knowing the effect of hypoglycemia in calling forth adrenalin, we always take great precautions to change diets slowly and to begin insulin in very small doses in diabetics susceptible to cardiac complications.

2. **Angina Pectoris and Coronary Arteriosclerosis.—Incidence.** —The occurrence of 410 cases of angina among 10,000 cases of diabetes gives a conservative idea of its frequency for the reason that among the 10,000 patients were many cases in whom the duration of diabetes was too short to give full opportunity for its effect upon the coronary vessels to become manifest. Furthermore, cases with sudden cardiac death without known antecedent cardiac pain have not been included. This frequency, exceeding so markedly the incidence of angina in a general hospital population, is the first indication of the specific influence of diabetes.

From 1940 to 1945 inclusive, the total number of patients diagnosed at the New England Deaconess Hospital as having diabetes and coronary arteriosclerosis with angina pectoris or coronary occlusion was 413. This figure is to be considered in relation to the total number of diabetic admissions to the hospital in the six years, which numbered about 11,000. However, in considering this relationship, it must be noted that among the diabetic admissions to the New England Deaconess Hospital the percentage of young patients is unusually high. Thus, in the year 1941, among 1856 diabetic admissions, 404 were under twenty-four years of age and 141 were between twenty-five and thirty-four years of age.

In the six years 1940 to 1945, acute coronary occlusion occurred in 96 patients at the Deaconess Hospital. Females numbered 50 and males 46. In Table 61 this series is summarized. Forty-two

---

[1] Liebig: Ztschr. f. d. ges. exp. Med., **109**, 715, 1941.
[2] Ellis and Faulkner: Am. Heart Jour., **17**, 542, 1939.
[3] Himwich, Goldfarb and Nahum: Am. Jour. Physiol., **109**, 403, 1934.

deaths occurred in the hospital and an additional ten deaths occurred soon after discharge.

TABLE 61.—CORONARY OCCLUSION IN 96 DIABETICS, 1940–1945.

Age.	Male.	Female.	Average age, yrs.	Average duration of diabetes, yrs.	Died in hospital.	Died after discharge.
20–29	1		27	14	1	
30–39						
40–49	3	2	45	8		
50–59	10	11	54	11	7	3
60–69	20	26	65	9	20	7
70 and over . . .	12	11	75	15	14	
Total	46	50			42	10

A second suggestion of the diabetic influence is the sex distribution of the cases. In Table 62, the 1223 deaths certified from coronary occlusion or angina pectoris occurring between 1898 and May 15, 1946 are summarized to indicate the slight difference in incidence between males and females. Coronary arteriosclerosis caused 44.5 per cent of the total (651) deaths in the Charles H. Best era.

TABLE 62.—DEATHS FROM CORONARY OCCLUSION AND ANGINA PECTORIS BY SEX.

	Females.	Males.	Total.
Naunyn era, 1898–1914	3	2	5
Allen era, 1914–1922	7	10	17
Banting era, 1922–1936	226	263	489
Hagedorn era, 1937–1943	270	286	556
Charles H. Best era, 1944–1946 . . .	77	79	156
Totals	583	640	1223

The sex ratio corresponded with the almost equal distribution of diabetes between the sexes in marked contrast to the incidence of angina in non-diabetic patients. In Nathanson's series of 100 diabetic autopsies the proportion of males to females with advanced coronary disease was 1.8 to 1. In 210 diabetic cases analyzed by Root and Graybiel, the proportion of males to females was 1.4 to 1. These figures contrast with the proportions given by Osler of 7 to 1 and an average proportion of 3 males to 1 female in other series of angina pectoris.[1] In Willius' series of coronary thrombosis in non-diabetics the proportion was males 7 to females 1.[2]

The average age at onset of diabetes was fifty-one years for the 210 cases analyzed by Root and Graybiel. The average age at onset for angina was sixty years. Diabetes had been present nine years before the onset of angina pectoris. In 188 cases diabetes preceded angina and in only 9 cases did the angina precede the diabetes. In 13 cases the two diseases were discovered at the same

[1] White: Heart Disease, 3d ed., New York, Macmillan Co., 1944, p. 825.
[2] Willius: Jour. Am. Med. Assn., **106**, 1890, 1936.

time. For a recent summary of the relationship between angina pectoris and coronary arteriosclerosis, see Levy[1] and Levine.[2]

That the frequency of angina pectoris in diabetes depends upon the duration of diabetes is supported by the occurrence of cases early in life among young adults with diabetes of long duration. Two cases occurred between twenty and thirty, and 4 between thirty and forty years. Three of these cases died suddenly after diabetes of 5.6 to 8 years' duration, and in 2 instances postmortem examination revealed acute coronary thrombosis. Anderson[3] reported a white male dying at the age of thirty-three years of cardiac decompensation. Diabetes had been present fourteen years. The descending branch of the left coronary artery showed marked sclerosis and the lumen was almost obliterated. There was a thrombus in the sclerotic right coronary vessel. Klingenberg[4] found 2 cases between the ages of twenty and thirty years, and in 1 autopsy showed an area of healed infarction in the left ventricle. Cullinan and Graham[5] describe a young man, aged twenty-seven years, with diabetes of eight years' duration, who died with coronary occlusion. Extensive atheromatous plaques occurred in the coronary arteries, aorta, arteries of the legs and brain. Although diabetes develops most frequently at fifty-one years, diabetic angina occurs most frequently in the decade where ten-year cases of diabetes are most common; namely, the seventh decade. P. D. White's[6] series shows the greatest frequency of onset of non-diabetic angina in the sixth decade. The later development of angina in diabetes seems to depend upon the fact that an exposure to diabetes of several years' duration is an important factor in the etiology. The frequency of angina pectoris trebles in the second ten years of diabetes. The susceptibility of the arteries later in life to the development of arteriosclerosis under the influence of a metabolic disorder is greater than in the earlier decades of life.

Heredity.—Among 210 cases of diabetes with angina,[7] 26 patients gave a family history of both diabetes and vascular disease; 47 patients of diabetes without vascular disease, making a total of 73 with diabetic heredity. Ninety-nine patients had a history of vascular disease in the family. If the inheritance of poor arteries were the outstanding etiological factor, one would expect more frequently the occurrence of arteriosclerotic heart disease before diabetes. Furthermore, the occurrence of hypertension before the onset of diabetes would be more frequent. As a matter of fact, the

[1] Levy: Diseases of the Coronary Arteries and Cardiac Pain, Macmillan Company, New York, pp. 119, 194, 273, 1936.
[2] Levine: Clinical Heart Disease, 3rd ed., Philadelphia, W. B. Saunders Company, 1945.
[3] Anderson: Minnesota Med., **12**, 484, 1929.
[4] Klingenberg: Norsk Mag. f. Lægevidensk., **95**, 940, 1934.
[5] Cullinan and Graham: Jour. Path. and Bacteriol., **38**. 167, 1934.
[6] White: Nelson Loose-Leaf Med., 1st ed., **4**, 502, 1926; p. 824, loc. cit., p. 507.
[7] Root and Graybiel: Loc. cit., p. 504.

figures collected by Root and Sharkey[1] indicate that among diabetic patients examined at postmortem within a year of the onset of diabetes the amount of arteriosclerosis in the aorta is rather less than it is among non-diabetic patients of similar age. On the other hand, among diabetic patients who have had the diabetes for a long period the amount of arteriosclerosis is very much in advance of non-diabetics of the same age, clearly indicating that the excessive arteriosclerosis found in diabetics takes place after the onset of the diabetes rather than before.

Hypertension.—Among 210 patients with angina 110 had a systolic blood-pressure over 150. The longer diabetic patients are observed, the more frequent is the development of hypertension among patients who originally had normal blood-pressures. Bell and Clawson[3] considered that hypertension was five times as common among diabetics as non-diabetics and Nathanson[3] in his autopsy series also found that hypertension was more frequent in diabetics than in non-diabetics. Donhoffer and Szabo,[4] in studying 420 patients with diabetes, conclude that there is no difference in the incidence of hypertension in diabetic and non-diabetic persons.

Pathogenesis.—The amount and extent of coronary arteriosclerosis in diabetic subjects examined postmortem is astonishingly great. In Table 63 are given the comparative frequencies by decade of coronary occlusion, recent or old, found in 349 diabetic and 3400 non-diabetic autopsies summarized by Root, Bland, Gordon and White.[5] Acute thrombosis with infarction of the heart was present in 21 per cent of 175 autopsies of diabetic subjects at the Deaconess Hospital.[6] Necropsy in 77 cases of diabetes reported by Blotner[7] showed marked disease of the coronary vessels in 45 per cent, while in 10 per cent death was due to cardiac infarction. Nathanson[3] found severe coronary arteriosclerosis in 41 per cent of 100 diabetic autopsies. Rupture of the heart occurred twice and aneurysmal dilatation of the wall of the left ventricle twice in the Deaconess Hospital series. This extraordinarily high incidence may be compared with the observations of Benson and Hunter,[8] in whose series of 1750 patients most of whom were coroners' cases, coronary infarction plus cardiac aneurysms formed 4 per cent of the whole. The experimental production of coronary atherosclerosis by Leary[9] should be studied in relation to diabetes. (See page 493.) The development of anastomoses following coronary thrombosis is

[1] Root and Sharkey: Loc. cit., p. 483.
[2] Bell and Clawson: Arch. Path., **5**, 939, 1928.
[3] Nathanson: Loc. cit., p. 483.
[4] Donhoffer and Szabo: Klin. Wchnschr., **17**, 1938.
[5] Root, Bland, Gordon and White: Loc. cit., p. 504.
[6] Root and Sharkey: Loc. cit., p. 495.
[7] Blotner: Loc. cit., p. 483.
[8] Benson and Hunter: Northwest Med., **24**, 606, 1925.
[9] Leary: Loc. cit., p. 218.

the rule both in diabetics and non-diabetics and has been carefully studied by Schlesinger,[1] using a method of injection followed by dissection of the vessels.

TABLE 63.—CORONARY OCCLUSION IN DIABETIC AND NON-DIABETIC PATIENTS IN PERCENTAGE OF CASES IN AGE GROUPS.[1]

	Males.				Females.			
	Diabetic.		Non-diabetic.		Diabetic.		Non-diabetic.	
Age groups.	Cases with occlusion.	Per cent of total.	Cases with occlusion.	Per cent of total.	Cases with occlusion.	Per cent of total.	Cases with occlusion.	Per cent of total.
41–50	2	15	23	7	3	11	2	1
51–60	13	33	47	10	13	25	8	3
61–70	28	48	52	11	26	40	17	7
71–80	9	41	24	11	13	43	9	10

Enklewitz[3] found coronary thrombosis in 26 of 92 diabetic cases studied at autopsy. Coronary thrombosis was twice as frequent in diabetics as in non-diabetics of both sexes.

The intima of the coronary arteries is much thicker in males than in females and this fact explains the greater frequency of coronary atherosclerosis in the male, according to Dock.[4]

Tobacco.—The effects of tobacco smoking upon the cardio-vascular system of diabetic patients are similar to those observed in non-diabetics. The existence of vasoconstriction in the peripheral blood vessels has been reported by various observers and determined by a decrease in the cutaneous temperature of the extremities, or by a decrease in the velocity of blood flow. The substances contained in tobacco smoke absorbed by the body are pyridine bases, carbon monoxide and nicotine. The amount of the first two substances is so small that it is doubtful that they can cause harmful effects. Nicotine has been regarded as the most toxic substance in tobacco smoke. The largest amount of nicotine is obtained from cigars and pipes, and the smallest from cigarettes owing to the fact that in the cigarette the combustion of the nicotine is more nearly complete. Roth[5] states that the effects of tobacco may be summarized as follows: In some persons smoking of tobacco produces pain somewhat like that of angina pectoris. In some persons a rise of blood-pressure precedes the onset of the pain. The pain produced by smoking is different from angina pectoris in its greater violence and longer duration. Furthermore, it occurs at rest. Electrocardiographic changes following smoking include tachycardia, arrhythmia, increased heart rate, lowering or inversion of the T waves, and in one case, sinoauricular block. Some evidence suggests that increased work of the heart is the cause of these changes, but the effect of

[1] Schlesinger: Am. Heart Jour., **15**, 528, 1938.
[2] Root, Bland, Gordon and White: Loc. cit., p. 504.
[3] Enklewitz: Am. Heart Jour., **5**, 386, 1934.
[4] Dock: Jour. Am. Med. Assn., **131**, 875, 1946.
[5] Roth: Modern Concepts of Cardiovascular Disease, Amer. Heart Assn., **14**, 1, 1945.

stimulating the sympathetic nerves or paralysis of the para-sympathetic nerves cannot be excluded. While coronary vasoconstriction has been regarded as a possible cause of angina pectoris, there is some evidence indicating that small amounts of tobacco or nicotine actually increase the coronary flow and that really large toxic doses are necessary to produce vasoconstriction in the heart of rabbits. Apparently the vasoconstriction of the peripheral blood vessels produced by smoking cigarettes is similar to that produced by a similar amount of nicotine injected intravenously. Weinroth and Herzstein[1] found in 301 male diabetic patients a higher incidence of thrombosed peripheral arteries in smokers than in non-smokers. The smoking of tobacco is most likely only a contributory factor in the production of cardiovascular disorders, but its relation to vasospasm and arteriosclerosis in the extremities as well as to tobacco poisoning of the optic nerve compel us to advise diabetic patients not to use tobacco.

Clinical Features.—Coronary occlusion may be regarded as a sign of underlying diabetes in many cases. Goldberger, Alesio and Woll[2] studied 14 patients with myocardial infarction by means of the Exton-Rose glucose tolerance test over a period extending up to thirteen months after the infarction. Of 11 patients tested in the first two weeks after infarction, 4 gave abnormal results. However, the findings in 5 patients who had normal values during the acute phase of the illness became progressively abnormal, finally reaching diabetic values after a period of months. During the years 1938 to 1942, Spühler[3] saw 113 cases of cardiac infarction, and in 1942 studied the carbohydrate metabolism in 38 of the patients aged from thirty to eighty-nine years. Those under fifty years showed only slight increases in sugar content of the blood and urine and in no case could definite diabetic changes be diagnosed. In older patients marked hyperglycemia and glycosuria were observed, and the blood-sugar curves in response to administration of large amounts of sugar were of diabetic type. Evidence of pancreatic damage was also shown by the raised diastase values of the urine and in a few cases by so-called pancreatic apoplexy.

The manifestations of coronary disease are varied and puzzling, as Herrick has noted.[4]

(a) Infarction of the Heart and Coma.—Acute infarction of the heart may simulate diabetic coma if unconsciousness is present with the hyperglycemia and depression of the blood CO_2 characteristic of shock in a diabetic. Case 24095, aged seventy-one years, developed severe pain in the chest on one day and was admitted to the Deaconess Hospital late at night on the day following, pulseless,

[1] Weinroth and Herzstein: Jour. Am. Med. Assn., 131, 205, 1946.
[2] Goldberger, Alesio and Woll: New York State Jour. Med., 45, 391, 1945.
[3] Spühler: Schweiz. med. Wchnschr., 73, 1458, 1943.
[3] Herrick: Ann. Int. Med., 11, 2084, 1939.

with a blood sugar of 656 mg. and blood CO_2 of 12 volumes per cent. Respiration was not characteristic of diabetic coma. Examination of the blood and urine showed no ketone bodies. At autopsy bilateral coronary occlusion was found. However, the association of infarction of the heart with severe diabetic acidosis and actual coma has occurred three times among 495 patients with coma treated at the Deaconess Hospital. Among 67 deaths subsequent to discharge after recovery from coma, seven were due to coronary thrombosis, two to coronary sclerosis, one to angina pectoris and one was probably coronary occlusion.

Medical shock, as in pneumonia, meningitis, coronary occlusion, may be responsible for extraordinary changes in the blood, especially if severe peripheral vascular failure is present. Davidson, Lewis, Tagnon, Adams and Taylor[1] show in 12 patients examples of blood-sugar values from 178 to 332 milligrams and a decline in some instances of the CO_2 of the blood to 8 to 12 milliequivalents per liter. This explains the occasional case of coronary occlusion with shock where CO_2 of the blood is at the coma level and yet the blood is free from acetone bodies.

Case 1794, aged thirty-three years, diabetes of eight years' duration, had taken insulin for nearly three years. She had gained 50 pounds. On June 4, 1925, she weighed 122 pounds and was taking 80 units of insulin. She had had slight precordial pressure and pain in the left shoulder at intervals for six weeks only. At 4 P.M. on June 8, 1925, her urine was sugar-free and blood sugar 0.11 per cent. In the absence of her nurse she broke her diet at supper and at 1 A.M. awakened with pain in the left shoulder and vomited. By noon the next day acidosis was extreme as shown by plasma CO_2 of 22 volumes per cent and blood sugar of 0.66 per cent. During the next twenty-four hours pain over the sternum, repeated vomiting, and Stokes-Adams seizures were followed by collapse and death. At autopsy coronary calcification and occlusion with infarction of the interventricular septum and the wall of the left ventricle were found.

Master, Dack and Jaffe,[2] in a study of 890 attacks of coronary artery occlusion, noted that 3 occurred during diabetic acidosis and 2 during the injection of insulin.

(b) Coronary Disease and Gall Stones.—Surgical removal of gall stones with relief of precordial pain is not rare, but more often the combination offers a serious therapeutic question. Thirty-five cases presented this combination, often a problem in diagnosis. Case 870, a clergyman, aged fifty-two years, duration of diabetes seventeen years, had had no recognizable angina. He had had a number of severe attacks of gall-stone colic. A gall-bladder filled with

---

[1] Davidson, Lewis, Tagnon, Adams and Taylor: New England Jour. Med., **234**, 279, 1946.
[2] Master, Dack and Jaffee: Am Heart Jour., **18**, 434, 1939.

stones was removed. Fourteen days after operation, he had symptoms of coronary occlusion, and died three days later. At autopsy both fresh infarctions and extensive old infarctions were found.

(c) **Angina Pectoris and Heart-block.**—Heart-block was found in a patient of Dreyfuss[1] who presented at necropsy remarkably mild arteriosclerotic changes especially in the coronary circulation. Many severe Adams-Stokes attacks had occurred, accompanied by ventricular standstill and finally by ventricular fibrillation. The unusual feature of the attacks was that they were controlled largely by good treatment of the diabetes. Only insulin and dextrose were effective in controlling seizures. Atropine, ephedrine and other drugs were of no avail. Dreyfuss considered that the condition might be designated as "nutritional heart disease." Case 20052, aged fifty-five years, with diabetes of seven years' duration, has had left bundle branch block with increasing edema of the feet. Following treatment with a liberal amount of vitamin B complex and a period of bed rest, he has remained free from edema. Cases 3569 and 4652 recovered from coronary occlusion, but auricular-ventricular block remained. Mohler[2] described a diabetic who developed heart-block during acidosis and recovered. Blaisdell's[3] diabetic patient with acute coronary thrombosis developed transient heart-block. Case 13309, male, aged forty-eight years, had had a diagnosis of duodenal ulcers five years previously. While bowling, he had sudden, severe pain in the epigastrium (not over the sternum) but also with pain in the neck and a little later pain in the left wrist. At the Deaconess Hospital four days later his chief complaint was of indigestion, discomfort in the epigastrium. However, the pulse-rate was 52 and an electrocardiogram showed complete dissociation of the auricles and ventricles, with inversion of T_1. Six days later the block was gone, although the P-R interval was 0.24 second. Deep inversion of T-waves in second and third leads developed together with a deep Q_3 during the next few days, but the P-R interval returned to 0.18 second. Incidentally, roentgen-ray examination showed no peptic ulcer. Case 12011, aged seventy-three years with diabetes of 1.7 years' duration, had attacks of dizziness as the only clue to his heart-block. The electrocardiogram showed a ventricular rate of 44. Case 9913, aged forty-seven years, had complete heart-block with congestive failure.

(d) **Coronary Sclerosis and Congestive Failure.**—Among diabetic patients congestive failure is increasingly common as the duration of life increases and other fatal diabetic complications, such as acidosis, are eliminated. With onset of congestive failure, the blood sugar often rises and the insulin used increases. But when cardiac or nephritic decompensation is established, oftentimes the

[1] Dreyfuss: Brit. Heart Jour., **7**, 128, 1945.
[2] Mohler: Jour. Am. Med. Assn., **81**, 1342, 1923.
[3] Blaisdell: Jour. Am. Med. Assn., **105**, 1518, 1935.

diabetes becomes so mild that actually the blood sugar may fall to normal and insulin may be given up. Case 16568 developed edema toward the end; her blood sugar, postmortem, was 0.02 per cent. Glycosuria may return when, under the influence of diuretics, such as salyrgan, edema disappears, as in cases described by Grote[1] and Lyon.[2] Probably variations in liver function and glyconeogenesis underlie these changes. In fact, Evans[3] has observed in animals subjected to low atmospheric pressure that an increase in the glycogen content of the liver takes place. Apparently this is a conversion of protein or fat into glycogen, in some way due to the slight degree of dyspnea present. Whenever the heart of a diabetic is acutely decompensated and dyspnea is present, usually there is an increased difficulty in controlling sugar of the blood and urine.

Auricular fibrillation occurred in 13 patients treated at the Deaconess Hospital during the three years, 1943 to 1945. It was the result of a recent acute coronary occlusion in three cases, of whom one died. A seventy-two year old male received quinidine for rapid fibrillation with acute infarction, and recovered.

(e) **Infarction of the Heart with Recovery.**—Healed infarcts were found in 31 cases at autopsy with 14 more cases showing both fresh and healed infarcts. In Case 2296 the onset of angina was obscure. He died suddenly at the age of fifty-one years and had diabetes for 21.6 years. Autopsy showed 8 separate, distinct areas of healed infarction.

(f) **Coronary Occlusion with Lowered Blood Sugar.**—Case 1520, aged seventy years, was brought to the Deaconess Hospital at midnight unconscious and rigid. Her blood sugar was 0.03 per cent. She had been given insulin three times a day elsewhere without testing the urine. She died after a few days and a fresh infarction of the heart was found in addition to several old healed infarctions.

(g) **Coronary Occlusion and Embolectomy.**—Embolism following coronary infarction is of frequent occurrence. Case 22183, aged thirty-two years, had had diabetes for thirteen years when he developed severe pain in the upper sternum nine days before admission. On the sixth day of his hospital stay an embolus lodged in the left femoral artery and was successfully removed by Dr. L. S. McKittrick. Unfortunately later pulmonary embolism resulted in death on the sixteenth day. At autopsy infarction had involved the interventricular septum as well as the left portion of the apex.

(h) **Coronary Occlusion and Other Complications.**—The increasing frequency of hypertension, albuminuria and chronic nephritis in young diabetics of long duration has been associated with frequent instances of coronary occlusion in patients less than thirty-five years of age. In Case 4746, aged thirty years, with diabetes of

1 Grote: Ztschr. f. Kreislaufforschung, **26**, 922, 1934.
2 Lyon: Gastroenterologica, **70**, 338, 1945.
3 Evans: Am. Jour. Physiol., **110**, 273, 1934.

fifteen years' duration, coronary occlusion occurred in association with intercapillary glomerulosclerosis and retinitis proliferans. In 2 patients coronary occlusion was associated with repeated vomiting of gastric contents containing old blood and actual intestinal obstruction was suspected until postmortem examination which showed bilateral coronary occlusion in 1 patient and both old and recent coronary infarction in the other.

Electrocardiogram.—Abnormalities in the electrocardiogram are frequent in diabetic patients in middle and late life and not always explainable on the basis of coronary disease. Levitt[1] studied 100 non-diabetic men and women over the age of seventy years with apparently normal hearts, who showed a surprising number of abnormalities in the electrocardiograms. Twenty-six of Levitt's 100 cases showed changes in the T-wave, prolongation of the $Q-R-S$ with or without notching or slurring, the Pardee Q_3 wave, auricular fibrillation or bundle branch block. Hegglen[2] found that in coma, insulin shock, and following large doses of insulin in the treatment of coma, electrical systole is lengthened and mechanical systole shortened. This demonstrates that electrical and mechanical events in the heart are not synchronous. Faulkner and Hamilton[3] studied 15 diabetic patients in coma at the Deaconess Hospital. Considering that in experimental animals slight changes in the pH of the blood toward the acid side caused changes in rhythm and conduction with also marked changes of the ventricular complexes, it seemed possible that in diabetic coma changes would occur. In 6 of the 15 records some abnormalities appeared such as a diphasic T-wave in one or more leads. The changes were not extensive and they concluded that in diabetic coma the only changes were minor T-wave abnormalities not likely to be confused with the picture of coronary occlusion. Transient changes in the T-waves, usually twenty-four hours after admission, were noted by Bellet and Dyer[4] in 17 patients in diabetic coma and 6 in pre-coma.

Definite changes in the electrocardiogram occurred in 60 per cent of a series of cases of angina reported by Root and Graybiel. Inversion of the T-wave in Leads I and II or the Pardee sign were present in 23 cases. Inversions of the T-wave in first and second leads or the second and third leads have had the usual grave significance. If we include cases with only inversion of the T-wave in the first lead, 20 per cent of the cases were dead within a year. Undoubtedly if electrocardiograms were obtained routinely on all patients regardless of cardiac symptoms or signs inversions of the T-waves would be found so much earlier in the clinical course of the disease that the present unfavorable prognosis would be greatly improved. Frequently changes observed during acidosis improve as the patients

[1] Levitt: Am. Heart Jour., **18**, 692, 1939.
[2] Hegglen: Cardiologia, **2**, 170, 1938.
[3] Faulkner and Hamilton: Am. Heart Jour., **8**, 691, 1933.
[4] Bellet and Dyer: Am. Heart Jour., **13**, 72, 1937.

improve under treatment and one must not be misled in attributing such changes to coronary thrombosis unless they are typical of the pattern known to represent coronary occlusion.

The common electrocardiographic evidences of occlusion, consisting of changes in the Q-wave and changes in the R–S–T complexes are occasionally not obtained or are obscured because of various reasons. Multiple areas of infarction as illustrated in Case 2296 or the presence of bundle-branch block, as in Case 13329, not infrequently have obscured the typical changes. In Case 13330 the amplitude of deflections in Leads I and II was so small that changes in the R–S–T were hardly recognizable.

In animals with insulin hypoglycemia inversions of T-waves were obtained by Costedoat and Anjaleu[1] and by Soskin, Katz and Frisch[2] which did not always revert to normal with glucose administration, according to the latter. In eviscerated animals the T-waves returned to normal when glucose was injected. Hence they concluded that insulin affects the electrocardiogram in two ways: (a) by producing hypoglycemia and (b) a specific action.

In 25 cases in childhood and youth Root[3] compared electrocardiograms taken during hyperglycemia and hypoglycemia. The changes observed in the young patients following insulin were slight and few.

Transitory characteristic changes do at times follow the administration of insulin. There is a flattening and a lowering of the T-wave, a broadening of the Q–R–S complex and appearance of a sinus arrhythmia, various extrasystoles, A–V rhythm, auricular fibrillation, and prolongation of the conduction time, according to de Chatel and Palisa.[4] One cannot definitely say whether the cause is a lack of glycogen or some injurious action of insulin. Against the glycogen theory is that rabbits, even with great doses of insulin, do not become glycogen poor. Further, the electrocardiographic changes are not relieved by the administration of grape sugar.

Their practical conclusions were: (1) that insulin does not exert on the healthy heart the anticipated harmful action which in general has been accepted; (2) even after months of induced severe hypoglycemic attacks in treatment of schizophrenia permanent changes are not observable (the experience of Goldman[5] agrees); (3) all of their observations relate exclusively to patients with completely healthy myocardia, and they cannot be considered as contradicting in any way results obtained in coronary disease after the administration of insulin, such as inversion of the T-wave observed by Schönbrunner[6] in a seventy-three-year-old diabetic woman. Under

[1] Costedoat and Anjaleu: Bull. et mém. Soc. méd. de hôp. de Paris, **48**, 876, 1932.
[2] Soskin, Katz, and Frisch: Ann. Int. Med., **8**, 900, 1935.
[3] Root: Ann. Int. Med., **11**, 1340, 1938.
[4] de Chatel and Palisa: Klin. Wchnschr., **14**, 1784, 1935.
[5] Goldman: Arch, Int. Med., **66**, 93, 1940.
[6] Schönbrunner: Klin. Wchnschr., **15**, 36, 1936.

these circumstances the adrenalin secreted under the stimulus of hypoglycemia may be expected to induce an anginal attack.

Non-diabetic glycosuria and coronary occlusion occur together. Raab and Rabinowitz[1] studied 21 patients with coronary occlusion and glycosuria. Abnormal glucose tolerance curves occurred during and immediately after the occlusion, but became normal later. They consider the possibility, suggested by Gottsegen,[2] that glycosuria during coronary thrombosis means that the patient is potentially diabetic, that during the attack vascular spasm in the pancreas causes the glycosuria, which may be temporary or permanent if irreversible changes occur in the pancreas. Raab and Rabinowitz believe that the transient glycosuria of coronary occlusion is due to a disturbance in the vegetative centers of the brain rather than to true diabetes.

Differential Diagnosis of Coronary Occlusion.—So frequent is acute coronary occlusion in diabetic patients that one is tempted to make that diagnosis with too great assurance. Thus, Case 12559, aged forty-three years, with sudden, severe, persistent substernal pain and pericardial friction, had acute purulent pericarditis rather than coronary occlusion. Case 6868, aged sixty-eight years, had previously suffered a coronary occlusion. During a court session, pain at the lower end of the sternum with collapse was recognized as due to a perforated duodenal ulcer by reason of muscle spasm and obliteration of liver dullness. In a woman with known pulmonary tuberculosis severe pain across the sternum was due to the rupture of an adhesion and spontaneous pneumothorax. In 1 case the final attack of pain was due to a pulmonary embolus rather than to coronary occlusion although she had previously had an attack of coronary occlusion.

Vander Veer[3] describes a diabetic patient whose angina pectoris began with pain in the right forearm and right infraclavicular region, and who subsequently died with coronary occlusion.

Dittler and McGavack[4] describe a bartender, aged fifty-three years, in whom acute pancreatic necrosis was associated with auricular fibrillation. The patient had a blood sugar of 206 mg. which in a few days rose to 375. These findings, together with a trace of sugar in the urine, were regarded as being due to coronary thrombosis, but insulin was given. The blood sugar, done seven times, never fell below 157 mg. Autopsy did not show any change in the heart and, therefore, the fibrillation was regarded as caused by reflexes originating within the abdomen.

In estimating the functional integrity of the diabetic heart, changes in size are much less significant than the history or than

---

[1] Raab and Rabinowitz: Jour. Am. Med. Assn., **106**, 1705, 1936.
[2] Gottsegen: Arch. f. Verdauungskr., **53**, 36, 1933.
[3] Vander Veer: Med. Clin. North America, **23**, No. 6, 1561, 1939.
[4] Dittler and McGavack: Am. Heart Jour., **16**, 354, 1938.

the electrocardiographic findings. Calcification in the aorta is shown by roentgen-ray with great frequency. In the last 200 films of the heart taken in our laboratory, 29 cases showed definite calcification in the arch of the aorta. Occasionally, calcification of the aortic cusps or of the mitral cusps is shown by roentgen-ray, as in Case 13328.

Prognosis.—The diabetic patient with angina has a poorer prognosis than the non-diabetic patient. The average duration of life from the first attack of angina to death was only two years in 136 fatal cases recorded by Root and Graybiel. Of these deaths 52.5 per cent occurred during the first year after the onset of angina. Cases in this series dying in the first year were, however, patients with conspicuously little treatment for the diabetes. By contrast, death after angina of fifteen years' duration occurred in a dentist and a physician, both of whom were faithful to the best diabetic treatment available. In 50 recent cases the average length of life after onset of angina pectoris was 1.6 years.

The largest series of non-diabetic patients with angina pectoris studied for a long period of time is that of Paul D. White.[1] This series of 497 patients observed from 1920 to 1943 consists of 445 patients who had died, and 52 who were still living in 1943. The average duration to death was 7.0 years and the average duration of disease in the living was 18.0 years, an average for the whole group of 8.4 years. The final report, however, including the cases living at present, is bound to give an average close to ten years for the entire series.

With moderate diets and earlier use of insulin treatment, the onset of coronary disease is being postponed, as indicated in Table 64 by the advancing age at death of patients.

Treatment.—Cardiac drugs are of limited value. Weight reduction by means of a low-calorie diet in order to restrict the vascular bed is important. Vasodilators such as nitroglycerine or aminophylline are commonly used, but patients tend to omit them and to rely upon restriction of activity and rest. Whiskey does not shorten the attacks or increase the capacity of the patient with angina for work.[2] The attacks are rarely so severe and the degree of coronary sclerosis usually so advanced that surgical measures have seldom been recommended and carried out in only 2 cases. Case 18491, female, age fifty-seven years, underwent bilateral thoracic sympathectomy performed by Dr. James Poppen. Relief was complete for one and a half years. Case 14045 took nitroglycerine thirty to forty times a day prior to sympathectomy performed by Dr. Poppen. Death followed from hepatic failure due to hemochromatosis.

Cardiac asthma is conspicuously rare in diabetic patients, even in patients in whom hypertension and hypertensive heart disease

---

[1] White: P. 830, loc. cit., p. 507.
[2] Stearns, Riseman and Gray: New England Jour. Med., **234**, 578, 1946.

are present. In an occasional case, the application of a tourniquet to the extremities reduces the amount of blood entering the lungs by way of the right side of the heart and will relieve an attack. It is necessary to remove the tourniquet slowly, however, or another attack will occur.

If good treatment for chronic cardiac disease requires the elimination of burdens and the very best treatment of existing complications, then the best treatment of the diabetes should prove advantageous for the diabetic patient with coronary disease. That the use of insulin properly managed prolongs his life is well shown in the following table.

TABLE 64.—DIABETIC PATIENTS DYING FROM CORONARY DISEASE.
THE ADVANCING AGE AT DEATH DURING THE INSULIN ERA.

	1923–1926.	1927–1929.	1930–1934.	1935–1936.	1937–1939.	1940–1943.	1944–1946.[1]
Average age at death, yrs.	60.9	62.7	65.4	65.2	66.2	66.2	64.4
Average duration of diabetes, yrs. .	11	13	12	13	13	14	13
Number of cases	55	56	242	126	254	302	156

It is evident from Table 64 that in the six successive periods between 1923 and 1943 the ages of the gatients dying of coronary disease advanced along with the duration of the disease and the use of insulin.

In accidental cases of insulin poisoning there is no evidence of harmful effect upon the heart. Case 12882, seen in consultation, aged twenty-seven years,[2] died after an accidental overdose of insulin. At autopsy the heart muscle showed only slight edema and some perivascular fibrosis. The edema was well explained by the fact that the patient had had a constant intravenous infusion of glucose solution for twelve hours before her death. Although it is difficult to demonstrate a direct and immediate effect exerted by diabetic treatment on the frequency and character of anginal attacks, a variety of facts indicate that metabolic factors are of importance. Middleton and Oatway[3] found definite depression of the T-wave in 100 per cent of cases of insulin shock with true hypoglycemia. Experimentally Cruickshank[4] found that although the isolated normal heart responds to insulin by storing glycogen, the diabetic heart stores glycogen better if the blood sugar is maintained well above normal. After diabetes of eight or more years' duration, the heart may become accustomed to an elevated blood sugar. Sudden reductions in the blood sugar brought about by reductions in diet or by insulin are not well borne. In Case 1520, fatal coronary thrombosis, proved at autopsy, occurred during insulin hypoglycemia. In Blotner's series,[5] death from cardiac infarction occurred in 3 cases shortly

[1] Deaths reported through May 15, 1946.
[2] Root: Loc. cit., p. 516.
[3] Middleton and Oatway: Am. Jour. Med. Sci., **181**, 39, 1931.
[4] Cruickshank, quoted: New England Jour. Med,, **201**, 600, 1929.
[5] Blotner: Loc. cit., p. 483.

after a rapid fall in blood-sugar concentration following the administration of insulin. Strouse et al.[1] found that some of their patients with coronary disease grew worse as the diabetes improved under treatment, and they warned against too rapid reduction in the level of the blood sugar. On the other hand, it is familar experience that the patients who have a large amount of sugar in the urine with anginal pain frequently are much improved when the diabetes is controlled. The dangerous effects of overdoses of insulin with hypoglycemia have been explained by Ernstene and Altschule[2] by an increase in the amount of cardiac work due to a rise in the venous pressure, minute-volume, output of the heart, pulse-pressure, blood flow and ventricular-rate. In some instances increase in the arterial blood-pressure was found.

Dicoumarol has been used in acute coronary thrombosis, but we have used it only in phlebitis at the New England Deaconess Hospital. In 48 attacks reported by Nichol and Page,[3] the mortality was 12.5 per cent. However, no deaths occurred in patients having their first attack of coronary occlusion.

The use of dextrose solution, administered intravenously in amounts of 20 cc. of a 50 per cent solution, sometimes gives relief of anginal pain and in one case gave much greater subjective comfort than any other means. During coronary thrombosis, especially if congestive failure is present, a marked loss in carbohydrate tolerance occurs and during this period the use of insulin is of value. Collens et al.[4] recommend insulin for coronary disease in elderly diabetics. Hepburn and Latchford[5] showed that insulin increased the average sugar consumption of the heart from the normal rate of 0.87 mg. per gram per hour to 3.06 mg. per hour. Lymburner's case[6] from the Mayo Clinic with a severe attack of angina, possibly really coronary occlusion, was given 250 units in twelve hours with excellent results. Case 11991, whose diabetes had done so well during the preceding six months that she had reduced insulin to 25 units daily, had an acute coronary occlusion with a fall of blood-pressure from 180 to 90, delirium and congestive heart failure; she received 65 units of insulin and during the next three weeks made a complete recovery. Her carbohydrate tolerance rose from 75 to 150 grams and she was able to leave the hospital without taking insulin. Such cases of recovery clearly indicate that during coronary occlusion, if uncontrolled diabetes is present, it should be relieved by the judicious use of insulin.

3. **Rheumatic Heart Disease.**—The frequency of rheumatic heart disease in diabetics is probably greater than is indicated by the fact

[1] Strouse, Soskin, Katz, and Rubinfeld: Jour. Am. Med. Assn., 98, 1703, 1932
[2] Ernstene and Altschule: Jour. Clin. Invest., 10, 521, 1931.
[3] Nichol and Page: Jour. Florida Med. Assn., 32, 365, 1946.
[4] Collens, Stoliarsky and Netzer: Am. Jour. Med. Sci., 191, 503, 1936.
[5] Hepburn and Latchford: Am Jour. Physiol., 62, 177, 1922.
[6] Lymburner: Proc. Staff Meet., Mayo Clinic, 8, 235, 1933.

that in 429 autopsies upon diabetics at the Deaconess Hospital there have been 13 cases of rheumatic heart disease. Case 11772 developed diabetes in 1919 at the age of twenty-four years during service in World War I. He had had rheumatic fever as a child. From February 2 to April 6, 1933, he was in the Deaconess Hospital with acute rheumatic fever, endocarditis and pericarditis with effusion. Pleural effusion was also present. Although his condition seemed desperate he made a recovery and in August, 1940, he was chief of police in a small community, taking from 25 to 30 units of insulin a day. His death occurred in 1945 from pneumonia and heart failure. Clinically, rheumatic fever has been even less frequent in the hospital wards. Case 3194 developed diabetes in 1922 at the age of fifty years. Later she became bedridden with a progressive form of atrophic arthritis and died on August 23, 1934, with terminal bacterial endocarditis developing on the background of a chronic rheumatic mitral and aortic valvular disease. At one time she took 100 units of insulin a day and at autopsy the pancreas weighed 15 grams. Case 2989, with mitral stenosis and auricular fibrillation, successfully underwent a gastro-enterostomy under local anesthesia. In the three years, 1943 to 1945, 4 male and 8 female diabetics with rheumatic heart disease, entered the Deaconess Hospital. Combined aortic and mitral disease were found in 2 men, aortic regurgitation in 1 case, mitral stenosis with fibrillation in 5 and compensated mitral disease in 4 patients.

4. **Pericarditis.**—Pericarditis, like renal infections, appears in diabetics chiefly as a blood-borne infection arising in some other septic focus. Three instances of rheumatic pericarditis occurred in Case 2197, Case 5983, and Case 11772. Case 2197, a housewife, aged fifty-seven years, following tonsillitis developed acute arthritis with pericardial and pleural effusion. She was in bed nine months with arthritis and made a complete recovery. Case 5983, aged thirty-nine years, female, died with rheumatic carditis and pericarditis with many Aschoff nodules in the myocardium. Case 11772, aged thirty-eight years, has been described in the preceding section. Pericarditis was associated with diabetic coma and pneumonia in Case 2988, stenographer, aged fifty-five years, and Case 7021, housewife, aged seventy-one years. Pericarditis was incidental to septicemia secondary to a gangrenous foot in Case 4507, housewife, aged fifty-seven years and secondary to a cellulitis of the scalp in Case 10804, housewife, aged seventy-six years. In 4 cases (4304, 12559, 13150, 13331) the pericarditis was associated with renal abscesses or chronic pyelonephritis. In Case 11167, clerk, aged fifty-five years, pericarditis was a terminal event in a patient with hemochromatosis, infected chylous ascites, retrocecal abscess and a perforated duodenal ulcer. Case 7763, aged sixty-nine years, died December 7, 1938 with coronary occlusion and infarction of the kidney, but at autopsy chronic adhesive pericarditis was present.

5. Bacterial Endocarditis.—In Case 15297, age sixty years, at admission on June 30, 1943, the explanation for her fever and anemia was found in the positive blood culture for streptococcus viridans. Within two weeks an aortic diastolic murmur developed. Embolic episodes with hemiplegia occurred, and she died two and one-half months after admission. Case 23567 developed diabetes at the age of fifty years. At her first examination the heart showed only a systolic murmur. Later a loud diastolic murmur developed and the blood cultures were positive on two occasions for staphylococcus aureus. She received intensive treatment with penicillin 300,000 units daily. The blood cultures became negative and have remained so for a year. When last seen in May, 1946 the diastolic murmur was still present, but she had been without fever for ten months.

6. Periarteritis Nodosa.—Periarteritis nodosa is generally regarded as an inflammatory lesion affecting the medium sized and small arteries in various parts of the body and probably of infectious origin. Whether it may properly be regarded as related to streptococcus infection or belonging in the rheumatic group is not as yet clear. Case 16353, aged forty-five years, developed diabetes in November 1937 and entered the Deaconess Hospital November 1, 1945 with fever, weakness and increasing pain in the legs. He had neuritic signs which finally included wrist drop. No eosinophilia, asthma or hematuria occurred. Death occurred after a series of convulsions. At autopsy the characteristic lesions were most extensive in the arteries within nerve trunks as well as in the heart, prostate and kidneys.

CHAPTER XVI.

INFECTIONS IN DIABETES.

REVISED BY ALEXANDER MARBLE, M.D.

THE inter-relationship of diabetes and infections has always been involved and puzzling. All students of the disease agree that diabetes is made temporarily more severe by an infection, that the uncontrolled diabetic clinically has less than normal resistance and that an infection has often been the cause of death in a diabetic, particularly prior to the introduction of the sulfonamides and penicillin. It is doubtful, however, that diabetes can be *caused* by an infection or made permanently more severe by one, except by certain rare infections of the pancreas itself. Moreover, the exact nature of the lowered resistance to infection which is common in uncontrolled diabetes, remains a problem about which little is known.

The diabetic is particularly susceptible to pulmonary tuberculosis and to infections of the urinary tract and skin. The decreased resistance to the tubercle bacillus is probably related to the bodily insult of acidosis. (See pages 447 and 649.) This is a possible explanation, too, for the high incidence of urinary tract infections. The increased susceptibility of the skin to infection is probably not dependent upon its high sugar content, although conceivably may be related to a low glycogen content.[1]

Throughout the present discussion, comments regarding resistance to infection apply in general to uncontrolled diabetes since with proper treatment, the response of the diabetic to infection approaches the normal. Williams,[2] in an analysis of present-day experience in doctors' offices and in general hospitals, concluded that pyogenic skin infections occur no more frequently in diabetic than in non-diabetic individuals. He stated his opinion that "it is extremely doubtful that diabetes increases the susceptibility of the diabetic appreciably to pyogenic skin infections." One would agree with this statement if control of diabetes is assumed.

In the course of serious prolonged infections such as osteomyelitis there may be a gain rather than a loss in carbohydrate tolerance, just as in diabetes complicated by tuberculosis. Examples are cited by Root[3].

A. INFECTION AS AN ETIOLOGICAL FACTOR.

Published reports vary considerably as to the relative frequency of acute infections prior to the onset of diabetes. In our juvenile

---

[1] Bayne-Jones: Bull. New York Acad. Med., 12, 278, 1936.
[2] Williams: Jour. Am. Med. Assn., 118, 1357, 1942.
[3] Root: New England Jour. Med., 210, 127, 1934.

cases, in whom one would expect the highest correlation, 90 out of 100 children had no significant infection within a year of onset. Severe and prolonged infections under close observation in general hospitals, especially in surgical wards, are common and yet the development of diabetes in such cases is so rare as to be an occasion for great surprise. These are practical reasons why we do not consider infections of great etiological importance. Lande,[1] writing from Umber's Clinic, recorded the same belief. (See page 742.) In contrast to this view John[2] found that 20 per cent of his juvenile cases had an infection within two months of onset. Barach,[3] too, found a high incidence of infection. An increasing incidence of diabetes after epidemics of influenza was reported by Jones.[4] Lierle and Potter[5] found that low-grade tonsillitis and colds occurred frequently prior to onset. Bertram[6] stated that in a large percentage of his cases diabetes became manifest during an infection. However, one must consider the possibility that if an individual has an infection he is more apt to go to a doctor, and in consequence a hitherto undiagnosed and latent diabetes may be brought to light.

John[7] has reported a case of interest in this connection. A twenty-three year old soldier with severe atypical pneumonia developed glycosuria for the first time eight days after admission at a time when fever had begun to abate and when the patient was showing slight improvement. The fasting blood sugar was 153 mg. per cent and blood sugar values of 210 mg. per cent and slightly above, were obtained. Insulin in dosage as high as 40 units daily was given for almost four weeks. Following this, glycosuria and hyperglycemia disappeared and remained absent even after the discontinuance of insulin. A glucose tolerance test about ten weeks after the original discovery of glycosuria, was entirely normal. Somewhat similar cases were reported by Marie, et al.[8] in two children with scarlet fever and infectious jaundice, respectively. All will agree that such patients should be watched carefully throughout life.

B. CAUSE OF LOWERED TOLERANCE FOR CARBOHYDRATE DURING AN INFECTION.

A lowered tolerance for carbohydrate during infections either in the diabetic or non-diabetic theoretically might be due to one of four causes: (1) lessened production of endogenous insulin; (2) increased production of hormonal antagonists; (3) destruction of insulin; (4) interference with the storage of glycogen.

[1] Lande: Klin. Wchnschr.. 10, 359, 1931.
[2] John: Ann. Int. Med., 8, 198, 1934.
[3] Barach: Arch. Int. Med., 39, 636, 1927.
[4] Jones, quoted by von Noorden: Die Zuckerkrankheit und ihre Behandlung. 8th ed., Berlin, Julius Springer, 1927.
[5] Lierle and Potter: Arch. Otolaryngol., 14, 432, 1931.
[6] Bertram: Med. Welt, Nos. 30, 32, 1936.
[7] John: South. Med. Jour., 37, 625, 1944.
[8] Marie, Seringe, Rouèche and Maurice: Semaine d. hôp. Paris, 22, 338, 1946,

1. Lessened Production of Insulin.—Lessened production of insulin has been suggested by some as the cause for the occurrence of glycosuria and loss of tolerance during infections in non-diabetics. This can be demonstrated by random blood sugar and tolerance tests. Thus, Williams and Dick[1] found that glycosuria occurred in 41 per cent of patients with acute infectious diseases. The largest average amount occurred with influenza. Diminished tolerance for carbohydrate after the ingestion of glucose is shown by sugar tolerance curves in acute infectious diseases and in experimental inoculation in animals. (See page 164.) Labbé[2] has demonstrated a lowered carbohydrate tolerance in pneumonia, and MacLean and Sullivan[3] in encephalitis, tuberculosis, meningitis and measles.

These observations have been thought to suggest an injury to the islands of Langerhans with lessened production of insulin in the presence of an infection. At such periods as during the course of pneumonia, both insular necrosis and regeneration are reported to occur.[4]

2. Increased Production of Hormonal Antagonists.—Hypersecretion of the thyroid and adrenal glands, producing hormonal antagonists was suggested by Lawrence and McCance.[5] Their patient, a girl, aged sixteen years, with septicemia, had a decrease in the requirement for insulin after an initial increase in dosage at the time when the sepsis became progressively worse. The reduction coincided with a falling temperature and failing reactive powers. It is suggested that this reaction may be due to increased activity of the suprarenals and thyroid. If their reaction fails or diminishes, then the antagonism to insulin is removed and the dose of insulin required becomes less in spite of increasing sepsis. On the basis of this reasoning, ergotamine was tried in cases of sepsis, but its toxic properties showed it to be undesirable. Greene and Swanson[6] reported that hyperglycemia and glycosuria in hyperthyroidism without diabetes can be abolished by a high carbohydrate diet and reproduced by one low in carbohydrate and high in fat.

3. Destruction of Insulin.—The actual destruction or chemical inactivation of insulin in circulation is believed by some to be possible. Trypsin or toxins produced by leukocytes, pus and bacteria may destroy it. *In vitro* pus cells destroy insulin but this has not been proved *in vivo*.

Rabinowitch[7] suggested that an insulin-destroying enzyme is produced during infections. On the basis of studies of sugar toler-

[1] Williams and Dick: Loc. cit., p. 165.
[2] Labbé: Bull. et mém. Soc. méd. d. hôp. de Paris, **49**, 1358, 1925.
[3] MacLean and Sullivan: Am. Jour. Dis. Child., **37**, 1146, 1929.
[4] Root and Warren: Boston Med. and Surg. Jour., **194**, 45, 1926.
[5] Lawrence and McCance: Brit. Med. Jour., **1**, 749, 1931. *See also* Lawrence and Buckley: Brit. Jour. Exp. Path., **8**, 58, 1927; and Evans and Zeckwer: Brit. Jour. Exp. Path., **8**, 280, 1927.
[6] Greene and Swanson: Jour. Lab. and Clin. Med., **26**, 360, 1940.
[7] Rabinowitch: Canad. Med. Assn. Jour., **26**, 551, 1932.

ance tests of diabetic patients during infection with and without fever and with varying degrees of fever, he concluded that it is the infection, not the fever, that causes the impaired tolerance.

4. Interference With the Storage of Glycogen.—Experimental evidence in favor of glycogen depletion as a cause of loss of tolerance for carbohydrate during infections is afforded by the experiments of Fetzer[1] upon the relation between carbohydrate metabolism and experimental staphylococcus infection in rabbits. He administered to rabbits for twelve days, twice daily, 10 grams of dextrose by stomach tube. On the fifth day of the experiment these rabbits as well as several control animals were infected with a culture of Staphylococcus aureus. Fetzer found that whereas the controls showed only a comparatively slight infection, in the animals that received the dextrose the infection was much more extensive. He interpreted this to indicate that the increased sugar content of blood and tissues favored the growth and the spread of the staphylococci. (See p. 527 for general comments regarding this interpretation.) To another group of animals a larger dose of infectious material was administered. To this more severe infection the dextrose animals showed a greater resistance, for they survived, whereas the control animals died less than twelve hours following the infection. In order to determine the behavior of the glycogen content of the liver, a new group of animals was infected with staphylococci. It was found that in the animals treated with dextrose the glycogen content was reduced to about one-fourth of the normal, whereas in the controls it was reduced to one-tenth. This suggests that the toxins of the staphylococci reduce the glycogen content of the liver. Fetzer thinks that the increased resistance of the dextrose animals against the toxins of the staphylococci may perhaps be due to their greater glycogen reserves, and he suggests that this may explain the good results obtained in toxic and infectious complications following administration of dextrose.

In a discussion of insulin resistance due to infection, Greene and Keohen[2] mention various theories which have been advanced to explain such resistance. These factors listed may, in general, be classified under the four headings above. Studies were carried out with human diabetic patients in an attempt to ascertain the effect on the insulin requirement of infections, idiopathic fever, administration of foreign proteins, hyperthermia produced in a fever cabinet and the administration of histamine and epinephrine. The results were inconclusive in that an increase in insulin requirement did not develop in all cases of infection or fevers or in response to histamine or epinephrine. Its occurrence was not related to sex, age, height and duration of fever, or to the apparent toxemia. Despite these findings, all would agree that in general an acute infection defi-

[1] Fetzer: Arch. f. Hyg., **107**, 255, 1932.
[2] Greene and Keohen: Loc. cit., p. 383.

nitely tends to make diabetes worse and that an increase in insulin requirement may be anticipated.

C. DECREASED RESISTANCE TO INFECTION IN DIABETES.

Since the introduction of insulin, and particularly protamine zinc insulin, treatment has been so improved that excellent control of diabetes is possible with almost all patients. In those with whom this is obtained and to whom an adequate diet is supplied, clinical resistance to infection appears to approach the normal.[1] However, even today in those patients whose diabetes is poorly controlled, the decreased ability to overcome infections cannot be denied. In their article on this subject, Marble, White and Fernald[2] discussed certain factors as *possible* causes of the lowered resistance to infection in diabetes; these are as follows:

(1) Increased sugar content of blood and tissues. (2) Decreased activity of blood elements associated with resistance to infection; (*a*) subnormal activity of complement; (*b*) subnormal phagocytizing capacity of leukocytes; (*c*) subnormal bacteriostatic and bactericidal action of whole blood. (3) Inadequate functioning of fixed tissue cells. (4) Lowered capacity of tissues to react to antigenic stimuli. (5) Lowered state of general cellular nutrition.

Formerly it was thought that the increased sugar content of the blood and tissues seen in diabetic patients favored the growth of bacteria, particularly staphylococci. Present-day opinion does not favor this explanation. Handmann[3] found that *in vitro* staphylococci grew no better on blood containing 0.5 to 1 per cent sugar than on normal blood; furthermore, the addition of glucose to blood within the limits found in diabetes did not decrease the bactericidal power of the blood or affect its opsonic index. Hirsch-Kauffmann and Heimann-Trosien[4] observed that streptococci, pneumococci and influenza bacilli grew better on blood agar plates made with blood from a patient in diabetic coma than on ordinary blood agar, but there was no effect from hyperglycemic blood from non-coma cases, from the addition of dextrose and acetone *in vitro*, or from cases of experimental hyperglycemia, lipemia and acidosis. Moen and Reimann[5] consider the liability to infections of patients with poorly controlled diabetes to be due not to hyperglycemia but to glycosuria and polyuria, *i. e.*, to extraordinary and long-continued loss of sugar and water. This is in keeping with the results of Pillsbury and Kulchar,[6] who found that when a disturbance in the fluid balance of rabbits was produced by parenteral injections of large

---

[1] Wohlenberg: München. med. Wchnschr., **88**, 883, 1941.

[2] Marble, White and Fernald: Jour. Clin. Invest., **17**, 423, 1938.

[3] Handmann: Deutsch. Arch. f. klin. Med., **102**, 1, 1911.

[4] Hirsch-Kauffmann and Heimann-Trosien: Klin. Wchnschr., **5**, 1655, 1926.

[5] Moen and Reimann: Arch. Int. Med., **51**, 789, 1933.

[6] Pillsbury and Kulchar: Am. Jour. Med. Sci., **190**, 169, 1935.

amounts of glucose or sodium chloride, a very marked increase in the extent of an experimental staphylococcic skin infection was noted. Likewise Mosenthal[1] regards polyuria and dehydration accompanying prolonged and marked glycosuria as responsible for the diminished resistance to infection seen in diabetes. He, as well as Bayne-Jones[2] and Richardson,[3] considered hyperglycemia *per se* as of little or no significance, although it usually indicates uncontrolled diabetes. Richardson, studying diabetic patients, and Horster,[4] depancreatized dogs, found that the amount and activity of the complement of the blood serum did not differ from that of normal blood. However, Bayer and Form[5] stated that following removal of the pancreas there occurred a decrease in hemolytic complement which could be temporarily restored to normal by the injection of insulin and glucose.

Moen and Reimann,[6] in the study previously referred to, found that the production of typhoid agglutinins was lower in patients with diabetes than in normal individuals. In proportion to the severity of the disease, similar results were reported by Richardson.[3] On the other hand, Wale and Madders[7] found that blood from diabetic patients had essentially the same amount of natural staphylococcal antitoxin and that following toxoid treatment antitoxin increased to practically the same degree as in normal individuals.

Richardson[3] found that diabetic blood had, in general, a lower bactericidal power than normal blood. The differences obtained by him were not great, however. In later work[8] he studied the relative importance of the nutritional state and the blood-sugar level in influencing the development of agglutinins after typhoid vaccine. He produced hyperglycemia in rabbits by injecting adrenalin and lowered the nutritional state by starvation. He concluded that the state of cellular nutrition was more important than the level of blood sugar in determining the antibody response. Richardson[9] observed in normal rabbits and depancreatized cats a significant correlation between the amount of glycogen in the liver and the survival time of the animals after intravenous inoculations with bacteria, including especially the staphylococcus aureus. In poorly nourished, depancreatized cats with a decreased liver glycogen, a low agglutinative titer was found after injection of typhoid vaccine. Alterations in the sugar, cholesterol, protein, and albumin content

[1] Mosenthal: Jour. Am. Med. Assn., **105**, 484, 1935.
[2] Bayne-Jones: Loc. cit., p. 523.
[3] Richardson: Jour. Clin. Invest., **12**, 1143, 1933.
[4] Horster: Deutsch. Arch. f. klin. Med., **176**, 502, 1934.
[5] Bayer and Form: Deutsch. med. Wchnschr., **52**, 1338, 1926.
[6] Moen and Reimann: Loc. cit., p. 527.
[7] Wale and Madders: Brit. Jour. Exper. Path., **17**, 279, 1933.
[8] Richardson: Jour. Clin. Invest., **14**, 389, 1935.
[9] Richardson: Jour. Clin. Invest., **19**, 239, 1940.

of the blood did not influence the dissemination of bacteria. Acidosis appeared to increase the frequency of this dissemination.

Marble, White and Fernald[1] found that fresh defibrinated blood and heparinized whole blood of diabetic patients possessed essentially the same phagocytic, bacteriostatic and bactericidal power against selected strains of streptococci as blood from normal controls. The results in individual patients could not be correlated with the duration, severity or state of control of the diabetes. Their findings suggested that diabetic patients who successfully overcome infections thereby develop specific immunity to approximately the same extent as individuals without diabetes.

In summary, it must be conceded that the causes for lowered resistance to infection in diabetes are still not apparent. It is certainly related to the malnutrition, lowered glycogen content of the liver, dehydration and acidosis which characterize the patient with poorly controlled diabetes. As to the exact mode and site of operation of these factors, little information is available.

D. THE MANAGEMENT OF INFECTIONS IN DIABETES.

An infection makes a diabetic worse. This rule is so exact that one can often make a safe prediction upon the condition of the infection by the course of the diabetes and, conversely, whenever a diabetic does badly, one must search for an infection, and incidentally for hyperpituitarism, hyperthyroidism, hemochromatosis or cancer of the pancreas. The effect of a carbuncle upon the diabetic process is an excellent example. With its advent a diabetes almost quiescent for years may become intensely severe, but with its subsidence resume its mild character. See page 683 for instructive cases.

TABLE 65.—A TEMPORARY SUBSTITUTE FOR STANDARD DIET.

Useful in the Treatment of Patients With Infections or Digestive Disturbances.

Food.[1]	Carbohydrate, gm.	Protein, gm.	Fat, gm.
Milk, 960 cc. (1 quart)	48	32	32
20 per cent cream, 120 cc. (¼ pint)	4	4	24
Bread, 90 grams (3 slices)	54	9	0
Oatmeal, 30 grams (1 large saucerful)	20	5	2
Egg, 1	0	6	6
Butter, 30 grams	0	0	25
Orange juice, 240 grams	24	0	0
	150	56	89
	4	4	9
Total calories	600	224	801

[1] For a child cream could be omitted and butter reduced.

1. **Diet and Insulin.**—Unless promptly and adequately treated, an infection may lead to acidosis, due largely to the fever with its

[1] Marble, White and Fernald: Loc. cit., p. 527.

resulting increase of metabolism. The insulin dosage will almost invariably need to be increased. Sufficient insulin should be given to secure satisfactory control of the diabetic condition. The diet should be simple and must often be more concentrated than usual because of the patient's illness. From 100 to 200 grams of carbohydrate should be taken daily.

Carbohydrate in the form of oatmeal gruel, orange juice and even puréed vegetables, protein as white of eggs, oysters, fish and chicken, and fat in the form of cream will tide over many emergencies. A simple diet is given in Table 65.

During active infections insulin should be given in doses large enough to keep the diabetic condition under good control although during the short period of acute infections, absolute sugar-freedom is not necessary or indeed, wholly desirable, since at almost any moment during an infection, recovery may begin and the need for insulin quickly abate. If the patient has not been followed closely, a hypoglycemic attack may be produced. Rapidly acting insulin may be administered at frequent intervals, every three or four hours according to some such schedule as the following:

If Benedict test is	Red	Orange	Yellow	Yellow-green
Give units	20	16	12	8

If the patient is already taking protamine zinc insulin, that type may be continued and rapidly-acting insulin added as needed, but usually in smaller amounts than just cited, such as

Red	Orange	Yellow	Yellow-green
10	8	6	4

every four to six hours or before meals.

2. **Sulfonamide Therapy.**—Diabetic patients with infections have shared with other sick persons in the better treatment and lower mortality rate made possible by the introduction of the sulfonamides several years ago. Sulfanilamide, sulfapyridine, sulfathiazole and, finally, sulfadiazine were used successively with benefit in diabetics as in non-diabetics. At present when sulfonamides are used, sulfadiazine is regarded as the drug of choice in most infections, using it in the same dosage and with the same precautions as for non-diabetics. Attention to the blood level of the drug, to an adequate fluid intake and output, and to examinations at suitable intervals of the blood and urine for possible toxic manifestations, are even more important in the diabetic than the non-diabetic. On the other hand, with proper care, particularly as to fluid intake (to allow at least 1500 cc. urine daily), diabetics tolerate sulfonamide therapy equally as well as non-diabetics and suffer no greater inci-

dence of nausea, vomiting, hematuria, crystalluria, dermatitis, leukopenia, neutropenia, anemia or other toxic effects occasionally seen in any group of patients receiving sulfonamides even though, as in our series, accompanying alkalis are not routinely given. This was the experience early reported by Styron, Bromley and Root.[1] No evidence of acidosis was observed following sulfathiazole or sulfadiazine.

3. **Penicillin.**—Although the sulfonamides were an extremely valuable addition to the armamentarium, the introduction of penicillin in 1943 and 1944 marked an advance which, in certain infections in diabetics, was revolutionary. Not only has penicillin changed the outlook as regards infections in general but in at least two types of lesions encountered in diabetics it has altered treatment radically. The first of these lesions is the carbuncle, usually on the back of the neck. Up until the advent of penicillin, treatment by our surgical colleagues consisted of heat and perhaps x-ray applications until such time as there was sufficient localization to allow a wide crucial incision. Often weeks and months elapsed from the onset of the infection until complete healing of the operative wound occurred. Experience with penicillin indicates that if the drug is started early enough and used in large enough doses (500,000 units intramuscularly daily), the infection may be overcome in the early stages and subsidence of the process take place with the necessity of little or no surgery. Without question penicillin has lowered mortality and shortened the hospital stay.

A second condition benefited by penicillin is infection of the feet. The use of penicillin has enabled the surgeon to be less drastic in amputations than formerly. In certain patients hitherto uncontrollable infections have been overcome and amputation avoided entirely. In others, it has been possible to carry out amputations through the metatarsals rather than through the leg or thigh, thus giving the patient a much more serviceable leg.

For a more complete discussion of penicillin in surgical infections and agranulocytosis, see pages 612, 701 and 705.

4. **Streptomycin.**—At the present time (August 1946), streptomycin has not been made available for general civilian use, so that we have had opportunity to try it in only a very few patients. From reports in the literature it should prove a valuable aid in the treatment of certain urinary tract infections to which the diabetic is liable, particularly those due to *E. coli*. One had hoped that it would be helpful in the treatment of tuberculosis, but reports to date have not been greatly encouraging; it is too early, however, to render a final opinion in this regard.

[1] Styron, Bromley and Root: Jour. Am. Med. Assn., **118**, 1423, 1942.

CHAPTER XVII.

THE DIGESTIVE SYSTEM IN DIABETES.

Revised by C. Cabell Bailey, M.D.

A. THE TEETH.

It is regrettable that the teeth of adult diabetic patients are often very poor. This is important because poor teeth can complicate the treatment of diabetes and infected teeth may make diabetes worse. An average of 1000 diabetic patients have been examined yearly since 1932 in the dental clinic at the New England Deaconess Hospital under the direction of Dr. Harold A. Kent and about 1 in 8 of these patients has had three or four teeth removed because of oral sepsis. The chief functions of this clinic have been to teach diabetic patients how to care for their mouths, to impress them with the importance of professional dental care, and to eliminate infected or hopelessly carious teeth. Miss Madelyn Lendall, dental hygienist, aids in this work.

The high incidence of caries in diabetic patients, however, is no greater than in non-diabetic patients. Surveys, made among large groups of individuals in the general population, have invariably shown an extraordinarily high incidence of dental abnormalities.

On the other hand, it is encouraging to examine so many younger diabetic patients who are comparatively free from dental disease. In a study of 43 patients from eleven to twenty-five years of age with diabetes of ten to twenty years' duration, Dr. Kent found 18 with no fillings or cavities, and in the entire group only 20 teeth, including 12 third molars, had been extracted. In Dr. Kent's opinion these young patients have teeth which are in as good or better condition than those of non-diabetic individuals of the same age group. The age of onset of diabetes in these patients ranged from six months to fourteen years. It so happened that all those with mouths free from caries or fillings had had diabetes since the age of eight years or younger. This is significant, because in spite of the high caries susceptibility of most young adults between the ages of seven and twenty, these diabetic patients had no caries. It also has been observed that if the onset of diabetes occurs during the middle or latter part of this high caries susceptibility period, many carious and infected teeth are found, but that this process is often arrested when the control of diabetes is satisfactorily maintained. The destruction of teeth and the supporting structures is very active just prior to the onset of diabetes.

In patients admitted in diabetic coma the mucous membranes of the mouth are usually dehydrated and have a dull cherry-red appearance. The teeth may become loose during and immediately follow-ing coma, but tighten when the diabetes is brought under control.

Rudy and Cohen[1] reported upon a two-year experience in the diabetic clinic of the Beth Israel Hospital in Boston. Of 403 patients, 138 were edentulous. Among the remaining 265 there were 4 children and 3 young adults with diabetes of long standing. Six of these 7 had excellent teeth with very little caries and no abnormal tartar formation.

It is not difficult to understand why a patient with uncontrolled diabetes of long standing should be susceptible to dental caries and pyorrhea. Added to the influence of acidosis and dehydration there is the factor of lowered resistance to infection which occurs in uncontrolled diabetes. With this and with lowered vitality of tissue, the gums may become unhealthy, pyorrhea and absorption of the alveolar soft tissue may take place and peridental infection develop. However, with proper treatment and control of the diabetic condi-tion the teeth and gums should remain in as good condition as those of a non-diabetic person.

Although tartar deposits, gingivitis and pyorrhea are commonly found in the mouths of adult patients whose diabetes is controlled, these changes are not as progressive as in those patients with poorly controlled diabetes. In the well controlled group the susceptibility to caries seems low. The teeth can be removed or minor operations performed in the mouth without fear of complications.

At the present time, using insulin if necessary, it is possible to allow adequate diets which are the equal or the superior of average, unselected diets in their completeness. It is possible, and indeed necessary, to include milk and other dairy products in the dietary of every diabetic, young and old. To insure an adequate calcium intake we insist that the diet of every adult diabetic contain at least 0.7 gram of calcium per day and that of every juvenile diabetic 1 gram of calcium a day. By this means and by the liberal use of sunlight, cod-liver oil and foods containing vitamin C, one can hope to build and maintain strong teeth and bones.

There is another reason why good treatment of diabetes should automatically include proper care of the teeth. Perhaps more than any other large group of individuals in the country, diabetics visit their doctors frequently and have frequent physical examinations. If both doctor and patient are alive to their responsibilities, early defects are noted and treatment instituted before irreparable damage is done.

One must consider that in attacking the problem of the building and maintaining of strong teeth and healthy gums there are two sides to be considered. First, on the metabolic side, the diet must contain sufficient vitamins and minerals and the diabetic condition must be kept under control. Second, patients must be drilled in the

[1] Rudy and Cohen: New England Jour. Med., **219**, 503, 1938.

proper local care of their teeth and gums. They must be taught to brush their teeth properly twice daily and see their dentist every three months.

Care of the Mouth and Teeth.

1. Use a small toothbrush with tufts well separated. Have two brushes and alternate each time you brush your teeth. Replace brush when bristles become soft.
2. A mixture of equal quantities of bicarbonate of soda and table salt is a satisfactory tooth powder.
3. Brush your teeth at least twice daily, morning and night, spending two minutes each time. Be sure that you do this properly. Ask the dental hygienist to show you how if you are not sure.
4. After brushing the teeth, massage the gums with your fingers, working fingers toward the teeth in a rotary motion. This is particularly important for diabetics.
5. Have your teeth cleaned and examined by a dentist or dental hygienist every three months. Keep all cavities filled.

For the extraction of teeth, local anesthesia should almost always be used since it does not necessitate the omission of food prior to its administration nor does it interfere with the scheduled use of insulin. For the protection of the patients and themselves, dentists should insist that the patient bring a recent report from his physician regarding the degree of control of his diabetic condition.

In their experience with the extraction of 252 teeth from 125 diabetic patients Blaustein and Ferguson[1] found that the percentage of postoperative sequelæ was not higher than that among non-diabetic individuals. The dental extractions caused no significant change in the levels of the blood sugar. Healing took place satisfactorily. They greatly prefer local to general anesthesia.

This agrees with the experience in the dental clinic at the New England Deaconess Hospital, except that it has been found that following the extraction of infected teeth the amount of sugar in the urine may increase temporarily and additional insulin be required for a short time. Consequently out-patients are instructed to test the urine three or four times daily for two or three days following extractions and to adjust the insulin dosage accordingly.

B. CONSTIPATION.

Although constipation is probably no more frequent among diabetic patients than among a similar group of non-diabetic individuals, it is a common complaint especially among older patients. The diabetic diet is not in itself constipating. The liberal amount of roughage afforded by 5 per cent vegetables along with the use of fruits at each meal encourage intestinal peristalsis. The diabetic is encouraged to exercise, since physical activity not only tends to

---

[1] Blaustein and Ferguson: Jour. Lab. and Clin. Med., **25**, 47, 1939.

lower the blood sugar when there is an adequate insulin supply but also is beneficial in maintaining regular bowel habits.

It is unfortunately true, however, that among diabetics, as among non-diabetics, one sees too many people who are, or who fancy that they are, constipated. Patients may consider themselves constipated, failing to realize that it may be perfectly normal to have only one bowel movement every day or every two days. When for any reason a patient begins with purgatives, often such drugs are employed in increasing amounts with the eventual result that a cathartic habit is established. That patients who have been constipated and have taken laxatives regularly for years and years can be cured of their difficulties and their bowels returned to normal function has been amply shown by Jordan,[1] Brailey,[2] Bauer[3] and others.

In the treatment of constipation as in the management of most diabetic problems, regularity is the keynote. Regularity in eating, in the taking of fluids, in sleeping, in exercise, in the time of going to the toilet—this is the most helpful, single direction that one can give. Constant repetition of advice by the physician is necessary. Patients unless continually encouraged are apt to drift back into slipshod habits of living, because for the moment such a course seems easier.

As stated above, the present diet of diabetic patients is, in a good many ways, an ideal one from the standpoint of regulation of the bowels. The abundance of vegetables and fruits is extremely helpful. Raw vegetables and coarse vegetables are, of course, useful. Great pains, however, should be taken to impress upon patients the necessity of preparing coarse vegetables in a simple manner. It is possible to cook cabbage, cauliflower, turnips, parsnips, and onions so as to be non-irritating to the digestive tract and yet preserve their laxative qualities. Diarrhea should be carefully avoided.

Physical exercise is a splendid aid in the prevention and treatment of constipation. The following exercises were prepared for the use of patients by the late Mr. Gustaf Sundelius.

1. **Abdominal Kneading and Stroking.**— *Kneading.*—Lying down, with knees slightly drawn up, place hands one on top of the other on the abdomen at the right groin; with small circular movements and deep pressure work upward until the ribs are met, then across toward left, following the boundary line of the chest, then downward to the left groin. Repeat 20 to 50 times. *Stroking.*—With hands similarly placed, make long, steady and deep strokes following the same route. Repeat 25 to 100 times.

2. **Leg Rolling.**—Grasp both legs just below knees, press knees close to abdomen, then carry them apart, then down and inward

[1] Jordan: New England Jour. Med., **203**, 826, 1930.
[2] Brailey: Ibid., **210**, 1116, 1934
[3] Bauer: Am. Jour. Digest. Dis. and Nutrition, **7**, 210, 1940.

until they meet again, thus letting the knees describe two circles. Repeat 10 to 20 times.

3. **Abdominal Compression.**—Standing against the wall with hands clasped behind neck, draw abdomen forcibly in, using the abdominal muscles, hold a second and then let go. Repeat 10 to 40 times.

4. **Trunk Rolling.**—Standing with hands on hips, feet apart and legs well stretched, roll the upper body in a circle on the hips by bending forward, to the left, backward and to the right. Then reverse, and repeat 6 to 12 times each way.

In addition to diet, exercise and regular habits it is often helpful to have the patient take 1 or 2 glasses of warm or hot water, flavored with a little table salt if desired, in the morning twenty to thirty minutes before breakfast. Often the stimulus from this, plus the gastro-colic reflex provided by the meal, will enable the patient to secure shortly after breakfast an evacuation if sufficient time is regularly left for this.

When upon special indication a cathartic is desired, any of the standard laxatives may be used. We ordinarily use the compound rhubarb pill. Often $\frac{1}{2}$ to 1 ounce of mineral oil at bedtime is helpful. Cascara sagrada, senna, magnesia, aloes or any of the other standard laxatives may be used if desired. In certain rhubarb pills the presence of peppermint or salicylate may lead to the excretion in the urine of an acid which may be confused with diacetic acid and thus lead to unwarranted alarm. Citrate of magnesia in liquid form is contraindicated. In one preparation examined there was found 11 per cent of sugar or 35 grams in one bottle.

As in non-diabetic patients one must be cautious about a change in bowel habits for such may signify a malignancy of the colon or rectum. Though probably of infrequent occurrence a thiamin deficiency may at times produce constipation as evidenced in experimentally induced thiamin deficiency in humans.[1] Case 20644, a male aged twenty-three years, with multiple vitamin deficiencies complained of extreme constipation which, after several months of treatment with large amounts of vitamins entirely disappeared.

C. DIARRHEA.

Diarrhea is a serious as well as a distressing complication in diabetic patients for with it there is loss of fluid and electrolytes, starvation or semi-starvation and a tendency to acidosis since fat catabolism is necessarily increased. Particularly if accompanied by vomiting, diarrhea may lead to coma because with abstinence from food there is often neglect to take insulin; patients often erroneously reason that they should not take any insulin because they do not eat. On the other hand, diarrhea may provoke a severe insulin reaction because the effectiveness of insulin is increased by the low

[1] Williams, Mason, Smith and Wilder: Arch. Int. Med., **69**, 721, 1942.

metabolism and the non-absorption of carbohydrate. Therefore, regard diarrhea in a diabetic seriously. One common cause is that of the irritation of coarse, bulky vegetables in a patient who has lived on a concentrated diet before the onset of diabetes or the institution of diabetic treatment. With such patients the return to a concentrated diet for a few days usually clears up the difficulty. One must not forget, however, that the diarrhea may have no such simple and easily remedied cause. In diabetics as in non-diabetics diarrhea may suggest cancer of the lower bowel, the onset of an ulcerative or a mucous colitis, an amebic dysentery, typhoid fever or other serious complicating diseases. In any diarrhea which does not respond quickly to simple measures, one should try to ascertain the true cause. If symptomatic treatment gives prompt relief, probably the diarrhea is of little consequence, but other possibilities should always be kept in mind.

Absence of free hydrochloric acid from the gastric juice may in some individuals—diabetic or non-diabetic—be associated with diarrhea, and for this reason one must consider the incidence of anacidity in diabetes and the possible rôle which this may play in any given patient. Bowen and Aaron[1] examined 10 diabetics with diarrhea and in no instance was hydrochloric acid present. Furthermore, it is true that most investigators have found among diabetics generally an increased incidence of anacidity. If one combines the published data of Bowen and Aaron,[1] McPherson,[2] Wiechmann and Elzas,[3] Root,[4] Rabinowitch, Fowler and Watson,[5] Wohl,[6] Moore[7] and Klein,[8] one finds that among 399 diabetic patients there were 131, or 32.8 per cent, with complete anacidity. These data are of great value but the anacidity alone may well bear no causal relation to diarrhea when it occurs. Bloomfield and Pollard,[9] after a careful and extensive study of gastric anacidity, concluded that this secretory defect probably does not cause diarrhea and that "in the occasional case associated with diarrhea, it is probable that coincident bowel lesions or disorders play an important part."

Pancreatic insufficiency resulting in poor digestion and inadequate absorption of food theoretically may lead to diarrhea and in several cases this has appeared to exist.

Jones and co-workers with our cases,[10] Labbé and Rechard,[11]

[1] Bowen and Aaron: Arch. Int. Med., **37**, 674, 1926.
[2] McPherson: Glasgow Med. Jour., **107**, 340, 1927.
[3] Wiechmann and Elzas: Deut. Arch. f. klin. Med., **164**, 163, 1929.
[4] Root: Jour. Am. Med. Assn., **96**, 928, 1931.
[5] Rabinowitch, Fowler, and Watson: Arch. Int. Med., **47**, 384, 1931.
[6] Wohl: Jour. Lab. and Clin. Med., **17**, 22, 1931.
[7] Moore: Brit. Med. Jour., i, 363, 1932.
[8] Klein: Deutsch. Arch. f. klin. Med., **173**, 359, 1932.
[9] Bloomfield and Pollard: Gastric Anacidity, New York, The Macmillan Company, p. 86, 1933.
[10] Jones, Castle, Mulholland, and Bailey: Loc. cit., p. 225.
[11] Labbé and Rechard: Arch. d. mal. de l'app. digest., **16**, 865, 1926.

Okada[1] and Walodin[2] have shown that impaired external secretion of the pancreas may be found in diabetes. Despite these findings, one must agree with Falta[3] that in the great bulk of diabetic patients, even in those with the disease in severe form, the digestion and absorption of food seem to take place in a completely normal fashion. Falta points out that in the pre-insulin days patients were fed enormous amounts of fat and protein with astonishingly little difficulty therefrom.

Coffey, Mann and Bollman,[4] from experiments on dogs, concluded that gross alterations in the digestive functions appear only in the *complete* absence of the external pancreatic excretions. Small amounts of pancreas were adequate to maintain complete digestion. These authors interpret their findings as making it seem rather probable that, because of the enormous factor of safety, rarely is there any disturbance in digestion due to disease of the pancreas.

When severe diarrhea occurs, the patient should be put to bed immediately, kept warm and for a few hours given only water, hot weak tea and oatmeal gruel, made with water, which is thoroughly cooked and strained. A half ounce of dry oatmeal will make $\frac{1}{2}$ pint of gruel, 4 per cent carbohydrate. Remaining without food for a few hours is allowable, but this should not go on for long. Then the carbohydrate of the diet should be resumed with simple foods such as gruel, crackers, toast, rice, macaroni, grapejuice or gingerale. For the carbohydrate content see Food Tables, page 810. See also Table 30 for the equivalent of the standard diet in simple and non-irritating forms. The return to the diabetic diet is rendered easy by the use of cottage cheese, soft cream cheese, lean meat, oatmeal, milk, cream, biscuits, eggs and puréed vegetables. Carefully prepared tender vegetables are frequently better borne than a diet containing considerable quantities of albuminous and fatty foods.

If liquid is not retained by mouth, it may be necessary to give physiologic solution of sodium chloride with or without 5 per cent glucose subcutaneously or intravenously. If there is any undigested food remaining in the stomach, this should be removed by lavage. The lower bowel should be cleared with an enema. In obstinate cases a teaspoonful of bismuth subcarbonate or as a last resort, an opiate, may be given before each meal and after each loose movement.

Diarrhea may necessitate the decrease or increase of insulin. If more insulin is required it is safer to give it in smaller doses more frequently.

Bargan, Bollman and Kepler[5] reported several cases of diarrhea of undetermined origin and referred to the condition as the "diarrhea of diabetes." In these cases no failure of external pancreatic secre-

[1] Okada *et al.*:   Proc. Imperial Acad. (Japan), **4**, 134. 1928.
[2] Walodin: Arch. f. Verdauungskrankh., **49**, 168, 1931.
[3] Falta: Loc. cit., p 389.
[4] Coffey, Mann and Bollman: Jour. Digest. Dis. and Nutr., **7**, 144, 1940
[5] Bargan, Bollman and Kepler: Proc. Staff Meet. Mayo Clin., **11**, 737, 1936.

tion could be demonstrated and the administration of pancreatic juice did not correct the abnormality as was the case in patients with steatorrhea caused by pancreatic insufficiency. Owens[1] also noted persistent and unexplained diarrhea in several diabetic patients at the Cincinnati General Hospital. All of these cleared up with careful diabetic control except for one patient, a man aged forty years whose nocturnal diarrhea continued.

Recently 40 cases of this unusual type of diarrhea occurring in diabetic patients at the George F. Baker Clinic were reported by Sheridan and Bailey.[2] The characteristic symptomatology in this series consisted of diarrhea occurring chiefly or entirely at night. There might be little or no diarrhea during the day, yet the patient might have 10 to 15 brown, watery stools during the night. It tended to occur intermittently in 34 patients (85 per cent) with remission lasting for several days followed by relapse. Nocturnal incontinence of feces occurred in 31 cases (78 per cent).

In this series the age of onset varied from twenty to seventy-nine years with an average duration of diabetes of nine years. There were 23 males and 17 females. Roentgenological examination of the upper gastro-intestinal tract in 17 cases and a barium enema in 28 cases were all negative except for increased spasticity of the colon observed in 6. Fifteen cases studied proctoscopically had normal mucosa. Achlorhydria, even after histamine, occurred in 14 of 29 patients.

Only 2 of the 40 cases had erythrocyte counts below 4 million per c.mm. and these had 3.94 and 3.82 million respectively. The hemoglobin averaged 90.6 per cent. Blood Hinton tests were negative in 39 and doubtful in 1.

Previous poor diabetic control as evidenced by hyperglycemia and glycosuria was outstanding in each of the 40 cases and diabetic neuritis preceded the diarrhea in 23 patients. Seventeen of 18 cases showed a definite elevation of the spinal fluid protein averaging 88 mg. per 100 cc. whereas in 6 cases values of over 100 mg. per 100 cc. were found.

Therapy consisting of chemotherapy (sulfasuccidine and sulfa-guanidine), hydrochloric acid, vitamins and drugs exerting a costive effect, has proven of little value. A low residue, non-irritating diet is always prescribed. It was found, however, that crude liver extract given parenterally was of definite benefit in controlling the diarrhea in 26 of 28 cases in which it was used. Injection of 2 to 4 cc. of the extract daily for a few days, followed by a maintenance dose of 1 to 2 cc. weekly, usually proved adequate. Lapses in treatment is usually followed by a relapse of diarrhea.

Despite the unexplained symptomatic improvement with liver extract, it is believed that this diarrheal syndrome probably repre-

[1] Owens: Personal communication.
[2] Sheridan and Bailey: Jour. Am. Med. Assn., **130**, 632, 1946.

sents a nerve disturbance of the bowel, possibly involvement of the sympathetic nerves, on the basis of diabetic neuropathy. Only 2 cases have recovered completely; both had diabetic neuritis and with cure of the neuritis the diarrhea disappeared.

Dr. Wayne Rundles in a personal communication reports that he has studied over 40 patients with diabetic neuropathy associated with gastro-intestinal symptoms by small intestinal roentgen examination and found motility not simply increased or decreased but really disorganized. He further points out that in addition to diarrhea, which is frequently nocturnal, a number of diabetics have alternating diarrhea and constipation. We, too, have noticed the alternating diarrhea and constipation in a few patients of which Case 10015 is an excellent example.

D. ULCER: GASTRIC OR DUODENAL.

From 1934 to 1944 among 12,000 diabetic patients observed in the George F. Baker Clinic at the Deaconess Hospital, peptic ulcer was diagnosed in 94 cases, an incidence of 0.89 per cent. A summary of this series has been made by Wood.[1] The disease occurred in 68 males and 26 females whose age ranged from twenty-three to seventy-four years at the beginning of ulcer symptoms. However, ulcer symptoms began usually in the older age groups and actually 73 patients were past the age of forty when symptoms first were noticed. The series includes 74 patients with single duodenal ulcers and 11 with single gastric ulcers. The presence of both gastric and duodenal ulcers were found in three instances by x-ray. Surgical specimens revealed an additional 5 cases with both gastric and duodenal ulcers. One of the surgical specimens had 4 ulcers and another 3,

Fifty-nine patients had diabetes for varying periods of time before the onset of ulcer symptoms and the remaining 35 patients had peptic ulcer first and developed diabetes later. A striking feature of the series was the fact that in 50 patients typical ulcer pain with respect to severity, relationship to food and localization of pain was lacking. In 4 no pain whatever was admitted. Symptoms consisted of vague, generalized, abdominal discomfort, without relation to meals and the patient often described the symptoms as "mild indigestion which didn't really bother me at all." Forty-four described definite pain, well localized and associated with food relief but rarely was the pain severe enough to awaken the patient at night.

Gastric acidity was determined in 58 cases. In 21, no free hydrochloric acid was obtained in the first specimen, in 18 cases the value was under 20 degrees, in 12 cases between 21 and 40 degrees and in

[1] Wood: To be published.

7, over 40 degrees. Five patients revealed no free hydrochloric acid even after the injection of histamine.

Among the 94 patients with peptic ulcer the diabetes was considered mild in 58 cases requiring from 0 to 25 units a day, moderate in 30 cases requiring 26 to 50 units, and severe in 6 cases requiring 51 to 75 units a day. A total of 7 cases in this series had diabetic coma subsequently to the onset of the ulcer.

The development of severe ulcer complications was unusually frequent and occurred at an average age of 61.6 years when the ulcer had been present an average of 6.0 years. Thus 54 individuals developed either massive hemorrhage, obstruction, perforation or gastric carcinoma.

Gross or massive hemorrhage occurred in 24 cases, in 2 of which it was fatal. In 8 others strongly positive tests for occult blood in the stool in addition to anemia indicated that some bleeding had occurred. Generalized arteriosclerosis was recognized in 42 patients not merely from palpation of the radial arteries but by study of the heart, kidney function and cerebral symptoms. Undoubtedly the age of the patient and the presence of generalized arteriosclerosis in the vessels supplying the region of the ulcer is an important factor in the frequency of severe hemorrhage. Case 14416, a female aged sixty years, developed a massive hemorrhage from a duodenal ulcer which required operation. Dr. L. S. McKittrick found a rigid artery projecting from the posterior wall of the duodenum illustrating well the special hazard to which arteriosclerotic vessels subject these patients. Her recovery from the emergency operation was complete.

Perforation occurred in 10 cases or 10.6 per cent of the series; in 2 cases perforation preceded the onset of the diabetes. Double or triple perforations occurred in 2 cases.

Gastric obstruction and retention was the largest single serious complication. In 32 cases or 34 per cent of all the diabetics with ulcers, obstruction was demonstrated by x-ray or operation. Five of these cases required a subtotal gastrectomy and 1 a posterior gastro-enterostomy. Major operations were performed in 13 cases among the whole series of 94 cases.

Five deaths occurred in the hospital, 2 from acute hemorrhage, 1 with an acute perforation and peritonitis and 2 postoperatively from embolism and from peritonitis.

Subsequent follow-up of these 94 patients revealed that 40 were completely relieved of symptoms, when last seen, as a result either of medical or surgical treatment and 20 were improved but were not wholly free from symptoms. In 34 cases a definite recurrence of symptoms in the form of hemorrhage, perforation or other symptoms had occurred.

The incidence of peptic ulcer among diabetics has provoked considerable discussion. Among Lande's[1] 2100 diabetic patients there were 22 with ulcers of the stomach or duodenum. Falta[2] had not encountered a single case of peptic ulcer among his 1403 diabetic patients. Among 2584 diabetic patients seen at the Mayo Clinic[3] in the three years 1935 to 1937 the diagnosis of peptic ulcer was made in 61 or 2.3 per cent, whereas, among patients of all types seen in 1937 the incidence of duodenal ulcer was 3.7 per cent. Rothenberg and Teicher[4] found peptic ulcer in 9 or 0.25 per cent of 3525 diabetic patients as contrasted with an incidence of 1.49 per cent among 130,500 total hospital admissions. A recent report by Spiegelman and Marks[5] shows that throughout the country approximately three-quarters of the diabetic patients are over fifty years of age. Peptic ulcer on the other hand is known to be most prevalent in younger individuals. It may be that if age differences and duration of life are considered the incidence of peptic ulcer in diabetic patients may equal that in the whole population.

Treatment of peptic ulcer in diabetics follow the same general scheme as in non-diabetics with the following exceptions: (1) The diabetic diet of necessity does not contain highly concentrated carbohydrate foods. (2) Hyperglycemia and glycosuria must be controlled. (3) Extremely high fat with very low carbohydrate diets are limited to a very few days or avoided entirely. Strict adherence to the program of rest, frequent bland feedings and control of the diabetic condition is essential in treatment.

E. DIVERTICULA OF THE DUODENUM.

Cases 3782 and 13253 were found on roentgen-ray examination to have diverticula of the duodenum and reported by Thorning and Root.[6] Since then 16 more cases have been recognized. The 2 published cases had had previous operations for gall stones and Case 13253 had a nodular enlargement of the liver due presumably to metastatic carcinoma. The possibility that inflammation in or about diverticula such as these can by extension cause chronic pancreatitis and diabetes[7] was not demonstrable in these cases.

F. GASTRO-INTESTINAL HEMORRHAGES IN THE DIABETIC.

Hemorrhage into the gastro-intestinal tract of diabetic patients occurs very readily. As mentioned above, gross hemorrhage from peptic ulcers occurred in 26.6 per cent of our cases.

[1] Lande: Klin. Wchnschr., 10, 359, 1931.
[2] Falta: Loc. cit., p. 389.
[3] Wilder: P. 303, loc. cit., p. 55.
[4] Rothenberg and Teicher: Am. Jour. Digest. Dis. and Nutrition, 5, 359, 1931.
[5] Spiegelman and Marks: Loc. cit., p. 29.
[6] Thorning and Root: Am. Jour. Digest. Dis. and Nutrition, 2, 17, 1935.
[7] Fulde: Deut. Arch. f. klin. Med., 173, 404, 1932.

In diabetic coma the stomach is often found to be distended with fluid containing changed blood. A third, although uncommon, cause of gastric hemorrhage in the diabetic is a severe insulin reaction. In an adult with convulsions after an overdose of insulin there was a gastric hemorrhage, and in several children a gastric hemorrhage has been observed in the course of a severe reaction in which the child was unconscious several hours.

Case 6562 had three massive hemorrhages from her upper gastro-intestinal tract, vomiting large amounts of blood. Roentgenological examinations have repeatedly failed to show an ulcer or cancer, but a gastroscopic examination by Dr. Edward Benedict revealed an extensive gastritis of undetermined origin.

G. CANCER OF THE GASTRO-INTESTINAL TRACT.

Cancer of the gastro-intestinal tract and particularly cancer of the pancreas in association with diabetes are of great interest. A full discussion will be found in Chapter XXIV.

H. SPECIFIC DISORDERS OF THE LIVER IN DIABETES.

1. **Hepatitis.**—Hepatitis may occur in diabetic as in non-diabetic patients. Droller[1] reported 63 cases of hepatitis occurring among diabetic patients at the Royal Hospital, Sheffield during a time when there was a high incidence of the disease in the general population. The injection of the gamma globulin fraction of blood may afford protection from this disease.[2]

Root[3] reported the striking case of a young woman (Case 6533), aged thirty-four years, with diabetes of seven years' duration with severe, acute hepatitis and jaundice, acidosis without ketonuria, anuria, nitrogen retention and macrocytic anemia. Recovery took place with the use of insulin, parenterally administered glucose, carbohydrate by mouth as permitted, concentrated salt solution intravenously to aid urinary secretion, and liver extract.

2. **Cirrhosis of the Liver.**—Cirrhosis of the liver has not been a common complication. In the five year period from 1940 through 1945 among 10235 diabetic admissions to the George F. Baker clinic there were 52 cases of cirrhosis of the liver—an average of 10.4 cases each year, or an incidence of 0.51 per cent. When it has occurred, it has usually resulted in an increase of the severity of the diabetes, due presumably to the disturbance of the glycogenic function of the liver. Rarely, however, the influence of the cirrhosis may be the exact opposite as in the case reported by Bordley.[4] This patient, a sea captain, was studied over a period of years at the

[1] Droller: Brit. Med. Jour., 1, 623, 1945.
[2] Stokes and Neefe: Jour. Am. Med. Assn., 127, 144, 1945.
[3] Root: New England Jour. Med., 212, 545, 1935.
[4] Bordley: Bull. Johns Hopkins Hosp., 47, 113, 1930.

Johns Hopkins Hospital and required at intervals abdominal tapping to relieve ascites. At the beginning he had undoubted diabetes, but as the years went on and the process in the liver developed, the diabetes became milder and milder and finally could not be demonstrated by sugar-tolerance tests. A somewhat similar case in an elderly man was described by Strieck[1] while working in Grafe's Clinic in Würzburg and another discussed in the Cabot Case Series of the Massachusetts General Hospital.[2] The last-named patient died with multiple abscesses of the kidneys.

Hart and Lisa[3] report the case of a confirmed alcoholic who developed cirrhosis of the liver with ascites. Diabetes was discovered at the same time and controlled with diet and insulin. Following tapping of the abdomen at the first visit there was no further evidence of ascites for seven years nor was there any further sign of progression of the cirrhosis. Following death from bronchopneumonia, autopsy showed a hob-nail liver with a surprisingly small amount of scarring. The authors regard the fact that ascites was arrested shortly after the diabetes was brought under control as more than coincidental. Schleusner,[4] of the Barmbeck General Hospital in Hamburg, analyzed 355 autopsy protocols of diabetic patients dying between the years 1930 and 1936. Among these there were 45 patients, 24 men and 21 women, who showed macroscopic evidence of cirrhosis of the liver. This incidence of 12.7 per cent is extraordinarily high. Schleusner states that in only one-third of the cases was the cirrhosis so outspoken that it could be diagnosed clinically. In 6 cases rupture of esophageal varices caused death. Schleusner was able to study carefully the histories of 20 of the 45 cases; in all instances the onset of diabetes seemed to antedate that of cirrhosis of the liver. The high incidence in Schleusner's series contrasts with that reported by Wilder[5] who states: "Cirrhosis is very uncommon. Evidence of it or of hepatitis was encountered at the Mayo Clinic in only 17 (0.7 per cent) of our 2584 separate cases of diabetes in the years 1935, 1936 and 1937, and when hepatic disease was found it seemed rarely to be related to the diabetes or to affect it seriously."

3. **Enlargement of the Liver.**—In the several years just prior to the introduction of protamine zinc insulin we came to regard hepatomegaly as one of the outstanding complications of juvenile diabetes. Sixty cases, occurring among 1077 children, were reported.[6]

[1] Strieck: Deut. Arch. f. klin. Med., **178**, 167, 1935.

[2] Kranes, Jones, Root, and Mallory: New England Jour. Med., **214**, 1314, 1936.

[3] Hart and Lisa: New York State Jour. Med., **38**, 1158, 1938.

[4] Schleusner: Ueber die Zusammenhänge zwischen Diabetes mellitus und Erkrankungen der Leber und der Gallenwege, Marburg-Lahn, Herman Bauer, 1938.

[5] Wilder: Page 309, loc. cit., p. 55.

[6] Marble, White, Bogan and Smith: Arch. Int Med., **62**, 740, 1938.

Similar cases had been described by Hanssen[1] and by Mauriac.[2] Our patients all had severe, poorly controlled diabetes and approximately one-third of them were true diabetic dwarfs. The enlargement of the liver was well-marked, with the lower edge of the organ to be found not infrequently in the pelvis. An enlarged spleen was noted in 31 cases. The abdomen was usually enlarged to gross inspection and bouts of abdominal pain were common. To abdominal palpation the edge of the liver was soft or rapidly became soft and difficult to palpate when the diabetes had been brought under control. Moderate hypercholesterinemia was the rule; little or no decrease in the percentage of combined (ester) cholesterol was present. Because of Best's[3] work with animals, we treated these patients with betaine over periods as long as eight months but without added benefit of striking degree, although in 50 per cent of cases there was a gradual diminution in size. With the good control of the diabetic condition, made possible by protamine zinc insulin, decrease in the size of the liver occurred in 79 per cent of cases.[4]

We have assumed that the enlargement of the liver in these children with poorly controlled diabetes is due primarily to gross fatty infiltration.[5] The condition certainly should be regarded as distinct from glycogen storage (von Gierke's) disease, although it is probable that the amounts of glycogen may in some cases approach the normal. A possible contributory factor in the enlargement is hydropic degeneration with retention of water. It is more difficult than one might suppose to find the report of an autopsy on a diabetic child with gross hepatomegaly apart from complicating diseases known to produce enlargement of the liver. In the case reported by Brian, Schecter and Persons[6] it seemed likely that the enlargement of the liver was not due to fat, although conclusions in this case were difficult to draw because chemical studies were not carried out until after eighteen months' storage in a dilute solution of formaldehyde. Furthermore, we know of only one report in the literature of a biopsy in such patients. This was the account of Stetson and Ohler[7] whose patient was a twelve-year-old boy with diabetes, enlargement of the liver and spleen, ascites, jaundice and mild fever; microscopic examination of biopsy material showed a tremendous amount of intracellular glucogen. (See page 133.)

One of our own cases was noteworthy in this regard.

Case 6884, a young woman, aged twenty-five years, with diabetes of eleven years' duration reentered the New England Deaconess Hospital

[1] Hanssen: Jour. Am. Med. Assn., **106**, 914, 1936.
[2] Mauriac: Paris Med., **2**, 525, 1934.
[3] Best: Lancet, **1**, 1274, 1934.
[4] White, Marble, Bogan and Smith: Loc. cit., p. 134.
[5] Marble, White, Bogan and Smith: Loc. cit., p. 134.
[6] Brian, Schecter and Persons: Arch. Int. Med., **59**, 685, 1937.
[7] Stetson and Ohler: New England Jour. Med., **217**, 627, 1937.

March 9, 1940 because of abdominal pain. Throughout most of her diabetic life her condition had been under poor control; she had had diabetic
coma several times and had had many admissions both at the Boston City
Hospital and the New England Deaconess Hospital. At this admission the
liver was found to be greatly enlarged. For other reasons which made the
procedure justifiable abdominal exploration was carried out, and in the course
of this a biopsy of the liver was taken. The finding of a large amount of
fat, 10.15 per cent, was not unexpected, but we were surprised to find the
glycogen content to be extraordinarily high, 12.1 per cent. The cause of
the high glycogen content was not clear although it may have been a manifestation of temporary hyperinsulinism, a carry-over from the protamine
zinc insulin given the day before. This idea is strengthened by the fact
that the fasting blood sugar on the morning of the operation was very low,
0.03 per cent. Incidentally, it is of interest that the patient suffered little
or no subjective hypoglycemic symptoms. Of significance was the normal
respiratory quotient, 0.82, obtained just before the operation with the
patient in the postabsorptive state. The patient died October 5, 1944, of
pneumonia. (See pages 175, 212, 220, 394, 573 and 758.)

Changes in the liver lipids can take place rapidly after the administration of insulin, as stated by Loubatieres and Monnier,[1] who
found that following removal of the pancreas from a dog the fat
content of the liver rose from 6.8 to 12.1 per cent. Yet within
twenty-four hours after insulin was given the fat content had
returned to almost the original value, 8 per cent.

4. **Liver Function in Diabetes.**—Gray, Hook and Batty,[2] using
the serum colloidal gold reaction, which they considered sensitive in
detecting early liver disease, report a positive test in 91 of 247
patients with diabetes, an incidence of 36.8 per cent. Evidence of
liver disturbance was found in 43.2 per cent of 148 patients receiving
irregular diabetic care as compared, with 27.1 per cent of 99 patients
under constant supervision. Furthermore, a positive test occurred
in 62 (49.9 per cent) of 123 patients with severe diabetes in contrast
to 29 (23.3 per cent) of 124 patients with mild diabetes, and in 26.3
per cent of diabetics with their diabetes under good control in contrast to 57.1 per cent of patients with poorly controlled diabetes.
No significant difference in the frequency of liver involvement was
apparent between the younger and older age groups.

Meyer[3] studied by various tests the liver function in 100 diabetic
patients at the Philadelphia General Hospital. Twenty-eight per
cent gave laboratory evidence of hepatic dysfunction. A review of
the literature including that of liver function tests in general is
given. Strikingly similar to the results of Meyer were those of
Rabinowitch.[4] Among 3000 analyses of the blood of diabetic
patients he found excess quantities of bilirubin in 27.4 per cent
(assuming the normal range to lie between 0.2 and 0.5 unit) and
among an equal number of analyses of urine he found excess quan-

[1] Loubatieres and Monnier: Compt. rend. Soc. de biol., **130**, 854, 1939.
[2] Gray, Hook and Batty: Ann. Int. Med., **24**, 72, 1946.
[3] Meyer: Arch. Int. Med., **47**, 182, 1931.
[4] Rabinowitch: Brit. Jour. Exp. Path., **17**, 249, 1936.

tities of urobilinogen in 27.5 per cent (assuming that detection in dilutions greater than 1 in 20 is abnormal). Rabinowitch regarded these data as proof of a high incidence of liver disease among diabetics. Somogyi[1] interpreted a high incidence of subnormal and borderline values for blood diastase among 382 diabetic patients as indicating disturbed liver function.

Schleusner[2] apparently considered that liver damage occurs commonly in diabetic patients citing as evidence the frequently elevated values for bilirubin. He stated that among 80 diabetics studied from July to September 1936 an average value of 1.15 units was found. It is difficult to understand this high incidence of disturbed liver function and of cirrhosis of the liver which Schleusner reports. In the authors' experience it is not common to find striking evidence of such among patients whose diabetes is under good control and whose diets contain 100 to 150 or more grams of carbohydrate a day.

I. HEMOCHROMATOSIS.

Hemochromatosis with diabetes is an uncommon disease. John[3] encountered only one case among 4491 diabetic patients. Only 30 cases were observed at the Mayo Clinic in fifteen years.[4]

Marble and Bailey[5] have analyzed the records of 24 cases of hemochromatosis proven either by autopsy or skin biopsy, seen in the George F. Baker Clinic among approximately 21500 diabetic patients since 1922. This series of cases is especially interesting since (a) 2 of the cases were women and hemochromatosis is rare in females, (b) 4 of the patients are still living, the duration of diabetes being 15.3, 11.0, 3.7 and 1.7 years respectively, (c) 1 case, 6247, developed marked insulin resistance and died in diabetic coma despite having received 1600 units of insulin daily for the three days prior to the day of death, (d) another case, 12069, diagnosed hemochromatosis in 1933 is alive and working thirteen years later. Careful iron metabolism studies have been reported in this patient by Marble and Smith.[6] (e) Five cases failed to show skin pigmentation but had other characteristic signs and symptoms. Four of these were proven by autopsy and one by skin biopsy.

The outstanding symptoms and signs among the 24 cases were (1) brownish or grayish-brown pigmentation in 19 cases, (2) hepatomegaly in all cases, (3) splenomegaly in 17, (4) loss of weight and weakness in all cases, (5) abdominal pain in 10 and (6) ascites in 8. A diabetic heredity was detected in 7 cases.

Four patients took alcohol moderately or excessively, 6 rarely and

[1] Somogyi: Jour. Biol. Chem., **134**, 315, 1940.
[2] Schleusner: Loc. cit., p. 544.
[3] John: Jour. Am. Med. Assn., **112**, 2272, 1939.
[4] Butt and Wilder: Arch. Path., **26**, 262, 1938.
[5] Marble and Bailey: To be published.
[6] Marble and Smith: Ann. Int. Med., **12**, 1592, 1939.

13 were abstainers. Of the total number, 20 are fatal cases of which the diagnosis of hemochromatosis was confirmed at autopsy in 11.

In addition to the 24 proven cases of hemochromatosis described above 13 cases have enlarged livers, diabetes and skin pigmentation highly suggestive of the disease. Ten of these have splenomegaly. In 7 of the 13 cases the skin biopsy did not show the deposition of iron pigments but it is known that a negative skin biopsy may occur in definite cases of hemochromatosis. Nine of the 13 patients are still alive.

The etiology of hemochromatosis itself remains obscure. Mallory's[1] suggestion, based on laboratory studies, regarding chronic poisoning with copper as the important cause of hemo-chromatosis, has not found general acceptance clinically. Dry[2] considered from his studies that there is no evidence to show that the excess of iron in hemochromatosis is the result of excessive hemolysis or that the retained food iron is itself the cause of the disease. He suggested that it may be an "inborn error of metabolism expressing itself as a disturbed intracellular circulation of iron leading to increase in the amounts normally present with ultimate destruction of the cell and replacement by fibrous tissue." Since this process goes on so slowly, it does not usually become marked enough to cause symptoms until the patient is in middle life. Much the same conclusion was stated by Sheldon[3] in an excellent monograph on hemochromatosis in which he considered the condition from every possible angle and based his statements on an analysis of 311 cases collected from the literature. He pointed out that the metabolic error evidences itself in two ways, (1) by a disturbance in the metabolism of melanin with deposits of hemofuscin in smooth muscle and connective-tissue cells and a great increase in the normal deposit of melanin in the deeper layers of the epidermis and (2) by the formation of an iron-containing pigment in nearly all the tissues.

One of our own patients, Case 12069, a man, aged fifty years, was studied carefully from the standpoint of his iron metabolism.[4] During four periods of three days each with an average intake of 16.9 mg. of iron a day, there was an average excretion of 0.4 mg. per day in the urine and 14.7 mg. per day in the feces, making a total output of 15.1 mg. per day and an average daily retention of 1.8 mg. The small amount of iron retained daily is in keeping with the theory that in hemochromatosis the accumulation of iron in the tissues takes place over years of time, probably a lifetime. Sheldon[3] states that the total iron content of the body of individuals dying with hemochromatosis varies from 25 to 50 grams as compared with the normal of about 3 grams. Taking the figures obtained with our patient as an example, if 1.8 mg. of iron were retained daily during a lifetime of fifty years, a total of slightly less than 33 grams would accumulate. It is

[1] Mallory, Parker and Nye: Jour. Med. Res., **42**, 461, 1921.
[2] Dry: Minnesota Med., **18**, 301, 1934.
[3] Sheldon: Hæmochromatosis, London, Oxford University Press, 1935.
[4] Marble and Smith: Ann. Int. Med., **12**, 1592, 1939.

possible, of course, that at certain stages of the disease iron is retained in excessive amounts not demonstrable later. This possibility is suggested by the results of Fowler and Barer.[1]

The outstanding features of hemochromatosis are diabetes, cirrhosis of the liver and pigmentation of the skin. The characteristic symptoms are increasing weakness, fatigability, loss of weight and strength, impotence, increasing pigmentation of the skin and abdominal distress or pain. Physical examination reveals, besides the signs of weight loss, atrophy of the prostate gland and testes, scanty axillary and pubic hair and the brown or bronze color of the skin which is more striking on the exposed surfaces and particularly prominent upon the exterior surface of the lower end of the forearms and the backs of the hands. In Case 12069 the pigmentation was so marked that after he had spent a summer in the sun at a bathing beach, he was taken for a negro. The abdomen is usually enlarged, distention is present and in the later stages large quantities of free fluid may be present and require paracentesis. The liver is large and may be tender, and often the spleen is palpable. There may be distention of the superficial veins along the costal margin and over the lower chest. Secondary anemia usually is present. The blood-pressure may be low but usually does not reach the level so characteristic of Addison's disease with which at times hemochromatosis may be confused.

Campbell, Adler and Hart[2] report a case of biliary cirrhosis with diabetes mellitus and pigmentation of the skin. Microscopic examination of a piece of liver removed at biopsy showed definite cirrhosis with marked pigmentation of the hepatic cells and particularly deep pigmentation of the epithelium of the bile ducts in the portal canals; there was no pigmentation of the connective tissue. Campbell and co-workers regard the distribution of the pigment as characteristic of biliary cirrhosis and not hemochromatosis. They suggest that some of the cases of hemochromatosis reported in the literature may have been falsely diagnosed. Beardwood and Rouse[3] believe that a diagnosis of hemochromatosis is justified only if iron pigment is actually demonstrated in the skin or internal organs.

Labbé, Boulin and Uhry[4] report 4 cases, 1 of whom was a woman. They state that evidences of involvement of endocrine glands other than the pancreas are often seen in cases of hemochromatosis. In 2 cases, postmortem examination showed degenerative changes in the testicles and in the thyroid and hypophysis. In 2 of them, loss of hair, especially over the pubes and in the axilla with atrophy of the testicles and impotence were prominent. In a woman, aged forty years, there was premature amenorrhea, atrophy of the breasts, and loss of the axillary and pubic hair. In all the cases, the skin

[1] Fowler and Barer: Jour. Lab. and Clin. Med., **23**, 47, 1937.
[2] Campbell, Adler and Hart: New York State Jour. Med., **38**, 1342, 1938.
[3] Beardwood and Rouse: Clinics **3**, 251, Aug. 1944.
[4] Labbé, Boulin and Uhry: Presse méd., **27**, 537, 1936.

was dry, brown and scaly.   Although the thyroid gland was involved, there was no lowering of the basal metabolism.

It is noteworthy that hemochromatosis occurs so seldom in women, but this is a finding reported by all observers.   Sheldon[1] found reports in the literature of only 16 cases in females and in 3 of these there was no postmortem examination.   One of the 2 cases reported recently by Harrington and Aitkenhead[2] was a woman with a large cirrhotic liver, moderate ascites, marked pigmentation, and severe diabetes, who finally died of sepsis.   Two of our own patients were women; an autopsy was done in 1 case and in the other a positive test was obtained upon biopsy of a bit of skin.   Lawrence[3] describes a family of nine in which two brothers had hemochromatosis.   Three other brothers and the mother, but none of the sisters, had some signs of the disease.

Boulin[4] reported 70 cases of bronze diabetes seen in a period of fifteen years among 4266 diabetic patients.   Fifty-nine cases were in men and 11 in women.   Five of his patients failed to show cirrhosis of the liver or diabetes.   He reports that insulin resistance may develop quickly and may be progressive.

Patients with hemochromatosis may require extraordinarily large amounts of insulin, although this is by no means an invariable rule. Among our 24 patients the daily dosage ranged from zero to 1680 units a day (Case 6247 reported by Root).[5]   In 11 of the 24 cases the daily dosage was under 50 units.   Cases requiring enormous amounts of insulin have been reported by Miller and Heinmark[6] and by Allan and Constam.[7]   John's[8] patient was relatively insensitive to insulin, especially to the protamine zinc variety, and at times as much as 140 units a day were given.

Diagnosis, particularly in an early case, may be verified by the findings of intracellular granules of hemosiderin in the urinary sediment[9] and by removal of a small bit of skin for examination of evidences of deposited iron pigment.   Care must be used not to take the skin from the axillæ or groin or from any part of the body where normally small amounts of iron pigment may accompany the characteristically large amounts of melanin.   The bit of skin must be dropped immediately into 80 per cent alcohol or formalin so that it can be kept in suitable condition for histological study.   Fishback[10] has suggested the intradermal injection of a small amount of

1 Sheldon: Loc. cit., p. 548.
2 Harrington and Aitkenhead: Glasgow Med. Jour., **14**, 61, 1939.
3 Lawrence: Lancet, **2**, 1055, 1935.
4 Boulin: Presse Med., **53**, 326, 1945.
5 Root: New England Jour. Med., **201**, 201, 1929.
6 Miller and Heinmark: Minnesota Med., **14**, 260, 1931.
7 Allan and Constam: Med. Clin. North America, **12**, 1677, 1929.
8 John: Jour. Am. Med. Assn., **112**, 2272, 1939.
9 Rous: Jour. Exp. Med., **28**, 645, 1918.
10 Fishback: Jour. Lab. and Clin. Med., **25**, 98, 1939.

fluid made up of equal parts of a sterile 0.5 per cent solution of potassium ferrocyanide and N/100 hydrochloric acid. If abnormal amounts of iron are present in the skin the wheal may turn a slight blue almost immediately; this darkens to a deep blue within five minutes. To demonstrate hemosiderin in the urine a fresh sample is centrifuged and the sediment suspended in 10 cc. of a fresh mixture containing equal parts of a 2 per cent potassium ferrocyanide and 1 per cent hydrochloric acid. After standing for ten minutes this is centrifuged and a drop of 1 per cent hydrochloric acid is added to a drop of the sediment on a slide. Blue intracellular granules indicate the presence of iron.

Liver function tests are valuable but in early cases may yield normal results due to the great margin of safety of the liver. Sachs, Levine and Griffith[1] determined the iron content of the blood, finding in normal men an average of 50 mg. per 100 cc., whereas in 3 men with hemochromatosis the values ranged from 88.9 to 74.4 per cent of these figures. However, an increase in the content of iron in the blood by no means invariably occurs in hemochromatosis. In Case 12069 already referred to, values for iron in the blood were found on several occasions to be well within normal limits, ranging from 43 to 47 mg. per cent. Recently Dr. Priscilla White has detected a marked reduction in the excretion of 17-ketosteroids in the urine of patients with hemochromatosis and in some the excretion has been essentially zero in twenty-four hours.

Treatment of hemochromatosis is unsatisfactory. Control of the diabetic condition may in some cases be difficult because of the large amounts of insulin required, but this is of little moment in comparison with the fact that one usually is able to delay very little the progress of the disease. Nevertheless in some patients (as in Case 12069) progression may take place very slowly, indeed. Gray[2] reports a man who lived eleven years after the diagnosis had been definitely established by biopsy of the skin and thirteen years after the first appearance of skin pigmentation.

During the past two years Dr. Priscilla White, on the basis of low 17-ketosteroid excretion in the urine and atrophy of the testes and prostate has treated several male patients with hemochromatosis with testosterone parenterally with gratifying results. There has been a return of strength, partial regrowth of axillary and pubic hair, increased potency and an improvement in general health.

It is preferable because of the lowered liver function to give a diet liberal in carbohydrate (at least 180 grams a day) and relatively low in fat because of the well-known difficulty which the liver has, when damaged, to deal with this substance. The use of concentrated

[1] Sachs, Levine and Griffith: Proc. Soc. Exp. Biol. and Med., **35**, 332, 1936.
[2] Gray: Ann. Int. Med., **19**, 501, 1943.

vitamin preparations, especially those containing vitamins A and B, may be helpful, as has been emphasized by Wilder.[1]

Abdominal paracentesis may be necessary to relieve the distention and distress caused by ascites. The food should, of course, be concentrated rather than bulky to avoid distention of the bowel and the formation of gas. The patient's activity must of necessity be somewhat curtailed.

J. APPENDICITIS.

For discussion, see page 707.

K. GALL STONES AND GALL-BLADDER DISEASE.

1. **Incidence of Gall Stones Among Diabetics.**—That disease of the gall-bladder is more common in the diabetic than in the general population seems definitely established. Warren[2] found at autopsy cholelithiasis in 139, and cholecystitis without stone in 28, of 453 diabetics over thirty years of age as contrasted with 107 and 14 instances, respectively, in 500 non-diabetics in the same age-group. Thus the incidence of gall stones alone was 30.7 per cent in the diabetic as compared with 21.4 per cent in the non-diabetic group. In 197 autopsies on diabetic patients at the Mayo Clinic between 1919 and 1936, gall stones either were present or had been removed at an operation in 66 or 33.5 per cent of the cases.[3]

Although approximately 1 in 4 diabetic patients are found to have gall stones at autopsy, by no means are all the cases recognized during life. In 1928, 5400 cases, including 4003 true diabetics over twenty years of age, were studied with this point in mind. Data were compiled from clinical histories, surgical operations and autopsies. One hundred ninety-nine cases, or 5 per cent, were found in 4589 cases of true diabetes. The average age at diagnosis of cholelithiasis in 189 cases was 47.7 years and of the diabetes in 199 cases was 51.3 years, thus showing a definite but not marked precedence of gall stones. A common etiology might be inferred by some from such data. Forty of the patients were males and 159 females, thus again emphasizing the need for the prevention of diabetes in females.

Gall-bladder disease has not been prominent as the chief cause of death in our patients. Of 4507 deaths from 1922 to 1940, only 21 were ascribed by the attending physician to gall-bladder disease. Among 1852 diabetic admissions to the George F. Baker Clinic in 1938 there were recognized 21 cases of gall-bladder disease. Our youngest patient was a girl, Case 10646, whose gall stones were removed in 1931, eighteen months after the onset of diabetes at thirteen years.

---

[1] Wilder: P. 325, loc. cit., p. 55.
[2] Warren: P. 106, loc. cit., p. 196.
[3] Wilder, p. 311; loc. cit., p. 55.

Among 68 unselected cases of diabetes at the Massachusetts General and New England Deaconess Hospitals, Jones and co-workers[1] found a diminished pancreatic enzyme activity in nearly one-half of the cases. Bile pigment elimination in the duodenal contents was abnormally high in about three-fourths of the cases. In nearly one-third of the cases there were associated enzyme and pigment abnormalities. The greatest alterations in enzyme activity were noted in the lipolytic and proteolytic ferments. Efficient insulin therapy with its associated increase in food intake and improvement of tissue function seemed to be associated with a reduction in pancreatic and hepatic abnormalities. Acidosis produced a marked disturbance of pancreatic enzyme activity and liver function. Cholelithiasis, as diagnosed by examination of the duodenal sediment, occurred in 19 per cent of their cases. In addition, several other patients had histories or operative findings consistent with the diagnosis of gall stones. Jones and his collaborators believed that the existing figures for the incidence of gall stones in diabetes were far too low.

According to Rabinowitch,[2] 80 per cent of patients with symptoms of cholelithiasis showed hyperglycemia, though not of sufficient degree to produce glycosuria. He found at the Montreal General Hospital that "nine times as many patients with disease of the gall-bladder and its passages had diabetes as would be expected if the influencing factors were completely independent. . . . The incidence of diabetes was greater in cholecystitis than in cholelithiasis and that in acute pancreatitis the incidence was forty times greater than chance would allow." With cholecystograms Tedstrom *et al.*[3] showed that 44 per cent of 70 diabetic patients past the age of forty years had abnormalities in the gall-bladder. The percentage in males was 24 and in females 49. It is also of interest that Barber[4] observed a lowering of the tolerance for carbohydrate as demonstrated by hyperglycemia in cholecystitis experimentally produced in animals. Ophüls[5] found pancreatic lesions associated with gall stones at 14 of 214 autopsies in which gall stones were present. The lesions consisted of focal necroses, chronic pancreatitis, and acute hemorrhagic pancreatitis.

Schleusner[6] cites the following from the literature: Singer[7] found 61 cases of gall-bladder or liver disease among 450 diabetics; Ferger[8] found gall-bladder histories in 19.4 per cent of a series of 160 diabetic patients, and in 16, or 10 per cent of the total, he believed there was a definite connection between disease of the gall-bladder and the

[1] Jones, Castle, Mulholland, and Bailey: Loc. cit., p. 225.
[2] Rabinowitch: Canad. Med. Assn. Jour., **14**, 296, 1924.
[3] Tedstrom, Bond, Olmsted, and Moore: Jour. Am. Med. Assn., **87**, 1603, 1926.
[4] Barber: Ibid., **87**, 1635, 1926.
[5] Ophüls: Stanford Univ. Pub., **1**, 131, 1926.
[6] Schleusner: Loc. cit., p. 544.
[7] Singer: Ztschr. f. klin. Med., **114**, 497, 1930; Med. Klin., **24**, 1858, 1928.
[8] Ferger: Ztschr. f. klin. Med., **119**, 81, 1931.

appearance of diabetes; Lande[1] found histories of gall-bladder disease in 219, or 9.6 per cent, of 2100 cases. Schleusner himself analyzed 355 autopsy protocols of diabetic patients dying in the Barmbeck General Hospital in Hamburg between the years 1914 and 1936. In 119 of these patients stones were found and in 6 other patients the gall-bladder had been removed. Consequently, in 35.2 per cent, gall stones had been found or cholecystectomy carried out. The average age at death of these patients was sixty-two and two-tenths years. Schleusner regards this percentage so great as to demonstrate without question the increased incidence of gall stones in diabetes.

2. **Incidence of Gall Stones Among Non-diabetics.**—Published reports as to the occurrence of gall stones among the general population vary so widely that accurate comparison of diabetic and non-diabetic groups is difficult. At one extreme we have White's[2] statement that in only 3 per cent of 11,031 autopsies at Guy's Hospital were gall stones found, and at the other, Mentzer's[3] finding that in 21 per cent of 600 autopsies at the Mayo Clinic stones were noted. Kaufmann[4] reported the presence of stones in 10.9 per cent of 16,025 autopsies at Basle. Ophüls[5] found 206 cases, or 8 per cent, among 2492 autopsies performed on patients over twenty years of age. Schleusner[6] quotes Achoff as finding gall stones 100 to 150 times among 1000 autopsies on non-diabetic individuals.

3. **Relationship Between Gall-bladder Disease and Diabetes.**— If we grant that cholelithiasis and cholecystitis are more common in diabetics than non-diabetics, are we justified in assuming an etiological relationship? Katsch[7] stated that diabetes is often the consequence of chronic gall-bladder disease, manifest or silent, and this was a belief commonly held in the past. However, in view of the recent emphasis of the common hereditary basis of diabetes we believe that one can no longer assign to gall-bladder disease a primary etiological rôle.

Probably Terbrüggen[8] is correct in stating that the occurrence of gall-bladder disease and diabetes in the same individual is explained by the obesity which is so commonly present in such a person. This was the conclusion reached also by Bowen, Vaughan and Koenig,[9] who compared 23 cases of diabetes and 12 of alimentary glycosuria by means of liver function tests and cholecystograms. Although they found a higher incidence of positive liver-function tests and positive cholecystograms in the diabetic group, they do

[1] Lande: Loc. cit., p. 542.
[2] White: Clin. Jour., 30, 273, 1907.
[3] Mentzer: Arch. Surg., 14, 14, 1927.
[4] Kaufmann: Lehrbuch der Speziellen Pathologischen Anatomie, 8th ed., Berlin, p. 779, 1922.
[5] Oph_ls: Loc. cit., p. 553.
[6] Schleusner: Loc. cit., p. 544.
[7] Katsch: Arch. f. Verdauungskr., 43, 224, 1928; Deutsch. med. Wchnschr., 54, 1508, 1928; Jahresk. f. ärztl. Fortbild., (Hft. 3), 21, 1, 1930.
[8] Terbrüggen: Klin. Wchnschr., 16, 161, 1937.
[9] Bowen, Vaughan and Koenig: Buffalo Gen. Hosp. Bull., 6, 41, 1928.

not consider as satisfying the evidence in favor of cholecystitis as a cause of diabetes. They believe that the higher incidence of gall stones found in diabetics may be accounted for by the obesity commonly present.

In a study of 2100 diabetic patients Lande[1] was unable to demonstrate a definite influence of gall-bladder or stomach disease upon the onset of diabetes except in those rare cases in which inflammatory conditions of the biliary system had by extension affected the pancreas and there led to marked involvement of islet tissue.

By approaching the problem from the other direction, Dublin, Jimenis and Marks[2] of the Metropolitan Life Insurance Company were also able to demonstrate little or no connection between gall-bladder disease and the development of diabetes. They studied the records of 2720 applicants accepted for insurance during the years 1912 to 1928 and traced to their policy anniversary in 1933. There were 159 deaths in the group. Despite the inclusion of a large number of females of more than average weight there were no deaths from diabetes among them and only three among males.

Dr. William R. Jordan,[3] formerly of our group, studied the records of 154 patients with diabetes (including 3 who had glycosuria not proven diabetic) complicated by gall-bladder disease. One hundred and seven of the group had been operated upon. His conclusions were as follows:

1. The incidence of gall-bladder disease discovered during life in diabetics is only a fraction of the incidence at postmortem examination.

2. Among diabetics, gall-bladder operation fails to effect a permanent cure of the gall-bladder condition in a considerable percentage of cases.

3. Based on longevity, gall-bladder operation was of no obvious advantage in this series of diabetics.

4. The gall-bladder disease preceded the diabetes twice as often as the reverse was true, and its average duration was 12.9 years prior to the onset of diabetes.

5. A significant number of patients developed diabetes after drainage or removal of the gall-bladder; but, in those cases with known weight between the operation and the diabetes, almost all were obese and the few exceptions had positive diabetic heredity. This emphasizes the importance of subsequent observation and treatment in postoperative gall-bladder cases over a long period of years.

6. Gall-bladder drainage or removal did not cause improvement of the diabetes as compared with a control group with gall-bladder disease and no operation. The only obvious exceptions occurred in patients with prolonged or frequently recurrent acute or subacute

[1] Ladne: Loc. cit., p. 542.
[2] Dublin, Jimenis, and Marks: Proc. Assn. Life Ins. Med. Directors Amer., 21, 34, 1934.
[3] Jordan: Unpublished data.

inflammation of the gall-bladder, and this is in accordance with the improvement of diabetes following the treatment of any active infection such as a carbuncle.

In summary, it seems fair to conclude that although cholelithiasis and cholecystitis occur more frequently in diabetics than in non-diabetics, gall-bladder disease cannot be regarded as a primary factor in the causation of diabetes.

4. **Surgery in Gall-Bladder Disease.**—Eisele[1] analyzed the findings in 67 of our diabetic patients at the New England Deaconess Hospital who had gall-bladder surgery between 1926 and 1942. The average age at operation was fifty-eight years with the youngest patient fourteen and the oldest seventy-nine years of age. Dr. L. S. McKittrick performed all except two of these operations. The operative mortality was 3.9 per cent for the entire group and 4.6 per cent for those with benign gall-bladder disease alone.

Complete relief of symptoms was obtained in 77 per cent, partial relief in 12 per cent and no relief in 11 per cent of the cases, a result equally as good as that obtained in similar series reported in non-diabetic patients.

The striking danger of perforation of the biliary system by calculi was illustrated by its occurrence in 8 of 65 patients coming to operation without neoplasm, an incidence of 14 per cent (Cases 6435, 8929, 10803, 12778, 15273, 15497, 15919, 17466). Three of the perforations were in acutely inflamed gall-bladders and 3 were in gall-bladders with empyema. The high incidence of gall-bladder perforation is consistent with the well known fact that the diabetic patient cannot limit infection in a normal manner. Commonly quoted statistics in all biliary tract disease are from 1 to 3 per cent perforation, in contrast to the 14 per cent in this series. Eradication of the diseased gall-bladder did not influence the severity of the diabetes as measured by the insulin requirement one year before as compared with one year after operation.

Rabinowitch[2] reported upon the operative treatment of chronic gall-bladder disease in 50 diabetics as compared with 179 non-diabetic cases. The mortality in the diabetic group (4 per cent) was less than in the non-diabetic (5.5 per cent). The average age of the diabetic was 51.8 years as compared with 47.2 for the control group.

Our own advice both to diabetic and non-diabetic patients with gall stones is to be operated upon when the conditions of time, place, surgeon and physician are propitious. Delay and neglect may permit repeated attacks of gall stone colic with the danger of perforation, may allow the subsequent development of a carcinoma and, in the opinion of certain clinicians, may favor the development of diabetes in the hereditarily predisposed non-diabetic.

[1] Eisele: Ann. Surg., **118**, 107, 1943.
[2] Rabinowitch: Ann. Surg., **96**, 70, 1932.

CHAPTER XVIII.

THE NERVOUS SYSTEM AND DIABETES.

Revised by C. Cabell Bailey, M.D. and Jean Murray, M.D.

The two most striking disturbances of the nervous system in diabetes mellitus are (1) neuritis, and (2) changes caused by hypoglycemia.

Hypoglycemia in diabetes is most frequently associated with overdosage of insulin, inadequate food intake or excessive exercise and is discussed in Chapter XI.

A. NEURITIS

The occurrence of specific disorders of the nervous system as a complication of diabetes mellitus has been recognized for almost a century.[1] Nevertheless, much still remains unknown about the etiology and pathology of diabetic nerve lesions.

Diabetic neuritis may manifest itself in many ways. A forty-two year old man, Case 21297, was admitted to the hospital by stretcher because of almost complete paralysis of both lower extremities, yet twelve months later he had completely recovered. Another man, referred by his local physician with a tentative diagnosis of angina pectoris, proved to have a neuritis involving especially the nerves of his left chest wall and eventually recovered. Case 16368 developed a bladder paralysis—a so-called cord bladder—and Case 19678 developed a bilateral external rectus paralysis of his eyes. A man aged fifty-six years (Case 27225) was unable to dress because of marked hypersensitivity of the skin. A man aged fifty years had such marked anesthesia of his feet that he received a second degree burn on stepping into a bath tub, yet the water felt "just right" to his feet. A woman who normally was quite stable emotionally cried all night because of pains in her legs, yet was essentially free from pain during the day. All of these patients had diabetic neuritis but well illustrate the diversified presenting neuritic symptoms one may encounter.

As emphasized by Root and Rogers[2] and by Rudy and Epstein,[3] diabetic neuritis is not limited exclusively to the peripheral nerves but involves the entire nervous system, including the central, peripheral and autonomic parts with an especial predilection for the peripheral nerves. Rundles,[4] in one of the most outstanding articles

1 deCalvi, M.: Recherches sur les accidents diabetiques, Paris, P. Asselin, 1864.
2 Root and Rogers: New Eng. Jour. Med., 202, 1049, 1930.
3 Rudy and Epstein: Jour. Clin. Endocrinology, 5, 92, 1945.
4 Rundles: Medicine, 24, 111, 1945.

in recent years on diabetic neuropathy, likewise stresses this point. He states that patients with diabetic neuropathy may develop evidence of peripheral sympathetic nerve damage as revealed by sweating deficiencies, loss of vasomotor and pilomotor control, dependent edema and certain types of skin alterations. He further illustrates this with 8 cases of orthostatic hypotension and orthostatic tachycardia, in some of whom change from the supine to the erect position produced a fall in systolic blood pressure of 50 or more mm. of mercury with resulting syncope.

1. **Symptoms and Signs.**—The most outstanding symptom of diabetic neuritis is pain which is characteristically worse at night. The pain may be superficial or deep, aching, grinding, darting, or lancing. Not infrequently sleep is prevented throughout the night until the discomfort subsides in the early morning hours. Thereafter the pain may not recur until the following night. No adequate explanation for the nocturnal character of the pain has been advanced.

Paresthesias are very frequent, occurring in 70 per cent of Jordan's[1] series, and like the pain are often more prominent at night. Burning sensations are particularly common along with numbness, tingling, a feeling of coldness of the extremities and a sensation as if the patient were walking on wool. Hyperesthesia may be so marked that the weight of the bedcovers may be unbearable. Mental depression and emotional instability are not uncommon but do not seem out of proportion to the discomfort experienced.

Abnormal neurological signs are usual and may at times be the first or only manifestation of the disorder. In Rundles' series of 125 cases he found diminished or absent tendon reflexes the most common neurologic abnormality. The achilles tendon reflex was absent in 101 cases (81 per cent) and greatly diminished in another 15, whereas the patellar reflexes were absent on one or both sides in 70 cases (56 per cent) and greatly diminished in an additional 29. The biceps and triceps reflexes were diminished or absent in one-third of his patients. Pronounced muscle tenderness was detected in 46 cases. Decreased skin sensitivity occurred in approximately one-half and 9 patients revealed areas of complete anesthesia. The vibratory sense at the ankle was diminished in 37 cases and absent in 20.

Muscular paresis and paralysis are frequently observed and complete foot drop and less frequently wrist drop may develop. Rundles reports 10 cases of foot drop and emphasizes that the peroneal nerve is more vulnerable than the tibial and the ulnar nerve more vulnerable than the radial or median.

2. **Classification of Neuritis.**—Attempts to subdivide diabetic patients with pain simulating neuritis into various groups present difficulties, especially since the groups may tend to overlap. It,

---

[1] Jordan: Arch. Int. Med., **57**, 307, 1936.

however, helps one to study individually the groups with similar symptoms, to determine their prognosis, and to separate the cases with true neuritis from those with pseudoneuritis.

Jordan subdivided 226 cases admitted to the Deaconess Hospital with symptoms suggesting neuritis under the following headings: (1) hyperglycemic, (2) circulatory, (3) degenerative, (4) neuritic.

In the first group he placed 34 cases with neuritic symptoms but usually with no signs other than tenderness along the nerve or muscle affected. All of these had hyperglycemia, and in all cases the symptoms of neuritis disappeared completely within a few days after adequate diabetic management and normal blood sugars had been attained. Whether or not these cases would eventually develop true neuritis if not treated is of course unknown.

The second group includes 27 cases with considerable circulatory deficiency of the legs and in addition pain, paresthesia and signs such as hyporeflexia and hyperesthesia. Intermittent claudication was present in some.

The degenerative group included 45 cases with rather mild neuritis symptoms and signs which begin insidiously and tend to progress slowly over a period of years. Decreased or absent tendon reflexes are common and mild pain or paresthesia is usually acknowledged if one questions the patient, but the symptoms of neuritis are rarely a major complaint.

Jordan often found it difficult to separate the patients with the circulatory type from those in the degenerative group. In fact, they seemed to overlap in many instances with similar symptoms, signs and course. Hence in his final analysis he grouped these two types as one group.

The final group of 120 cases, the neuritic group, includes those cases ordinarily described as having diabetic neuritis. Here pain and paresthesias were marked with weakness progressing in some cases to paralysis with foot drop and quadriceps paralysis.

Pain, characteristically worse at night, was present in 83.3 per cent and of the remaining 20 cases with no pain, muscular paresis was present in 16, paresthesia in 2, optic neuritis in 1 and absence of reflexes in 1, with return of one knee jerk almost to normal in one year. Paresthesias occurred in 70 per cent of the cases and like the pain was usually worse at night. Paresis, varying from slight to complete paralysis, was present in 65 per cent. The neuritis involved the legs in 81 cases and the arms in 8. In 32 cases the sites of involvement were multiple or limited to special nerves such as the cranial nerves. The optic, oculomotor, facial, auditory and recurrent laryngeal nerves were included. Abnormal sensation, as detected by pinprick, was found in 51 per cent of these cases. The prognosis for recovery in this group is good.

Treusch[1] uses a very similar classification. He designates Jordan's

[1] Treusch: Proc. Staff Meet. Mayo. Clin., 20, 393, 1945.

hyperglycemic group as "diabetes with pain." He combines the circulatory and degenerative groups and calls this group ischemic neuropathy. The neuritic group of Jordan he terms "diabetic polyneuritis." Treusch adds a fourth division called "diabetic visceral neuritis," in which he includes cases with involvement of the vasomotor fibers of the autonomic system and the corresponding peripheral visceral sensory fibers. These patients have burning paresthesia of the feet in the absence of objective neurologic signs and in the presence of such objective vasomotor changes as would occur after sympathectomy.

TABLE 66.—CLASSIFICATIONS OF DIABETIC NEURITIS USED BY VARIOUS AUTHORS.
Modified from table by Treusch.[1]

Author.	Group 1.	Group 2.	Group 3.
Treusch[1]	Diabetics with pain	Ischemic neuropathy	Diabetic polyneuritis
Woltman and Wilder[2] .	. . . . .	8 cases	2 cases; diabetic pseudotabes
Root and Rogers[3] . .	Abnormal nutrition	Neuritis with deficient blood supply	Diabetic neuritis with paralysis
Jordan[4]	Hyperglycemic type	Degenerative and (circulatory) type of neuropathy	Diabetic neuritis; diabetic tabes; neuritic type
Swartz[5]	Diabetic neuritis without signs	Diabetic neuritis with signs	

Group 4: Diabetic visceral neuritis (Treusch)

3. Analysis of Cases Recently Seen.—Recently the records of 50 cases with typical diabetic neuritis at the New England Deaconess Hospital were analyzed. No sex difference was found as 26 were males and 24 were females. The average age at onset of the neuritis was 50.8 years, the oldest case being seventy-seven and the youngest twenty-five. Diabetes had been present an average of 5.9 years.

Pain was usually the presenting symptom and was found in 45 cases involving most commonly the feet and legs and described as cramping, aching, darting and boring. The pain was much worse at night in 41 of the 45 cases and often prevented sleep. In some the pain was not limited to the lower extremity but included superficial abdominal pain and chest pain. In 2 cases pain in the arms was conspicuous.

Paresthesias noted in 41 cases included especially burning of the feet but also numbness, tingling, formications, anesthesia and

[1] Treusch: Loc. cit., p. 559.
[2] Woltman and Wilder: Arch. Int. Med., 44, 576, 1929.
[3] Root and Rogers: Loc. cit., p. 557.
[4] Jordan: Loc. cit., p. 558.
[5] Swartz: Thesis, Mayo Foundation, 1940.

hyperesthesia. In some, hyperesthesia was so marked that the patient could not bear the weight of even the bed cover upon his legs.

Weakness of one or more extremities was present in 27 cases. Peroneal paralysis (foot drop) was detected in 8 cases and quadriceps paralysis in 5. Absent patellar reflexes were noted in 28 cases. The Achilles tendon reflex was absent in only 11 cases but in many it was not tested.

The striking finding in the spinal fluid was an elevation of the total protein in 26 of the 30 cases so examined. In one the total protein reached 320 mg. per cent, whereas in 10 cases values of over 100 mg. per cent were obtained. In 16 cases determinations between 50 and 100 mg. were found and in only 4 cases were normal values noted.

Colloidal gold determination in 25 cases revealed normal values in 11, elevation of the curve to the left in 12 and a midzone rise in 2 cases. Spinal fluid Hintons in the 25 cases examined were all negative and the blood Hinton was negative in all 50 cases.

The severity of the neuritis tends to parallel the level of the spinal fluid protein and clinical improvement is usually accompanied by a decrease in the spinal fluid protein.

The duration of symptoms was quite variable, ranging from two months to seven years. In some instances prolonged neuritis seemed to be associated with continued poor diabetic control. The duration of the neuritis was less than a year in 21 cases, although 6 were not entirely well on the last report; the duration was one to two years in 13 cases with 4 not relieved when last heard from, whereas in 11 cases the neuritis lasted from two to seven years. In the last group the majority (7) had still not completely recovered.

Large doses of vitamins, including the B complex and especially thiamin chloride, were administered in nearly all cases, but there was no evidence that this therapy altered the course of the disease.

TABLE 67.—PROTEIN CONTENT IN CEREBROSPINAL FLUID IN DIABETES.[1]

Protein content (mg. per 100 cc.).		Diabetic neuropathy (per cent).	Surgical infections of feet (per cent).	Syphilis (per cent).	Others* (per cent).
Low to Normal:	15–50 . . .	13	57	42	58
Moderate:	51–70 . . .	29	26	17	19
High:	71–120 . . .	44	17	33	12
	121–390 . . .	14	0	8	11
Number of cases		84	53	24	74

* Others included meningo-encephalitis (6), tumors (4), epilepsy (6), cerebral hemorrhage (17), miscellaneous (41).

4. **Spinal Fluid.**—The striking and often only abnormality of the spinal fluid in diabetic neuritis is an abnormal elevation of the spinal fluid protein. In 1930 Root and Rogers[1] analyzed the spinal fluid findings in 84 patients with diabetic neuropathy and compared the

[1] Root and Rogers: Loc. cit., p. 557.

results with 53 cases of diabetics with surgical infection of the feet, 24 cases of syphilis and 74 miscellaneous cases including brain hemorrhage and others.   Table 67 shows this comparison and Table 68 compares the ages at the time of the occurrence of the neuropathy.   Among the 84 cases of diabetic neuropathy, 18 were regarded as severe, 14 moderate and 52 of mild character. As seen in Table 69, of the 84 cases of diabetic neuropathy, 84.5 per cent had a definite elevation in spinal fluid protein.

Rundles, Merritt and Freemont-Smith[1] and Rudy and Muellner[2] and Needles[3] have reported similar results in fewer cases.

TABLE 68.—AGE INCIDENCE OF DIABETIC NEUROPATHY.

Years.

10–19	1
20–29	2
30–39	13
40–49	5
50–59	32
60–69	25
70–79	5
80–	1
	84

The cellular content, pressure and spinal fluid dynamics are characteristically normal in diabetic neuropathy and the globulin usually increased.   The colloidal gold curve may be elevated, often in the midzone, but may simulate the paretic gold curve with elevation to the left.

5. **Ocular Paralysis.**—Case 19678, admitted to the hospital, developed successive bilateral external rectus paralysis within two days.   Spinal anesthesia had been used, however, at the time of a transmetatarsal amputation of an infected foot twelve days before the first ocular palsy.   No other signs of central nervous system disturbances or any evidence of meningeal irritation were detected. In 5 cases of cranial nerve paralysis reported by Root[4] a double paralysis of each internal rectus muscle occurred in 1, the third nerve was involved in 2 cases and the sixth nerve was involved in 2 others.

Jordan reports 1 case of ocular palsy and stresses that the onset is usually abrupt and recovery rapid and complete in some instances. The case of Schick and Silbermann,[5] a diabetic with three separate attacks of paralysis of the third nerve, had a large area of calcification in the center of the sella turcica.   Double vision due to hypo-

[1] Merritt and Freemont-Smith: The Cerebro-spinal Fluid, Philadelphia, W. B. Saunders, 1937.
[2] Rudy and Muellner: Jour. Urol., **45**, 844, 1941.
[3] Needles: Jour. Am. Med. Assn., **121**, 914, 1943.
[4] Root: Med. Clin. North Amer., **16**, 985, 1933.
[5] Schick and Silbermann: Wien. klin. Wchnschr., **45**, 1255, 1932.

glycemia is always to be considered, but it is quickly relieved and therefore of temporary duration.

Facial paralysis occurred twice in Case 6876, a lawyer, aged sixty-five years, one side being involved in 1925 and the other in 1928. The youngest patient with facial paralysis was Case 5257, aged fifty years with diabetes for sixteen years whose facial paralysis occurred in March, 1940. The condition developed in Case 16836 at the age of sixty-two years with diabetes for six years, in Case 18835 at the age of sixty-six years and in Case 15518 at the age of 55.7 years after diabetes of 21.7 years' duration.

6. **Pupillary Reactions.**—Abnormal pupillary reactions have been reported in many cases of diabetes. Jordan found 20 such cases among 120 patients in his so-called "true neuritic group." True Argyll-Robertson pupils were noted in 5 instances, and in 8 others sluggish responses were observed. These cases were all non-syphilitic so far as could be determined by history, physical examination, blood Wassermann reaction and in 5 instances spinal fluid examination. Rundles also reports 2 cases with Argyll-Robertson pupils in whom no evidence of syphilis could be detected. In others with sluggish light reflexes, he noted their return to normal with general neurologic improvement.

7. **Genito-urinary Disturbances.**—Among 115 patients with diabetic neuropathy, Rundles found 32 (25.6 per cent) with genito-urinary or sphincter disturbances. Complete lack of sexual potency was recorded in 19 patients. An atonic type of bladder paralysis was found in 18 patients, 15 of whom were males. This type of so-called cord bladder has been reported several times as a manifestation of diabetic neuropathy. McKittrick and Root[1] reported 3 cases, Jordan and Crabtree[2] 7 cases, Jordan[3] an additional 5 cases and Rudy and Muellner[4] 11 cases. As emphasized by Jordan, this type of bladder disturbance is usually irreversible.

Gill[5] reported 2 cases of marked paralysis of the urinary bladder in patients with mild arteriosclerosis and long-standing severe diabetes mellitus. Both patients died; in one an autopsy was permitted. The spinal cord pathologically in this case showed a mild diffuse gliosis of the dorsal columns with vacuolization, rarefaction and loss of substance. Sheppe's[6] patient with a similar paralyzed bladder, ataxia, areflexia, disturbance of sensation and diabetes of 8 years' duration, showed at autopsy scattered areas of degeneration (non-inflammatory) in the spinal cord and nerve roots. In Case 4023, female, whose paralysis of the bladder persisted from 1926

---

[1] McKittrick and Root: Diabetic Surgery, Philadelphia, Lea and Febiger, 1928.
[2] Jordan and Crabtree: Arch. Int. Med., **55**, 17, 1935.
[3] Jordan: Loc. cit., p. 558.
[4] Rudy and Muellner: Loc. cit., p. 562.
[5] Gill: Jour. Urol., **36**, 730, 1936.
[6] Sheppe: West Virginia Med. Jour., **321**, 1, 1936.

until her death in 1938, no definite pathological change was found in the spinal cord.

8. **Chemistry of Diabetic Nerves.**—Chemical analyses of 52 nerves of diabetic patients and 23 nerves of non-diabetics at the Deaconess Hospital have been carried out in the laboratory of Prof. W. R. Bloor, and the results reported by W. R. Jordan, L. D. Randall, and W. R. Bloor.[1] In their two papers the literature is reviewed. Their results show that the average phospholipid, cholesterol, and cerebroside content of diabetic nerves was much lower than that of the nerves used for control. In Table 69 are shown the values for nerves from diabetic patients with arteriosclerosis as compared with normal averages.

A third report by Randall[2] also demonstrated that the peripheral nerves from such subjects showed marked decreases in phospholipids, cholesterol and cerebrosides and an increase in neutral fat. The posterior tibial nerve showed more extensive change than the sciatic and the latter more than the femoral. The greater extent of change in the more distal parts of the nerves suggested an inadequate blood supply and anoxemia. Vascular disease was not the sole cause for these changes in chemical structure of the diabetic nerves. Previous inadequate control of the diabetes seems to affect the nerve unfavorably, although a constant correlation between the severity and duration of the diabetes and the extent of the chemical changes was not shown.

TABLE 69.—LIPID CONTENT OF NORMAL AND DIABETIC NERVES. AVERAGE VALUES WITH RESPECT TO ARTERIOSCLEROSIS.

Arteriosclerosis.	No. of cases.	Phospholipid, per cent.	Cholesterol, per cent.	Cerebroside, per cent.
1 + (slight) . . .	1	3.85	1.15	1.60
2 + ...	6	1.69	0.64	0.69
3 + ...	12	1.67	0.60	0.77
4 + (advanced) . .	1	1.40	0.45	1.46
Normal average		**4.40**	**1.36**	**1.73**

9. **Pathology of Diabetic Neuritis.**—Since typical diabetic neuritis is reversible and not fatal, it is not surprising that very little is known about its pathology. Biopsies of nerves are not feasible because of resulting paralyses. As Warren[3] states, the rapidity of recovery in some cases of diabetic neuritis practically precludes any marked pathological change. Fraser and Bruce[4] studied the posterior tibial nerve of a man with diabetes and neuritis and described demyelinization of the nerve.

The degenerative or circulatory type of neuropathy has been studied by Woltman and Wilder,[5] who described areas of degenera-

[1] Jordan, Randall and Bloor: Arch. Int. Med., 55, 26, 1935.
[2] Randall: Jour. Biol. Chem., 125, 723, 1938.
[3] Warren: Loc. cit., p. 196.
[4] Fraser and Bruce: Edinburgh Med. Jour., 42, 300, 1896.
[5] Woltman and Wilder: Loc. cit., p. 560.

tion in the peripheral nerves, more marked distally and associated with thickening of the walls of the nutrient vessels. They therefore attributed the nerve changes to arteriosclerosis, which probably explains the irreversibility of this type of nerve lesion. Spinal cord studies were also reported, but only slight changes, which were most marked in the posterior columns and attributed to arteriosclerosis, were found. Kauvar[1] believes there is a striking similarity between the lesion found in the nerve changes associated with arteriosclerosis and those found in diabetic neuritis, but the fact that neuritis occurs often in young persons without appreciable arteriosclerosis and the fact that it is completely reversible is evidence that the typical case of acute diabetic neuritis is not due to arteriosclerosis.

Most other reports on diabetic nerve and spinal cord lesions were published fifty years or more ago. Certainly this aspect of neuritis deserves a careful study with modern techniques.

10. **Etiology.**—Although the etiology of diabetic neuritis has been attributed to many causes, the outstanding fact remains that true diabetic neuritis, in almost if not all instances, follows a period of uncontrolled diabetes. Rundles states that he has seen this complication only after months or even years of grossly uncontrolled diabetes, and none of his 125 cases reported had regularly attended the diabetic clinic or had been under the adequate supervision of competent physicians. Seventy-five per cent of his cases had lost 20 or more pounds in weight within a few months before the onset of the neuritis, which he felt was not due to dietary restrictions but usually to excessive food consumption. A third of his cases had lost over 40 pounds. Joslin and Root[2] emphasize that symptoms practically always develop during a time of uncontrolled diabetes and assert that all patients with true diabetic neuritis recover if diabetic control is sufficiently well maintained over a period of from one to five years. Treusch[3] in a recent report from the Mayo Clinic concurs in their view.

Arteriosclerosis has long been incriminated as a probable etiological factor and, as shown by Woltman and Wilder, may well be associated with the neurological factors in the ischemic type of neuropathy. Kauvar points out that if a tourniquet is applied to an extremity and the circulation occluded, symptoms and signs of peripheral neuritis are soon apparent. Any association, however, between arteriosclerosis and the typical acute reversible neuritis often found in young diabetics seems very remote.

The rôle of vitamins, especially that of a thiamin deficiency in relation to diabetic neuritis was discussed by Root[4] as early as

[1] Kauvar: Jour. Clin. Endocrinology, **1**, 955, 1941.
[2] Joslin and Root: Trans. Assn. Amer. Phys., **54**, 251, 1939.
[3] Treusch: Loc. cit., p. 559.
[4] Root: Med. North Am. Clin., **5**, 1433, 1922.

1922 but is still unsettled. Although vitamin deficiencies may occur in diabetic patients just as in non-diabetic patients, and the mild neuritic symptoms in the 8 patients apparently cured with thiamin chloride by Fein, Ralli and Joliffe[1] may well represent a vitamin deficiency, we strongly concur with the opinion expressed by Rundles that he has "never seen clinical improvement in diabetic neuropathy by any treatment regimé in the absence of effective diabetic control."

The diet of 63 patients with diabetic neuropathy was found adequate by Jordan[2] in all but 1 case, and Needles[3] reports similar findings in 2 patients. The possibility of a decreased absorption or an increased utilization or excretion of the vitamin in these cases must be considered. Robinson, Melnick and Field,[4] however, found normal excretory values for thiamin in 4 patients with diabetic neuritis given a test dose of thiamin. Pollack, Ellenberg and Dolger[5] carried out similar studies upon 139 diabetics and found values possibly indicating a thiamin deficiency in only 13, which was a lower percentage than they found among a group of non-diabetic individuals.

Jordan was unable to attribute an etiological rôle in his cases of neuritis to anemia, alcohol, dietary deficiency, drugs, infection, or lead poisoning.

11. **Treatment.**—Unless the diabetes is brought under control by insulin and diet, all other therapy is of no avail; hence the salient point in treatment should be to acquire and maintain meticulous diabetic control. Initial hospitalization is usually necessary in order to obtain the best results. Insulin should always be given.

The use of vitamins is unsettled but certainly does no harm unless one substitutes their use for attempts to control the diabetes. The whole B complex supplemented with thiamin chloride is most frequently used, but striking improvement with their use must not be expected or promised. In some patients with neuritis, the pain may at times interfere with the adequate intake of food and in these cases especially the use of vitamins may prove rational.

Ordinarily the relief of pain is the main concern of the patient and this requires immediate attention. Salicylates in the form of aspirin or sodium salicylate gr. 5 to 10, repeated frequently, may prove adequate, but salicylism must be watched for. Local warmth with blankets may help, but electric pads and hot water bottles must be used cautiously, for burns are frequent since the feet may be partially anesthetic. Warm tub baths are often soothing but some obtain more relief from ice packs or cool baths. A cradle over the foot of the bed to suspend the covers over the lower extremities

[1] Fein, Ralli and Joliffe: Jour. Am. Med. Assn., **115**, 1973, 1940.
[2] Jordan: Loc. cit., p. 558.
[3] Needles: Arch. Neurol. and Psychiat., **41**, 1222, 1939.
[4] Robinson, Melnick and Field: Jour. Clin. Investigation, **19**, 399, 1940.
[5] Pollack, Ellenberg and Dolger: Arch. Int. Med., **67**, 793, 1941.

is helpful when hyperesthesia is marked. Opiates must be used very cautiously but when needed codeine should not be withheld.

When the painful neuritis is well localized or restricted to the territory of a single peripheral nerve, Rundles considers the advisability of local anesthesia, nerve crush or nerve section, but feels that results obtained have not been encouraging and we must warn against such strenuous measures.

If foot drop is present, support for the plantar surface of the foot is supplied and a wire hoop placed over the foot of the bed to counteract the pull of the covers, in an effort to prevent contractures of the calf muscles.

Mild cases usually respond to therapy in a few weeks; moderate cases take several months to a year and severe ones may require one to several years for complete recovery. For the severer cases, encouragement is needed and it is well worth while to show the patient a cured case as proof of recovery. Patience both on the part of the doctor as well as patient is necessary.

B. UNUSUAL MANIFESTATIONS OF DIABETIC NEUROPATHY.

1. **Neuropathic Foot.**—The occurrence of bone changes in the foot as a complication of diabetes has been pointed out by Root,[1] and by Jordan.[2] Recently Bailey and Root[3] have studied 16 diabetic patients with foot lesions simulating Charcot joint yet with no evidence of central nervous system syphilis. These changes are believed to represent a manifestation of diabetic neuropathy. The earliest gross change detected in the foot is a thickening of the tarsal region which tends to progress slowly and eventually to become a thickened deformed foot with a tendency to eversion, external rotation and a flattening of the longitudinal arch.

By x-ray the neuropathic foot is quite similar to the Charcot joint of syphilis except that the destruction is usually limited to the tarsal and proximal ends of the metatarsal bones. One such foot studied pathologically by Dr. Shields Warren at the Deaconess Hospital revealed a complete loss of bone structure with numerous spicules of bone scattered throughout the area of involvement, undergoing various stages of absorption with an attempt being made by the remaining periosteum to form new bone.

In Bailey and Root's series there were 8 males and 10 females with an average age of fifty-six at the time the foot lesion was discovered, the oldest being sixty-nine years and the youngest thirty years. Diabetes had been present an average of eleven years.

Spinal fluid examination in 12 cases revealed a negative Wassermann but a definite elevation in spinal fluid proteins in 10 of the 12

[1] Root: Jour. New York Med., **42**, 2296, 1942.
[2] Jordan: Loc. cit., p. 558.
[3] Bailey and Root: To be published.

cases, averaging 69 mg. per cent.   The blood Hinton was negative
in 14 cases and positive in 2, both of whom had negative spinal
fluid tests for syphilis.   There was no clinical evidence of syphilis in
any case.

Evidence of neuritis was found in 13 of the 16 cases including
absent knee reflexes, foot drop, anesthetic feet, loss of sensation and
vibratory sense, bladder paralysis and paresthesias.   Only 2 patients
complained of nocturnal pain in the extremities.

Hypertension was present in 14 cases, significant albuminuria
(over 100 mg. per cent) in 6 and diabetic retinitis in 9 cases.   Two
had diabetic nocturnal diarrhea.

It is believed that the bone destruction represents a trophic
change resulting from diabetic neuropathy and is similar to the
arthropathies which result from neurosyphilis, syringomylia or from
the neural form of leprosy.   No case has shown any tendency to
improve and the only treatment that has proved helpful is the use of
orthopedic applicances in an effort to relieve weightbearing and
thereby help to prevent further deformity.

2. **"Diabetic Nocturnal Diarrhea."**—Another condition believed
to represent an unusual manifestation of diabetic neuropathy is
diabetic nocturnal diarrhea.   Details of this condition are given in
Chapter XVII.

C. DISEASES OF THE NERVOUS SYSTEM AS COMPLICATIONS OF DIABETES.

1. **Epilepsy.**—The evidence of epilepsy among uncomplicated
adult diabetics is no higher than in unselected normal persons in
corresponding age groups.

According to Lennox,[1] cerebral dysrhythmia is found in 8 to 10
per cent of non-diabetic persons.   This parallels the incidence of
8 per cent noted in routine electroencephalography in our uncomplicated adult diabetics.   This material was presented in a recent
paper by Greenblatt, Murray and Root.[2]   Fifty-one per cent of
patients who complained of frequent severe insulin reactions, however, had abnormal electroencephalograms.   This would seem to
indicate that some diabetics who seem unduly difficult to regulate
may have cortical instability, and that relatively minor drops in
blood sugar may give marked clinical reactions.   The character of
these "reactions" varies widely, from dizziness, speech disturbances,
paresis and temper tantrums to attacks of petit mal, spells of unconsciousness and generalized convulsions.   The electroencephalograph
has proved invaluable in differentiating these attacks from true
epilepsy, and we have been fortunate in the past few years to have
available the facilities and coöperation of the electroencephalo-

[1] Lennox: Science and Seizures: New Light on Epilepsy and Migraine, New York
and London, Harper Bros., 1941, pp. 166–169.
[2] Greenblatt, Murray and Root: New England Jour. Med., **234**, 119, 1946.

graphic department of the Boston Psychopathic Hospital in studying many of our patients.

Case 23586, aged twenty-seven years, who had had diabetes since age fourteen, had an electroencephalogram consistent with epilepsy but no convulsions except with low blood sugar. He had no sedation and did well with more careful control. Case 19893, aged twenty-four years, with diabetes of eight years' duration had no convulsions but developed many "temper tantrums," during which she cut window screens with scissors and threw books at her family. Her electroencephalogram was consistent with grand mal epilepsy and she was treated with phenobarbital and dilantin simultaneously but with only slight success. Case 17083 showed the grand mal type of epilepsy at the age of sixteen, four years after developing diabetes mellitus. Her convulsions were often precipitated by low blood sugar but she usually recovered with little or no hypoglycemic treatment. Her convulsions were controlled with dilantin.

The possible rôle of repeated hypoglycemia due to insulin in the production of permanent cerebral damage, and possibly epilepsy, must be considered. Bix[1] believes that severe hypoglycemic reactions can produce lesions of the brain. In severe hypoglycemic shock, small hemorrhages may occur in the brain and conceivably these could be responsible for epilepsy. Himwich[2] has found that prolonged hypoglycemia may produce permanent brain damage. In insulin-sensitive rats, Gellhorn and Kessler[3] found the effect of hypoglycemia on the electroencephalogram to be the same as that produced by anoxia. It is established that diabetics are more sensitive to hypoglycemia than normal individuals. A low blood sugar does not precipitate attacks in non-diabetic patients with grand mal or psychomotor epilepsy, although it may increase the electrical abnormality in patients with petit mal, according to Gibbs *et al.*[4] Most of our patients with true epilepsy receive sodium dilantin. A few whose only evidence of epilepsy has been manifested by routine electroencephalogram are taking phenobarbital. In the group of unstable diabetics with frequent severe insulin reactions and some degree of cerebral dysrhythmia, phenobarbital has been useful. One patient noted that after starting phenobarbital he had warning of his impending reactions, whereas previously he has experienced a sudden onset of hypoglycemic convulsions without premonitory symptoms.

2. **Hysteria.**—Hysteria is seldom seen among our diabetic patients. Case 10863, housewife, aged fifty-one years, with diabetes of one years' duration, following a slight auto accident and an operation, developed an unsteady gait and emotional changes. Anesthesia

[1] Bix: Jahrb. f. Kinderh., **151**, 176, 1938.
[2] Himwich: Am. Jour. Digest. Dis., **11**, 1, 1944.
[3] Gellhorn and Kessler: Am. Jour. Physiol., **136**, 1, 1942.
[4] Gibbs, Gibbs and Lennox: Arch. Neurol. and Psychiat., **41**, 1111, 1939.

of the glove-and-stocking type was present at times. In addition
to an impending law suit, there were important complications in her
family life. Case 5461, school girl, aged seventeen years in January,
1930, with diabetes of four years' duration, was depressed and
troubled with ideas of self accusation but was not retarded. A
diagnosis of psychoneurosis with hysteria was made. Later the
basal metabolism was 18 per cent below normal, the plasma cholesterol was 78 mg. per cent and she was regarded as a case of pituitary dysfunction. In 1934 she graduated from a girl's school and in
June 1939 still seemed to be doing well. In September 1940, however, she was regarded as a schizophrenic and was in a mental
hospital.

3. **Psychoses.**—The frequency of diabetes among patients in
state hospitals with definite mental disorders deserves study. Dr.
Clifton T. Perkins has courteously provided data from Massachusetts Mental Hospitals and State Schools. Among 2341 patients in
State schools, diabetes occurred in 6 cases, or 0.25 per cent. For
23,690 patients in State hospitals the incidence of diabetes was 0.89
per cent, consisting of 124 females and 89 males. Among 1416 older
patients with a diagnosis of cerebral arteriosclerosis the incidence
of diabetes was 2.18 per cent, whereas among 12,300 cases of
dementia præcox, the incidence of diabetes was 0.68 per cent, consisting of 57 females and 27 males.

Through the kindness of Dr. Charles Bolduan the data for 3685
admissions at the Manhattan State Hospitals are available. For
1056 cases from fifteen years to forty-five years of age, 1.4 per cent
of the males and 2.3 per cent of the females had glycosuria. For
the age period from forty-five to sixty-five years 3.5 per cent of the
males and 4.5 per cent of the females had glycosuria.

(a) *Manic-depressive.*—Case 18321, a housewife, aged forty-seven
years, with diabetes of four years' duration and pernicious anemia,
of two years' duration, which had responded well to liver extract,
developed a marked depression in January 1943. She was given
electric shock therapy by Dr. O. J. Raeder and made a rapid
recovery.

Case 9823, a female, aged forty-nine years, with diabetes for
sixteen years, developed a marked depression in October 1943.
She received four electric shock treatments within a period of ten
days and made a complete and rapid recovery. Case 24551, a
diabetic woman, aged fifty-four years, likewise made a rapid recovery
with this form of therapy.

(b) *Senile Dementia.*—Senility, often premature, is a common
and an extremely important problem. Not infrequently elderly
diabetic patients with cerebral arteriosclerosis show mental confusion for the first time in the hospital, especially following surgical
procedures and particularly at night. Among the early symptoms of
senility are changes in business judgment and the power of decision

which, when combined with irritability, may lead to consequences most distressing to business associates, family and friends. The diagnosis, therefore, of the onset of changes which are destined to be progressive is one of great practical importance. Dr. O. J. Raeder in consultation has helped with a number of such problems. Case 7596, engineer, aged fifty-nine years, with diabetes of three years' duration, and Case 12778, business man and executive, aged fifty-seven years, with diabetes of only one years' duration, showed depression, irritability, headaches, and in the second case the problem was complicated by attacks of acute alcoholism. Both men were loath to give up the idea of returning to business although it was obvious that to do so would be only to court disaster. When cerebral hemorrhage or thrombosis has occurred, even though recovery takes place, depression and emotional instability are often prominent features as in Case 13026.

4. **Hemichorea.**—Case 4529, aged sixty-one years at onset, in 1912, recovered from hemichorea in 1925 but died in 1927 of gangrene. Case 4166, aged sixty-one years at onset in 1912, lived but eight weeks after choreic symptoms developed and died in 1924. Case 6043, a female, aged seventy-five years, with diabetes of eighteen years' duration developed leg pains suggestive of diabetic neuritis. The pains persisted for one year, at the end of which time she developed choreiform movements of the right arm on voluntary effort, which disappeared after twelve days. One month later she developed severe hemichorea of the entire right side.

5. **Paralysis Agitans.**—Parkinson's disease is not infrequent in the elderly diabetic. Four new cases per year on the average have been seen in the George F. Baker Clinic. Kuckens[1] observed paralysis agitans in 5 generations and in the same family diabetes was present four times, being grave in 2 univitelline twin boys, aged fifteen years.

6. **Meningitis and Encephalitis.**—The discovery of the sulfonamides and of penicillin has completely changed the prognosis of meningitis in diabetics as in non-diabetics. Case 14045, a man, aged twenty-one years, with diabetes for eight years was admitted to the hospital with acute meningococcus meningitis and a spinal fluid cell count of 17,000. He received large doses of sulfadiazine intravenously and orally and made a rapid recovery.

Case 18961, thirty-three years of age, developed meningococcemia and meningococcus meningitis (type 2) two months postpartum. She also made a complete recovery with sulfadiazine orally and intravenously.

Encephalitis probably explains the development of epilepsy and mental deterioration in Case 3019. This little boy whose diabetes began at the age of fourteen months, developed epileptic attacks a few weeks after he had measles. At the time, the diagnosis of en-

[1] Kuchens: Klin. Wchnschr., 4, 2289, 1925.

cephalitis was not made but subsequently as he deteriorated this diagnosis was forced upon us.

Case 11098, aged sixty-four years with diabetes of two years' duration, entered the Deaconess Hospital in June, 1934, having had a severe cold about ten days before from which she thought she had recovered. Gradually weakness of the eyelids developed and when she entered the hospital double ptosis, inability to move either eye to right or left and up or down were present. Dr. G. C. Caner and Dr. W. P. Beetham saw her in consultation and placed the lesion as somewhere in the midbrain or at the base of the brain. To our great pleasure she has made a complete recovery and all the neurological signs disappeared in January, 1935. Her condition was good in October, 1939.

7. **Herpes Zoster.**—This seems to be a frequent lesion in diabetic patients. Whether the diabetic's susceptibility to infection applies to the central nervous system is not clear.

8. **Multiple Sclerosis.**—Case 18100, male, a school principal, aged twenty-five years, with diabetes for eighteen years, complained of recurrent bouts of difficulty in walking, diplopia and weakness. An examination revealed positive Babinski reflexes bilaterally, nystagmus, absent abdominal reflexes, a positive Romberg test, hyperactive knee jerks, inability to perform fine movements with his hands and a spastic gait. He received large doses of vitamins. A remission followed in a few months, but one year later he again developed difficulty in walking and nystagmus returned. In December 1945 another remission had occurred. Case 10355, female, aged twenty years at onset of diabetes in January, 1925, had hyperthyroidism August, 1931 for which a subtotal thyroidectomy was done. In March, 1933 her gait was ataxic, reflexes were hyperactive, the Babinski reaction was positive in both sides and sphincter disturbances were present as well as nystagmus and slight ptosis. The abdominal reflexes were absent and the serological examination of the blood and spinal fluid was negative. On March 23, 1933, she was taking 24 units of insulin a day. In October, 1934, she walked with great difficulty. The spinal fluid Wassermann was negative, but the gold sol curve was 4555552000 which has been reported consistent with multiple sclerosis. In may 1941 her right leg was almost completely paralyzed. Vitamin E therapy had not improved the condition.

9. **Friedrich's Ataxia.**—Dr. C. E. Richards, of Cincinnati, Ohio,[1] described 3 cases of Friedrich's ataxia in one family, the second, third and twelfth children, of whom 2 were diabetic. The oldest, a white male, aged thirty-two years, was admitted to a hospital in diabetic coma and died. His ataxia had begun about the age of eight years and had progressed, resulting in paraplegia and cord-bladder. The second, a male, aged twenty-nine years, showed a blood sugar of 310 mg. per cent an hour after the taking of 100

[1] Richards: Personal communication.

grams of glucose. He had bilateral pyramidal signs, ataxia, nystagmus, staccato speech, etc. The third is a female, aged eleven years, and at present has ataxia, nystagmus and a loss of patellar reflexes. The glucose-tolerance test is still normal.

The 2 diabetic sisters with Friedrich's ataxia described by Schlezinger and Goldstein[1] also presented evidences of multiple endocrine dysfunction.

Curtius, Störring and Schönberg from Umber's Clinic in Berlin[2] report two diabetic sisters with Friedrich's ataxia. Among a large number of the relatives of these two sisters, evidences of abnormalities in bony structure and in the central nervous system occurred frequently. They point out that the diabetes is not nervous diabetes but true pancreatic diabetes as shown in the case of Meltzer; this patient, at autopsy, showed marked changes in the islands of Langerhans and throughout the pancreas. Rossi (quoted by Curtius, *et al.*) described an eighteen-year-old sister and sixteen-year old brother who both had Friedrich's ataxia and diabetes. They mention eight other authors who have described cases of the combination of the two diseases. The study of 25 relatives of these two sisters by blood sugar analyses did not show any cases with latent diabetes. They felt the combination of Friedrich's ataxia and diabetes was not a coincidence but rather depended upon pathological genes.

10. **Suicide.**—Case 6884, a woman aged twenty-nine years, with diabetes for sixteen years with severe neuritis was found unconscious with three empty vials of U-80 insulin and a wet syringe beside the bed. Her blood sugar was 27 mg. Despite large doses of glucose, permanent cerebral damage was present and no evidence of higher cerebral function returned. She succumbed to pneumonia four and a half weeks later. (See page 394 for further details.)

Case 6523, aged fifty-five years, with diabetes of fourteen years' duration, attempted suicide by means of illuminating gas. During the fifteen years that followed she was at times somewhat depressed but did not make a second attempt. Her death occurred in February, 1940, from hypertensive heart disease. In all, 29 cases of suicide are known in this series. Secher[3] reports one unsuccessful attempt at suicide with insulin, and Beardwood[4] describes two others.

11. **Cerebral Hemorrhage.** — Cerebral vascular accidents in marked contrast to arteriosclerotic gangrene or to coronary occlusion apparently do not occur with any greater frequency in diabetic than in non-diabetic patients. Jordan and Watters[5] studied 70 such cases. The age at onset of the apoplexy varied from forty-six to seventy-seven years with an average of 62.2 years. Of the 70 cases,

[1] Schlezinger and Goldstein: Arch. Neurol. and Psychiat., **42**, 586, 1939.
[2] Curtius, Störring and Schönberg: Relation of Friedrich's Ataxia and Diabetes, Ztschr. f. d. ges. Neurol. u. Psychiat., **153**, 719, 1935.
[3] Secher: Ugesk. f. Laeger, **89**, 365, 1927.
[4] Beardwood: Jour. Am. Med. Assn., **102**, 765, 1934.
[5] Jordan and Watters: Am. Jour. Med. Sci., **186**, 488, 1933.

31 were dead at the time of the report.   Of these only 4 died within a short time from the shock and 2 others died of heart trouble within a week.   Of the 39 living cases none was completely incapacitated. Fifteen cases had more than one attack of apoplexy, and of these, 5 were still alive.   Arteriosclerosis and hypertension were the outstanding etiological factors.   On the whole diabetics seem to tolerate cerebral hemorrhage as well as non-diabetics.

Among 5669 fatal cases between 1898 and March 29, 1940, 472 cases have succumbed to cerebral hemorrhage, thrombosis or allied conditions.

15. **Miscellaneous.**—Byrom and Russell[1] describe a case with ependymal cyst of the third ventricle.   Fleming, Herring and Norris[2] describe three children aged eleven years, two years and one year and eleven months, respectively, entering the hospital in coma. The urine contained sugar, and in each case glucose-tolerance tests showed a blood sugar rise to well above 200 mg. per 100 cc.   However, the blood sugars became normal and the urine sugar-free.   In 2 cases there was a lesion of the pituitary with tumor and in 1 instance the development of a typical Fröhlich syndrome.   The third case died and was found to have atrophy of the cerebral cortex. The one striking clinical point was that with the coma, glycosuria and ketonuria, there was no definite Kussmaul respiration.   Cerebral lesions must be considered in the diagnosis of coma.

Subarachnoid hemorrhage may simulate diabetes.   Case 8517, aged eleven years, waked at 1 A.M. with headache and became unconscious at 3 A.M. on December 1, 1929.   In a nearby hospital the urine contained much sugar and the spinal-fluid sugar was 408 mg. per 100 cc.   The urine gave a red test for sugar every hour from 4.30 A.M. to 9.30 A.M. and insulin was given so that she received a total of 157 units in the first thirteen hours.   A second test of the cerebrospinal fluid sugar showed 419 mg. per 100 cc.   The fluid was bloody.   After the first day all urine tests were sugar-free.   The only blood-sugar test was 0.08 per cent after she had received 100 units of insulin.   One year later a second hemorrhage occurred.   Since that time she has been entirely well, according to her family physician (March, 1940).

Myasthenia gravis occurred in Case 11122, a physician, aged fifty-nine years, with diabetes of eleven years' duration in September, 1936.   Although he had been unable to swallow by the afternoon of each day, the use of ephedrin and glycocoll brought about some improvement, and prostigmine gave dramatic relief.   He was alive in April 1946.

Von Recklinghausen's disease occurred in Case 16327, housewife, aged thirty-eight years, in 1937, with diabetes of two years' duration. The neurofibromata were present along nerves of the arms, legs, feet and trunk.

[1] Byron and Russell: Lancet ii, 278, 1932.
[2] Fleming, Herring and Norris: Arch. Dis. Childhood, 10, 397, 1935.

CHAPTER XIX.

THE GENITO-URINARY SYSTEM IN DIABETES.

Revised by Charles W. Styron, M.D.

A. INFECTIONS OF THE URINARY TRACT.

The vulnerability of the diabetic to infection is evident in a study of the complications of the genito-urinary system. In 422 autopsies from 1919 to December 1, 1945 infection of the genito-urinary tract was found in 85 cases, or 20 per cent. The youngest, Case 11499, male, aged twelve years, with diabetes of six years' duration died of septicemia, paranephric abscess, and aspiration pneumonia. Of 212 deaths (hospital deaths plus deaths occurring at various intervals after discharge) in patients treated at the George F. Baker Clinic from August 1, 1939, there were 40 patients, or 19 per cent, with genito-urinary disease. In these 40 patients the genito-urinary complication was considered the primary cause of death in 16 cases and a secondary cause in 24 cases. There were 27 males and 13 females with an average age of sixty-seven years and an average diabetic duration of ten years.

In recent years significant changes have occurred in the management of urinary tract infections. Introduction of the chemotherapeutic agents, particularly the sulfonamides, penicillin and streptomycin[1] (the last named agent is not as yet generally available) has revolutionized the treatment of urinary infections. Numerous conditions formerly refractory to treatment are now managed successfully. Pyelonephritis of pregnancy, Proteus vulgaris, Streptococcus fecalis, and Pseudomonas æruginosa urinary infections formerly very difficult to cure are sensitive to the agents mentioned above. Treatment has become so simplified, in fact, that danger exists in the temptation to treat before making an accurate diagnosis. It is a simple matter to give the patient a trial of treatment with the idea of doing necessary studies later if treatment is unsuccessful. If such a course is taken, an infection may be ostensibly cured, whereas actually there remains serious underlying disease.

Proper management depends on (1) identification of the organism, (2) exact information regarding the morphology of the urinary tract, and (3) knowledge of any systemic disease affecting cure.

In the great majority of urinary infections in the present series and in those cases reported by Sharkey and Root[2] and by Baldwin and Root[3] the organism was the colon bacillus. On occasion it was found

---

[1] Helmholz: Proc. Staff Meetings Mayo Clinic, **20**, 357, 1945.
[2] Sharkey and Root: Jour. Am. Med. Assn., **104**, 2231, 1935.
[3] Baldwin and Root: New England Jour. Med., **223**, 244, 1940.

in association with the Staphylococcus aureus, Staphylococcus albus, Proteus vulgaris, Streptococcus hemolyticus, Streptococcus fecalis, Aerobacter ærogenes, Pseudomonas æruginosa, and at times the organisms named were found in pure culture or as mixed infections.

It is essential to know whether the route of invasion of the urinary tract is hematogenous or retrograde. In hematogenous infections the organism usually found is the Staphylococcus aureus. Frequently the hematogenous urinary tract infection is preceded by furuncles, carbuncles, foot infections with gangrene and cellulitis, and septicemia. Of 85 autopsies in which genito-urinary infection was present, 55 per cent were of hematogenous origin. Septicemia was demonstrated in 31 of these cases though bacteremia was certainly present in some others. Ascending urinary tract infection was present in 30, or 35 per cent, of the 85 autopsy cases. The common causes were calculi and prostatic hypertrophy. Carcinoma, paresis of the bladder, and urethral stricture were also found. There were 8 cases of the series in which no etiological factor for urinary infection could be found.

B. PYELONEPHRITIS.

From August 1, 1939 to December 1, 1945, 78 cases of pyelonephritis were treated. There were 72 females and 6 males. The cases of prostatic disease with urinary infection are not included. The average age of the group was forty-six years, and the average duration of diabetes was eleven years. The youngest patient was a female aged six, and the oldest a male, aged eighty-one. Severity of diabetes based on insulin dosage varied from very mild to quite severe. The records of these patients indicate that control of the diabetes was only fair. The organisms cultured from the urine were as follows: Escherichia coli in pure culture 22, mixed 19; Staphylococcus aureus hemolyticus, pure culture 6, mixed 12; Staphylococcus aureus non-hemolyticus pure culture or mixed 10; Streptococcus non-hemolyticus 4; Streptococcus hemolyticus 3; Pseudomonas æruginosa 3; Proteus vulgaris 3; Klebsiella pneumoniæ 2; Streptococcus fecalis 2; miscellaneous mixed infections of three or more organisms 6. The routes of infection were hematogenous 16 cases, obstructive 21, retrograde 27, unknown 14. The route was classified hematogenous only when the presence of a condition causing bacteremia and secondary renal infection was known and the etiologic organism was cultured from both the original lesion or the blood and the urine. The obstructive route was designated only when a structural defect was found by urological investigation and no definite evidence of hematogenous infection could be demonstrated. The retrograde classification was used for the most part in old patients or patients with urinary stasis due to debility or cachexia, but in whom no obstruction could be found.

Unknown was used for certain young or middle aged individuals who developed urinary tract infection without demonstrable cause.

Cases of pyelonephritis were classified as acute, recurrent, or chronic. There were 35 acute cases and 43 combined recurrent and chronic cases. It seems clear that a patient who is kept free of symptoms by urinary prophylaxis, but who has an exacerbation of acute pyelonephritis when the prophylaxis is stopped for a short while, is in reality a chronic case but one in whom the infection is kept at a minimum. Such examples are Cases 21073 and 10600, females of sixty and sixty-four years each with diabetes of many years' duration, who were able to keep asymptomatic on small doses of sulfadiazine. If the dose were omitted for a few days, symptoms would quickly arise.

The policy of immediate treatment of infection and aggressive eradication of its source is particularly necessary in pyelonephritis. Harrison and Bailey[1] have called attention to the significance of necrotizing pyelonephritis in diabetes mellitus. They stated that bacteria in the urinary tract are potential hazards and to be seriously regarded. When pyuria is present, it may be assumed that the focus of infection has been set up in the urinary tract and that destruction of tissue has already begun. It is true in our cases that those patients who have had pyelonephritis for any length of time before treatment is instituted, can hope to keep the infection under control and to remain asymptomatic only as long as chemotherapeutic agents are used. In fact the recurrence of symptoms, unless the patient has been treated from the earliest symptom, is the rule rather than the exception. The initial steps in the pathogenesis of the disease must be taken care of to avoid disasastrous results. Such early symptoms as frequency and dysuria are oftentimes not present in the diabetic of long-standing. It is therefore often necessary to depend upon urine culture and sediment, and urological procedures to make an early diagnosis.

The relationship of pyelonephritis to its most common complication, hypertension, is a much discussed but as yet unsettled, problem. Interest in the pyelonephritic contracted kidney was revived by the article of Weiss and Parker[2] who called attention to the high incidence of severe hypertension following pyelonephritis. Bowen and Kutzman[3] carried out complete urological examination in 84 unselected diabetic women. Only 7 of these 84 women had normal urinary tracts. Fifty-one patients had abnormalities of the kidneys, ureters, or bladder and of these 34 had active infection in the bladder and in one or both renal pelves. Twenty-two patients had a reduction of function on one or both sides, and 81.8 per cent of these had hypertension.

[1] Harrison and Bailey: Jour. Am. Med. Assn., **118**, 15, 1942.
[2] Weiss and Parker: Medicine, **18**, 221, 1939.
[3] Bowen and Kutzman: Ann. Int. Med., **17**, 427, 1942.

37

In the 78 cases of pyelonephritis in the authors' series, there were 29, or 37 per cent, with a blood-pressure of 150 or above systolic, and 90 or above diastolic. Of these 29 cases there were 20 who had chronic pyelonephritis. The average age of the hypertensive group was fifty-six, and the average age of the non-hypertensive group was thirty-nine years. Of the 43 cases with chronic or recurrent pyelonephritis, therefore, there were 20, or 47 per cent, who had hypertension. There were 4 patients who had a non-functioning kidney, 2 of whom had hypertension. Case 10775, male, aged twenty-one with diabetes of ten years' duration, had a non-functioning right kidney due to pyonephrosis and left pyelectasia. The blood-pressure was 130ı80. A right nephrectomy was done and the post-operative course was complicated by a 50 per cent pneumothorax on the right. In 1942 he had diabetic coma with a blood sugar of 1232 mg. per 100 cc. and CO_2 content of 7 volumes per cent. His treatment required 1820 units of insulin. In 1945 with diabetes of fifteen years' duration the remaining kidney functioned normally and the blood-pressure was 120/80. Case 17060, female, aged sixty-seven with diabetes of eleven years' duration had a non-functioning right kidney due to chronic pyelonephritis for a period of eight years. Yet the blood pressure remained unchanged at 160/90 through the years.

Treatment of Pyelonephritis.—The steps usually taken in the management of patients with pyelonephritis were the following in this order: (1) urine culture, (2) intravenous pyelogram, (3) treatment of acute infection, (4) urological consultation, and (5) retrograde pyelogram if the first steps indicated further study. The experience was that acute cases responded readily to small doses of sulfadiazine, and maintenance of adequate (1500 cc. a day) urine volume. Ordinarily 2 grams daily in divided doses gave adequate urinary drug concentration to combat most infections. For Proteus vulgaris and Streptococcus fecalis infections, doses up to 4 grams daily were used for higher concentration. Mandelic acid was also used in Streptococcus fecalis infections. If the response to treatment was not prompt, a course of penicillin was used in coccal infections. Any obstructive condition or malformation found by the urologist was corrected if the condition of the patient warranted operative procedures. Of equal importance in management of the infection was the best possible diabetic control, for without good control of the diabetes satisfactory results are not obtained. In this series a number of operative procedures were performed in an attempt to remove the cause or the source of infection. Operations performed were nephrectomy in 3 cases, nephrolithotomy in four cases, and miscellaneous procedures such as ureteral band excision, ureteral extraction of stone, urethral dilatation, drainage of paranephric abscess, and repairs of cystoceles and rectoceles. Patients were followed at frequent intervals after discharge for reappearance of pyuria. Oftentimes in acute primary infections and always in the chronic infections they were advised to take 1 to 1½ grams of sulfadiazine daily, and to keep the urine volume up to 1500 cc. daily. There were no instances of reactions or complications as a result of this small sulfadiazine dosage despite constant medication over a period as long as six months. *Any risk taken in prolonged chemotherapy is not as great as the risk of allowing recurrence of pyuria*

C. RENAL CALCULI.

Renal calculi were not a frequent cause of renal infection. From August 1, 1939 to December 1, 1945, 28 patients were seen with renal calculi. Of these, 6 had pyelonephritis. The colon bacillus was cultured from the urine in 5 cases and the Staphylococcus aureus hemolyticus in 1 case. The average age of the patients was fifty-nine years and the average duration was ten years. The youngest patient, Case 8949, a male, aged twenty-nine. had had diabetes eighteen years and the oldest patient, Case 14102, male, aged eighty years, had had diabetes ten years. There were 17 males and 12 females. Eleven of the patients were operated on by Dr. Harvard H. Crabtree. There were 4 nephrectomies and 4 patients with bilateral stones operated on twice. There was one death following operation. Case 21180, female, aged seventy-five, with diabetes of nine years' duration died following right nephrectomy for renal stones.

Calcium and phosphorus determinations of the blood were done on each patient and no abnormal levels were found.

D. CYSTITIS.

In 104 recent cases of cystitis treated, 84, or 81 per cent, were females. Escherichia coli was found in the majority of cases. The infections, as a rule, were secondary to a variety of conditions, among which were neoplasm of the bladder, pelvic cellulitis, cervicitis, bladder calculi, urethritis, benign prostatic hypertrophy and catheterization, although there were a few patients in whom no apparent cause was present. The infection was cleared in the majority of cases with as little as 1½ grams of sulfadiazine daily, provided the primary abnormality was corrected.

Catheterization should be carried out with great care. A sample of urine for culture should be obtained on the first catheterization, and following the procedure urinary prophylaxis should be used. The use of 1½ grams of sulfadiazine daily for three days will afford ample protection. If constant drainage is used, sulfadiazine should be given daily, and for at least three days following the removal of the catheter. We have seen one case with the bladder full of air due to improper use of the catheter. Pneumaturia has been reported[1]

[1] Riley and Bragdon: Jour. Am. Med. Assn., **108**, 1596, 1937.

due to yeast infection of the bladder, probably the result of catheri-zation. Gas was expelled at the end of micturition and the patient could void only when erect.

Kretschmer[1] states that the triad of symptoms, frequency, dysuria and pyuria frequently results in diagnoses of cystitis, few of which are substantiated, and that, oftentimes, the serious under-lying disease is allowed to progress until conservative surgery becomes impossible. A trial of treatment without urological studies, if ever permissible, is so only when the patient can be watched for recurrence. Otherwise an intravenous pyelogram and possibly cystoscopy should be performed together with any acces-sory studies required for a diagnosis.

E. PARANEPHRIC ABSCESS.

Although the frequency of renal cortical abscesses and pyelone-phritis would seem to predispose to paranephric abscesses,[2] these have been uncommon. Following an attack of furunculosis, Case 16593, male, aged forty-five years was placed on sulfadiazine in February 1944, because of sepsis and right costo-vertebral angle tenderness. Blood cultures showed Staphylococcus aureus. Several days later a large paranephric abscess was drained and Staphylo-coccus aureus cultured from the exudate. In April 1944, a large subfascial abscess of the right shoulder was drained. In November 1944, he was readmitted because of fever, emaciation, and pain in the lumbosacral region. An x-ray showed osteomyelitis of the 5th lumbar vertebra and calculi in the left kidney. Penicillin was given for thirty days and gradual improvement ensued without surgical treatment of the osteomyelitis. In June 1945, an x-ray of the back was taken. There was no acute infection apparent, but instead evidence of an old healed process in the 5th lumbar vertebra. The general improvement of the man was so great as to make him hardly recognizable.

Aside from the remarkable cure of osteomyelitis without drain-age, this case is notable because it emphasizes the chronicity of Staphylococcus infection and the absolute necessity for constant supervision following apparent recovery. Case 2008, male, aged forty-six years, with diabetes of eighteen years' duration died of Staphylococcus aureus septicemia following drainage of a para-nephric abscess in September 1938. The patient had been treated some months previously in another institution for pyuria. Unre-mitting follow up and treatment might have saved his life. Case 9543, aged twenty-two years with diabetes of six years' duration died following drainage of a paranephric abscess as a result of bilateral pyelonephritis. Case 4289, female, aged twenty-nine years

[1] Kretschmer: New England Jour. Med., **233**, 339, 1945.
[2] Boyd: Textbook of Pathology, 4th ed., Philadelphia, Lea & Febiger, p. 611, 1943.

with diabetes of two months' duration entered the hospital in December 1924 in diabetic coma and acute thyroid storm. She recovered from these conditions, but later a furuncle of the labium was found, a paranephric abscess followed and was incised, but she died of septicemia. Case 4142, male, aged forty-seven years with diabetes of three years' duration entered the hospital and died of Staphyloccus aureus septicemia. Autopsy disclosed a paranephric abscess of moderate size. Case 2720, male, aged nineteen years with diabetes of ten months' duration, entered in July 1922 with acidosis and died of a paranephric abscess which extended through the diaphragm and caused an abscess of the lung. Case 2988, female, aged fifty-six years with diabetes for four years died in 1926 with diabetic coma, a paranephric abscess and bronchial pneumonia.

F. PARESIS OF THE BLADDER.

Paresis of the bladder is an unusual finding associated with reflex changes and paresthesiæ due to diabetic neuritis. The condition occurs in both young and old, and the diabetes may be of recent or of many years' duration. There is no evidence that the cause of the atonic bladder is old age, combined system disease, lues, tumor, or injury. It is commonly seen in cachectic females with infection and gangrene of the extremities in whom the expectancy of life is short. The condition has occurred in one patient, male, aged thirty-two, Case 16571, and has persisted for as long as thirteen years. The total spinal fluid protein may be elevated, and this fact is of some diagnostic significance provided other causes of elevation are carefully eliminated. Treatment has consisted of closed drainage with frequent trials for spontaneous micturition. Parasympathetic stimulators (mecholyl and doryl) have been helpful, and in one case doryl injections produced voiding of 1000 cc. at a time. In addition to urological treatment all patients with bladder paresis should receive vitamin B complex. Recovery is expected if diabetic control is maintained over a period of one to five years. Secondary infections are frequent sequelæ, and it is advisable to use sulfadiazine in small doses as a urinary prophylactic while the patient is under treatment. Temporary atony of the bladder may occur in diabetic coma when as much as 2000 cc. of urine may be present in the bladder. Usually there is associated areflexia. Recovery parallels recovery from coma.

Case 4023, female, aged seventy-two years with diabetes of fifteen years' duration had been treated for paresis of the bladder for eleven years at death in 1937. In 1927, 2600 cc. of urine were obtained by catheter. It was possible to reduce the residual urine to a few ounces when she was first under treatment, but if the patient became excited or nervous, the residual would oftentimes exceed 2000 cc. The last two years of life the residual was seldom under 1500. Urinary antiseptics were constantly necessary for pyuria. Autopsy showed bladder dilatation, cystitis and right hydronephrosis.

G. DIABETIC COMA AND URINARY TRACT INFECTION.

Genito-urinary infection is a subtle and not infrequent precipitant of diabetic acidosis. The diabetic, as a rule, is trained to watch for and to have treated the simplest of infections. The merest abrasion, the smallest infected hair follicle, the common cold are all immediately evident and the patient is forewarned. Oftentimes the earliest symptoms of urinary tract infection are overlooked or more commonly misunderstood. Frequency and dysuria, for example, are thought by the patient to be due to two much sugar until extension of the process causes fever and pain. If the patient is accustomed to make only infrequent visits to the doctor, the focus of infection may have such a head start that irreparable damage is done. This is particularly true of pyelonephritis. Any condition causing urinary stasis, such as a cystocele or silent kidney stone, should be watched carefully and corrected as soon as possible. Confinement of older patients in bed is oftentimes a cause of urinary stasis and infection.

In 121 cases collected by Sharkey and Root[1] and Baldwin and Root,[2] 14 patients entered the hospital with diabetic acidosis, 10 of whom were in coma. Nine patients had pyelonephritis, 3 paranephric abscesses, and 2 acute cystitis. It is often necessary to catheterize patients in diabetic coma and unless measures are taken to prevent urinary infection, it will surely occur. The measures used at the George F. Baker Clinic are outlined under cystitis. Case 18521, female, aged thirty-two with diabetes of eight years' duration is an excellent example of the occasional clinical course of a diabetic with pyuria. While under treatment she developed diabetic coma and was transferred to the New England Deaconess Hospital. On admission the blood sugar was 368 mg. per cent, and the CO_2 content 15 volumes per cent. Following treatment for coma an intravenous pyelogram revealed poor kidney function on the left side with dilated pelvis and calyces. This patient has since been followed, and has invariably shown pyuria due to the colon bacillus. The infection has been controlled to the point of keeping the patient asymptomatic with sulfadiazine in small doses.

H. DISEASES OF THE PROSTATE.

1. **Benign Prostatic Hypertrophy.**—From August 1, 1939 to December 1, 1945, 101 patients with benign prostatic hypertrophy were treated. Of these patients, 5 died as a direct result of the disease. The average age was sixty-eight years and the average duration of diabetes twelve years. The youngest patient was forty-six years old and the oldest patient eighty-four years. One patient in three of the group had hypertension. Forty patients had symptoms which varied from mild nocturia to acute retention; 35 of

[1] Sharkey and Root: Loc. cit., p. 575.
[2] Baldwin and Root: Loc. cit., p. 575.

these had residual urine from one ounce upwards. There were 28 with non-protein-nitrogen levels over 40 mg. per cent, the highest of which was 133 mg. per cent. Thirty-two patients had urinary infection mostly of slight degree, although a few had serious acute ascending infections. Three entered the hospital in acute retention and 2 patients developed acute retention following admission, 1 in the course of treatment for pneumonia and 1 following a toe amputation.

Operation was carried out on 30 of the 101 patients. Their average age was sixty-eight years. Fourteen had hypertension. In addition, arteriosclerotic and hypertensive heart disease, severe peripheral arteriosclerosis, retinal hemorrhages and nephrosclerosis were common findings. In general, therefore, they were poor operative risks. Transurethral prostatic resection was done in 24 cases and a two-stage suprapubic prostatectomy in 6. There was no death as a result of the prostatectomies, but Case 22363, aged fifty-six, on whom a transurethral resection was planned, died of a pulmonary embolus following cystoscopy. Case 2545, aged eighty-four, entered the hospital for prostatectomy and died of a cerebral hemorrhage before any operative procedure was carried out. Case 22191 was discharged on the seventh postoperative day but the average postoperative hospital course was sixteen days for the transurethral resections and thirty-seven days for the suprapubic operations. The preoperative preparation was often prolonged, particularly in the 10 patients who entered with urinary infection, and in those requiring vasectomy or gradual decompression. The final results of operation were satisfactory. Five patients of the 30 continued to have frequency or nocturia, but to a less degree than previously. In several, bladder symptoms were probably due to low grade infection or to diabetes. Management of the diabetes was not difficult as a rule since the disease was not usually severe.

2. **Carcinoma of the Prostate.**—In addition to the 101 cases of benign hypertrophy of the prostate there were 7 cases of prostatic carcinoma. Their ages ranged from sixty-two to eighty-four. The most satisfactory results were in Case 5398, aged seventy-five, who had a transurethral resection for prostatic obstruction in 1940. In 1943, he developed low back pain and bladder symptoms due to extension and metastasis of an adenocarcinoma of the prostate and a bilateral orchidectomy was done. In the summer of 1945, he was getting along satisfactorily at the age of eighty with diabetes of thirty-eight years' duration. Case 17211, aged seventy-eight, with duration of diabetes of thirteen years had a transurethral resection in March 1943. The resection was followed by orchidectomy, which he survived for thirteen months having had only temporary relief. Case 21741, aged seventy-five, with diabetes of five years' duration had only slight bladder symptoms due to a low grade urinary infection three years following an orchidectomy. Only 2 cases of

prostatic carcinoma were operated on in the preceding five year series. Case 3345, aged seventy-six years, underwent a successful prostatectomy by Dr. G. G. Smith for carcinoma in 1931. He died of tuberculosis in 1938.

3. **Infections of the Prostate.**—Fourteen cases of prostatitis were treated from August 1, 1939 to December 1, 1945. Case 5390, aged forty-six with diabetes of twenty years' duration had iridocyclitis in 1941 thought to be related to a non-specific chronic prostatitis. Case 12086, aged fifty, had chronic prostatitis which was followed by an iritis. Case 21260, aged fifty-nine, with diabetes of two years' duration, survived a furuncle on the upper lip, a large abscess of the left thigh, an abscess of the prostate, and Staphylococcus aureus septicemia. He was treated with sulfadiazine and incision and drainage of the thigh abscess. The prostatic abscess fortunately ruptured into the urethra and required no surgery.

In 86 cases of genito-urinary infection prostatic abscesses occurred 8 times. They were the focus of septicemia on four occasions and in five instances the direct cause of death. The prostate of the diabetic in particular is likely to be the source of metastatic abscesses. The secondary abscesses may appear before the prostatic abscess has given rise to symptoms. On a few occasions patients have run an intermittent septic fever for days before local symptoms have occurred.

I. MISCELLANEOUS.

1. **Tumors.**—The prostate has been by far the most common site of tumor, but not of carcinoma. Of 219 cancer deaths prior to 1934, 14 were primary in the bladder and 8 in the prostate. Case 9195, female, aged eighty-one, with diabetes of fourteen years' duration had a papilloma of the ureter with marked hydroureter and hydronephrosis for eight years prior to death in 1944 of cerebral hemorrhage. Case 7678, male, aged sixty, with diabetes of fifteen years' duration had a nephrectomy for carcinoma of the kidney after symptoms for one year. In 1944, two years postoperative, there was no recurrence. Case 4609, male, aged sixty-eight, with diabetes of twenty-one years' duration, showed no evidence of recurrence four years after removal of a carcinoma of the bladder. Case 26286, male, aged fifty-nine with diabetes of one year duration had suprapubic excision of two epidermoid carcinomas of the bladder in 1945. There was no recurrence in six months. Case 3654, male, aged seventy-six, with diabetes of twenty-one years' duration had excision of a highly malignant carcinoma of the bladder in 1944 without recurrence in a follow-up one year later.

2. **Malformations.**—Case 4506, female, aged thirty-four with diabetes of twenty years' duration has an infected right kidney, an infected accessory right kidney and ureter removed at operation in

1943. Case 7016, aged sixty-three, female, with diabetes of seventeen years' duration had a horseshoe kidney with pyelonephritis.

3. **Calcification of the Vas Deferens.**—Calcification of the vas deferens is occasionally seen in patients with long-standing diabetes. Case 17801 aged sixty-seven years, with diabetes of eighteen years' duration died of pneumococcus septicemia. At autopsy each vas deferens was found to be calcified and the lumen obliterated. Case 18685, aged thirty years, with diabetes of twelve years' duration had vas deferens calcification, retinal hemorrhages, calcification in the arteries of the legs and albuminuria. Case 15635 died in uremia of chronic nephritis at age forty-eight. Calcification occurred in Case 13982, aged sixty-four years, with diabetes of only $3\frac{1}{2}$ years' duration. There was no genito-urinary infection in any of these patients.

4. **Incidental Cases.**—Case 16470, female, aged thirty, had an infected right kidney and right ureteral stricture. When ureteral dilatation and retrograde pyelogram was performed the dye extravasated to the perinephric tissues. On nephrectomy, a tuberculous pyelonephritis was found, the first such case in this series.

Case 22548, aged thirty-eight, with diabetes of two years' duration had extensive gangrene of the scrotum due to Staphylococcus aureus hemolyticus. Following partial excision, drainage, and sulfadiazine therapy, healing was uneventful. Case 7972, aged eighty-three, with diabetes of ten years' duration had gangrene of the scrotum and testicle followed by two ischio-rectal abscesses. After amputation of the scrotum and testicle prompt healing occurred. Case 8313, aged thirty-eight, with diabetes of thirteen years' duration developed left orchitis and necrosis with epididymitis and prostatitis. Recovery was rapid following orchidectomy. Case 22571, aged fifty-three, with diabetes of ten years' duration had bilateral epididymectomy for chronic infection.

Case 7686, aged thirty, duration of diabetes sixteen years, had severe mixed fusiform and anærobic streptococcus balanitis which responded readily to dorsal slit, irrigations and penicillin. Two other cases of balanitis have occurred recently. Circumcision would seem to be indicated in diabetics.

Infarction of the kidney occurred in Case 10205, aged fifty-one, male, with diabetes of ten years' duration due to embolism from a fibrillating heart. Case 8903, female, aged sixty-two, had kidney infarction following an operation for hyperthyroidism. Case 7763, female, aged sixty-nine, had adhesive pericarditis and coronary occlusion followed by infarction of the kidney.

J. PRINCIPLES OF MANAGEMENT.

In management of the diabetic patient there are frequently so many factors to consider that one may fail to heed the danger of pyuria. We try to keep in mind the following principles of management.

1. The first physician who sees a patient with urinary tract infection has the best chance of eradicating that infection before the development of complicating features.

2. Since no single medication is effective against all organisms, identification of the infecting organism is essential.

3. Along with treatment for pyuria, search for an obstructive lesion is made. Chemotherapeutic agents are so effective that pyuria is easily cleared up in most cases. However, without definitive treatment of the cause of the pyuria, recurrence and extension of the infection is almost certain to occur.

4. Delay in investigation of pyuria is dangerous. In the diabetic, destructive changes may occur in a few weeks which will make the infection incurable.

5. Distention of the bladder in the aged, the postoperative, and in the comatose patient should be avoided. Failure to use the catheter may do more harm than its use. Once a patient has been catheterized, the use of sulfadiazine 1½ to 2 grams daily as a prophylactic and administration of fluid by mouth or by needle to insure an output of 1500 cc. urine daily are important.

6. Any diabetic patient who has had a urinary tract infection needs follow-up and treatment for an extended period.

CHAPTER XX.

DISORDERS OF THE SKIN IN DIABETES.

REVISED BY PRISCILLA WHITE, M.D.

THERE are no diseases of the skin which are absolutely unique to diabetes. However, certain affections are more common in diabetics than non-diabetics; among these are infections with furuncles, boils, carbuncles; pruritus of the external genitalia seen particularly in female patients with marked glycosuria; xanthosis; xanthomata; and necrobiosis lipoidica diabetica.

A. HYPERGLYCEMIA AND DISEASES OF THE SKIN.

There is by no means agreement that an increase of sugar in the blood predisposes to disease of the skin. Goldsmith[1] believes that "carbohydrate disturbances are not known to give rise to any specific dermatoses. Moreover, their relationship to any disorder of the skin is very uncertain." Rost[2] states that a "disorder of carbohydrate metabolism is occasionally connected with skin disease. Whether certain groups of skin diseases are regularly connected with hyperglycemia is doubtful." Urbach[3] describes skin diabetes, a syndrome characterized by furunculosis, sweat gland abscesses, eczema and pruritus resistant to therapy. High fasting skin sugar level is demonstrated along with normal blood sugar. Improvement, clinical and chemical, follows low carbohydrate diets with or without insulin. As far as infections are concerned, experiments *in vitro* have shown that blood to which 0.5 to 1 per cent dextrose has been added is no better culture medium for staphylococci than normal blood and that adding dextrose does not diminish the blood's bactericidal power. For further discussion see page 527.

Tauber,[4] comparing a group of diabetics with one of non-diabetics, found twice the number of infections of the hands and feet in the non-diabetic group. In the common diseases of the skin, the blood sugar was normal almost without exception. He reports that in furunculosis, pyoderma and ecthyma, beneficial results quickly followed the use of a high-carbohydrate diet, liver extract and injections of 500 cc. of 5 per cent glucose intravenously daily for six successive days. This agrees with the experience of Crawford and Swartz[5] who believed that glucose intravenously improved

[1] Goldsmith: Recent Advances in Dermatology, Philadelphia, P. Blakiston's Sons & Co., p. 170, 1936.

[2] Rost: Brit. Jour. Dermat. and Syph., **44**, 157, 1932.

[3] Urbach: Jour. Am. Med. Assn., **129**, 441, 1945. See also Urbach: Skin Diseases, Nutrition and Metabolism, New York, Grune and Stratton, 1946.

[4] Tauber: Arch. Dermat. and Syph., **27**, 198, 1933.

[5] Crawford and Swartz: Arch. Dermat. and Syph., **33**, 1035, 1936.

cases of acne vulgaris.   Although Loeb,[1] in a series of 462 cases, found an absolute increase in the blood sugar of patients with certain skin lesions, in others a definite hypoglycemia was present. Darnet[2] advises investigation of the blood sugar in all cases of chronic skin lesions, suggesting that if a high content is found insulin should be tried.

As stated on page 151, Trimble and Carey[3] found that the average true sugar content of skin in non-diabetic subjects was 56 mg., and in diabetic subjects, 144 mg. per cent; among the diabetic group the average true sugar of the blood was 226 mg. per cent.   These figures are similar to those of Urbach et al.[4] who found in normal human beings an average of 61 mg. per cent of "free" sugar in the skin and 103 mg. per cent in the blood; in 1 patient with diabetes whose fasting blood sugar was approximately 220 mg. per cent, the corresponding skin value was approximately 135 mg. per cent.

Talbert and Silvers[5] found sugar in the sweat of 28 non-diabetics in amounts varying from 5.6 to 40 mg. per 100 cc., the average being about 15 mg.   Likewise Usher and Rabinowitch[6] showed that dextrose is a normal constituent of sweat.

B. INCIDENCE AND VARIETY OF SKIN DISEASE IN DIABETES.

1. **General.**—A comparison between the incidence and variety of skin affections in a group of 500 diabetic patients at the New England Deaconess Hospital and various series of non-diabetics was made by Greenwood.[7]   Twenty-five per cent of the diabetics gave a history of skin disease.   Skin lesions were actually present in 11.4 per cent of the number, as compared with 10 per cent for the general clinic at the Out-Patient Department of the Massachusetts General Hospital and 5 per cent in the private practice of Dr. C. G. Lane.[8]

In the group of 500 diabetics, furunculosis, carbuncles, erysipelas, psoriasis, xanthoma palpebrarum and Dupuytren's contractures showed higher percentages than in the non-diabetic series, in contrast to eczema, the incidence of which was lower.

Rudy stated that in his experience, "skin manifestations of the pellagrous type are not infrequently observed in diabetic patients, especially when they are markedly debilitated."[9]

[1] Loeb: Arch. f. Dermat. u. Syph., **152**, 529. 1926.
[2] Darnet: Semana méd., **34**, 769, 1927.
[3] Trimble and Carey: Loc. cit., p. 151.
[4] Urbach and Rejtö: Arch. f. Dermat., **166**, 478, 1932; Urbach, Depisch and Sicher: Klin. Wchnschr., **16**, 452, 1937.
[5] Talbert and Silvers: Quoted by Greenwood.[7]
[6] Usher and Rabinowitch: Arch. Dermat. and Syph., **16**, 706, 1927.
[7] Greenwood: Jour. Am. Med. Assn., **89**, 774, 1927.
[8] Lane: Quoted by Greenwood.[7]
[9] Rudy: Endocrinology, **27**, 206, 1940.

2. **Pruritus.**—Pruritus appeared in 33 cases of Greenwood's series, approximately 1 case in 15. This was localized in type in 17 patients. Pruritus pudendi frequently occurs in uncontrolled diabetes, especially in females. It will usually vanish within a few days, but occasionally not until two weeks after the disappearance of sugar from the urine. General pruritus, fortunately less common, may be annoying and persist for weeks, and resist all forms of treatment. If pruritus pudendi does not clear up promptly, as the urine becomes sugar-free, an examination will probably disclose a local cause, such as a prolapse, leucorrhea, urinary incontinence, trichomonas, or skin diseases such as herpes, psoriasis, or urticaria. Rest in bed, absolute cleanliness, simple douches and the simplest ointments are indicated. The free use of oil to prevent irritation during micturition is helpful. There may be cases in which $\frac{1}{4}$ skin unit doses of roentgen-ray become necessary to allay the itching. In Hédon's depancreatized dog this was only accomplished when he received cystine. Pruritus is a frequent symptom in the latent stage of diabetes, according to Marañon. Hesseltine[1] has made a special study of vulvovaginitis in diabetic patients. He found that fungicidal therapy cures diabetic pruritus and synthetic glycosuria does not produce either pruritus or vulvitis. Although glycosuria does not cause the condition, it provides an adequate medium for the fungus.

TABLE 70.—A COMPARISON OF CERTAIN AFFECTIONS OF THE SKIN IN DIABETICS IN THE OUT-PATIENT DEPARTMENT OF THE MASSACHUSETTS GENERAL HOSPITAL, AND IN A GENERAL PRACTICE. (FROM GREENWOOD.[2])

Disease.	Diabetics.		Mass. Gen. Hosp., per cent.	Lane, per cent.
	No.	Per cent.		
Furunculosis	7	1.4	0.9	0.24
Carbuncle	3	0.6	0.12	0.2
Erysipelas	2	0.4	0.04	0.11
Psoriasis	12	2.4	0.23	0.1
Eczema	14	2.8	4.0	0.5
Seborrheic dermatitis	1	0.2	0.27	0.2
Xanthoma palpebrarum	9	1.8	0.02	
Dupuytren's contractures	8	1.6	0.016	

Experimentally it has been proved that the diabetic skin is more easily infected with monilia than the normal. The reason is, however, obscure since the course of an infection does not run parallel with the degree of hyperglycemia.[3] It has been the experience of Dr. A. M. Greenwood and Dr. E. M. Rockwood that monilial infection in diabetics is primarily of the vulval mucous membranes with possible extension to the skin, whereas in non-diabetics monilial infection has been intertriginous, affecting the submammary regions, groins and axillæ.

[1] Hesseltine: Jour. Am. Med. Assn., **100**, 177, 1933.
[2] Greenwood: Loc. cit., p. 588.
[3] Goldsmith, p. 346, loc. cit., p. 587.

Rudy and Hoffmann[1] describe the pronounced cutaneous eruptions in diabetic patients not unlike that of pellagrins, frequently due to vitamin deficiencies, especially of nicotinic acid. In this condition, the vulnerability to any kind of irritation, mechanical, chemical or thermal, and to infection, is greatly increased. They consider the vulvitis as well as pruritus vulvae and pruritus ani in diabetes as evidences of vitamin deficiency. Also, violaceous color and the shiny surface as well as fine peeling or scaliness, or ridging with edema, blistering or maceration are variations in the picture. Frequently superinfection with monilia on certain regions suggest intertrigo. The deficiency is notable and aided only by vitamin administration.

Dosa[2] found that borax promptly stopped the growth of fungi even in weak concentrations and most efficiently with a pH around the neutral point or slightly toward the acid side. Dr. E. M. Rockwood advises for pruritus pudendi due to infection with monilia, compresses and Sitz baths of 0.5 per cent sodium borate (20 Mule Team Borax, 1 teaspoonful to 1 quart of water) followed, when the acute condition subsides, by 1 per cent aqueous solution of gentian violet. Silver nitrate, 0.25 per cent, may also be useful.

Menopausal or senile vulvitis (kraurosis) may be best treated as in others by estrogen orally, by injection or inunction.

Pruritus ani in diabetics, according to Greenwood, can be separated into three types: (1) those in which the skin around the anus is definitely infected with bacteria; (2) those in which it is definitely infected with fungi; and (3) those in which the skin shows no change. It is almost impossible to tell from appearances alone how to distinguish between the first two. The only way it can be done accurately is by careful microscopic search for fungi. In general, the mycotic infections are apt to show outlying lesions and also a peculiar white macerated appearance back of the anus in the intergluteal fold.

As treatment Greenwood has used mercurochrome or a similar substance in the bacterial types. For the second type, he prescribes Whitfield's ointment, or more commonly an ointment of salicylic acid and sulphur, āā 2; petrolatum 30—or strong potassium permanganate up to 30 grains to the ounce (2 grams in 30). For the last type, local anti-pruritic methods and roentgen-ray are used. At times he uses roentgen-ray for all types, but unless there are very definite results after four treatments of 75 roentgen it should be discontinued. The total dosage should not exceed 1000 r. If at all possible in these cases take every means to prevent scratching, even going so far as to splint the arms at night.

General measures may be adopted while the attack of pruritus is acute. These include bed rest, cold compresses of water, boric

[1] Rudy and Hoffmann: New England Jour. Med., **227**, 893, 1942.
[2] Dosa: Arch. f. Dermat. u. Syph., **176**, 261, 1937.

or sodium bicarbonate antipruritic substances, ointments with novocain or cocain. Nerve sedatives may be necessary.

3. **Epidermophytosis.**—Epidermophytosis was the most common disease in the patients studied by Greenwood. Including all types, there were 198 cases, 40 per cent, in which this was present in the feet. Every other patient over twenty years of age had a fungus infection of the feet. This is about the same percentage which Hulsey and Jordan[1] found among university students, 67 per cent, but above the percentage for men in the United States naval service.[2] In diabetes these epidermophytotic infections are most serious. They give to the skin a parboiled appearance between the toes with, at times, open fissures in the depths of the interdigital spaces or on the plantar surfaces of the toes or at their junction with the soles. Since 100 per cent of the interdigital spaces in diabetics give cultures of staphylococcus such fissures may give portals of entry for serious infection and many a diabetic patient has subsequently lost a toe or a foot from resulting osteomyelitis.

Greenwood thinks the danger of treating epidermophytosis with strong proprietary preparations of unknown make-up should be particularly stressed. It is probably true that at least one-half of the cases seen by dermatologists show severe dermatitis due to such treatment and quickly subside under the simplest methods, such as boric acid soaks and compresses, and bland applications. In addition, too vigorous treatment of fungus infections is at times followed by a generalized eruption, an epidermophytid, which is most disagreeable. Such an eruption should not, of course, be treated by fungicidal applications. This applies particularly to the hands where such allergic reactions to fungus infections elsewhere are most frequent.

4. **Infections of the Skin.**—Infections of the skin demand immediate, thorough, yet gentle, treatment. One of the first duties of the physician is to tell diabetic patients to keep the skin exquisitely clean and to report the beginning of an infection at once. Patients should be warned of the danger from slight wounds, should specifically be advised not to allow manicurists or chiropodists to draw a drop of blood and cautioned to report promptly any injury to the skin. Finger and toe nails should be cleaned with a blunt, not sharp, tipped file or, better, an orange stick. Tincture of green soap is recommended for children. Absolute cleanliness of the body is essential.

A diabetic is particularly prone to infections if he has a dry skin, and his feet are so commonly infected by fungus diseases that they deserve particular care.

Subcutaneous injections can be given as in any normal individual, but scrupulous asepsis should be practised.

[1] Hulsey and Jordan: Am. Jour. Med. Sci., **169**, 267, 1925.
[2] Butler, Houghton and Cooper: U. S. Naval Med. Bull, **21**, 615, 1924.

In Greenwood's series the percentage of furunculosis rose from 1.4 to 6.6 per cent, of carbuncles from 0.6 to 1.8 per cent and of erysipelas from 0.4 to 1 per cent when the histories of the patients as well as what they presented upon examination were combined.

5. **Furunculosis.**—If there is the slightest tendency to furunculosis at once adopt simple measures analogous to those described by Bowen.[1] The patient is advised to wash the whole body twice a day with soap and water, using a fresh piece of sterilized gauze and powdered or liquefied soap and to dry the skin with a freshly boiled towel without rubbing, so as to avoid breaking open any pustule; the whole body is then bathed with a saturated solution of boric acid in water, with the addition of a small proportion of camphor water and glycerin. We have often advised a solution of 2 parts medicated alcohol No. 1 and 1 part water to advantage, but Bowen, in his second paper, still prefers the boric acid. Individual furuncles may be treated with the following ointment, according to Bowen:

Boric acid	4
Precipitated sulphur	4
Carbolated petrolatum	30

One should be careful, however, not to overtreat the skin. Harm may result from frequent dressings. The simplest lotions should always be employed. In severe cases the patient should be put to bed, all linens changed twice daily and the patient treated in an aseptic manner. In a few cases, vaccines have appeared to be of a marked benefit. "This procedure—thorough bathing and soaping, the application of the borated solution and the dressing of the individual furuncles—is repeated, as has been said, morning and night. A further point of vital importance relates to the clothing that is worn next to the skin. Every stitch of linen worn next to the skin should be changed daily, and in the case of extensive furunculosis all the bed-clothing that touches the individual, as well as the night-clothing, should be subjected to a daily change. Naturally, the treatment must be continued for several weeks after the last evidence of pyogenic infection has appeared, and this fact must be emphasized to the patient at the outset."[1]

For the management of infections and carbuncles in diabetes, see pages 529 and 683.

6. **Xanthochromia.**—Xanthochromia (xanthosis) is a yellow discoloration of the skin frequently seen in diabetes, but this common appearance is not to be confused with xanthoma diabeticorum. It is particularly noticeable on the palms of the hands, soles of the feet and nasolabial folds. It may be seen on the face, but more rarely over

---

[1] Bowen: Jour. Am. Med. Assn., **55**, 209, 1910; Boston Med. and Surg. Jour., **176**, 96, 1917.

the body generally.   The pigment which causes it may also be found in the blood.   It is a lipochrome and the discoloration must be considered due to an excess of lipochrome in the blood and tissues, which in turn is derived from food.   One of the pigments is carotin, as demonstrated by Palmer.   Writers quite generally agree that the lipochrome, found so constantly in the blood of diabetics, is due to their food which is especially rich in lipochrome. Green vegetables, spinach, salad, egg-yolk, carrots and butter all contain a large portion of it.   Stoner[1] has written a concise article on carotinemia and summarized the literature to which Hess was an early contributor.   See page 217 for data from autopsy.

However, the diet is not the only factor responsible.   There is evidently some disturbance in the patient's ability to excrete or destroy lipochrome as shown by Ralli and co-workers.[2]   Xantho-chromia occurs in severe, not mild diabetes, and this a priori is usually associated with disordered fat metabolism.   Klose[3] encoun-tered it more commonly in the obese child.   A peculiar color of the skin due to vegetables is noticed with the Laps and in a certain section of Japan.

Xanthosis is not confined to diabetic patients.   Boeck and Yater[4] observed it in 9 per cent of 100 patients with diabetes, in 9 per cent of 22 patients with renal disease and in 3 per cent of 23 other hospital patients selected at random.

The treatment of xanthosis consists in (1) adequate control of the diabetic condition; (2) temporary restriction of the intake of pig-mented fruits and vegetables and occasionally of eggs and butter; (3) supplementary medication with vitamin concentrates and min-erals as indicated to replace those ordinarily obtained in the foods restricted.

Pigmentation of the skin in diabetes (brown or slightly grayish) first suggest hemochromatosis.   However, Peck and Sage[5] report another case of Albright's syndrome associated with diabetes mel-litus.   In addition to the osteitis fibrosa disseminata, areas of skin pigmentation and endocrine dysfunction, mild exophthalmus were observed together with insulin resistance.

7. **Xanthoma Diabeticorum.**—Xanthoma diabeticorum is a dis-ease of considerable frequency in a diabetic clinic, but apparently not very common in dermatological clinics.   Thus, C. J. White, in 1920, wrote he had encountered but 3 or 4 cases.   Major[6] described 3 cases and collected 74 from the literature.   The lesions are tumors often brilliant yellow, and associated with a red periphery which differentiates them from all other types of xanthomata.   The erup-

[1] Stoner: Am. Jour. Med. Sci., **175**, 31, 1928.
[2] Ralli, Brandaleone and Mandelbaum: Jour. Lab. and Clin. Med., **20**, 1266, 1935: Stueck, Flaum and Ralli: Jour. Am. Med. Assn., **109**, 343, 1937.
[3] Klose: München. med. Wchnschr., **66**, 419, 1919.
[4] Boeck and Yater: Jour. Lab. and Clin. Med., **14**, 1129, 1929.
[5] Peck and Sage: Am. Jour. Med. Sci., **208**, 35, 1944.
[6] Major: Bull. Johns Hopkins Hosp., **35**, 27, 1924.

tion may appear somewhat suddenly and may extend over the body generally. The tubercles are most numerous on the outside and back of the forearm, and especially about the elbows and knees where they are confluent. They are usually absent from the flexures of the larger joints. The tubercles are of various sizes, some being as large as a small pea.

The presence of xanthomata is recorded in 12 of our patients. Three of these cases were males and 9 cases were females. The age of the youngest patient was twelve years. The duration of the diabetes when the patient was first seen varied between one and twenty-one years.

The blood fat in xanthoma diabeticorum is usually reported to be increased. This was true of Major's cases. In the 2 cases observed by Nicholson[1] among his 600 diabetics the cholesterol was 1.26 per cent with one and the creamy blood of the other showed 4.4 per cent (Bloor) blood fat. The latter case confirms C. J. White's favorable prognosis of the condition in that, with the improvement of the diabetes, there was a disappearance of the xanthoma.

The highest level of cholesterol of the blood prior to the lesion is shown in Table 71. The average age at recognition was 29 years; duration of diabetes, five years. The average blood sugar was 0.28 per cent and average cholesterol, 756 mg. per 100 cc. Four patients had lipemia retinalis, 1 gall stones, 2 marked retinitis, 1 heart disease, and 1 gangrene.

TABLE 71.—CHOLESTEROL IN THE BLOOD IN PATIENTS WITH XANTHOMA DIABETICORUM.

Case No.	Sex.	Onset. Age.	Onset. Date.	Discovery of lesion. Age.	Discovery of lesion. Date.	Cholesterol, mg./100 cc.	Blood sugar, per cent.	Complications.
1705	M	21	1919	25	1923	..	0.31	Lipemia retinalis
1707	F	46	1917	53	1924	214	0.20	Arteriosclerosis
1753	F	8	1916	12	1920	..	0.12	Blood fat, 1.1 per cent.
2980	F	56	1916	62	1922	..	0.35	Arteriosclerosis
3785	F	12	1924	33	1945	1150	0.32	
4568	F	12	1922	19	1929	344	0.29	Arteriosclerosis, retinitis proliferans
6767	F	10	1925	16	1931	710	0.36	Arteriosclerosis
7833	F	41	1925	45	1929	794	0.28	Gall stones
9250	F	32	1925	40	1933	644	0.12	Lipemia retinalis
10439	F	35	1929	37	1931	675	0.28	
10601	M	19	1931	19	1931	695	0.37	
12383	M	13	1931	16	1934	1600	0.25	Lipemia retinalis
18540	F	19	1939	19	1939	1125	0.36	Coma; lipemia retinalis
21367	F	10	1941	13	1944	1150	0.24	Vit. A deficiency thyroid deficiency
Average		24		29		827	0.28	

The rarity of the lesion, its association with lipemia, to localization extensor surfaces, elbows, knees, palms and tendon sheaths, have been reëmphasized by Diamond.[2]

[1] Nicholson: Clifton Med. Bull., 9, 12, 1923; Lyon: Edinburgh Med. Jour., 28, 168, 1922.
[2] Diamond: Med. Bull. Vet. Admin., 20, 225, 1943.

Peculiar processes of involution of xanthoma diabeticorum have been described by Goldstein and Harris.[1] Following the use of insulin, the lesions on the palms disappeared completely, those on the elbows coalesced and left large pigmented patches, while those on the legs and thigh passed through degenerative changes resulting in extensive scar formation.

For incidence of xanthelasmata, see page 621.

Montgomery and Osterberg[2] and Thannhauser and Magendantz[3] have written excellent articles regarding the different types of xanthomatous diseases. Xanthoma tuberosum is usually associated with the high value of cholesterol in the blood and an increase in total lipoid. Often there is severe cardio-vascular damage, especially coronary sclerosis and intermittent claudication. Curiously enough, in disseminate xanthomatosis there is often a high incidence of diabetes insipidus, and in this condition oftentimes the lipoids of the blood are within normal limits. These lesions frequently do not change no matter what kind of dietary change is made. In the xanthoma tuberosum, however, the skin lesions may undergo partial or complete involution, the lipoids can be brought to normal by a low-calorie diet. In both conditions, however, there is often a definite increase in the cholesterol content of the lesions. Juvenile xanthoma may occur in the disseminate form. Xanthoma diabeticorum occurs in cases of severe diabetes with chronic acidosis and marked increase in fat content of the blood.

McGavack and Shepardson[4] report xanthoma and hypercholesteremia in a case of acromegaly and diabetes. A similar case is reported by Grau Triana.[5]

Treatment of xanthoma diabeticorum consists of excellent control of the diabetic condition together with, in some cases, a diet low in fat of animal origin.

8. **Necrobiosis Lipoidica Diabeticorum.**—In 1928, Oppenheim observed a hitherto undescribed skin condition in a diabetic patient. In 1932, Urbach reported the study of a similar lesion to which he gave the name of necrobiosis lipoidica diabeticorum, and others have been described since by Galewsky, Gottron, Balbi, Zeisler and Caro, and Michelson and Laymon.[6] The last named writers reviewed the literature, giving an excellent summary and reported their own case in a child, aged ten years. Since this report we have reviewed our cases and believe that we have had 25. See Table 72.

Lesions of this nature were originally considered by us as tuberculides of the skin and later thought to be symbiotic infections but were not proved to be such.

[1] Goldstein and Harris: Am. Jour. Med. Sci., **173**, 195, 1927.
[2] Montgomery and Osterberg: Arch. Dermat. and Syph., **37**, 373, 1938
[3] Thannhauser and Magendantz: Ann. Int. Med., **11**, 1662, 1938.
[4] McGavack and Shepardson: Ann. Int. Med., **7**, 582, 1933.
[5] Grau Triana, Arguelles Casals, Romero Jordan and Bulle Merry, Vida nueva, **53**, 274, 1944.
[6] Michelson and Laymon: Jour. Am. Med. Assn., **103**, 163, 1934.

TABLE 72.—TWENTY-FIVE CASES NECROBIOSIS LIPOIDICA DIABETICORUM.

No.	Sex.	Onset D.M. Age.	Date.	Onset Necrob. Age.	Date.	Site.	Chol. Blood mg./100 cc.	sugar, (%).	Complications.	Present Status of Lesion.
2052	M	17	1920	35	1938	Foot	172	0.16	.....	Improved
3040	F	10	1922	20	1932	Leg	216	0.32	Ulcer (leg)	Healed
4250	M	8	1923	19	1934	Leg	195	0.28	Traumatic ulcer leg, AS	?
5661	F	11	1925	11	1925	Leg	510	0.26	Tracheo-bronchial adenitis	Unchanged
5844	F	9	1927	20	1939	Leg	?	0.29	Pregnancy	?
6310	F	9	1927	14	1932	Leg	232	0.35	Art. sclr.	Healed
6767	F	11	1925	28	1942	Legs	213	0.15		?
7067	M	18	1925	32	1939	Arms, back	172	0.28	TBC.	Died 11-21-41
7311	F	24	1928	25	1929	Feet	240	0.33	Pregnancy, neuritis	Improved
7312	F	17	1928	23	1934	Leg	195	0.20	.....	Unchanged
7313	F	64	1928	72	1936	Leg	220	0.18	Ca. uterus and breast	Much improved
7993	F	18	1929	24	1935	Feet	258	0.29	.....	Healed
8711	M	11	1930	18	1937	Legs	190	0.24	Dwarfism; enlarged liver	?
9538	M	10	1930	16	1936	Skin, foot	196	0.26	.....	?
10276	F	22	1930	31	1936	Ankles, feet	291	0.14	Pregnancy	
10899	M	9	1918	28	1937	Leg	174	0.31	.....	Healed
11328	F	5	1930	20	1945	Foot	150	0.19	Coma	
12036	F	39	1933	43	1937	Feet, arms, hands	237	0.28	.....	Improved
12723	F	50	1934	50	1934	Abdomen	295	0.27	Art. scler.	?
12997	F	6	1933	9	1936	Legs	214	0.15	Coma	Healed
13959	M	9	1935	12	1938	Ankles	...	0.24	.....	Unchanged
17332	F	32	1937	33	1938	Foot	180	0.15	Pancreatic cyst	Unchanged
18958	F	12	1937	11	1936	Leg	...	0.14		
24635	F	16	1933	28	1945	Hip	...	0.30	Pregnancy	
27442	F	6	1942	9	1945	Legs	...	0.44	.....	Unchanged

The earliest lesions described by Urbach and Oppenheim are sharply bordered, distinctly elevated red papules, from 1 to 3 mm. in diameter, which may be capped by a slight scale and do not disappear under glass pressure. One of our patients mistook them for mosquito bites. Later the areas are round, oval or irregular plaques with well-defined borders, firm consistency, and smooth glistening surface which looks "as if it were covered with a layer of tightly stretched cellophane." Still later there is a depressed area with atrophy and ulceration.

The pathogenesis is a matter of debate. Endarteritis is probably the origin of the lesion. Oppenheim considered it fatty degeneration of connective tissue. Urbach considers it necrobiosis of the connective tissue (due to damage in the blood-vessel walls) followed by imbibition of lipoids. Michelson and Laymon believe that in the absence of xanthoma and giant cells the dermatosis is not an atypical form of xanthoma diabeticorum, but is more closely allied to diabetic gangrene.

That this condition is not limited to diabetics is proven by its appearence in non-diabetics.[1] Goldsmith's case[2] had a normal blood-sugar curve and normal blood cholesterol. Greenwood and Rockwood's case[3] had a normal blood sugar curve but high blood lipids. Goldberg[4] finds that 10 per cent of the cases occur in non-diabetics

[1] Dowling (Discussion by Freudenthal and Goldsmith): Proc. Roy. Soc. Med., 39, 95, 1945.
[2] Goldsmith, p. 167: Loc. cit., p. 587.
[3] Greenwood and Rockwood: Personal communication.
[4] Goldberg: Ohio State Med. Jour., 39, 1009, 1943.

and Cannon[1] also comments on the fact that necrobiosis lipoidica diabeticorum may be found months or years prior to the onset of diabetes.

Wilder[2] points out that necrobiosis lipoidica diabeticorum occurs more commonly in females than in males. In our own series of 25 cases, 7 are males and 18 are females. It is most common in juvenile diabetics; the average age at onset of diabetes in our 25 patients was 17.7 years. A history of trauma may be obtained in some patients. The lesions may be single or multiple and occur most commonly on the lower legs or about the ankles. At times two lesions, one on each extremity, may appear in surprisingly symmetrical locations.

No treatment is available except excellent control of the diabetic condition and ordinary care of the lesions if they become ulcerated or secondarily infected. The condition appears to be self-limited, the lesions tend to disappear, leaving white scars or even no traces whatsoever.

9. **Dermatitis Gangrenosa.**—Gangrene of the skin of the trunk or arms occurring during or after diabetic coma is described by Riven.[3] His patient, aged forty years, developed blebs on the back, thighs and legs, associated with fever, and necrosis with gangrene followed. The presence of staphylococci in the blebs suggests skin infection to which the patient's resistance was lowered by acidosis. One such case occurred at the Deaconess Hospital when a coma patient developed a gangrenous slough at the site of a hypodermic injection.

10. **Dupuytren's Contracture.**—We have noted that contraction of the palmar fascia seems to occur more frequently among older diabetic, than non-diabetic, persons. (See Table 70.) This has also been Wilder's[4] impression. Although surgical treatment may be applied, rarely is it necessary.

11. **Lanugo.**—Downy hair often appeared upon the backs of patients in the days of treatment by undernutrition. When improvement took place with insulin, it gradually disappeared and one never sees it today save in neglected cases and dwarfs.

12. **Tumefactions Due to Insulin (Insulin Lumps).**—(See page 377.)

13. **Lipodystrophy.**—Lipodystrophy, or atrophy of subcutaneous fat, presents a distinct problem in the treatment of diabetic patients with insulin. It is most commonly seen in children of both sexes among whom it occurs frequently. It is seen occasionally in adult females but almost never in adult males. Its predilection for children and females probably is due to the relatively greater deposition of fat. Atrophies may be noted first from within several weeks to many months after the institution of treatment with insulin; the

[1] Cannon: South. Med. Jour., **38**, 105, 1945.
[2] Wilder, p. 296–297: Loc. cit., p. 55.
[3] Riven: Am. Jour. Med. Sci., **189**, 550, 1935.
[4] Wilder, p. 299: Loc. cit., p. 55.

average interval from the onset of therapy is about six months. The lesions are seen almost always at the site of injections, although in rare instances we have noted what seemed to be typical atrophies in remote parts, as in the face (Case 5127), submental region (Case 8189) and breast (Case 22003). Spiegelman's case[1] unlike most cases showed atrophy in one site only. Wilder[2] states that he has not observed atrophies in areas remote from the sites of injection.

Various causes have been suggested for the disappearance of the subcutaneous fat. These were summarized in part in a publication[3] from this clinic as follows: (1) The tricresol which formerly was used as the preservative in insulin distributed commercially;[4] (2) assumed lipase content of insulin;[4] (3) trauma of mechanical[5] nature due to the repeated injections, particularly in a restricted area; it has been thought that possibly there occurs damage to "the delicate protoplasmic cell envelope of the fat cells so that fat globules are released, and, acting as foreign bodies in the tissue, result in the formation of histiocytes which take on lipophagic activity;"[6] (4) low-grade inflammation;[7] (5) Nichols'[8] suggestion was that "the strong initial concentration of insulin . . . causes an active local oxidation of carbohydrate, which in turn causes an active combustion of local fat;" (6) nerve injury; (7) antiseptics such as alcohol, at times used in sterilizing the needle and syringe; (8) androgen insufficiency.

Few of the above-mentioned possibilities have found adequate support in fact. Thus Rabinowitch[9] found no lipase in insulin; he and Avery[6] did not believe that the method of sterilization of the needle was at fault; Mentzer and DuBray[10] and Price[11] found no evidence of inflammatory changes in sections from lesions. Most of the other explanations do not lend themselves well to proof or refutation. In the early days of the use of the protamine and protamine zinc insulin it seemed to us that fewer insulin atrophies were seen. This suggested that lipodystrophy had been due to the acidity of regular insulin. (The pH of regular insulin is 2.5 to 3 whereas that of protamine zinc insulin is about 7.3.) Since that time we have had numerous instances of atrophy due solely to protamine zinc insulin and suspect that if the frequency of atrophies due to this type of insulin is less, it is probably because fewer injections are

[1] Spiegelman: New York State Jour. Med., 44, 2723, 1944.
[2] Wilder, p. 95: Loc. cit., p. 55.
[3] Joslin, Root, White, Marble and Joslin: Med. Clin. North America, 22, 711, 1938.
[4] Priesel and Wagner: Klin. Wchnschr., 9, 1548, 1930.
[5] Carmichael and Graham: Lancet, 1, 601, 1928.
[6] Avery: Brit. Med. Jour., 1, 597, 1929.
[7] Fischer: Am. Jour. Dis. Child., 38, 715, 1929.
[8] Nichols: Am. Jour. Med. Sci., 180, 90, 1930.
[9] Rabinowitch: Canad. Med. Assn. Jour., 18, 560, 1928.
[10] Mentzer and DuBray: California and West. Med., 26, 212, 1927.
[11] Price: Lancet, 1, 1015, 1930.

required daily. The frequency of the lesion in young children and females suggests that androgen may protect the adult male and lack of it accounts for the frequency in children and women. Hypogonadal adult males such as patients with hemochromatosis or cirrhosis of the liver have had insulin lipodystrophy.[1]

Marble and Smith[2] studied 500 cases of insulin treated diabetes and found the total incidence to be 18.4 per cent: among patients under twenty years of age 32 per cent, over twenty years of age 15 per cent. In this group there were no males over twenty. Biopsies of the areas showed a diminution of neutral fat.

Lipodystrophy due to insulin is a harmless complication since no important structure is damaged. It is annoying solely because of the cosmetic effect. Treatment consists in avoidance of areas of atrophies for many weeks or months. In a fair percentage of patients redeposition of subcutaneous fat will take place; in others the depressed areas seem to change very little year by year. In prophylaxis one must insist upon varying the site of injection from day to day according to a definite schedule so that no one area 2 cm. in diameter receives insulin oftener than once a month. High strength insulin as U-80 or U-100 should be used to keep down the volume of fluid injected. Care should be taken to blow out all traces of alcohol from the syringe used. The insulin should be deposited in the subcutaneous spaces well beneath the skin and not given superficially. Finally in those patients in whom atrophies continue despite observance of all these rules, areas of the body may be chosen such as the abdominal wall which are not exposed to public view and in which the loss of subcutaneous fat might be welcomed rather than deplored.

14. **Allergy to Insulin.**—See Chapter XIV.

15. **Rôle of the Skin in Carbohydrate Metabolism.**—Urbach and co-workers[3] have attempted to evaluate the rôle of the skin in the intermediary metabolism of carbohydrate. They found that in a group of normal human subjects the skin sugar averaged 61 mg. per 100 cc., or 59 per cent of the corresponding blood sugar value (103 mg. per cent). In diabetes the fasting skin sugar, as well as the blood sugar, is above normal and bears the same relationship one to the latter as in normal individuals. However, after the administration of glucose the percentage of sugar in the skin rises more slowly and subsequently falls more slowly than that in the blood; hence at about the fourth hour after the administration of sugar the ratio of the skin to the blood sugar increases so that the skin value is about 80 per cent of the blood value. Similar findings may be obtained with depancreatized dogs.

In diabetic patients with skin disease (furunculosis, eczema,

---

[1] Waldenstrom: Personal communication.
[2] Marble and Smith: Proc. Am. Diabetes Assn., **2**, 173, 1942.
[3] Urbach and Rejtö; Urbach, Depisch and Sicher: Loc. cit., p. 588.

pruritus, urticaria) the ratio of skin to blood sugar is much higher than in diabetic patients without skin manifestations. The average quotient (ratio of skin to blood sugar) in the former group is 69 per cent as opposed to 59 per cent, as stated above.

Urbach and associates determined not only the free but also the "bound" sugar in the skin of diabetic and non-diabetic individuals with and without disease of the skin. The free sugar is largely glucose; by bound sugar is meant those substances which are determined by the usual blood-sugar methods after acid hydrolysis. The amount of bound sugar was 15 times greater than that of free sugar in the skin. The fact that skin contains such large amounts of bound sugar leads one to regard it as an important organ for intermediate carbohydrate metabolism and for the storage of sugar. This is borne out also by the observations of Folin, Trimble and Newman[1] and of Warren.[2] Folin *et al.* found that following the giving of sugar to animals, a surprisingly large part of it was stored, at least temporarily, in the skin. Warren has pointed out that whereas the skin of normal persons may contain large amounts of glycogen, that of patients with diabetes may contain little or almost none.

Urbach states, in apparent contradiction to the above, that in human diabetic patients the content of bound sugar is much higher than in normal individuals. The administration of sugar raises the content of bound sugar still more. Experiments on dogs show that in diabetes large amounts of carbohydrate are stored in the skin but further administration of sugar increases the amount of bound sugar very little.

[1] Folin, Trimble and Newman: Jour. Biol. Chem., **75**, 263, 1927.
[2] Warren, p. 89; loc. cit., p. 196.

CHAPTER XXI.

BLOOD COMPLICATIONS IN DIABETES.

REVISED BY HOWARD F. ROOT, M.D. AND ELEANOR A. WASKOW, M.D.

A. ANEMIA.

THE concept of the erythron, attributed by Castle and Minot[1] to Boycott,[2] establishes the circulating blood together with the tissue from which it arises as a single organ susceptible to many influences, metabolic as well as infectious and toxic. The cytology of the blood in diabetes is therefore important not merely because of the frequency of pernicious anemia in diabetics, but because the blood cells are no longer regarded merely as elements with variations in age, size and shape but as objects reflecting the results of certain definite chemical processes in the bone-marrow, liver and elsewhere. The presence of anemia in a diabetic has been regarded as indicating a complicating disease but not until recent years has the frequency of anemia of both the primary and secondary types has appreciated.

The size of the red blood corpuscles in diabetes mellitus has been studied carefully by Mohr, utilizing a series of patients at the New England Deaconess Hospital in Boston and in the metabolic ward of the Johns Hopkins Hospital.[3] Hematocrit determinations were made with the Wintrobe hematocrit. The 64 cases were divided into three groups: (1) uncomplicated diabetes, (2) diabetic acidosis, (3) diabetic dwarfs. Of 42 cases of uncomplicated diabetes, 6 had a mean corpuscular volume of 95 cubic microns or over; 11 had a corpuscular volume of 93 cubic microns or over. Diabetic dwarfs with large livers were studied, but in only one of these was the corpuscular volume above 95 cubic microns. Apparently actual acidosis did not affect the volume of red blood cells and yet there was a variation in size. Thirty-five per cent of the cases of acidosis had a mean corpuscular volume above 95 cubic microns, a value which is above the normal range from 85 to 95 cubic microns.

Anemia frequently occurs in even mild infections and sometimes constitutes a difficult problem in the more severe and long-standing infections of the extremities, of the kidneys or of the superficial tissues as in multiple abscesses. Infections with extensive areas of necrosis result in prolonged drainage and loss of plasma and hemoglobin. In 281 consecutive diabetic patients, 45, or 16 per cent,

---

[1] Castle and Minot: *Pathological Physiological and Clinical Description of the Anemias*, Oxford Medical Publications, p. 3, 1936.

[2] Boycott: Pathology of the Blood, Chap. II, Textbook of General Pathology, Pembrey and Ritchie, New York, 1913.

[3] Mohr: Am. Jour. Med. Sci., **196**, 67, 1938.

had red blood counts of less than 4,000,000. Of this group, 2 had pernicious anemia, 10 had only arteriosclerosis and hypertension as complications, 10 were apparently uncomplicated and the complications in the remainder of the group included carcinoma, cirrhosis of the liver, cholecystitis, infection of the urinary tract; tuberculosis, gangrene and cystitis.

Among these patients lack of free hydrochloric acid in the stomach was a frequent finding.

In 3 successive cases of coma a high color index of the blood reaching 1.49 and 1.6, was observed by Lawrence, Lucas, and McCance.[1] The explanation of the increased color index they believed to lie in a true megalocytosis due to a change in the activity of the bone-marrow. Leukocytosis, at times of extreme degree, is the rule in coma. (See page 441.) A white count of 92,000 was present in a girl, aged twelve years, in coma March 9, 1939 (Case 13074) and white counts of 30,000 to 50,000 are frequent in coma. Young leukocytes, myelocytes and even myeloblasts are occasionally encountered. Bertram[2] describes a constant leukocytosis, a shift to the left in the leukocyte formula and absence of eosinophiles in coma.

It is possible that the apparent disappearance of eosinophiles in diabetic coma may be explained by the fact that the eosinophiles do not decrease in coma, but are simply concealed by the large number of other polymorphonuclear cells. Bertram[3] mentions the lymphocytosis, sometimes reaching 60 per cent, in insulin hypoglycemia, indicating an increased discharge of epinephrin. The explanation of leukocytosis in coma, granting that anhydremia or a concomitant infection may play a part, should be consistent with a cause for gastric hemorrhage which is so frequently an associated symptom.

B. PERNICIOUS ANEMIA

The report by Root[4] of 79 cases of pernicious anemia combined with diabetes indicates that the former rarity of the association of these two diseases no longer holds true. In the literature 19 more cases are mentioned. Forty-two new cases at the 'Deaconess Hospital bring the total to 140.

Of these 140 cases of combined diabetes and pernicious anemia, 65 were observed at the Deaconess Hospital. To this number should be added certain patients presenting anemia and achlorhydria but in whom we have not yet been able to establish satisfactorily the diagnosis of pernicious anemia. Explanations of the increased frequency of this combination must take account of the marked prolongation of life brought about in each disease by the discoveries

[1] Lawrence, Lucas and McCance: Brit. Med. Jour., ii, 145, 1932.
[2] Bertram: Ergebn. d. inn. Med. u. Kinderh., 43, 258, 1932.
[3] Bertram: P. 78, loc. cit., p. 87.
[4] Root: New England Jour. Med., 208, 819, 1933; Jour. Am. Med. Assn., 69, 928, 1931.

of insulin and liver extract. The review of hematology by Bethell *et al.*,[1] should be consulted for data regarding pernicious anemia, although diabetes is not mentioned.

Greater opportunity for the simultaneous occurrence of the two diseases certainly exists, but the frequency of pernicious anemia among diabetics of long duration suggests the existence of some specific relationship. Heredity stands out as important in each disease. Thus in 13 per cent of the cases with combined pernicious anemia and diabetes, anemia was known to exist in the family and diabetes was known to exist in 33.3 per cent of these families. In 1500 consecutive cases of diabetes, pernicious anemia was present in a parent, brother or sister in 15 instances. The accuracy of family histories for each disease errs on the side of understatement.

Pernicious anemia and diabetes were frequently encountered in the ancestry of a patient of Dr. George R. Minot. "Patient, aged about fifty-nine years, has undoubted pernicious anemia. Brother, aged about fifty-nine years has often had sugar in urine and is said to have pernicious anemia with mild cord symptoms. Sister, aged fifty-five years, anemic for eight years, has undoubted pernicious anemia now. Brother, aged about fifty years, has undoubted diabetes from history given. Brother, aged about forty-nine years, well. Mother died of diabetes. Father 'showed sugar in urine in last illness and died of infected foot that became gangrenous.' Father's brother 'had anemia and died of it.' Father's sister died in thirties of pneumonia. No other brothers or sisters. Mother's sister had diabetes. Definite information given concerning this. Mother's brother died of old age. No other brothers or sisters. Patient's paternal grandfather probably died of pernicious anemia. He was said to have been very pale in last two years of life and had difficulty in walking. An ill-defined history of this man's brother suggests that he had anemia."

In Root's 79 cases with sufficient clinical data, diabetes preceded the pernicious anemia in 56 cases and in only 11 was pernicious anemia first in development. The youngest person to develop pernicious anemia was aged thirty-two years and the oldest seventy-six years. The average duration of the diabetes before the development of the pernicious anemia was 5.3 years. In contrast, the duration of anemia before the development of diabetes in the 11 cases where it took precedence was only three years. Indeed, in 6 of these 11 cases the duration of anemia was estimated at one year or less. There has been no comparable increase in other blood diseases associated with diabetes at the Deaconess Hospital. In the 2 cases of pernicious anemia associated with diabetes mellitus reported by McGregor,[2] in one the diabetes preceded the anemia and in the other the reverse was true.

[1] Bethell, Sturgis, Rundles and Myers: Arch. Int. Med., **77**, 80, 1946.
[2] McGregor: Brit. Med. Jour., **2**, 617, 1937.

Beckert[1] states that in the City Hospital of Dresden-Friedrich-stadt, among 900 ambulant diabetics there were 9 patients with pernicious anemia (1 per cent of the cases). About 3 per cent of the women included had hypochromic anemia. Of the 9 patients with both diabetes and pernicious anemia, 7 ranged in age from thirty to fifty years; 2 were older. In 3 cases the diabetes was severe and in the remaining mild. The combination of the two diseases was known by the author in 6 of the patients to exist for over four years, in 5 cases pernicious anemia being diagnosed three to seven years after the diabetes. In the remaining patients it could not be so exactly determined which disease was primary. His impression was that only the cord symptoms in the diabetics appeared more frequently and to a greater degree than in non-diabetics with pernicious anemia.

Benjamin[2] described 3 cases of associated diabetes mellitus and pernicious anemia. The first was a twenty-three year old woman, the second was a woman aged sixty-four years, and the third was a man, aged forty-six years. The degrees of anemia were severe and in the two younger patients insulin was used for treatment of the diabetes. He discusses the various theories of the relationship between the two diseases. In 2 of the patients hereditary diabetes was present.

Pathology.—The pathological changes in combined diabetes and pernicious anemia have been little studied. Only 7 autopsies were summarized in Root's 1931 article. An eighth autopsy in Neuburger's first case, female, aged fifty-three years, with diabetes for twenty years, showed regenerative bone-marrow, atrophy of gastric mucosa, hemosiderosis of liver and chronic pancreatitis with atrophy.

A ninth autopsy is given by Clay and Lawrence[3] in the case of an insulin resistant man, aged fifty-three years, who had been treated for pernicious anemia and coronary occlusion. During the last five days of his life in the hospital, his insulin dose had to be steadily increased from 190 units a day to 960 units and his blood sugar was never recorded below 0.294 per cent. Ketonuria continued to the end. He was not anemic. Autopsy showed moderate atheroma and old thrombosis of the anterior descending branch of the left coronary artery. The liver and kidneys were essentially normal, except for slight fatty degeneration of the liver, four soft gall stones and pale, congested kidneys. The bone-marrow showed predominantly normoblastic activity and a few megaloblasts were seen. The endocrine glands were normal. The islands of Langerhans seemed normally abundant.

Clinical Features.—The extent of the anemia has been variable. In Table 73 are listed 18 cases discovered since our last report. In

[1] Beckert: München. med. Wchnschr., **87**, 230, 1940.
[2] Benjamin: Folia Hæmatol., **52**, 113, 1934.
[3] Clay and Lawrence: Brit. Med. Jour., **1**, 697, 1935.

TABLE 73.—EIGHTEEN CASES OF COMBINED DIABETES AND PERNICIOUS ANEMIA

Case No.	Sex.	Age at onset, years.		Gastric Free HCl.	Discovered since 1940. Date.	Blood.			Spinal cord changes.	Treatment.		Alive in 1945, age.	Cause of death.	Age at death.	Notes
		D.M.	P.A.			Hgb. %.	R.B.C. mill./cmm.	Sugar. %.		Liver.	Insulin. C.I.P.Z.I.				
2095	M	27	48	0	1942	60	3.01	.333	+	+	20+40	Yes 51	....	..	Carbuncle; diarrhea in 1940
5851	F	49	68	0	1944	65	3.40	.270	+	++	16+32	No	Coronary occlu.	69	Free HCl 1936
14074	M	68	72	0	1940	86	4.28	.230	0	++	8+28	No	Cerebral hem.	78	
15990	F	62	71	0	1943	..	3.99	.240	?	++	10+28	No	Cerebral throm.	73	
18321	F	43	43	0	1942	80	3.85	.250	+	++	12	Yes 50	....	..	Psychosis
18929	F	55	55	0	1940	82	4.39	.300	+	++	6+40	...	....	..	
19683	F	52	52	0	1940	90	3.31	.190	0	++	10	Yes 58			
19725	M	27	31	0	1940	68	3.34	.240	+	++	20	Yes 36			
20742	F	59	69	0	1932	80	4.09	.333	+	++	10+34	No	....		
20981	M	76	79	0	1941	50	1.59	.203	+	++	0	? ?	Cardiac	81	
21133	M	47	42	0	1935	100	5.00	.208	?	++	10+32	No ?	....	..	Deficient circulation
22407	F	70	70	0	1943	73	3.9	.200	+	+++	14	Yes 72	....	..	Pellagra
22549	F	53	38	0	1928	100	5.41	.290	?	++	12	Yes 54	....	..	
22894	F	48	48	0	1943	78	3.95	.253	0	++	30	Yes 54	....	..	Taking lextron; diarrhea 6 mos.; incontinence
23020	M	78	79	0	1944	76	3.99	.085	0	++	30	Yes 83			
24018	F	42	42	0	1944	75	3.44	.206	0	++	12	Yes 43			
24569	F	28	48	0	1944	55	3.81	.238		++	40+80	Yes 49	....		Nephritis
25494	F	54	54	0	1934	84	4.04	.150	+	+	12+28	Yes 65			

2 only was the anemia discovered before the diabetes. In 1 case the count was 1,590,000, in 8 cases from 2,000,000 to 3,000,000 and in 8, 3,000,000 to 4,000,000. Females numbered 12 and males 6.

Two of our patients with diabetes and pernicious anemia have had diabetic coma.

Case 12887, aged forty-eight years, housewife, entered the Deaconess Hospital on July 2, 1934, diabetes having been discovered one month before. She was in deep coma with a CO_2 combining power of 2 volumes per cent and a blood sugar of 0.45 per cent. With 130 units of insulin given in the first eight hours after admission, she improved and left the hospital, taking 40 units of insulin a day and 2 cc. of liver extract intramuscularly twice a week. Her red blood count of 2,530,000 increased to 4,340,000. The red blood count of 2,530,000 during severe acidosis may have been higher than would have been true without the dehydration of coma. She reported that she was in good condition on October 1, 1945. Case 14793, housewife, aged fifty years upon admission to the Deaconess Hospital in August, 1936 in diabetic coma had had diabetes four years. At this time the CO_2 combining power of the blood was 5 volumes per cent and the blood sugar was 0.53 (530 mg.) per cent. With 170 units of insulin given during the first five hours of her stay she recovered. At this time her red blood count was 4,970,000. In September, 1939, the red cells numbered 2,900,000. The white count was 5050 and the red cells showed characteristic alterations in size and shape. She was alive on June 26, 1945.

Spinal cord changes were present in 46 of the 140 cases in the literature. Case 18321, Jewish housewife, aged forty-three years at discovery of diabetes and pernicious anemia in 1942, was unable to stand because of weakness, spasticity, and ataxia. Recovery from the cord symptoms occurred rapidly after the use of liver extract. Later she made a rapid recovery from an acute depression treated by means of electric shock therapy and is alive in August, 1946.

Ca e 9819, with the classical symptoms and findings of combined system disease, developed as the result of a paralyzed urinary bladder, a severe pelvic phlebitis from which she gradually recovered.

The 140 cases have occurred in many different localities, indicating the wide distribution of this combination.

Murphy and Howard[1] found 9 cases of diabetes among the complications developing in 440 cases of pernicious anemia. Each case was over forty years of age when the diabetes developed and the disease ran a mild course except that it became more severe in 2 patients who had been under liver treatment for eight or ten years, respectively, and who had developed complications. In these 2 it was necessary to institute insulin treatment.

Jolliffe, Brandaleone and Most[2] studied 2 patients who had com-

[1] Murphy and Howard: Review of Gastroenterology, **3**, 105, 1936.
[2] Jolliffe, Brandaleone and Most: Jour. Clin. Invest., **143**, 362, 1935.

bined diabetes and pernicious anemia. When they were given a high-protein diet, the carbohydrate tolerance was much reduced and this reduction could not be explained by the increase in calories or by the extra carbohydrate. Even insulin did not prevent this loss of tolerance for protein.

Schwab and Schwab[1] describe a woman who had eaten almost no meat for sixty years and developed diabetes at sixty-five years, at which time the blood counts were normal. Her sister also had diabetes. Four years later, the red blood cells numbered 1,800,000. Signs of combined system disease with typical Parkinsonian tremor were present. The absence of muscular rigidity led the authors to regard the Parkinson's syndrome as the result of the pernicious anemia affecting the lenticulostriate region.

Diagnosis.—The appearance of the skin and mucous membranes in diabetic patients is often misleading. The skin frequently is lax, pale and cool suggesting an anemia which is not found upon examination. In acidosis the flushed cheeks serve to disguise true anemia as was illustrated in Case 10893 who, though only twenty-three years of age, following coma proved to have a red cell count of 2,960,000 and achlorhydria. A yellowish tint to the skin due to carotinemia may suggest pernicious anemia. Carotinemia is easily differentiated by its intensity upon the soles of the feet and the palms of the hands as well as by the lack of the lemon-yellow tint of true pernicious anemia. In hemochromatosis the skin may show a slight brownish pigmentation and the pigmentation of hyper-thyroidism is to be considered.

Paræsthesias such as numbness and tingling in hands and feet are common to both diseases. In more severe stages of development diabetes leads to pain and motor paralysis whereas pernicious anemia is accompanied by spasticity and ataxia associated with subacute combined sclerosis. The changes in the central nervous system due to diabetes are usually temporary, responding to treatment, and relief can be promised. In pernicious anemia, however, the spinal cord lesions are difficult to improve. On the other hand, in our experience every case who has received adequate liver treatment and adequate diabetic treatment has shown no increase whatever in the symptoms due to central nervous system involvement.

Both diabetes and pernicious anemia bring about variations of the lipoid content of the blood varying with the stage of severity of the disease. In severe or inadequately treated diabetes an increase not only in cholesterol but also in lecithin, fatty acid and free fat of the blood occurs. This increase is relieved by adequate diabetic treatment and especially by means of insulin. In pernicious anemia, on the other hand, during severe stages, the concentration of cholesterol in the blood plasma is below normal. Thus in a typical case the cholesterol varied between 50 and 70 mg. per 100 cc. and thir-

[1] Schwab and Schwab: Arch. Neurol and Psychiat., **35**, 126, 1936.

teen days after beginning liver treatment it reached the normal value of 135 mg. Variations in the blood sugar in anemia produced by bleeding and in pernicious anemia have been recorded. Goudsmit[1] reports that 8 dextrose tolerance tests using 50 grams of dextrose showed in 5 cases a rise of blood sugar to over 0.17 per cent. Rennie[2] found abnormal glucose tolerance curves in 58 per cent of a series of 90 cases of pernicious anemia.

The reticulocyte response following the use of liver or liver extract requires careful study. Where a typical response following either intramuscular or oral administration of sufficient liver extract is observed, that is, a rise of the reticulocytes to 20 or 25 per cent in five to seven days with a fall to normal at the end of fifteen days, one can feel that the result is due to the specific material. On the other hand, as Minot[3] points out, maximal responses occurring within forty-eight hours or after a delayed period suggest that the response is due to something else than the specific liver extract. Frequently in diabetic patients one observes a rise of reticulocytes to 5 or 6 per cent occurring four or five days after the administration of liver extract and particularly where the level of the red cells has not been low. In the presence of certain complications the diagnosis of pernicious anemia may become difficult.

Sturgis and Goldhamer[4] cite 10 cases of macrocytic anemia not due to pernicious anemia. Cases of cirrhosis of the liver or even of acute hepatitis developed macrocytic anemia for the reason that in these conditions there is a deficiency in the power of the liver to store the erythrocyte-maturing factor. Their cases showed typical response in reticulocytes in such cases of liver disease, as also occurred in a diabetic reported by Root,[5] who had acute hepatitis, developed a macrocytic anemia and was much helped by the use of liver extract intramuscularly.

Treatment.—Treatment at present is based on the use of intramuscular injections of liver extract. The concentrated forms of the extract are so potent that the injection of 15 units every two to four weeks may be sufficient after the acute relapse. A standing order at the Deaconess Hospital requires that all diabetic patients with hemoglobin below 75 per cent shall receive iron. Instead of Blaud's pills, at present 12 to 18 grains a day of ferrous sulphate are being used.

The amount of liver extract required to prevent changes in the spinal cord is of utmost importance. It would seem, when two diseases each of which has the power of producing degenerative changes in the spinal cord occurred together, that the treatment of anemia would require more and larger amounts of liver extract. In Case

[1] Goudsmit: Nederl. Tijdschr. v. Geneesk., **74**, 1447, 1930.
[2] Rennie: Jour. Lab. and Clin. Med., **16**, 557, 1931.
[3] Minot: Trans. Assn. Am. Phys., **49**, 287, 1934.
[4] Sturgis and Goldhamer: Ann. Int. Med., **12**, 1245, 1939.
[5] Root: New England Jour. Med., **212**, 545, 1935.

4374, aged fifty-eight years at onset of pernicious anemia after nine years of diabetes, the evidences of change in the spinal cord consisted of marked numbness and tingling of hands, fingers and toes with overactive knee jerks. Red cells numbered 2,500,000 in August, 1933. During the ensuing years his red blood count was kept at 5,000,000 with the administration of liver extract intramuscularly, at first once a week and later once in ten days. No progression of symptoms occurred up to the development of his terminal illness from carcinoma of the stomach and death, in February, 1945. Concentrated liver extract (Lilly) has been given in doses of 1 cc. In other cases, an injection of liver extract has been reduced to once in two to four weeks. Cheney and Niemand[1] point out that in pernicious anemia there is a marked insufficiency of pancreatic enzymes, notably trypsin, in addition to the gastric achylia. In their feeding experiments they found that beef digested by hydrochloric acid, pepsin and trypsin yielded the factors necessary to produce the blood changes characteristic of a remission in pernicious anemia. They hold that the deficiency in pernicious anemia is due to a lack of both peptic and tryptic digestion, both of which deficiencies occur in certain cases of diabetes.

Ralli[2] could demonstrate no beneficial effect upon the carbohydrate metabolism after a period of a month to a year of treatment in diabetic children or diabetic adults, from the taking of liver extract. In Bowen's case[3] of combined diabetes and pernicious anemia, no evidence of a blood sugar lowering effect of the liver or liver extract was found.

C. PURPURA HÆMORRHAGICA.

One case has occurred at the George F. Baker Clinic, Deaconess Hospital. Case 8045, male, aged thirty-one years with diabetes of three years' duration, entered the hospital on June 11, 1929. He had taken insulin for three years. One week before admission he noticed discoloration of the skin about the needle pricks from his insulin. Hemorrhages from the gums followed. The hemoglobin was 65 per cent and the red cells numbered 2,240,000. Preparations were made for a splenectomy. However, on the morning of the operation he developed an acute throat infection and did not at any time regain strength sufficient for operation. At autopsy there was found an acute intestinal obstruction due to intussusception and a massive hemorrhagic clot in the intestine.

D. LEUKEMIA.

Only occasional cases of leukemia complicating diabetes have been reported in the literature. In an article published in December

[1] Cheney and Niemand: Arch. Int. Med., **49**, 925, 1932.
[2] Ralli: Jour. Lab. and Clin. Med., **17**, 1204, 1932.
[3] Bowen: Jour. Am. Med. Assn., **95**, 30, 1930.

39

1941, Levi and Friedman[1] state that there were then 14 reported cases[2,3] of associated diabetes mellitus and leukemia. One can be certain, however, that the cases reported in the literature do not constitute a complete list. Among the 14 cases, the types of leukemia were represented as follows: chronic myeloid leukemia, 4; chronic lymphatic leukemia, 8; acute myeloid leukemia, 1; and monocytic leukemia, 1. The case reported by Levi and Friedman was one of chronic lymphatic leukemia in a sixty-four year old man who died in acidosis and in congestive cardiac failure forty-seven days after admission to the hospital. He was extremely insensitive to insulin; during the forty-seven days, 76,195 units of insulin were administered. On 4 successive days, the patient received 4000 units in each twenty-four hours.

In our own series, case 392 was extraordinary for the long duration of leukemia. He was fifty-two years of age in January, 1911, when diabetes was discovered. At this time the white blood cells numbered 23,200. His differential count showed 93 per cent lymphocytes. Dr. C. W. McGavran[4] followed him for many years and noted variations in the white blood count from 40,000 to 79,000. In May, 1926, Dr. G. R. Minot found 88 per cent of lymphocytes. He had diarrhea at this time probably due to leukemic involvement of intestinal glands. After attacks of angina pectoris for ten years death came on November 29, 1935 as a result of his second coronary occlusion. At autopsy both an old area of cardiac infarction and a fresh area of infarction in the left ventricle were found. Changes characteristic of chronic lymphatic leukemia were found in the lymph nodes, the spleen, bone-marrow, lungs, pericardium, liver, bladder and prostate.

Case 24076, housewife, aged sixty-three years, entered the Deaconess Hospital on January 8, 1944 with chronic myelogenous leukemia. The white blood count of 132,500 was reduced by X-radiation to 2700 by January 19. She was reported to be in good condition in April, 1945.

Case 12678, male, mill-worker, aged thirty-seven years, developed diabetes in January, 1934. On April 16, 1934, the urine contained only 0.3 per cent sugar, and the blood sugar was 0.12 per cent. The white blood cells numbered 77,000 and the lymphocytes were 84 per cent. With deep Roentgen-ray therapy at the Palmer Memorial, suggested by Dr. Wyman Richardson, the white count rapidly fell, and on April 24, 1934, the white blood cells numbered 12,800. He died on July 19, 1938, of chronic lymphatic leukemia.

Monocytic leukemia occurred in Case 12587, a merchant, whose diabetes began in November, 1930, at the age of forty-one years.

[1] Levi and Friedman: New England Jour. Med., **225**, 975, 1941.
[2] Rapaport: Calif. and West. Med., **27**, 802, 1927.
[3] Hart, Lisa and Riedel: Jour. Am. Med. Assn., **113**, 1222, 1939
[4] McGavran: Ann. Int. Med., **12**, 396, 1938.

He entered the Deaconess Hospital on March 8, 1934, complaining of weakness, fever, dyspnea, loss of weight, and pain in the back. The red cells numbered 1,800,000 and white cells 12,300. The hemoglobin was 33 per cent. During the next three weeks the white count steadily increased to 30,000 and the character of the cells changed. The predominant cells were large with indented reniform nuclei, containing a large amount of cytoplasm, finely granular in appearance. Vacuolation was frequent. The bone-marrow examination was compatible with monocytic leukemia. He died on April 27, 1934.

Case 17765, aged seventy years, died in March, 1939 with aleukemic myeloid leukemia. Carcinoma was suspected because of the large number of nucleated red cells in the smear.

Three other patients, Cases 1983, 7260 and 10018, died of leukemia; in the first two it was of the chronic lymphatic, and in the third, chronic myeloid type.

E. BENZOL POISONING.

Case 17891, male, aged fifty-six years, was found at routine examination on May 15, 1939 to have a white blood count of 23,500 per c.mm. and a myeloid blood picture. He had worked for twenty years for a company manufacturing rubber-shoe machinery. The degree of exposure to benzol was difficult to assay. He was seen in consultation by Dr. Wyman Richardson and Dr. F. T. Hunter and his case report included in a paper by the latter.[1] The diagnosis was believed to be chronic benzene poisoning or chronic myeloid leukemia. The patient has been kept under close observation; in August, 1940 his general condition was excellent despite a continued elevation of the white blood count (20,000 to 30,000 per c.mm.). In April, 1944, the white blood cells numbered 204,000. Three courses of X-radiation were given. On April 12, 1946, the white blood count was 11,500. The diagnosis of myeloid leukemia seems clear.

F. POLYCYTHEMIA.

Case 4551, a Jewish merchant, aged fifty-three years at the onset of diabetes in September, 1924, with 5 per cent sugar in the urine, had a red blood count of 8,760,000 and white blood count 29,600 in April, 1925. His diabetes continued to be mild. The typical red cheeks and smooth hairless skin of the hands had been present for twenty-five years he said. He died December 5, 1933.

Hemoconcentration in diabetic coma may give an increased red blood count. See page 442.

G. HODGKIN'S DISEASE.

Cases 5951, 6868 and 13998 are the only instances. Case 6868, a judge, developed diabetes at the age of sixty-five years in 1928.

---

[1] Hunter: Jour. Indust. Hygiene and Toxicol., **21**, 331, 1939.

In May, 1931, he had coronary occlusion. Complications included a renal calculus, duodenal ulcer and Hodgkin's disease diagnosed in January, 1932. Diagnosis, therefore, was puzzling when he collapsed with severe pain during a court session on June 10, 1932. The perforation of a duodenal ulcer was repaired by Dr. L. S. McKittrick. He did well for two days, then died almost instantly from a fresh coronary occlusion. At autopsy healed infarcts of the heart as well as the recent coronary thrombus were found in addition to a stone in the left kidney, duodenal ulcer and lymphomatous infiltration of pancreas, prostate and kidney.

Case 13998, a factory worker, age twenty-five years, had developed diabetes at the age of fourteen years. In April, 1945, he was found to have Hodgkin's disease with a large mediastinal mass. Repeated x-ray treatment controlled fever and severe pain. However, he died in January, 1946.

H. AGRANULOCYTOSIS.

Recovery from critical agranulocytosis with the use of constant intravenous administration of penicillin occurred in Case 5672, who entered the Deaconess Hospital at the age of nineteen on September 3, 1943 in diabetic acidosis, and with bilateral axillary abscesses. She was given emergency coma treatment, x-ray therapy to the abscesses, and sulfadiazine, 5 grams, intravenously, in a single dose followed by daily administration of sulfadiazine until she received in the next thirteen days a total of 58 grams. The blood sulfadiazine levels on two occasions were 7.4 and 9.7 mg. Sulfadiazine was omitted on September 16, thirteen days after admission, and three days later she was discharged in satisfactory condition. She returned to the hospital five days after discharge because of a chill, fever, and generalized malaise. Her temperature was 103.2 degrees. The throat was sore, but no ulcerations and no severe inflammation was present. The white blood count was only 1350 and the smears on two occasions showed no granulocytes. The use of pentnucleotide every four hours was begun but no improvement was noted. During the next twenty-four hours the throat became swollen, edematous, and swallowing became impossible. During the next three days, constant intravenous administration of penicillin was carried out and she received a total of 350,000 units. Her temperature fell the second day of treatment and the throat improved on the third day. Within the next three days the white count returned to 8450 with 65 per cent polymorphonuclear cells. The leucopenia was regarded as probably due to sulfadiazine. Absence of granulocytes for three consecutive days with high fever and advancing infection of the throat presented a critical condition. However, the control of the infection by means of penicillin made possible rapid improvement. The patient had been a diabetic for sixteen out of her nineteen years of life.

Prior to the introduction of penicillin, fatal agranulocytosis developed in 4 women coincidentally with severe infections. A large cervical abscess, gangrene of a foot with septicemia, erysipeloid infection of a leg, and a mastoid infection together with primary endothelio-hemangioma of the middle ear were the complications.

Case 17292, female, aged fifty-six years, seen in consultation, died in December, 1938 with pneumonia and agranulocytosis. Her white blood count fell from 11,800 to 700 in forty-eight hours. She had had phenacetin in small doses for only three days.

I. APLASTIC ANEMIA.

Two patients have presented aplastic anemia. Case 5327 developed diabetes at the age of thirty-eight. In 1941, at the age of fifty-three years, examination of his blood revealed the hemoglobin 50 per cent, red blood count 2,600,000, white cells 1800 with a scarcity of platelets. In spite of repeated transfusions, improvement was temporary and he died in August, 1941.

Case 27222, with onset of diabetes at the age of thirty-nine years, was first examined on July 15, 1945, at the age of sixty-five years with a complaint of angina pectoris, weakness and numbness in the legs. Examination of his blood revealed hemoglobin 58 per cent (9.0 grams), red blood count 2,440,000, white cells 2900, platelets 32,620, and reticulocytes, 1.8 per cent. He died on October 12, 1945 with coronary thrombosis.

J. BANTI'S SYNDROME.

A group of 5 patients have shown enlargement of the spleen which has persisted over a period of years. No cirrhosis of the liver has developed, leukopenia is usually present although the patients have sometimes entered the hospital with infection, and at that time a leukocytosis has occurred. As a group they have developed anemia rather easily, and gastrointestinal hemorrhage has occurred in Case 17240. Severe anemia developed in Case 20126 with infection. So far none of this group has developed fluid in the abdomen. In one case, a young veteran seen through the courtesy of Dr. John King of Baltimore, Md., splenectomy was performed successfully and the pathological examination of the spleen showed Banti's disease.

CHAPTER XXII.

THE SPECIAL SENSES IN DIABETES.

REVISED BY HOWARD F. ROOT, M.D.

A. THE EYES.

THE ocular complications in diabetes are frequent, distressing and present a challenging problem. Information as to the number of blind persons in the community has at best been incomplete. Among 12,652 blind persons in Canada surveyed by Aylesworth[1] diabetes was present in 234 cases. Among 1176 blind persons known to the Division of the Blind in Massachusetts, Riemer[2] found 45 with diabetes. Plans for further investigation by the Massachusetts Division of the Blind in coöperation with the U. S. Public Health Service under the direction of Major H. L. C. Wilkerson are under way. The recent discovery that alloxan diabetes results in the rapid development of cataracts affords a new opportunity for the study of methods of treatment and prevention of cataract. (Page 190.) However, the outstanding ocular danger today is the specific diabetic retinopathy which begins with retinal hemorrhages and develops progressively the proliferative changes characteristic of retinitis proliferans.

From 1929 until 1933 an investigation of the ocular condition of diabetic patients was carried out at the Deaconess Hospital by Dr. J. Herbert Waite and Dr. W. P. Beetham together with chemical investigation of diabetic lenses in the chemical laboratory of the Deaconess Hospital under the direction of Miss Hazel Hunt and the late Dr. Helen Updegraff (Carey). Grateful acknowledgment is made to the Chemical Foundation and especially to Mr. and Mrs. F. P. Garvan for financial assistance which made this extended study possible. We appreciate being allowed to quote freely and to extract tables from the report of Waite and Beetham.[3] We are fortunate also in having the conclusions of Wagener, Dry and Wilder[4] for reference as well as the analysis by Wagener[5] of 312 cases of retinopathy among 1021 diabetics in 1944.

1. **Retinitis Proliferans.**—Among young patients with diabetes of more than ten years' duration retinitis proliferans presents an increasingly serious problem and deserves primary consideration. Some writers give two types: first, in which following hemorrhage

[1] Aylesworth: Canadian Med. Assn. Jour., **54**, 30, 1946.
[2] Riemer: Arch. Ophth., **32**, 304, 1944.
[3] Waite and Beetham: New England Jour. Med., **212**, 367 and 429, 1935.
[4] Wagener, Dry and Wilder: New England Jour. Med., **211**, 1131, 1934.
[5] Wagener: Proc. Am. Diabetes Assoc., **5**, 203, 1945.

a dense, white membrane forms anywhere in the fundus but chiefly at the disc; and second, in which dependent upon circulatory impairment and degenerative vascular disease, the new formation of blood vessels occurs chiefly at the disc apparently in an attempt to clear away foreign material by development of collateral circulation. The contraction of scar tissue in the vitreous sac may cause separation of the retina. The spontaneous hemorrhages often occur at night. A protein-rich transudate may be poured out from the capillaries with a resulting rise in ocular pressure from the normal level of 20 to a level approaching the systolic blood-pressure, and consequent glaucoma of the hemorrhagic type.

Duke-Elder[1] finds the majority of cases in young people because of the frequency of infection in the background. However, chronic vascular disease in nephritis as well as diabetes has long been regarded as an etiologic factor. The series originally studied by Waite and Beetham[2] has been increased until up to December 1, 1945 retinitis proliferans had been recognized in 110 patients involving 194 eyes. Of these 41 were male and 69 female, a sex distribution not far different from the distribution of diabetes in mortality tables at the present time. Twenty-one patients developed diabetes before the age of ten years, and thirty-three, or just one-third of the series, developed diabetes before the age of twenty years, in contrast to the fact that only 10 per cent of all cases in this series of diabetics had their onset in the first two decades of life. The onset of retinitis proliferans did not occur in any case during the first ten years of life, but did occur in three patients in the second decade. Retinitis proliferans developed in 30 cases before the thirtieth year. In contrast to the statement of Duke-Elder about the youth of patients, however, is the fact that in this diabetic group, 57 cases, or 51.8 per cent, developed retinitis proliferans after the age of fifty years.

TABLE 74.—AGE AT ONSET OF DIABETES AND RETINITIS PROLIFERANS.

Age at onset.	Male.		Female.	
	Diabetes.	Retinitis proliferans.	Diabetes.	Retinitis proliferans.
0–10	11	0	10	0
11–20	7	1	5	2
21–30	3	17	8	10
31–40	9	3	15	4
41–50	8	5	17	11
51–60	3	10	12	28
61 and over	0	5	2	14
Total	41	41	69	69

The duration of diabetes was less than two years in only 2 cases. In 15 cases the duration of diabetes was from two to five years.

---

[1] Duke-Elder: Textbook of Ophthalmology, St. Louis, C. V. Mosby Co., 3, 2604 1941.

[2] Waite and Beetham: Loc. cit., p. 614.

The striking feature, however, is the fact that in 93 cases, the duration of diabetes was more than five years and in 53 cases the diabetes was of more than fifteen years' duration. Actually 23 of the patients had never taken insulin or, in 1 case, had omitted insulin for seven years. In 9 cases insulin had been taken for less than two years and yet the average duration of their diabetes was ten years. Yet 25 cases had taken insulin for more than fifteen years, and the average duration of their diabetes was nineteen years. The important point is not merely the duration of insulin treatment but the character of the dietary control. Although insulin may be used, irregularity in following diet results in hyperglycemia, glycosuria, ketonuria, disturbances in vitamin and mineral metabolism. Actually in only 3 cases who were elderly patients, intelligent and with mild diabetes, could one say that dietary instructions had been closely followed with satisfactory blood and urine tests. In 35 cases dietary control was graded B, meaning that the patient had only intermittently followed dietary instructions carefully and that blood and urine tests had seldom been normal. In group C were found 35 patients who were known to have had acidosis or coma who had frankly given up any attempt at approximating a careful diet. A common statement of this group particularly the young patients was that the food was carefully measured the first few years of diabetes and then for a period of six or more years, very little if any dietary restriction had been carried out. In 38 patients our evidence was not sufficiently clear to justify classifying them but none of this group could possibly have been considered in group A with excellent dietary control. The mechanism by which lack of control of diabetes by reason of dietary error can effect the retinal vessels inducing hemorrhage is a mystery. The occurrence of neuropathy in a few of these younger patients might suggest that the disordered metabolism of diabetes in some way interfered with the efficiency of vitamins even though the intake of vitamin A, B, C and D unquestionably had been adequate. The severity of the diabetes varied greatly. In 8 cases no insulin was required in the hospital. These were mild patients late in life. In 11 cases less than 10 units of insulin was sufficient under hospital conditions and a great majority of the group required from 11 to 60 units a day with 12 patients requiring 61 units or more.

The blood-pressure at or near the discovery of retinitis proliferans varied. A normal systolic pressure of 140 or less was observed in 32 cases and diastolic pressure of less than 90 in 49 cases. However, 78 patients had a systolic blood-pressure from 140 to 245 millimeters and 61 patients showed diastolic pressures from 90 to 126 millimeters. More significant, however, than the blood-pressure are the evidences of nephritis. In 35 cases, albuminuria was present prior to discovery of retinitis for periods varying from months to several years, and in 42 cases albuminuria was present at the time the patient first came for examination with retinitis proliferans. However, in 33 cases, albuminuria was absent and had been known to be absent both prior to and at the time of the discovery of retinitis. Albuminuria, therefore, either preceded or developed soon or about the time of the onset of retinitis proliferans in two-thirds of the cases. However, in one-third of this series, albuminuria had been absent. It is true that in a small group of younger patients, albuminuria has been known to precede the onset of hypertension which then was associated with progressive nephritis. However, there is another group in which hypertension has preceded the albuminuria. Of the two, the first group is more numerous.

The quantitative measurement of albuminuria indicated that although there were 33 patients in whom albuminuria was absent at the discovery of retinitis proliferans, there were only 22 patients in whom albuminuria continued absent during the period of observation. In 17 patients albuminuria varied from 50 milligrams to 200 milligrams. In 23 patients albuminuria was from 200 to 1000 milligrams per 100 cc. and in 5 cases the amount exceeded 1000 milligrams. It is true that such excessive albuminuria was not always present even in the advanced stages. Renal function was good as shown by the non-protein nitrogen of the blood of 20 to 40 milligrams per 100 cc. in a total of 57 patients. Elevation of the non-protein nitrogen of the blood above 40 milligrams occurred in 49 patients. The phenolphthalein excretion in two hours was above 50 per cent in 28 cases; from 30 to 50 per cent in 17 cases; and from 0 to 30 per cent in 10 patients. No test was made in 55 cases.

Increased plasma cholesterol values from 220 milligrams to 262 milligrams were observed in 25 cases in the series with only 15 normal values and no reading obtained in a total of 70 cases. Similarly our data on the albumin globulin ratio is insignificant since only 15 analyses were made and in only 3 cases was the ratio less than 1. It is clear that no very extensive search was made for the nephrotic syndrome but it must be stated that in the cases with inversion of the albumin-globulin ratio, increases in plasma cholesterol, and edema relieved by transfusion or by treatment with acacia, the clinical features were convincing that vascular nephritis with a nephrotic stage, or so-called intercapillary glomerulosclerosis with malignant hypertension plays a more prominent part in the complete course than these figures would indicate.

The common lesions of the kidney in diabetic patients include pyelonephritis, chronic vascular nephritis leading to a contracted kidney with nitrogen retention, and third, glomerular nephritis with a nephrotic phase including edema, great albuminuria, and hypercholesterinemia. Intercapillary glomerulosclerosis, characterized by hyaline deposits within the glomerulus, hypertension, edema, increased cholesterol in the blood is found in some non-diabetic patients, but its advanced form seems to be much more frequent in diabetic patients. Rosenbusch,[1] reporting the late complications in a series of 80 diabetic children observed over a period of twenty years, emphasizes the close relation between retinitis and the characteristic diabetic nephropathy, or intercapillary glomerulosclerosis. Among 35 of his children, retinal hemorrhages developed in 8 cases. He maintains that the hemorrhages do not follow but precede the hypertension and arteriosclerotic changes. The retinitis and nephropathy are due to the sum total of the metabolic changes in diabetes, including endocrine imbalance. In our series Case 9500 died at the age of twenty-seven years after diabetes of fourteen years. He had retinitis proliferans in both eyes, had suffered cataract extractions and had had coma three times. Albuminuria was excessive (1060 milligrams) and the non-protein nitrogen was 108 milligrams in the last stages. The plasma cholesterol had been 363 milligrams. The postmortem examination showed chronic pyelonephritis with also arteriosclerosis involving the coronary vessels.

A recent patient, Case 22,303, fifty-two years of age, with diabetes beginning in November, 1941, had a blood-pressure of systolic 210, diastolic 114 in December, 1942. At that time she had 200 milligrams of albumin, and yet in March, 1946, the urine was free from albumin, while retinitis proliferans had advanced to the point where she was completely blind.

In this group of 110 patients, glaucoma occurred in 15 cases and in three instances hemorrhagic glaucoma required the removal of an eye. Vitreous hemorrhages were recorded in 38 cases and detachment of the retina in 11 cases. Loss of eyesight is usually progressive in the patient once it has started, but so far only a few patients have become completely blind. The progression of associated vascular disease usually leads to fatality before complete blindness occurs.

Seventeen male and 20 female cases have died after an average duration of diabetes from onset of fourteen years for the males and eighteen years for the females. The duration of retinitis proliferans was three years for the males and four years for the females. The causes of death are tabulated in Table 75.

TABLE 75.—CAUSES OF DEATH IN THIRTY-SEVEN CASES OF RETINITIS PROLIFERANS.

	Male.	Female.
Arteriosclerotic nephritis	8	6
Cerebral and/or coronary arteriosclerosis	7	8
Tuberculosis	1	1
Hypoglycemia	0	1
Gangrene	0	1
Uremia	1	2
No cause given	0	1
	17	20

[1] Rosenbusch, Ann. Pædiatrica: **164**, Nos. 5 and 6 and **165**, No. 1, 1945.

Arteriosclerotic nephritis was responsible for 14 deaths and cerebral or coronary arteriosclerosis for 15 deaths. Other causes included tuberculosis, 2 cases; hypoglycemia, 1 case; gangrene, 1 case; and uremia, in 3 cases which may have been due to chronic pyelonephritis. The significance of arteriosclerosis as a cause of death in these cases becomes much enhanced when it is realized that 10 of the 29 arteriosclerotic deaths occurred in patients less than thirty-five years of age at the time of death.

Two deaths occurred in young men twenty-five to thirty years of age following sympathectomy planned to relieve hypertension. Shock with fall in blood-pressure apparently was the chief factor in one death but in the other coronary occlusion was the cause. Against this dark picture of the unfavorable prognosis attending the diagnosis of retinitis proliferans in diabetic patients may be placed a group of 13 patients, 10 female and 3 male, who are alive ten years and more after the recognition and diagnosis of retinitis proliferans. These patients belong in the older age group and possibly illustrate the fact that the females survive hypertension for much longer periods on the average than do males.

Treatment has thus far been disappointing. Early diagnosis of diabetes and prolonged control with faithful observance of dietary rules seems of prime importance.

2. **Clinical Material.**—Waite and Beetham examined, consecutively, the eyes of 2002 diabetics from the New England Deaconess Hospital, and, as a control group, examined similarly 457 non-diabetics from the Massachusetts General Hospital. Special equipment, including all necessary instruments and a slit-lamp, was established in rooms set aside in the Palmer Memorial Branch of the Deaconess Hospital. Comparison of the ocular data was made with such clinical data as heart size, determined by percussion and roentgen-ray plates, condition of the arteries, blood-pressure, chemical analyses of the blood, insulin, the electrocardiogram, and basal metabolic-rate.

In this series were included 297 juvenile[1] cases under the age of twenty years, and 2162 adults. All the juveniles were diabetic. Division according to ages is shown in Table 76.

Forty per cent of the diabetic patients were male and 60 per cent were female. With the non-diabetics, 51 per cent were male and 49 per cent were female. With the diabetic patients, hypertension with systolic pressure above 160 mm. mercury was present in 486 cases and the diastolic was above 90 mm. mercury in 465 of the 2002 diabetic patients. Diagnoses of tuberculosis were made in 54 of the diabetic group and of syphilis in 33 of the group. Among the non-diabetic patients diagnoses of tuberculosis were made in 30 cases and of syphilis in 29. The other diseases present included

---

[1] Juvenile in this section applies to patients under twenty years of age.

heart disease, gastro-intestinal disease, 57 cases of blood disorders, and a variety of other conditions.

TABLE 76.—AGES OF DIABETIC AND CONTROL GROUPS.[1]

Age.	Diabetics.		Non-diabetics.	
	No.	Per cent.	No.	Per cent
Under 20	297	15		
20–39	302	15	75	16
40–59	776	39	269	59
60–up	627	31	113	25
	2002		457	

In Table 77 are summarized the ocular abnormalities found in the entire series.

TABLE 77.—OCULAR ABNORMALITIES IN DIABETES.[1]

	4001 eyes of diabetics.		914 eyes of non-diabetic.	
	No.	Per cent.	No.	Per cent.
Wrinkles of posterior cornea	1040	26.0	96	10.5
Weakness of accommodation	165[2]	21.0		
Deep retinal hemorrhages	730[3]	18.0	34[4]	3.7
Waxy exudates in retina	420[3]	10.0	7[4]	0.8
Depigmentation of iris epithelium	258	6.0	21	2.0
Transitory refractive changes	246[5]	6.0		
Cataracta complicata	246[6]	6.0	75	8.0
Iritis	52	1.3	12	1.3
Atrophy of optic nerve	27[3]	0.6	4[4]	0.4
Homonymous hemianopsia	22	0.5		
Flocculi cataract, juvenile diabetics	22	0.5		
Glaucoma	21	0.5		
Argyll-Robertson pupils	20	0.5	2	0.2
Paralysis of extrinsic muscles	16	0.4	1	0.1
Tobacco amblyopia	14	0.3		

3. **Transitory Refractive Changes.**—Dr. J. H. Waite states that the incidence of transitory refractive changes in diabetes ranges from 6 per cent in an unselected chronological series,[1] to over 50 per cent in a selected freshly-treated group.[7] These changes are bilateral, have dramatic onset, and they may last from a few days to a few weeks. The magnitude of the change usually amounts to 2 diopters or less, but in young diabetics the shift in refraction may amount to 8 diopters. (1) The sudden appearance of myopia in any

[1] Waite and Betham: Loc. cit., p. 614.
[2] Only 759 eyes had accommodation measured.
[3] Only 3893 fundi of diabetics visible. (Fundi not seen in 108 eyes because of opacities in media.)
[4] Only 901 fundi of non-diabetics visible. (Fundi not seen in 13 eyes because of opacities in media.)
[5] Transitory refractive changes picked up by history only in majority of cases, and incidence figure, therefore, is not complete or accurate.
[6] Complicated cataracts in diabetics over twenty years, 235.
  " under twenty years, 11.
                      246.

[7] Granström: Acta Ophth., **11,** 1, 1933.

patient should raise the question of possibility of an unsuspected diabetes; (2) the appearance of hyperopia in a treated diabetic should suggest too rigorous insulinization; (3) alteration in the patient's glass equipment should be delayed until osmotic equilibrium between the crystalline lens and the ocular fluids is attained, a period which may require four weeks.

4. Eyelids.—The eyelids of diabetics show lesions of the skin and mucous membranes of the same type and frequency as those found in non-diabetics of similar age. Only two exceptions to this generalization were found in the eye series, namely, in adult diabetics a slight predonderance (diabetic, 1.4 per cent and non-diabetic, 0.8 per cent) of xanthelasmata,[1] and in juvenile diabetics the frequent presence of elongated eyelashes. No xanthoma diabeticorum lesion was observed in the entire series.

5. Cornea.—In the cornea the frequency of arcus was the same in diabetics and non-diabetics, but a striking difference appeared in the frequency with which wrinkles involving Descemet's membrane occurred. Thus, in the diabetic, such wrinkles were found in 26 per cent, whereas in non-diabetics they occurred in only 10.5 per cent. These wrinkles are invisible with the ophthalmoscope, but were seen with the aid of the slit-lamp and corneal microscope. They appear earlier, are more frequent and numerous in the diabetic eye, occurring in 60 per cent of the gangrene patients and in 51 per cent of the cases with deep retinal hemorrhages. No definite correlation between these wrinkles and the blood sugar, the insulin dose or the pressure within the eye could be found. Paresis of accommodation was especially frequent, occurring in 165 of 759 eyes of diabetics. The explanation was not entirely clear although it seemed possible that excessive glycogen deposition in the pigment epithelium of the ciliary bodies might hamper accommodation. Depigmentation of the epithelial layer of the iris was found three times as frequently in diabetics as in non-diabetics. A possible explanation for this was suggested by Waite and Beetham in the facile release of pigment from the uveal tract of the diabetic, due to an alteration in iris pigment epithelium through selective glycogen storage in diabetics.

6. Pupils.—Pupillary abnormalities occurred in 2.8 per cent of the diabetic eyes. Ten diabetic patients presented Argyll-Robertson pupils without history, clinical or serological evidence of syphilis in the blood or spinal fluid. That such pupillary reactions are not always pathognomonic of syphilis is supported by the view of

---

[1] *Xanthelasmata* (not synonymous with xanthoma diabeticorum). Xanthelasmata are benign, slowly growing, flat yellowish tumors of the skin of the nasal portion of each eyelid, at times unilateral, but more frequently bilateral and symmetrical. They occur in both sexes after the fiftieth year, but they predominate in females. High blood cholesterol has been invoked as a cause by some authors, but quantitative determinations of cholesterol in xanthelasmata patients fail to substantiate this theory. Fifteen such patients in our series in whom cholesterol was quantitated showed only 7 patients running a cholesterol over 229 mg. per 100 cc.

Duke-Elder;[1] Perry, Wartis, Ricarde and Fair[2] who report cases showing Adie's syndrome[3] with pupillary reactions resembling those of the
Argyll-Robertson pupil, not due to syphilis. (See p. 563.)

7. **Lens.**—In the lens two types of abnormality stood out in the
series of Waite and Beetham, refractive changes and lenticular
opacities. The first consisted of transitory refractive changes occurring with blurred vision in 123 cases. Fifty-eight patients were
under fifty years of age. Although the explanation for these changes
was not clear, they must be due to changes in the index of refraction of the lens nucleus, resulting from changes in salt retention
and osmotic interplay associated with rapid shifts in blood sugar.

Lens opacities were studied through dilated pupils with a slit-
lamp and the corneal microscope. The curve of incidence of opacities in the lens showed a somewhat earlier appearance of wheels and
spokes in the diabetics than in the non-diabetics in spite of the fact
that for the series as a whole the diabetics showed a larger percentage
of lenses entirely free from opacities in the anterior cortex than the
non-diabetics. Similarly, when the curve for the frequency of
cholesterin crystals in the anterior cortex of diabetics was compared
with the incidence by age with non-diabetics, the curve practically
interlaced showing no striking differences. Thus at the age of fifty
years both diabetics and non-diabetics showed such cholesterin
crystals in 13 per cent of the cases. Counting all types, lens
opacities were found in 1732 lenses among 3407 diabetic eyes, an
incidence of 50 per cent. In the non-diabetics over twenty years
of age, the incidence was 57 per cent. Shepardson and Crawford[4]
report lenticular opacities in 54 per cent of 68 diabetic patients
ranging in age from eighteen to seventy-nine years, the average age
being fifty-four years.

Cataracta complicata[5] has usually been regarded in the literature
as more frequent in diabetics than in non-diabetics. Table 78
summarizes the incidence of complicated cataracts. In general,
the frequency of complicated cataracts increased with the duration

[1] Duke-Elder: Textbook of Ophthalmology, St. Louis, C. V. Mosby Co., **1**, 562,
1934.
[2] Perry, Wartis, Ricarde and Fair: Arch. Ophth., **19**, 68, 1938.
[3] Costello: New York State Jour. Med., **39**, 781, 1939.
[4] Shepardson and Crawford: California and West. Med., **35**, 111, 1931.
[5] In contradistinction to the usual uncomplicated cataract in which there is
degeneration of the crystalline lens without evidence of disease in any other ocular
tissue, the term "complicated cataract" denotes that type of cataract which commonly complicates other ocular diseases, such as irido-cyclitis, chorio-retinitis, retinitis pigmentosa, high myopia, or detached retina. Having no direct blood supply,
the lens is nourished by food products and oxygen which pass through the semi-
permeable lens capsule from the ocular fluids. Toxic fluids appear first to affect the
most vulnerable portion of the capsule, the thin and cell-free posterior capsule.
Here appears the first sign of "complicated cataract" in the form of an opacity consisting of vacuoles and edema of the lens-fiber system. The opacity extends involving the entire posterior cortex, later the anterior cortex, and finally producing a
mature cataract. In the diabetic series, the incidence of "complicated cataract"
was found to be no greater than in non-diabetics.

of the diabetes. Thus, of patients with diabetes of less than one year's duration, only 2 per cent had such cataracts, whereas among those in whom the duration exceeded three years, the percentage was 9. When the diabetes was from five to ten years' duration, the percentage was 5, and from ten to fifteen years 7 per cent had complicated cataracts. With durations over fifteen years cataracts occurred in 10 per cent of the cases. However, in this last group the average age was 61.8 years as compared with an average age between forty and fifty-five years for the other age groups. No definite correlation was found between complicated cataract and the amount of insulin given, blood-sugar content or other eye complications such as diabetic retinitis. The average blood-sugar value for 100 true diabetics with complicated cataract was 234 mg.

Flocculi occurred in 11 patients or 4 per cent of 297 juvenile diabetics. They were always bilateral and in 7 cases were associated with fine iridescent crystals. In one-half the patients presenting flocculi the diabetes was not controlled at the time the patient first came under supervision. This point was also brought out by O'Brien, Molsberry and Allen.[1] In these 11 patients with flocculi, 3 had had coma, 1 with fatal termination later. All had uncontrolled diabetes and two developed tuberculosis. Six of the 11 had some evidence of endocrine disturbance apart from diabetes. Three of the 11 had a blood non-protein nitrogen above 39 mg., and 1 had a blood cholesterol over 229 mg. per 100 cc. Nine of the 11 had suggestive sclerosis of the peripheral or of the retinal vessels.

TABLE 78.—CATARACTA COMPLICATA IN DIABETICS AND NON-DIABETICS (DISTRIBUTION BY AGE).[2]

Age	Diabetics.			Non-diabetics.		
	Eyes examined.	Cataracta complicata	Per cent	Per cent	Eyes examined.	Cataracta complicata.
Under 10	130	0				
10–19	464	11	2			
20–29	284	12	4	..	20	0
30–39	319	8	2	1	130	2
40–49	520	16	3	3	306	9
50–59	1032	55	5	10	232	24
60–69	999	102	10	18	170	31
70 up	253	42	16	16	56	9
	4001	246	6	8	914	75

Braun[3] has tabulated 21 cases of true diabetic cataracts from the literature occurring in patients from eleven months to forty-nine years of age. Large doses of insulin not only have nothing to do with causing cataracts, but can cause diabetic lens opacities to disappear.

Until more careful diagnostic study is made of the cases with cataract operated upon in the various ophthalmological clinics it

[1] O'Brien, Molsberry, and Allen: Jour. Am. Med. Assn., **103**, 892, 1934.
[2] Waite and Beetham: Loc. cit., p. 614.
[3] Braun: Klin. Wchnschr., **14**, 222, 1935.

will be impossible to settle the primary question as to whether diabetes does actually produce more cases of cataracts than are found in non-diabetics. Kirby, Estey and Wiener[1] analyzed 88 cases of diabetes, finding arteriosclerotic changes in 38 per cent of the patients. The crystalline lens was clear in 36 per cent of the patients, but in the remaining 64 per cent various types of cataract were present. Lens opacities were found in 70 per cent of the diabetics who showed in addition a recognized condition of general vascular hypertension. The frequency of lens changes increased with the duration of diabetes from 22 per cent in whom diabetes was known for one year to 70 per cent of the cases in whom diabetes had been known to exist for more than five years. They performed glucose tolerance tests on 56 patients with cataracts admitted to the eye department of the Vanderbilt Clinic. In 14 cases, 35.9 per cent of the group, a definite curve with a high peak and delayed return to normal pre-glucose level was obtained. In addition to these definite diabetic curves they had abnormal curves in 7, with a high peak but prompt return to normal, and 10 cases, or 25 per cent, with a lag type of curve, indicating a slowing up in the removal of glucose from the blood by the tissues. Such careful examinations if carried out routinely among the cataract patients in eye clinics would probably show a much higher incidence of diabetes than is generally assumed. Kirby, Estey and Wiener also studied variations in the dextrose content of the primary aqueous humor and of the regenerated aqueous humor as well as the blood sugar level of the capillary and venous blood in 75 cases, among whom 23 patients were diabetic with cataracts and 25 were non-diabetic with cataracts. Although the concentration of dextrose in the aqueous humor tends to follow the concentration of dextrose in the blood there is a definite lag so that the changes appear in the aqueous considerably later than they occur in the blood sugar following the administration of dextrose. Also following an injection of insulin the fall in blood sugar is more rapid than the fall in the concentration of dextrose in the aqueous humor.

Anthonisen[2] shows statistically the close relationship between cataract and diabetes. Among eye patients admitted to the Rigshospital in Copenhagen in twenty years 1717 cases were operated for mature cataract and 349 cases operated for primary glaucoma. Congenital cataracts were excluded. The number of diabetics in Denmark is known by means of a registry of cases under treatment for purposes of insulin distribution. He calculated the number of diabetics per 100,000 population by decade and then the number of diabetics among 100,000 cataracts, finding that the number of diabetics among cataract cases was from 15 times as great as expected in the age period sixty-five years to seventy-four years, to

[1] Kirby, Estey and Wiener: Trans. Am. Acad. Ophthal., **37**, 196, 1932.
[2] Anthonisen: Acta Ophth., **14**, 150, 1936.

202 times as great as expected in the period from twenty-five to thirty-four years.

He points out that he has included only cataracts sufficiently advanced to require surgery. If every lens opacity discoverable with magnifying glass and mydriasis is counted then the number of cataracts in aged people of the general population becomes so large that the diabetics as a group form too small a portion of the population to afford a fair test.

Salit[1] analyzed 191 senile cataractous lenses extracted by the intra-capsular method for sugar content. Significantly, only 0.85 per cent of the incipient, 2.4 per cent of the mature, 12.5 per cent of the intumescent cataracts came from diabetics. Inclusive of diabetics, the average sugar value increases from 40.1 milligrams per cent in incipient cataracts to 47.1 milligrams per cent in intumescent cataracts, then decreases to 37.1 milligrams per cent in mature cataracts. Exclusive of diabetics, the value increases from 39.5 milligrams per cent to 42.2 milligrams per cent, then decreases to 35.1 milligrams per cent respectively. The average sugar value of the six cataracts from diabetics is 103.1 milligrams per cent. The intumescent cataract is, therefore, intimately associated with general disturbances in sugar metabolism.

The average sugar value of the crystalline lens, exclusive of diabetics, decreases rather uniformly with age from 40.0 milligrams per cent in the fourth and fifth decades to 36.2 milligrams per cent in the eighth decade. On the other hand, that of the blood increases from 112 milligrams per cent to 145 milligrams per cent respectively.

Cataract is much more frequent in diabetic patients than in non-diabetic patients as reported by Shah.[2] He examined the eyes in 36 untreated diabetic patients and 24 showed lenticular opacities. The greatest frequency was among patients from sixty to seventy years of age with moderately severe diabetes. The cataracts were of the senile cortical type.

Foglia and Cramer[3] found that in all rats with 5 per cent pancreas remaining after partial pancreatectomy, cataracts appeared after a period of time which varied from 50 days onward.

Chemical differences between diabetic and non-diabetic cataractous lenses consist chiefly in the changes in the calcium-phosphorus ratios according to the investigations of Carey and Hunt.[4] Working in the chemical laboratory at the Deaconess Hospital they analyzed 10 normal lenses, 13 cataractous lenses of diabetic patients, 30 cataractous lenses of non-diabetic individuals, 1 dislocated calcified lens and 1 lens from a glaucomatous eye. Carey and Hunt found that the normal lens contained per 100 grams approximately

[1] Salit: Am. Jour. Ophth., **27**, 612, 1944.

[2] Shah: Indian N. Gaz., **78**, 71, 1943. (Abstr. from Nutr. Abstr. and Rev., **13**, 468, 1944.)

[3] Foglia and Cramer: Proc. Soc. Exper. Biol. and Med., **55**, 218, 1944.

[4] Carey and Hunt: New England Jour. Med., **212**, 463, 1935.

9.5 milligrams calcium, 16.5 milligrams phosphorus, and 400 milligrams cholesterol. The calcium content of the cataractous lens was 30 milligrams per cent, or three times the normal lens or blood value. The cataractous lens contained 525 milligrams per cent cholesterol or about 20 per cent more than the normal lens. The phosphorus (non-lipid) found in the normal lens was 16.5 milligrams and the calcium phosphorus ratio was 0.6. In the cataractous lens of the non-diabetic the average phosphorus value was 19.7 milligrams per cent and the calcium-phosphorus ratio was somewhat higher than normal. In the cataract of the diabetic, on the other hand, the phosphorus value was much lower than in the cataract of the normal lens or of the lens of the non-diabetic individual, the average value being 6.2 milligrams per cent. Therefore, the calcium-phosphorus ratio was correspondingly high. The important point is brought out, therefore, that although in general the cataract forming in the eye of the diabetic appears chemically similar to the classical senile cataract, the phosphorus metabolism was markedly different. This may be an important clue inasmuch as the relation between phosphorus and the dextrose metabolism in blood and tissues is already under intensive study.

In properly prepared and carefully followed diabetics, Waite holds that hemorrhage is no more frequent in diabetics than in non-diabetics following cataract surgery. Proper care includes:

1. Pre-operative and postoperative recognition and control of vascular hypertension. For safety, diastolic pressure must be under 100 mm. Hg.
2. Pre-operative recognition and removal of focal infection.
3. Pre-operative recognition and removal of infection in the conjunctiva or tear apparatus.
4. Hemostasis and control of blepharospasm at the operating table can be accomplished through injection of novocaine and adrenalin into the orbit in the vicinity of the ciliary ganglion, and into the eyelids blocking the VII nerve terminals.
5. Attention pre- and postoperatively to adequate intake and proper utilization of vitamins.

Finally, in an eye exhibiting both glaucoma and cataract, for safety, the ocular pressure should first be reduced to normal level by glaucoma surgery, and the cataract should then be extracted later. Otherwise one does meet with ocular hemorrhage, even expulsive hemorrhage.

8. **Vitreous.**—In the vitreous, opacities occurred with about the same frequency in both diabetics and non-diabetics.

9. **Retina.**—The retinal abnormalities are summarized in Table 79.

In this summary appears the most striking difference between diabetics and non-diabetics. Deep retinal hemorrhages and waxy exudates often mark the primary stage of the progressive diabetic retinopathy. The increasing frequency of retinal hemorrhages in recent years is explained partly by the longer duration of diabetes. Wagener[1] recently stated that 60 per cent of cases of diabetes of more than 10 years' duration show retinal hemorrhages. One point seems clear from these studies of Waite and Beetham and from the studies of Wagener, Dry and Wilder[2] and Folk and Soskin,[3] namely, that the deep retinal hemorrhages of diabetes are not due solely to hypertension or to retinal sclerosis. Although debated for many years, the observations at the Mayo Clinic, at the Michael Reese Hospital in Chicago, in Hamburg and in Boston make it clear that this correlation does not explain their frequency.

TABLE 79.—RETINAL ABNORMALITIES.[4]

	Diabetics in 3915 visible fundi.		Non-diabetics in 101 visible fundi.	
	No.	Per cent.	No.	Per cent.
Deep retinal hemorrhages .	730	18.6	34	3.0
Waxy exudates	420	10.7	7	0.7
Nerve fiber layer hemorrhages	196	5.0	33	3.0
Cotton-wool exudates . . .	168	4.3	35	3.0
Cholesterin crystals . . .	28	0.7	4	
Proliferation of capillaries in retina	26	0 7		

Lawrence[5] speaks more hopefully of the fact that in some diabetics retinal hemorrhages disappear.

Two types of sclerosis are found in the retinal arteries. In the larger vessels of the disk, the atheromatous type involving the endothelium is the rule and it leads to occlusion. In the smaller branches which contain no elastic lamina, the more common type is the hyaline thickening of the media without complete obliteration of the lumen. It is difficult to distinguish the two types according to Waite and Beetham. When they graded the arteries of the retina in four groups and classified them according to grade and age, they came to the surprising conclusion that there was no greater amount of sclerosis of the retinal arteries in the diabetics than they observed in the non-diabetic control series. No close correlation is shown between these deep hemorrhages and the blood-pressure.

Diabetes of long duration was associated with the greatest increase in retinal hemorrhages. When the diabetes had existed over ten years a sharp rise in the curve took place with the result that 59 per cent of the patients with diabetes of fifteen years or over had retinal hemorrhages. Careful analysis led Waite and Beetham to conclude that the only dangers from insulin, so far as retinal hemorrhages were concerned, lay in withholding it.

[1] Wagener: Jour. Omaha Midwest Clin. Soc., **7**, 43, 1946.
[2] Wagener, Dry and Wilder: Loc. cit , p. 614.
[3] Folk and Soskin: Am. Jour. Ophth., **18**, 432, 1935.
[4] Waite and Beetham: Loc. cit., p. 614.
[5] Lawrence: Brit. Med. Jour., **2**, 312, 1943.

Lawrence, Madders, and Millar[1] analyzed the serum calcium of 10 cases of diabetes with retinitis and like Waite were unable to find that a low blood calcium was associated with diabetic retinitis.

The frequency of waxy exudates followed closely the frequency curve for deep retinal hemorrhages, increasing with age. The similarity of their location and frequency would seem to indicate that the waxy exudates may arise through hyalinization of deep retinal hemorrhages. Waite and Beetham distinguished the hemorrhages in the nerve fiber layer from the deeper hemorrhages and point out that in the nerve fiber layer hemorrhages do not occur with any greater frequency in the diabetics than in the non-diabetics. Miscellaneous fundus abnormalities such as druses in the fundus, crystals, atrophy of the optic nerve and so forth are listed by Waite and Beetham, but seem to have no direct connection with the diabetes.

Bedell[2] presented an analysis of the fundus changes in 205 diabetics, seen in consultation because of eye symptoms. Besides a general examination, a fundus photograph was made in all patients. In only 40 cases were the fundi negative in both eyes. Most patients were in the fifth and sixth decade; 72 per cent were women. Because serial photographs accurately record the fundus changes, Bedell recommends them for their clinical and prognostic value, especially in cases of diabetic retinitis.

Clinical study of 195 cases of retinal changes in 966 diabetic patients examined in the Copenhagen Hospital between the years of 1928 and 1938 leads Hanum[3] to divide the retinal manifestations into four types: (1) exudative diabetic retinitis, (2) circinoid diabetic retinitis, (3) hemorrhagic diabetic retinitis, (4) proliferative diabetic retinitis. Sixty per cent of the patients had the first type, but he considered the fourth type in the greatest detail, although there were only 12 patients in this group. He believes that in this group capillary resistance is lowered and that usually ascorbic acid and vitamin P (citrin) are indicated as treatment. He could not support Volhard's thesis: "Without hypertension no retinitis in diabetic patients." He concluded that hyperglycemia, acidosis and cholesterinemia could not be related etiologically to retinitis. The prognosis of sight was apparently good except in cases of proliferative retinitis. The mortality for diabetic patients with retinitis was considerably greater than that for diabetics without retinitis.

Increased capillary fragility is especially marked in cases of diabetic retinitis although some diabetics show increased capillary fragility before retinitis has appeared. The effect of rutin upon the capillary fragility in a few of our diabetics is being studied. At the Deaconess Hospital Dr. Raphael Rodriguez measured the capillary

---

[1] Lawrence, Madders and Millar: Brit. Med. Jour., 2, 559, 1930.
[2] Bedell: Trans. Ophthal. Soc. United Kingdom, 59, 219, 1939.
[3] Hanum: Acta Ophth., Suppl. XVI, Copenhagen, 1939.

fragility of 100 diabetics. The index of fragility measured by the technic of Gothlin was greatly increased in 26 cases of retinitis, moderately increased in 12 hypertensive diabetics without retinitis and in 3 diabetics with normal blood-pressure and eyes and normal in 59 diabetics. In the normal group were included 4 diabetics with retinal hemorrhages. Similar studies have been made by Mallery[1] and by Beaser, Rudy and Seligman.[2] The latter authors studied 54 adult patients of whom 15 were hypertensive. The diabetics showed a greater incidence of increased capillary fragility at each age decade than the non-diabetic controls. In 10 diabetics a higher incidence of increased fragility was found at the higher levels of pressure, *i. e.* midway between diastolic and systolic, than at lower levels. Searborough and Steward[3] administered hesperidin successfully to reduce the number of hemorrhages in patients with vitamin P deficiency. The hemorrhages appeared to be independent of the ascorbic acid in the diet.

Messinger[4] reports the eye findings of 200 diabetics. Retinal arteriosclerosis was present in the majority of cases and senile cataract present in 86 cases. Eight instances of eye-muscle paralysis and 9 cases of glaucoma were included.

Leopold[5] describes the ocular findings in patients with diabetes mellitus observed for 10 or more years. Of the 100 cases 20 showed superficial hemorrhages and all showed at least grade two sclerosis on the retinal vessels. Only two of these showed no evidence of hypertension or renal damage or had blood-sugar levels below 150 milligrams.

Elwyn[6] has restated his views that hemorrhages in the retina must be considered as a result of prestasis, that is, the result of slowing of the blood flow through dilated terminal vessel units. He regards the hyperglycemia as the causal factor in diabetic retinitis, and in all probability for the capillary dilations, or "micro-aneurysms."

Ballantyne[7] distinguishes between the fundus picture of diabetes and that of hypertension although both are composed of vascular changes, hemorrhages and exudates. In diabetes the lesions affect primarily the venous and in hypertension the arterial side of the retinal circulation. In diabetes, these changes point to venous stasis and hemorrhages with exudates, congestion of the veins and micro-aneurysms of the capillaries. The earliest recognizable change of the diabetic patient takes the form of minute fatty granules in the vascular endothelium whereas in hypertension these granules are seen more frequently in the media. He conceives that toxic

[1] Mallery: Univ. Hosp. Bull., Ann Arbor, **11**, 33, 1945.
[2] Beaser, Rudy and Seligman: Arch. Int. Med., **73**, 18 and 23, 1944.
[3] Searborough and Steward: Lancet, **2**, 610, 1938.
[4] Messinger: Rhode Island Med. Jour , **27**, 643, 1944.
[5] Leopold: Am. Jour. Med. Sci., **209**, 16, 1945.
[6] Elwyn: Arch. Ophth., **33**, 315, 1945.
[7] Ballantyne: Arch. Ophth., **33**, 97, 1945.

factors may be responsible for the early changes in both conditions but regards them in part at least specific points.

Among the Chinese, hypertension and arteriosclerosis are considered to be less frequent than in Western countries, and the diabetes seems less severe. However, Bock[1] reports that of 183 diabetic patients whose fundi were examined, 49 or 26.4 per cent showed diabetic retinitis, consisting of deep round hemorrhages and white patches.

10. **Lipemia Retinalis.**—In addition to the 2 cases reported by Gray and Root[2] 9 other patients have been observed at the Deaconess Hospital. Case 1705, male, aged twenty-one years who had lipemia in 1923, in 1934 had cataracts and the eyes showed retinal hemorrhages; Case 2296, a clergyman, aged forty years; Case 5114, male, aged twenty-eight years; Case 9250, housewife, aged thirty-three years at onset in 1925 had multiple xanthomata on the heels and hands in 1933 with a plasma cholesterol of 644 milligrams; Case 9629, an Italian woman, aged twenty years, with coma and sepsis; Case 12383, a boy, aged fifteen years; Case 12384, a boy, aged eight years; Case 14971, male, aged thirty-four years, with diabetes of only three months' duration and plasma cholesterol of 1086 milligrams on October 20, 1936. Case 18540, a girl aged nineteen years, showed on December 20, 1939, retinæ with a typical creamy color which made retinal arteries and veins indistinguishable. Acidosis was present and the plasma cholesterol value was 1125 milligrams per cent. Rapid improvement occurred with insulin and diet. A girl, aged sixteen years in diabetic coma, described by Dr. L. M. Pepper[3] of the Kansas City General Hospital, is the fifty-second case in the literature. The 7 cases occurring among 108 cases of diabetic coma reported by Baker[4] bring the total number to 59.

Marble and Smith[5] made serial determinations of the total blood fat, total cholesterol, ester cholesterol and phospholipins in 2 of our cases (12383 and 12384). One case had an initial blood fat of 14.1 and the other of 7.5 per cent. The greatest increase took place in the fatty acid fraction. Next in order of relative increase were the cholesterol and, lastly, the phospholipin fractions.

Kauffmann[6] described 2 cases of lipemia retinalis, one of whom was a colored male twenty-five years of age without diabetes. The blood cholesterol was 960 milligrams. The pallor of the vessels disappeared the day following admission. The second case, a woman aged twenty-two years, had been in coma on many occasions but was not in acidosis on admission. The blood cholesterol value

[1] Bock: Arch. Ophth., **29**, 919, 1943.
[2] Gray and Root: Jour. Am. Med. Assn., **80**, 995, 1923.
[3] Pepper: Personal communication.
[4] Baker: Loc. cit., p. 421.
[5] Marble and Smith: Arch. Ophth., **15**, 86, 1936.
[6] Kauffmann: Arch. Ophth., **29**, 693, 1943.

was 1216 milligrams per 100 cc. The retinæ were studded with exudates and a dozen or more small, round hemorrhages.

The ages of development in 50 of the 60 cases of lipemia retinalis were less than twenty years in 20 cases, between twenty and thirty years in 17 cases, between thirty and forty years in 10 cases and above forty years in only 3 instances.

Formerly lipemia retinalis was regarded as a reflection of a hopelessly fatal condition occurring in the young person destined soon to die, but Case 1705 taught school eleven years following the lipemia retinalis but died in March, 1938 of multiple abscesses and septicemia. Case 2296 lived eleven years to die of coronary occlusion, and Cases 2842, 9250, 12,383, 12,384, 14,971 and 18.540 were alive December, 1944 after having diabetes for periods varying from three to ten years. The remaining 3 cases are dead, average duration of diabetes 2.9 years.

11. **Optic Tracts.**—In the optic tracts three types of abnormalities were observed by Waite and Beetham; (1) sector defects, 48 cases; (2) homonymous hemianopsia, 24 cases; and (3) toxic amblyopia, 14 cases. The susceptibility of older diabetics to tobacco poisoning should be emphasized according to Waite. "Careful tangent screen measurements constitute the only way in which the amblyopia can be recognized. The defect at first does not involve the fixation point, and therefore there is no defect in reading vision. The defect starts as an enlargement of the normal blind spot of Mariotte, especially for red and green, but not for blue or white. The poisoning is cumulative, and the ceco-central scotoma extends to involve the fixation point, and then central vision (reading vision) is suppressed. The peripheral visual field is never affected unless optic atrophy supervenes. The greater portion of the ceco-central scotoma is absolute for red-green and relative for blue-white but there are cores of absolute defect for white-blue tangent to and even involving the fixation point.

"The prognosis is good if the patient will omit tobacco completely, provided optic atrophy has not already set in. Recovery is complete in several months in light poisoning but takes longer in severe cases. Alcohol tends to keep the recovery in check, and it should be omitted also. Free elimination by bowel, bladder, and sweat glands, and the use of vitamin B in the form of yeast are indicated. Sedatives should be used the first few weeks to tide the patient over a very difficult period.

"The exact explanation of what toxic agents produce tobacco amblyopia is still lacking (nicotine, CO, etc.). It is thought that the toxic agents poison the retinal ganglion cells, rather than the fibers of the optic nerve itself." (Waite.[1])

DeSchweinitz and Fewell[2] first in this country called attention

[1] Personal communication.
[2] DeSchweinitz and Fewell: Therap. Gaz., **42**, 623, 1926.

to the frequency of tobacco amblyopia in diabetics. Shannon and McAndrews[1] describe a diabetic with toxic amblyopia.

Waite and Beetham saw 16 eyes with paresis or paralysis of one or more ocular muscles, the most common one being the external rectus. (See p. 562.) Glaucoma occurred in 21 eyes and abnormally low ocular pressures were observed in coma cases of which there were 113 cases.

Optic atrophy occurred in 4 children of the same family described by Wolfram.[2] Although the economic status of the family made the diet quite inadequate in vitamins, since the food consisted chiefly of potatoes, bread and oatmeal with an occasional serving of meat, nevertheless, the diet of the healthy children of the family was even less adequate. Probably lack of vitamins did not explain the condition. No central scotomata were present. The condition did not seem to be the same as Leber's disease. In the 1937 edition von Noorden[3] states that simple optic atrophy occurred in 4 per cent of 477 diabetic patients. Grafe stated that simple primary optic atrophy should not be considered as purely a diabetic affection.

12. **Tumor.**—Melanotic sarcoma, originating in the retina, occurred in Case 6871, whose diabetes began three years later in March, 1928, at the age of nineteen years. In 1925 at the age of sixteen years an injury to the eye led to the discovery of melanotic sarcoma originating in the retina, and the removal of the eye. During the winters of 1932 and 1933 this young man played on a professional hockey team and during this same summer he played professional baseball. In September, 1933, he developed pain in the abdomen, and after a lingering illness died with sarcomatous metastases in the liver.

B. THE EARS.

A frequent and troublesome complication particularly in middle-aged or elderly diabetic patients is the combination of symptoms resembling Ménière's disease. Usually the onset is fairly sudden with dizziness of severe type, frequently with vomiting, the patient is forced to go to bed and the condition may continue for weeks. Pain and deafness are absent, but the dizziness and frequent tinnitus are most distressing. Genuine Ménière's disease occurred in Case 1245, housewife, aged forty-four years, at onset of diabetes in 1913. Although afflicted with angina pectoris and high blood-pressure, as well as gall stones, in January, 1933, a sudden attack began with severe pain in the ear, deafness and extraordinary dizziness. She was confined to her room and bed for nearly a year and never recovered her hearing in the right ear. Death occurred on February 18,

[1] Shannon and McAndrews: Arch. Ophthal., **11**, 757, 1934.
[2] Wolfram: Proc. Staff Meet. Mayo Clin., **13**, 715, 1938.
[3] Von Noorden: Die Zuckerkrankheit und ihre Behandlung. Berlin, Hirschwald, p. 307, 1937.

1934, from coronary occlusion. Case 5525 developed Ménière's in 1934 at the age of forty-seven years, eight years after onset of diabetes. She was successfully operated upon by Dandy in 1935.

Infections of the Mastoid.—In 18 cases mastoidectomy has been performed with 3 deaths following operation, two from meningitis and one with septic neutropenia. Mastoid infections have also caused the deaths of 6 children. In 1939, mastoidectomy was performed successfully in 4 cases (10128, 17683, 17991 and 10893), all of whom showed necrosis and destruction of mastoid cells far out of proportion to the clinical evidence of fever, leucocytosis and pain. Childrey and Gray[1] report a diabetic, aged twenty-seven years, with mastoiditis without any apparent otitis media. The absence of preceding otitis media was shown by the normal drum. No pus was obtained after myringotomy. A zygomatic abscess was present.

Otogenous meningitis resulted fatally in Case 523, male, aged sixty-three years, who entered the Deaconess Hospital for treatment of suspected coma. Although diacetic acid was present in the urine, the plasma CO_2 was 46 volumes per cent. A stiff neck, Cheyne-Stokes respiration and a cloudy spinal fluid containing many streptococci indicated the cause of his unconscious condition.

Diabetic coma can be precipitated by acute otitis media, as illustrated by Case 11726, aged eleven years, who entered the Deaconess Hospital on December 31, 1934 with diabetic coma and subnormal temperature. As she recovered from coma her temperature rose to 105° F. and the red bulging ear-drum soon burst. Recovery was uncomplicated. Operations upon the mastoid have become rare since the introduction of the sulfonamides and penicillin.

[1] Childrey and Gray: Jour. Am. Med. Assn., **98**, 2199, 1932.

CHAPTER XXIII.

TUBERCULOSIS.

By Howard F. Root, M.D.

A. INCIDENCE OF TUBERCULOSIS COMPLICATING DIABETES.

THE susceptibility of the diabetic to pulmonary tuberculosis depends largely upon the control of the diabetes. It has been shown that the incidence of pulmonary tuberculosis in diabetic patients treated with the high caloric diet in 1898–1914 was about the same as when the diabetes was treated with under-nutrition prior to the discovery of insulin, whereas the rate of development of pulmonary tuberculosis in relation to the years of exposure fell to one-third during the years following the use of insulin.[1] The susceptibility of the uncontrolled diabetic to tuberculosis deserves continued emphasis. Two hundred and two cases have been discovered up to January 1946 since our report of 364 cases[2] of pulmonary tuberculosis recognized in 15,072 diabetics between 1898 and January 31, 1938. Early recognition of tuberculosis will require the extension on a large scale of case-finding mass surveys as recommended by the Tuberculosis Control Division of the U. S. Public Health Service,[3] and at present being carried out in Philadelphia.[4]

Aretaeus, in the second century, A.D., whose name is associated with the history of diabetes, also gave an accurate clinical description of tuberculosis and suggested good treatment, according to Moorman.[5] Prior to 1900, pulmonary tuberculosis was found in nearly 50 per cent of diabetic autopsies performed upon patients dying in the public hospitals of large European cities. These figures can hardly be compared with the autopsy statistics in a somewhat later period when the segregation of tuberculous from non-tuberculous patients had become more general. However, Thiery[6] studied 95 cases of pulmonary tuberculosis in diabetics observed in Labbé's Clinic in Paris. He states that pulmonary tuberculosis is the cause of death in 40 per cent of the diabetic patients and this percentage rises to 60 per cent in severe diabetes with malnutrition. Ponteva[7] reports that among 731 diabetics treated in Finland, pulmonary tuberculosis caused 18.8 per cent of the deaths occurring

[1] Root: Am. Jour. Med. Sci., **200**, 53, 1940.
[2] Root and Bloor: Am. Rev. Tuberc., **39**, 714, 1939.
[3] Hilleboe and Morgan: Mass Radiography of the Chest, Chicago, 1945.
[4] Proposed Diabetic Survey: Jour. Am. Med. Assn., **129**, 758, 1945.
[5] Moorman: Jour. Oklahoma State Med. Assn., **32**, 204, 1939.
[6] Thiery: Jour. Am. Med. Assn., **104**, 330, 1935.
[7] Ponteva: Acta Med. Scan., Suppl., **88**, 1, 1938.

subsequent to discharge. Vartiainen[1] recently compared 166 diabetic autopsies with a similar number of non-diabetics from Finland. Active pulmonary tuberculosis was present in 46 of the diabetics and 39 of the non-diabetics. Wiener and Kavee[2] studied 218 cases of pulmonary tuberculosis and diabetes observed at the Montefiore Hospital and its sanatorium during the decade ending December 31, 1932. It is striking that among 3385 tuberculous patients admitted diabetes mellitus also was present in 6.4 per cent. In 1944 among 232 tuberculous patients on the Pulmonary Division of the Montefiore Hospital 33, or 14.2 per cent had diabetes. These are much higher percentages than have ever before been reported for tuberculosis patients, and probably due, as Wiener and Kavee first stated, to the fact that at the Montefiore Hospital there is special interest in diabetes and the population is almost exclusively Jewish.

Interpretation of autopsy figures is difficult. Among 51,705 non-diabetic autopsies an incidence of active tuberculosis of 22.9 per cent was found by Root,[3] whereas among 1121 diabetic autopsies active tuberculosis was present in 28.4 per cent. Considering that two diseases occur in association with less frequency than either one alone is found in a series of autopsies, it appears that tuberculosis is about two or three times as frequent at autopsy as would be expected in diabetics. A review of 1138 necropsies with active pulmonary tuberculosis at the London Chest Hospital by Gloyne[4] revealed 16 diabetics, or 1.4 per cent of the total. Among 1688 necropsies with non-tuberculous disease in the same hospital and the same period only 4 were diabetics. The chief criticism of autopsy figures depends upon the fact that until recently diabetics examined at autopsy were apt to be patients with diabetes of short duration, who died of coma or an acute infection before they have lived long enough with diabetes to demonstrate whether or not they would have developed tuberculosis. The true importance of pulmonary tuberculosis for diabetes of today and the future is best shown by the fact that deaths from pulmonary tuberculosis still make up nearly 3 per cent of all diabetic deaths.

The incidence of pulmonary tuberculosis in adult diabetics is diminishing. The development of tuberculosis in the juvenile diabetic formerly occurred more than twelve times as frequently as among non-diabetic Massachusetts grade and high school children. Pulmonary tuberculosis developed in 8 per cent of diabetic patients within three years after recovery from coma, between 1923 and 1929. Among 97 patients treated for coma between February, 1929 and November, 1932, 24 died of other causes within a year or two. Of the remaining 73 patients, 13 have developed tuberculosis within

[1] Vartiainen: Acta. Med. Scan., **118**, 579, 1944.
[2] Wiener and Kavee: Am. Rev. Tuberc., **34**, 179, 1936.
[3] Root: New England Jour. Med., **210**, 8, 1934
[4] Gloyne: Brit. Med. Jour., **2**, 163, 1938.

five years. In 83 per cent of these cases the development of progressive tuberculosis appeared to follow the onset of diabetes.

The improvement in the incidence of pulmonary tuberculosis among diabetic patients is best shown by comparing the mortality from pulmonary tuberculosis in three different periods of diabetic treatment. Thus in the period 1898 to 1922 the mortality rate from pulmonary tuberculosis among diabetics was 7.8 per 1000. During this period the death rate was not affected by the change from overfeeding to underfeeding. With the introduction of insulin in 1922 in spite of the prolongation of diabetic life and therefore possible exposure, the mortality rate fell to 3.7. From 1929 to 1939 again mortality from pulmonary tuberculosis was halved, reaching 1.8 per 1000. Improvement in mortality rate appears to be due chiefly to better control of the diabetes brought about through the use of insulin.

	1898 to Aug. 7, 1922.	1922 to Jan. 1, 1929	1929 to Jan. 1, 1939.[1]
Death rates from pulmonary tuberculosis	7.8	3.7	1.8

B. CHANGING MORTALITY RATES.

Although the primary infection of the diabetic is no more frequent than in the non-diabetic, since it depends upon contact with a tuberculous case, evidently diabetes lowers resistance and favors the subsequent development of pulmonary tuberculosis. The longer the duration of diabetes, the greater the opportunity for contact with active cases and therefore of infection. The less well controlled the diabetes, the greater the susceptibility to infection becomes. All students have agreed that tuberculous patients do not develop diabetes with any greater frequency than non-tuberculous. In attempting to estimate the probabilities of tuberculosis in diabetes in the future one must bear in mind the changing death-rate from the two diseases and the many social factors influencing the contagion and spread of tuberculosis. The falling death-rate from tuberculosis in the community undoubtedly means a lessening of the frequency of infection. In the Southwest high death rates from tuberculosis are largely due to the high frequency of tuberculosis among Negroes, Indians, Mexicans and Oriental race stocks, and can be attacked by expanding diagnostic and curative facilities.[2] The provision of sufficient sanatorium beds for active cases removes the infective cases from the community. Another public health measure is the extended use of pneumothorax treatment which by closing cavities has reduced infections. On the other hand, the steadily rising age at death from diabetes means a larger number of diabetic patients in the community, who, because of longer life, are more frequently exposed to infection.

[1] Based upon the follow-up of 25 cases in each 100.
[2] Dublin: National Tuberculosis Association, 37th Meeting, 1941.

Dr. Dublin's prophecy in 1930 that within ten years the death-rate from diabetes would exceed that from tuberculosis is approaching fulfillment. It appears that in Massachusetts in 1939 deaths from diabetes and pulmonary tuberculosis were almost identical, 1505 accredited to pulmonary tuberculosis and 1506 to diabetes (State figures). In 1943 the diabetes mortality in 13 states of the United States exceeded that from tuberculosis and Mr. Herbert Marks points out the fact that white females show more deaths from diabetes than from tuberculosis in a majority of the states.

In 1943 the death rates per 100,000 population for pulmonary tuberculosis in the United States were 39.1 and for tuberculosis of other forms 3.4. In Massachusetts the rate for pulmonary tuberculosis was 39.9 and other tuberculosis 2.9, an unexplained increase of 189 deaths, or 11.6 per cent over the previous year. However, this rate fell to 34.4 per 100,000 in 1945. The rate for pulmonary tuberculosis in the Middle Atlantic States was 46.5 and in the East South Central States 47.9. For diabetes the United States rate was 27.1 but for Massachusetts it was 38.2. Indeed the rate for the Middle Atlantic States was 41.1 and the East South Central States was only 13.7. The difference in rates is probably largely a difference in the accuracy in reporting diabetes.[1]

In Boston the annual death rates for pulmonary tuberculosis have varied from 61.3 in 1942, to 62.5 in 1945. In the same period the allocated deaths and rates for diabetes have varied from 36.2 in 1942, to 36.5 in 1945. At present we plan to continue the practice of trying to secure a roentgen-ray examination of the lungs with repetition annually, especially in youthful diabetics, to those who have had coma, and to cases with known exposure to tuberculosis, and we hope beginning July 1 to roentgen-ray every diabetic hospital admission. The evidence of infection with tuberculosis in childhood diabetes is clear cut. In 201 children, only 1 case of pulmonary tuberculosis and 1 early acute case were found in the initial roentgen-ray examination. These children were not acutely ill and therefore the series is not comparable with a general hospital series. Nevertheless 42 per cent of the cases in the first decade and 70 per cent of the cases in the second decade showed some calcification of tracheo-bronchial glands.

Tests for tuberculous infection by means of the skin test have been carried out at the Deaconess Hospital on children, sometimes using the Mantoux test with old tuberculin, but more recently the purified protein derivative of tuberculin and the Patch test have been employed. In adults we have carried out tests up to the age of forty years, using the purified protein derivative. Positive tests with the tuberculin in childhood diabetics have varied from 30 to 45 per cent.

From the group with calcified glands in the lungs have come 5 cases of pulmonary tuberculosis within four years. Among 1430

[1] National Summaries, Vital Statistics, Department of Commerce, **21**, 147, 1945.

diabetics with onset of the disease before fifteen years of age, 21
have subsequently developed pulmonary tuberculosis of the adult
type; 9 were girls and 12 boys. An even higher rate was found in
diabetics with onset between fifteen and twenty years. Pope[1] found
in a follow-up of 5000 Massachusetts school children that pulmonary
tuberculosis developed in 0.6 per cent. This group of 5000, selected
from 140,000 children examined, were classified as having calcified glands, childhood tuberculosis, or as suspects. Therefore, the
incidence in the school population was 0.12 per cent in contrast to
an incidence among the 1126 diabetic children of 1.5 per cent.
Although no case of tuberculosis in any of our diabetics under
twenty years of age occurred during the three years ending with
January, 1940, 3 cases developed between 1940 and 1946, with an
additional death from tuberculosis of the maxillary sinus in Case
21,585. Between 1941 and 1946 among 76 deaths in diabetics
originating in childhood, 6 deaths were due to pulmonary tuberculosis. (See page 768.)

Of Umber's[2] 107 diabetic children, 5 had died, 4 of tuberculosis
and 1 of coma. In tracing the deaths of 104 diabetic children,
Joslin[3] found that among the 10 dying after ten to fifteen years of
diabetes, tuberculosis caused 40 per cent of the deaths. A similar
excess of tuberculosis in diabetic adults was found in a series of
1659 roentgen-rays of diabetics consecutively examined at the New
England Deaconess Hospital. Forty cases were found, or an incidence of 2.8 per cent for adults. These patients were not bed-
patients, but were admitted for dietary treatment and instruction.
The series should be compared with the result of community surveys
and draft-board examinations where the usual incidence found is
less than 1 per cent.

The frequency of diabetes in tuberculosis sanatoria is increasing.
Between 1916 and 1931 only 4 cases of combined diabetes and
pulmonary tuberculosis entered the Trudeau Sanatorium, whereas
between 1931 and 1936 such cases numbered 10. In Massachusetts, whereas 1 person in the State out of 200-250 has diabetes, in
1934, 0.7 per cent of the sanatorium population had diabetes. This
percentage is growing because, according to Dr. Alton S. Pope,
Director, Division of Tuberculosis, it is 2.4 per cent in 1945 in our
State and County Sanatoria for pulmonary tuberculosis.

C. PATHOLOGY OF TUBERCULOSIS IN DIABETES.

It is easy to point out certain peculiarities of tuberculosis in diabetes, but difficult to explain them. Steinbach, Klein and Deskowitz[4] have set a worthy example in studying experimental diabetes

---

[1] Pope: Jour. Am. Med. Assn., **97**, 846, 1931.
[2] Umber: Deutsch. med. Wchnschr., No. 30, p. 1197, 1936.
[3] Joslin: Ann. Int. Med., **11**, 1348, 1938.
[4] Steinbach, Klein and Deskowitz: Am. Rev. Tuberc., **32**, 665, 1935.

and tuberculosis in a dog. Study of the pathological findings at autopsy should be encouraged. Root tabulated 126 autopsies upon tuberculous diabetics including 15 cases from the New England Deaconess Hospital series. Although these 15 included all the tuberculous cases from 150 autopsies, only 7 cases were sufficiently advanced to be a cause of death. Three showed small active lesions, not the cause of death, and 5 showed only healed lesions. This low incidence again must be interpreted with caution, since it is the custom at the Deaconess Hospital to transfer immediately any patient with active pulmonary tuberculosis to a hospital in which such cases receive specialized treatment for their disease. From this series of 126 autopsies it was evident that healing had occurred frequently. In 8 cases only healed processes were present, but in many others small areas of pleural thickening and calcified foci indicating old healed lesions were noted. In 50 per cent of the cases, described in detail, cavities were present. Cases 7041, boy, aged 14.8 years, with diabetes of 8.5 years' duration and 2 boys of Naunyn's series had large cavities. Rapidly developing caseation has been considered characteristic of diabetic tuberculosis. In caseation there is a coagulation of tissue protein associated with the deposition of considerable quantities of fat. Again one is reminded of the disordered fat metabolism of the diabetic. Caseation occurred in 60 per cent of the autopsies of this series. A "non-sensitized" tuberculosis resembling the overwhelming primary tuberculosis of the child has been considered characteristic of adult diabetic tuberculosis. This form occurs in negroes rather frequently. In the 7 Deaconess Hospital cases 4 showed caseating bronchial or abdominal glands together with advanced pulmonary tuberculosis. These cases were 7041, aged 14.7 years, 6791, aged 41.5 years, 1977, aged eighty years, and 11471, aged forty-eight years. The apices were involved in all the Deaconess Hospital cases.

Mayer,[1] in discussing the complications of diabetes in the upper air passages, states that tuberculosis of the tongue or the upper air passages tends to quick progress and caseation.

Wiener and Kavee[2] give an excellent comparison of the pathological findings of 48 diabetic and 48 non-diabetic patients with pulmonary tuberculosis. Thick pleural adhesions of both lungs were twice as frequent in non-diabetics as in diabetics. This comparative lack of adhesions is an important explanation of the fact that in diabetic patients collapse therapy can often be carried out with excellent results. This fact also is consistent with the observed more rapid development of tuberculous processes in the diabetic. They emphasize the seriousness of prognosis. Twenty per cent of the cases died in less than one year. Tuberculosis outside the lungs

[1] Mayer: Monatschr. f. Ohrenheilk., **79**, 397, 564, 1935.
[2] Wiener and Kavee: Loc. cit., p. 635.

and especially of the serous surfaces is rare in diabetes, except in combination with pulmonary tuberculosis.

Little[1] describes a white woman, aged sixty years, who died of advanced pulmonary tuberculosis and a tuberculous abscess in the head of the pancreas. The abscess was filled with creamy purulent fluid in which were demonstrated acid-fast organisms by direct smear. Large tuberculous lesions of the pancreas are exceedingly rare according to Van Valzah,[2] who reported a case and reviewed the literature. It is assumed that the pancreas possesses a relative immunity to tuberculosis. Indeed, as early as the 18th century this fact was used as an illustration of local immunity to tuberculosis. It has been thought that lipase would destroy the fatty envelope of the tubercle bacillus and thus render destruction easy.

Among the etiological factors, contact with active cases in the family or in the neighborhood takes first place. The factors of poverty, race, housing, alcohol, seemed to play no more part than in non-diabetic cases.

D. METABOLIC INFLUENCES AND GROWTH OF THE TUBERCLE BACILLI.

Many students have stated that the tubercle bacillus is found less frequently in diabetic than in non-diabetic tuberculous cases. The variations in form of the tubercle bacillus, studied by Petroff and others, raise the question whether the metabolic changes in diabetes might favor some peculiarity of form in the tubercle bacillus which would render it difficult to find. In the Deaconess Hospital cases the usual forms occurred and positive sputa were found with the usual frequency. The cultural and metabolic characteristics of the tubercle bacillus have been the subject of intense chemical investigation. Long[3] brought out many points which bear upon the susceptibility of the diabetic to tuberculosis. The bacillus obtains its nitrogen from the amino group and this can be supplied on artificial media. In the diabetic the protein metabolism is seriously disturbed especially during periods of active diabetes where great losses of weight with wasting of the muscles occur. Especially during acidosis and coma is there excessive destruction of protein. Case 2448, aged 17.9 years at onset of diabetes, entered the Deaconess Hospital December 1, 1921. The twenty-four hour urine contained 30.8 grams nitrogen, and 2.2 grams acetone, as well as 660 grams sugar. Repeated attacks of acidosis occurred during the next few years. Pulmonary tuberculosis developed at the end of two years with death four years later.

Glycerol appears to be the only alcohol capable of acting as the sole source of carbon for the bacillus. Glycerol is present in the

---

[1] Little: New England Jour. Med., **222**, 135, 1940.
[2] Van Valzah: Am. Rev. Tuberc., **9**, 409, 1924.
[3] Long: The Harvey Lectures, p. 144, 1929–1930.

human body chiefly in the combined form of fat, but a certain amount must be circulating free at times. With the great changes in the fat metabolism of the diabetic the amount set free or the rate at which it is set free must vary greatly. Long and Finner[1] studied the effect of increasing the amount of glycerol upon the growth of tubercle bacilli in cultures and have shown that the yield of bacilli increased ten-fold when the concentration of glycerol was increased from 0.5 to 12.5 per cent. Furthermore, the proportion of the dry weight of the bacilli was thereby multiplied two and one-half times. Long[2] also injected glycerol intravenously into tuberculous rats daily for two months. Similarly infected but non-treated rats served as controls. The rats treated with glycerol developed a more rapid and extensive tuberculosis than did the control rats. Although the concentration of glycerol found in human tissues probably is never so great as can be induced experimentally, nevertheless, an increase taking place constantly throughout a period of time might easily affect the cultural conditions within the body and Long, therefore, feels that the disturbed fat metabolism of the diabetic may exert an important influence upon the susceptibility of the diabetic to tuberculosis.

As causes of the low resistance of diabetics, Banyai and Cadden[3] speak of possible changes in the reticulo-endothelial system and especially acidosis. It was shown by Smithburn[4] that the virulence of tubercle bacilli can be increased by increasing the acidity of the culture medium.

The study of immunity to tuberculosis in diabetes might give valuable data regarding the metabolic aspects of immunity. Native immunity in contrast to acquired immunity must vary greatly in different individuals. In diabetics as a group it is not low before the development of diabetes if one considers that (1) deaths from tuberculosis in diabetic children are rare; (2) the ages at death of tuberculous diabetics are not less than among non-diabetics; (3) the evidence of healing shown by calcified glands in diabetics routinely examined by roentgen-ray shows that many have been infected and partially, at least, healed. Nevertheless, this native immunity does not prevent the growth of bacilli in the tissues. Nor does the immunity conferred by the healing of a primary infection suffice for the protection of the diabetic. Something occurs after the development of diabetes, whether it is by reason of weight loss, or by reason of acidosis or other chemical changes, which reduces his normal resistance. The influence of diabetes is also indicated by the fact that control of the diabetes by active treatment does favor improvement of the tuberculosis.

[1] Long and Finner: Am. Rev. Tuberc., **16**, 523, 1927.
[2] Long: Arch. Path., **6**, 1138, 1928.
[3] Banyai and Cadden: Arch. Int. Med., **74**, 445, 1944.
[4] Smithburn: Nat. Tuberc. Assn. Tr., **31**, 161, 1935.

Scheel[1] believes that primary infection in young adults is becoming more frequent. Although often benign, it may be severe. He studied 202 cases of erythema nodosum, which he considered an evidence of primary tuberculous infection. This is certainly a rare condition in diabetics. We cannot recall a case.

The low resistance of diabetics to tuberculosis does not apply to other pulmonary infections. Delijannis[2] tabulated the occurrence of lobar and lobular pneumonia for diabetics and non-diabetics and found that both forms were conspicuously less common in diabetics than in non-diabetics, percentages being, at autopsy, 24.3 per cent for diabetics and 40 per cent for non-diabetics. At the New England Deaconess Hospital pneumonia has been rare in diabetics. Actually the clinical diagnosis of pneumonia was made 73 times in 13,188 diabetic admissions, or 0.5 per cent.

E. ONSET OF TUBERCULOSIS IN THE DIABETIC.

Clinically, it is an outstanding fact that in the past the discovery of tuberculosis in a diabetic in a truly incipient stage has been almost unknown. The hopeless prognosis and rapid progression of tuberculosis in the diabetic are probably due largely to the extra-ordinarily tardy diagnosis, usually established when the tuberculosis was so far advanced that nothing but a short course could have been expected. In our 566 cases there were only 25 in which the lesion was incipient according to the standards established by the American Sanatorium Association and the National Tuberculosis Association. The comparative ages of onset of tuberculosis and diabetes are shown in Table 80.

TABLE 80.—FIVE HUNDRED AND SIXTY-SIX CASES OF COMBINED TUBERCULOSIS AND DIABETES.

Years of onset.	Tuberculosis, No. of cases.	Diabetes, No. of cases.
0–9	4	10
10–19	34	55
20–29	78	73
30–39	103	109
40–49	78	114
50–59	140	128
60–69	93	64
70–79	32	13
80+	4	

Eighty per cent of the 566 cases had been more than 5 per cent overweight before the onset of diabetes. Great loss of weight was an outstanding feature. The average loss of weight for 219 cases was 42 pounds and in 19 cases the loss of weight was in excess of 75 pounds each.

[1] Scheel: Primary Infection With Tuberculosis in Adolescent and Adult, International Conference Against Tuberculosis, Libson, 1936.
[2] Delijannis: Wien. Arch. f. inn. Med., 27, 97, 1935.

The degree of glycosuria and the essential severity of the diabetes show the same range of variation as are found in other diabetics. When a diabetic is not doing well without an apparent cause, tuberculosis should be suspected. The fact that this old rule holds indicates that with advancing tuberculosis the effect upon the diabetes may be unfavorable. On the other hand, the opposite effect is frequently seen. When the tuberculosis is advancing rapidly, emaciation is occurring, then the diabetes may become so amenable to treatment that the glycosuria completely disappears, and a small dose of insulin may provoke a serious hypoglycemia. A gradual gain in tolerance even without insulin was well illustrated in Case 344. In the course of a year, as the tuberculosis advanced, the diabetes became extremely mild and all acidosis disappeared. Umber[1] noted 4 such cases among 143 tuberculous diabetics. Lundberg[2] based his belief that tuberculous tissue contains an insulin-like substance, para-insulin, upon improvements in tolerance which he observed. However, death from tuberculosis occurred in 9 of the 14 cases in his series. A similar gain in tolerance is seen in long-continued chronic septic infections of diabetic patients. Case 5608, with osteomyelitis of the hips, became sugar-free and developed a high tolerance during the months that the infection continued.

The blood sugar in tuberculous diabetics exhibits about the same variations as are found in the non-tuberculous except when, due to wide dissemination of the infection, the functions of the liver or of the adrenals are impaired. The cholesterol of the blood oftentimes may fall to a low level in tuberculous patients with cachexia and serve as a warning of impending hypoglycemia. Cases 2448 and 11471 in this series had cholesterol values of 78 and 72 mg. per 100 cc. respectively. Severe hypoglycemia occurred with only 15 units of insulin in Case 11471. Both patients died within a few days.

On the basis of insulin requirement, mild cases might be considered to take up to 20 units a day, moderate from 20 to 50 units and severe cases from 50 units upward. Among the 245 patients 16 cases left the hospital taking more than 50 units daily. The more severe diabetics are usually cases who have had coma, have lost much weight and frequently have had a more tardy diagnosis of tuberculosis. These facts must be considered in ascribing to the severity of the diabetes responsibility for the acutely fatal forms of tuberculosis. It is difficult to find a form of tuberculosis typical of diabetes.

The onset of tuberculosis in the diabetic is no more insidious than in the non-diabetic although the rapidly progressive form of tuberculosis is most frequently described. In general prognosis is as good as in non-diabetics if the diabetes follows the tuberculosis,

[1] Umber: Deutsch. med. Wchnschr., **58**, 241, 1932.
[2] Lundberg: Acta med. Scand., **62**, 1, 46, 1925.

but if the tuberculosis develops after the diabetes the outlook is more serious, according to Boller.[1] A large number of chronic cases pursuing a slow course do exist. Kennedy[2] agrees that the type of onset and the course of tuberculosis vary just as in the non-diabetics. Hemoptysis has been present in 45 of 245 cases. Pleurisy with effusion was uncommon. The most frequent type of onset was catarrhal, bronchitic and insidious. Actually, comparison with the series from the Trudeau Sanatorium analyzed by Lawrason Brown reveals more cases in his series with proven tuberculosis without physical signs than are found among the diabetics. The usual physical signs, râles and dulness, are found in diabetics if we but examine them frequently enough.

F. LIPID CONTENT OF DIABETIC LUNGS.

A striking feature in the tissues of diabetic patients is the remarkable alteration of the fat content of certain organs. The removal of fat from one tissue and its deposit in another have been correlated with certain well-recognized changes in the severity and intensity of diabetes. It is of some interest, therefore, to know whether or not the lipid content of lung tissue could be related in any way to the resistance of the diabetic lung to tuberculin infections. Analyses of lungs removed at autopsy at the Deaconess Hospital are reported by Root and Bloor.[3] Although few figures are available for the lipid content of lung tissue in animals or human beings, certain comparisons were made. Root and Bloor listed the clinical data and analyses of 26 diabetic and 2 non-diabetic patients together with the values for phospholipid and cholesterol content of the lungs. Among 12 cases whose phospholipid value exceeded 1.10 grams per 100 grams wet tissue, 5 showed evidences of tuberculous infection chiefly healed. One patient with a value of 2.44 grams had a fatty liver and indeed fat-filled livers with lipoidosis of the spleen were noted in 4 cases. Fifteen of the 26 diabetics had cholesterol values of 0.35 grams per cent or higher and in this group we find 6 of the patients with healed apical tuberculosis and again almost constant arteriosclerosis and fatty livers. A number of patients, however, had low phospholipid values, a fact which may well be considered together with the observation that diabetic cataracts also show a los phosphorus content as described by Carey and Hunt.[4] (See p. 625.) The frequent development of tuberculosis in diabetic patients who have true diabetic cataracts has been stressed by Himsworth.[5]

[1] Boller: Klin. Tuberk., **85**, 173, 1934.
[2] Kennedy: Canad. Med. Assn. Jour., **29**, 482, 1933.
[3] Root and Bloor: Loc. cit., p. 634.
[4] Carey and Hunt: New England Jour. Med., **212**, 463, 1935
[5] Himsworth: Quart. Jour. Med., **7**, 373, 1938.

G. ROENTGENOGRAMS IN TUBERCULOSIS IN DIABETES.

Roentgenograms of the lungs in 87 cases with proved tuberculosis showed multiple areas of calcification indicating former infection. Moderate and advanced processes formed 89 per cent of the cases. No special type of diabetic lesions was observed, although exudative, pneumonic types with cavitation frequently developed in patients with evidences of old infection. Kennedy,[1] in reporting active pulmonary tuberculosis in 41 cases among 2500 diabetics, noted that the tuberculosis in diabetes may be acute, chronic or a latent type detectable only by roentgenography, and the lesion may be of the apical or the hilus-pneumonic variety. Himsworth,[2] in a study of 230 consecutive diabetics upon their first hospital visit, found 15 cases of tuberculosis, of whom 13 could be diagnosed only by roentgen-ray examination. The incidence of pulmonary tuberculosis increases with the duration of diabetes. Thus, in our series of 1600 routine roentgen-rays, among 19 males with diabetes over twenty years in duration, 3, or 16 per cent, had active pulmonary tuberculosis. In 49 cases tuberculosis developed after the age of sixty years. Processes apparently latent for much of a lifetime developed activity after the onset of diabetes. The rate of progression can be measured only by roentgen-ray examination. On the other hand, remarkable improvement may occur. Case 4232, a schoolgirl with onset of diabetes, September, 1921, at thirteen years of age, had coma at the age of sixteen, and a cavity in the right lower lobe was found at the age of twenty years. A year later under sanatorium treatment, the process, after having extended throughout the middle portion of the lung, became quiescent. Gradually the left lung entirely cleared and the cavity closed on the right, but death occurred November, 1936, of tuberculosis.

H. COMPLICATIONS IN TUBERCULOUS DIABETICS.

The complications occurring in tuberculous diabetics are numerous. General paresis was present in Case 8967. Cirrhosis of the liver was the cause of ascites and edema in Case 6725. Silicosis was recognized in Case 10548, quarryman, aged sixty-five years. He also had primary hyperthyroidism, advanced arteriosclerosis and left bundle-branch block. Gangrene occurred sixteen times among the 245 cases. The youngest to develop gangrene was Case 6809 whose diabetes began at twenty-eight, tuberculosis at thirty and gangrene at thirty-three years; he died November, 1929, of bilateral pulmonary tuberculosis. Among the children with tuberculosis, cataracts, carbuncles, arteriosclerosis and coma have occurred.

[1] Kennedy: Loc. cit., p. 644.
[2] Himsworth: Loc. cit., p. 644.

Clayman[1] describes a case of primary carcinoma of the liver associated with diabetes and pulmonary tuberculosis.

Among 414 cases of pulmonary tuberculosis in patients between fifty and eighty years of age reported by Rubin[2], 72 were diabetics. In 90 per cent of these 72 cases, the tuberculosis was rapidly progressive. X-ray revealed much more extensive processes than were suspected from the physicial examination. Hemoptysis was three times as frequent in the diabetics.

Bertram[3] believes that hemorrhages are in no sense due to insulin but rather to a diet improperly balanced with regard to carbohydrate. He feels that the hemorrhages are far more likely due to overactivity of the opposing regulatory mechanism, which leads to an outpouring of adrenalin, increased tonus in the peripheral vessels and an increase in the minute volume in the lungs and so to increase of blood-pressure. Such hemorrhages occur in many other types of conditions as well as tuberculosis, indicating that the important thing is not tuberculosis but the susceptibility of the diabetic to vascular damage when the adrenalin response is too great.

Lobectomy and Pneumonectomy.—In Table 81 are summarized the records of 9 patients in whom advancing pulmonary tuberculosis was treated by surgical removal of one lobe in eight instances and total pneumonectomy in one case (6593). The indications for the operation accepted by Dr. Richard Overholt were the presence of active extending pulmonary tuberculosis limited largely to one lobe or to one side with cavities and in 2 cases a lesion which by x-ray resembled a tumor. No other cases of pulmonary tuberculosis in our diabetic patients have undergone this surgery at the Deaconess Hospital. Surgical recovery occurred in each case. Six of the 9 cases were females, and 4 of the 9 patients had the onset of diabetes before the twentieth year, the youngest at the age of 6.8 years. In this young group the duration of diabetes from its onset to the time of operation for pulmonary tuberculosis varied from six years to sixteen years. In the older group the tuberculosis was discovered within seven months after the discovery of the diabetes in one case and in ten years after the onset of the diabetes in Case 11,225. The diabetes was mild in 3 of the 9 cases and the insulin requirement in 3 cases varied from 52 to 90 units a day. Weight loss had been considerable in the majority of patients.

In Case 11,225 an apparently solid tumor in the right upper lobe proved at operation to be a tuberculoma with seeding throughout the lobe when it was removed. She did extremely well and was still actively at work until March, 1946. Then x-ray evidence

[1] Clayman: Jour.-Lancet, **65**, 144, 1945.
[2] Rubin: Am. Rev. Tbc., **26**, 524, 1932.
[3] Bertram: Ztschr. f. Tuberk , **78**, 13, 1937.

of recurrence required bed rest and death occurred in August, 1946. Cases 21,421 and 24,674 were quiescent in October 1945.

TABLE 81.—LOBECTOMY IN DIABETIC PATIENTS WITH TUBERCULOSIS.

Case No.	Sex.	Onset of diabetes. Age.	Date.	Insulin units.	Max. wgt. lbs	Weight before operation.	Date of operation.	Follow-up date L. or D.
6593	M	19.7	I '28	34	140	114	Dec. '42	L Mar. '46
9018	F	13.7	III '30	52	150	130	Feb. '45	L Mar. '46
11225	F	34.7	VI '32	30	135	112	Nov. '42	D Aug. '46
12997	F	6.8	X '33	80	142	136	Feb. '45	L Feb. '46
21421	F	52.2	IX '41	0	160	138	Apr. '42	L Nov. '45
23343	F	18.8	XII '39	94	184	139	Mar. '45	L Mar. '46
24674	F	44.2	VII '43	34	155	123	Mar. '44	L Apr. '45
26016	M	63.3	XI '42	20	185	133	Mar. '44	D Oct. '45
26614	M	54.6	XII '44	12	195	158	Aug. '45	L Dec. '45

Case 6593, operated in December 1942 has been back at work for many months in spite of the fact that the right lung which was removed showed extensive tuberculosis throughout and there was an early tuberculosis on the left side. X-ray examination in February 1946 by Dr. Overholt was satisfactory. Case 12,997 has shown further extension and in March 1946 entered a sanatorium. Case 26,016 also a year later after the operation showed extension to the other side and died of tuberculosis in October 1945. Admittedly the period of observation in these surgical cases is too short to permit conclusions to be drawn. However, the results in the cases operated upon in 1942 give some reason to believe that this type of surgery performed in properly selected patients may afford another ray of hope for the diabetic patients who develop pulmonary tuberculosis.

I. DIET, CRYSTALLINE INSULIN AND PROTAMINE ZINC INSULIN.

Diet.—The object of treatment in tuberculous diabetics should not be dictated by a slavish regard for sugar-free urine and a normal blood sugar, if that attitude leads to the use of a diet too poor in carbohydrate, to undernutrition or to the use of too large doses of insulin which may provoke an overactivity of counterregulatory and opposing influences in the body. Nevertheless, control of the diabetes with normal blood sugar values aids in controlling the tuberculosis.

Sample diets for use with tuberculous patients on the basis of a patient weighing 132 pounds may be classified as follows:

TABLE 82.—DIETS FOR TUBERCULOUS DIABETICS.[1]

	Carbohydrate, grams.	Protein, grams.	Fat, grams.	Calories.
1. Standard diet	150	80	100	1820
2. Surgical diet—before operation	200	75	70	1730
—day of operation	100	20–30	40–50	840–970
3. Diet to increase weight	250	100	120	2480

[1] From Root and Bloor: Loc. cit., p. 634.

In children and young adults insulin should be given as soon as the diagnosis of diabetes is made. The use of protamine insulin is advantageous, especially in sanatorium practice, since it reduces the frequency of injections from two to three times a day to a single treatment before breakfast. In case of exposure to an open case of tuberculosis, insulin should never be omitted unless the exposure is known to be slight, weight and general health are normal, and the urine and blood sugar are normal with an adequate diet. Among 144 cases the average insulin prescribed at discharge from the hospital was 28 units. The smallest daily dose was 2 units and the maximum 83 units. The distribution of the injections in various areas is important in order to avoid induration and consequent loss of efficiency of insulin. Atrophy of subcutaneous fat has not been noted in tuberculous cases. On the average, tuberculous cases do not require more insulin than non-tuberculous. These results indicate that the harmful effects of tuberculosis on diabetic tolerance are easily exaggerated. During periods of high fever and toxemia the insulin requirement will usually be increased. As a rule, however, when careful dietary treatment and adjustment of the insulin dose are carried out so that wastage is avoided, no evidence of a great increase in the insulin requirement appears.

Hypoglycemia is not rare in tuberculous diabetics undergoing dietary and insulin treatment. Patients with advanced tuberculous lesions and acute toxemia from pneumonia or generalized tuberculosis seem especially liable to insulin reactions. If Addison's disease is present, hypoglycemia may easily develop even with small doses, since the antagonistic action of the adrenals is absent. Spontaneous hypoglycemia without insulin occurred in Case 11419, whose diabetes began in January, 1932 at the age of fifty years. On October 12, 1932 he weighed 128 pounds and the blood sugar was 0.28 per cent. He then took 5 units of insulin a day. In February, 1934 he entered the hospital with anasarca, the blood sugar was 0.06 fasting, the non-protein nitrogen was 49 mg. and the cholesterol of the blood was 70 mg. per 100 cc. Insulin was immediately stopped and his diet increased to 220 grams carbohydrate. Two weeks later he was apparently dying at 7 A.M. with faint respiration and the blood sugar was 10 mg. per 100 cc. He recovered after 20 cc. glucose solution (50 per cent) were given intravenously. Death occurred within a week from tuberculosis and amyloid disease.

Foley and Andosca[1] report the treatment of tuberculous diabetics in a sanatorium with a high caloric house diet of at least 3000 calories with, in addition, minerals and vitamins. An example of an ordinary diet consists of 345 grams of carbohydrate, 120 grams of protein and 130 grams of fat. They urge strict control of the diabetes with the high caloric diet using as necessary large amounts of insulin.

[1] Foley and Andosca: Med. Clin. North America, **28**, 499, 1944.

Banyai and Cadden[1] reported that of 115 tuberculous diabetic patients at discharge 47 per cent with moderately advanced tuberculosis were classified as having the disease arrested, quiescent or improved.

Sattler[2] also reported a patient, aged fifty-six years, with diabetes for six years and tuberculosis for ten years, whose diabetes disappeared as he developed amyloid changes in the liver, the spleen, and the kidneys. He says that usually in a simple nephrosis a lowering of the sugar threshold is observed, whereas, in inflammatory and vascular contraction of the kidney a rise in the threshold occurs.

Rathery, Roy and Conte[3] followed the curve of the blood sugar during twenty-four hours in diabetic patients with and without tuberculosis. They found a wide range of variation in different diabetic patients. In certain tuberculous patients a spontaneous fall of blood sugar in the middle of the day made the giving of insulin at that time of the day hazardous. Allergic sensitiveness to insulin is described by Grishaw[4] whose patient, a man, aged thirty-eight years, had had tuberculosis for many years. Local reactions occurred with the beginning of insulin, but on the twenty-fifth day of treatment general urticaria with itching lasted four hours. He found that the patient could take only one brand of insulin without urticaria.

Remarkable improvement in nutrition has occurred among the tuberculous diabetics. Case 3775, male, aged sixty-four years, gained 20 pounds in a year with insulin 30 to 40 units daily, and roentgenograms showed reduction in the size of the cavities. Case 5448, male, aged fifty-one years, gained 30 pounds during the next six months in the sanatorium. Case 2274, aged six years at onset of diabetes in 1921, onset of tuberculosis at twelve years, grew 15 inches and gained 53 pounds between 1921 and 1931 under home treatment. Death occurred in 1934. Ten cases of active pulmonary tuberculosis received on the average at discharge from the Deaconess Hospital carbohydrate, 157 grams, protein, 83 grams, and fat, 116 grams; Calories 2004. The average calories per kg. of body weight were 34. Insulin was omitted in 1 case. The amount prescribed in the other 9 varied from 12 to 77 units. All 10 cases had tubercle bacilli in the sputum, and 9 were acutely ill with fever and cavities.

J. COMA IN TUBERCULOUS DIABETICS.

Coma and tuberculosis frequently occur in the same patient contrary to the former belief that coma was rare in the tuberculous diabetic. More important is the fact that pulmonary tuberculosis often develops after attacks of coma. Bertram[5] states that 80 per

[1] Banyai and Cadden: Loc. cit., p. 641.
[2] Sattler: Wien. Arch. f. inn. Med., **30**, 313, 1937.
[3] Rathery, Roy and Conte: Paris méd., **2**, 9, 1935.
[4] Grishaw: Jour. Am. Med. Assn., **97**, 1885, 1931.
[5] Bertram: P. 114, loc. cit., p. 87.

cent of his asthenic diabetics developed tuberculosis after having diabetic coma.

Between 1923 and 1929 pulmonary tuberculosis developed in 8 per cent of 105 diabetic patients within three years of recovery from coma. Among 97 patients treated for coma between February, 1929 and November, 1932, 24 died of other causes within a year or two. Of the 73 patients remaining, 13 developed tuberculosis within five years. Among 651 instances of coma in 495 patients treated at the Deaconess Hospital, up to January 1, 1946, 67 have died since discharge, and of these 15 died of tuberculosis. The development of tuberculosis in other cases of this coma series has already been recorded. (See page 646.) At present we try to secure roentgen-rays of the lungs of every coma case once a year. In January, 1944, Case 11256, aged thirteen years at onset of diabetes in 1931, had coma requiring 810 units in the first twenty-four hours. During the two years after his recovery, he continued to work but did not report for physical examination. In March, 1946 he complained only of weakness but a roentgenogram disclosed multiple tuberculous cavities.

K. PROGNOSIS OF TUBERCULOSIS IN DIABETES.

The duration of life in diabetic patients with tuberculosis is sometimes surprising. Case 10163, female, illustrates the development of pulmonary tuberculosis before diabetes. It occurred at the age of fifteen years, and she spent three years in a sanatorium. In 1918 diabetes was discovered when she had a miscarriage. In 1922 at the Boston Tuberculosis Hospital multiple cavities were present and the sputum was positive. Insulin was begun in 1924 at the Deaconess Hospital with 30 units daily. She died in November, 1933. Unusually rapid primary healing following thoracoplasty occurred in Case 13614, aged thirty years with diabetes of four years' duration in 1935. In February, 1946 he was at work, in good condition, taking 10 units of crystalline and 34 units of protamine zinc insulin daily. The effect of insulin is shown by the fact that fatal cases treated with insulin lived 8.9 years and those treated before insulin lived 5.2 years after the onset of diabetes. Among insulin-treated cases alive in 1945 pulmonary tuberculosis had been present in 25 cases for more than five years, the average being ten years. In fact, the prognosis for pulmonary tuberculosis in diabetics may be better than in non-diabetics, if they are discovered at relatively the same stage of tuberculosis.

Nevertheless, the combination is to be dreaded, as shown by Table 83, which summarizes the durations of diabetes and tuberculosis in 367 fatal cases. Clearly the duration of life has increased since the use of insulin. The duration of life after onset of diabetes has more than doubled and the same is true for tuberculosis.

Actually the average duration of diabetes before the onset of tuberculosis has also increased from 2.7 years in the period 1898–1914 to 6.1 years in the period 1938–1946.

TABLE 83.—DURATION OF DIABETES AND PULMONARY TUBERCULOSIS
IN 367 FATAL CASES.

Period.	No. of cases.	Diabetes, years.	Tuber-culosis, years.	Total diabetic deaths.	Per cent tuber-culosis.
1898–1914, August 7	19	5.4	2.7	342	5.6
1914, August 8–1922, August 7 .	47	5.2	3.0	805	5.8
1922, August 8–1930	87	6.2	3.1	1278	6.8
1930–1938, July 29	128	9.9	3.3	1880	5.6
1938, July 29–1946, Jan. 1[1] . .	86	11.6	5.5	2734	2.5

Only by the earlier discovery of tuberculosis in an incipient stage can the prognosis be greatly improved. In the aged, arteriosclerotic complications affect the course and shorten life. Nevertheless, in 49 cases where the diabetes began after the age of sixty years, the average duration of life after the onset of the diabetes in 36 fatal cases was eight years. The average duration of tuberculosis in this group, however, was less than one year, and represented the terminal stage of chronic tuberculosis. The earlier the diagnosis, the greater is the value of sanatorium treatment, and the more frequently can the advantages of collapse therapy and surgery be utilized.

Case 4261, with onset of diabetes at nine years, after repeated attacks of coma, developed pulmonary tuberculosis in 1933, aged nineteen years. Therapeutic pneumothorax on the left has maintained collapse for six years. In her second pregnancy she was delivered by cesarean section in February, 1938. Both mother and daughter were in good condition in January 1946, the mother taking 36 units of protamine zinc insulin. The use of surgical measures to attain collapse of the affected lung has strikingly favorable results in diabetics.

In some way the resistance to tuberculosis is lowered during emaciation. In obesity the trend of fat metabolism is predominantly synthetic. Fat tends to be stored up as neutral fat and this may mean that less of the intermediaries of fat metabolism, including glycerol, are in circulation. In diabetes with loss of weight, on the other hand, the fat metabolism is catabolic. Beware of too rapid weight reduction in a diabetic!

Tuberculosis is in considerable measure the penalty of neglected diabetic treatment. Among poorer patients and particularly among public hospital patients in contrast to private practice the incidence of tuberculosis is high.

Wessler and Hennell[2] report 8 cases of diabetes and pulmonary

---

[1] We are indebted for the tabulation of these data to Mr. Herbert Marks of the Statistical Bureau of the Metropolitan Life Insurance Company.

[2] Wessler and Hennell: Am. Rev. Tuberc., 27, 47, 1933.

tuberculosis in whom cavities healed. Three of the patients were under forty-five years of age. In spite of positive sputum and fever, with prolonged treatment, including insulin and a proper diet, the cavities were closed. In recent years no more dramatic change in diabetes can be reported than the improvement in the results of treatment of complicating pulmonary tuberculosis.

L. PREVENTION OF TUBERCULOSIS IN DIABETICS.

Prevention of tuberculosis in diabetic patients must constantly be borne in mind. Avoidance of contact with open cases must be brought about by the discovery and isolation of such cases in the families of diabetic patients. Good hygiene must include adequate rest, fresh air, outdoor life, regular exercise, and pasteurized milk. Summer camps should be utilized for diabetic children with calcified glands and positive skin tests. Diabetic girls should not become nurses. Early use of insulin and constant control of the diabetes are fundamental in maintaining nutrition and resistance.

Detection of tuberculosis in diabetics will never be made at a reasonably early period until routine roentgenograms are taken at frequent intervals and always upon the slightest suspicion of pulmonary disease. Indeed, in hospital routine roentgen-rays are more important than routine Wassermann tests.

CHAPTER XXIV.

CANCER COMPLICATING DIABETES.

By Alexander Marble, M.D.

A. INTRODUCTION.

There are but few reports in the literature which present data as to the incidence of cancer in diabetic patients. Consequently the paper of Ellinger and Landsman[1] in 1944 is of interest. These workers found that in 1933 to 1941, of 1280 diabetic patients seen at Montefiore Hospital in New York City, 39, or 3.04 per cent, had malignant disease. This incidence of cancer was six and one-half times as great as that of 0.46 per cent for cancer in the general population of the State of New York in 1941, although it must be admitted that the data are not entirely comparable. In the course of a statistical study of associated causes of death (as recorded on death certificates) in individuals dying with cancer in Massachusetts during a ten-year period, Wilson and Maher[2] observed that diabetes and cancer occurred together much more frequently than would be expected on the assumption that the two diseases are independent. They state that "it would appear that either diabetics tend to develop cancer or that cancer patients tend to develop symptoms recognized as diabetic." In Warren's[3] series of 527 diabetic patients on whom a postmortem examination was done (made up largely of patients of the George F. Baker Clinic) there were 47 patients, or 8.9 per cent, with malignant disease. Further indication of the incidence of cancer among our diabetic patients is afforded by the figures in Table 84, compiled with the aid of the Metropolitan Life Insurance Company.

TABLE 84.—Incidence of Cancer Among Deceased Diabetics, 1898–1946.
(Experience of Elliott P. Joslin, M.D., and associates.)

Period.	Deceased diabetics.	Cancer deaths.	Per cent cancer deaths of all deaths.
1898–1914	326	5	1.5
1914–1922	836	32	3.8
1922–1936	3988	350	8.8
1937–1943	2583	227	8.8
1944–May 15, 1946 . . .	651	58	8.9

In the ten years from 1936 to 1946, the mortality from cancer among diabetics has averaged 8.8 per cent of the total from all

[1] Ellinger and Landsman: New York State Jour. Med., 44, 259, 1944.
[2] Wilson and Maher: Am. Jour. Cancer, 16, 227, 1932.
[3] Warren: P. 65, loc. cit., p. 196.

causes. This represents a 132 per cent increase from the figures
for the period from 1914 to 1922. That this increase is much greater
than that in the general population in the same period of years is
evident from a study of Table 85, in which are shown the data for
Massachusetts. Here the increase of the ratio of cancer deaths to
total deaths from 1915 to 1944 was from 11.17 to 18.66, or 67.1 per
cent, in the age group forty to forty-nine; from 14.39 to 20.21, or
40.4 per cent, in the age group fifty to fifty-nine; and from 13.15
to 19.16, or 45.7 per cent, in the age group sixty to sixty-nine years.
Hence, the percentage of increase in cancer among diabetics was
three to four times that in the general population of about the
same age group.

TABLE 85.—RATIO OF CANCER DEATHS TO TOTAL DEATHS[1] IN MASSACHUSETTS.

Percentage of deaths due to cancer.

Year.	All ages.	40–49.	50–59.	60–69.
1895	3.49	7.54	10.32	8.87
1900	4.12	8.67	11.07	9.36
1905	4.94	9.42	11.87	10.59
1910	5.77	10.38	13.20	11.33
1915	6.92	11.17	14.39	13.15
1920	7.75	11.96	17.12	14.97
1925	10.10	14.04	17.83	16.74
1930	11.74	14.49	19.13	17.33
1935	12.79	15.44	18.46	17.71
1940	14.26	17.70	19.95	18.38
1944	14.68	18.66	20.21	19.16

If one considers the influence of the asserted tendency for two
major diseases not to occur in the same individual ("hypothesis of
independence"), a higher incidence of cancer among diabetic patients
would take on added significance. However, with modern methods
of treatment, the controlled diabetic now approaches the normal
individual more and more. His life expectancy at the time of development of diabetes is already more than half as great as that of the
non-diabetic and his length of life is steadily increasing. Therefore,
it seems logical to assume that at the present time this principle
can be applied to diabetes to a less extent than to other major
diseases.

One other consideration may account for the apparent greater
increase of cancer among diabetic individuals; the age at death of
diabetics has increased from 46.7 years in 1914 to 1922 to 64.5 years
in 1944 to 1946, thus bringing more patients into the cancer zone.
Although it is true that the average age at death of individuals in
the general population has increased (from 42.0 years in 1915 to
1919 to 55.9 years in 1940), this increase is less than that among
diabetic patients and places relatively more diabetics in the cancer

---

[1] Compiled from Table 102 of Bigelow and Lombard: Cancer and Other Chronic
Diseases in Massachusetts, Boston, Houghton, Mifflin Company, 1933. Figures
for 1930, 1935, 1940 and 1944 are available through the courtesy of Dr. Herbert
L. Lombard.

age zone. This becomes of great importance if one considers how much more common is death from cancer in the sixth and seventh decades than in the fifth decade of life.

The discussion above indicates that from data now available it is difficult to draw conclusions regarding the relative incidence of cancer among diabetics and non-diabetics. Certain evidence seems to indicate that cancer is more common in diabetes but, as pointed out above, there are serious objections to such a conclusion.

B. CASES OF CANCER AND DIABETES IN AUTHORS' SERIES.

1. **Series Studied in 1933.**—In 1933 a study was made[1] of the records of approximately 10,000 patients with proved diabetes who were included in a series of 12,000 individuals of all ages coming for diagnosis or treatment of glycosuria. Among this number 256 cases of malignancy, or approximately 2.6 per cent of the patients with true diabetes, were known to have occurred up to September, 1933. At that time 219 were dead and 37 living; up to April 1940, 24 of the 37 patients were known to have died, making a total of 243 fatal cases of this original study group. Among the fatal cases the average age at the onset of diabetes was 55.9 years and at death 63.4 years, making an average duration of diabetes of 7.5 years.

In only 185 of the fatal cases was it possible to estimate the duration of cancer symptoms up to death and in this group the average was 2.5 years. Allowing for inaccuracies, this figure is still so much less than that of 7.5 years for the duration of diabetes, as stated above, that one is forced to conclude that in most instances the onset of diabetes came well before that of cancer. Furthermore, of the 185 cases, in 159 the onset of diabetes preceded that of cancer symptoms, and in only 26 instances did the onset of cancer symptoms precede that of diabetes. In other words, one is dealing with a group of diabetic patients who later developed cancer, rather than with a group of patients with malignant disease who developed diabetes. The figure of 2.5 years, for duration of cancer symptoms from onset until death, is slightly greater than that of approximately two years found by Macdonald[2] in a study of cancer deaths in Massachusetts in 1932.

Ellinger and Landsman[3] believe that there is direct correlation between the virulence of the malignant growth and the severity of the diabetic condition. In their patients the duration of life after onset of tumor symptoms decreased from 4.6 years in mild diabetes to 0.9 years in severe diabetes. Nine of the 39 patients with cancer and diabetes lived for five or more years after onset of tumor symptoms; the severity of diabetes was rated as mild in all but one of these.

[1] Marble: New England Jour. Med., **211**, 339, 1934.
[2] Macdonald: Am. Jour. Pub. Health, **28**, 818, 1938.
[3] Ellinger and Landsman: Loc. cit., p. 653.

Among the total group of 243 fatal cases in the authors' series, the ten most common sites of cancer were as follows: breast 35 cases, pancreas 33, uterus 27, stomach 17, urinary bladder 15, liver 14, large intestine (exclusive of rectum) 13, skin 11, rectum 9, and prostate 9 cases. Autopsy was carried out in 26 of the fatal cases. As nearly as could be made out, the malignant disease did not differ in nature, type of metastases or in other characteristics from that found in non-diabetic individuals.

2. **George F. Baker Clinic Series, 1934 to 1938.**—In 1940 and again in 1946 we have studied the records of 101 diabetic patients with cancer treated at the George F. Baker Clinic in the five-year period from 1934 to 1938 inclusive. Of these, 34 were male and 67 female. In the 1946 follow-up study it was found that up to January, 1945, 85 of the 101 patients had died. Data regarding the series are presented in detail in Table 86.

TABLE 86.—SUMMARY OF DATA REGARDING DIABETIC PATIENTS WITH MALIGNANT DISEASE SEEN AT GEORGE F. BAKER CLINIC, 1934–1938 (INCLUSIVE).

	Living.	Fatal.	Total cases.
Number of cases	16	85	101
Age at onset of diabetes	50.5	57.2	56.1
onset of cancer	56.7	62.7*	61.7*
death, or January, 1945	67.7	65.5	65.9
Duration of diabetes, years	17.2	8.3	9.8
Duration of cancer, years	11.0	2.8*	4.2*
Cases operated upon	13	60	73
Duration of life after operation, years	9.4	2.3	2.6

Site of Malignant Disease:

	Living.	Fatal.	Total cases.
Lip, tongue and cheek	2	4	6
Esophagus	..	2	2
Stomach	..	2	2
Colon, including sigmoid	3	10	13
Rectum	1	8	9
Pancreas	..	12	12
Liver secondary, primary site undetermined	..	1	1
Gall-bladder and bile ducts	..	4	4
Kidneys	..	2	2
Bladder	..	2	2
Uterus	5	9	14
Ovary	1	..	1
Vulva and vagina	..	3	3
Prostate	..	4	4
Lungs and bronchus	..	3	3
Breast	2	12	14
Skin	2	3	5
Brain	..	1	1
"Carcinomatosis"	..	2	2
Melanotic sarcoma	..	1	1
Totals	16	85	101

* Data not available for all patients.

Study of the data shown in Table 86 yields findings which are in essential agreement with those mentioned above for the larger series of 256 cases.

In the group of 101 cases there were not included those patients with benign tumors, and patients with known cancer successfully treated elsewhere before coming to the George F. Baker Clinic for treatment of diabetes.

C. CANCER OF THE PANCREAS.

Cancer of the pancreas deserves special mention. Both in the series of 256 cases of cancer reported upon in 1934 and in the recent series of 101 cases presented in Table 86, carcinoma of the pancreas comprised a relatively high proportion of the total, forming 13 per cent of the former and 12 per cent of the latter series.

The above figures contrast sharply with that of 2.5 per cent for this type of lesion in the 5300 cases of cancer reported in Boston during 1920 to 1924 and studied statistically by Hoffman.[1] In a later paper, Hoffman[2] stated that "It is probably safe to assume that when all allowance is made for perfection of diagnosis, the present mortality from cancer of the pancreas is not less than 3 per cent of the total mortality for all forms of malignant disease in the United States." Bigelow and Lombard[3] found (see their Table 108) that 4.8 per cent of the cancer deaths in Massachusetts hospitals in 1928 to 1930 were due to cancer of the pancreas. Among 87,981 deaths from cancer during the five year period, 1940 to 1944, in industrial policyholders of the Metropolitan Life Insurance Company[4] there were 3007 deaths from cancer of the pancreas, an incidence of 3.4 per cent. In the United States from 1939 to 1943, inclusive, there were 802,355 deaths from cancer of all types reported; of these, 27,816, or 3.5 per cent, were due to cancer of the pancreas.

Among our own cases, the patients with cancer of the pancreas numbered 33 in the first series and 12 in the second series, a total of 44 cases (Case 11647 was included in both series). Of these, 18 were males and 26 were females. At the age at which cancer of the pancreas is most common, there are about twice as many females as males with diabetes, so that actually the sex incidence was higher in males than is apparent at first glance. In the literature the condition has been reported to occur almost twice as often in men as in women, although in Kiefer's[5] series there was almost equal distribution between the sexes. In our 44 cases the average duration of diabetes at death was 3.6 years, as opposed to an average duration of cancer symptoms of 1.0 year. The average age at death was

[1] Hoffman: San Francisco Cancer Survey, Third Preliminary Report, Newark, N. J., The Prudential Press, p. 29, 1925.

[2] Hoffman: New England Jour. Med., 211, 165, 1925.

[3] Bigelow and Lombard, p. 264; Loc. cit., p. 654.

[4] Figures for the Metropolitan Life Insurance Co. and for the United States were kindly furnished by Mr. Herbert H. Marks, Statistical Division, Metropolitan Life Insurance Co.

[5] Kiefer: Arch. Int. Med., 40, 1, 1927.

42

62.2 years. In 30 cases the diagnosis was proven either at operation or autopsy. In practically all cases the tumor occupied the head of the organ.

Symptoms.—The chief symptoms complained of were jaundice, abdominal pain, loss of weight and strength, nausea and at times vomiting, and anorexia. Most patients suffered pain or marked abdominal distress at some time or other during the course of their illnesses. The pain was usually epigastric or over the region of the pancreas, although at times, as with Case 11661, the chief discomfort was across the lower abdomen. Doubtless the location of the pain depends in large measure on the site of metastases. Loss of weight and strength was usually striking.

Diagnosis.—Preterminally, diagnosis may offer little difficulty, but in the earlier stages of the condition, exact diagnosis is difficult. In addition to the characteristic symptoms and signs, laboratory studies usually show a secondary anemia, often absence of free hydrochloric acid in the stomach contents, and often excess of fat and absence of bile in the stools. Roentgenograms of the gastrointestinal tract may accomplish two things: (a) rule out disease in the stomach or intestine, and (b) in a certain number of cases, show a wide sweep of the duodenum to the right, demonstrating pressure from the pancreatic tumor.

Relationship Between Cancer of the Pancreas and Diabetes.— The interesting question naturally arises as to whether in these cases diabetes may have arisen because of the involvement of the pancreas by the carcinomatous growth. The impairment of pancreatic function both as regards internal and external secretion by the encroachment of tumor tissue certainly affords an explanation for the occurrence of diabetes far more satisfying than one is accustomed to find. Although in the present series the fact that the onset of diabetes preceded by an average of 2.6 years the onset of symptoms referable to the pancreatic tumor is against such a conclusion, it must be admitted that the duration of diabetes among the cases of cancer of the pancreas, 3.6 years, is the shortest duration among any group of diabetics under observation. The consensus of other writers on the subject is that although glycosuria is not infrequent in cases of carcinoma of the pancreas, actual diabetes seldom occurs.

Among Kiefer's 33 cases from the Peter Bent Brigham Hospital in Boston, there were only 2 patients who excreted sugar in the urine and neither of these had diabetes. Among 251 cases which he collected from the literature, 43 or about 1 in 6 had glycosuria. In the carefully studied case reported by Urmy, Jones and Wood[1] mild diabetes mellitus developed during the last one and a half years of the life of a man with proved adenocarcinoma of the pancreas in whom symptoms of pancreatitis dated back five years

[1] Urmy, Jones, and Wood: Am. Jour. Med. Sci., 182, 662, 1931.

before death. In a case of this sort, the evidence seems quite conclusive that the diabetes was due to encroachment of the tumor tissue since at autopsy it was estimated that 95 per cent of the island-bearing tissue had been destroyed. In the case cited by Grafe,[1] the diabetic condition was mild despite the fact that at autopsy the entire pancreas was involved with a carcinomatous growth and microscopic examination failed to reveal any normal pancreatic tissue. Cases with such extensive involvement are rare, however. The patient of Labbé, *et al.*[2] had a carcinoma of the body of the pancreas which had reduced the pancreatic tissue to a small nodule and almost entirely destroyed the islet tissue. This sixty-seven-year old woman had had known diabetes for two years prior to the onset of symptoms of the cancer.

Carcinoma of the pancreas probably does not cause diabetes oftener because: (1) the tumor is usually situated chiefly in the head and body of the gland, whereas most of the islet-bearing tissue is in the tail of the organ. (2) Islet tissue seems capable of repelling invasion possibly because of its independent blood supply. In 2 of our cases, 5335 and 9853, a definite note was made by the pathologist that even in tumor-filled portions of the pancreas, certain groups of islet cells could be made out despite the fact that they were entirely surrounded by malignant tissue. (3) Approximately nine-tenths of the pancreas must be destroyed or removed in order to produce diabetes. Strangely enough, if the entire pancreas is removed in man, the resulting diabetes is not severe; in the few reported cases, not more than 40 to 50 units have been required daily for control.[3]

[1] Grafe: Metabolic Diseases and Their Treatment, Philadelphia, Lea & Febiger, p. 249, 1933.

[2] Labbé, Boulin, Uhry and Antonelli: Bull. et mém. Soc. méd. d. hôp. de Paris, 52, 320, 1936.

[3] Goldner and Clark: Loc. cit., p. 139.

CHAPTER XXV.

SYPHILIS AND DIABETES.

Revised by C. Cabell Bailey, M. D.

Syphilitic infiltration of the pancreas was believed to play an etiological rôle in the production of diabetes mellitus late in the nineteenth century when diabetes was frequently looked upon as being a "parasyphilitic" disease. After the discovery of the S. pallida and of the Wassermann reaction early in the twentieth century, and the development a few years later of laboratory procedures for the determination of blood-sugar levels as well as methods for the differentiation of types of sugars excreted in the urine, many problems in the diagnosis of syphilis and of true diabetes mellitus were clarified. Excellent reviews of the relationship of diabetes and syphilis have been published by Labbé and Touflet[1] from France and by Lemann[2] in the United States. In this country syphilis has been said to infect 1 person in 42[3] and diabetes has now become the eighth chief cause of death, being responsible in 1940 for 1 in every 40 deaths.[4] Although the incidence of diabetes is steadily increasing, the incidence of syphilis has been greatly reduced.

A. CRITERIA FOR ASSUMPTION OF "SYPHILITIC DIABETES."

In 1905, Troller[5] stated four postulates that must be fulfilled before diabetes could be said to result from a syphilitic infection: (1) diabetes must appear subsequent to the syphilitic infection; (2) diabetes should appear at the same time as other syphilitic manifestations; (3) antisyphilitic treatment alone should cause disappearance of both the syphilis and the diabetes, and (4) antidiabetic treatment alone should be ineffective. Proving these postulates is difficult. As Kitchell[6] has said, symptoms of syphilis may be overlooked until the more evident symptoms of diabetes appear. Also a tentative diagnosis of syphilis is frequently made today on the sole basis of repeatedly positive serological tests in the absence of visible syphilitic manifestations. Antisyphilitic treatment alone should have no effect on diabetes not caused by syphilis whereas such treatment should soon produce improvement in "syphilitic diabetes" unless the pancreatic fibrosis has ended in permanent damage to the

---

[1] Labbé and Touflet: Ann. de med., **13**, 367, 1923.

[2] Lemann: Am. Jour. Syph., **13**, 70, 1929.

[3] Parran and Vonderlehr: Plain Words about Venereal Disease, New York, Reynal and Hitchcock, 1941.

[4] Joslin: N. E. Jour. Med., **234**, 476, 1946.

[5] Troller: Essai sur le diabète sucre syphilitique, No. 138, Paris, 1905.

[6] Kitchell: Penna. Med. Jour., **41**, 587, 1938.

islands of Langerhans. For proper appraisal of the third and fourth postulates it is obviously necessary for a patient to be on a standard diabetic regimen.

B. CASES IN THE LITERATURE.

In spite of the fact that there is no longer much concern over a possible etiological relationship between syphilis and diabetes, each year several papers appear on this subject. In most of them only a single case report is given. A review of these cases has shown that the details presented are usually insufficient, not only as regards the diagnosis of either disease, but also as concerns the treatment and eventual outcome. The few promising cases are those reported by Perkins,[1] Paullin and Bowcock,[2] Elmer and Kedzierske[3] and Kitchell.[4] At the very root of the whole problem is the proof of cure[5] and practically none of the reported cases has been followed for a sufficient length of time.

Perkins[1] studied 42 definite and 12 probable cases of syphilis occurring in diabetic patients. Three cases reported in detail showed marked improvement in carbohydrate tolerance with a normal glucose tolerance test following antisyphilitic therapy with arsenic, bismuth and iodides. In two, diabetic tolerance curves were again evident in six and seven years respectively, whereas in the third case, two mildly diabetic curves were again obtained four years after treatment followed by a normal tolerance test four years later. He states that there is no evidence that syphilis alone will produce diabetes in a previously normal individual but believes that tertiary syphilis may be a precipitating factor in individuals with a latent or hereditary defect in their insulinogenic mechanism. Williams[6] could detect no improvement in carbohydrate tolerance following antisyphilitic treatment in 17 diabetics with syphilis. Naunyn,[7] in 1906, stated that because a diabetic may improve with antisyphilitic treatment is not particularly significant, because a diabetic will improve with treatment of any complicating, coëxisting disease. With so many factors involved in this problem, extremely careful study of a case would need to be done before one could say that antisyphilitic treatment "cured" diabetes. A few of the important points usually not considered are: (1) the quick response that many patients with newly acquired diabetes make with the first antidiabetic treatment, (2) that either purposely or unwittingly diabetic treatment is often instituted simultaneously with anti-

[1] Perkins: Ann. Int. Med., **21**, 272, 1944.
[2] Paullin and Bowcock: Jour. Am. Med. Assn., **82**, 702, 1924.
[3] Elmer and Kedzierske: Ann. de méd., **24**, 332, 1928.
[4] Kitchell: Loc. cit., p. 660.
[5] Root and Marble: New England Jour. Med., **218**, 918, 1938.
[6] Williams: New York State Jour. Med., **41**, 252, 1941.
[7] Naunyn: Der Diabetes Mellitus, Vienna, Alfred Hölder, 1906.

syphilitic treatment, (3) the factor of weight reduction in the amelioration of diabetic symptoms, and (4) that cases must be followed for years before a real cure can be said to have been attained.

C. PATHOLOGY OF SYPHILIS IN DIABETES.

Syphilis, if it could produce diabetes, would be most likely to do so by its action on the pancreas, and particularly upon the islands of Langerhans. Such involvement might result from the production of generalized sclerosis through perivascular and interstitial fibrosis, and by obliterative endarteritis. Thus it would appear that diabetes would be a late manifestation of syphilis brought about by a very dense fibrosis, resulting in a permanent choking destruction of the islands of Langerhans so that regeneration of its cells could not occur, unless only temporarily.

Excluding congenital syphilis Williams[1] states that syphilitic pancreatitis was not found a single time among 4800 routine necropsies.

D. SPECIFICITY OF SEROLOGICAL TESTS.

Because of the wide fluctuations that may occur, chiefly in blood-sugar and blood-cholesterol values, in controlled and uncontrolled diabetes, the problem of falsely positive serological tests has frequently been studied; some false reactions have been reported. In diabetic acidosis, acetone bodies are also present. Richards[2] believed that the presence of diacetic and betaoxybutyric acids might influence the specificity of the Wassermann reaction, but this has never been confirmed. Van Saun[3] and Williams[4] investigated diabetic sera in relation to the cholesterol content and found no evidence of false tests. After the introduction of the precipitation serological tests there was still no evidence that false tests would appear in diabetic subjects if the test had been properly done. From this diabetic practice in 1931, Root and Stuart,[5] in a study of the effect of variations in blood sugar, blood cholesterol, of acidosis, and of albuminuria upon 1078 Wassermann, Hinton and Kahn tests, found no false reactions. Since that report several thousand new diabetic patients have been observed and still no false tests have been recognized. Richardson[6] observed that some human sera specifically fixed complement in the presence of regular commercial insulin, but in applying this observation to diabetic patients he found no correlation between the reaction and the clinical condition.

[1] Williams: Loc. cit., p. 661.
[2] Richards: Jour. Am. Med. Assn., **60**, 1139, 1913.
[3] Van Saun: Jour. Med. Res., **37**, 205, 1917.
[4] Williams: Jour. Am. Med. Assn., **70**, 365, 1918.
[5] Root and Stuart: New England Jour. Med., **204**, 1179, 1931.
[6] Richardson: Proc. Soc. Exper. Biol. and Med., **38**, 874, 1938.

E. INCIDENCE OF SYPHILIS.

In 1940 McDaniel, Marks and Joslin[1] reported a detailed study made upon 17,500 glycosuric patients seen between 1897 and 1939. From this group 15,095 fulfilled the criteria of true diabetes mellitus. Of this number, 258 cases had proven syphilis. Therefore, the incidence of syphilis in this diabetic practice was 1.7 per cent. This incidence tends to be lower than that in diabetic groups reported in the world's literature, which vary all the way from 0.16 per cent to 11.5 per cent, but this is by far the largest group on record of proven diabetics with syphilis, and most of these cases have been followed over an extended period of time.

A diagnosis of syphilis was made upon the evidence of a positive serologic test or tests, usually performed in different laboratories, supplemented often by a history of acquisition of a syphilitic infection sometimes followed by specific treatment. Rarely syphilitic lesions were observed. The routine serological test employed has generally been the Hinton test,[2] but Kahn and Wassermann tests have been done frequently. Of the 258 cases, 51.6 per cent were identified by serology alone. No cases were included where a single doubtful test was obtained or where only the initial routine test was positive and was not confirmed by history or physical signs. Some cases were included where the serological test was negative but in whom there was a history of syphilitic infection followed by various amounts of antisyphilitic therapy.

It is significant to note that the incidence of 1.7 per cent of syphilis in diabetics is less than the minimal incidence of 2.7 per cent of syphilis in the general population[3] in this area of the country.

F. GENERAL STATISTICS.

Through the coöperation of the Statistical Bureau of the Metropolitan Life Insurance Company of New York, the records of these 258 cases were studied carefully.[1]

Of this number 188 were males and 70 were females. The average age of onset of the diabetic did not vary significantly from that of ordinary diabetic patients and the incidence of obesity in the group with syphilis was similar to that found in the regular diabetic practice.

Although syphilis definitely preceded the onset of the diabetes in 41.5 per cent and probably preceded it in another 43.4 per cent it is well known that syphilis is a disease usually acquired in youth whereas diabetes usually appears in middle age or later. On the average, men had syphilis twenty-one years and the women fifteen

[1] McDaniel, Marks and Joslin: Arch. Int. Med., **66**, 1011, 1940.

[2] Hinton and Davies: Suppl. No. 9 to Venereal Disease Information, Washington, Government Printing Office, p. 172, 1939.

[3] Merritt and Moore: New England Jour. Med., **219**, 874, 1938.

years before the onset of diabetes. Thus, 86.8 per cent had reached the latent stage of syphilis at the time of the first examination.

The diabetes was considered mild in 66 per cent, moderate in 19 per cent and severe in 9 per cent. No difference in diabetic heredity was apparent, for 26.7 per cent of the diabetics with syphilis had a positive heredity history as compared with 24.5 per cent in a group of 6357 diabetics.

Only 3 cases of congenital syphilis occurred among the 258 cases of syphilis and among the 1400 cases of childhood diabetics—an incidence of 1.2 per cent.

Sixty per cent of the entire series received some antisyphilitic treatment. There was no evidence, however, that treatment produced improvement in carbohydrate tolerance, although one case for some months did show some improvement. Such temporary improvement is not uncommonly seen among diabetics without apparent cause. In some, the diabetes became steadily more severe in spite of antisyphilitic treatment.

The cause of death in 130 diabetics with syphilis was compared with that of 4474 diabetics and no significant difference was detected in the two groups.

G. DOES SYPHILIS CAUSE DIABETES?

The careful study of 258 cases reported by McDaniel, Marks and Joslin[1] failed to show any etiological relationship between syphilis and diabetes. The history and mode of onset of the diabetes and the progression of the diabetes in diabetic patients with syphilis were just the same as for any patient with diabetes. They were unable to recognize any characteristics of such a clinical condition as "syphilitic diabetes." Clinicians of such experience as Labbé and Touflet,[2] Lemann,[3] Naunyn,[4] Moore,[5] Bertram,[6] von Noorden,[7] and Rosenbloom[8] have seen no definite cure of diabetes by antisyphilitic therapy. Stokes, Beerman and Ingraham[9] state that diabetes due to syphilis, if it exists at all, must be a rarity.

[1] McDaniel, Marks and Joslin: Loc. cit., p. 663.
[2] Labbé and Touflet: Loc. cit., p. 660.
[3] Lemann: Loc. cit., p. 660.
[4] Naunyn: Loc. cit., p. 661.
[5] Moore: The Modern Treatment of Syphilis, Springfield, Charles C Thomas, 1933.
[6] Betram: P. 32, loc. cit., p. 87.
[7] von Noorden and Isaac: Die Zuckerkrankheit und ihre Behandlung, 8th ed., Berlin, Julius Springer, p. 350, 1927.
[8] Rosenbloom: Am. Jour. Syph., 5, 634, 1921.
[9] Stokes, Beerman and Ingraham: Modern Clinical Syphilology, 3rd ed., Philadelphia, W. B. Saunders Co., 1944.

CHAPTER XXVI.

SURGERY AND DIABETES.

REVISED BY HOWARD F. ROOT, M.D.

A. NATURE AND INCIDENCE OF SURGERY IN DIABETES.

THE discovery of insulin inaugurated the modern surgical era in diabetes and the introduction of treatment with the sulfonamides and finally with penicillin, has vastly improved the prognosis for the surgical diabetic. Operative surgery and modern diabetic treatment have so prolonged the lives of patients with the dreaded infectious and gangrenous lesions of the feet that the duration of life after recovery from such operations has made the total duration of life after onset of diabetes almost equal to the average for that diabetic age. Substitution of the transmetatarsal for higher amputations is a significant advance (see page 700). Surgical cases in the wards do so well that when the urine has become sugar-free and the blood sugar normal, sometimes one has to be watchful lest, with improvement in the diabetic condition, insulin be taken unnecessarily.

Diabetic surgery foreshadows the preventive surgery of the future. An infection makes a diabetic worse, but it is the surgical procedure which removes the infected teeth and tonsils, appendix, gall-bladder or kidney, and brings to an end infections of the feet. An increased metabolism transforms a mild diabetic into a severe one, but the surgeon relieves the hyperthyroidism by removal of the thyroid and transforms the diabetic into his original and usually benign state. We hear much of preventive medicine; we should hear more of preventive surgery.

The frequency of surgery among diabetics is steadily increasing. In the year 1923 at the Deaconess Hospital there were 69 operations on diabetic patients. From January 1, 1923 until January 1, 1946 a total of 5004 operations (excluding dental surgery) were performed. An equal number of patients had operations elsewhere or possessed ailments requiring surgical treatment in the future. Every other diabetic will need surgical treatment before he dies, and its success will be measurably affected by the degree of diabetic control attained during the preceding years.

B. AGES OF SURGICAL DIABETICS.

Surgical diabetics fall into three age groups. About one-fifth (927) were under forty years of age, two-fifths (1980) were between forty and sixty years of age, and those in the remaining group (2097) were over sixty years of age. The youngest group is growing,

(665)

first, because these patients now live so much longer and, second, because improved medical methods make operations of election safe. The oldest surgical group should decrease because preventive measures are converting what formerly was major surgery into minor surgery or no surgery at all. In this fashion the doctors' better medical tillage of the diabetic soil is opening up for the surgeons more fertile surgical fields.

C. PROGNOSIS OF THE SURGICAL DIABETIC.

The prognosis for the surgical diabetic has steadily improved. The mortality for our surgical cases at the Deaconess Hospital for 1923 to August 1, 1926 was 11.5 per cent. The total operative mortality was 7.3 per cent for 3551 operations from 1923 to December 31, 1941. In 1939 the total mortality in 264 operations was 6.4 per cent, the lowest mortality for any period up to 1940. The surgical mortality for 1942 to January 1, 1946 reached a new low of 2.2 per cent.

In Naunyn's time few deaths were due to surgical diseases, probably because patients did not live long enough to acquire such. Among his autopsies only 12 per cent were diagnosed as such, in contrast to 71 per cent for the autopsies at the Deaconess as reported by Root and Warren.[1]

An important factor in determining the prognosis for the surgical diabetic is the presence or absence of diabetic treatment during the months that precede the development of surgical conditions. It is disastrous to develop a surgical disease if you have diabetes and do not know it or, knowing you are a diabetic, have been negligent.

The surgical diabetic requires more, far more, attention than the medical diabetic because his condition is more critical. Fairness to the surgeon and to the patient demands that he be treated in the medical wards where he can obtain the detailed and intimate treatment which the severest medical diabetics receive. A surgeon unfamiliar with insulin should not undertake alone the care of a diabetic. Cases of diabetes in coma are visited by a physician every hour; surgical cases need almost as much medical care. For this reason it is essential that surgical cases be grouped with medical cases. Border-line wards for medical and surgical diabetics should exist in every hospital. Seldom is the surgeon to blame for the surgical mortality. As a rule, the responsibility is medical and is more often remote than immediate in that preventive measures have not been instilled early enough into the minds of the patients.

Concentration of the surgical treatment in the hands of a single team is wise. "Better a youngster who has had special experience with the care of diabetics than the senior surgeon who includes diabetes with a hundred other interests."[2]

[1] Root and Warren: Boston Med. and Surg. Jour., **196**, 864, 1927.
[2] Churchill: Personal communication.

TABLE 87.—5004 DIABETIC OPERATIONS (JANUARY 1, 1923 TO JANUARY 1, 1946) NEW ENGLAND DEACONESS HOSPITAL.

	1923-1941. Age at operation.				1942-1946.
	0-39.	40-60.	60-89.	Total.	
Amputations, major	4	210	519	733	269
Amputations, fingers, toes	10	194	246	450	322
Carbuncles	6	65	45	116	18
Ulcers, abscesses	142	176	113	431	108
Thyroid	39	145	59	243	66
Tonsillectomy	137	43	6	186	48
Laparotomy	111	203	114	428	132
Genito-urinary	24	50	77	151	46
Pelvi-rectal	38	125	71	234	56
Ocular	27	53	68	148	49
Miscellaneous	113	176	142	431	339
Total	651	1440	1460	3551	1453
No. fatal	16	97	147	260	32
Per cent fatal	2.5	6.7	10.1	7.3	2.2

D. VARIETY OF OPERATIONS.

The striking change in the mortality for surgical operations in the period prior to 1942 as contrasted with the four years from January 1, 1942 to January 1, 1946 is brought out in Table 87. The general mortality has fallen from 7.3 per cent to 2.2 per cent, an improvement brought about by many factors of which the use of sulfonamides and of penicillin undoubtedly is one of the most important. Pulmonary embolism caused 6 deaths. The variety of operations has been altered chiefly by the inclusion among the major amputations of 56 transmetatarsal amputations through the foot with a single death. (See page 701.) Major amputations (1002) and of toes (772) constituted more than one-third (1774) of the 5004 operations upon our diabetics at the Deaconess Hospital up to January 1, 1946.

Next in frequency were superficial and deep septic processes (673) caused by infections gaining entrance through the skin, such as abscesses and ulcers (539) and carbuncles (134). These 2 groups, amputations and infections through the skin, made up nearly one-half of the total operations. Fortunately, the amputations and the infections are largely preventable, and, therefore, it becomes the duty of all medical men to warn their diabetic patients of the dangers to which they are exposed. The mortality from this lamentable, but compulsory, diabetic surgery constitutes one-half of the total surgical mortality.

Non-preventable surgical conditions and reparative surgery are responsible for the other half of the surgical cases, with cancer in various sites taking a leading position. Operations upon the thyroid gland (309) resulted in 6 deaths, but there were no deaths in 66 operations from 1942 to 1946. Tonsillectomies (234) were without a single fatality or even a significant hemorrhage. Diseases of the genito-urinary tract (197) are frequently associated with diabetes as

serious complications. The causes for operation range from nephrectomies for calculi and pyonephrosis to the removal of the prostate. (See Chapter XIX.)

Laparotomies (660) of a varied nature were undertaken with a
mortality of 13 per cent, a figure largely explained by the cause for
the operation. The remaining surgical procedures consisted of those
about the pelvis and rectum (290). Operations upon the eye (199)
consisted of removal of cataracts, of relief of glaucoma and excision
of the entire eye. Finally a group (770) of most miscellaneous
character included operations upon the mastoid, antra, the breast,
bones, etc. Case 17470, age fifteen years, is included in this group
for she recovered without complications when Dr. Betts repaired a
large diaphragmatic hernia and restored a portion of the stomach and
the intestinal tract to their proper abdominal position.

Dental extractions have not been classed as surgical operations.
The extractions in many instances were extensive and had they not
been performed with unusual dexterity, judgment and proper
medical supervision, they might easily have entailed disastrous
results, as happened years ago. No fatalities occurred following
removal of teeth or tonsils. Dental surgery is so common that we
do not appreciate its perfection. Probably there have been 5000
patients who have undergone extractions between 1925 and January
1, 1946. The delicate care required for surgical wounds in the
mouth was well described by Kent.[1]

E. DEATHS IN DIABETIC SURGERY.

In the present series (see Table 88) less than one-half the deaths
were due to gangrene and sepsis (59) plus gangrene with coronary
occlusion (13). Actually since January 1, 1942 in 269 major amputations only 10 deaths have occurred, or 3.7 per cent. In retrospect
it may be said that a few years ago our hope for a better future for
medical diabetics lay in the fact that most of the deaths were then
due to coma and coma was considered preventable. That hope has
been fulfilled. So now it is with surgery and septicemia. Deaths
from staphylococcus and streptococcus septicemia have ceased,
thanks to penicillin.

Reports of a lowered surgical diabetic mortality continue.
Palmer, Mangham and Booth[2] report 100 cases of gangrene and
infection of extremities in 1387 adult diabetics over a fifteen year
period. The surgical mortality for major amputation was 30.6
per cent and for minor amputation 14.6 per cent. They urge pre-
ventative measures, prompt and early treatment of minor lesions as
a means of lowering the mortality.

[1] Kent: The Apolloman, October, 1937.
[2] Palmer, Mangham and Booth: Northwest Med., 43, 74, 1944.

TABLE 88.—CAUSES OF DEATH OF SURGICAL DIABETICS—162 DEATHS.
(JANUARY 1, 1931 TO JANUARY 1, 1946.)

Gangrene and sepsis	59
Cancer	29
Gangrene and coronary occlusion	13
Carbuncle	7
Coronary occlusion	3
Kidney infections	7
Gall-bladder, perforation	5
Postoperative shock	2
Prostate	2
Pelvic phlebitis and thrombosis	1
Appendicitis and peritonitis	4
Septicemia·	
(1) Cellulitis of scalp	1
(2) Periostitis	1
(3) Gas bacillus, source unknown	1
(4) Friedländer's Bacillus, liver abscess	1
(5) Osteomyelitis	2
Pneumonia	3
Peritonitis, ruptured ovarian cyst	2
Intestinal obstruction	3
Strangulated hernia	1
Perforated duodenal ulcer	1
Mastoiditis	1
Pulmonary edema	1
Abscess of lung and empyema	2
Embolus, pulmonary	4
Diverticulitis	1
Splanchnicectomy	2
Brain tumor	2
Fractured hip	1
Total	162

Wilder[1] stated that at the Mayo Clinic the operative mortality has increased from 3.3 per cent between 1921 and 1932 to 7.5 per cent in 1937 and 6.2 per cent in 1938, but that the difference was due to the increasing proportion of operations for carcinoma and the advancing age of the patients.

Sprague and Wilder[2] give the operative mortality for 2607 operations upon diabetics at the Mayo Clinic in the years 1930 to 1939 as 4.3 per cent. Macey and Bickel[3] report a mortality of 11.4 per cent for 66 major amputations on 61 patients.

The elements which hinder or promote success in diabetic surgery can be easily summarized. Of the former, acidosis and a liability to infection are now largely eliminated. Coma has become only an accident. Old time surgery courted it (1) by the administration of chloroform and ether, only too frequently by untrained hands; (2) by the sudden restriction of carbohydrate prior to the operation with the desire to lower the glycosuria; (3) by the attempt to relieve the patient's hunger thus caused with an excess of protein and fat,

[1] Wilder, p. 210: Loc. cit., p. 55.
[2] Sprague and Wilder: Christopher, Textbook of Surgery, 3d ed., Philadelphia, W. B. Saunders Co., 1685, 1942.
[3] Macey and Bickel: Surg., Gynec. and Obst., **74**, 821, 1942.

wholly unmindful that in so doing acidosis was favored; (4) by the large doses of sodium bicarbonate which upset the digestion, making it still more difficult for the postoperative patient to take liquids or food freely, besides possibly releasing latent acid bodies whose excretion would irritate the kidneys.   Coma can be avoided by the administration of a diet of 100 grams or more of carbohydrate with the simultaneous use in three- to eight-hour intervals of insulin sufficient to enable the patient to utilize it.   Invariably in the twenty-four hours subsequent to operation the patient receives 150 grams carbohydrate by mouth, subcutaneously or intravenously.

The danger of a clean wound in a diabetic becoming infected is slight if the diabetes is properly controlled.   Given an infection, it is freely granted that the disease becomes worse; prevent the infection, and healing is prompt.   In so close a relation do both stand to each other that a loss of tolerance for carbohydrate may be recorded on the diabetic chart before the wound discloses a retrograde course. The presence of an excess of sugar in the blood may not be so serious as acidosis, but neither is desirable.   The skin, upon analysis, appears to be overloaded with sugar, but patients so often recover when large quantities of sugar are present in the blood that it is difficult to believe that hyperglycemia of itself is much of a factor predisposing to infection.   It is the infection which makes the diabetic worse and so favors hyperglycemia and acidosis.   Control this infection and then diabetes and the course of the patient become smooth.

The third handicap, old age with attendant arteriosclerosis and consequent slow healing of old tissues, is still a real obstacle to recovery.   Indeed, the age of the diabetic is largely accountable for the poor reputation he has acquired at the surgeon's hands. Gangrene, carbuncles and gall stones, the common diabetic surgical ailments, are conditions which attack the elderly.   The slow healing of diabetic wounds can hardly be attributed to vitamin C deficiency. The blood values are normal in almost all diabetic patients, although occasionally in patients in public wards values at the lower level are found.   The prevalence of damaged hearts, arteries and kidneys among the diabetics is to be blamed for the serious prognosis equally with the diabetes.   We almost dread to tell our surgical confrères that coronary disease exists in essentially all the patients with gall stones or gangrene for whom we beg their aid.

The presence of gall stones may result in serious damage to liver function.   This entails a hazard not only for operation upon the gall-bladder, but even for operation at a distance from the gall-bladder.   Coller and Jackson[1] regard as diagnostic of this damage to liver function the presence of hypoglycemia which was observed in 1 of their 3 cases when he was unconscious.

Case 10142 developed a critical "liver storm" after a simple

[1] Coller and Jackson: Jour. Am. Med. Assn., **112**, 128, 1939.

cholecystectomy. The explanation seemed clear when chemical analyses of an excised portion of liver showed at the end of the operation almost no glycogen present and a great increase in fatty acid.

The importance of the liver is demonstrated by the occasional cases in which with certain lesions of the liver the severity of the diabetes diminishes to a point where it may almost be said to have disappeared. Thus, Case 10861 was taking 12 units of insulin before operation. Because of jaundice due to a carcinoma at the head of the pancreas, cholecystgastrostomy was performed. During the next eight days she had continuous intravenous administration of glucose solution sometimes reaching 400 grams of glucose a day. Even with this large intake, the amount of glucose excreted in the urine varied from as little as 34 grams a day to a maximum of 95 grams on one day. Thus, with a daily dose of insulin varying from 15 to 30 units she utilized between 307 and 360 grams of glucose when given by vein. When she left the hospital she was taking 200 grams of carbohydrate a day without any insulin. At autopsy a few months later she had many metastases in the liver. A somewhat similar case is described by Unterhuber[1] whose patient had a carcinoma of the liver. The diabetes had been longstanding, but had almost disappeared as metastases developed in the liver and insulin was discontinued. The primary tumor was not discovered because of a limited autopsy. Leriche and Jung[2] reported a young woman whose insulin was omitted for some months during external biliary drainage. (See page 710.)

In diabetic patients the occurrence of shock, whether as a result of surgical operation or severe medical disease such as coronary occlusion, often provokes a great increase in the blood sugar, glycosuria, and a fall in the CO_2 of the blood. These effects are more readily understood in the light of the experimental studies of carbohydrate metabolism in traumatic shock carried out by Haist and collaborators,[3,4] as well as by other students. In shock caused in animals by anoxia of the extremities produced by tourniquets, the changes produced are in the glycogen stores, in the muscle, in the liver, and a marked change in the tolerance for administered glucose. Thus a rise of the blood sugar to 400 milligrams was observed in the shock animals who received glucose two hours after the shock was established. The liver failed to store glycogen in a normal fashion. Insulin lowers the blood sugar in those animals, but does not increase muscle or liver glycogen. Since, in most of the animals, if the tourniquet is reapplied to the leg, the changes are reversed, it seems evident that change produced in the animal tissues is due in some way to changes occurring in the damaged and anoxic tissues of the animals.

[1] Unterhuber: Wien. klin. Wchnschr., **52**, 815, 1939.
[2] Leriche and Jung: Ann. d'End., **1**, 3, 1939.
[3] Haist and Hamilton: Jour. Phys., **102**, 471, 1944.
[4] Haist: New York Diabetes Association, 1946.

The diabetic with a gangrenous toe needs exercise to help burn up his sugar. Therefore, teach him a set of movements to perform whenever the clock strikes the hour. Show him how to protect his lungs by long breaths and by turning over in bed. In short, keep him busy getting well. A masseur may be of great help to an elderly diabetic, especially if he combines massage with resistant motions, but self-massage is cheaper. Too often the pathetically low level to which these poor old men and women have been reduced is forgotten, simply because the laboratory reports a positive diacetic acid reaction or a trace of sugar in the urine. Be careful! Do not treat the laboratory test instead of the patient!

The factors which favor surgical success in diabetes are first of all an early diagnosis and an early decision to operate. The principle must be recognized that the surgical necessity determines the day (or night) and hour of operation. Today medical treatment is labile and can be adapted to the condition in hand, and the convalescence from the surgical complication utilized to free the patient from sugar and acidosis. The patient should be treated for the operation rather than for the diabetes. Get him successfully through the operation first, and then, if you like, treat him for the diabetes the rest of his life. Obviously for patients whose ailments are not urgent one would secure a sugar-free urine and a normal blood sugar before operation. Yet even in these cases if they are arteriosclerotic and of long duration one must be cautious not to lower the blood sugar rapidly or as low as in the younger diabetics.

The *second factor* which favors success in diabetic surgery is the *adjustment of the diet to the surgical requirements*. If there is no need for haste, any of the well-recognized systems recommended to get the patient free from sugar and acidosis will suffice. It is a great advantage to store carbohydrate in the body and particularly to fill the liver with glycogen before an operation. The storage of glycogen in the liver under the influence of diet and insulin makes the severest diabetic temporarily mild. Therefore, feed the patient up to within twelve hours before the operation begins, and never fast a patient before a surgical operation. As a corollary to the above advice, begin the administration of food as soon as possible after operating.

F. DIET IN DIABETIC SURGERY.

Malnutrition in diabetic surgical patients has long been recognized, but it is only within the last few years, particularly since the use of insulin, that a variety of methods for improving nutrition have been available for treatment of seriously ill patients. Long periods of uncontrolled diabetes, not merely produce loss of weight, dehydration and frequently acidosis, but during these periods there may have been significant loss in protein and base and disturbance in vitamin metabolism. In addition to the diabetes itself, other factors, such as achlorhydria, diarrhea, the symptoms associated with the surgical complication itself, such as pain and nausea, may have resulted in the arrival of the diabetic patient at the hospital in a partial or moderate state of starvation. Hypo-proteinemia with its harmful effects upon wound healing and sub-clinical vitamin deficiency more and more concern the surgeon, especially in gastro-intestinal surgery.

Vitamins.—The use of vitamins for a few days prior to operation is often indicated in diabetic patients, whose diabetes has long been uncontrolled, who show dehydration, emaciation, anemia, dry skin, and suggestive lesions such as cheilosis. When the clinical symptoms are definite, such treatment must necessarily be continued after operation. If the patient is unable to retain or absorb food, he should receive vitamins parenterally in such daily doses as 10 milli-grams of thiamin, 100 milligrams of ascorbic acid, 5 milligrams of riboflavin and 100 milligrams of niacin. Liver extract may be given by injection. Doses of vitamins commonly employed pro-phylactically are: Vitamin A 10,000 units, thiamin 10 milligrams, riboflavin 5 milligrams, nicotinamide 50 milligrams, vitamin K 2 milligrams.

Protein.—One of the most serious dietary deficiencies in surgical patients is deficiency of protein. Protein provides the necessary amino acids from which damaged tissue may be repaired as well as the amino acids necessary for the formation of hormones, anti-bodies, and enzymes. Protein is important also both in carbo-hydrate and fat metabolism. The usual measurement of protein stored in the body in the sick patient is the serum protein level. This measurement is open to difficulties in interpretations since in an acute phase such as bad burns or hemorrhage, or intestinal obstruction, it does not give an accurate picture of the stores of protein. In chronic disease a low serum level may indicate the loss of less important proteins in order to maintain more vital organs. There can be no doubt that a low level of protein in the blood interferes with proper healing, as has been shown experimentally and clinically. The low level of serum protein affects the osmotic pressure of the blood and causes edema. Actually a considerable degree of edema may exist before it is evident. Edema is not usually apparent until the weight of the affected part is increased by fully 10 per cent.

The treatment of hypoproteinemia in acute emergencies, such as caused by severe burns, intestinal obstruction, etc., usually requires prompt administration of blood plasma. Chronic protein deficiency is usually considered a dietetic problem, but frequently the possi-bilities of administering sufficient proteins to control a severe deficiency are remote. Elman, quoted by Ravdin and Zintel,[1]

[1] Ravdin and Zintel: Wohl's Dietotherapy, Philadelphia, W. B. Saunders Co., 875, 1945.

43

points out that if a patient weighing 60 kilograms, and therefore with 3000 cc. of plasma, requires a restoration of 2 grams per cent in his serum albumin, that is, from an observed value of 2.6 grams to the normal of 4.6 grams, he will need 60 grams serum albumin and thirty times that amount to restore the deficiencies of the rest of the body. If only one-half the ingested protein is retained, the amount required becomes 3600 grams. Add 25 grams protein for daily endogenous needs and the total required for a ten-day period is 3850 grams, or the equivalent of 385 grams of protein per day. The difficulty in administering so much protein is well illustrated in Case 27821, age fifty-seven years, who entered the Deaconess Hospital on July 19, 1945 with a large appendix abscess, which was operated on by Dr. C. C. Lund. Diabetes of seven years' duration had never been treated with insulin or diet and the urine contained 6.0 per cent sugar and 4 plus diacetic acid during the first week or ten days of her stay. A mixed infection of the abdominal wall with streptococcus and hemolytic staphylococcus aureus resulted in sloughing the entire abdominal skin and subcutaneous tissue from the pubes to the ensiform and from flank to flank. A continuous loss of protein from this area occurred during the period from late July until September. The patient was a large woman, her usual weight being 200 pounds. The plasma protein value varied from 3.8 to 4.8 grams per cent. In addition to repeated transfusions she received on certain days, 4000 cc. of 5 per cent amigen solution in glucose during the period when she could take nothing by mouth. About September 10 the infection having been controlled, her appetite returned and she was given protein by mouth in amounts planned to provide 250 grams consisting of steaks and other forms of meat, cheese, eggs, milk and aminoids. Actually her protein intake by mouth during this period exceeded 200 grams in a day on only four days. However, she took from 175 to 200 grams of protein on thirteen days. She was finally discharged on October 20, having made a complete recovery. The best proteins for restoring protein deficiency are meat, milk, eggs, wheat, and soy beans. A recipe first suggested by Stare and Thorn[1] provides a tomato soup which was used with this patient, and in other patients where concentrated protein and vitamins are desired.

High protein tomato soup.	Carbohydrate.	Protein.	Fat.	
Butter, 35 grams	0	0	28	
Casein, 15 grams	0	13	0	
Wheat germ, 15 grams	7	6	0	
Soy bean flour, 10 grams	5	5	2	
Milk, 240 cc.	12	8	10	
Tomato purée, 2 tablesp.	3	2	0	
Salt to flavor	—	—	—	
Total	27	34	40	Cal.—604

Melt butter in top of double boiler. Stir in casein, wheat germ, soy bean flour. Mix in tomato purée and bouillon (other flavorings for variety). Add milk gradually, cook ten minutes.

[1] Stare and Thorn: Jour. Am. Med. Assn., **127**, 1120, 1945.

Salt and Water Balance.—Water balance for the maintenance of the body fluid level is of utmost importance in surgical patients and is particularly easily upset in the diabetic. In diabetics who had diabetic acidosis or coma, the possibility of the most extreme dehydration exists. However, without actual acidosis, the polyuria of uncontrolled diabetes may produce more than a slight degree of dehydration and also a disturbance in the salt metabolism. Normal water intake by mouth varies from 800 to 3000 cc. a day. The food of the ordinary diet yields from 1000 to 1500 cc. of water and the oxidation of foodstuffs in the body tissues adds from 200 to 400 cc. The oxidation of one gram of carbohydrate or one gram of protein provides about 0.5 cc. of water and the oxidation of one gram of fat produces 1.0 cc. of water. The loss of water by insensible perspiration and vaporization amounts to between 1000 and 1500 cc. daily. When diabetic patients were compared with hyperthyroid patients by Benedict and Root[1] at the Deaconess Hospital, the amount of insensible perspiration was found to vary from an extremely low value, or 15 grams per hour, in a child with dehydration and acidosis to 100 grams per hour in a patient with hyperthyroidism. Water is lost through the lungs and skin easily. The kidneys, however, produce water largely in relation to the amount of water available. Normally, the kidneys excrete 35 grams of dissolved solid matter in twenty-four hours, and with a normal person the minimum of the amount of water to excrete this waste material is 473 cc. according to Lashmet and Newburgh.[2] With diseased kidneys, the amount of water required to excrete this amount of waste matter varies with the concentrating power of the kidney and may rise to a level of 1439 cc. when the specific gravity of the urine varies between 1.010 and 1.014. Under ordinary circumstances, therefore, the normal intake of water should vary from 2000 to 3000 cc. in twenty-four hours, and the surgical patient with normal kidneys should have at least 2000 and preferably 3000 cc. of fluid daily. If renal function is impaired, then alterations in this amount may be necessary. Actually, Ravdin[3] calculated that in seriously ill patients with drainage, the following figures would apply: For vaporization, 2000 cc.; for urine, 1500 cc.; bile drainage, 1000 cc.; Wangensteen drainage, 3000 cc.; total 7500 cc. fluid required. Actually, in diabetic patients, 7000 cc. of fluid is not an excessive amount to give provided acidosis has produced severe dehydration. In Case 24537, age seventy-five years, who entered the Deaconess Hospital with complete gastric obstruction due to a carcinoma of the pancreas which had obstructed the fourth portion of the duodenum, the plasma protein was 4.7 per cent, and plasma chloride was 76 m. eq. per liter. She required aspiration of the stomach twice daily for four days before all food remains could be

[1] Benedict and Root: Arch. Int. Med., **38**, 1, 1926.
[2] Lashmet and Newburgh: Jour. Clin. Invest., **11**, 1003, 1932.
[3] Ravdin and Zintel: P. 884, loc. cit., p. 673.

obtained. Auricular fibrillation was present. The patient received 1000 cc. of 5 per cent amigen solution in glucose and 1000 cc. of 5 per cent glucose in salt solution daily but on alternate days a third 1000 cc. of 5 per cent amigen in glucose was given. Plasma protein and plasma chloride did not, however, attain a normal value until ten days after a duodeno-jejunostomy was performed successfully. In her case also the high protein tomato soup proved acceptable in the diet.

When salt intake is greatly reduced or when there has been a great loss of salt by vomiting, then the kidneys conserve salt and the concentration of salt in the urine is greatly reduced. Thus, in diabetic coma when there has been a great loss of salt by vomiting or in the urine preceding coma, it will be found that the gastric content contains no free hydrochloric acid and the chloride content of the urine is low. When chloride is lost as in vomiting, the kidneys retain this element and excrete sodium. When basic elements are lost as in diarrhea, sodium is retained and the chloride is excreted. In surgical cases water and salt must be kept constantly in mind. In patients with high fever or hyperthyroidism additional amounts of fluid are lost steadily. Losses of fluid when continuous gastric drainage are carried out may be considerable. Dehydration may be evident clinically by the pinched expression, dry skin and tongue, increased thirst and low urinary output. Coller and Maddock[1] consider that when these findings are present dehydration is equivalent to at least 6 per cent of the body weight and the patient, therefore, should be given fluid equivalent to this amount in addition to the normal daily requirement. However, it must be pointed out that in elderly patients with cardiac complications caution should be observed. Actually in diabetic patients dehydration may often be much more severe, and following diabetic coma we have not infrequently given in the course of twenty-four hours 10, or even up to 15, per cent of a patient's body weight without the production of edema.

When hypochloremia is present, dullness, lethargy, muscular twitching, acidosis or alkalosis are commonly observed. Every patient about to be operated upon for a serious abdominal condition should have a determination of the plasma chloride. The amount of sodium chloride required to raise the serum chloride one milliequivalent per liter is 13.3 milligrams of sodium chloride per pound of body weight.

Excessive administration of saline solution leading to edema must also be warned against. Coller, Campbell, Vaughan, Iob and Moyer[2] emphasized the relatively high incidence of "salt intolerance" following a general anesthesia, and decry the use of isotonic salt solution or Ringer's solution during the day of operation

[1] Coller and Maddock: Surg. Gynec. and Obst , **70**, 340, 1940.
[2] Coller, Campbell, Vaughan, Iob and Moyer: Ann. Surg., **119**, 533, 1944.

especially in patients who are anemic, acidotic, or oliguric, or have low protein values in the blood.

The forcible introduction of *liquids* into the patient after operation is a familiar sight in any hospital, but it is wiser to supply him liberally with liquids the day before. These should include broths on account of the salts therein contained, coffee, tea, water, and if necessary, salt solution or tap water by rectum. It is a safe, routine procedure to inject salt solution subcutaneously before the patient leaves the operating table. Especially is this desirable if ether is used, because ether diminishes the excretion of urine, nitrogen and glucose, and what is still more important diminishes the excretion of acetone bodies. There are few diabetics who do not need an intravenous or subcutaneous injection of salt solution at the time of an operation.

The administration of glucose intravenously or subcutaneously to diabetic patients is often of great value, particularly under the following circumstances: (1) When prolonged undernutrition is present; (2) when slight acidosis has been present; (3) when there is dehydration; (4) when there is a supply of circulating insulin to insure either the utilization of glucose or its storage as glycogen. In a few diabetics studied at the Deaconess Hospital the intravenous administration of 50 grams of glucose in salt solution was not followed by a rise in the respiratory quotient or in the metabolism and yet, although the blood sugar rose, there was no loss of glucose in the urine. Similar results have been obtained in Case 17162, a patient with extraordinarily severe diabetes who, at one time, required 1500 units of insulin a day and later, after a period of six months, was in good equilibrium with only 100 units of insulin a day. The failure of the respiratory quotient to rise after the giving of glucose may be explained on the assumption that in those cases the action of insulin was to promote glycogen formation, rather than to increase carbohydrate combustion. In normal subjects Pijoan and Gibson[1] found that when 25 grams of glucose were given intravenously, within forty-five minutes most of the glucose had been removed from the blood stream. In their normal case the respiratory quotient rose from 0.77 to 0.81.

Of what shall the *diet for surgical diabetic patients before and after operation* consist? If the case is one which is to be prepared leisurely for operation, no special change need be made in the regular program to free the urine from sugar and acid, save that the food should be prepared in simpler form. Coarse diabetic foods should be omitted. If the situation is acute, and but a day or a few hours are available, sudden restriction of carbohydrate, particularly when dealing with severe diabetics or elderly patients, must be avoided, and great care taken not to upset the stomach. The simplest foods are, therefore, the best. Except when the nature of

[1] Pijoan and Gibson: Am. Jour. Physiol., 121, 534, 1938.

the operation requires special dietary regulations, liquids, such as oatmeal gruel made with water, hot tea or coffee (with crackers or toast) are given freely, and ginger ale and orange juice with egg white are given sparingly on the day after operation. On the second postoperative day milk and, if the patient desires, cooked cereals, junket or boiled custard are added to the diet. Thereafter the diet is increased according to the patient's tolerance and desires. If possible, 100 to 150 grams of carbohydrate are given daily, any amount not taken by mouth being supplied by parenteral adminis- tration in the form of 5 per cent dextrose by vein or 2.5 per cent dextrose in physiological solution of sodium chloride under the skin. Occasionally as much as 300 grams of carbohydrate may be given in cases of severe damage to the liver. Eventually a diet approxi- mating 160 grams of carbohydrate, 75 grams of protein and 90 grams of fat will be attained. This represents the average diet on discharge of 10 patients after amputation of a leg for gangrene noted by McKittrick and Root.[1]

If the food is not forced during convalescence, and if calories are kept at 20 to 25 per kilogram body weight, most any middle-aged adult diabetic will become sugar-free before he recovers from his surgical lesions. In fact, a surgical operation is ofttimes a blessing rather than a curse.

The *diet after operation* should certainly contain as a minimum between 0.66 and 1.25 gram of protein per kilogram body weight.

When dealing with infections, an over-vigorous attempt should not be made to get the patient sugar-free either before or after operation. With surgical treatment to remove or drain the infection, the tolerance for carbohydrate will improve. It is painful to look over the proto- cols of cases suffering from infections in years gone by, who were terribly undernourished with the purpose to make them sugar-free.

The advantage of a routine blood-sugar determination in prepa- ration of a diabetic patient for surgery is illustrated by one case in the excellent summary of 80 diabetic operations by Rabinovitz and Weisman.[2] A woman aged sixty years was admitted with renal sepsis. The urine was negative for sugar and after operation she developed diabetic acidosis. The diabetic condition was not known before operation due to renal insufficiency, which caused an absence of glycosuria with a high blood sugar.

If acidosis exists either before or after operation a vigorous attack upon it already will have been made by the inauguration of the diet above outlined and the use of insulin about to be described.

G. INSULIN IN DIABETIC SURGERY.

An early position on the surgeon's operating list is desirable in order to avoid hypoglycemia from the continuing action of protamine

---

[1] McKittrick and Root: Arch. Surg., **40**, 1057, 1940.
[2] Rabinovitz and Weisman: New England Jour. Med., **219**, 423, 1938.

insulin. If insulin has been used regularly by the patient, give the same total number of units in twenty-four hours, at the time of operation, but divide into smaller and more frequent doses, irrespective of meals. On the morning of operation approximately one-half the usual dose of protamine zinc insulin is given and supplementary doses of crystalline insulin are given after operation. If insulin has not been employed, give it when two successive specimens contain sugar and omit it when two successive specimens are sugar-free. Avoid worry by giving small doses every three or four hours, more rarely two or eight hours, rather than larger doses infrequently, until acquainted with the tolerance of the patient. During convalescence when the urine is sugar-free, often test the need for insulin by omitting or reducing a single dose, usually the noon dose first, then the evening dose. It is as important to have a blood-sugar test in the late forenoon as before breakfast for a guide to insulin administration.

Although many older surgical diabetics are relatively insensitive to insulin, the danger of reactions must not be forgotten especially if no food is taken and glucose solution is given by vein. Under these circumstances the total calories may be low and the effect of a moderate dose of insulin excessive.

Alterations in the metabolic rate, produced by artificial fever and sodium dinitrophenol, shortened the period of insulin activity but caused little change in the actual degree of depression of the blood sugar, according to Hayward and Duncan.[1] Other factors besides the fever and increased metabolism are necessary to produce the resistance found in diabetic patients with infection.

Allergy to insulin is sometimes associated with acute infection. The occurrence of generalized urticarial reactions following the administration of insulin in diabetic patients with insulin resistance has occasionally been observed in patients who, having once taken insulin and then stopped it for a considerable period, subsequently were forced to resume taking it. Case 11934, housewife, aged forty-four years at onset of diabetes in January 1933, first received insulin in June 1933. She gave it up subsequently and took no insulin until about July 20, 1943 when she developed an infection on one toe. Insulin was required because of glycosuria and rapidly extending infection. Generalized urticarial reactions occurred with three different types of insulin and she entered the Deaconess Hospital with gangrene of the foot, fever and acidosis in spite of the fact that she had received 120 units of insulin the day before. She required 250 units of insulin a day to control the acidosis in spite of the severe urticaria. Almost immediately following the amputation of the infected leg diacetic acid disappeared from the urine and the urticarial reactions ceased. A rapid reduction in insulin dose occurred so that she left the hospital with a

---

[1] Hayward and Duncan: Am. Jour. Med. Sci., **198**, 396, 1939.

normal blood sugar requiring only 16 units of protamine zinc insulin daily. Through the courtesy of Dr. Jacob Lerman studies of her blood showed a strongly positive test for antibodies by the passive transfer method. Her case was reported by Root.[1]

Protamine zinc insulin is generally used at the Deaconess Hospital. Table 89 summarizes the dosage in 447 cases receiving protamine zinc insulin. Patients who were admitted taking an average of only 18 units protamine insulin numbered 179, whereas at discharge 221 patients taking protamine insulin required only an average of 20 units. The group of 149 cases taking both regular and protamine insulin required an average of 39 units upon admission; at discharge 186 cases took an average of 12 units regular and 38 units protamine insulin. Obviously the diabetes was not controlled at entrance.

TABLE 89.—DIABETIC SURGERY IN 1937 AND 1938.

Adjustment of Insulin in 447 Patients Treated With PZI During Surgery.

	Number.	Average Dose
Admission:		
PZI only	179	18
RI and PZI	149	12 + 27
RI only	64	38
No insulin	55	
	447	
Discharge:		
PZI only	221	20
RI and PZI	186	12 + 38
RI only	26	25
No insulin	14	
	447	

H. ANESTHESIA IN DIABETIC SURGERY.

The *anesthetic*, including its method of application, contributes to the fortunate outcome of a surgical operation upon a diabetic. With the aid of insulin practically any type of anesthesia can be adopted, but one should remember the effect of anesthetics *per se* and utilize this knowledge so painfully acquired before the discovery of insulin. Every effort should be made to shorten the period of anesthesia, irrespective of the type of anesthetic or of the availability of the use of insulin. If a preliminary injection of morphine is given, this should be small. Avoid apprehension and excitement on the part of the patient. It is just as valuable to have an anesthetist accustomed to diabetics, as it is in thyroid operations to have both surgeon and anesthetist accustomed to their peculiarities. Details count and in diabetic surgery it is right to be meticulous.

The avoidance of anoxia during anesthesia should be a prime consideration, as Courville's[2] report so strikingly demonstrated.

[1] Root: Jour. Am. Med. Assn., **131**, 882, 1946.
[2] Courville: Medicine, **15**, 129, 1936.

McClure, Hartman, Schnedorf and Schelling,[1] participating in a symposium upon anesthesia, give analyses of the oxygen and carbon dioxide content of arterial and venous blood under various types of anesthesia. Morphine and barbiturates, as pre-operative medication, tend to produce anoxia. If added to nitrous oxide anesthesia, dangerous anoxia in debilitated patients may occur.

The effect of anesthesia of various types upon the diabetic heart must be considered. Experimentally, Brow and Long[2] found with ether and chloroform a great loss of glycogen in the heart muscle in a period of two and one-half hours anesthesia. The loss of glycogen was due to an increased break-down with the formation of lactic acid and other intermediaries. Amytal did not cause so rapid a loss of glycogen, but Long[3] has shown that resynthesis of glycogen in skeletal muscles is delayed under amytal anesthesia. Best, Hoet and Marks[4] found that amytal decreased the glycogen content of resting skeletal muscles. Clinically amytal has been under grave suspicion as an agent dangerous to diabetics. Remember that under some anesthetics overdosage with insulin may be causing grave hypoglycemia without any of the clinical symptoms such as convulsions, as shown by Horsters and Brugsch.[5]

In general the choice of anesthetic should be (1) local, (2) spinal, (3) general.

(a) **Chloroform.**—All agree that chloroform is harmful to the patient in diabetic surgery.

(b) **Ether.**—During etherization the formation of glycogen is said to cease. Bloor[6] has shown that ether given to normal dogs results in a marked rise, 40 to 100 per cent, in the concentration of the blood fat, and this has been explained on the basis of an increased solubility in the blood-ether mixture of fatty substances in the tissues. Perhaps interference with the carbohydrate metabolism might be as important a factor. We combat nausea immediately with subcutaneous or intravenous glucose, because all diabetics should have available 100 to 150 grams carbohydrate daily. The statement will bear repetition that ether anesthesia is a burden which a light case of diabetes may easily bear, which may change a moderate to a severe case, and to a severe case prove fatal, yet with the help of insulin the harmful effects may be averted.

(c) **Nitrous Oxide-oxygen.**—Nitrous oxide-oxygen anesthesia has rarely been employed in long operations. Frequently gas-oxygen induction has been followed by ether. In Case 2311, it was resorted to with success when spinal anesthesia was impossible on account of marked hypertrophic osteoarthritis.

[1] McClure, Hartman, Schnedorf and Schelling: Ann. Surg., 110, 835, 1939.
[2] Brow and Long: Anesth. and Analg., 9, 193, 1930.
[3] Long: Jour. Biol. Chem., 77, 563, 1928.
[4] Best, Hoet and Marks: Proc. Roy. Soc. London (B), 100, 32, 1926.
[5] Horsters and Brugsch: Arch. f. exp. Path. u. Pharm., 147, 13, 1930.
[6] Bloor: Jour. Biol. Chem., 19, 1, 1914.

The disadvantages of nitrous-oxide are the poor muscular relaxation, anoxia and the unusual skill and experience required of the anesthetist for abdominal surgery.

(d) **Ethylene.**—Ethylene has been used occasionally since 1923, chiefly during thyroid and abdominal operations. No accidents have thus far occurred at the Deaconess Hospital with diabetic patients.

(e) **Cyclopropane.**—Used frequently in thyroid operations, cyclopropane also was chosen by Dr. Lahey, for the removal of a large tumor of the left kidney region in Case 15370. The tumor proved to be a benign pheochromocytoma.

(f) **Spinal Anesthesia.**—In amputations of gangrenous legs and toes this method of anesthesia has been by far the most satisfactory at the New England Deaconess Hospital. No unfavorable incident has occurred during the last fifteen years as a result of its employment. Arachnoiditis and paralysis following spinal anesthesia such as described by Kennedy, Somberg and Goldberg[1] have not been seen at the Deaconess Hospital, but, deliberately, spinal anesthesia is rarely employed in young patients. Pontocain in the dosage required has little toxicity.

(g) **Novocaine.**—**Cocaine.**—Local anesthesia frequently works admirably, and often shortens the period of employment of one of the group of anesthetics previously discussed. In a region where the blood supply is good, one need not hesitate in clean cases to use novocaine. Cocaine is too dangerous for use in general surgery.

(h) **Miscellaneous.**—Chloral, morphine and urethane always cause hyperglycemia which is not lessened by the addition of scopolamine.[2]

Avertin has been used in few patients. It is less safe than some other anesthetics for aged patients and, indeed, Coleman[3] found avertin more toxic to the liver than other anesthetics.

The intravenously administered pentothal was most successful in an operation upon a metastatic tumor of the cauda equina in Case 13356.

A rise in blood sugar occurred abruptly twenty-four hours after pentothal sodium anesthesia in diabetic patients studied by Wilcox and Tovell.[4] They used the drug in 90 mild diabetics with satisfactory results.

The avoidance of trauma is a *potent element* in promoting surgical success. There are various kinds of trauma, not alone the trauma due to bungling surgery, the trauma due to unnecessary tourniquets, but trauma due to the employment of strong antiseptic solutions. Indeed, antisepsis often means trauma. Undoubtedly asepsis instead of antisepsis has contributed a great deal to the success of modern diabetic surgery.

[1] Kennedy, Somberg and Goldberg: Jour. Am. Med. Assn., **129**, 664, 1945.
[2] Pi Suner and Formiguera: Treballs de la Soc. de biol., **8**, 151, 1920–1921.
[3] Coleman: Surgery, **3**, 87, 1938.
[4] Wilcox and Tovell: Anesth. and Analg., **18**, 94, 1939.

I. CARBUNCLES AND DIABETIC SURGERY.

Today the use of penicillin is transforming the treatment of carbuncles. In the last two years among 16 carbuncles treated at the New England Deaconess Hospital 7 required no surgery. Even positive blood cultures for Staphylococcus aureus and a large carbuncle in Case 25035 yielded to penicillin without incision or drainage. In 9 instances, however, the unusual extent of the area of necrosis required drainage as well as the use of penicillin. We still dread the large carbuncle particularly, as in Case 13784, where penicillin resistant organisms apparently were present, and suspect that about every tenth patient with the large carbuncle will be a fatality, although during the ten years ending in 1939 only 4 (5.6 per cent) of 71 patients with large and small carbuncles operated on by Dr. L. S. McKittrick at the Deaconess Hospital died. In the past no sooner has one seen a few carbuncles do well than one was shocked by a death from septicemia. It was usually the neglected small carbuncle which eventually raised the mortality. Now with prompt and energetic use of penicillin the number of large carbuncles should be greatly reduced.

Radiation has helped early and small carbuncles, but it should be prescribed and supervised by both the surgeon and the roentgenologist. Many patients with small carbuncles undoubtedly recover both in and outside hospitals, but there are many insignificantly appearing infections which develop into enormous carbuncles, and their hosts suffer for weeks, waste away and die with metastatic abscesses or septicemia instead, as formerly, of coma.

Carbuncles like coma and gangrene are more apt to appear in the fat than in the thin diabetic. Scrupulous cleanliness is essential in order to avoid them. "The washed neck, like the watched pot, never boils" (Brigham).

Fischer,[1] writing from the Surgical Clinic of the University of Giessen, advocates surgical treatment of carbuncles, and particularly the use of the electrical cautery knife. This means that bleeding is prevented.

The diabetic condition is not extremely severe in many patients when the carbuncle develops, but it is made severe by the infection. Fortunately today with healing of the carbuncle, carbohydrate tolerance returns, sometimes very suddenly. Thus, Case 1129 entered the Deaconess Hospital with 7 per cent sugar and a bad carbuncle. With combined surgical and medical care he did well. He was discharged sugar-free with carbohydrate 119 grams and insulin reduced from 45 to 20 units. Case 5872 was a very mild diabetic, became severe with a carbuncle, requiring 60 units of insulin a day. When healing began, suddenly the insulin dose fell to 5 units.

[1] Fischer: Diabetes und Chirurgie, Vortrage aus der Praktischen Chirurgie, Stuttgart, M, 1937.

All diabetics should be warned against becoming infected from others in the household. The husband of Case 1245 had boils; his wife contracted a carbuncle. The length of one of the crucial incisions in her back was 10 inches, yet she recovered.

The success which the surgeons at the Deaconess Hospital have had in the treatment of large and broken-down carbuncles of our patients can be attributed to surgical intervention at the proper time. It is important that operation be not undertaken too soon. The diabetes should be under reasonable control.

Vaccines have not been employed in recent years.

J. GANGRENE AND DIABETIC SURGERY.

Gangrene was found by Morrison[1] to be a contributory cause of death in 23 per cent of 775 fatal cases of diabetes in Boston during the years 1895 to 1913. It was present in 7 per cent of all diabetic patients admitted to the Peter Bent Brigham Hospital, according to Blotner and Fitz,[2] and in 3.5 per cent at the Montreal General Hospital.[3] Gariépy[4] reported gangrene in 4.3 per cent of the diabetic admissions at Notre Dame Hospital, Montreal. Eliason[5] states that 175, or 13 per cent, of 1305 diabetics admitted to the Philadelphia General Hospital (1930–1933) developed gangrene requiring surgery. Walters, Meyerding, Judd and Wilder[6] report 150 cases of gangrene of toes or feet in 4800 diabetic admissions, or 3.1 per cent. In our series, the percentage of the total mortality has risen from 3.7 per cent prior to 1914 to 4.2 per cent between that period and 1922, to 9.3 per cent from then until 1926, and since that date has decreased steadily to 4.7 per cent. These figures represent a follow-up of deaths among patients seen one or more times since 1898, both in or outside the hospital. Four hundred and ninety-seven or 3.8 per cent of 12,864 diabetic admissions to the New England Deaconess Hospital from 1939 to 1946 were the result of gangrene or infection of an extremity requiring operation.

The season of the year influences the frequency of gangrene of the lower extremities; there are more such lesions in the winter than in the summer. We think this is simply due to the circulation in the feet being less good, their lessened sensitiveness to heat and cold, their liability to burns from hot-water bags, and other methods of artificial heating, and perhaps most of all to their being bathed less often. Lemann[7] in New Orleans has shown that although rare in private practice, gangrene is as frequent in hospital practice as in Boston. Therefore, it is the social status of the patient and con-

[1] Morrison: Boston Med. and Surg. Jour., **175**, 54, 1916.
[2] Blotner and Fitz: Boston Med. and Surg. Jour., **194**, 1155, 1926.
[3] Rabinowitch: Canad. Med. Assn. Jour., **17**, 27, 1927.
[4] Gariépy: Bull. d. l'Assn. méd. lang. franç., **1**, 136, 1935.
[5] Eliason: Am. Surg., **98**, 1, 1933.
[6] Walters, Meyerding, Judd and Wilder: Minnesota Med., **17**, 517, 1934.
[7] Lemann: Jour. Am. Med. Assn., **89**, 659, 1927.

ditions incidental to cold weather rather than the climate, *per se*, which make gangrene common.

A much better idea of the incidence of gangrene is seen by the study of Table 90, in which its frequency according to the age at onset of diabetes is recorded. Among 670 cases with onset of diabetes after the age of seventy years, 69 had gangrene treated at the Deaconess Hospital. The frequency was less in those who acquired diabetes a decade earlier, between the ages of sixty-one and seventy years, although in that decade the occurrence was more frequent than in any preceding decade.

TABLE 90.—GANGRENE IN RELATION TO AGE AT ONSET OF DIABETES.

Age at onset of diabetes.	1898–1922.	1923–1927.	1928–1935.	1936–1939.	July 1, 1939–Jan. 1, 1946.	Total.
20–29	4	3	4	0	1	12
30–49	26	20	69	23	52	190
50–59	23	26	108	47	66	270
60–69	23	25	69	35	57	209
70–79	8	5	15	12	26	66
80+	..	..	..	..	3	3
Total	84	79	265	117	205	750

The average age at which the gangrene developed was sixty-four years. Arranged by decades, as is done in Table 91, the percentage distribution according to age at onset of gangrene is still more plainly shown. The youngest patient to develop gangrene was aged thirty-two years and the age of the oldest patient was eighty-nine years.

TABLE 91.—AGE AT ONSET OF GANGRENE OF 750 DIABETIC PATIENTS—WITH SURGERY.

Age at onset gangrene.	1898–1922.		1923–1926.		1927–1939.		July 1, 1939–Jan. 1, 1946.		Tota	
	No. of cases.	Av. age at onset.	No. of cases.	Av. age at onset.	No. of cases.	Av. age at onset.	No. of cases.	Av. age at onset.	No. of cases.	Av. age at onset.
30–49	8	44	3	47	16	46	6	49	33	47
50–59	28	56	23	57	76	56	43	55	170	56
60–69	40	65	49	65	168	65	76	65	333	65
70–79	8	72	15	75	105	73	61	73	189	73
80–	0	0	1	80	5	84	19	83	25	83
Totals	84	61	91	64	370	64	205	64	750	64

It is usually precipitated by trivial infections, resulting from trifling traumata, which have been neglected. Epidermophytosis between the toes in recent years has become a predisposing cause of increasing frequency. On account of the impaired circulation of the extremity, due to sclerosed, narrowed and thrombosed vessels, rarely occluded by embolism, osteomyelitis and necrosis of bone results. Hines,[1] in a clinical study of 280 cases of thrombo-arteriosclerosis obliterans, found the ratio of men to women 6 to 1. He distinguished it sharply from thrombo-angiitis obliterans, in which

[1] Hines: Proc. Staff Meet. Mayo Clin., **13**, 694, 1938.

the sex difference is even greater. Twenty per cent of his cases had diabetes. In 8 per cent of this series ischemic neuritis was present. In the arteriosclerotic lesions of diabetes the two sexes are almost equal.

Embolic gangrene is not rare in diabetes. It may occur by the detachment of an arteriosclerotic plaque in the aorta. Kiefer, Brigham and Wheeler[1] report sudden infarction of the left foot in a boy, aged nineteen years, who was in diabetic coma complicated by pneumonia, and review 52 cases from the literature. Case 11692, aged forty-six years, suffered from embolus at the bifurcation of the aorta due to a fibrillating heart, and died of gangrene. The effect of digitalis upon the predisposition to clotting reported by Gilbert, Trump and DeTakats[2] may be important in cardiac cases. Case 127, aged sixty-four years, developed gangrene from an embolus arising from an intracardiac thrombus. Case 6707 suffered amputation of the arm because of gangrene resulting from an embolus in the axillary artery. Case 22806, age 56.3 years, with auricular fibrillation had a riding embolus at the bifurcation of the aorta. Both legs became suddenly cool, pale, paralyzed and painful. At operation the pelvic vessels were too calcified and rigid to permit opening. Heparin 150 mg. was injected and treatment with both heparin and dicoumerol was continued for a week. Treatment was successful and she left the Deaconess Hospital August 2, 1946 without gangrene. Silbert[3] warns against the application of heat and elevation of the extremity in the treatment of arterial embolism.

Embolism from venous thrombosis occurs occasionally after operations upon the lower extremities. Bauer[4] records 2874 cases of thrombosis with 16.6 per cent fatal pulmonary embolism among 178,252 surgical operations in the literature. In the Mariestad Hospital, Sweden, he found a decline from 18 per cent to 1.4 per cent in the mortality among thrombotic cases following the use of heparin treatment.

Raynaud's disease as a cause of gangrene has only occurred once in our diabetics. Trauma is of common occurrence in diabetics. Trauma may make the diabetes worse by leading to infection, although almost never may it be found to be the prime cause in initiating diabetes.[5]

A pulsating dorsalis pedis artery is a favorable prognosis sign in a diabetic foot, but its absence is not a contraindication for reparative surgery. The painful foot is the foot with a poor circulation and poor prognosis according to McKittrick, who also adds that the hypesthetic foot is often the one with a good circulation.

Gangrene seldom occurs in the young diabetics or in the early

[1] Kiefer, Brigham and Wheeler: Boston Med. and Surg. Jour., **194**, 191, 1926.
[2] Gilbert, Trump and DeTakats: Jour. Am. Med. Assn., **125**, 840, 1944.
[3] Silbert: Bull. N. Y. Acad. Med., **22**, 397, 1946.
[4] Bauer: Lancet, **1**, 447, 1946.
[5] Joslin: Loc. cit., p. 83.

years of diabetes. Its frequency under the age of fifty years has diminished. (See Table 92.) Out of the first 84 cases there were but 8 who acquired gangrene in the first half century of life, and all but 1 of these cases were seen prior to 1917. By comparing Table 90 with Table 91, it will be found that none of the 12 patients whose diabetes began under the age of thirty years developed gangrene before thirty-one years of age, that of 202 cases whose diabetes began prior to the age of fifty years, there were but 33 who developed gangrene before fifty-one years of age, but that when the sixth decade is reached, the interval between onset of diabetes and onset of gangrene is short. Upon studying our data in detail there were discovered but 67 cases out of 545 who developed gangrene during the first year of diabetes. (Table 93.) With 179 the duration was between one and five years. Two hundred and ten of the patients had the disease five to ten years, 239 ten to twenty years and there were 50 patients whose diabetes extended over twenty years. There were 5 whose durations were unknown.

TABLE 92.—PERCENTAGE OF CASES DEVELOPING GANGRENE BEFORE THE AGE OF FIFTY YEARS, BY PERIODS.

	1898–1922.	1923–1926.	1927–1939.	July 1, 1939–Jan. 1, 1946.
Total cases	84	344	117	205
Per cent under fifty years	10	5	3	3

TABLE 93.—DURATION OF DIABETES PRECEDING GANGRENE.[1]

Years of diabetes.	1898–1923.	1923–1926.	1927–1939.	July 1, 1939–Jan. 1, 1946.	Total. No.	Per cent
Under 1	13	8	35	11	67	8.9
1–5	16	16	100	47	179	23.8
5–10	24	11	121	54	210	28.0
10–20	23	22	116	78	239	31.9
20–30	3	3	26	10	42	5.6
30–40	0	1	2	4	7	1.0
40+	0	0	0	1	1	0.1
Uncertain	5	0	0	0	5	0.7
Total	84	61	400	205	750	100.0

A serologic test for syphilis was recorded for 323 of the cases and in 1.9 per cent was positive in contrast to 1.7 per cent of positive reactions in 15,095 cases in our general series of diabetic patients. (See page 663.) Rabinowitch[2] cites a case in which the institution of antiluetic treatment was most useful.

The cholesterol was determined in the blood of 16 of the gangrene cases of Rabinowitch. Only 2 of the patients had normal amounts of cholesterol. This corresponds to the views expressed on page 493 upon the dependence of diabetic arteriosclerosis on cholesterol. Among an equal number of non-diabetic sclerotics, Rabinowitch

[1] Includes 33 cases with amputation of second leg.
[2] Rabinowitch: Ann. Clin. Med., **7**, 1478, 1934.

found 6 with a normal cholesterol. The average was for the diabetics 0.344 per cent and for the non-diabetics 0.249 per cent.

Tetanus.—No cases of tetanus have occurred in our patients. Among 3 known cases, one reported by Boulin, Uhry and Charousset[1] is distinguished by the fact that the use of 60,000 units of tetanus antitoxin on the third day and a total of 240,000 units of antitoxin injected by the subcutaneous and intramuscular route resulted in cure.

Gas Bacillus Gangrene.—Lehnhoff, Rynearson and Bickel[2] compare the pre-insulin and insulin eras with respect to diabetic gangrene and find that immediate high guillotine amputations are not nearly so frequently indicated as formerly. However, the dangers from gas gangrene have not been obviated in their experience by the new sulfonamide drugs and penicillin. They recommend guillotine amputation for gas gangrene and particularly stress the fact that every patient with diabetic gangrene needs an individual appraisal before treatment is decided.

A gas bacillus infection occurred in 1945 for the first time in fifteen years at the Deaconess Hospital among our diabetic patients following an amputation in Case 14547, age fifty-nine years. This patient had suffered a progressive thrombosis of the large vessels of her left leg and finally underwent amputation of the thigh. A few days after operation she suddenly developed some swelling of the thigh and in a few hours massive induration spread from the thigh to the abdominal wall. She went into collapse and died in twelve hours. At autopsy acute coronary occlusion was discovered so that the death was not due solely to the gas bacillus infection. In the treatment of diabetic gangrene, Lehnhoff, Rynearson and Bickel[2] state that a prophylactic dose of tetanus and gas gangrene antitoxin is always given.

Gangrene in an upper extremity occurred in 5 cases requiring amputation of the arm, secondary to severe infection. In a sixth case gangrene of a finger developed following a minor operation performed elsewhere, using a tourniquet and novocaine. Avoid the tourniquet!!

Amputation of Both Legs.—The malignant and progressive character of vascular disease in the diabetic is indicated by the involvement of the second leg. Both lower extremities were affected with gangrene in 73 instances, and amputation of both legs was required. (See Table 94.) In only 7 cases were both legs amputated at a single hospital admission. An amputation of both legs is not necessarily of bad prognosis, because 32 of 58 such patients operated upon since 1926 are still alive, and only twice in the last twelve years has gangrene of the second leg ended fatally at the Deaconess

[1] Boulin, Uhry and Charousset: Jour. Am. Med. Assn., **109**, 144, 1937.
[2] Lehnhoff, Rynearson and Bickel: Med. Clin. North America, **28**, 978, 1944.

Hospital. Amputation of both legs for gangrene may result in improved efficiency and comfort. In 100 consecutive patients followed by McKittrick,[1] after amputation of one leg for gangrene 22 subsequently lost the second leg and 19 more had gangrene of the other foot but no operation.

TABLE 94.—DIABETIC GANGRENE WITH AMPUTATION OF BOTH LEGS.

Period.	No. of cases.
1898–1922	7
1923–1926	8
1927–1935	31
1936–1946	27

Diagnosis of Gangrene.—The causes of gangrene, arteriosclerosis and mild infections develop slowly, and consequently gangrene itself is usually preceded by a long duration of symptoms. Charcot pointed out intermittent claudication as a precursor of gangrene, and coldness of the extremities and numbness and pains in the feet are common signs of approaching danger.

Pain occurring only at night suggests neuritis. Nocturnal cramps may be relieved by the use of prostigmin, 15 milligrams by mouth. The important question in a given lesion is whether the primary cause is infection in a foot with good blood supply, or whether the cause is primarily deficient blood supply. Inspection of the legs may yield the following evidences of deficient circulation; (*a*) reddish areas, discrete and never numerous, on lower legs and feet, later replaced by pigmented areas or scars, as described by Kramer;[2] (*b*) blisters or blebs, developing especially on the toes without known trauma; (*c*) cadaveric pallor of the toes on elevation, and (*d*) redness ("rubor") or cyanosis of the foot when hanging down; (*e*) shiny red, slightly swollen toes; (*f*) atrophy of calf muscles on one side or atrophy of subcutaneous tissue or of the nail bed with short, thick nails. The examination clinically may reveal (1) absence of pulsation in femoral, popliteal, posterior tibial or dorsalis pedis arteries. Olmsted and Olch[3] have emphasized the prognostic value of pulsation in the posterior tibial artery. Hyman Morrison[4] in a study of 1000 normal individuals found in 191 cases absence of one or more of the four pulsations in the feet, due to anatomical anomalies and this point is also emphasized by Olmsted.[5] (2) With both legs bared, the hand passed downward from the thigh will detect a change of temperature. A gradual change is normal, but a definite level of change suggests deficient blood supply. (3) The oscillometer[6] gives quan-

[1] McKittrick: Arch. Surg., **40**, 352, 1940.
[2] Kramer: Med. Jour. and Rec., **132**, 338, 1930.
[3] Olmsted and Olch: Jour. Missouri Med. Assn., **30**, 427, 1933.
[4] Morrison: New England Jour. Med., **208**, 438, 1933.
[5] Olmsted: Int. Clin., **1**, Series 46, 195, 1936.
[6] Friedländer: Jour. Am. Med. Assn., **104**, 297, 1935.

titative evidence of the level at which large vessels are occluded, but for an estimation of the more important collateral circulation other tests must be utilized. (4) The use of surface temperature measurements after spinal anesthesia and other special tests such as the flare test and the use of acetylcholine have proven useful in special cases.

Systematic examinations of the feet of diabetic patients in diabetic clinics and in the office revealed a high incidence of abnormality in the joints with hammer toes or restricted joint motion and consequent pressure points, deficient blood supply and changes in the nails and skin. This is well shown in careful examination of a series of diabetics and controls at the Stamford University Diabetic Clinic reported by Gray and Close.[1]

Prevention.—The prophylactic treatment of gangrene is seldom preached, but it is important. Gangrene typically occurs in the elderly patient with mild diabetes of long duration and inadequate diabetic treatment. In Table 95 it is evident that in the years 1939 to 1942 just as in the period 1923 to 1929 a period of seven to nine years passed without insulin treatment and without careful dietary treatment in patients subsequently suffering amputations of toes or thighs. Earlier use of insulin is the first step in prophylaxis.

TABLE 95.—LACK OF INSULIN TREATMENT PRECEDING DIABETIC AMPUTATIONS.

Period.	Cases.	Duration of diabetes in years preceding surgery.	Insulin therapy in years preceding thigh amputation.
1923–1929 . . .	160	8.6	0
1939–1942 . . .	230	9.6	2.7*

* 39 cases out of 107 had never received insulin.

At one time, 1 diabetic in 5 who came for hospital treatment after the age of seventy years acquired gangrene and for eighteen years in Boston 1 diabetic in 5 died with it as a contributory cause. Already education of the patient has begun to tell. About one-third of the diabetics at the Deaconess Hospital with foot lesions come early enough now to avoid operation. Now less than one-fifth require amputation of a leg. Of 100 amputation cases (33 toes and 67 legs) the average maximum weight for females (51 cases) was 188 pounds. The average maximum weight for males (49 cases) was 213 pounds. The avoidance of obesity must be strenuously urged. Unfortunately, one cannot hold out this incentive to a diabetic, "if you keep sugar-free, you will avoid gangrene," but he can be told that if sugar-free there is less chance of his developing it. The emphasis in prophylaxis must be placed, first and foremost, upon treatment of the diabetes, which today is designed to prevent early disease of the arteries; second, upon cleanliness of the feet; third, upon those conditions which might predispose to an infection by abrasion of the

[1] Gray and Close: Medical Record, **154**, 445, 1941.

feet. New shoes should be worn but a few hours at a time, and blisters which may have formed pricked only under aseptic precautions; arch supports should be used with care; corns and toe nails are to be cut only after thorough cleansing of the part and with good instruments and in a good light. Strong liniments are to be avoided, and the dangers of hot-water bags and heaters made vivid to the patients; a stiff big toe is not uncommon and these patients must be taught to limber up their toes. Epidermophytosis must be checked, because it favors deep infections between the toes. (See page 591.) Patients must be drilled. Patients predisposed to gangrene must be urged to walk for short intervals each day, to go through such gymnastic exercise as will bring about a free flow of blood in the feet, and not to remain long in one position. The legs are not to be crossed and compressing garters should be avoided. Massage is useful. Warm foot baths should be encouraged, but the danger of heat even in the form of hot air is brought out by Starr[1] who found that with the temperature above 35° C. the feet become blue and painful.

It is important to bear in mind that the use of heat in any form may hasten gangrene in a foot with deficient blood supply. In such a foot, the application of heat increases the rate of metabolism and of oxygen need in a part in which the blood supply cannot keep pace with the increased requirements.

Treatment of Feet.

The following sheet of instructions is given to patients at the Deaconess Hospital.

Hygiene of the Feet:

1. Wash feet daily with soap and lukewarm water. Dry thoroughly, especially between toes, using pressure rather than vigorous rubbing.
2. When thoroughly dry, rub with lanolin as often as necessary to keep skin soft and free from scales and dryness, but never render the feet tender. If the feet become too soft, rub once a day with alcohol.
3. If nails are brittle and dry, soften by soaking in warm water one-half hour each night and apply lanolin generously under and about nails and bandage loosely. Clean nails with orange-wood sticks. Cut the nails only in a good light and after a bath, when the feet are very clean. Cut the nails straight across to avoid injury to the toes, and do not cut the nails too short. If you go to a chiropodist, tell him you have diabetes.

---

[1] Starr: Proc. Assn. Am. Phys., **47**, 339, 1932.

4. All patients with overlapping toes or toes that are close together should separate them by lamb's wool. Patients with large joints or cramped-up toes should wear shoes without box toes and only vici kid leather.
5. All patients over sixty years should have daily rest periods and remove their shoes. Every Sunday morning ask someone to examine your feet.
6. Do not wear bed-room slippers when you ought to wear shoes. Slippers do not give proper support. Do not step on floor with bare feet.
7. Wear shoes of soft leather which fit and are not tight (neither narrow nor short). Wear new shoes one-half hour only on the first day, increasing one hour daily.
8. Use bed socks instead of hot water bottles, bags, bricks or electric heaters.
9. After fifty years one hears less well, sees less well, and the sense of feeling is diminished. Remember this and be cautious about the feet.

Treatment of Corns and Calluses:

1. Wear shoes which fit and cause no pressure.
2. Soak foot in warm, not hot, soapy water. Rub off with gauze or file off dead skin in or about callus or corn. Do not tear it off. Do not cut corns or calluses. Do not try to remove corns or calluses with patent or other medicines.
3. Prevent calluses under ball of foot,
    (a) by exercises such as curling and stretching toes twenty times a day,
    (b) by finishing each step on the toes and not on the ball of the foot.

Aids in Treatment of Imperfect Circulation:—Cold Feet:

1. Exercises. Bend the foot down and up as far as it will go six times. Describe a circle to the left with the foot six times and then to the right. Repeat morning, noon and night.
2. Massage with lanolin or cocoa butter.
3. Do not wear circular garters or sit with knees crossed.
4. If you have had gangrene or been threatened with it, keep off your feet five or more minutes each hour of the day, and if an amputation, fifteen or more minutes.

Treatment of Abrasions of the Skin:

1. Proper first-aid treatment is of the utmost importance even in apparently minor injuries. Consult your physician immediately.

2. Avoid strong irritating antiseptics, such as sulpho-naphthol and iodine.
3. At once after injury some surgeons recommend applications of sterile gauze saturated with medicated alcohol or hexyl-resorcinol (S.T. 37). Keep wet for not more than thirty minutes by adding more of the antiseptic solution. Sterile gauze in sealed packets may be purchased at drug stores.
4. Elevate, and, as much as possible until recovery, avoid using the foot.
5. Consult your doctor for pain, redness, swelling, or any inflammation.

Buerger[1] has suggested that certain passive exercises may be of value in inducing hyperemia or rubor in the affected limb, and therefore, therapeutically beneficial in increasing the blood supply. If the method is carried out daily for a long period, it is of great value in improving the circulatory conditions and in increasing the blood supply.

Buerger's Passive Exercises.—"The affected limb is elevated with the patient lying in bed, to from 60 to 90 degrees above the horizontal, being allowed to rest upon a support for thirty seconds to three minutes, the period of time being the minimum amount necessary to produce blanching or ischemia. As soon as blanching is established, the patient allows the foot to hang down over the edge of the bed for from two to five minutes, until reactionary hyperemia or rubor sets in, the total period of time being about one minute longer than that necessary to establish a good red color. The limb is then placed in the horizontal position for about two to five minutes, during which time an electric heating pad or hot-water bag[2] is applied, care being taken to prevent the occurrence of a burn. The placing of the limb in these three successive positions constitutes a cycle, the duration of which is usually from six to ten minutes. These cycles are repeated over a period of about one hour, some six to seven cycles constituting a seance."

The Buerger boards as used at the Deaconess Hospital consist of two boards, each ¾ inch thick, 30 inches long, and 11 inches wide, hinged at one end. In the middle of one board is a hinged tongue with a cleat on the other board so that the boards can be opened at an angle of 30 degrees, 45 degrees or 60 degrees as desired. Patients may spend from three to six hours daily in doing these exercises.

So convincing are the effects of treatment that a special nurse has been placed in charge of the care of the feet of all the surgical diabetics at the Deaconess Hospital. She also supervises the "Beauty Parlor for Diabetic Feet" given the hospital by Mr. and

---

[1] Buerger: Surgical Diagnosis and Treatment by American Authors, edited by A. J. Ochsner, Philadelphia, Lea & Febiger, **4**, 810, 1920.

[2] Experience with diabetics has taught us never to advise a patient to apply heat in any form to the feet.

Mrs. William L. Shearer in which Dr. John Kelly is the chiropodist. In fact, now we have two foot rooms and two surgical diabetic nurses who work in conjunction with the regular ward nurses.

Pathology.—The pathological findings at autopsy performed upon diabetic patients often reveal more extensive changes than had been anticipated and, in general, emphasize the great susceptibility of the surgical diabetic to general infection. The existence of generalized arteriosclerosis in the older patients is well shown in a series of 82 autopsies performed upon patients dying subsequent to surgical operations at the Deaconess Hospital.

The condition of the arteries and veins of extremities amputated for diabetic gangrene has been described by Buerger[1] as differing in no way from the lesions of the arteries in senile gangrene. With this statement, we cannot entirely agree.

Certainly arteriosclerosis is the basis for gangrene, but differences are found. In legs amputated for gangrene the arteriosclerosis is characterized by the fact that although the arteries of the leg are of the muscular type, the changes found are predominantly of the type which in non-diabetic patients is found in the elastic arteries, such as the aorta. In the legs of non-diabetic patients the changes consisting of calcification, necrosis and sclerosis, occurring chiefly in the media, form the so-called Mönckeberg type of arteriosclerosis. No great narrowing of the lumen occurs until, through degeneration of the intima, a suddenly formed thrombus completely occludes the artery. Typical senile gangrene, usually of the dry type, then develops. Such senile changes may be present in the arteries of persons developing diabetes in the late middle life, and hence senile arteriosclerotic gangrene may occur in a diabetic person. Characteristically, however, in the arteries of diabetic persons there is found marked intimal involvement[2] consisting of a heaping up of intima with deposition of fatty material in which many cholesterol crystals are seen. The heaping up of intima results in an early and gradual narrowing of the lumen with a limitation in the amount of blood supply. This process is usually of slow development, but may progress fairly rapidly in the course of a few months. As a result of this slowly progressive occlusion of the lumen, there tends to develop a compensatory collateral circulation, so that in time in a foot in which the large arteries are partially or completely obstructed, the blood supply may still be sufficient to keep the foot alive and in apparently satisfactory condition for the ordinary burdens of life. Gangrene develops when a sudden occlusion or thrombosis occurs for which the foot is not adequately prepared, or more frequently when the edema and inflammation, due to trauma or infection, cause thromboses of small arteries. The infection

[1] Buerger: Arch. Diag., April, 1915. See also articles by Silbert and Samuels Jour. Am. Med. Assn., 88, 1780, 1927; 89, 964, 1927; 90, 831, 1928.
[2] Root: Arch. Surg., 22, 179, 1931.

spreads rapidly, due to the lack of resistance in the diabetic patient, and gangrene follows. Owing in part to the collateral circulation, diabetic gangrene is usually moist, and the foot frequently warm. Evidence of the effect of diabetes upon the arterial wall is discussed on pages 216 and 221.

Chronic phlebitis is commonly found in diabetic legs. Phlebo-thrombosis[1] has been responsible for numerous pulmonary emboli and involved the vena cava in Case 21180, as demonstrated at autopsy. Ligation of femoral veins for the prevention of embolism is frequently employed, although in younger patients dicoumarol has been occasionally used.

We have never seen thrombo-angiitis obliterans in a diabetic at the Deaconess Hospital proved by pathological section, although on clinical grounds we have often suspected its presence.

If one needs to be convinced of the uselessness of attempting to save most gangrenous legs, the specimens removed at operation should be injected and studied. These show how hopeless it is to expect the arteries to regain their function. Regret is felt, not for the removal of the leg at the time, but rather that it had not been removed earlier.

The value of the roentgen-ray in reaching a conclusion as to the desirability of operation is considerable, when one desires evidence as to the existence of bone or joint destruction. The inspection of roentgen-ray plates of the lower extremities for arteriosclerosis is not simple, because one may err by considering visible vessels arteriosclerotic, or by not using a magnifying glass and so failing to notice punctate deposits of calcium. Visible calcification of arteries is of little help in determining the adequacy of the blood supply. Visualization of the arteries in the living body by means of Thorotrast in order to recognize the site of occlusion has been carried out by Allen and Camp.[2]

Treatment.— *Diet.*—The dietetic treatment of cases with gangrene is simple and along the lines already described for surgical cases in general. (See page 672.) The diabetes of these patients is essentially mild, as is commonly the case in those over sixty years of age. The chief precautions are not to make it worse by rigid curtailment of carbohydrate and calories on the one hand, or by overnutrition on the other.

One is anxious to prevent gain in weight in order to protect the stump when the artificial leg is worn. Persistence in a moderately low diet will prove an apparently severe diabetic to be mild. Healing may take place in the presence of a high blood sugar.

Insulin.—The use of insulin with cases of gangrene is the same as with any elderly arteriosclerotic diabetic of long duration having an infection. The decrease in the need for insulin during the hospital

[1] Wilkins and Friedland: New England Jour. Med., **229**, 17, 1943.
[2] Allen and Camp: Proc. Staff Meet. Mayo Clin., **7**, 657, 1932.

stay is striking, especially since the introduction of protamine insulin which, contrary to Jacobi,[1] we have found to work well with our surgical cases.

Exercise.—Exercise both before and after operation, except in the presence of an active infection, is essential. The muscles burn sugar. They must be utilized to maintain the diabetes in a mild state. Bed gymnastics therefore are carried out under the supervision of a trained technician. These exercises lessen pain and, incidentally, are at the same time a good prevention against pneumonia as they improve not only the local circulation but the pulmonary circulation as well. Also they protect against venous stasis and pulmonary embolism. In the presence of fever, avoid exercise.

Passive Vascular Exercise.—Through the work of Herrmann and Reid[2] mechanical apparatus has been devised which will automatically bring about rhythmic alteration of the environmental pressure of an extremity from any desired amount of negative pressure to any desired amount of positive pressure. Herrmann designed his Pavaex unit to bring about gradual change in pressure. Collens and Wilensky[3] have reported the use of intermittent venous occlusion in the treatment of peripheral vascular disease in 34 diabetics with open lesions and 14 without open lesions with excellent results. Certainly at the Deaconess Hospital this type of treatment has been employed in non-infected cases with sluggish lesions of the extremities and deficient blood supply with better results than any other mechanical apparatus has given. The oscillating bed for the treatment of cardiovascular disease (Sanders) has given good results according to Barker.[4] Our experience with it did not warrant continued use.

For impending ischemic gangrene Katz[5] has used intravenous injections of 10 cc. ether in saline daily for vasodilation and relief of pain. Good results were obtained in 58 of 66 cases.

Ultra-violet Ray.—Light treatments are employed in the winter. They exert a favorable action locally, but perhaps are more important as a general tonic. We must confess that when the ultra-violet ray apparatus broke down and we continued to turn patients *every two hours* on their side for a few moments the effects were so good, the ultra-violet ray was not resumed.

Surgery.—The treatment of actual gangrene demands the closest coöperation between a physician and an expert surgeon. Eliason feels that the responsibility for diabetic surgery should be placed with a single surgeon in each hospital. It is heart-rending to listen to the histories. We will cite one instance. A patient, having devel-

[1] Jacobi: Am. Jour Digest. Dis. and Nutr., **3**, 908, 1937.
[2] Herrmann and Reid: Jour. Med., **14**, 524, 1933. Herrmann: Passive Vascular Exercises, New York, J. B. Lippincott, 1936.
[3] Collens and Wilensky: Jour. Am. Med. Assn., **109**, 2125, 1937
[4] Barker: Proc. Staff Meet. Mayo Clin., **14**, 618, 1939.
[5] Katz: New Orleans Surg. Jour., **98**, 542, 1946.

oped gangrene in November, was treated by her local physicians and the surgeons of two well-known hospitals whom she said advised her to wait until the affected part dropped off. She entered the hospital penniless in June at 7 P.M. The leg was so foul smelling that by 9 P.M. all were glad to have it removed and the patient after a good night smilingly met a group of visiting doctors in the morning. Think of those months of suffering!

F. M. Allen[1] had applied refrigeration to gangrenous or infected extremities. By this means tissue metabolism may be reduced to a level consistent with the diminished blood supply, infection is checked, pain is reduced and amputation can be done without anesthesia. Patterson[2] compared amputation in 7 cases of diabetic gangrene with 14 diabetic limb amputations performed before the advent of refrigeration. The mortality rate of diabetics was zero with refrigeration technic. Shock was practically non-existent.

Gangrene deserves aggressive treatment on the part of physician and surgeon from start to finish. This does not mean that all gangrenous infected legs should be immediately amputated or partially amputated, but it does mean first, that their inherent possibilities for causing a fatal issue shall be appreciated, and second, that the lesions shall have expert surgical care. As long as the consulting surgeon agrees that satisfactory progress is taking place, well and good, but, if this referee is in doubt, operate immediately.

Indications for Operation in Gangrene.—Many factors must be taken into account, but the most important is the evident improvement or non-improvement of the patient. In cases with the dry type of gangrene which is plainly becoming localized, decision to defer operation is clearly indicated. It is easy to decide to advise immediate operation when there is a history of rapidly progressing moist gangrene. If the condition is remaining stationary, an operation favors safety, because in the course of a day or two an old focus, quiescent for weeks, can light up and lead to septicemia. Such flare-ups occur more frequently with vessels which are moderately sclerotic than extremely sclerotic. In general, the younger the patient, the more aggressive the surgical treatment.

To the mere presence of sugar or acid in the urine we attach little importance, because these can be controlled with or without operation by diet and insulin, but only effectively provided the infection is subsiding.

Procrastinating medical methods do more damage than prompt surgical intervention. The chief task of the medical or surgical consultant is to bring to an end dangerous delays and to secure action.

Pain is an indication for operation, and we have been thankful that the operation was performed for this reason in certain diabetics whose gangrene was comparatively slight. The pain attendant

[1] Allen: Am. Jour. Surg., **52**, 225, 1941.
[2] Patterson: Proc. Am. Diabetes Assoc., **4**, 143, 1944.

on the marked arteriosclerosis in the leg was too great to witness, much more to bear, and it was a relief to see the change in the comfort of these elderly people after the leg had been removed. It led one Jewish patient to return to have his remaining leg removed while the beginning gangrene was at a much earlier stage of development.

The financial aspect of gangrene is a serious factor. The medical treatment of gangrene during weeks and months in home or hospital is far more expensive and exhausting than early surgery. Subsequently patients regret the postponement of their operation and returning to the hospital advise other patients to be operated upon earlier. An infected gangrenous foot before it is healed costs, in our opinion, at least $400, quite apart from medical, surgical or special nursing fees or loss of wages.

Convalescence is often prolonged, but since the amputated stumps have been closed tight and without drainage, has been much shortened. Extraordinary precautions must be taken to protect the sound leg after operation. A woolen sock is placed on it before the patient leaves the operating table to guard it against undue pressure and for the same purpose a frame with supports by which the patient can lift himself is put over the bed.

Results of Treatment for Gangrene.—To our surprise, a follow-up in 1939 of 380 patients operated upon for gangrene when compared with 308 patients operated upon for infections of the feet revealed almost the same duration of life in each group.

The 206 deaths in the gangrene group represent 54 per cent of all the gangrene operations performed with recovery, whereas 147 deaths following operations for infection represent 47 per cent of the operations for infections of feet. This difference is clearly due to the fact that in general the group with infections are distinctly younger than the group with gangrene. Among the 206 gangrene cases, 48 died in the first year after operation but the average length of life was 2.9 years after operation. Among the 147 cases operated upon for infection, 23 died during the first year after operation but the average length of life was 3.4 years. It is evident that if patients pass the first year they can look forward to a considerable period of living.

Nearly all cases dying within a few days of operation died because operation was performed too late. To reduce mortality from gangrene and sepsis, therefore, we must (a) prevent lesions of the feet, and (b) if they occur (1) educate the patient to report them at once, (2) reach an earlier decision as to when to operate, (3) perform a more radical operation, and (4) build up more energetically the vitality of the patient by dietetic and other means.

A sharp distinction must be made between lesions of the feet due chiefly to infection, and those due to deficient blood supply. The latter patients suffer from wide-spread arteriosclerosis with a correspondingly shortened life expectancy and have a greater danger of septicemia.

It is inappropriate here to discuss in detail the surgical treatment of gangrene. Constant improvement has taken place in the methods of procedure employed by surgeons. The use of pinch grafts after amputations of two or more toes and for other large open areas has expedited healing. The use of the strong war antiseptics led to a very careful protection of the skin adjacent to the area involved by means of liquid rubber cement and sterile boric acid dressings. Unnecessary manipulation of the part is sternly prohibited. One in 6 amputations for gangrene and about 1 out of 6 major amputations necessary for infection are done below the knee. So sure are these operators of their technic that the wounds are closed without drainage. Far more radical attempts to save a major amputation by the removal of a toe or by the transmetatarsal amputation, even in the absence of dorsalis pedis pulsation, are made now than formerly. The oldest patient to have amputation through the lower leg is Case 5690, age seventy-six years. The Gritti-Stokes operation which preserves the patella is preferred if the infection has not extended too high and the patient's condition will permit. A guillotine operation has been employed with good effect in certain cases of early septicemia and subsequently the stump has been reamputated and closed.

Painful amputation stumps are a problem chiefly in patients who have had long periods of deficient blood supply and pain before amputation is performed. The persistence of pain is assumed to be due to chronic long-standing irritation of centrally conducting axons which produce an impression on the censory cortex and are projected back to the area of irritation. White[1] discusses various procedures for the elimination of the phantom limb pain such as resection of a painful neuroma, sympathetic block, sympathectomy and finally even frontal lobotomy. In 1 case at the Deaco es Hospital a painful neuroma was removed with relief. Usually in diabetic patients the phantom pain subsides after varying periods of time and is rarely of extreme severity. DeTakats and Fowler mentioned the resection of neuromas and their implantation into bone marrow as giving satisfactory results.

If the diabetic kept his feet as clean as his face, gangrene would seldom occur. Gangrene is responsible for 5 to 8 per cent of all diabetic deaths, and all diabetics above fifty years of age should be taught how to avoid it.

If the beginning of gangrene were as noisily ushered in as an attack of biliary or renal colic the results of treatment would be far different. Death from gangrene today is usually the result of procrastination on the part of the physician and patient, and in the past was often associated with the inauguration of a fat-

[1] White: Jour. Am. Med. Assn., **124**, 1030, 1944.

protein diet and ether anesthesia. Surgery often receives, but seldom deserves, the blame of a fatal issue.

Gangrene in Other Tissues.—Diabetic gangrene of the skin and other tissues such as the nose, tongue, lungs, vulva and glans penis have repeatedly been reported. In most instances severe staphylococcus or streptococcus infection with thromboses of small arteries is the probable cause of gangrene.

An extensive staphylococcus cellulitis of the neck with some areas of gangrene recovered with the use of penicillin, as described by Millett and Darby.[1]

Diabetic gangrene of the nasal septum and turbinate have been described by Goldberg[2] and Speidel,[3] of the nose by Wood,[4] in whose case spontaneous amputation of the nose occurred. In the case of Riven,[5] the skin of the entire body was involved, and the author gave the condition the name "Dermatitis Gangrenosa." In another case described by Millett,[6] gangrene of the face was present. Gangrene of the penis was reported by McCrea[7] and Townsend and Flagg.[8]

K. TRANSMETATARSAL AMPUTATION.

A considerable number of diabetic patients have circulatory, neurologic, or orthopedic condition in their toes such that an open lesion on one toe will be followed within months or a year by recurring lesions on other toes. The chief cause of the lesion in the toe is deficient blood supply due to arteriosclerosis, but complicating factors may be rigid arthritic joints and impaired sensations due to diabetic neuropathy. The transmetatarsal amputation is done primarily for gangrene of a part of one or more digits when the gangrene and infection is limited to the toes, or for other lesions of the toes where the extent of the infection or the lack of circulation renders satisfactory healing unlikely should the removal of the digit alone be attempted. In addition, the operation may be done for those patients with satisfactory circulation, but who have recurring ulcers on the distal portion of the foot on a neurogenic basis. In this latter group the operation has been done more or less as a measure of desperation to save the patient frequent hospital admission.

One reason for this procedure for lesions in one toe is the fact that occasionally following the amputation of one toe, within a year or two a patient has returned with a lesion on another toe which had

[1] Millett and Darby: New Eng. Jour. Med., **235**, 12, 1946.
[2] Goldberg: Arch. Otol., **32**, 16, 1940.
[3] Speidel: Kentucky Med. Jour., **42**, 184, 1944.
[4] Wood: Ann. Otol., Rhinol. and Laryngol., **46**, 1112, 1937.
[5] Riven: Am. Jour. Med. Sci., **189**, 550, 1935.
[6] Millett: Jour. Am. Med. Assn., **112**, 1143, 1939.
[7] McCrea: Clinics, **4**, 796, 1945.
[8] Townsend and Flagg: Jour. of Urol., **40**, 464, 1938.

been allowed to progress and to extend into the foot or leg so that, at his second admission, a major amputation at the level of the knee was required which might have been avoided had all the toes been removed at the first operation.

Moore[1] discussed the first seven transmetatarsal amputations done at the Deaconess Hospital and emphasized the part played by virulent infection in increasing the local metabolic requirement of tissues in an arteriosclerotic foot, and thus decreasing the blood supply by edema and venous thrombosis with resulting gangrene. Penicillin has been of inestimable value in this group of patients and was used in 48 of the 56 cases in Table 96, both in the pre-operative period and afterward for periods varying from five days to three weeks. The total dosage has varied from a minimum of 500,000 units to a maximum of 7,440,000 units.

The transmetatarsal amputation, when successful, gives a foot which enables the patient to walk successfully and to carry on usual activities, provided the blood supply is sufficient to enable healing of the operative wound, and further provided that the neurotrophic anesthesia and the associated susceptibility to pressure are not present. It is obvious, therefore, that patients should be selected for this surgery with care. Operations should not be done to active extending infections in the foot, and, therefore, in some patients with lymphangitis or active infections extending to the ankle or above, a considerable period may be necessary for the treatment by means of penicillin and local measures to bring about the subsidence of that infection. This does not mean that in every case all infections must have been cleared away from a point beyond the base of the toe, but no active extending infection should be present. The most careful assessment of the circulatory supply is fundamental. In this group of patients, 56 in number, shown in Table 96 absence of pulsation in the dorsalis pedis artery was a feature in the majority of cases. In nearly all the patients circulatory impairment in the toe was such that an amputation of the toe alone probably would not have succeeded. The better blood supply at the level of the transmetatarsal amputation was a necessary condition for success. Even so in fully half the patients, the operation could only be offered to the patient with a distinct understanding and a clear explanation of the fact that with the impaired blood supply success was not certain and that the patient's acquiescence in a higher amputation might be necessary. In all these patients, infection was present, and all but the first 8 cases received treatment with penicillin, usually 300,000 units a day, but sometimes 500,000 units a day for periods varying from three or four days, to as much as two weeks before operation. This same treatment was continued following operation for periods varying from five days to three or four weeks. Unquestionably, control of infections and the edema associated with

[1] Moore: Am. Jour. Digest. Dis., **11**, 398, 1944.

infections by means of penicillin has been an important factor contributing to success.

In the selection of patients, age has not been a decisive factor. Of the four patients between forty and forty-nine years of age, recurring infection in pressure areas and in the foot with neurotrophic lesions were present. Although all four healed, one patient now in Mexico is reported by mail, to be suffering from a pressure area in that foot and also a lesion in the other foot. He illustrates the serious risk with any kind of treatment for patients with diabetic neuropathy of the feet. Two patients over eighty years of age were healed successfully. One patient, Case 25878, had a successful transmetatarsal amputation on one foot, but a year later, when the second foot was involved, arteriosclerosis had progressed during that year so that the transmetatarsal amputation failed and a low thigh amputation was necessary. A total of 9 patients have required a higher amputation, failure coming in each case due to a greater deficiency in blood supply and lower resistance to infection, than had been anticipated. The long duration of diabetes is an outstanding fact, in this group, as in gangrene cases in general. A long period, averaging 11.6 years of mild diabetes treated without insulin and without careful dietary control precedes the development of the foot lesion. In March 1946, one patient, operated on one year before, had returned with a fresh area of gangrene and had a thigh amputation.

In discussing the future of this operation, McKittrick insists that judgment must be withheld until a longer period of observation of the patients who have been operated upon is possible. Further investigation of the possibility that longer periods of pre-operative preparation, with bed exercises, may bring about a better circulatory balance, and improve the chances of success in those patients in whom the combinations of infection and borderline blood supply makes healing uncertain. At present the point of greatest weakness where the operative incision is most likely to break down is on the dorsum of the foot in the center. The explanation is not clear, but the success in healing this area would overcome one of the major difficulties at present.

TABLE 96.—FIFTY-SIX TRANSMETATARSAL AMPUTATIONS, 30 FEMALE—26 MALE.

Age, years.	Case No.	Healed success.	Higher amputation subsequently.	Duration diabetes.
40–49	4	4	0	15.0
50–59	16	14	3	9.3
60–69	23	18*	3	11.2
70–79	11	8†	3	14.7
80+	2	2	0	1.3

* One patient had 2 transmetatarsal amputations in successive years—one failed.
† One fatal.

L. INFECTIONS OF THE EXTREMITIES.

The importance of the recognition and early treatment of infections of either the lower extremities or of the hands of the diabetic patient rests upon the fact that, in these patients the presence of adequate blood supply gives an excellent prognosis, with prompt treatment, for many years of usefulness. On the other hand, delay in treatment favors the development of septicemia and inevitable death. The diagnosis of adequate blood supply rests upon (1) the presence of good pulsations in the dorsalis pedis artery, or (2) excellent collateral circulation as shown by a foot of normal appearance, nutrition and temperature in the absence of pulsations in the dorsalis pedis or posterior tibial arteries. If gangrene is present it is secondary to infection and local impairment of blood supply, rather than to primary arterial occlusion. It is in this group that the deceptive lack of normal sensation and sometimes actual anesthesia frequently leads the patient to conclude that the absence of pain means safety and therefore to receive delayed or half-hearted treatment. Infection beginning under a corn or a callus leads to osteomyelitis of the phalanx which may pursue a sluggish course for weeks or months before suddenly developing a rapidly ascending infection. In the following table are summarized operations since 1923 upon 695 diabetic patients.

TABLE 97.—INFECTIONS REQUIRING SURGERY OF DIGIT OR LIMB.
(January 1, 1923 to January 1, 1946.)

Ages of patients, by decades, at time of operation.

	0–14	15–29	30–49	50–59	60–69	70–79	80–	Total.
Incision of finger or hand	3	5	16	16	7	3	0	50
Amputation of finger.	0	3	6	9	8	1	0	27
Amputation of arm .	0	0	1	0	2	0	0	3
Incision of toe or foot	2	5	12	25	24	7	0	75
Amputation of toes .	0	7	44	127	164	56	3	401
Amputation of leg .	0	0	8	13	36	15	1	73
Incision or amputation of toe followed by amputation of leg .	0	0	3	19	14	2	2	40
Guillotine .	0	0	3	3	3	0	0	9
Guillotine followed by thigh	0	0	0	4	1	2	0	7
Transmetatarsal amputations .	0	0	2	4	2	2	0	10
Total .	5	20	95	220	261	88	6	695

The group with infected lesions is distinctly younger than the group with gangrene. Guillotine amputations numbered 16 cases and were done for serious and spreading infection. After control of from ten days to two weeks, a secondary amputation at a higher level above the knee joint was performed in 7 instances.

Defective sensation in diabetic feet occurs in various degrees, and influences the frequency of serious infections. It is particularly important with regard to the healing of operative wounds and the question of the ability of the foot to stand daily weight bearing in the future. The lack of pain often leads patients to delay coming for treatment until a slight infection in the corn or callus has extended and led to osteomyelitis. The degree of anesthesia is most striking in those patients in whom deep incisions for drainage or partial amputation of the toe can be done in bed without anesthesia. In patients where the anesthesia extends beyond toes into the mid-portion of the foot or higher, it is almost certain that the foot will break down under the pressure of weight bearing if operation or amputation is done at a point distal to the area of anesthesia. In its most advanced form this neuropathic condition is seen in the feet showing changes in the joints closely resembling the typical Charcot joints. These patients usually show a gradual, progressive thickening of the tarsus, swelling without pain or redness, and x-ray evidence of destruction of the joint surfaces. Sometimes infections of the toes or pressure areas are present. Unlike the classical arthropathy of Charcot, the condition does not begin with sudden spontaneous swelling of the foot and is rarely preceded by injury or pain. It is not luetic and in the 19 cases (see page 567) reported by Bailey and Root[1] none of the symptoms or reflex changes associated with syphilis were present.

Infection of a leg with gas bacillus occurred in 3 cases prior to 1930 and once in 1945. An infection simulating that with gas bacillus occurred in Case 27996, who underwent an amputation at the junction of the middle and lower third of the left leg because of a gangrenous great toe with lymphangitis above the ankle. After treatment of penicillin and the subsidence of the lymphangitis, the amputation was carried out with apparently excellent results until the twenty-first day. Then suddenly a rise in pulse rate was accompanied by swelling and discoloration of the stump. A smear showed gram-positive bacilli. These organisms were found at amputation to have invaded the tissues to a distance of 3 inches from the wound. They proved to be Bacillus subtilis. This is the first time in a diabetic patient at the Deaconess Hospital that this organism has been found to have invaded tissues for some distance and apparently to have possessed pathogenicity.

Infections of the hand or arm numbered 80 cases and amputations of the arm were done in 3 cases, with death from septicemia in 2 instances and metastatic abscess of the lung in one. These cases occurred prior to 1930. Two deaths from streptococcus septicemia occurred in patients receiving only incision, giving a total mortality of 6 per cent. The serious character of these infections was well brought out by Fredet and Jeanneney.[2] The extensive necrosis and the difficulty of controlling abscesses, particularly in the palmar region, was striking in these cases as in the cases described by Bothe.[3] Garrey and McKittrick (quoted by McKittrick[4]) studied 70 diabetic patients admitted to the New England Deaconess and Massachusetts General Hospitals between January 1, 1933 and Janu-

[1] Bailey and Root: To be published.
[2] Fredet and Jeanneney: Rapport, 48th Congres français de chirurgie, 1936. See also Fredet: Journ. de Chir. **48**, 499, 1936.
[3] Bothe: Pennsylvania Med. Jour., **37**, 661, 1934.
[4] McKittrick: Surg., Gynec. and Obst., **68**, 508, 1939.

ary 1, 1937, with infections of the hand. Of these, 7.1 per cent died and another 7 per cent survived an amputation through or above the forearm. Thirty per cent of the patients lost all or part of one or more fingers. They stress as important causes for these poor results late hospitalization and inadequate incision, especially after ambulatory treatment and secondarily the presence of a mixed infection.

Varicose ulcers are comparatively infrequent in diabetic patients although varicose veins requiring injection or ligation, are not uncommon. Case 18918, a male aged fifty-six years, is the only diabetic patient who developed acute thrombophlebitis of the thigh after an operation performed upon the foot.

The sensitization of local tissues to bacteria or fungi contributes to chronicity, to the acute flare-ups in patients with recurrent ulcerations and especially those with fungus infections.[1]

Antibiotics and Chemotherapy of Pyogenic Infections.—The increasing use of penicillin and sulfa drugs, and the intensive bacteriological and laboratory studies of these substances have shown their extreme value in certain types of infections. The use of penicillin for treatment in infections in diabetes mellitus has been fully as dramatic in its results as in non-diabetic patients. It has almost entirely replaced the sulfonamides. The reactions seem to be no more frequent and the incidence of bacterial resistance to penicillin seems no greater among the diabetics. It might be supposed that in the presence of diabetes some metabolic factors might be present which would interfere with the action of penicillin. Unfortunately, the exact mechanism of the action of penicillin is not yet understood. It is presumed that penicillin acts by interfering with some essential process in the metabolism of susceptible bacteria. Penicillin is active only when bacteria are in the phase of growth and multiplication, and seems to have no action on bacteria that are in the resting stage according to Keefer and Anderson.[2]

TABLE 98.—ORGANISMS SENSITIVE TO PENICILLIN.

Staphylococcus albus	Clostridium novyi
Staphylococcus aureus	Clostridium œdematis maligni
Streptococcus pyogenes	Clostridium perfringens
Non-hemolytic streptococci	Clostridium tetani
Anaërobic streptococci	Corynebacterium diphtheriæ
Diplococcus pneumoniæ	Treponema pallidum
Neisseria gonorrhæ	Treponema pertenue
Neisseria intracellularis	Streptobacillus moniliformis
Bacillus anthracis	Spirillum minus
Clostridium botulinum	Borrelia novyi
Clostridium histolyticus	Actinomyces bovis

The table above taken from Keefer and Anderson includes the organisms which are ordinarily susceptible to penicillin although it

[1] Thompson: Yale Jour. Biol. and Med., **16**, 665, 1944.
[2] Keefer and Anderson: In Oxford Medicine, New York, Oxford University Press, vol. 4, Part 4, p. 938, 1945.

45

must not be forgotten that certain pathogenic organisms are affected by minute concentrations of the drug whereas others are not influenced even by high concentrations. In diabetics, the frequency of mixed infections with hemolytic staphylococcus aureus, streptococci and colon bacillus presents a difficult problem involving symbiosis and local metabolic changes as yet little understood.

Attempts to give penicillin by mouth have met with three obstacles. First was the fact that the free hydrochloric acid in the gastric juice inactivated the penicillin, and secondly the rate of absorption from the upper bowel must be rapid since penicillin is so quickly excreted by the kidney. Third, penicillin is destroyed in the lower intestine by penicillinase-producing organisms in the bowel. Penicillin, therefore, has been given by mouth in tablets buffered with such substances as aluminum hydroxide, magnesium oxide, etc.; as capsules of penicillin in oil and penicillin combined with aluminum hydroxide gel for streptococcus and staphylococcus infections. A minimum of 20,000 to 40,000 units of penicillin should first be given parenterally. After the acute phase has been reduced oral treatment may be continued with dosages of 40,000 to 50,000 units each two or three hours. As prophylaxis against secondary infections following tonsillectomy or tooth extraction, particularly in patients with a history of rheumatic fever or rheumatic heart disease, 100,000 to 200,000 units daily may be given before and for three or four days after surgery. The statement concerning penicillin products by Keefer et al.[1] should be consulted.

Among the points constantly to be considered in order to obtain effective penicillin therapy may be mentioned: (1) Sufficient prolongation of therapy to prevent relapses. (2) Sufficient dosage to produce an effective blood concentration. (3) Intramuscular injection is the method of choice for acute and severe infections. (4) Effective blood levels usually range from 0.02 to 0.16 units per cc. of blood requiring approximately 25,000 units every two hours. (5) Penicillin is generally superior to the sulfonamides and, although toxic infections do occur they are less frequent and less serious. Patients with staphylococcus bacteremia from carbuncle, osteomyelitis and prostatic abscess have all recovered. Penicillin resistant infections do occur, but are not common. Case 13784 with a tremendous carbuncle is the most outstanding example of apparent penicillin resistance in the carbuncle series, and a few cases with severe foot infections have been resistant. Every diabetic with an infected foot, with or without gangrene, receives penicillin 200,000 to 500,000 units per twenty-four hours before operation and for at least five days after operation. In tissues ischemic from arteriosclerosis, larger doses are indicated and the intravenous route may be recommended especially in severely necrotic lesions, as suggested

[1] Keefer, Herwick, Van Winkle and Putnam: Jour. Am. Med. Assn., 128, 1161, 1945.

by Naide and Sayen.[1] Intra-arterial injection of penicillin for infections of the extremities has been recommended by Glasser, Herrlin and Pollock.[2] Streptomycin may prove more effective in selected cases. Herrell and Nichols[3] describe a diabetic with severe bacteremia due to Escherichia coli, who recovered after receiving 20,000,000 units in thirteen days.

It is evident that many types of bacteria are practically unaffected by the sulfonamides. Thus certain hemolytic streptococci are not affected. In the diabetic patient we occasionally deal with streptococci situated in throat or tonsils or else localized in the kidneys, prostate or skin, where it has always been difficult to eradicate the organism and the danger of severe infection with necrosis has been genuine. Nevertheless, the greatest danger in the diabetic patient from the streptococcus has been the danger of invasion of the blood stream, and it is exactly at this point at which sulfadiazine has been most valuable in saving both life and limb.

Unfortunately in diabetic patients streptococcus infections form only a small percentage of the serious infections of the extremities or of the kidneys. It is the staphylococcus, hemolytic or non-hemolytic, which is the most serious and frequent invader. It is true that infections of the feet, accompanied by gas formation in the tissue, frequently show in cultures not only staphylococci, but streptococci and colon bacilli, and in these patients sulfonamide therapy has been less useful than pencillin. The dangers of treatment with sulfonamides are no greater in diabetic patients than in non-diabetic patients, if the usual care is taken to watch for anemia, leucopenia, and hematuria due to deposition of crystals in the kidneys. Our rule is to give intravenous fluid immediately if the twenty-four-hour urine secretion falls below 1200 cc.

The use of sulfadiazine and sulfathiazole was compared in 100 consecutive diabetics by Styron, Bromley and Root.[4] None but mild toxic reactions were observed and these were less frequent in patients receiving sulfadiazine.

The sensitivity to sulfonamide drug which results in weakness and prostration can be combatted by the use of large doses of vitamin C, such as 200 to 500 milligrams, according to Holmes.[5]

M. APPENDICITIS AND DIABETIC SURGERY.

Appendicitis in the diabetic may be insidious, almost symptomless, may simulate coma or conversely coma may simulate it. The syndrome of abdominal pain, vomiting, spasm of the abdominal muscles and leukocytosis often associated with diabetic acidosis

[1] Naide and Sayen: Jour. Am. Med. Assn., **129**, 869, 1945.
[2] Glasser, Herrlin and Pollock: Jour. Am. Med. Assn., **128**, 796, 1945.
[3] Herrell and Nichols: Proc. Staff Meet. Mayo Clin., **20**, 449, 1945.
[4] Styron, Bromley and Root: Loc. cit., p. 531.
[5] Holmes: Ohio State Med. Jour., **41**, 923, 1945.

may lead to a variety of surgical diagnoses. Operation can be carried out successfully even though acidosis and peritonitis are present. The weakness and sweating of a protracted recovery may be due to an insulin reaction rather than to shock or pocketed pus.

Case 10775, aged twenty-one years, with diabetes of nine years' duration, entered the Deaconess Hospital on August 8, 1939 with a history of pain of twenty-four hours' duration. He was drowsy, dyspneic, the blood CO_2 was 18 volumes per cent and the blood sugar 600 mg. Nevertheless, with unquestioned diabetic coma present, the local signs were definite and within two hours a gangrenous appendix was removed with recovery. Do not sacrifice a patient to appendicitis just because he has diabetes and approaching coma. If in doubt, operate, although you may rarely do so needlessly.

The appendix may be located high under the liver in the diabetic due to congenital failure of rotation. In two cases this fact led to difficulty and delay in diagnosis of acute appendicitis.

N. GALL STONES AND DIABETIC SURGERY.

Of 88 diabetics operated upon for gall stones from 1923 to July 1, 1939, there were 6 deaths. In a total of 70 operations upon the biliary tract between January, 1934 and June, 1938, McKittrick reported 5 deaths, or a mortality of 7.1 per cent.[1] In 10 of the 70 cases the operation consisted of joining the gall-bladder to the stomach or duodenum because of carcinoma of the pancreas. During the four years ending January 1, 1946, cholecystectomy was performed upon 39 diabetics without a fatality.

Jaundice in a diabetic may mean gall stones, hepatitis, carcinoma or cirrhosis, and the effects produced upon the diabetes may vary from hypoglycemia to severe acidosis. Bade[2] considers that jaundice develops more easily in diabetics than in non-diabetics. McCabe and Hart's[3] diabetic woman had jaundice and ascites but recovered. Notwithstanding severe and longstanding jaundice and relatively inadequately followed diet the tolerance does not get worse. Verger[4] cites 10 such cases, of whom several had enlargement of liver with blood bilirubin values as high as 6 milligrams and yet after several weeks, gained tolerance and gave up insulin. Is it due to failure of fat to enter the liver and thus to allow larger glycogen deposits?

Fatal perforation of the gall-bladder has occurred in Cases 6435, 8929, 10803, 15273, 15497, 15919, 17466, and these cases, all observed at the Deaconess Hospital, have influenced us to advise any diabetic patient to have his gall stones removed when conditions are most favorable.

[1] McKittrick: Loc. cit., p. 704.
[2] Bade: München. med. Wchnschr., **83**, 171, 1936.
[3] McCabe and Hart: Jour. Am. Med. Assn., **105**, 859, 1935.
[4] Verger: Ztschr. klin. Med., **127**, 166, 1934.

We are grateful to the surgeons for repeatedly emphasizing the importance of the use of glucose and protein in postoperative conditions, particularly in gall-bladder disease to protect the liver. Ravdin[1] studied 127 patients operated on for biliary tract disease, of whom 37 received a special diet of 74 per cent carbohydrate, 20 per cent protein and 6 per cent fat for five days or more before operation. In 90 patients not on the special diet, liver tissue showed 3.0 per cent glycogen and 5 per cent fatty acids as compared with a normal average of 4 per cent fatty acids; obese patients showed higher amounts up to 10 per cent. In 10 patients with severe disease not on a controlled diet the liver showed 3.3 per cent glycogen and 4.2 per cent fatty acids. It is pointed out that glucose administration is not enough to protect liver parenchyma and promote regeneration. Adequate protein intake is also essential.

O. DISEASE OF THE THYROID GLAND AND DIABETIC SURGERY.

Here again surgery not only improves the symptoms due to the thyroid but frequently the diabetes. This subject has twice been reported in detail in association with F. H. Lahey.[2] In the first report 63 operated cases were reported with a mortality of 4.8 per cent. To this series were added 102 operated cases with a mortality of 2.6 per cent, or a mortality for the combined series (165 cases) of 3.4 per cent. The mortality-rate was first reduced by doing multiple stage operations on diabetics with hyperthyroidism, but now thiouracil has still further reduced the operative risk. A series of 76 cases without a postoperative death (1940–1946), is now included. (See page 725.)

P. PROSTATECTOMY AND DIABETES.

Sixty-three cases were operated upon and all recovered but 3. The use of transurethral resection in selected cases has been advantageous. For discussion of other urological conditions, see Chapter XIX.

Q. SURGICAL TREATMENT OF DIABETES AND PANCREATIC SURGERY.

Operations performed to ameliorate or cure diabetes have been attempted both in animals and in human beings.

(a) Grafts of pancreas obtained either from animals or human beings fail to grow. Dr. Harvey Stone, of Baltimore, has succeeded in growing cells of the thyroid and pancreas, making use of human

---

[1] Ravdin, Thorogood, Riegel, Peters and Rhoads: Jour. Am. Med. Assn., **121**, 322, 1943.

[2] Joslin and Lahey: Am. Jour. Med. Sci., **176**, 1, 1928; Ann. Surg., **100**, 629, 1934.

serum. All hope that he will find a solution of the problem by making grafted islands of Langerhans grow in a human body.

(b) Total thyroidectomy has been performed in order to lower the total metabolic rate, and 2 cases reported, one from the Mayo Clinic by Wilder[1] and one in Boston by Rudy.[2] Results did not justify repetition. (See page 126.)

(c) Severance of splanchnic nerves results in slightly increased sensitivity to insulin. (See page 124.)

(d) Denervation of the adrenals has increased the sensitivity to insulin. (See page 124.)

(e) Hypophysectomy in depancreatized animals and in human acromegalics ameliorates the diabetes. (See page 121.)

(f) Ligation of the submaxillary or parotid ducts has been attempted experimentally without striking results.

(g) Prolonged drainage of the biliary tract has been used experimentally and in 1 human case by Leriche and Jung.[3] Their patient was a young woman, aged thirty-one years, who had required 80 to 100 units of insulin a day. With prolonged drainage of the biliary tract from April, 1937 to July, 1937, her diabetes seemed almost to disappear. When the drainage was discontinued, however, the diabetes returned. They concluded that further study may show the possibility of drainage by way of attaching the gall-bladder to the jejunum for relief of diabetes.

Operations upon the pancreas for the treatment of spontaneous hypoglycemia in non-diabetics have now been reported in a sufficient number of cases to keep this clinical condition before the attention of every surgeon. (See Chapter XII.)

Hüttl[4] performed the Mansfeld ligation of the pancreas in 3 diabetics and 4 cases of carcinoma with increase in size of the islands observed at autopsy.

Removal of the pancreatogenic factor by hypophysectomy was reported by Chabanier.[5] A boy, aged fifteen years, developed diabetes in October, 1927. The diabetes became severe so that by 1932 he was taking 140 to 150 units of insulin daily. At this time he developed pulmonary tuberculosis. In 1934 the tuberculosis was active and he was having serious hypoglycemic reactions, taking about 150 to 170 units of insulin a day. Therefore, it was decided to remove the anterior lobe of the hypophysis in the hope that the diabetes would be controlled with less difficulty and smaller amounts of insulin. The operation was carried out without difficulty and a normal pituitary gland removed. After the operation he continued to have insulin reactions but they were less severe, and he required only 70 to 80 units a day. The patient developed

[2] Wilder, Foster and Pemberton: Loc. cit., p. 126.
[3] Rudy, Blumgart and Berlin: Loc. cit., p. 126.
[3] Leriche and Jung: Loc. cit., p. 671.
[4] Hüttl: Bruns Beitr., 163, 206, 1936.
[5] Chabanier, Puech, Lobo-Onell and Lelu: Presse médicale, 44, 938, 1936.

a more active form of tuberculosis, however, and died in April, 1935. The hypophysis, stained by the special stain of Dr. P. Bailey was entirely normal. The case did show, however, that it is possible to remove the pituitary and to produce in that way some amelioration of the diabetic condition.

Acute interstitial pancreatitis must be remembered in cases of diabetic coma which do not do well with insulin. In 3 cases at the Deaconess Hospital failure to recover from coma was proved at autopsy to be associated with acute septic pancreatitis.[1] Foord and Bowen[2] described 2 cases, aged twenty-three years and eighteen years respectively, with fatal fulminating coma and pancreatitis. In one case a large liver with extreme fatty metamorphosis, deposition of lipid substances in the abdominal lymph nodes, spleen, and kidney, and lipemia were present. Lewis[3] emphasizes care in giving glucose solutions in acute pancreatitis, since the intravenous administration of glucose may increase the damage by stimulating a further flow of pancreatic juice.

Cancer of the pancreas seems far more frequent today than in the past. Among 101 cases of malignant disease seen from 1934 to 1938 inclusive, there were 12 cases of carcinoma of the pancreas. (See page 657 for discussion.) Case 24332 after pancreatectomy for carcinoma on June 26, 1944, became sugar-free and was able to discontinue a previous dose of 28 units of insulin. On September 26, 1945 the blood sugar was 128 milligrams after lunch, without insulin.

R. FRACTURES AND DIABETES.

Fractures of bones in middle-aged or elderly diabetics are frequent, occur with slight trauma and present a serious problem in the hospital care of the elderly diabetics. Among 165 instances of fractures in diabetic patients, certain types stand out with especial importance. Sixteen cases of crushing of the vertebræ with little or no trauma in elderly diabetics with generalized osteoporosis have occurred. A crushed vertebra has been found following a convulsion due to insulin hypoglycemia in 2 cases. Patients under care in hospitals especially with foot lesions who are having limited exercise, because of unsteadiness and weakness, may slip either getting into bed or when rounding a corner. Instances of fractured skull, fractured collar-bone and fractured femur have occurred. Root, White and Marble[4] noted the following factors which might influence the calcium and phosphorus metabolism in diabetic patients: (1) age of patient, (2) activity, (3) amount of lime salts in the diet, (4) great excess in the diet of calcium over phosphorus and *vice versa*, (5) achlorhydria and diminished or lacking pancreatic lipolytic

[1] Root: Jour. Am. Med. Assn., **108**, 777, 1937.
[2] Foord and Bowen: Am. Jour. Med. Sci., **180**, 676, 1930.
[3] Lewis: New York State Jour. Med., **36**, 14, 1015, 1936.
[4] Root, White and Marble: Arch. Int. Med., **53**, 46, 1934.

ferment, (6) prolonged diarrhea, (7) prolonged acidosis, (8) excessive fat in the diet, particularly if unabsorbed, and (9) deficient supply of vitamin D.

Medical treatment must include an arrangement of the diet, particularly for middle-aged diabetic patients, such as will provide a minimum of 0.7 gram calcium daily and sufficient vitamin D substances.

S. BURNS.

Thermal injury to the skin and underlying tissues may have grave consequences in a diabetic. Experimentally, Clark and Rossiter[1] found that burning caused a rise in blood sugar of both rats and rabbits which was much greater in well fed rabbits than in starved animals. Taylor, Levenson and Adams[2] describe the frequent occurrence of hyperglycemia, lactacidemia and lowered carbon dioxide combining power of the blood in normal human subjects after thermal injuries.

Two diabetics treated at the Deaconess Hospital illustrate the most severe effects of thermal injury.[3] In an elderly housewife with mild diabetes under good control, who had previously suffered an amputation of the leg, the accidental spilling of boiling water on the body resulted in a third degree burn, nausea, vomiting and diabetic coma. She recovered from coma, but subsequently died from the infection of the burned areas. A young man received a sunburn which became infected with resultant paranephric abscess, metastatic osteomyelitis and amputation of the leg. In diabetic patients poorly controlled, normal glycogen stores are greatly reduced, but the amount of glucose present in blood, tissue fluid and skin is increased. The danger of burns in diabetic patients is vastly greater than in non-diabetic patients, partly because in a non-diabetic patient endogenous insulin is available whereas in diabetic patients the lack of insulin reserve makes possible the rapid development of serious disturbances in carbohydrate metabolism and even acidosis.

When a surgical diabetic is not doing well, do not blame the diabetes. The treatment of diabetes now rests upon so sure a scientific foundation that if the course of the patient is not favorable, one must suspect a complication. Where is the pus? Was the poor old man exposed to tuberculosis in his youth and has it now come to the fore? Has the frail old lady a carcinoma of the pancreas, which you could not detect when, forced by emergency, you removed her gall stones under novocaine? Has there been an advent of hyperthyroidism, hyperpituitarism or a tumor adjacent to the hypophysis? Remember that diabetes is a good disease, but has bad companions and these have injured her reputation. Attack them, not her.

[1] Clark and Rossiter: Quart. Jour. Exper. Physiol., **32**, 279, 1944.
[2] Taylor, Levenson and Adams: New England Jour. Med., **231**, 437, 1944.
[3] Root: New England Jour. Med., **232**, 279, 1945.

CHAPTER XXVII

CLINICAL DISORDERS OF THE GLANDS OF INTERNAL SECRETION COMPLICATING DIABETES.

REVISED BY HOWARD F. ROOT, M.D. AND PRISCILLA WHITE, M.D.

REFERENCE has been made repeatedly throughout the text to the close interrelationship between the various glands of internal secretion and the influence particularly of the pituitary, thyroid, and adrenal glands upon diabetes. The outstanding feature is the experimental production of diabetes by means of injections of anterior pituitary extract. (See page 121.) In this chapter will be considered certain of the clinical disorders of these glands (other than the pancreas) occurring in association with diabetes.

A. THE PITUITARY AND DIABETES.

Thirst with a history of being a "water drinker as long as I can remember" is a symptom not uncommonly volunteered by diabetic patients. This symptom together with the known tendency of diabetic children to be above height for their age at the onset of diabetes, the proved development of their bones a year in advance of their age, the peak of incidence of diabetes in children being at maturity—twelve years for our cases—the occurrence of glycosuria in pregnancy, the general frequency of obesity prior to the onset of diabetes in adults, and the onset of diabetes during the menopause, all suggest that the pituitary may be concerned in the development of diabetes.

1. **Hyperpituitarism.**—(a) **Incidence of Glycosuria.**—This view of the connection of the pituitary with the pancreas is strengthened by the fact that in disease of no other organ save the pancreas are glycosuria and diabetes so common. In 100 cases of proved acromegaly Davidoff and Cushing[1] found glycosuria in 25 per cent and diabetes in 12 per cent. Coggeshall and Root,[2] in a follow-up of these 100 cases with an addition of 53 later cases of acromegaly made possible through the courtesy of the late Professor Harvey Cushing and the Peter Bent Brigham Hospital, found that actually the incidence of glycosuria was 36 per cent. Analysis of these cases is given in further detail in later pages. Among these 153 acromegalics, 26, or 17 per cent, developed diabetes.

(b) **Character of Diabetes in Acromegaly.**—Since the first description of acromegaly by Pierre Marie, the development of diabetes in

---

[1] Davidoff and Cushing: Loc. cit., p. 120.
[2] Coggeshall and Root: Loc. cit., p. 86.

acromegalic patients has been frequently noted. The common impression is that the diabetes which is found in connection with acromegaly or other pituitary disease does not differ essentially at any given date from ordinary diabetes,[1,2,3] but that it varies from time to time according to the activity of the pituitary and in consequence a spontaneous, temporary or permanent cure of the diabetes may be effected. With the development of hyperthyroidism or myxedema in a diabetic patient the course of the diabetes is markedly altered, but no such clear dependence of the pancreas upon the thyroid is presented as is met with in disease of the pituitary. Practically the only temporary or permanent cures of diabetes recorded are those cases in which a pituitary factor has been present. The article by Davidoff and Cushing is replete with suggestive evidence.

Among these 29 cases of acromegaly with diabetes reported by Coggeshall and Root (26 from Cushing's series and 3 from the Deaconess Hospital), certain features stand out. Since acromegaly is often a fluctuating but progressive disease, usually of long duration, the time interval between the onset of acromegaly and the onset of diabetes might indicate to some degree the influence of hyperpituitarism as an etiological factor in diabetes. Also, the effects of treatment, either surgical or by means of roentgen-ray, in contrast to those patients receiving no treatment, might be significant. The evaluation of treatment, however, was difficult, since in cases presenting intracranial pressure, a high mortality-rate interfered with the period of observation. The average interval between the onset of acromegaly and that of diabetes was 9.5 years, but there were actual intervals of from one to twenty-two years with a majority of cases of diabetes occurring within fifteen years. In this series, 10 cases had some treatment directed toward the pituitary gland, but no characteristic difference in the time of appearance of diabetes in these cases was evident. Ten were males and 19 females; the average age at onset of diabetes was 38.8 years in both males and females, an age quite different from the median age at onset of 6357 diabetics, for whom it was 46.5 years for males and 49.2 years for females. The duration of the diabetes from onset to death or last observation varied from none to seventeen years, with an average of 8.6 years. Jews form 27 per cent of the acromegalic series, in contrast to the Jewish percentage of 11.6 per cent for all males and of 16.3 per cent for all females in the series of 6357 diabetics. (See page 47.)

A history of diabetes in the family was obtained in 6 of the 29 cases, whereas in the acromegalics without diabetes a family history of diabetes was found in only 3 of 124 cases.

The clinical course of the diabetes varied greatly. Three of the

[1] Colwell: Medicine, **6**, 1, 1927.
[2] John: Arch. Int. Med., **37**, 489, 1926.
[3] Yater: Arch. Int. Med., **41**, 883, 1928.

16 fatal cases are known to have died in coma. Twelve individuals in this series displayed no evidence of sterility, although it must be admitted that most of the children of these patients were born in the early years after the onset of the acromegaly. The common complications of diabetes were frequent. Arteriosclerosis and pyogenic infections occurred in 7 of the cases; thyroid enlargement was a common finding. One case had a thyroidectomy performed because the basal metabolism was plus 74 per cent. Dietary management was difficult because of the remarkable polyphagia present in some cases. In general mere restriction of carbohydrate seemed to have little effect on the fasting blood sugar. However, as a whole, the severity of the diabetes observed, while varying in degree, showed no greater variations than are seen in a large diabetic clinic.

The opinion that acromegalic diabetes does not differ essentially from ordinary diabetes has been challenged by several workers, including Davidoff and Cushing,[1] Hantschmann,[2] Lucke[3] and Meythaler and Schroff.[4] The action of insulin was thought to be normal by many other writers, including Blum and Schwab,[5] Colwell,[6] Labbé, Escolier and Dreyfus[7] and Peremy.[8]

Acromegaly of long duration is described in 4 cases with postmortem examinations by Goldberg and Lisser.[9] Ages at death range from thirty-seven to fifty-eight years, and the duration of the acromegaly from six to twenty-six years. Diabetes was present in 3 of the 4 cases, but had developed in 1 case only a few months before death, in the seventeenth year of the disease. This illustrates again the fact that the usual statistics upon the incidence of diabetes during acromegaly are unreliable since diabetes may not develop and usually does not occur for some years after the beginning of the disease. Those patients who have died from intercurrent infections or after operation, might well have developed diabetes had life been prolonged. All 4 cases in this series were given x-ray treatment, but the microscopic picture in 3 of the pituitary adenomas was that of actively functioning tissues. The insulin requirement in the first case was 50 units a day; the third case showed increasing insulin resistance, and required 50 units a day which had to be increased to 90 units in spite of a carefully weighed diet. She discontinued the insulin and was brought back to the hospital in diabetic acidosis. The patient later committed suicide. Irradiation of the pituitary seems to the authors to be the most effective form of treatment. Improvement in headache and vision should occur promptly. If no improvement occurs, the treatment should be repeated in

[1] Davidoff and Cushing: Loc. cit., p. 120.
[2] Hantschmann: Deutsch. med. Wchnschr., **60**, 498, 1934.
[3] Lucke: Ztschr. f. klin. Med., **122**, 23, 1932.
[4] Meythaler and Schroff: Klin. Wchnschr., **14**, 893, 1935.
[5] Blum and Schwab: Compt. rend. Soc. de biol., **89**, 195, 1923.
[6] Colwell: Loc. cit., p. 714.
[7] Labbé, Escolier and Dreyfus: Ann. de méd., **29**, 722, 1931.
[8] Peremy: Klin. Wchnschr., **14**, 92, 1935.
[9] Goldberg and Lisser: Jour. Clin. Endocr., **2**, 477, 1942.

two or three months. If then no remission is produced, the tumor should be considered as radio-resistant. The use of sex hormones in treatment was regarded as beneficial.

Cushing's syndrome has been recognized twice, Cases 13999 and 25930, the former consulting us for diabetes, the latter for obesity. Both had characteristic signs and symptoms of overactivity of baso- and eosinophilic cells, the presence of diabetes, hypertension, high excretion of 17-Ketosteroids, hirsutism, amenorrhea, loss of libido, purple striæ, lymphocytosis and osteoporosis. Both were treated with radiation. Case 13999 died August 24, 1939, four years later, of cerebral arteriosclerosis. A small tumor of the pituitary was found at autopsy.

Case 25930, aged twenty-three years, had gained 27 pounds during the two years that followed her marriage. Spontaneous compression fractures of the thoracic vertebræ occurred with persistent severe pain. Headache and rapid progression of weakness occurred. Exploration of the adrenals did not reveal any tumor. Trial with hormonal treatment was refused in favor of operation upon the pituitary gland. The anterior lobe of the pituitary was removed. Death followed within thirty-six hours. At autopsy a small basophilic tumor was found in the pituitary. The diabetes in this patient was mild in contrast to the patient of Pullen and Sodeman[1] who presented many symptoms of Cushing's syndrome, obesity, changes in the sex organs, hirsutism, and hypertension. Their patient received 260 units of crystalline insulin daily without any pronounced effect upon the carbohydrate metabolism and without insulin reactions. Four cases of Cushing's syndrome with alkalosis, low blood potassium, no tumor, no hyperplasia of adrenal cortex and transient diabetes are reported by Claxton, Bennett, Power and Kepler.[2]

TABLE 99.—THE BEHAVIOR OF THE BLOOD SUGAR IN 3 CASES OF ACROMEGALY UPON THE SIMULTANEOUS INJECTION OF INSULIN AND PITUITRIN. (DAVIDOFF AND CUSHING.)

	Case I.	Case II.	Case III.
Fasting . . .	0.33 per cent, 20 units insulin and 1 cc. pituitrin subcutaneously	0.13 per cent, 20 units insulin and 1 cc. pituitrin subcutaneously	0.15 per cent, 20 units insulin and 1 cc. pituitrin subcutaneously.
After two hours .	0.32	0.14	0.142
After four hours .	0.30	0.12	0.112

(c) **Antagonism of Pituitary Extracts and Insulin.**—The antagonism of pituitrin and insulin, first pointed out by Burn[3] and confirmed in Cushing's clinic, has been explained recently by Cori's experiments. (See page 115.) Davidoff and Cushing cite the following experiments. In 3 of their patients with acromegalic diabetes who had been shown to respond normally to insulin, 20 units of insulin

[1] Pullen and Sodeman: Jour. Clin. End., 3, 345, 1943.
[2] Claxton, Bennett, Power and Kepler: Jour. Clin. End., 5, 61. 1945.
[3] Burn: Jour. Physiol., 57, 318, 1923.

combined with 1 cc. of pituitrin were injected. The results are given in Table 99 and show that the expected fall in blood sugar at the end of a two-hour period had not occurred.

Ulrich[1] described a man, aged twenty-four years, in whom a pituitary tumor was discovered; a few months later glycosuria and hyperglycemia were so marked that within a few days the insulin requirement was increased to 360 units a day. Within a month, however, so rapid was the disappearance of glycosuria and the fall of the blood sugar that the urine remained sugar-free without the use of any insulin, and with a non-diabetic diet. Later he did require insulin again and he died after an operation for pituitary adenoma. Clearly the severity of diabetes associated with acromegaly fluctuated greatly and it may well be argued that the rapid change in the severity of the diabetes is due solely to the change in the anterior pituitary activity. Actually the results obtained in Ulrich's case with three or four weeks' treatment by use of insulin and diet were much better than are seen in ordinary patients with diabetes.

A new interpretation of the results obtained in this case is well supported by the fact that Best[2] has been able to show that the development of diabetes by means of daily injections of anterior pituitary extract can be prevented if the animal receives at the same time with the injections of pituitary extract sufficiently large amounts of insulin. It is clear that in some way insulin is able to neutralize the diabetogenic effect of injections of the pituitary extract. Cori's demonstration that insulin removes the inhibiting effect of the anterior pituitary upon the action of the enzyme hexokinase, which with adenosine triphosphate converts glucose to glucose-6-phosphate could explain this phenomenon. (See page 115.) In Ulrich's case, therefore, it seems reasonable to assume that at the time when 360 units of insulin a day were required, the effect of this large dose of insulin was to prevent serious damage to the islands of Langerhans which might have resulted from the excessive strain imposed by the temporary hypersecretion of a diabetogenic substance of the anterior pituitary gland.

The fluctuating character of acromegalic glycosuria is its striking feature. Hyperpituitarism as expressed by acromegaly is not a steadily progressive disorder any more than is hyperthyroidism. Davidoff and Cushing write as follows: "There are distinct waves of what the patient recognizes as more or less intense periods of 'acromegalism.' Some pronounced acromegalics go through a long life very little troubled by these symptoms; others are continually more or less miserable from the toxic effects of the disease. Still other patients may never have more than a single primary wave of transient hyperpituitarism, and such evidences of overgrowth as may have been occasioned remain barely discernible. Indeed, the

[1] Ulrich: Arch. Int. Med., **43**, 785, 1929.
[2] Best: Loc. cit., page 99.

acidophilic adenoma which is unquestionably the underlying lesion may become completely degenerated and cystic, just as may a thyroadenoma, and signs of actual pituitary insufficiency come to be superimposed on the relics of a once active acromegaly. With these peculiarities of acromegaly in mind one can appreciate how it happens that acromegalics may show waves of melituria, even periods which justify the designation of actual diabetes and yet spontaneously recover from them, irrespective of any dietary restrictions or treatment by insulin."

Young's experiments show that in dogs slight to severe and temporary to permanent changes in the islands of Langerhans can be produced by varying the amounts of the anterior pituitary extract which is injected.

Young[1] suggests that the diabetogenic action of anterior pituitary extract in normal animals might be due to a combined action of as many as three different factors. Thus, Long has found prolactin is particularly effective as a diabetogenic agent when the dog has had a surgical removal of the hypophysis and the pancreas. A second substance is the ketogenic pituitary substance. It may be required when ketonuria is produced. The third factor is a labile factor, essential for the production of glycosuria in the dog, and this factor is less stable than the ketogenic factor.

(d) **Effect of Irradiation of the Pituitary Gland**—Pijoan and Zollinger[2] studied the carbohydrate metabolism of patients undergoing massive radiations of the pituitary regions because of the menopausal syndrome before and after the radiations. Ten patients, whose ages varied from twenty-nine to fifty years, received a total of 1400 to 1600 R skin doses over a period of fourteen days. Their blood-sugar curves were obtained after the oral administration of 1 gram dextrose per kilogram body weight. The results showed no essential difference between the curves obtained before the radiation and after. They conclude, then, that such radiation of the pituitary gland caused no change whatever in carbohydrate metabolism.

Weinstein[3] describes a white woman who developed acromegaly at the age of twenty-three years. At the end of six years the evidence of a tumor of the pituitary was so impressive that radiation of the pituitary was carried out. The result was prompt and brilliant. The headache and eye symptoms disappeared and after a childless marriage of ten years' duration the patient gave birth to a healthy infant in 1936, eight years after the roentgen-ray treatment.

Attempts have been made to suppress the activity of the anterior lobe of the pituitary gland and thereby to reduce the severity of human diabetes by the administration of estrogenic substances. In depancreatized dogs some diminution in the glycosuria following

---

[1] Young: Proc. Roy. Soc. Med., **31**, 45, 1938.
[2] Pijoan and Zollinger: Endocrinology, **21**, 357, 1937.
[3] Weinstein: Ann. Int. Med., **13**, 720, 1939.

such estrogenic substances has been reported. Attempts, however, to treat diabetic patients with such injections of estrogenic substances have met with slight or indifferent success. At present there is no adequate evidence that the administration of such substances, capable of depressing one function of the pituitary, has any significant effect on human diabetes mellitus. (See page 126.)

(e) **Illustrative Cases.**—Various clinicians have from time to time reported groups of cases of hyperpituitarism and diabetes. Thus Yater[1] studied 79 acromegalic patients, finding glycosuria in 10 per cent of them. Marañon and Morros[2] observed 4 cases of glycosuria in 26 acromegalic patients (15 per cent). Ortiz and Rothmann[3] report 3 cases of diabetes with tumors of the pituitary, 2 of whom had acromegaly. They noted the aggravation of the diabetes during the period of active development of the hyperpituitarism. John[4] has described 3 cases of acromegaly with diabetes, in 2 of which the onset of acromegaly preceded the onset of diabetes. Ralli[5] has reported an interesting case of a woman, aged thirty-seven years, suffering from acromegaly with diabetes and xanthoma diabeticorum. The hypercholesteremia and lipemia responded well to insulin and diet, but in spite of this the xanthomatous tumors regressed slowly.

Grau,[6] *et al.* report a similar case in a fifteen year old girl. Squires and Thannhauser[7] report a cure of acromegaly with secondary multiple endocrine insufficiencies. Rocca and Peres[8] report an acromegalic treated with estradiol with some success. Daugherty,[9] among 425 cases of diabetes, found one with hyperpituitarism.

In addition to the 29 cases of acromegaly and diabetes reported by Coggeshall and Root, the following 2 were observed at the George F. Baker Clinic recently.

Case 19000, Italian housewife, aged fifty-three years at her first visit in 1940. About 1926 the hands, feet and face began to enlarge gradually. In 1931 she began to have a beard, her hair became thin and her voice husky. Menses began at sixteen years and were always regular, menopause at forty-seven years. She began the use of insulin in December 1937, and required 55 units in 1940. For five years she had had poor vision in the left eye. The hair was sparse and dry, the skin wrinkled, jaw prognathous, eyebrow ridges thick, ears large. Mental state was good. Fundi: primary atrophy in the left eye, right eye normal. Bitemporal hemianopsia to gross

---

[1] Yater: Loc. cit., p. 714.

[2] Marañon and Morros: Endocrinology, **13**, 564, 1929.

[3] Ortiz and Rothmann: Anal. Ateneo clin. méd., **1**, 274, 1931.

[4] John: Arch. Int. Med., **37**, 489, 1926.

[6] Grau Triana, Arguelles Casals, Romero Jordan and Bulle Merry: Loc. cit., p. 595.

[6] Grau, *et al:* Vide Nueva, **53**, 274, 1944.

[7] Squires and Thannhauser: Bull. N. E. Med. Center, **3**, 335, 1941.

[8] Rocca and Peres: Dia. Mid., **17**, 66, 1945.

[9] Daugherty: Penn. Med. Jour., **45**, 229, 1941.

tests. Muscle power reduced. No atrophy or spasticity. Sensations normal, reflexes active, equal and normal. Coördination good. Hands and feet were large, spatulate, with thick pads and subcutaneous tissue. Hirsutes on the face. The tongue was large and beefy.

Roentgenograms showed (1) a tumor of the pituitary with calcification in the tumor mass and compression of the floor of the sella; (2) tufting of the terminal phalanges. B.M.R. was +30, cholesterol 256 mg. The diabetes was controlled on a diet of carbohydrate 216, protein 96 and fat 85 grams with 40 units of protamine zinc insulin plus 14 units of crystalline insulin every morning. Blood-sugar values ranged from 160 to 260 mg. In April, 1941 she required 80 units of protamine zinc insulin daily She died July 6, 1945 with gangrene of one foot and uremia.

Case 27129, German housewife, aged forty-two years at onset of diabetes, had developed acromegaly five years previously. Although her blood sugar was 616 mg. on September 17, 1945, the diabetes was soon controlled with a single dose of 20 units of protamine zinc insulin. A large adenomatous goiter with intrathoracic extension was removed by Dr. S. F. Marshall on December 3, 1945.

The possibility that hyperpituitarism may exist for brief periods or without very obvious evidences and may thus be the cause of the diabetes, must lead to a thorough search for symptoms and signs. Coggeshall and Root tabulated 100 cases of acromegaly and 100 cases of diabetes with a comparison of the symptoms and signs recorded in the two groups. It is evident that certain symptoms, such as the disturbances of the menstrual cycle, headaches, diminished libido, amenorrhea, increased basal metabolism, visual disturbances, excessive perspiration, obesity and polydipsia occur with rather striking frequency in both conditions. However, until more accurate diagnostic procedures are known, we can only entertain suspicions as to the actual faults of the pituitary in cases that do not show the outspoken evidences of overgrowth of skeleton or soft tissue.

Weight of Visceral Organs in Acromegaly and Diabetes.—The clinical course of acromegaly has been divided into three periods by Davidoff: (1) the early period with general overgrowth, gain in weight and menstrual disturbances; (2) the middle period with neighborhood symptoms from pressure, visual disturbances, increases in the sella turcica; and (3) the final period with polyphagia and polydipsia, etc., due to visceral splanchnomegaly and secondary effects upon the other endocrine organs. The splanchnomegaly of acromegaly is a true overgrowth of all tissues and not due merely to laying down of excess fat or to increased water in the tissues. It is assumed that the enlargement of acra as well as the splanchnomegaly is due to excessive production of a hormone secreted by the acidophilic cells of an anterior pituitary adenoma. One must suppose that excessive development of diabetes in such patients is also due to this same agent acting either directly or indirectly upon the islands of Langerhans. In either case under the influence of such a substance, we would expect to find some relation between the weight of the pancreas and the weight of other organs of diabetic patients as occurred in acromegaly. To test this hypothesis, Coggeshall and Root, therefore, tabulated the weights of tissues in 11 acromegalic patients in Table 100, together with the weights of tissues in groups of diabetics and in cases of Simmonds' disease.

It will be seen that the acromegalic patients are divided into three groups: (1) those without diabetes; (2) those in whom the acromegaly was fugitive, in the sense that the overgrowth in the acra and jaw developed at ages varying from seventeen to thirty-eight years, but no further changes followed; and (3) those with diabetes and acromegaly. Definite acromegaly was present both in the patients with acromegaly alone and in those with diabetes in addition to acromegaly. It is true that the average weight of the heart was 605 grams in patients with diabetes in contrast to 743 grams in acromegalics without diabetes. The liver of the diabetics on the average weighed 2645 grams, whereas the liver of the acromegalics without diabetes weighed 2937 grams. The kidneys of the diabetics weighed 671 grams, whereas the kidneys in acromegalics without diabetes weighed 633 grams. Similar differences appeared in the weights of the spleen and adrenals. Unfortunately, there is a record of the weight of the thyroid gland in only one of the acromegalics with diabetes, although in two others the thyroid was noted as being large. It is of interest that the weight of the pancreas averaged 149 grams both in the acromegalics without, and those with, diabetes.

The group classified as fugitive acromegalics requires some further explanation. In each at autopsy a mixed tumor of the pituitary was found. The tumors contained both chromophobe and chromophilic tumors. Case IV died of a subdural hemorrhage. Case V died of myocarditis and chronic interstitial nephritis, and thus an adequate explanation for the enlargement of the heart was found. Case VI died of a hemorrhage into a pituitary cyst or a cystic area in the pituitary tumor. Case VII died of congestion of the lungs, probably cardiac in origin. Possibly the excessive function of the acidophilic cells of the tumor had been checked after a period by some influence such as the pressure of the chromophobe portion of the tumor.

In all the acromegalic patients, with and without diabetes, acidophilic tumors were found. The size of the tumors varied from a tumor so small that as in Case I, who suffered to the fullest extent from the classical picture of acromegaly, it had produced no enlargement of the sella turcica, to tumors which had extended far beyond the confines of the sella turcica as in Case II.

The diabetic patients are divided into three groups, according to pancreas weights. From the 14 cases in which the pancreas weighed more than 120 grams is excluded one case with a large carcinoma of

46

the pancreas, weighing 450 grams. In the others fatty invasion largely accounted for the excessive weight. In the diabetic group with small pancreases weighing 40 grams or less is included one

TABLE 100.—COMPARATIVE WEIGHTS OF ORGANS IN DIABETES AND PITUITARY DISEASE.[4]

	Autopsies.	Ht., cm.	Wt., kg.	Heart.	Liver.	Kidneys.	Spleen.	Thyroid.	Adrenals.	Pancreas.
	Normal male	172	70	350	1500	300	200	25	12	80
Acromegalics without diabetes	I. Male, age 52 Duration 30 years[1]	185	97	1050	3150	853	535	310	43	225
	II. Male, age 40 Duration 13 years[1]	198	122.4	480	3380	565	385	105	43	83
	III. Female, age 39 Duration 26 years	164.5	62.1	700	2280	480	260	20	33	140
	Average	183	94	743	2937	633	393	145	39	149
Fugitive acromegalics	IV. Male, age 63 Duration 25 years	177	66.2	280	1545	200	200			
	V. Female, age 55 Duration 23 years	..	..	500	1700	350	205	140		
	VI. Male, age 57 Duration 40 years	182	70.6	300	1720	300	220			
	VII. Male, age 42 Duration 13 years	172	98.6	330	2015	360	450			
	Average	177	78	352	1745	303	269			
Acromegalics with diabetes	VIII. Male, age 35[1] Duration 15 years	173	100	1000	2480	650	..	100	30	150
	IX. Female, age 51[1] Duration 21 years	157	68	460	2500	695	240	..	18	
	X. Male, age 58 Duration 23 years	168	91	600	2900	460	330	'enlarged'	28	180
	XI. Male, age 42 Duration 17 years	187	108	360	2700	880	240	'enlarged'	..	117
	Average	171	92	605	2645	671	270	..	25	149
Diabetics:	Group I (14 cases) more than 120 gm.	168	88	410	1978	382	269	20	normal	152[2]
Large pancreas	Group II (23 cases) between 100–200 gm.	165	88	272	1645	375	156	21	normal	106
Small pancreas	Group III (13 cases) 40 gm. or less	164	78	359	1630	312	115	19	normal	32
Simmonds' disease		..	..	175	982	237	85	20	19	67
		170	50	200	850	150	..	13.5	6	40[3]
		157	50	290	1400	260	..	17	8	100[3]

[1] See Cushing, Harvey, and Davidoff, L. M.:   Monograph 22, Rockefeller Institute for Medical Research 1926; for complete discussion of these autopsies.
[2] Excluding 1 case with carcinomatous masses.
[3] Gallavan and Steedman: Arch. Int. Med., 59, 865, 1937
[4] Coggeshall and Root: Loc. cit., p. 86.

pancreas weighing only 15 grams, of a woman who died in the Deaconess Hospital after observation for nearly ten years. There was no very close correlation between the weight of the diabetic patient and the weight of the pancreas. The average maximum weight of the diabetic patients with large pancreases was 175 pounds and average height 65 inches. The average weight of the diabetic patients with small pancreases was 141 pounds and the average height 63 inches. The striking features in the diabetic group are, therefore, the lack of correlation between the weight of the pancreas and the weight of the heart, liver, kidneys, spleen or thyroid. As a matter of fact, in the first group of diabetic patients with large pancreases the average weight of the liver, 1978 grams, is due to the inclusion in this group of 6 patients who had a definite reason for congestion and enlargement of the liver, including chronic cardiac failure and cirrhosis of the liver. In contrast 2 cases of Simmonds' disease showed great reduction in weight of all organs.

From the Mayo Clinic Wilder[1] reports 20 cases of acromegaly among 9377 diabetics. He also points out that these 20 instances of diabetes occurred in 218 cases of acromegaly and included 13 frank cases of diabetes, an incidence of only 6 per cent. The thyroid was adenomatous in one-half the cases and in some the diabetes preceded the acromegaly. He holds that "the hypophysis is not of such great importance in the production of clinical diabetes as has been supposed."

Peck and Sage[2] implicate the pituitary in the case of diabetes and Albright's syndrome (osteitis fibrosa disseminata, areas of skin pigmentation and endocrine dysfunction with precocious puberty in females) which they report.

Houssay and Foglia[3] find meta hypophyseal diabetes similar to pancreatic diabetes.

Summary.—From this comparison of the actual weights of organs in diabetes and pituitary disease, one must conclude that there is no suggestion of any influence upon the weight of tissues of the diabetic patient by any substance such as is responsible for the enlargement of the skeleton and the visceral organs in patients with acromegaly.

The outstanding fact is the great rarity of acromegaly or gigantism in the diabetic clinic. Thus, only 5 cases of acromegaly and 3 of gigantism have occurred in some 17,000 diabetic patients. On the other hand, 17 per cent of 153 acromegalic patients developed diabetes. Acromegalic diabetics may develop coma and, therefore, require the same careful adjustment of diet and insulin as non-acromegalic diabetics of similar severity.

Basophilic adenomata have been proven in 2 cases.

[1] Wilder, pp. 263, 264; Loc. cit., p. 55.
[2] Peck and Sage: Am. Jour. Med. Sci., **208**, 35, 1944.
[3] Houssay and Foglia: Rev. de la Biol., **20**, 247, 1944.

2. Hypopituitarism. — Just as with increased secretion of the anterior lobe glycosuria appears, with decreased secretion the tolerance for carbohydrate is raised. This is shown in the animal experiments of Houssay already discussed on page 121.

Cushing has called attention to the abnormally low level of the blood sugar in dystrophia adiposogenitalis, as have also Marañon and Morros,[1] who state that in conditions of underfunctioning of the pituitary, particularly in Froelich's syndrome, diabetes is very rare and an increase in carbohydrate tolerance is almost always observed. In their own series of 115 hypopituitary patients of all kinds they found spontaneous glycosuria in only 2 cases, a father and son. They mentioned also the fact that extirpation of the hypophysis raises the carbohydrate tolerance and increases the individual's sensitiveness to insulin. The association of clinical diabetes and hypopituitarism should be rare, but Wilder[2] states that it is not uncommon with newer techniques of determining such pituitary hormones as FSH and 17-ketosteroid excretion to find that the incidence of hypopituitary diabetes decreases. We have observed *one* such case—pituitary myxedema. Daugherty[3] reports one in 425 diabetics.

The opposite—increase in tolerance for carbohydrate and sensitivity to insulin is the rule. Heinbecker[4] reports loss of eosinophilic cells and adrenal cortical atrophy in insulin sensitivity.

3. Diabetes Insipidus and Diabetes Mellitus. —Allan and Rowntree[5] have described 2 cases in which diabetes insipidus with diabetes mellitus occurred together and 1 case in which transitory glycosuria preceded diabetes insipidus. The relationship of these two diseases is still uncertain. It is stated that the disturbance of carbohydrate metabolism encountered can usually be controlled by diet and insulin and the use of pituitary extract for control of polyuria does not interfere with the effectiveness of insulin. Association of the two diseases has been described by Lawrence and McCance,[6] by Moloney,[7] whose patient, a woman aged sixty-three years was dramatically relieved by the use of posterior pituitary extract, and by Rutledge and Rynearson,[8] whose patient, an obese woman, had mild diabetes mellitus and whose symptoms of diabetes insipidus were relieved by nasal insufflation of powdered posterior pituitary glands. The development of diabetes insipidus in a woman aged twenty-five years at the onset of diabetes mellitus and who later became pregnant and had diabetic coma, is described by Greene and

[1] Marañon and Morros: Loc. cit., p. 719.
[2] Wilder, p. 265; Loc. cit., p. 55.
[3] Daugherty: Loc. cit., p. 719.
[4] Heinbecker and Rolf: Am. Jour. Physiol., 141, 566, 1944.
[5] Allan and Rowntree: Endocrinology, 15, 97, 1931.
[6] Lawrence and McCance: Lancet, 1, 76, 1933.
[7] Moloney: New Zealand Med. Jour., 38, 263, 1939.
[8] Rutledge and Rynearson: Proc. Staff Meet. Mayo Clin., 14, 441, 1939.

Gibson,[1] who found in the literature up to 1939 only 20 cases in which diabetes mellitus and diabetes insipidus coexisted. They quote Soule,[2] who found only 37 incidences of pregnancy in cases of diabetes insipidus.

McPherson's[3] case, a sixty-year-old man, had moderately severe diabetes which later became mild as symptoms of diabetes insipidus appeared. He died after a femoral thrombosis and at autopsy relative hyperplasia of the eosinophilic cells of the pituitary was reported. However, diabetes insipidus has not been a characteristic feature of cases of acromegaly where known eosinophilic tumors were present. At the post mortem examination of the 53 year old man reported by Gray and Moffat,[4] certain pathological changes consistent with current concepts of diabetes insipidus were noted in the pars intermedia and pars neuralis of the pituitary gland.

Case 16762, male, had an extraordinary history of diabetes insipidus for six years with spontaneous relief. At the age of fifty-nine years he began to drink every five to fifteen minutes and passed urine at the same rate. He could not leave the house and had to give up his work. He drank about 5 gallons a day. This continued for six years and then gradually disappeared. True diabetes mellitus came on three years later. He died of cerebral hemorrhage August 16, 1939, at the age of seventy years.

B. THE THYROID AND DIABETES.

1. **Hyperthyroidism.**—Before the days of insulin and modern surgery the association of two such dynamic diseases as diabetes and hyperthyroidism was a catastrophe, because each accentuated and accelerated the downward course of the other. Even today, although the combination of diabetes and hyperthyroidism is amenable to treatment, it requires little imagination to perceive that one is dealing with a highly powered, highly geared machine, which is always traveling at an excessive rate of speed. Any trifling defect in the machine soon makes itself apparent, and even a slight divergency from the routine pathway of treatment which would be negligible with the diseases apart can promote disaster when they are combined. The dramatic physical improvement noted in the hyperthyroid diabetic a few weeks after operation, if uncontrolled by chemical tests, would be most deceptive. The casual observer would conclude that the large majority of these patients had been cured and it is with some disappointment that one must record that complete recovery has, as yet, not taken place in any case in our experience. The effect of hyperthyroidism is probably dual, according to Wilder.[5] There is an adrenergic-like action which interferes

[1] Greene and Gibson: J. Lab. and Clin. Med., **24**, 455, 1939.
[2] Soule: Am. Jour. Obst. and Gynec., **33**, 878, 1937.
[3] McPherson: Glasgow Med. Jour., **131**, 220, 1939.
[4] Gray and Moffat: Endocrinology, **27**, 430, 1940.
[5] Wilder; p. 246. Loc. cit., p. 55.

with the storage of glycogen or increases the release of glycogen and, secondly, there is an antagonism to the action of insulin. The fact that the requirement for injected insulin increases in the diabetic with hyperthyroidism suggests that in the non-diabetic patient the pancreas must be stimulated by hyperthyroidism to provide a larger amount of insulin. Glaser[1] noted hydropic degeneration and atrophy in the pancreatic islands of mice after injections of thyroxin which suggests the exhaustion by stimulation such as Young obtained with repeated injections of extract of the anterior lobe of the pituitary. It was striking that the pancreas of Case 4289, who died after a thyroid storm, showed rather large islands of Langerhans. On the other hand, some postmortem studies of pancreases in cases of exophthalmic goiter have shown a decrease in the amount of islet tissue. Wilder believes that in the non-diabetic patient with hyperthyroidism the supply of insulin from the pancreas is sufficiently increased to maintain normal utilization of dextrose, but, even so, complete stabilization of liver glycogen in the face of a hyperirritable sympathetic nervous system may be impossible.

The series of diabetics with hyperthyroidism reported in 1928 and 1934 with Dr. F. H. Lahey[2] have been brought up to January 1, 1946, by the addition of 76 cases shown in Table 101, a total of 256 cases. The first report concerned 43 patients with primary and 28 with secondary hyperthyroidism, of whom 63 were operated upon (there were in addition 2 operative cases and 2 non-operative cases with hyperthyroidism with type unknown). A second study was made[3] of 33 cases of primary and 30 of secondary hyperthyroidism, of whom 56 were operated upon. Reviews have been published in this country on this same topic by Fitz[4] and by Wilder.[5] In the series of the former there were described 39 thyroid diabetics, and in that of the latter 99 cases. John[6] has contributed various articles. Foster and Lowrie[7] report 42 cases of diabetes associated with hyperthyroidism at the Henry Ford Hospital from 1925 to 1938.

(a) Incidence of Glycosuria.—Hyperthyroidism is the fundamental factor in disease of the thyroid which leads to glycosuria. This is evident from the incidence of glycosuria in 500 cases of disease of the thyroid in the Lahey series: primary hyperthyroidism 38.6 per cent, adenomatous goiter with secondary hyperthyroidism 27.7 per cent, non-toxic goiter 14.8 per cent.

In John's series[6] of 100 dextrose-tolerance tests in 82 cases of hyperthyroidism and 10 cases of colloid goiter there was fasting

[1] Glaser: Arch. f. Entwicklngsmech. d. Organ., 107, 98–128, 1926.
[2] Joslin and Lahey: Loc. cit., p. 709.
[3] Joslin and Lahey: Loc. cit., p. 709.
[4] Fitz: Arch. Int. Med., 27, 305, 1921.
[5] Wilder: Arch. Int. Med., 38, 736, 1926; p. 244, Loc. cit., p. 55.
[6] John: Ann. Surg., 87, 37, 1928; Endocrinology, 11, 497, 1927; Jour. Am. Med Assn., 99, 620, 1932; Am. Jour. Dig. Dis. and Nutr., 4, 4, 1937.
[7] Foster and Lowrie: Endocrinology, 23, 681, 1938.

glycosuria in 19 per cent. Hatlehol[1] performed glucose tolerance tests on 17 patients suffering from hyperthyroidism and 7 patients with hypothyrosis. Each group was tested both before operation or treatment with thyroid extract and afterwards. Abnormalities appeared in the carbohydrate metabolism during thyrotoxicosis, but they disappeared after operation upon the thyroid gland. He found no good proof that thyrotoxicosis prediposes to diabetes. Neither did he find any evidence which proved that in hypothyrosis the carbohydrate metabolism deviated from normal.

(*b*) **Incidence of Hyperglycemia.**—In hyperthyroidism the fasting blood sugar is usually normal. Evidently the changes in carbohydrate metabolism occurring in connection with the thyroid gland are concerned more with its function than with its anatomical structure, and this suggests that a similar relation may hold with the pancreas. In other words, the removal of nineteen-twentieths of the pancreas is a gross method of producing diabetes. A far more natural method would be a procedure which would influence the function of the gland. This is accomplished temporarily in diabetes by an infection. An infection similarly intensifies hyperthyroidism.

(*c*) **The Diagnosis of Diabetes in Thyroid Disease.**—Acknowledging the disturbance of carbohydrate metabolism in hyperthyroidism as shown by the frequency of glycosuria and hyperglycemia, one wonders about the closeness of the relation between the two diseases or symptom complexes, diabetes and hyperthyroidism. Are these totally distinct diseases, fortuitously occurring together on rare occasions? Does one cause the other or is either an etiological factor in the development of the other?[2] Does true diabetes ever occur in hyperthyroidism unless there has been the diabetic "anlage" in the Naunyn sense? Moreover, is the disturbance of carbohydrate metabolism of hyperthyroidism any more than one might obtain as a result of increased metabolism from any other cause, such as that which occurs in fever or after exercise? Recognizing the disturbed carbohydrate metabolism in hyperthyroidism, how far can it proceed before one must classify it as diabetes? These questions illustrate the complexity of the problem which is, furthermore, increased by the circumstance that after operation and cure of the hyperthyroidism a slight disturbance of carbohydrate metabolism may return to normal. It is evident that one must be cautious or one will find himself making many diagnoses of diabetes and attaining many cures of a disease in which as yet one hesitates to advance such claims. For this reason the diagnosis of diabetes in hyperthyroidism must rest on a different basis from that usually adopted. Ordinarily a patient is said to have diabetes who has certain charac-

---

[1] Hatlehol: Acta med. Scandin., **77**, 558, 1932.

[2] Labbé (Ned. Tidj. v. Gen., **81**, 237, 1937) held that the frequency of diabetes in association with exophthalmic goiter is so great as to indicate clearly an endocrine relationship.

teristic symptoms, a glycosuria varying with the diet and a blood sugar of 0.13 per cent or higher fasting, or 0.17 per cent or higher after a meal. For the present, therefore, and to avoid premature diabetic cures, we have raised the standard for a diagnosis of diabetes in hyperthyroidism to a blood sugar of 0.15 per cent fasting, or 0.2 per cent or more after meals in addition to glycosuria. Wilder[1] was evidently forced to a similar conclusion and, like Fitz[2] and ourselves, has been extremely careful to exclude any but true diabetics.

(d) **The Incidence of Associated Diabetes and Hyperthyroidism.**— Our 256 cases of combined diabetes and hyperthyroidism occurring in 25,148 true diabetics constitute an incidence of 1.0 per cent. Certainly allowance must be made for some errors of diagnosis and also for the fact that hyperthyroidism may have been present and treated elsewhere subsequent to the patient's observation at the Deaconess Hospital. Furthermore, among this large number of diabetic patients many have as yet had diabetes for so short a period of time that opportunity has not been sufficiently great to allow for the occurrence of hyperthyroidism.

The incidence of diabetes at the Mayo Clinic in all cases of hyperthyroidism increased from 1.1 per cent among 3471 cases during the years 1923–1926, to 3.3 per cent among 1882 cases in the years 1935–1938, an increase which Wilder attributed to the mounting incidence of diabetic morbidity in the population. He also points out that the incidence of diabetes among patients with adenomatous goiter and hyperthyroidism was 5.6 per cent in the later period, whereas the incidence of diabetes among patients with exophthalmic goiter at the same time was only 1.7 per cent. It is obvious that the incidence of diabetes in cases of hyperthyroidism is much lower than the incidence of diabetes in acromegaly which Coggeshall and Root[3] found to be 17 per cent in their series.

(e) **Priority in Appearance of Diabetes or Hyperthyroidism.**—If a marked priority in the appearance of symptoms of diabetes or hyperthyroidism could be demonstrated, it would be of significance in the relation of the two conditions to one another. Such a demonstration, however, is not so simple as might be thought, because of the uncertain onset of each. Of the two the period of onset of diabetes is rather more easily determined. With some reservation as to their real value, the statistics of the series of Wilder and our own can be interpreted.

The earlier series of thyroid diabetics indicated that hyperthyroidism preceded the diabetes in cases of primary hyperthyroidism in from 75 to 85 per cent of the cases. In cases of adenoma with hyperthyroidism the hyperthyroidism preceded the diabetes in from 47 to 62 per cent of the cases. However, in the report by Regan

[1] Wilder: p. 249, loc. cit., p. 55.   [2] Fitz: Loc. cit., p. 726.
[3] Coggeshall and Root: Loc. cit., p. 86.

and Wilder[1] the hyperthyroidism preceded the diabetes in only 52 per cent of the cases of primary hyperthyroidism and 62 per cent in the cases of adenoma with secondary hyperthyroidism. In our third series, hyperthyroidism was first to develop in 6 and apparently at the same time in 8 of 29 cases of primary hyperthyroidism and was primary in only 8 of 17 cases of adenoma with secondary hyperthyroidism. A similar relationship holds in our fourth series. The question whether hyperthyroidism therefore commonly provokes the onset of diabetes is still not very well answered. An important point in our two recent series is the fact that a known heredity of diabetes was present in the family in 52 per cent. This is a higher incidence than is ordinarily found in adult series.

TABLE 101.—INCIDENCE OF HYPERTHYROIDISM WITH OPERATION IN 25,148 CASES OF TRUE DIABETES MELLITUS.

	No. of cases.	Cases operated upon.	Sex.		Av. age, onset of diabetes.	Av. age at operation.
			Male.	Female.		
Series 1928:[1]						
Primary hyperthyroidism	43	37	10	33	40.5	43.7
Adenoma and secondary hyperthyroidism	28	26	4	24	47.8	51.5
Total	71	63	14	57		
Series 1934:[2]						
Primary hyperthyroidism	33	30	9	24	42.0	43.0
Adenoma and secondary hyperthyroidism	30	26	5	25	55.0	58.0
Total	63	56	14	49		
Series 1939:[3,4]						
Primary hyperthyroidism	29[4]	29	7	22	42.3	46.0
Adenoma and secondary hyperthyroidism[5]	17[4]	17	4	13	52.4	58.1
Total	46	46	11	35		
Series 1940—Jan. 1, 1946						
Primary	45	45	14	31	40.5	45.7
Adenoma and secondary hyperthyroidism	30	30	3	27	50.2	51.0
Cancer	1	1	..	1		
Total	76	76	17	59		

[1] Joslin and Lahey: Loc. cit., p. 709.
[2] Joslin and Lahey: Loc. cit., p. 709.
[3] Cases from January 1, 1934 through June 16, 1939.
[4] Includes operated cases only.
[5] Excludes 12 non-toxic adenomatous goiters, and 1 case of abscess of thyroid.

(*f*) **Physiological Considerations.**—Hyperthyroidism and a disturbance of sugar metabolism, and even diabetes, are distinctly related, as shown by statistical evidence. Thus, in 38.6 per cent of cases

[1] Regan and Wilder: Arch. Int. Med., **65**, 1116, 1940.

of primary hyperthyroidism and in 27.7 per cent of cases of secondary hyperthyroidism there was glycosuria, and diabetes was present in 2.5 per cent of the former and 4.3 per cent of the latter.

Diabetes[1] with acute lesions of beta cells may result from thyroid feeding of animals with pancreas reduced to one-fifth of normal or those treated with anterior pituitary extract. Diabetic symptoms follow the administration of thyroid to diabetic animals.

Thyroidectomy in normal animals increases the tolerance for carbohydrate, may lead to hypoglycemia, and causes a definite increase in sensitivity to insulin for ten to twenty days after operation. In the following ten days this returns to normal and eventually there is a heightened tolerance toward insulin.[2] Yet Richardson, Levine and DuBois[3] found that the glycogen reserves of 2 patients with exophthalmic goiter were apparently as great as normal. The problem is confused by an increase of the blood-sugar threshold found as a result of thyroid feeding, which makes it difficult to determine the carbohydrate utilization.[4]

Althausen *et al.* showed a difference in the blood galactose curves following oral administration in contrast to intravenous administration. (See page 153.)

The work of Burn and Marks[5] and that of Bodansky[6] throws additional light on the relationship of the thyroid and the pancreas. They found that either by the feeding of thyroid gland or by injections of thyroid substance the liver is made hypersensitive (overresponsive) for the discharge of its sugar, as a result of some stimulation which favors the conversion of glycogen into sugar. If the discharge of glycogen is prevented by section of the splanchnics, a dose of insulin, which was without effect before the operation, now produces severe symptoms.

Similarly should thyroidectomy be performed instead of severing the splanchnics, convulsions would be produced with one-third, one-fifth or even one-sixth the dose of insulin necessary before the operation. Here, too, the conversion of glycogen into sugar and its discharge from the liver as sugar is prevented as a result of the thyroidectomy and in consequence less insulin is required to reduce the sugar in the blood and convulsions result.

If thyroid is fed, insulin acts less well. If, however, thyroid feeding is continued for more than ten days the reserve of glycogen in the liver becomes exhausted. Should insulin be injected at this time, convulsions are produced with less than the usual dose of insulin. The glycogen in the liver shows no change in the early

[1] Houssay and deFinis: Jour. Am. Med. Assn., **123**, 50, 1943.
[2] Britton: Am. Jour. Physiol., **84**, 133, 1928.
[3] Richardson, Levine and DuBois: Jour. Biol. Chem., **67**, 737, 1926.
[4] Kawashima: Jour. Biochem., **7**, 361, 1927.
[5] Burns and Marks: Loc. cit., p. 125.
[6] Bodansky: Proc. Soc. Exp. Biol. and Med., **20**, 538, 1923; **21**, 46, 1923.

days of feeding, but later is decreased and finally disappears from the liver at the end of eighteen days.

Thus from the physiological standpoint one gets an explanation of what is observed clinically. In disease of the thyroid gland, glycosuria and hyperglycemia are neither casual phenomena nor dependent alone upon the increased metabolism of hyperthyroidism. There is a certain relation between the thyroid and pancreas through glycogen storage just as there is between the pituitary and pancreas. One can hardly fail to reach the conclusions that if the diabetic "anlage" were present only to a slight degree in a patient, hyperthyroidism would bring a latent diabetes to the fore. One lesion associated frequently with hyperthyroidism, namely, chronic parenchymatous hepatitis, deserves emphasis because of its possible relationship to the disturbed carbohydrate metabolism in thyroid disease. John does not agree with previous authors that the liver is the chief factor in producing hyperglycemia in hyperthyroidism. On the other hand, Wever and co-workers[1] conclude from their studies that the liver is the chief seat of the disturbance of carbohydrate metabolism seen in hyperthyroidism. On this basis, treatment with glucose, especially preoperatively, is indicated.

(*g*) **The Pathology of the Pancreas.**—Definite anatomical changes in the pancreas are said to result from the administration of thyroid but the whole question deserves further investigation. Shields Warren, in a study of the pancreas in 3 of our cases with hyperthyroidism, 4289, 5176, and 5335, found no abnormalities which could be considered specific or characteristic for thyrotoxicosis.

(*h*) **Age.**—Diabetics with primary hyperthyroidism are relatively young diabetics. Case 377, aged thirteen years at onset of diabetes in 1910, developed exophthalmic goiter in 1910 and died in 1912. Cases 10713, 14148 and 14064 were operated upon at thirteen, sixteen and eighteen years, respectively, for primary hyperthyroidism. As may be seen in Table 101, the average age at onset of diabetes in cases of primary hyperthyroidism has averaged 41.5 years, as compared with that of 43.8 years in 4592 consecutive cases of true diabetes. The difference is not great, however, and the data bear out the finding of John, that the curves of age incidence of diabetes with and without hyperthyroidism are quite parallel.

In the patients with adenoma and hyperthyroidism, the average age of onset of diabetes was considerably greater, being 47.8 years in the 1928 series, fifty-five years in the 1934 series, 52.4 years in 1939, and 50.2 years in the 1940 to 1946 series.

(*i*) **Sex.**—The female sex greatly predominated both in the cases of primary hyperthyroidism, 110 out of 150 cases, and still more in the cases of secondary hyperthyroidism, 89 out of 105 cases. This is due, of course, to the fact that a much greater number of women

[1] Wever, Althausen, Biskind and Kerr: Am. Jour. Dig. Diseases and Nutrition, **2**, 93, 1935.

than men have hyperthyroidism. The preponderance of females in the general series of diabetic patients of comparable age groups is definitely less. (See pages 35–37.)

(*j*) **Duration of Life.**—The duration of life of patients successfully operated upon has been as long as that of diabetics without hyperthyroidism. Among 50 cases operated upon between 1923 and 1931 the average duration of diabetes to death in 20 cases was 10.1 years. Patients alive January, 1939, number 30, and their average duration is 15.3 years, or 12 years since operation. So long as hyperthyroidism is present, the hazards of diabetic coma and of cardiac damage especially in older patients with coronary disease, must be borne in mind. With the aid of modern surgery and insulin we would predict that the duration of life would be greater than that of the average diabetic (for these figures see page 318).

(*k*) **Causes of Death.**—One death from coma (15656) has occurred among the 29 recent cases of primary hyperthyroidism. Among the primary hyperthyroid cases of the 1928 series there were 4 deaths from coma, or 33.3 per cent of the total deaths in this group, and among the 6 fatal cases of secondary hyperthyroidism, 4 cases. This relatively high percentage shows how seriously one must regard the hyperthyroid diabetic, because in general coma is characteristic of severe diabetes. The other causes of death were cardiac, 2; pneumonia, 2; postoperative hyperthyroidism or shock, 4; and septicemia, cancer, inanition and cerebral arteriosclerosis, 1 each. Postoperative deaths in the 1939 series were 2 (15989 and 16209), both due to coronary occlusion. No postoperative deaths occurred in the 76 cases of the last series.

Coma is by no means always fatal in the hyperthyroid diabetic. Indeed, the diagnosis of diabetes was first made in Case 4306, when she was found in diabetic coma. Cases 5346 and 5649 also survived coma. In Case 13172, diabetic coma and acute thyrotoxicosis ("thyroid storm") combined to form a remarkable clinical picture. Cases 4289 and 13173 were reported in detail.[1]

(*l*) **Basal Metabolic Rate.**—An increase in the basal metabolism of 20 per cent or more above normal, not due to some other cause, is usually considered necessary for the diagnosis of hyperthyroidism. Mild grades of hyperthyroidism may easily be unrecognized, especially since certain symptoms, loss of weight, weakness and nervousness commonly occur in both diabetes and hyperthyroidism. The normal metabolism of undernourished patients with diabetes may be from 12 to 25 per cent below the level for normal individuals of similar height and weight. Therefore, a basal metabolic rate of 10 to 20 per cent above normal may in such a case be due to hyperthyroidism. Our surgical confrères have repeatedly commented upon the discrepancy between a high metabolic rate in certain thyroid diabetics and the comparative mildness of their clinical symp-

[1] Root, loc. cit., p. 431.

toms. Such discrepancies do occur in non-diabetic thyroid cases also, especially in the older age groups. It is an important point in relation to treatment, since such patients may react after operation with such a "storm" as indicates the true severity of the thyrotoxicosis. Severe diabetic acidosis may mask the symptoms of grave thyrotoxicosis, as in the cases cited by Wilder.[1]

Before operation 35 patients with primary hyperthyroidism showed an average basal metabolic rate of +61 per cent, in contrast to +49 per cent for 1000 cases of primary hyperthyroidism before operation in the Lahey Clinic. After operation the basal metabolic rate fell to +7.4 per cent in 33 of the thyroid diabetic patients, as compared with +5 per cent for 850 cases of uncomplicated hyperthyroidism, who reported for basal metabolism estimations three months after operation in the Lahey series. Partial thyroidectomy, therefore, produces identical results in the diabetic hyperthyroid as in the hyperthyroid patient alone. The data above regarding the basal metabolic rate apply to the cases reported in 1928.

(*m*) **Gain in Weight Following Operation.**—There is a twofold reason for the loss of weight in the hyperthyroid diabetic, namely, that caused by increased metabolism and that due to the loss of sugar in the urine. But the condition is aggravated still more, because overeating, which is so generally associated with a high metabolism, makes a diabetic worse and often leads him to coma. In hyperthyroidism the overeating is continuous. Therefore, the removal of the cause of overeating, namely, the high metabolism of hyperthyroidism, by surgical procedures, yields striking results in diabetes.

(*n*) **Relief of the Hyperthyroidism.**—The favorable influence of iodine in hyperthyroidism with diabetes was observed by Labbé.[2] It has been difficult to estimate it in our cases, because insulin, diet and iodine or thiouracil have been begun simultaneously in our zeal to ameliorate the condition of the patient. About all we can say is that the three as thus combined work well.

(*o*) **Treatment Before and After Operation.**—No radical attempt has been carried out before operation to make the urine completely sugar-free with diet or insulin. The carbohydrate has been maintained at 150 or more grams daily, the protein at approximately 1 gram, and the total calories at not far from 30, per kilogram body weight. Insulin has been given in adequate doses, one, two, three or more times a day. On the morning of operation neither food nor insulin is given preoperatively, because it was found that even if three hours had elapsed since food in the form of orange juice or gingerale, occasionally vomiting took place during the operation or was increased following the operation, due undoubtedly in part to delay of passage of food from the stomach. By the plan followed recently, one can begin to feed the patients sooner after operation.

[1] Wilder, pp. 247, 248: loc. cit., 55.
[2] Labbé: Ann. de méd., **7**, 95, 1920.

Following operation great effort is made to give as much as possible of the carbohydrate of the original diet. Urine specimens are obtained every three or four hours for twenty-four or forty-eight hours, and the amount of insulin to be given gauged by the character of the Benedict test. Except in the very severe cases, we have found the sudden increase in glycosuria after operation was temporary and unattended with obvious harm.

The quantity of iodine given daily before operation is 10 minims, three times a day for eight to ten days. The dose is then increased to 20 minims, three times a day, the day before operation. After operation Lugol's solution is given during the stay in the hospital, usually eight days and often for a few weeks subsequently. With patients who vomit postoperatively, the Lugol's solution may safely be given intravenously with glucose and salt solution insuring thereby the constant effect of iodine regardless of postoperative gastric upsets.

In patients with postoperative reactions of any severity or whose preoperative course is such that a postoperative thyroid reaction is anticipated, intravenous infusions of glucose with normal saline solution are given once or more during the immediate postoperative period. Fifty to 150 grams of glucose may be given in this way in a twenty-four-hour period.

(*p*) **Surgery.**—The combined series of 241 operated cases of hyperthyroidism shows a mortality rate of 2.4 per cent. This is considerably higher than the average mortality-rate figures in patients with primary and secondary hyperthyroidism unassociated with diabetes, the average rate in primary being 0.6 per cent and in secondary hyperthyroidism, 1.7 per cent, and the average rate for both being approximately 1 per cent. These comparative figures may be taken to indicate that the combination of diabetes with hyperthyroidism increases the risk of operation and demands a more conservative operative approach. Dr. Lahey ascribed the lowered mortality in the second series to the fact that there have been 50 to 100 per cent more multiple stage operations on patients with diabetes and hyperthyroidism than are done on patients with uncomplicated hyperthyroidism. Operation in cases of hyperthyroidism should be performed when a full effect has been obtained from the administration of thiouracil and iodine and when the diabetes is under good control. Thiouracil has been given 0.6 gram daily for five to seven weeks, then both thiouracil and Lugol's solution for one week and Lugol's solution alone for one week prior to operation. Multiple operations have become unnecessary. In emaciated patients with thyroidism of long duration it is especially important to study hepatic function. If liver tests are below normal, diets high in carbohydrate, supplemented with vitamin A and concentrate of vitamin B complex are recommended by Wilder. Frequent injections of insulin sometimes every two to three hours may be necessary especially if a thyroid "storm" follows operation.

(q) **Results of Operation.**—No instance of a cure of the diabetes has been observed among patients with primary or secondary hyperthyroidism following operation. Thyroidectomy does not modify pancreatic diabetes in the dog.[1] In general, a gain in tolerance for carbohydrate has been greater with the secondary than with the primary hyperthyroid. Each group of cases appears to do rather better than the ordinary diabetic, but it is clearly evident that end-results must be awaited until a longer period of time has elapsed.

Diabetes developed subsequent to an operation for hyperthyroidism in 8 of our 75 hyperthyroid diabetics. Such cases are mentioned by Wilder,[2] Holst,[3] and Labbé.[4] In 2 of Holst's cases, diabetes occurred after a partial thyroidectomy, but in both of these cases the symptoms of hyperthyroidism had persisted. Wilder reports 2 cases of diabetes developing in thyroidectomized patients. The hyperthyroid who has been operated upon, therefore, should be warned of the possibility of developing diabetes later, even though the disease may not be so likely to appear as if he had not been operated upon at all. Progressing longevity increases the incidence of diabetes in the community and this progressing longevity of the hyperthyroid, brought about by operation, may also be a factor in that it brings him into the diabetic age zone.

2. Myxedema and Diabetes.—Myxedema is commonly thought to be rare in diabetes. Shepardson and Wever,[5] in a review of the subject, however, conclude that "the coincidental occurrence of myxedema and diabetes mellitus is no more nor less than could be predicted from the occurrence of either disease alone." They found in the literature 12 cases which they consider authentic, and to this group add a carefully studied case of their own. The case recorded by Wilder[2] is included in the list compiled by Shepardson and Wever. Escamilla, Lisser and Shepardson[6] describe a patient with advanced myxedema whose sugar tolerance curve was markedly influenced by the giving of thyroid extract.

McCullaugh[7] reports 5 cases of myxedema and diabetes. Daugherty[8] reports 1 case of severity.

A summary of our 7 cases follows: Case 2899 noticed an enlarged thyroid in 1920, hoarseness in Ocotber, 1921, and at her first visit, in February, 1922, aged fifty-three years, weight 213 pounds dressed, the symptoms of myxedema and a large multiple adenomatous goiter

[1] DeFinis and Houssay: Rev. Soc. argent, de biol., **19**, 94, 1943.
[2] Wilder: Loc. cit., p. 726.
[3] Holst: Schweiz. med. Wchnschr., **53**, 725, 1923.
[4] Labbé: Loc. cit., p. 733.
[5] Shepardson and Wever: Internat. Clin., **4**, 133, 1934.
[6] Escamilla, Lisser and Shepardson: Ann. Int. Med., **9**, 297, 1935.
[7] McCullaugh: Cleveland Clin. Quart., **9**, 123, 1942.
[8] Daugherty: Loc. cit., p. 719.

were noted. The urine was sugar-free and the blood sugar 0.1 per cent. The metabolism was −32 per cent. With thyroid extract she promptly improved. Upon November 16, 1922, she reported that her eyesight had failed a month before and that polyuria and pruritus vulvæ had developed. The urine contained 8.4 per cent sugar. With dietetic treatment she promptly became sugar-free and could easily keep so upon about 100 grams carbohydrate. Thyroid medication had been continued by herself according to her symptoms. At her visit on March 28, 1928, the urine contained 3.1 per cent sugar, the blood sugar was 0.31 per cent fasting, metabolism − 9 per cent and weight 178 pounds dressed. Because of the marked glycosuria, she was induced to spend a few days in the hospital, where treatment with insulin was begun. She was operated upon for a cataract of the left eye. On November 10, 1936, she came with a superficial infection between the first and second toes of the right foot and lymphangitis of the foot and lower leg. No pulsation could be felt in the arteries to the foot. Amputation through the right lower thigh was performed on November 17th. She continued to take 5 grains of thyroid extract (Burroughs and Wellcome) daily. Death occurred September 16, 1939 from coronary occlusion.

Case 14850, girl, aged ten years at onset of diabetes in 1936, developed obesity and mental slowness in 1938. The basal metabolic rate was −42 per cent and plasma cholesterol was 454 milligrams per 100 cc. With 1 grain Armour's thyroid extract daily, the basal metabolic-rate rose to −20 per cent and the plasma cholesterol value fell to 137 milligrams per 100 cc. In June, 1945, at the Deaconess Hospital, her weight was 122 pounds and basal metabolism −21 per cent. Her insulin dose was 14 units regular and 36 units protamine insulin. She required 3 grains Armour's thyroid extract daily.

Case 28866, housewife, aged fifty-four years, in August, 1946 presented typical myxedema with enlargement of all chambers of the heart and an electrocardiogram with markedly lowered complexes and almost flat T waves. Clinical improvement was rapid with one grain Armour's thyroid extract.

Cases 10444 and 11362 died of cerebral hemorrhage and myocardial failure respectively.

Cases 16787, 21367 and 19560 also have myxedema.

It is important to consider the possibility that hypopituitarism may underlie apparent myxedema. A low metabolic-rate with emaciation would immediately suggests Simmonds' disease.

One case of hypothyroidism has followed operation in the last 46 cases of hyperthyroidism and diabetes. Holst[1] has reported one such case.

Some of the apparent recoveries of normal tolerance after thyroidectomy may be due to the development of myxedema, especially

Holst: Loc. cit., p. 735.

when exophthalmic goiter is accompanied by thyroiditis, according to Wilder.[1] An extraordinary case of myxedema in a child of seven years is described by Wilder. The basal metabolism was −45 per cent. When the rate was raised by means of thyroid extract, glycosuria appeared and the fasting blood sugar reached 145 milligrams per cent. The child gained weight and strength, but glycosuria continued in spite of a rigid diet and the use of insulin. Such cases support Wilder's belief that the effectiveness of insulin is determined largely by the level of the basal metabolic rate. The tissue cells, with a metabolism accelerated by thyroxin required for a given amount of dextrose an amount of insulin which is greater than would be necessary when the metabolic exchanges are performed at a more leisurely rate. Possibly insulin is more rapidly destroyed when hyperthyroidism exists. When oxidation is proceeding at a rapid rate a catalyst such as insulin may undergo rapid decay.

Wilder *et al.*[2] have reported the results of total ablation of the normal thyroid in 1 case of severe diabetes in a man aged twenty-six years. Operation caused a marked increase in the sugar tolerance of a degree which roughly paralleled the decrease in the metabolic rate. Despite this, the symptoms of myxedema were so disturbing to the patient that it was felt that the amelioration of the diabetes did not justify the operation, and the authors do not advise it for other patients. (See also paper by Rudy, Blumgart and Berlin[3] for the effect of complete thyroidectomy in a diabetic with pulmonary tuberculosis.)

C. THE SUPRARENAL AND DIABETES.

Hypoglycemia is produced experimentally by adrenal cortical insufficiency and in addition a diminution in the glycogen content of liver and muscles occurs, according to Grollman.[4] Also the glycosuria following experimental pancreatectomy may be reduced by excision of the adrenal cortex. The physiological relationships have been studied experimentally by Long.[5] (See page 124.)

Hypoglycemia was first noted in Addison's disease by Porges, in 1910. Stenström[6] recorded a case of spontaneous hypoglycemic coma, relieved by adrenalin, and of pleuriglandular origin. Bloomfield's[7] case, a thirty-year-old American, had uncomplicated diabetes requiring 56 units of insulin a day, but one year later when asthenia, skin pigmentation and other evidences of Addison's disease developed, his insulin requirement fell to 10 units a day. Care-

[1] Wilder, p. 258: Loc. cit., p. 55.
[2] Wilder, Foster and Pemberton: Proc. Staff Meet. Mayo Clinic, **8**, 720, 1933.
[3] Rudy, Blumgart and Berlin: Loc. cit., p. 126.
[4] Grollman: Am. Jour. Physiol., **122**, 460, 1938.
[5] Long: Medicine, **16**, 215, 1937.
[6] Stenström: Deutsch. Arch. f. klin. Med., **152**, 173, 1926.
[7] Bloomfield: Bull. Johns Hopkins Hosp., **65**, 456, 1939.

ful study showed that although desoxy-corticosterone acetate failed to produce an increase in glycosuria or blood sugar, eschatin given in large doses for three or four days did cause a definite increase in the blood sugar and in the glycosuria.

One case of Addison's disease has been recognized in this series. Case 1546 died elsewhere on March 2, 1933, at the age of sixty-nine years, twenty-eight years after the onset of diabetes. His attending physician recorded Addison's disease as a cause of death. Since details concerning his last years are not available, this diagnosis cannot be considered proved. Indeed, in the entire literature, Arnett[1] found, in 1927, only 5 cases of Addison's disease in diabetics, and the diagnosis was questionable in each. He himself reported 1 case in detail and summarized the literature.

Nix[2] believes that only 8 unequivocal cases of Addison's disease and diabetes have been found. Armstrong[3] reports a case of diabetes, Addison's disease and hypothyroidism. Desoxycorticosterone, thyroid, insulin and testosterone improved the appetite, well-being and activity. McCullagh[4] reports a case of diabetes, Addison's disease and necrobiosis.

The onset of diabetes mellitus in a patient with Addison's disease who had been intensively studied and had received adrenal cortical hormone therapy for four years was characterized by progressive anorexia, weakness, loss of weight, fall in blood pressure, and increase in the requirement for hormones. In describing the patient, Thorn and Clinton[5] emphasized the modifying effect of each disease on the other. Spontaneous hypoglycemia occurred, particularly during intercurrent infection, after fasting or exercise. The decrease in glucose tolerance was observed before actual clinical diabetes was noticed. Marked improvement in appetite followed the institution of insulin treatment, and the food chosen changed from carbohydrate exclusively to include fatty foods. A marked alteration in personality occurred with the development of diabetes. The administration of a single dose of Compound E (Kendall) was followed by a loss of glucose tolerance. No changes in sodium and chloride excretions occured with Compound E treatment. However, when insulin was withdrawn, a striking increase in potassium excretion occurred. They concluded from the studies on this patient that the inability of patients with uncomplicated Addison's disease to maintain a normal fasting blood-sugar level was not dependent solely upon deficiency of the adrenal cortical hormone.

Selye and Dosne,[6] using adult male rats in the fasting state, found that both hyperglycemia caused by adrenalin and (2) the hypogly-

[1] Arnett: Arch. Int. Med., **39**, 698, 1927.
[2] Nix: Canad. Med. Assn. Jour., **49**, 189, 1943.
[3] Armstrong: Jour. Clin. Endocrin., **4**, 23, 1944.
[4] McCullagh: Loc. cit., p. 735.
[5] Thorn and Clinton: Jour. Clin. Endocrin., **3**, 335, 1943.
[6] Selye and Dosne: Proc. Soc. Exper. Biol. and Med., **42**, 580, 1939

cemia following insulin administration might be inhibited, though not completely suppressed, by cortin.

Rogoff, Ferrill and Nixon[1] have tested the hypothesis of Zuelzer that epinephrine and insulin were antagonistic and that suppressing the secretion of the adrenal medulla would ameliorate diabetes. Their experiments were carried out by removing one adrenal and denervating the other and then removing the pancreas. It was found that the insulin requirement of these animals bore no relation to the rate of secretion of the epinephrine. However, they made another interesting discovery, namely, that in animals in whom the pancreas is removed there is a spontaneous suppression of epinephrine production. In such animals stimulation of the splanchnic nerve led to increase of secretion to the normal rate, showing that the gland had retained a large measure of its capacity to respond to stimulation. This work does not support the idea of treating diabetes by interfering with the function of the adrenal gland.

Among 30 or more adrenal cortical steroids are 4 characterized by the presence of oxygen at carbon atom 11 of the sterol ring, which exert the metabolic effects of the adrenal cortex. They are described as "diabetogenic" because they increase the glycosuria of depancreatized rats. They are not known to cause clinical diabetes, according to Lukens.[2]

In discussing the diabetes of bearded women (suprarenal tumor, diabetes and hirsutism) occurring in 18 cases, Shepardson and Shapiro[3] refer first to the classification by Broster:[4] (1) cases with pseudohermaphroditism, (2) cases with virilism and (3) the Achard-Thiers syndrome in which the adrenal lesion is but one component of a multiple glandular disturbance. Their own case, a thirty-year-old woman, only developed diabetes some years after the other symptoms of the syndrome. Her father had diabetes, again emphasizing the importance of the diabetes heredity even when other glandular disorders are present in the diabetic. Parts of each adrenal were removed surgically, but only after death was the adenoma found. The diabetes was refractory to insulin chiefly because of the marked disturbance in metabolic processes resulting from the disease in the suprarenal cortex.

Kepler and Wilder[5] summarized 8 cases of tumor and 2 of hyperplasia of the adrenal cortex. In all 8 cases the tumors were removed. Four were dead within a year. The other 4 recovered, virilism disappeared and no diabetes developed. The 2 cases with cortical hyperplasia and 1 girl with cortical tumor had frank diabetes.

---

[1] Rogoff, Ferrill and Nixon: Arch. Int. Med., **60**, 805, 1937.
[2] Lukens: Med. Clin. North America, **26**, 1803, 1942.
[3] Shepardson and Shapiro: Endocrinology, **24**, 237, 1939.
[4] Broster: Arch. Surg., **34**, 761, 1937.
[5] Kepler and Wilder: Acta med. Scandin., (Suppl.) **40**, 87, 1938.

Sprague, Priestly and Dockerty[1] report diabetes without other endocrine manifestations in a case of tumor of the adrenal cortex.

Case 11129, female, died of infection, but at autopsy had an adenoma of the adrenal cortex. She also had a large heart, hirsutism, obesity and high blood-pressure.

One case of diabetes with pheochromocytoma is reported by Duncan, Semans and Eager.[2]   Disappearance of diabetes followed removal of the tumor.   Another case of pheochromocytoma with hypertension and diabetes reported by Green[3] had a normal glucose tolerance test one month after removal of the tumor.   In Case 15370, removal of a large pheochromocytoma in 1938 had not been followed by a change in severity of diabetes up to 1945.

A case of adrenocortical hyperplasia, aged forty-six years, female, is described by Wilder,[4] who had, in addition to frank adrenal virilism and intense alkalosis associated with hypochloremia, a thymic tumor 5 cm. in diameter. Sixty-five units of insulin were required. Periods of tetany occurred in her terminal illness. The changes described by Crooke were present in the basophilic cells of the pituitary but no adenoma was found.

D. THE THYMUS AND DIABETES.

In Major's[5] case, a child, aged eleven years, with diabetes of two years' duration, and occasional attacks of asthma becoming increasingly infrequent, was brought into the hospital in deep coma, with stertorous respiration, blood sugar 0.645 per cent and carbon dioxide tension about 4.5 per cent. She survived but four hours.

The necropsy showed edema of the lungs, an unusually large thymus covering the entire surface of the pericardium anteriorly and weighing about 50 grams. The abdominal lymph glands were enlarged. In the pancreas the islands were strikingly reduced in number but were without evidence of degeneration.

Large doses of thymus hormone increased alimentary hyperglycemia, a result similar to that following anterior pituitary extract and failure of the anterior pituitary extract to produce results if the thymus is removed has suggested a significant rôle for the thymus in diabetes origin.[6]

[1] Sprague, Priestly and Dockerty: Jour. Clin. Endocr., 3, 28, 1943.
[2] Duncan, Semans and Eager: Ann. Int. Med., 20, 815, 1944.
[3] Green: Jour. Am. Med. Assn., 131, 1260, 1946.
[4] Wilder: p. 268; Loc. cit., p. 55.
[5] Major and Helwig: Jour. Am. Med. Assn., 86, 1766, 1926.
[6] Bombskov and Stein: Ztschr. f. Klin. Med., 139, 96, 1941. Bomskov and Schweiger: Ztschr. f. Klin. Med., 139, 102, 1941.

CHAPTER XXVIII.

DIABETES IN CHILDHOOD.

By Priscilla White, M.D.

The juvenile form of diabetes is characterized by greater severity than the adult form. It is complicated more often by coma and hypoglycemia. It can retard growth and development. It can predispose the child to sepsis terminating in septicemia. It can favor the early development of occlusive vascular disease. The purpose of this chapter, therefore is to review the data pertaining to 2191 diabetic children, to point out certain fundamental differences between juvenile and adult diabetes and to present data suggesting the cause, prevention and correction of the complications of child-hood diabetes.

Definition.—In this discussion the diabetic child is defined as any patient in whom the onset of diabetes has occurred at 15.0 years of age or under. Among the 2191 patients are 8 (pre-insulin survivors) now in the fifth decade of age, 206 patients in the fourth and 741 in the third decade. This continued separation of patients with onset of diabetes in childhood is valuable, because it permits the study of the nature of diabetes in young patients and its eventual course and consequences.

Our 2191 patients classified as diabetic children have been observed for nearly fifty years, namely, from 1898 to 1946. A follow-up ending January 7, 1946 showed that 1774, or 81 per cent, are living, 385, or 18 per cent, have died, 28, or 1 per cent, are untraced and 4, having been untraced for years, are considered lost.

TABLE 102.—STATUS OF 2191 DIABETIC CHILDREN SEEN BETWEEN 1898 AND 1946.

	Total.	Living.	Dead.	Untraced.
1898–August, 1922	290	126	164	
August, 1922, to January, 1946 . .	1901	1648	221	32
Total	2191	1774	385	32

A. Incidence of Diabetes in Childhood.—The total prevalence of diabetes of the childhood type is great. In the United States today there are some 37,000 such patients, of whom about 13,000 are under fifteen years of age.[1] The sex incidence in our series of juvenile patients is even, whereas in older decades females predominate. Girls, however, contract diabetes at a slightly earlier age than do boys. The peak of incidence is found at age eleven in girls and at

[1] Spiegelman and Marks: Loc. cit., p. 29.

(741)

age thirteen in boys, suggesting puberty and pituitary influences. Three peaks in the age at onset of diabetes occur in childhood, namely, at ages three, six and twelve. Jewish children comprise 8 per cent of our cases.

B. Etiology.—The juvenile patient whose family history may be rechecked yearly for many years has added much evidence in favor of the theory that the tendency to develop diabetes appears to be inherited. At the onset of diabetes, 20 per cent of the children have diabetic relatives, after twenty years of diabetes, 55 per cent have found diabetics in their families. The total incidence of heredity in our 2191 cases is 35 per cent, 33 per cent hereditary, 9 per cent familial. Among Jewish children the heredity is 49 per cent.

(*a*) **Inheritance.**—The evidence in favor of the hereditary transmission of diabetes is as follows: First, the high incidence of diabetes in similar twin mates, namely, 50 per cent; second, the statistically significant excess of diabetics in the close blood relatives of patients, amounting to seven times the incidence in the control population; third, the demonstration of Mendelian ratios of the recessive type in cases reporting in sequence; fourth, the demonstration of Mendelian ratios of the recessive type in families tested with glucose tolerance tests; fifth, the occurrence of diabetes in like sexed siblings; and sixth, in the tendency toward anticipation. (See Chapter III, pages 54 to 68.)

Secondary factors permitting the expression of the gene are presupposed, because clinical signs and symptoms of diabetes occur at any age and are not evident at birth or soon thereafter. Infections, trauma, past dietary habits, psychosomatic disturbances and endocrine imbalance, all known to favor hyperglycemia, have been evaluated in the consideration of possible inciting causes of diabetes in our juvenile diabetics in the discussion which follows.

TABLE 103.—INFECTIONS IN THE YEAR OF ONSET OF 504 DIABETIC CHILDREN.

Pertussis	. . . 12	Tonsillitis	. . 5	Adenitis	. . . .	2
Measles	. . . 10	Mumps .	. . 3	Appendicitis	. . .	1
Chickenpox	. . 8	Influenza	. . 3	Diphtheria	. . .	1
Scarlet fever	. . 7	Jaundice	. . 2	Rheumatic fever	. .	1
Coryza	 7					

(*b*) **Infections.**—Acute infection appeared to play no rôle in the etiology of our diabetic children. Whereas, 10 per cent of 504 of our cases reviewed with this in mind had an infection of severity in the year of onset, 90 per cent had none. The experience of Grishaw, West and Smith[1] is similar. They report an incidence of infection in 20 per cent of their cases in the year of onset. John[2] and Lande,[3] however, found a relatively high incidence of infections prior to

---

[1] Grishaw, West and Smith: Arch. Int. Med., **64**, 787, 1939.
[2] John: Loc. cit., p. 524, ref. 2.
[3] Lande: Loc. cit., p. 524.

onset of the disease. The relative frequency of infections in the year of onset of 504 of our children is shown in Table 103. Chronic foci of infection such as diseased teeth and tonsils were not conspicuous on first examination.

(c) **Trauma, Psychosomatic Disturbance, Obesity.**—Trauma, important from the medico-legal point of view, did not precede diabetes onset in more than 3 of the cases and can thus be considered to have a coincidental rather than causal relationship. Psychosomatic disturbances were the exception rather than the rule. Only 5 per cent of the children at onset of diabetes had exceeded their expected weight for age.

(d) **Endocrine Overactivity.**—An appraisal of the diabetic child at onset was made to determine the presence or absence of disturbance of normal endocrine balance. This has included, in addition to the physical examination, an x-ray examination for bone age, basal metabolism tests, and in a few cases the determination of serum follicle-stimulating hormone and urinary 17-keto-steroids.

Overheight, measured within three months of the onset of the disease, was found in 86 per cent of 417 of our diabetic children. These 417 children exceeded the Baldwin and Wood standard of height for age by 2.5 inches. In order to evaluate the effect of modern diets and improved hygiene on growth in stature, 114 cases seen between 1938 and 1939 were analyzed separately. The average height of the 66 boys exceeded the standard by 3.2 inches and the average height of the girls exceeded the standard by 2.8 inches. Whether the Baldwin and Wood, the Englebach and Schaefer, or the Meredith standard was used, the stature of the diabetic child exceeded the normal. The 114 children were representative of all socio-economic levels, but included few really privileged children.

The average bone development was found by Bogan and Morrison[1] to be eighteen months in advance of the chronological age at the time of onset and the dental development was found by Robinson[2] to be twelve months in advance. The basal metabolism was on the average, plus 12 per cent. In a study by Wagner, White and Bogan[3] the hip and breast development, appearance of puberty and axillary hair and age at onset of first menstruation occurred earlier in the diabetic than in the normal controls. The growth of testes, penis, pubic and axillary hair, lowering of voice and growth of body hair of the diabetic boy occurred at an earlier age in this same study than in the normal controls.

The level of follicle-stimulating hormone (FSH) was measured at onset of diabetes in the serum of 31 of our children. Among these

---

[1] Bogan and Morrison: Am. Jour. Med. Sci., **174**, 313, 1927.
[2] Robinson: Personal communication.
[3] Wagner, White and Bogan: Am. Jour. Dis. Child., **63**, 667, 1942. White: Diabetes in Childhood and Adolescence, Philadelphia, Lea & Febiger, 1932.

fresh cases of diabetes 70 per cent reacted positively with 3 cc. or less of prepared serum compared with 13 per cent of 22 non-diabetic controls of comparable age.

Forty diabetic children had 17-keto-steroid determinations done at or near onset of diabetes and showed a tendency to develop higher levels than did the non-diabetic controls.

TABLE 104.—17 KETO-STEROID EXCRETION IN 40 DIABETIC CHILDREN.

17 keto-steroid, mg. per 24 hrs.

Age, yrs.	Diabetic, boys.	Normal, boys.	Diabetic, girls.	Normal, girls.
2			0.7	
3	0.8			
4	1.5			
5	6.0			
6		0.5	0.8	0.5
7		0.7	2.8	0.7
8	1.5	1.3	2.6	1.3
9	3.0		3.0	3.0
10			5.0	4.0
11	7.0	4.0	2.3	
12		3.0	3.3	
13	12.0	5.0	8.0	3.5
14	14.0	6.0	8.0	5.0
15		7.0	5.0	6.0

(e) **Congenital Defects.**—Congenital anomalies were reported by Wagner, White and Bogan, to occur more often in the diabetic than in the control children. These anomalies were usually slight and as follows: Dupuytren contracture, curved fifth finger, brachydactylia, brachycephalus, ear nodule on the lateral aspect of the auricle.

Correlation of Experimental and Clinical Data.—Pancreatectomy, hormones, namely, anterior pituitary extract, adrenal cortical extract, possibly thyroid and estrogens, and chemical agents, alloxan and alloxan-like derivatives, have produced diabetes experimentally. Hemosiderin has been thought to cause diabetes found in cases of hemochromatosis.

No clinical counterpart to hemosiderin diabetes is found in the child. None of our own juvenile diabetics has hemochromatosis, and we are unaware of a juvenile case having been reported in the literature. Alloxan diabetes in the human patient waits chemical proof. Congenital hypoinsulinism corresponding to ablation of the pancreas is suggested by the small size of pancreas with poor islet development found at postmortem examination. Gene linkage of anomalies is thus suggested. Thyroid or estrogen diabetes in childhood is not borne out any more than in the adult by physical or laboratory examination. A mechanism through the adrenal is suggested by the severity of diabetes, and the elevation of 17-keto-steroid excretion. A mechanism through the anterior pituitary is suggested by the high elevation of FSH, 17-keto-steroid, basal metabolic rate, advanced bone and gonad development and the early appearance of body hirsutism. The following theory is therefore postulated, that the gene induces hyperactivity of the pituitary which then produces the diabetes complex by reducing insulin output and increasing gluconeogenesis.

Type of Onset and Early Course.—Acute, rapid, and gradual types of onset occur more often in the child than in the adult, the onset of whose diabetes is most often indefinite. Thus 18.0 per cent of the 2191 children had a sudden or rapid onset. The early course of diabetes in the child is often virulent. The first recognition of the disease may be in coma. Thus, in 500 consecutive cases in children the diagnosis of diabetes was made in coma in 69, or 14 per cent, and in all except one of the 13 children whose diabetes occurred under one year of age. In these children as in Young's[1] pituitary diabetic dogs, the sign of nascent diabetes was ketosis.

Symptoms and Signs.—The characteristic symptoms of diabetes are invariably present in the child. Those most frequently reported are polyuria, polydipsia, polyphagia, loss of weight, loss of appetite, pruritus, furunculosis, alternating near and far vision, pains in the legs, muscle cramps, change in disposition and school failure. The signs are those of loss of weight and dehydration in the typically tall child with advanced bone and dental development.

C. Diagnosis of Diabetes.—Errors in the diagnosis of diabetes in childhood arise from the fact that glycosuria is very common in children. Children may thus be treated with dietary restriction and insulin before an accurate diagnosis is established. The diagnostic criteria for diabetes are the same in all age groups, namely, the presence of hyperglycemia and glycosuria. The diagnostic levels for blood sugar in this clinic are as follows: 130 milligrams fasting, 170 milligrams postprandial, venous, and 200 milligrams postprandial, if capillary blood.

Glucose tolerance tests are used if the diagnosis of diabetes is not established by random blood and urine analysis. The preparation of the child for glucose tolerance test is as important as preparation of the patient for a basal metabolism test or for x-ray examinations. Fever, past restrictions of total calories or of carbohydrate, past administration of insulin and possibly emotional factors, favor hyperglycemia, whereas excess of carbohydrate such as repeated administration of glucose and exercise favor relative hypoglycemia. At the time of the test, the child must be afebrile. The diet of the weeks prior to the test should be of normal composition. Insulin should not have been administered during this same period and the patient should be at rest during the test.

The normal utilization of glucose under age two is 3 grams per kilogram of body weight.[2] For all other age groups the normal utilization is 1.8 grams per kilogram of body weight. Such amounts

---

[1] Young: Loc. cit., p. 121.
[2] Livingston and Bridge: Jour. Am. Med. Assn., **119**, 117, 1945.

of glucose are prescribed for juvenile patients who weigh less than 100 pounds. To children weighing over 100 pounds, the adult quantity, 100 grams of glucose, is given. Obese children who have abnormal curves when they have received glucose according to actual body weight are retested with that quantity of glucose which is based upon their ideal weight for height and age. For practical purposes we use 1 gram of glucose per pound of body weight. The blood sugar is then obtained fasting, after one-half, one and two hours, for venous curves and preferably an additional hour for capillary curves. The diagnosis as with the adult patient is based upon the peak rather than upon the fall of curve. If the popular Exton-Rose test is employed the quantity of glucose is again calculated on the basis of body weight. The total quantity is divided into equal parts, one administered fasting, the other one-half hour later. (See page 160.)

Unclassified glycosuria, renal glycosuria, and potential diabetes designate the same types of glycosurias as they do in the adult population. (See page 788.) Of some importance in the juvenile population are the meliturias with excretion of sugars other than glucose, namely, pentose, levulose, lactose and galactose. Renal glycosuria has been demonstrated in 12 children, 4534, 6676, 6708, 6709, 14040, 15032, 15855, 16089, 22499, 25737, 7157 (at eleven months) and 15117. Essential levulosuria has been identified in 2 children and essential pentosuria in 5, 4 males, 1 female, all juvenile, 1484, 6767, 7995, 18070, 18217. Lactosuria has not been sought in our patients. It is a physiological finding in the nursling. Galactosuria may be found in children with digestive disturbances.

D. Pathology.—The study of the pathology of the juvenile diabetic is logically divided into 2 parts. The first part is concerned with the pancreas and the second part is concerned with the body as a whole. The latter is further divided as follows: (1) disturbance of normal sugar-fat relationship; (2) sepsis; (3) occlusive vascular disease.

Pancreas.—The growth of the islands of Langerhans under age two parallels the rate of growth of the total pancreas. From age four to twelve, it falls to almost half the rate and in adolescence the rates are equal again. After age three, the numbers of islets remain constant. The growth variation lag appears to coincide with peaks of age at onset. (See page 742.) The weight of the pancreas at birth averages 2.6 grams and increases to an average of 66 grams at twenty-one years. Warren has reported the changes in the islets of 19 juveniles as follows: few islets, 7 cases; hydropic degeneration, 5; lymphocytic infiltration, 5; fibrosis, 3; pyknotic nuclei, 2; hyalinization, 2; hypertrophy and sclerosis of islets, 1 each. As in the adult, Warren[1] emphasized that the chief character-

---

[1] Warren: P. 167, loc. cit., p. 131.

istic is the wide variety of lesions observed in a single pancreas suggesting a toxic agent destroying islets and permitting regeneration.

Glycogen—Fat Deposition.—The disturbance of carbohydrate-fat relationship was characteristic of the autopsies of the pre- and early-insulin era. Fatty infiltration of Kupffer's cells of the liver, spleen pulp and the intima of the aorta and skin was shown along with depletion of fat in the central nervous system. Abnormal deposition of glycogen was found in liver cell nuclei, Henle's loops and convoluted renal tubules and in the heart. Depletion of glycogen stores occurred in structures normally containing it, namely, the skin and muscle.

Sepsis.—With the widespread use of insulin and especially after the use of long acting insulins the above changes became less conspicuous and postmortem examinations from 1930 to 1940 showed the ravages of sepsis including pyelonephritis, abscesses of liver, heart, lung, spleen, brain. Chemotherapy has altered the fatal course of sepsis in the diabetic child, as it has in the general population. Thus, a preponderance of vascular changes became evident in young diabetics surviving many years of diabetes, and coming to autopsy in the present decade.

Arteriosclerosis.—Of the 4 types of arteriosclerosis, (1) atheromatous, involving the aorta, coronaries and extremities, (2) Mönckeberg—universal, (3) arteriolar, involving the kidney, and (4) senile; the first three have prevailed in the young diabetic. Characteristic of diabetes in youth as elsewhere in diabetes, atheromatous lesions may involve arteries commonly involved in other types of sclerosis. What ever the type the end result here appears to be occlusive vascular disease.

Since nephritis is replacing other causes of death in young diabetics (see page 767), the kidney pathology may be discussed in more detail. Under age forty severe grades of intercapillary glomerulosclerosis were found in 13 of 40 cases with postmortem examinations.

Diabetic glomerulosclerosis, the term used by Spuehler and Zollinger[1] described the intercapillary glomerulosclerosis seen in these cases. The process alters the glomerularplexus. Diffuse hyalinosis of the mesoangium, a senescent process paralleling arteriosclerosis occurs. Spuehler and Zollinger describe a fusion of fibroid lipoproteins throughout the homogenous hyaline membranes, namely, in capsular membrane, and capillary membrane, basement membrane of the tubules and boundary membrane of the arterioles. The same condition is found not only in the kidneys but also to an unusual extent in the eyes.

It is their interesting and logical conception that diabetic glo-

[1] Spuehler and Zollinger: Loc. cit., p. 487.

merulosclerosis is a metabolic disturbance commonly accompanied by arterio- and arteriolar sclerosis. Infection manifests itself in diabetes as a localizing factor. It is possible that these changes which are the basic cause of the membrane injuries express themselves in infiltrations during disturbances of lipoid and protein metabolism.

Infections, disturbances of steroid, especially sex endocrine steroids would seem to be possible toxic agents capable of local or hematogenous kidney damage or retinal damage.

E. Management of Juvenile Diabetes.—The management of the juvenile patient includes four essentials: (1) regulation of diet; (2) replacement of insulin; (3) timing of exercise and (4) training in anticipation for emergencies.

Dietary Treatment.—The caloric prescription for the juvenile patient must be adequate. Undernutrition, a useful adjunct in the treatment of the adult, is harmful for the child. Total calories may be prescribed by many standards. Perhaps the simplest are based as follows: first, upon height, namely, 35 calories per inch; second, by age and weight, for infants, 100 calories per kilogram, at age five years, 75 calories per kilogram, age ten years, 50 and at age fifteen, 40 calories per kilogram. The simplest of all standards is that based upon age, namely, 1000 calories for age one year, 100 calories added for each year until the completion of growth at about age thirteen in girls, nineteen in boys. Thus the maximum diet for a diabetic girl is 2200 calories; boys require well up toward 3000. The adolescent diabetic girl prone to obesity, may require the adult prescription of 30 calories per kilogram of ideal body weight.

The composition of the diet in childhood is normally as follows: carbohydrate 50 per cent of the total calories, protein 15 per cent, fat 35 per cent. The composition of the diet prescribed for our diabetic children is carbohydrate 40 per cent, protein 20 per cent, fat 40 per cent. For rapid calculation the carbohydrate in grams is 10 per cent of the figure for the total calories, and the protein and fat approximately half the figure of the carbohydrate. For example, according to our rule for age, the child of nine requires 1800 calories, 10 per cent of that figure gives carbohydrate 180, halved for protein and fat gives 90 (or 1890 calories). The maximum carbohydrate prescribed is 225 grams. After age thirteen the protein and fat portions of the diet are increased for diabetic boys. (See sample diets in Table 105.)

The carbohydrate for the day may be divided into even thirds or one-fifth at breakfast, two-fifths at noon and night. Thirty grams of carbohydrate are subtracted to be given as 3 small lunches in mid-morning, mid-afternoon and at bedtime.

Supplementary doses of vitamins are added for although the diabetic diet is liberal in all vitamins except vitamin D, faulty utilization may occur. Freston and Loughlin[1] reported the vitamin deficiencies at Camp Nyda to be 27 per cent in 93 children. The report of Mosenthal and Loughlin[2] showed vitamin A deficiency in 68 per cent, B in 25 per cent and C in 4 per cent. Hypercarotinemia was present in 28 per cent. At Clara Barton Camp, all 130 children were tested for vitamin C in 1938, and no subnormal values were found. During years of depression, we found clinical signs of vitamin A deficiency; during war restriction, vitamin B deficiencies were found to predominate. Dark adaptation was normal in a small group of our children tested; none has given a history of night blindness, but characteristic skin lesions occur. Faulty utilization of vitamin A has been suspected because of hypercarotemia and hepatomegaly. Since vitamin A is formed in the liver by the splitting of carotene, a lack may be inferred.

TABLE 105.—SAMPLE DIETS.

Carbohydrate, 140; Protein, 60; Fat, 70.

Egg.	Meat.	Bacon.	Vegetables. 5%.	Vegetables. 10%.	Oat-meal.	Butter.	Cream.	Milk.	Orange.	Potato.	Bread.
1	..	..	..	..	15	5	60	120	100	..	15
..	45	..	150	..	..	10	..	180	100	..	15
..	30	..	150	..	..	10	..	180	100	45	15

Carbohydrate 10 gm. at 10, 3, and 9.

Carbohydrate, 160; Protein, 70; Fat, 80.

1	..	15	..	..	15	5	60	240	100	..	20
..	45	..	150	..	..	10	..	240	150	..	20
..	45	..	150	..	..	10	..	240	150	45	20

Carbohydrate 10 gm. at 10, 3, and 9.

Carbohydrate, 180; Protein, 80; Fat, 90.

1	..	15	..	..	30	10	60	120	100	..	15
..	60	..	150	..	..	10	..	180	150	..	30
..	60	..	150	..	..	10	..	180	150	90	15

Carbohydrate 10 gm. at 10, 3, and 9.

Carbohydrate, 200; Protein, 100; Fat, 100.

1	..	15	..	..	30	10	60	180	100	..	30
..	90	..	150	150	..	10	..	180	150	..	30
..	90	..	150	150	..	10	..	180	150	90	15

Carbohydrate 10 gm. at 10, 3, and 9.

Diet for day of illness: Milk 1 quart, eggs 3, orange juice 1 quart or parenteral glucose 100 grams.

The calcium content of our diets exceeds 1 gram. If adequacy can be measured by incidence of osteoporosis our diets are adequate. Bone atrophy has been exceptional since 1926. Serum determinations for calcium and phosphorus show the former to be normal, the latter usually slightly below normal.

Emergency Diets.—The diet during acute infections may be reduced to carbohydrate 150, protein 50, fat 50 grams, consisting

[1] Freston and Loughlin: New York State Jour. Med., **42**, 1833, 1942.
[2] Mosenthal and Loughlin: Arch. Int. Med., **73**, 391, 1944.

of eggnogs, milk, fruit juices. A simple rule is an alternate glass of fruit juice or eggnog every two hours for seven feedings. The surgical patient should receive 75 to 100 grams of glucose parenterally preferably as a 5 per cent solution.

For other plans for treatment, see Barach,[1] Boyd,[2] Escudero,[3] Wilder,[4] Stolte,[5] Lichtenste n,[6] Colwell *et al.*,[7] and Jackson and McIntosh.[8]

Insulin.—All diabetic children require substitutional insulin therapy continuously from the day of recognition of the disease. The guide for the prescription for the initial dose of insulin may be based upon the age of the patient rather than upon the degree of glycosuria as follows: Under age five years, 10 units; five to ten years, 20 units; ten to fifteen years, 30 units. Readjustments are then made according to premeal tests of blood or urine.

At the present writing a choice among four types of insulin or insulin mixtures is possible, namely: (1) regular, (2) crystalline, (3) protamine zinc, (4) globin and mixtures of crystalline and protamine zinc or crystalline and globin insulin. For the management of the juvenile diabetic the knowledge of the following three properties of the four types of insulin is essential: (1) the time of availability after injection, (2) the duration of action, (3) the time of maximum hypoglycemic effect.

	Available after injection, hours.	Maximum hypoglycemia, hours.	Duration of action, hours.
RI	1	3– 4	8
CI	1	3– 4	10
PZI	8	20–24	24–72
GI	2	6– 8	24

Overlapping, slow release and nocturnal hypoglycemia are the defects of PZI. Slow release, mid-afternoon hypoglycemia and failure to overlap are the defects of globin insulin. The former protects the diabetic population from ketosis, the latter perhaps to some degree from nocturnal hypoglycemia. Since in juvenile diabetes coma is more feared than hypoglycemia, protamine remains the insulin of our choice. Short duration of action and need for multiple doses are the obvious defects of crystalline and regular insulin.

Nocturnal hyperglycemia prevents the successful use of two daily doses of rapidly acting insulin in the childhood case. Postprandial glycosuria prevents the successful use of slowly acting insulin alone.

[1] Barach: Am. Jour. Digest. Dis., 11, 350, 1944.
[2] Jackson, Boyd and Smith: Am. Jour. Dis. Child., 59, 332, 1940.
[3] Escudero: Inst. Nac. Nutricion, Buenos Aires, Recop. Tirab. Acnt., 5, 200, 1940.
[4] Wilder: P. 121, 202; loc. cit., p. 55.
[5] Stolte: Med. Klin., 28, 831, 1931.
[6] Lichtenstein: Nord. med. Wchnschr., 10, 1329, 1935.
[7] Colwell, Isso and Stryker: Arch. Int. Med., 69, 931, 1942.
[8] Jackson and McIntosh: Proc. Cent. Soc. Clin. Res., 17, 74, 1944.

Therefore, separate injections of protamine and crystalline insulin are usually administered before breakfast, the protamine insulin increased to render the true fasting specimen sugar-free or green, the crystalline insulin increased to render the prelunch and pre-supper tests sugar-free or green. Increases and decreases of 2 units of CI and 4 of PZI are suitable for the juvenile patient. The typical ratios of CI to PZI vary with the age of the patient as follows: Under age five, CI, 1.5; PZI, 1. At age five, CI, 1; PZI, 1. Older children CI, 1. PZI, 2.

Supplementary insulin, CI, is administered according to urine tests at four hour intervals during infections and after surgery.

A novel scheme for desugarization has been suggested by Brush,[1] as follows: The number of units of insulin should be $\frac{2}{3}$ the number of grams of fat. A dose of insulin is given at 4 A.M. After the 4 A.M. dose of insulin is administered the rest is divided $\frac{4}{7}$ before breakfast, $\frac{1}{7}$ before noon and $\frac{2}{7}$ before supper. On this scheme shocks occur on the fourth and fifth day. The insulin is reduced 1 unit the first day, 2 the second and thereafter 7.5 per cent of the original dose daily until a 30-unit level is reached.

Complications of Insulin Therapy in Childhood.—Complications of insulin therapy in childhood are: (1) hypoglycemia, (2) lipodystrophy, (3) allergy, (4) resistance, (5) induration, (6) sepsis, (7) epilepsy (page 568).

Insulin hypoglycemia constitutes a major problem in management of the juvenile patient. From the child's point of view it is a source of physical discomfort, social embarrassment and of failure in school or athletic progress. It represents a serious hazard, for it may result in irreversible cerebral changes or rarely in a fatal outcome.

Mild reactions in the child are caused: (1) by errors in the time and amount of exercise, (2) by errors in the time or the quantity of food intake and (3) by errors in the administration of insulin such as overdose, change in site of injection, change in strength or type of insulin, change in type of syringe. Blameless reactions result from variation of the rate of absorption of insulin or of food or following bouts of nausea, vomiting and diarrhea.

Although the blood sugar in mild or severe hypoglycemia is low, 60 milligrams or below, the urinary sugar may represent a lag and, therefore, vary from sugar-free to a maximum reduction. A second specimen will be free from sugar, or nearly so.

The manifestations of mild reactions are related to the vegetative nervous system or the adrenalin effect and include hunger, faintness, tremor, vomiting and paresthesia. The physical signs are sweating, pallor, tremors, twitching, rise of blood-pressure, fall of pulse rate and leucocytosis. Prevention of mild reactions is sought in the training of the patient. The child requires regular timing of

[1] Brush: Am. Jour. Dis. Child., **67**, 429, 1944.

insulin, diet and exercise. Quantitative sugar analyses may show that an increase in insulin is not necessary. Postmeal exercise is preferred to premeal exercise. Anticipatory lunches may be necessary. Simple substitutes for the usual diet during sickness must be available. The correct dosage of units, correct type and strength of insulin and type of syringe must be known.

The treatment of insulin reactions is elevation of the blood sugar by carbohydrate orally, anti-insulin hormones, adrenalin, dosage 0.3 cc., pituitrin, pitressin subcutaneously, or concentrated glucose (50 per cent) intravenously.

The symptoms and signs of severe hypoglycemia are described in detail elsewhere. They include unconsciousness, stupor, catatonia and dementia, convulsions, involuntary micturition and defecation, compulsive and ridiculous behavior and instability of temperature, an early fall and late rise. The severe reactions may develop during sleep, or if hypoglycemia has become chronic, through errors in diagnosis, an effort to obtain attention or even a suicidal attempt.

Nearly all of the severe reactions respond to repeated 20 cc. doses of 50 per cent glucose administered intravenously, but some patients require more aggressive treatment. Such treatment for the entire twenty-four hours includes: (1) constant venoclysis 150 to 300 grams of glucose, (2) adrenalin in 5 cc. doses, (3) nasal oxygen or oxygen under positive pressure, (4) suction and airway, (5) transfusion of fresh whole blood, (6) sedation such as sodium luminal, (7) dehydration, (8) lumbar puncture.

Fat Atrophy at, near, or remote from the site of injection of insulin occurs in one-third of all diabetic children. The cause is unknown. Local hypoglycemia has been suggested and also endocrine factors because the lesion is limited to children, female adults or hypogonadal male adults. The treatment is unknown but a good prognosis for recovery may be given. Spontaneous regeneration occurs in two to eight years.

Urticaria at the site of injection of insulin is common but spontaneous desensitization usually occurs in three to four weeks.

True resistance to insulin has not been encountered in any juvenile patient in our series.

Single or Multiple Abscesses follow errors in aseptic technic. Contamination of the insulin probably accounts for the multiple abscesses, more common in children than in adults.

Induration of the tissues at the site of the injection occurs in children. Absorption is decreased and hypoglycemia may follow change in the site of the injection.

Examination of the Blood and Urine in the Diabetic Child.—The minimum number of tests essential in the management of diabetic children is seven, as follows: (1) sugar—qualitative (Benedict); (2) sugar—quantitative; (3) acetone or diacetic acid; (4) albumin; (5) micro blood sugar, such as Folin ferricyanide; (6) tests for alveolar air or alkali reserve such as is possible with the Van Slyke apparatus; (7) x-ray of the chest.

Desirable, but not absolutely essential tests include quantitative blood lipids, acetone, non-protein nitrogen, chloride, albumin-globulin ratio, x-ray for calcified blood vessels, intravenous pyelogram, electrocardiogram, electroencephalogram. The patients or families should have material for the qualitative test for sugar, test for acetone or diacetic acid, and many can be taught simple quantitative tests for glycosuria.

Exercise should be timed for after meal rather than premeal periods. The amount varies with the level of fatigue. Swimming and horseback riding may be hazardous because of the danger of hypoglycemia.

Home Management.—Prebreakfast, prelunch and/or presupper urine tests may be used to guide the patient in the daily regulation of insulin. The bedtime sugar-free specimen serves as a warning against night hypoglycemia. Meals should be spread far apart. Quantitative twenty-four hour tests may be done once in one or two weeks. The child should be weighed at least once a month. Monthly visits to the physician are recommended for the first three months and then every three months thereafter.

Summer Camps have been used to provide safe vacations and readjustments of treatment after the original hospitalization, but reëducation of the child, preferably in the hospital is recommended after the age of sixteen.

The first camp for diabetic children was started by the late Dr. Wendt in Detroit. Our own camp program had its simple beginning when a Deaconess nurse took one child to her home in Maine for the summer. The result was excellent and in the subsequent year, 1927, she was persuaded to take 5 children and gradually expanded her work until the time when her own health failed. In 1932 our first group of children was sent to the Clara Barton Camp in North Oxford. Fifty-five children can be cared for at one time, for two weeks each, or a total of 170 children, during July and August. This camp is supported by the Universalist Church, the Diabetic Fund and the children. Similar units have been used for our boys at Prendergast and at Hawthorne House. This year the Social Service of the Massachusetts Unitarian Women helped organize Camp Tonawandah for boys in New London, New Hampshire. Diabetic units of 8 to 12 girls have been cared for at Camp Teela-Wooket at Roxbury, Vermont and 8 to 12 boys at Camp Idlewild at Lake Winnipesaukee, New Hampshire. For other camps for diabetic children, see Joslin.[1]

Standards for the Control of Diabetes.—Perfect control, good control of diabetes, or indifferent control of glycosuria without ketosis, have all been advocated as the ideal standards for this

---

[1] Joslin: New England Jour. Med., **234**, 442, 476, 1946.

48

disease. Perfect control of juvenile diabetes is almost impossible outside of institutional care. The aglycosuric active child develops hypoglycemia and refuses to tolerate its discomfort and embarrassment. If diabetes could be perfectly controlled without hypoglycemic shock, all clinicians would strive for perfection. Good control, a loss of less than 10 per cent of the carbohydrate intake, is our ideal, in order to retain calories for growth and comfort, a positive nitrogen balance, vitamin B_1, and the anti-infection protein fractions, and also to avoid dehydration, disturbed acid base balance and further islet degenerations.

The complete standard for control of the juvenile patient is glycosuria less than 10 per cent of the carbohydrate intake, freedom from ketosis, blood-sugar levels normal before meals, average gain in weight, normal energy and happiness.

Behavior Problems.—Close adherence to the prescribed routine is the rule in the first year of treatment. The child may have pride in hypodermic injections, testing outfits, etc. After the first year, the routine of treatment palls. Indiscretions occur. Up to the time of adolescence the child may be coaxed back to routine, but in adolescence, medical rejection parallels parental rejection. The diabetic routine does not favor the social success of the patient. Unity of behavior pattern and fastidiousness conflict with the prescribed diabetic treatment. Complete break in the control of diabetes occurs only too often. With the normal diabetic child the rejection rarely lasts more than two years. If the rejection is long and bizarre, psychiatric investigation is indicated. Abnormal electroencephalograms suggesting psychomotor behavior, grand and petit mal, occur. Such patients become more coöperative with appropriate sedation therapy. The following behavior should be investigated: self-induced hypoglycemia or coma, pseudo cures, and repeated hospitalization. Incorrectly kept (perfect) urine charts, the substitution of water for a specimen of urine, the substitution of an obliging normal friend's urine for the patient's own, while annoying to the physician, should not be considered abnormal behavior for the juvenile diabetic. Such acts do not require a psychiatric consultation but a remembrance of the spirit which pervades Angelo Patri's writings.

Intelligence of the Diabetic Child.—Intelligence tests have been made by Louise Cone on 169 of our diabetic children and found to be higher by 10 on the average, than a control series whose median age was the same. Others, Brown and Thompson[1] and McGavin, Schultz, Peden and Bowen,[2] have not found evidence of mental superiority.

Physical Examination.—The physical examination of the diabetic child after several years' duration, compared with normal children,

[1] Brown and Thompson: Am. Jour. Dis. Child., **59**, 238, 1940.
[2] McGavin, Schultz, Peden and Bowen: New England Jour. Med., **223**, 119, 1940

reveals that the diabetic has a wider range of height and weight, short and obese children occurring less frequently in the control population studied and reported by Wagner, White and Bogan.[1] Fisher, Macklen and Marks[2] report similar deviations of height and weight for a diabetic group.

The skin except for xanthosis shows no common difference. The teeth had less evidence of caries, hardly more than physiological caries of the sixth and twelfth molar were observed. Pyorrhea, usually of only slight degree, occurred more frequently in the diabetics than in the non-diabetics. Systolic heart murmurs are more often heard. These are functional, not organic. The liver is more often palpable, and there is more evidence of congenital anomalies of the mesenchymatous tissue, such as ear nodules, clubbed fingers, curved fingers, web toes.

Of the secondary sex characteristics, the early ones are often precipitated and the late ones postponed. The measurement of the follicle-stimulating hormone and of 17-keto-steroid shows the same behavior especially in reference to the latter, the excretion of which is high at onset of diabetes and later falls to subnormal values. The follicle-stimulating hormone is elevated at onset, falls to low values and then may rise again.

F. Complications of Diabetes in Childhood.—The diabetic child may develop coma, infections, skin lesions such as xanthosis, xanthoma, necrobiosis lipoidica diabeticorum, neuropathies, epilepsy, retardation of growth and development, nephritis, hypertension, arteriosclerosis, cataracts and retinopathies.

1. **Diabetic Coma.**—The incidence of diabetic coma in the juvenile diabetic population is relatively great. Yearly, 40 per cent of the coma admissions at the George F. Baker Clinic are childhood diabetics. The intercurrence of an infection, omission of insulin and overeating are the inciting causes. Similar irregularities in the diabetic adult do not incite coma as easily as they do in the child, who has a smaller total quantity of glycogen stored. This deficiency in storage of glycogen has been demonstrated experimentally by Mirsky and Nelson,[3] who administered phloridzin, 15 to 20 grams, to diabetic children and produced hypoglycemia and ketonemia. This did not occur in the adult.

The signs and symptoms of diabetic coma are the same in the child and the adult. The onset, however, may be more rapid in the child because coma has been known to occur within twelve hours of hypoglycemia. The warning signs and symptoms are malaise, increasing weakness, intense thirst, pains in legs, abdomen and back, nausea, vomiting, air hunger, drowsiness often preceded by excitability. Physical examination shows the signs of dehydration,

[1] Wagner, White and Bogan: Loc. cit., p. 743.
[2] Fisher, Macklen and Marks: Am. Jour. Dis. Child., **64**, 1833, 1942.
[3] Mirsky and Nelson: Jour. Am. Med. Assn., **67**, 100, 1944.

acidosis, and medical shock: the color is flushed and the papillæ of the tongue prominent, a membrane may extend from the tonsillar region into the larynx, the pulse is rapid, the respiration Kussmaul in type, the blood-pressure low, the heart sounds weak, the apex may be displaced, harsh breath sounds and sometimes crepitant râles are heard, the abdomen may be rigid, diffusely tender and spastic, the eyeballs are soft, the odor of acetone prevails, reflexes may be diminished or absent.

The chemical signs of coma are the lowering of the alkali reserve, the elevation of the blood sugar and non-protein nitrogen. The white count is elevated, the urine contains sugar, acetone and diacetic acid, albumin, and showers of granular casts. The gastric content often consists of old blood.

Treatment.—The treatment of coma in the child differs little from that of the adult except in simplicity and consists largely of three measures: insulin to combat diabetes, fluid to combat dehydration, and lavage to correct gastric dilatation. The size and frequency of the dose of insulin depend upon the clinical severity of the case. Of all single determinations, as a guide for the prescription of insulin, the level of the blood sugar is of greatest value. From five to fifteen years, if the blood sugar is less than 500 milligrams, 100 to 150 units in six hours are usually adequate. If the range of blood sugar is from 500 to 750 milligrams, 150 to 200 units; if 750 to 1000 milligrams, 200 to 250 units; over 1000 milligrams, 300 units or more. Infants and children under five years of age require from 25 to 100 units. The rate of administration and the size of the individual dose vary from 5 units every hour for the infant to 50 units every half hour for the severe adolescent. Combined subcutaneous and intravenous injections are indicated if the patient is unconscious.

Fluid is second in importance to insulin; from 500 to 5000 cc. of normal salt solution have been administered in twelve hours.

Repeated gastric lavage and enemata are often necessary to counteract gastro-intestinal stasis; constant venoclysis, caffeine, ephedrine, epinephrine and blood transfusion are indicated in case of circulatory collapse which, however, seldom occurs in the child. Ten per cent saline solution, 30 to 90 cc., may correct renal block.

Pre-coma and coma in childhood must be differentiated from hypoglycemia, uremia, pneumonia, acute appendicitis and diphtheria. Complications of convalescence are infections of the skin, infections of the urinary tract, and edema.

The prognosis for recovery is 100 per cent except for patients *in extremis* at the beginning of treatment. (See Chapter XIII, page 420.)

2. **Infections.**—Until recently a variety of infections have been second in importance to coma as the cause of death in young diabetics. The sites of the infection and the types of the invading organ-

isms are almost specific. Abscesses and carbuncles, osteomyelitis, pyelonephritis, all usually due to staphylococcus infections, and pulmonary tuberculosis are characteristic of diabetes. Delayed development of antibody to staphylococcus toxin in diabetic children was observed by Bates and Weiss,[1] who compared 14 normal children with diabetics given 7 or 8 weekly injections of unmodified staphylococcus toxin. There was no effect upon the diabetes, but there was a delay in the development of antibody after intradermal injection of staphylococcus toxin in diabetic children. Not only was there slower production of alpha antistaphylolysin, but the maximum titers attained after several weeks of immunization were lower than those of a similar group of normal children. Lack of control of diabetes retarded and diminished the production of antihemolysin. (See Chapter XVI, page 523, for discussion of long resistance to infection in diabetes.) Eight per cent of our children are known to have had severe skin infections (178). Three per cent had pyelonephritis (53 cases). Two per cent (41 cases), pulmonary tuberculosis, and five-tenths of 1 per cent (11 cases), osteomyelitis. Chemotherapy has altered the course of sepsis in the young patient.

The outcome of tuberculin or Mantoux tests does not indicate increased susceptibility to tuberculosis, because 13 per cent of the children tested between 5.0 and 9.9 years of age were positive reactors, 39 per cent between 10.0 and 14.9 and 22 per cent between 15.0 and 19.9 years. The mortality in the 41 cases of tuberculosis was high, 50 per cent. Control of diabetes and sanatorium care are indicated. Surgical removal of the diseased area process has been attempted in two, but the total number of cases operated upon is too few and the period of postoperative observation is too short for conclusions as to the advantage of the radical approach.

3. **Hepatomegaly.**—Hepatomegaly has been recorded in 110 of our diabetic children. The livers so classified were palpated 4 fingers or more below the costal margin and by roentgen-ray were frequently found to extend into the pelvis. Such children exhibit protuberant abdomens, have bouts of abdominal pain and are often dwarfish in stature. The nature of the enlargement is not known because of lack of autopsy and biopsy material. The most probable explanations are fatty infiltration, glycogen deposition or hydropic degeneration. Estimation of blood fat and response of the blood to adrenalin have revealed no deviation from the normal. Liver function tests were also normal.

In experimentally produced diabetes hepatomegaly results. The depancreatized dog exhibits fatty infiltration of the liver, but the depancreatized dog has been deprived of external as well as internal pancreatic elements. There is a possibility that the child has a congenitally small pancreas lacking in external as well as internal

[1] Bates and Weiss: Am. Jour. Dis. Child., **62**, 341, 1941.

factors. The anterior pituitary injected dog of Young had hepato-megaly associated with an increase of glycogen.

Stetson and Ohler[1] report a most valuable case, the only juvenile at that time with biopsy findings. The liver showed essentially normal structure. The nuclei contained no glycogen but there was a large amount of intracellular glycogen. There was no increase in fat deposit. The amount of glycogen laid down as glycogen was tremendous. Impairment of glycogenolysis rather than glycogenesis was considered responsible.

In March, 1940, Case 6884, age at onset of diabetes 13.3 years, duration 11.7 years, was explored for a possible tumor in relation to the liver. None was found, so a biopsy of the liver was done. The liver substance was studied histologically and chemically. The fat content was 10.5 per cent, the glycogen 12.1 per cent. At the time of operation the blood sugar was 33 milligrams, yet there were no symptoms of hypoglycemia. Lack of comparable material from control subjects makes interpretation of the data difficult. The patient was receiving crystalline insulin 20 units plus protamine zinc insulin 60 units. (See page 545.)

The phosphatase was 9 Bodanski units. She was not acidotic at the time. Is this a blocking of glycogen due to the low blood sugar and liberation of adrenalin? Is it an example of overproduction of sugar and of fat? Or does it merely represent a transition from poorly controlled diabetes with an excess of depot fat toward con-trolled diabetes with glycogen replacing fat?

Raw pancreas, betaine and protamine insulin were all used in therapy of these cases. Raw pancreas probably had no effect in 2 cases, but we must admit that we have confessions of much dis-carded therapy. Betaine, in 50 per cent of those treated with it, was followed by a significant reduction in the size of the liver and complete reduction in all was noted when protamine zinc insulin was employed. Grayzel and Radwin[2] report reduction of the size of the liver when the patients were treated with pancreatic extract. They believe the enlargement due to fatty infiltration and found instances resistant to protamine zinc insulin, a situation we have not observed. Lipocaic and choline have also been advocated. We consider the prognosis for recovery with protamine zinc insulin is 100 per cent. Protamine zinc insulin corrects this complication when found and we believe usually prevents its development.

4. **Lesions of the Skin.**—The skin lesions include xanthosis, xan-thoma and necrobiosis lipoidica diabeticorum. Xanthosis is the yellow to orange discoloration of the nasolabial fold, plantar and palmar surfaces. It appears to be due to the high carotin content of the diet

---

[1] Stetson and Ohler: Loc. cit. p. 545.
[2] Grayzel and Radwin: Loc. cit. p. 134.

or its faulty utilization in diabetes. Omission of vegetables with high carotin content, carrots, tomatoes and peas, promotes recovery.

Xanthoma diabeticorum (see page 593), a rare lesion, has been recognized in 5 juvenile patients. The lesions disappear when faulty fat metabolism indicated by hypercholesterolemia, has been corrected.

Of greatest interest is the lesion of necrobiosis lipoidica diabeticorum. Its incidence is almost exclusively in young patients, with females predominating. (See Chapter XX, page 595.) Seventeen juvenile patients have been known to have it; 12 are girls. The cause and treatment are unknown but the lesions tend to fade, often leaving a white scaly scar and, sometimes, no trace whatsoever.

5. **Neuropathies.**—Epilepsy proved with abnormal electroencephalograms has occurred in 50 cases. Petit or grand mal and, sometimes, both occur. Hyper- and hypoglycemia have been suspected as causes. It is possible that hypoglycemia merely reveals the latent case. A few cases have had serious progression. More have apparently subsided with sedation therapy which has been followed with improvement in electroencephalographic tracings.

Of some interest is Case 15322, whose similar twin does not have diabetes. The electroencephalograms reveal similar deviations from the normal. The diabetic has epileptiform attacks in the absence of hypoglycemia. The non-diabetic twin has had none.

Neuropathies have been relatively infrequent in childhood. One patient only has had a neuropathic joint, 40 have had severe neuronitis, 7 have had typical nocturnal diarrhea. Although the neuropathies appear to follow bouts of uncontrolled diabetes, resumption of control and replacement of large quantities of vitamin B have not resulted in prompt recovery.

6. **Retardation of Growth and Development.**—One hundred forty-five of the diabetic children in this series of 2191 are known to have retardation of growth and development. The classification of retardation was made when the height deviated 4 or more inches below the Baldwin and Wood standard for age. This series includes the 118 reported by Wagner, White and Bogan.

The child who is most susceptible to retardation is the one whose age at onset of diabetes occurs under five years. Boys constituting 92 of the total are more susceptible than girls. Although at onset of retardation the child is often of subnormal weight, eventually obesity usually occurs. One hundred forty-four of the 145 were normal or above height at onset of the disease. One child was 4 inches below height at onset of diabetes.

An appraisal of the retarded child shows infantile proportions, normal intelligence, range of I.Q. from 65 to 130, immature behavior, protuberant abdomen, hepatomegaly, retardation of sexual development, delay of osseous development, elevation of basal metabolism with normal specific dynamic action, elevation of serum FSH in 18 of 22 tested and lowering of 17-keto-steroid in 8 of 9 tested, low calcium in 2 of 11 cases and phosphorus, low in 3 of 17 tested.

Cataracts, infections, caries and pyorrhea occurred with slightly greater frequency than in other diabetic children.

The control of diabetes in the retarded child in our series was good—excellent (90 to 100 per cent retention of ingested carbohydrate) 70 per cent of the time, good (80 to 90 per cent retention) 23 per cent of the time and poor only 7 per cent of the time.

In addition to typical diabetic pseudo-dwarfism which occurred in 92 of these cases, 63 appeared to belong to different classifications as follows: transitory infantilism 32, constitutionally small individuals 14, undernutrition 3, congenital anomalies 2, neglect 1, tertiary lues 1.

Faulty nutrition, hypopituitarism and hypogonadism have been offered as possible causes of retardation. The obesity characteristic of most, does not favor the theory that undernutrition *per se* is the cause. The high titers of follicle-stimulating hormone measured in some, indicates that the pituitary is not inactive. The low level of excretion of 17-keto-steroid suggests a mechanism through gonadal failure and its possible effect on nitrogen metabolism. Chesler and Tislowitz[1] found stunting in young alloxan rats who had distended abdomens and infantile primary and secondary sex organs. Miller and Mason[2] have observed diminished excretion of 17-keto-steroid in retarded diabetic children.

The therapy of diabetic pseudo-dwarfism in our patients has passed through four stages: dietary, thyroid, anterior pituitary extract and sex hormones. Dietary treatment was difficult because these children have small appetites. Thyroid feeding was followed by growth in some, but not all cases. Presumably it resulted from stimulation of the eosinophilic cells of the pituitary as in the congenital dwarf mouse so treated. Good results were obtained when pituitary extracts were administered intramuscularly with or without thyroid. So long as the epiphyses were open, response occurred at any age, but after seventeen years of age, puberty was precipitated and the period of growth short, resulting in an adult who still had infantile proportions. Puberty was not precipitated in the younger cases and the end result is one of more proportionate growth. The growth curve, the yearly percentage rate, and the velocity measured by Brodes' formula all show that accelerated growth followed the administration of anterior pituitary extract.

The greatest acceleration of growth followed the use of tetosterone in retarded boys. Masculinization followed its use in girls who responded somewhat to estrogen therapy. The usual prescription was oreton 25 milligrams intramuscularly, twice or three times weekly for two or three years.

[1] Chesler and Tislowitz: Science, 101, 468, 1945.
[2] Miller and Mason: Jour. Clin. Endocrinology, 5, 220, 1945.

The criteria for selection of cases for treatment is bone age, two or more years less than the chronological, open epiphyses, height 4 or more inches below the standard for age.

The diet for the retarded group must be adequate in calories, high in protein, 2 grams per kilogram of body weight and supplemented with vitamins.

No harmful growth effects were observed. There was no evidence of anti-hormone production. The probable effect upon the course of diabetes is of interest. Measured by units of insulin per kilogram, the retarded child treated with growth hormone has the greatest requirement of any group studied, *i. e.*, tall children, ten-year duration children, untreated dwarfs and thyroid-treated dwarfs. No attacks of coma were precipitated. Whether or not diabetes remains severe after cessation of treatment, we do not know.

Nutritional rather than an endocrine origin is the view of McCullagh[1] and Herron and Shepardson.[2] Isolated reports of dwarfism have been made by Villanerde[3] and Oakley.[4]

7. **Cataracts** have been identified in 31 of our 2191 juvenile cases or 1.5 per cent. Not all of the 2191 cases have been examined routinely with the slit lamp. Most of these cataracts occur early in the course of the disease, even at the time of the diagnosis of diabetes; often they are observed in patients whose disease is under three years' duration and are rarely first diagnosed after five years of diabetes. Opacities occur in the posterior subcapsular area and showers of fine cholesterol crystals can be demonstrated. Not all progress. Nine of our 31 patients have been operated upon and the treatment is surgical when vision is sufficiently impaired.

O'Brien[5] reports cataracts in 14 per cent in 260 cases examined. Wachs[6] reports reversal of the cataract, a case in a sixteen year old diabetic. Boyd, Jackson and Allen[7] report posterior subcapsular opacities in one-third of 69 diabetics related to episodes of poor control of diabetes. In contrast to this latter view, Karlstrom[8] reports 38 children treated with the free diet without cataracts.

Our own experience with these patients who have developed cataracts correlates them with poor control of the disease. A common history is of unrecognized diabetes, active symptoms of diabetes for a year, recognition of diabetes in coma and signs of vitamin B deficiency.

8. **Retinal hemorrhages**, small, round, deep and near the disc have been found in 129. Moccasin venom has been used. The results

[1] McCullagh: Rev. Psychiat. Progress Related to Exceptional Child, pp. 49–55, Oct., 1944.
[2] Herron and Shepardson: Clinics, 1, 782, 1942.
[3] Villanerde: Vide Nueva, 18, 42, 1944.
[4] Oakley: Proc. Roy. Soc. Med., 35, 450, 1942.
[5] O'Brien and Allen: Jour. Am. Med. Assn., 120, 190, 1942.
[6] Wachs: Am. Jour. Ophth., 25, 336, 1942.
[7] Boyd, Jackson and Allen: Jour. Am. Med. Assn., 118, 694, 1942.
[8] Karlstrom: Sveno Ratak Tidning, 38, 2623, 1941.

are difficult to evaluate because the hemorrhages may be absorbed spontaneously.

Increased capillary fragility and disease of the retinal vein are attracting attention as factors of greatest importance as the cause of small retinal and large preretinal hemorrhages. Advanced venous and capillary disease may exist in the presence of normal arteries. A mechanism similar to that of menstrual bleeding and pre-eclampsia, suggested by Smith and Smith[1] should be considered. The disturbance of fluid balance caused by the fall of the sex hormones results in cell destruction. This in turn releases a toxic substance, necrosin. In the premenstruum, in preëclampsia, in diabetes, a decrease in steroid hormones is found and hemorrhage characterizes all. Replacement of these substances is being made to see what effect it will have upon the occurrence and course of retinal lesions.

9. **Retinitis proliferans** is known to have occurred in 51 juvenile patients. All except one have nephritis. (See Pathology.) Vitamin therapy, x-ray, moccasin venom and rutin have been employed in this group, but without favorable results.

10. **Nephritis** has been recognized in 165 of our children. At any time, but rarely before ten years' duration of diabetes, albuminuria, edema, hypertension, retinitis, and reversal of the albumin-globulin ratio, may be observed. Hypercholesterolemia complicates many. Others have evidence of pyelonephritis. Heart failure or uremia terminate the course of this nephritis. Pyelonephritis or intercapillary glomerulosclerosis and sometimes both are found at postmortem examination.

The plan for treatment of this group is as follows: First, infection is sought and if found, standard chemotherapy is administered; *E. coli* is treated with sulfonamides, mandelamine or streptomycin; streptococcal infections with sulfadiazine or penicillin; staphylococcal are treated with penicillin parenterally; and *Streptococcus fecalis* with mandelamine. Large doses of vitamin A may be prescribed.

High protein diets are used when low serum protein values are found. Salt is restricted, ammonium chloride, potassium nitrate and mercupurin are employed. If the NPN is high, low protein diets are advised.

Acacia, plasma and salt-free albumin have been used. Successful relief and failures have followed the use of acacia and plasma. Subjective and, at least, temporary chemical improvement followed the administration of albumin. Steroids are being employed, stilbesterol in the female and testosterone in the male, partly because they were found to be deficient and partly because of the experimental work of Selye[2] that steroids promote renal growth. Choline

[1] Editorial, Jour. Am. Med. Assn., **129**, 805, 1945. See also Smith and Smith: J. Clin. Endocrinology, **6**, 483, 1946.
[2] Selye, Hall and Rowley: Lancet, **1**, 30, 1945.

should be considered because it has reversed the hemorrhagic nephritis found in the experimental diabetes of the dog.

Splanchnicectomy was performed upon 3 of the children, Case 5000, Case 6346 and Case 8405. None survived. Postoperative shock terminated Cases 5000 and 8405, and cerebral hemorrhage and myocardial infarct Case 6346. All were poor surgical risks but intercapillary glomerulosclerosis is, in our opinion, not an indication for splanchnicectomy.

11. **Arteriosclerosis** has been demonstrated by opththalmoscopic or *x*-ray examination in 186 children. (See below.)

G. Children Surviving Twenty Years of Diabetes.—In order to evaluate the course of diabetes in childhood, long duration cases have been reported in series, the Fifteen Year Duration Case by White,[1] (150 cases), the Twenty Year Duration Case (73 cases) by Eisele.[2] These patients are again reviewed in the section which follows.

Of the 249 patients who had survived twenty or more years of diabetes on January 1, 1946, 237 were living and 12 had died.

The sex distribution in this group is almost even, 128 males and 121 females. Fifty-five per cent had other members of the family with diabetes. The peak of the age at onset is earlier in this group, being at age five, compared with age twelve for the entire series. Complications were as follows: Coma was known to have occurred in 94, or 38 per cent. Skin infections of severity had occurred in 63, or 25 per cent, pyelonephritis in 22, or 9 per cent, tuberculosis in 6, or 2.5 per cent, osteomyelitis in 3, or 1 per cent. Retardation of growth and development occurred in 37, or 15 per cent, hepatomegaly in 40, or 16 per cent, neuritis in 37, or 15 per cent. Diarrhea occurred in 2 cases. Necrobiosis occurred in 4, or 1.6 per cent, xanthoma in 4, or 1.6 per cent, epilepsy in 3, or 1.5 per cent, cataracts 4, or 1.6 per cent. The significant and disturbing complications were arteriosclerosis, retinitis and nephritis. Arteriosclerosis was found in 106 of 154 cases examined for it, or 70 per cent. Retinal hemorrhage occurred in 51 of 79 cases examined, or 65 per cent. Retinal exudate occurred in 35 of 72 cases examined or, 50 per cent. Hypertension occurred in 49 of 128 cases examined, or 40 per cent and albuminuria in 46 of 138 cases examined, or 35 per cent. Nineteen, or 8 per cent had retinitis proliferans.

It is thus evident that with the number of years of exposure to diabetes occlusive vascular disease and hemorrhage are the chief enemies of the young diabetic. The possible etiological factors are, first, diabetes *per se* through disturbed cellular nutrition, dehydration, trauma from change in osmotic pressure due to fluctuating blood sugar or from disturbed pH. Hypercholesterolemia is a pos-

---

[1] Joslin, Root, White and Marble: Treatment of Diabetes Mellitus, 7th ed., Philadelphia, Lea & Febiger, 1940.
[2] Eisele: Jour. Am. Med. Assn., **120**, 188, 1942.

sibility. Actually in this group 82 patients had repeated determinations for cholesterol. Arteriosclerosis even occurred in all 39 whose cholesterol values were normal. An error in fat metabolism, such as has been suggested by Peters, Kendrick, Keaton and Paul,[1] however, is possible. They believe that since choline furnishes labile methyl groups for the synthesis of phospholipids from fatty acids, inadequate choline results in accumulation of cholesterol and cholesterol esters. In blood phospholipids accumulate until extra supplies of choline are furnished and lead to unloading of fatty acids in the tissues. The rôle of choline in transportation of fatty acids is definite but secondary to that of phospholipid. Choline is, therefore, a suggested form of preventive therapy.

Abiotrophy must be considered. Seventy per cent of parents of diabetics in a series analyzed by Root[2] had vascular disease.

Since occlusive vascular disease progresses (physiologically) with alteration of sex endocrine factors this must be considered. We have evidence that estrin, progesterone and 17-keto-steroid are all lowered in the body of young diabetics and may be replaced. A specific toxin such as necrosin is still another possibility. Infection and sex endocrine abnormalities may be related to its release and their control result in prevention.

Economic Status.—Nearly all of the 249 twenty-year cases have been self supporting. Eighty-three attended college. The occupation of 158 of them are listed below.

6 physicians	1 reporter	1 cashier
4 lawyers	2 photographers	11 factory workers
4 engineers	2 social service workers	27 clerks
9 teachers	3 accountants	13 secretaries
3 musicians	2 technicians	7 salesmen
4 artists	2 dental assistants	6 mechanics
3 chemists	12 business men	2 farmers
1 physicist	5 students	2 salesgirls
1 nurse	1 advertising man	4 chauffeurs
1 architect	1 radio operator	1 glassblower
3 dietitians	1 radio announcer	1 dressmaker
1 librarian	1 draftsman	1 plumber
1 entomologist	1 waiter	1 electrician
1 journalist	2 waitresses	1 game warden
	1 bookkeeper	1 mail carrier

One hundred twenty-six were married and 52 living offspring have been reported by the males and 43 living offspring resulted from 72 pregnancies in the females of this group.

An excellent analysis of the complications of juvenile diabetes has been made by Hans Rosenbusch.[3] He reports 88 cases carefully studied and emphasizes especially the nephropathies and tuberculosis, polyneuritis, eye complications, and retardation of growth and development. Organic nervous disturbance was prevalent in his

[1] Peters, Kendrick, Keaton and Paul: Jour. Am. Med. Assn., **124**, 733, 1944.
[2] Joslin, Root, White and Marble: Treatment of Diabetes Mellitus, 7th ed., Philadelphia, Lea & Febiger, 1940.
[3] Rosenbusch: Loc. cit., p. 618.

group. He believes that early and carefully increasing insulinization will prevent serious disturbances in metabolism and endocrine balance, and that infection may be the inciting cause of nephropathies.

Forty of our cases are, or are becoming, incapacitated because of failing vision.

Diseases of the Other Endocrine Glands and Diabetes.—Deficiency of the posterior lobe of the hypophysis has not been recognized. Posterior pituitary extract is useful in the treatment of the disease, however, for we use it in hypoglycemic insulin reactions in the form of pitressin and pituitrin.

(a) *Adrenal.*—The endocrine gland which is third in rank in connection with carbohydrate metabolism is the adrenal. Marked clinical evidence of hyperactivity of the adrenal occurred in none of our children. Truly precocious puberty or a Hercules child was not known. One of our dwarfish children had a calcified adrenal. High levels of 17-keto-steroid excretion is characteristic of diabetes at onset followed by subnormal levels in many cases after ten years' duration of the disease.

(b) *Thyroid.*—The incidence of thyroid disease in juvenile diabetes is somewhat accidental. Thus among 2191 children there have been 4 (Cases 377, 3428, 10713, 14148) with typical primary hyperthyroidism. There was nothing remarkable about them. Diabetes was aggravated until the patients were relieved of their hyperthyroidism by operation. Three of our children have been treated for hypothyroidism (Cases 5560, 14850, 21367).

(c) *Gonads.*—The rôle of the gonads in diabetes is of interest because of the possible etiological relationship—the greatest incidence of onset occurring at twelve years, and the effect of catamenia on the course of the disease. Removal of the gonads does not prevent the onset of diabetes in the depancreatized animal. An increased sensitivity and finally increased resistance to insulin is reported.

The cycle of 24 girls was studied at camp in 1939. With an almost unchanged diet and insulin dosage, the glycosuria appeared to be greatest in the pre-menstrual and menstrual periods falling to low levels between seven and twenty-one days. Blood-sugar determinations were not made. Whether this is a change in severity or threshold, we do not know.

Low level of 17-keto-steroid in diabetic boys and young male adults suggests hypogonadism after years of duration of the disease. The levels fall below that which might indicate adrenal insufficiency alone.

Amenorrhea, meno- and metrorrhagias and chronic cystic mastitis complicate diabetes. A syndrome of edema, amenorrhea accompanied by low level of 17-keto-steroid excretion and often with high level of FSH, has been observed in 22 of our diabetic girls this past year.

TABLE 106.—FSH AND 17-KETO-STEROID VALUES IN HYPO-MENORRHEIC DIABETIC GIRLS.

Age.	Case No.	17-keto-steroid.	FSH M.U./100 cc. serum.	Menses.
18	24516	0.32	+33	Amenorrhea 3 years' duration
28	11032	0.36	<33	Irregular amenorrhea—long periods
32	20814	1.60	+*	Irregular
14	24060	1.60	<33	Not established
20	10628	2.30	..	Irregular, every 6 weeks
14	12824	2.40	..	Not established
18	20358	2.60	+*	Amenorrhea
18	27888	2.90	<33	Irregular
18	18935	3.00	<33	Amenorrhea
22	20332	3.50	+33	Amenorrhea
22	24586	3.70	N.D.	Amenorrhea
18	11420	3.70	+33	Irregular
19	16332	3.80	+50	Amenorrhea
20	24626	4.20	<33	Onset 18—every 4 months
28	27467	4.40	+33	Regular

* Urine 20 milligrams.

Amenorrhea in this group is corrected, but presumably with anovulatory cycles, by the administration of stilbesterol 0.5 milligrams daily for fourteen days followed by the administration of pranone 10 milligrams daily for seven days and omission of therapy for seven days. Thyroid, 1 grain of Armour's extract, is given continuously, but thyroid alone has rarely corrected amenorrhea in this group. If the 17-keto-steroid excretion is low, the hypogonadism in boys has been treated with testosterone.

(*d*) *Pancreas.*—None of our diabetic children has developed hyperinsulinism.

(*e*) *Hypothalamus.*—Obesity is a problem of the female adolescent diabetic. Since the distribution has resembled Fröhlich's syndrome a pituitary hypothalamic deficiency has been suspected.

Diabetes in Infancy.—A most complete report of diabetes in infancy (onset under twelve months) was made by Limper and Miller.[1] Thirteen of our children had onset on or before their first birthday. Of these 11 are alive with durations of diabetes ranging from two to twenty years. Case 5459 at the age of thirteen had the physical development of a boy of eighteen years and had the highest I.Q. ever observed by an examiner with much experience in private schools.

Complications such as acidosis, skin lesions, and gangrene have been reported with relatively great frequency in this group. In our series coma was the rule, one had tuberculosis, hepatomegaly and dwarfism, and one died probably of coronary heart disease.

Course of Diabetes.—Based upon the behavior of the blood sugar and the total dosage of insulin, juvenile diabetes appears

[1] Limper and Miller: Loc. cit., p. 206.

progressively severe. But based on units of insulin per kilogram of body weight, the increasing severity is not so apparent. Although the absolute number of units of insulin increases with age and duration, the units per weight (kilogram) are nearly constant, there being a rise in the twelfth year, perhaps indicating puberty (pituitary) changes.

Attempts at Alleviation of Diabetes.—In the recent past serious attempts other than dietary have been made to alleviate the course of the diabetes. These attempts, unsatisfactory to date, are the natural outcome of the experiments of Young and Houssay. Inhibition of pituitary activity has been attempted through surgery, p. 709, radiation, p. 123, estrogen, p. 127, and androgen[1] treatment. No dramatic cures have been reported but clinical experiments should be continued. This seems especially true when one remembers the carefully controlled experiments of Professor Zondek who demonstrated that the estrogens were capable of inhibiting certain of the pituitary factors, namely growth and gonadotropic, the growth factor inhibited to the extent of producing symmetrical dwarfism. A theoretical objection is raised here, however. If it is only a brief period of hyperactivity of the pituitary which is capable of producing permanent and irreversible changes, such therapy would have less value in the management of actual than in the potential diabetics. These latter can be classified today only on a genetic basis, the similar twin of a diabetic or the offspring of conjugal diabetics. This is not a contradiction of the Houssay experiments, because the mechanism of hypophysectomy after pancreatectomy is conceded to be one of increased utilization of glucose, and inhibition of glucose production. Lacking insulin, these animals have no diabetes when fasted; they have mild diabetes when fed. Best has added another successful method of preventing the development of experimental diabetes, for the disease does not follow the simultaneous administration of insulin and pituitary extract. (See page 123.) No spontaneous cures have occurred in our juvenile series.

H. Mortality.—Of the 2191 diabetic children 1774 are living and 385 have died, 221 in the insulin era. As deaths from coma and sepsis are falling, those due to vascular disease, especially nephritis and to a less extent coronary heart disease, have increased. (See Table 108.) Deaths from coma are commonest in short duration cases accounting for more than half of the deaths occurring under five years of the disease. After fifteen years of diabetes half of the deaths are due to

[1] Through the courtesy of Dr. Herbert Pollack we are allowed to give his experience. On September 10, 1940, he wrote as follows: "My associates and I have given up to 150 milligrams of testosterone propionate, intramuscularly, each week, to a group of patients with diabetes mellitus over a period of months. There was no detectable effect on the diabetes *per se*, even though there was some relief of the impotence in half of the male patients treated. This work was presented at the Graduate Fortnight of the New York Academy in 1939. We are continuing further experiments with larger doses."

nephritis. Until 1930, coma deaths far out-numbered all others. From 1930 to 1936 deaths due to infections approached those due to coma. Between 1940 and 1946, nephritis has become the chief cause of death in patients with onset of diabetes in childhood.

TABLE 107.—CAUSES OF DEATH ACCORDING TO DURATION OF DIABETES.

	Total.	Coma.	Nephritis.	Tuberculosis.	Sepsis.	Hypoglycemia.	Accident.	Pneumonia.	Heart.	Miscellaneous.
Less than 1 yr.	12	10	1	0	0	0	0	0	0	1
1– 4.9	66	46	2	1	0	3	1	4	1	8
5– 9.9	59	21	3	13	6	2	3	1	0	10
10–14.9	36	9	8	4	2	2	2	1	1	7
15–19.9	36	2	17	3	2	1	2	2	1	6
20+	12	0	6	0	1	0	1	0	3	1
Total	221	88	37	21	11	8	9	8	6	33

TABLE 108.—CAUSES OF DEATH ACCORDING TO PERIODS OF TREATMENT.

	Total.	Coma.	Nephritis.	Tuberculosis.	Sepsis.	Hypoglycemia.	Accident.	Pneumonia.	Heart.	Miscellaneous.
1922–1929	49	39	2	0	0	0	1	3	1	3
1930–1935	45	20	3	6	6	2	3	2	0	3
1936–1940	51	15	6	7	4	3	2	1	1	12
1941–1946	76	14	26	8	1	3	3	2	4	15
Total	221	88	37	21	11	8	9	8	6	33

Conclusion.—The course of juvenile diabetes after twenty-five years of insulin therapy is in most respects a favorable one. Survival is assured. Seven hundred forty-nine children in this series have had the disease fifteen years or more, 249, twenty years, 93, twenty-five years and 5 for over thirty years. Coma, sepsis, hepatomegaly, cataracts, skin complications, failure of growth and development, are largely preventable or correctible. Vascular disease alone remains the chief enemy of the young diabetic surviving more than fifteen years' duration of the disease. Correction of all abnormalities in the diabetic should be attempted in an effort to prevent vascular disease in our generations of diabetic children.

CHAPTER XXIX.

PREGNANCY COMPLICATING DIABETES.

By Priscilla White, M.D.

The forty thousand potentially child-bearing diabetic women of the United States are concerned with the following problems: their chances (a) for conception, (b) for surviving pregnancy, (c) for reproducing living children and (d) for transmitting the tendency to develop diabetes.

A. FERTILITY IN DIABETES.

Prior to insulin therapy, few diabetic women conceived. Thus, Bouchardat,[1] the great French clinician, saw no cases of pregnant diabetics and Naunyn[2] in his wide experience saw only one. They wrote as follows: "Dans le nombre si considérable de diabétiques qui sont venus me consulter je n'ai pas mémoire d'avoir vu une seule femme enceinte", and "Ich kenne aus eigner Erfahrung nur einer Fall, der hierer gehört."

Statistics from obstetrical hospitals imply that diabetic women are not fertile. Chicago Lying-in Hospital and Boston Lying-in Hospital in their annual reports show one diabetic pregnancy in about every 1000 deliveries. Barns[3] reports 1 diabetic in every 930 in a study covering fourteen years. This, however, is the expected rate, since only about 1 woman in 1000 of child-bearing age is a diabetic. Observations in diabetic clinics suggest a high fertility rate. The number of pregnant diabetics under observation at any single time in our clinic now never falls below 20 undelivered women and often rises as high as 40. The diabetic woman today who requires investigation for sterility is the exception rather than the rule.

Control of diabetes, however, may be an important factor in fertility and lack of control of diabetes may favor sterility. Thus Zondek[4] has shown that 18 per cent of all sterility cases can be explained on the basis of glycopenia uteri. Increase in the fertility rate in diabetes has followed the course of improved control of the disease. The first increase followed the use of insulin in 1922 and a greater increase in the number of diabetic pregnancies followed the use of slowly acting insulins which control the disease for longer periods of time.

---

[1] Bouchardat: De la Glycosurie ou Diabete Sucre, Paris, Bailliere, 1875, p. 176.
[2] Naunyn, p. 234; Loc. cit., p. 56.
[3] Barns: Jour. Obst. and Gyn., Brit. Emp., **48**, 707, 1941.
[4] Zondek: Genital Functions and their Hormonal Regulation, Baltimore, Williams and Wilkins Co., p. 224, 1941.

49

TABLE 109.—OUTCOME OF 309 PREGNANCIES AMONG 202 DIABETIC WOMEN SEEN
BETWEEN 1898–1936.

	Pre-insulin era.	Insulin era.
Births—Living births		
Number	57	97
Per cent	53	60
Neo-natal		
Number	0	8
Per cent	0	5
Stillbirths		
Number	23	23
Per cent	21	14
Deaths—Miscellaneous:		
Number	23	13
Per cent	21	8
Extrauterine		
Number	0	1
Per cent	0	1
Therapeutic abortion:		
Number	5	20
Per cent	5	21

B. MORTALITY—MATERNAL AND FETAL.

1. **Maternal Mortality.**—The maternal mortality in diabetic
pregnancies should be low. Between January, 1936 and March,
1946 our maternal mortality rate was 0.4 per cent in 271 cases.
There was 1 death eight weeks after delivery, due to infectious
hepatitis.

2. **Fetal Mortality.**—Fetal wastage has been the great problem
in obstetrical diabetes. Recent publications[1] indicate that the fetal
mortality rates have ranged from 25 to 60 per cent, depending on
the length of the pregnancy observed. If the study is limited to
the third trimester, 30 per cent; if the entire period of pregnancy
has been observed, it is as high as 60 per cent. Between 1922 and
1936 the case histories in this clinic show that only 60 per cent of
diabetic pregnancies delivered viable infants, 13 per cent of the
total number of pregnancies terminating in abortion or miscarriage,
14 per cent in stillbirths. If late pregnancies only are included,
the survival is 75 per cent.

Prolonged observation shows that there are five significant abnormalities when pregnancy complicates diabetes. These may be
simply designated as: (1) maternal, (2) obstetrical, (3) chemical,
(4) fetal and (5) placental.

---

[1] Barns: Loc. cit., p. 769. Lawrence and Oakley: Quart. Jour. Med., 11, 45,
1942. Ronsheim: Am. Jour. Obst. and Gyn., 35, 256, 1933. Potter and Adair: Am.
Jour. Obst. and Gyn., 35, 256, 1938. Herrick and Tillman: Surg., Gyn., and Obst.,
66, 37, 1938. Skyper: Quart. Jour. Med., N. S., 2, 353, 1933. Brandstrup and
Okkels: Acta. Obst. and Gyn. Scand., 18, 136, 1938. Lavietes, Leary, Winkler and
Peters: Yale Jour. Biol. and Med., 16, 151, 1943. Miller, Hurwitz and Kuder:
Jour. Am. Med. Assn., 124, 271, 1944. Mosenthal: Bull. New York Acad. Med.,
18, 217, 1942. Smith, Smith and Hurwitz: Am. Jour. Med. Sci., 208, 25, 1944. Bill
and Posey: Am. Jour. Obst. and Gyn., 48, 405, 1944. Cameron: Jour. Oklahoma
Med. Assn., 37, 443, 1944. Ewald: Lancet, 65, 13, 1945. Gaspar: West. Jour.
Surg., Obst. and Gyn., 53, 21, 1945. Johnstone: Brit. Med. Jour., 1, 765, 1938.
White: Jour. Am. Med. Assn., 128, 181, 1945.

The purpose of the discussion which follows is to describe these abnormalities, to evaluate them in relation to fetal deaths, to indicate our attempts to correct them and to alter fetal survival. This analysis includes 271 pregnancies observed between January 1936 and March 1946. Only cases carried to the twenty-fourth week are included. In this series there were 1 maternal and 47 fetal deaths.

C. ABNORMALITIES OF DIABETIC PREGNANCIES.

1. **Maternal Abnormalities.**—Maternal abnormalities complicating obstetrical diabetes are two, vascular disease and hypoovarianism. Diffuse vascular disease manifested clinically by nephritis, coronary heart disease, calcified vessels and retinopathies has occurred in 70 per cent of our diabetic children who have survived twenty years of the disease. The clinical evidence of vascular disease is usually first recognized more than ten years after the onset of diabetes. Up to five years of duration of diabetes, therefore, the young diabetic obstetrical patient may be considered the same as the non-diabetic. After five years' duration of the disease, the status of the vascular pattern may be evaluated by adding the duration of diabetes to the chronological age and, when the duration of diabetes exceeds fifteen years, by doubling the chronological age.

Hypo-ovarianism is suggested clinically by amenorrheas, meno- and metrorrhagias, chronic cystic mastitis and a type of retardation of growth seen in young diabetics. The patients with menstrual abnormalities and growth failures have characteristically normal or high titres for FSH and low levels for excretion of 17-ketosteroids suggesting normal pituitary function with gonad and (or) adrenal failure. This disturbance of endocrine balance is not characteristic at onset of diabetes where the levels of FSH are high and 17-ketosteroid excretion high, but are observed with increasing duration of the disease. Atrophy of the ovary with poor follicular development has been reported at postmortem examination. Thus, in spite of an outward appearance of youth and vigor, the young diabetic woman must be considered a physically and gynecologically aging individual.

2. **Obstetrical Abnormalities.**—The obstetrical course in diabetes includes many abnormalities, the first of which may be uterine irritability. Contractions are present throughout pregnancy. Early spontaneous rupture of membranes without delivery but with loss of amniotic fluid for months occurred in 1.5 per cent of our cases. Miscarriage occurred in 25 per cent, pre-eclampsia in 40 per cent and breech presentation in 33 per cent. Uterine inertia and shoulder dystocia are common. A normal obstetrical course in diabetes in our experience has thus been conspicuous.

3. **Chemical Abnormalities.**—The chemical abnormalities in diabetic pregnancies are three: (1) the low renal threshold for glucose;

(2) water retention, and (3) imbalance of the sex hormones of pregnancy.

The low renal threshold for glucose physiological for pregnancy complicates a co-existing diabetes. If untreated, it favors acidosis and if overcorrected with insulin treatment, favors hypoglycemia. Thus, in spite of nearly normal levels for blood sugar, the excretion of sugar may amount to 50, 100 or 150 grams per day. Carbohydrate deprivation is further increased by the demands of the fetus (up to 50 grams a day), the blockage of glycogen in tissues which results from over-insulinization (exogenous) and the occasional low food intake to which the capricious appetite of pregnancy predisposes the diabetic as well as the normal woman. These four causes of carbohydrate deprivation in the simplest type of pregnancy in the diabetic favor the utilization of fat and early development of ketosis. Therapeutic ammonium chloride to correct edema, lowered efficiency of the liver in storage of glycogen, lowered efficiency of the kidney in excreting acids when toxemia complicates a diabetic pregnancy enhance the easy development of acidosis.

Profound disturbance of water balance is one of the most characteristic features of pregnancy in the diabetic. This is shown by the abnormal gain in weight, edema (85 per cent of all cases),[1] hydramnios (24 per cent), hydremia and fetal edema.

The imbalance of the sex hormones was found in 227, or 80 per cent, of the 271 patients in this series of diabetic pregnancies. This imbalance consisted of low excretion of pregnandiol, low serum level of estrin, high serum level of chorionic gonadotropin and disappearance of basophilic navicular cells from the vaginal smear. The underlying mechanism appears to be faulty production of progesterone with poor production or metabolism of estrogens and compensating high levels of chorionic gonadotropin.

The techniques for determinations and the standards for classification of cases are as follows:

The serum to be tested for chorionic gonadotropin is precipitated with ethanol and stands overnight. It is then extracted with ether and the residue suspended in 6 cc. of normal saline. Since we are attempting to routinize procedures, low levels of gonadotropin are not determined. The following amounts of sera are used: 0.5, 0.3, 0.2, 0.15, 0.1 and 0.075 to give readings on 200, 333, 500, 775, 1000 and 1500 rat units per 100 cc. of serum. Twenty-one day-old rats weighing 35 to 45 grams are injected twice daily for three days. The morning of the sixth day the rats are necropsied. The end point sought is the macroscopic demonstration of mature corpora lutea. The tests are made in duplicate, one positive reading out-weighing a negative. Animals whose weights exceed 59 grams at the time of exploration are discarded.

As in any test in which the determination of the end point is objective, accuracy and consistency in detecting the presence of corpora lutea in the ovary are the result of experience. Ovarian and uterine weights have not been used as criteria in the cases reported here. Whereas ovarian weights usually parallel the end point of macroscopic corpora lutea in a few

[1] White and Hunt: Jour. Clin. Endocrin., 111, 500, 1943.

instances, these have not been present in large ovaries and, conversely, have been present in some small ones. The uterine weights were inconsistent, frequently the largest uteri (cystic) were observed in rats with the smallest ovaries and likewise in some cases the smallest uteri were seen in animals with large ovaries.

Pregnandiol: The method of Venning and Browne[1] was first used and later that of Astwood[2] for determination of pregnandiol. The curves published by Venning and Browne were used as standards.

Estrogen: Few estrogen assays were made because in the past the procedure has been time-consuming and fetal death or termination of the pregnancy may occur before significant data are accumulated. It was also found that the values for estrogen were usually in indirect proportion to the gonadotropins and the test for the latter is more simple and practical from the chemical point of view, 5 or 10 cc. of blood being necessary, in contrast to the 40 or 50 cc. for the established estrogen assays. Newer methods using minute quantities of blood recently have been described.

Vaginal smears taken according to the technique of Papanicolaou and Traut[3] have been done on 27 delivered cases. The smears have been graded:

0	all navicular, basophilic cells
0–0.5	few squamous acidophilic cells
0.5	$\frac{1}{8}$ acidophilic
1	$\frac{1}{4}$ acidophilic
2	$\frac{1}{2}$ acidophilic
3	$\frac{3}{4}$ acidophilic
4	all acidophilic cells

4. Fetal Abnormalities.—The fetal abnormalities are physical, chemical and pathological. The physical abnormalities include (1) the large size; (2) jaundice; (3) atelectasis, and (4) congenital defects. A birth weight exceeding the expected normal for the period of gestation occurs in 80 per cent of the infants of diabetic mothers.[4] The body length also exceeds the average for the chronological age. The body weight of the infants is influenced by three factors: (a) fat, (b) edema and (c) large size of the organs. The gross appearance and the depth of the adipose tissues measured at autopsy were evidence of the nutritional obesity. Edema occurred commonly in the infants. It is evidenced by pitting, diuresis and total weight loss. The maximum weight loss in our infants was 2 pounds in three days and a near maximum 1 pound in twelve hours. The weight loss in seventy-two hours of 60 of the infants in whom data were available was on the average 10.5 ounces as compared with 6.3 ounces for 60 infants of non-diabetic mothers delivered during the same interval at the Faulkner Hospital. The range of weight loss was 0.5 to 25 (32 not included) ounces for infants of diabetics and 1 to 12 ounces for non-diabetics.

Splanchnomegaly: The most striking observation in autopsy protocols has been visceral enlargement. Hertig[5] had previously

[1] Venning: Jour. Biol. Chem., **119**, 473, 1937.

[2] Astwood and Jones: Jour. Biol. Chem., **137**, 397, 1941.

[3] Papanicolaou and Traut: Diagnosis of Uterine Cancer by the Vaginal Smear, New York, The Commonwealth Fund, 1943.

[4] Fischer: Zentralbl. f. Gynäk., **59**, 241, 1935.

[5] Hertig: Personal communication.

reported cardiac enlargement in infants of diabetic mothers. Over a period of years isolated reports of splanchnomegaly occurring in infants of diabetic mothers have appeared. White,[1] White and Hunt,[2] and Miller and Wilson[3] reported series of such infants in 1943. The enlargement is marked in the liver, spleen and heart, less so in lungs and kidneys, variable in the adrenals, pancreas and the thymus. The brain did not equal the expected weight for the normal in any of our infants. Advanced bone development and more mature genital development have also been observed. Schretter and Nevinny[4] observed changes in the fetal hypophysis.

Jaundice with normal blood counts and no tendency to bleed has occurred in all the infants in our series. *Atelectasis* has been observed in one-third of the living and all of the fatal cases.

Congenital anomalies have often been reported[5] and occurred in 12 per cent compared with the expected incidence of 1.8 per cent. They include syndactylism, dwarfism, pancreatic cysts, short tendon, kidney cysts, defects of the skull, heart, claw hand, club foot, web toes, congenital hip, cretinism, feeblemindedness, Mongolian idiocy, ovarian cyst, angioma, cysts of the mouth and varices of the heart. Similar anomalies usually of mesenchymatous tissue have been noted in diabetics. Genetic origin appears to be the most logical explanation. One patient whose infant had a congenital heart had profound vitamin B deficiency treated with parenteral vitamin B throughout pregnancy. Vitamin B deficiency and hormonal imbalance have produced anomalies in the experimental animal.

A tendency for the infants of the diabetic mother to develop *hypoglycemia* has been much emphasized in the obstetrical and pediatric literature. Case reports by Platou,[6] Bigby and Jones,[7] Woodrow,[8] Rynearson and Randall,[9] Dubreuil and Anderodias,[10] Wiener,[11] Gray and Feemster,[12] Lawrence,[13] Nevinny and Schretter,[14] Schretter and Nevinny,[4] Sennenwald,[15] Ehrich,[16] Gordon,[17] and Higgons[18] are referred to.

1 White: Virginia Med. Monthly, **70**, 436, 1943.
2 White and Hunt: J. Clin. Endocrinology, **3**, 500, 1943.
3 Miller and Wilson: Jour. Pediat., **23**, 251, 1943.
4 Schretter and Nevinny: Arch. Gynäk, **143**, 465, 1930.
5 Skyper: Loc. cit., p. 770.
6 Platou: Lancet, **62**, 348, 1942.
7 Bigby and Jones: Brit. Med. Jour., **1**, 360, 1945.
8 Woodrow: Brit. Med. Jour., **1**, 721, 1942.
9 Rynearson and Randall: Jour. Am. Med. Assn., **107**, 919, 1936.
10 Dubreuil and Anderodias: Compt. rend. Soc. deBiol., **83**, 1 490, 1920.
11 Wiener: Am. Jour. Obst. and Gynec., **7**, 710, 1924.
12 Gray and Feemster: Arch. Path. and Lab. Med., **1**, 348, 1926.
13 Lawrence: Quart. Jour. Med., **22**, 191, 1929.
14 Nevinny and Schretter: Arch. f. Gynäk, **140**, 397, 1930. See also Schretter and Nevinny: Ztschr. f. Geburtsh. u. Gynäk., **98**, 258, 1930.
15 Sennenwald: Zentralbl. f. Gynäk, **54**, 817, 1930.
16 Ehrich: Klin. Wchnschr., **13**, 584, 1934.
17 Gordon: Jour. Mich. Med. Soc., **134**, 167, 1935.
18 Higgons: Am. Jour. Dis. Child., **50**, 162, 1935.

Instability of blood sugar rather than hypoglycemia is, we believe, characteristic of the infant of the diabetic mother. The level of blood sugar at birth is above the average normal; this falls precipitously to low normal or slightly subnormal levels in four hours and is then followed by a spontaneous rise. Such behavior is not unlike what is seen during glucose tolerance tests. Indeed the infant may theoretically have been given one—through the spontaneous maternal hyperglycemia or that produced by the glucose administered to the mother during delivery.

The average blood sugar for 38 cases at birth was 100 milligrams, in four hours in 31 cases 70, and in eight hours for 26 cases 80. The range was 30 to 260 milligrams per cent in birth, 9 to 120 milligrams in four hours and 40 to 130 milligrams in eight hours. The lowest blood sugar, 9 milligrams per cent, was associated with signs of hypoglycemia, pallor, sweating and twitching. Glucose relieved the infant instantly.

The minimum, average and maximum blood sugars for the first day of life for the normal infants of normal mothers were found by Lucas et al[1] to be 40, 50, and 60 milligrams per cent respectively. Kitteringham and Austin[2] found the level of blood sugar of the newborn (normal) to be 55 to 75. McKittrick[3] demonstrated the same behavior and reports a normal infant whose blood sugar fell to 28 milligrams but who remained asymptomatic. Comparative blood sugar studies in the parturient woman and the newborn were made by Hanley and Horn.[4] The average maternal macro blood sugar was 106 and micro 128.7 and 126.8. Umbilical venous blood at birth macro was 111.3 and micro 111.7 milligrams. Umbilical arterial blood was macro 88.3 milligrams, micro 95.8 and 96.4. One hour after delivery heel or finger blood was 80.3, six hours after delivery fontanelle 66.1 macro, heel or finger 77.1, 77.5.

Barnes[5] likewise discountenances hypoglycemia in the infants of diabetic mothers and the experimental data of Himwich, Fazekas and Homburger[6] indicate that low blood sugar levels were well tolerated in infancy. Infant rats survive hypoglycemia longer than do adults because of their lower cerebral metabolic requirements.

Pathological characteristics of the infants of diabetic mothers. Excessive hematapoiesis of liver and spleen,[7] glycogen infiltration of the heart, islet hyperplasia,[8] and evidence of gonadotropin stimulation,[9] corpora hemorrhagica in female ovary and advanced bone

[1] Lucas, Dearing, Hoobler, Cox, Jones and Smyth: Am. Jour. Dis. Child., **22**, 525, 1931.
[2] Kitteringham and Austin: Am. Jour. Med. Sci., **195**, 318, 1938.
[3] McKittrick: Personal communication.
[4] Hanley and Horn: Am. Jour. Obst. and Gynec., **46**, 502, 1943.
[5] Barnes: Loc. cit., p. 769.
[6] Himwich, Fazekas and Homburger: Endocrinol., **33**, 96, 1943.
[7] White: Loc. cit., p. 774.
[8] Miller and Wilson: Loc. cit., p. 774.
[9] Banner: Arch. Path., **32**, 818, 1941.

development are the pathological characteristics of the infants of diabetic mothers. So closely does this resemble erythroblastosis that by some the condition is thought to be erythroblastosis without anemia and with positive Rh mothers. Excessive gonadotropin is, I believe, a more logical explanation because chorionic gonadotropin is capable of stimulating hematapoiesis and gonad development. High titer of gonadotropin was found in the infant of Case 10663.

Atelectasis has been an important lethal factor in our cases. Farber[1] describes alveolar changes consistent with intrauterine respiration.

5. The **placenta of the diabetic** pregnancy usually deviates from the normal in size; it is notably large, the cord thickened abnormally and infarcts may be present. A very small placenta occasionally occurs.

6. **Evaluation of the Abnormalities.**—Although all of the factors contribute to fetal fatalities, some we can exclude as not of prime importance, some we must include as being of prime importance.

Maternal acidosis per se is not important as a lethal factor in producing infant deaths as is shown by the slight increase of 6 per cent in the fetal survival rate following the inauguration of insulin treatment. Our clinical observations since 1922 have shown that some fetal deaths occurred in cases of diabetes which were clinically controlled while viable infants were delivered subsequent to treatment of diabetic coma and prolonged acidosis. Diabetic coma complicated pregnancy in 5 of the cases reported here and was followed by delivery of a living child in all instances. Coma did not complicate the course of pregnancy in the 47 patients whose fetuses died.

Hypoglycemia: In our clinical experience we have not seen cases in which maternal hypoglycemia caused fetal fatalities. The most striking example was that of Case 13215 who by mistake received 210 units of protamine zinc insulin in a single injection. At this time she had toxemia and was in the thirty-first week of pregnancy. In spite of continuous administration of glucose she became hypoglycemic to the point of unconsciousness but was delivered of a healthy infant six weeks later. Another patient in the twelfth week of pregnancy, Case 3040, whose case is not included in this series, was admitted to the hospital hypoglycemic and unconscious. She delivered of a healthy infant at term. Case 11872 contracted hypoglycemia in the fourth month of pregnancy and severe acidosis in the third month with survival of the infant.

Whether or not the placenta is permeable to insulin has not been clearly established. Snyder and Hoskins[2] presented evidence of failure of passage of insulin from fetal to maternal circulation.

[1] Farber: Personal communication.
[2] Snyder and Hoskins: Anat. Rec., **35**, 23, 1932.

Britton[1] showed that the administration of insulin to pregnant cats failed to reduce the blood sugar level of the fetuses near term. A species difference in fetal resistance to insulin is shown by the experiment of Schlossman[2] and Parsmore.[3] The fetal dog, sheep and goat are resistant to insulin; the two latter scarcely respond to doses as great as 415 units per kilogram (administered directly into the fetus). In contrast to these animals, fetal rats are susceptible even when insulin is injected into the mother.

Placental glycopenia as a cause of fetal death in pregnancy complicating diabetes is an interesting possibility. Theoretically, placental glycopenia may result from uncontrolled diabetes or more probably the reverse condition, hypoglycemia, whereby there is a blockage of glycogen in the placental cells leading to glycogen insufficiency. Although the placenta plays an important rôle in fetal glycogen metabolism, the fetal liver can function. Since the fetus is not diabetic its liver should respond to the stress and strain produced by placental glycopenia. Our clinical experience does not favor the theory that the disordered carbohydrate metabolism of uncontrolled diabetes or hypoglycemia produced fetal deaths. That good control of diabetes favors successful outcome of diabetic pregnancies is still advanced by Lawrence and Oakley. Cameron, Jordan, Palmer, Rice, Tolstoi and many others now agree with us that diabetes may be well controlled and yet the fetus can die and vice versa.

Congenital anomalies contributed to but one neonatal and two infancy deaths.

The imbalance of the sex hormone of pregnancy appeared to be the most important single harmful factor. The hormonal balance was classified as normal in 64 cases. The fetal survival in this group was 97 per cent (62 cases), the incidence of premature deliveries 0 and of toxemia 2 per cent (1 case).

Fifty cases were classified as having an abnormal hormonal balance. Fetal survival was 52 per cent (26 cases); preëclampsia occurred in 50 per cent and premature delivery in 40 per cent. In this group of cases we saw the behavior we had thought characteristic of diabetic pregnancies; namely, abnormal gain in weight, edema, hydramnios, hypertension and albuminuria and either an intrauterine death or premature delivery with neonatal death. We did not observe this abnormal course when the hormonal balance was normal. Since this suggested a causal relationship an attempt was made to supply the progesterone and estrin to see what effect it would have upon fetal survival, preëclampsia and premature deliveries. This was done in 157 cases.

Results: The fetal survival (corrected) rose to 90 per cent (uncorrected 88 per cent). Premature deliveries fell to 15 per cent,

---

[1] Britton: Am. Jour. Physiol., **95**, 178, 1930.
[2] Schlossmann: Jour. Physiol., **92**, 219, 1938.
[3] Parsmore and Schlossmann: Jour. Physiol., **92**, 459, 1938.

preëclampsia in cases treated early to 5 per cent and the majority of the infants were normal in size and appearance. If we correct for erythroblastosis (1) and a group of patients who received a different progesterone without a single fetal survival, the fetal survival is 90 per cent. Confirmatory studies on the hormonal imbalance in diabetic pregnancies are reported by Hellbaum and Keltz,[1] Jordan,[2] Rice[3] and Bowen.[4]

D. MANAGEMENT OF DIABETIC PREGNANCIES.

Rules for the management of diabetic pregnancies have been evolved during the ten years in which these patients have been studied. Not all have been treated precisely as outlined here. The rules include maternal, obstetrical, chemical and pediatric care.

The diabetic management of our patients during pregnancy is not difficult. The diet must be adequate. Calories are prescribed by weight; namely, 30 per kilogram of increasing body weight. The carbohydrate allowance is liberal, 200 grams. The protein intake should be high, 2 grams per kilogram of body weight, and sufficient fat to complete the caloric requirement. The diet is supplemented with vitamins A, B, C, D, E, and K.

Insulin is prescribed primarily according to blood sugar levels rather than urinary sugars in order to avoid the pitfalls resulting from the lowered renal threshold. The usual routine for insulin treatment in our clinic is maintained, namely, simultaneous administration of protamine zinc insulin and crystalline insulin before breakfast. A pregnant diabetic has the same prescription based on blood sugar levels, but in addition often small to larger doses of crystalline insulin are given before lunch and the evening meal. The amount of insulin for the small later doses is determined by the result of blood rather than urinary sugars. The small doses prevent the excretion of glucose which, as previously stated, may be excessive with nearly normal blood sugar levels. Total insulin requirement increases with each trimester.

The obstetrical management of the pregnant diabetic included the decisions for the time, the type of delivery, the anesthesia and medication (sedation) to be employed.

Early delivery was first recommended by Titus[5] and the time elected in our patients between 1928 and until 1945 was the thirty-seventh week. A gain in confidence has encouraged us to add another week and our present choice is the end of the thirty-seventh week or the early part of the thirty-eighth week. Lawrence and

1 Hellbaum and Keltz: Personal communication.
2 Jordan: Virginia Med. Monthly, **70**, 441, 1943.
3 Rice: Personal communication.
4 Bowen: Jour. Am. Med. Assn., **126**, 18, 1944.
5 White, Titus, Joslin and Hunt: Am. Jour. Med. Sci., **198**, 482, 1939.

Oakley recommend delivery thirty-sixth to thirty-eighth, Woodrow the thirty-sixth to thirty-seventh, Palmer the thirty-sixth to thirty-eighth, Kilkenny eight lunar months. The indication for early delivery is prevention of late intrauterine death characteristic of diabetic pregnancies.

Of our 271 deliveries, 80 per cent have been by cesarean section and 20 per cent by the normal route. Unless the patient is multiparous, has had diabetes for a short period of time and has had a pregnancy which is normal clinically and chemically, we believe she is best delivered by cesarean section. Uterine inertia, contraction bands, shoulder dystocia occur too frequently, breech presentations are too common and the infants too often abnormal in structure and behavior. Cesarean section was first recommended by Titus in 1928. Fraser[1] points out that endocrine disturbances other than diabetes often result in fetal death during delivery. It is true our cases are unique in that they will return to us for future obstetrical care and one obstetrical team handles all. Diabetics tolerate surgical procedures well and early delivery by induction is not practical if the cervix has not been effaced. Fraser, Palmer, Lawrence and Oakley, Woodrow, Rice and others haveor sorgical delivery. Individualization of cases is the logical suggestion of Bill and Posey.

If cesarean section is performed no preliminary sedation is administered. In our practice spinal anesthesia is the one of choice. If normal delivery is feasible minimum sedation is presctibed consisting of not more than 3 grains of seconal or nembutal and $\frac{1}{150}$ grain of scopolamine. Caudal, spinal or nitrous oxide anesthesia may be used during the third stage of labor or for episiotomy.

The pre-operative preparation of the diabetic includes 1000 cc. of 5 per cent glucose in distilled water. Insulin is prescribed after delivery and given 2 to 3 times during the day according to reduction of the urine with the Benedict test. The intravenous, 5 per cent glucose in distilled water, is repeated on the day of surgery and twice daily for three days. Carbohydrate as warm liquids is permitted up to 100 grams by mouth. On the fourth day a suitable soft solid diet of carbohydrate 180, protein 60, fat 60 to 90 grams is tolerated and gradually the normal diabetic diet resumed.

Glucose as 5 per cent solution may be indicated during normal delivery and insulin prescribed at 4 hourly intervals according to tests, 12 units if red or orange by the Benedict test, 8 if yellow, none if better than yellow green.

The chemical management of the diabetic pregnancy includes the use of ammonium chloride 60 to 120 grains daily for edema, restriction of salt, prohibition of sodium bicarbonate and the prescription

---

[1] Fraser: Personal communication.

of the high protein diet. The latter is possible with meat, eggs, milk (skim), cottage cheese and egg white.

The need for hormonal therapy was shown by the fact that an unsuccessful pregnancy appeared to follow one of two general courses: (a) following the hormonal imbalance the mother would deliver prematurely of an infant which was mature in appearance but which would die of atelectasis, (b) during the period of hormonal imbalance the mother would gain weight abnormally, develop visible edema, hydramnios, albuminuria and hypertension. Intra-uterine fetal death would occur followed by the disappearance of the clinical signs of toxemia and later there would be a delivery of a macerated giant.

Diabetes of long standing and severity appears to favor the occurrence of hormonal imbalance in pregnancy and at the present time if a patient presents a history of an obstetrical accident or on physical appraisal appears to have hypogonadal stigmata, such as periods of amenorrhea, menorrhagia, chronic cystic mastitis, edema, or high titres for follicle stimulating hormone, therapy may be instituted prior to the demonstration of a hormonal imbalance. Usually, however, weekly analyses for pregnandiol, chorionic gonadotropin and vaginal smears are made in order to determine if hormonal therapy is indicated. If the pregnandiol falls below the minimum normal according to the curve of Venning and Browne,[1] progesterone and estrogen therapy are started. If the results of two tests during the critical period, the twenty-fourth to thirty-sixth week, exceeds 200 rat units of chorionic gonadotropin per 100 cc. of serum combined therapy is inaugurated. Also if the classification of the vaginal smear is 2 to 4, combined therapy is started. Smith et al.[2] are influenced by low estrin and pregnandiol.

Parenteral hormonal therapy appeared to give better results than oral therapy. There seemed to be no difference in the response to natural or synthetic estrogens. Progesterone preparations did not appear to be equally effective. When therapy with progesterone and estrogen was instituted it was maintained daily or every other day until delivery. The present scheme for treatment is stilbestrol and proluton daily or every other day as follows:

Week of Pregnancy.	Progesterone Proluton mg.	Estrogen Stilbestrol mg.
20	5	5
20–24 . . .	10	10
24–28 . . .	15	15
28–32 . . .	20	20
32–36 . . .	20	25
36	15–50	30–50

[1] One hundred and fifteen milligrams in the twelfth week, 15 in the sixteenth week, 19 in the twentieth, 28 in the twenty-fourth, 40 in the twenty-eighth, 50 in the thirty-second, and 55 in the thirty-sixth week of pregnancy.

[2] Smith, Smith and Hurwitz: Loc. cit., p. 770.

Pellet implantations with crystalline progesterone were used in 5 cases in this series requiring corpus luteum hormone therapy. The results appeared to be satisfactory.

Even with oral stilbestrol in 200 mg. daily doses there were no side reactions. Abscesses have occurred in 8 cases and urticaria requiring discontinuance of treatment in one who subsequently had an intrauterine death.

Bilirubin excretion tests have been normal. No evidence of carcinogenesis has been found. Hyperplastic endometria with prolonged post partum staining has occurred and for this reason the dose of estrogen has been reduced.

Delay in inauguration of treatment, inadequate dosage, failure to double dosage during bouts of fever, failure of absorption of oral therapy, use in hopeless cases, incorrect estimation of the duration of pregnancy account for the majority of the few unsuccessful cases. Only one patient was adequately treated with unsuccessful outcome. Others, Palmer, Rice, Bowen and Cameron, are reporting the successful treatment of pregnant diabetics with estrogen and progesterone.[1]

The ante natal care of the infant includes good treatment of maternal diabetes and hormonal therapy. The natal care includes the choice of the least traumatizing type of delivery. The brain and other structures are not normal and are easily traumatized unless favored. Oxygen is administered to the mother during the delivery. Respiratory depressants which may be transferred from mother to infant are prohibited.

The post natal care of the infant is directed against atelectasis and includes the use of oxygen and insurance of its delivery. The air passages are drained through suction and by posture. The infant of the diabetic certainly has more amniotic fluid in the air passages than the normal. Two possible explanations occur. Windle has shown that the fetuses into whose amniotic sacs sugars have been introduced swallow the fluid. The amniotic fluid of the diabetic was shown long ago by Grafe to contain an excess of glucose. It is not illogical to think these infants swallow and therefore have amniotic fluid in their upper air passages. The uterus of the diabetic is irritable and the change in pressure due to uterine contraction may favor the onset of intrauterine breathing. Farber found evidence suggesting ante natal respiratory efforts in several cases examined by him.

The infant is placed in an oxygen incubator Hess bed immediately after birth. It is stimulated to cry at frequent intervals and if sluggish, stimulated with the Emerson resuscitator. The infant is dehydrated by omission of fluid for three to five days. Magnesium

[1] Palmer and Barnes: West. Jour. Surg., **53**, 195, 1945. Rice: Personal communication. Bowen: Loc. cit., p. 778. Cameron: Loc. cit., p. 770.

sulfate could be used. Alpha-lobelin and adrenalin may be used as respiratory stimulants. Glucose has not been given since 1940.

E. POST PARTUM COMPLICATIONS AND TREATMENT.

Eclampsia is treated as in the non-diabetic. We have seen it twice, in both instances in the post partum period. One patient had received estrogen and progesterone therapy, the other had not. Glucose, oxygen under positive pressure, suction, sedation and magnesium sulfate may be employed. The great difficulty is in differential diagnosis between eclampsia and hypoglycemia. Fortunately the treatment is essentially the same for both conditions.

Pyelonephritis complicates pregnancy and the puerperium more often in the diabetic and is the chief cause for post partum fever. Appropriate chemotherapy, sulfadiazine for Streptococcus, penicillin for Staphylococcus, mandelamine for E. coli, corrects the complication.

Lactation rarely occurs. The chemical analysis of the milk of the diabetic woman is the same as that of the normal woman and nursing is recommended if possible.

F. PREGNANCY AS A CAUSE OF DIABETES.

Only 5 per cent of our female patients of childbearing age have onset of diabetes during pregnancy; pregnancy does not appear to be an inciting or, at least, a common inciting cause of diabetes. West suggests that the influence of pregnancy in this respect is latent since eventually twice as many women contract diabetes as do men.

G. ZONDEK TESTS.

False positive and negative tests occur in diabetes. The negative tests in our experience have been mostly due to submission of samples too early in pregnancy. The positive ones are probably confused with the high titers for FSH seen at onset of diabetes and in diabetic amenorrhea.

H. PREDIABETIC STATE.

The tendency of the diabetic to produce large infants and to follow an abnormal obstetrical course prior to the onset of diabetes has been emphasized by Bix,[1] Bowcock,[2] Bowen,[3] Woodyatt,[4] and Millar.[5] Dolger and Herzstein[6] did not confirm this in a recent review of diabetic women. The large infant produced by the pre-

[1] Bix: Med. Klin., **29**, 250, 1933.
[2] Bowcock and Greene: Jour. Am. Med. Assn., **90**, 502, 1928.
[3] Bowen: Personal communication.
[4] Woodyatt: Personal communication.
[5] Millar: New England Jour. Med., **233**, 376, 1945.
[6] Dolger and Herzstein: Jour. Am. Med. Assn., **125**, 931, 1944.

diabetic suggests a pituitary influence consistent with the high titres for FSH found early in the disease. Chorionic gonadotropin appears to be the growth factor in pregnancies occurring after onset. The serum of our patients injected into hypophysectomized rats did not produce maturation of the ovaries or uteri.

The tendency to develop diabetes is transmitted through mendelian recessive genes. Therefore, childbearing is not prohibited if one marital partner is diabetic, the other normal of a non-diabetic family. It is prohibited if both of the pair are diabetic, not advised if one is diabetic, the other a carrier (child of a diabetic) or a potential diabetic—similar twin of a diabetic or offspring of two diabetics. Three pairs of conjugal diabetics in this series have 4 children five to twenty years of age who at the present writing do not have diabetes.

There are no indications for abortion in diabetes which differ from those for the general population. Indications for sterilization are two, as follows: (1) Three or more cesarean sections and, (2) complicating nephritis, tuberculosis or vascular disease. Although there is no functional effect from sterilization it has a bad psychological one in the diabetic.

I. DIAGNOSIS OF GLYCOSURIA.

The criteria for the diagnosis of diabetes are the same as in any patient. Patients should be restudied after delivery and after cessation of lactation. Odell and Mengert[1] point out that glycosuria is the second most common complication to toxemia in the obese patient.

J. PROGNOSIS FOR CHILD AND MOTHER.

Five of the 255 infants died in their first year, two of congenital lesions namely of transposed heart and meningoencephalocele, one of pneumonia, one of malnutrition and one from a fall on a cement floor.

The prognosis for the mother is good. Two have died, the one referred to earlier whose death occurred eight weeks after delivery and appeared to be due to toxic hepatitis, the other eight years after delivery due to nephritis. Two patients developed psychoses; each had a family history of schizophrenia.

K. EFFECT OF PREGNANCY UPON THE COURSE OF THE DIABETES.

During the pregnancy insulin requirement increases, later after delivery it decreases. Sixty per cent of the cases who received hormonal treatment required less insulin after delivery. Thirty per cent of the cases receiving no hormonal treatment required less insulin after delivery.

[1] Odell and Mengert: Jour. Am. Med. Assn., **128**, 87, 1945.

L. SUMMARY.

The reason for the abnormal course in obstetrical diabetes may be sought in the maternal background, the abnormalities of which are vascular, chemical, endocrine and genetic. It is not illogical to think that these abnormalities predispose to rapid aging of the placenta in which the imbalance of the sex hormones is a correctible part. Hypo-ovarianism, primary or secondary to arteriosclerosis, might favor compensatory growth and early aging of the placenta. The sex hormone imbalance leads to miscarriage, toxemia, uterine inertia and the failure of lactation. Chorionic gonadotropin favors the splenomegaly, hematopoiesis, and advanced bone and gonad maturity evident in the infant. Fetal survival and the clinical course have changed with substitutional hormonal therapy. Spontaneous correction is possible in the normal woman but the diabetic with her vascular disease and poor hormonal production and metabolism can rarely correct this disturbance herself. Maternal survival in diabetic pregnancies is good, 99.5 per cent. Fetal survival varies with the balance of the sex hormones. When it has been abnormal 50, corrected 90 and normal 97 per cent, are our results, but only when the whole problem of vascular disease in diabetes is solved will the results be exactly comparable to normal pregnancies.

CHAPTER XXX.

NON-DIABETIC GLYCOSURIA.

By ALEXANDER MARBLE, M.D.

A. INCIDENCE.

THE finding of glycosuria in any patient must not be dismissed lightly, but pains should be taken to establish as soon as possible a definite diagnosis, that of diabetes or of non-diabetic glycosuria. Although it is imperative by careful treatment to protect any patient with true or potential diabetes, it is unfair, unjustifiable and in some instances may be actually harmful to impose diabetic treatment on an individual with "benign" glycosuria. The recognition of such a condition is, therefore, the duty of the physician.

Several years ago a study was made of 14,000 patients who had come for diagnosis or treatment of supposed diabetes in the thirty-eight years from 1897 to 1935. It was found that of these there were 2065 patients, or 14.8 per cent, who at the time of the original observation were thought not to be diabetic. As will be brought out in some detail later, over a period of years extending up to 1937, 119 of these 2065 patients were reclassified as diabetic, either because of actual progression of the disease or because of better methods of diagnosis. However, even after subtracting these cases of changed diagnosis, 1946 or 13.9 per cent of the total group remained in whom diabetes had not been proved.

Various studies have been made in an attempt to ascertain the incidence of glycosuria in the general population. Thus, Watson[1] found the incidence of glycosuria in routine examinations of college students to be 1.14 per cent with no appreciable difference between sexes. Evidence of definitely disturbed carbohydrate metabolism, as indicated by an abnormal glucose tolerance test, was present in 15.5 per cent of the individuals with glycosuria.

Short and Ley[2] studied the incidence of glycosuria at different age periods among 10,000 unselected individuals undergoing routine health examinations. When the figures were adjusted to the age and sex distribution of the population of the United States it was found that in 9.2 per cent of males and 7.9 per cent of females, urinary sugar to the extent of 0.15 per cent or more was noted. When, however, quantities of 0.5 per cent or less were excluded from consideration the percentages were much less and the incidence of glycosuria relatively much less in the younger, and greater in the older, age groups.

[1] Watson: Endocrinology, **25**, 845, 1939.
[2] Short and Ley: Proc. Life Extension Examiners, **1**, 134, 1939.

Blotner and Hyde[1] found in World War II that of 45,650 consecutive selectees and volunteers, aged eighteen to forty-five years, examined at the Boston Induction Station, 367 or 0.8 per cent had glycosuria. Among the 367 the following diagnoses were made: 208 cases of diabetes mellitus, 126 of transient glycosuria and 33 of renal glycosuria. In a second study which included 69,088 selectees, aged eighteen to thirty-seven years, Blotner[2] found an even higher incidence; approximately 2 per cent of the examinees, or 1.1 per cent of the total, had either clinical diabetes or sugar tolerance tests indicating impairment to a degree usually accepted as diagnostic of diabetes. In their study of 32,033 consecutive selectees at the New Orleans Induction Station, Spellberg and Leff[3] found a much lower incidence of glycosuria and diabetes. In their group there were only 37 cases of glycosuria and in only 9 of these was the diagnosis of diabetes made. The rates were, therefore, only 0.12 per cent for glycosuria and 0.03 per cent for diabetes. The wide discrepancy between the findings of the Boston and the New Orleans workers was thought to be due in part to a slightly lower average age of the New Orleans selectees, to the fact that one-third were negroes and, more likely, to a difference in the selection of material and diagnostic methods and criteria used. (See also paper of Wolman.[4])

In a health survey of nearly 150,000 young people employed or seeking employment in programs of the National Youth Administration during the first nine months of 1941,[5] sugar was found in the urine of 2.6 per cent of the youth. No variation with age and sex was noted but the incidence in negroes was slightly higher (3.5 per cent) than that for whites (2.4 per cent). Of the 147,813 young people, 2.2 per cent showed a "slight," 0.2 per cent a "medium," and 0.2 per cent a "marked" degree of positive test for sugar in urine. Diabetes mellitus was noted in 0.1 per cent.

B. DIAGNOSIS OF THE TYPE OF MELITURIA.

When sugar has been found in the urine, these questions arise: Has this patient true diabetes mellitus? If not, what is the cause of the urinary sugar? What is the nature of the sugar and what steps should be taken to establish its identity? What treatment should be prescribed? Naturally, if the patient presents the classical symptoms and signs of diabetes, or if in his case there is a family history of diabetes, it is likely that the presenting condition is one of true diabetes mellitus. This presumption is probably true also if the amount of urinary sugar found is large. The greatest aid in diagnosis is the level of the blood sugar. The rule which we have

[1] Blotner and Hude: Loc. cit., p. 42.
[2] Blotner: Loc. cit., p. 43.
[3] Spellberg and Leff: Loc. cit., p. 43.
[4] Wolman: Amer. Jour. Med. Sci., 212, 159, 1946.
[5] The Health Status of NYA Youth, Washington, U. S. Government Printing Office, page 40 and tables 33 and 34, page 76, 1942.

followed, although in infrequent instances it may be open to criticism, is to make the diagnosis of diabetes if, in an individual with glycosuria, the fasting blood sugar is 130 milligrams per cent or over or the postprandial blood sugar is 170 milligrams per cent or over (venous blood). If at random office visits the value is found to be 170 milligrams per cent or over, diabetes, in the usual case, may be considered present. Often, however, the patient presents himself three or more hours after a meal and at such a time a blood-sugar value may be obtained which is not definitely abnormal. In this instance, the patient is requested to report on the same or the following day one hour after a meal liberal in carbohydrate. At this time record is taken of the food eaten and a second examination of blood and urine made. If these tests are not conclusive, other examinations of blood and urine may be made subsequently, taking specimens as before, one hour after a liberal meal. Occasionally doubt still exists and one must resort to a formal sugar tolerance test. Our procedure in this regard has been described elsewhere. (See page 158.) If, by blood-sugar tests, it is shown that the melituria is non-diabetic, it is desirable, particularly when sugar is found constantly in the urine, to determine the *type* of sugar being excreted.

In any uncertain instance one must fall back upon clinical data to support the data obtained from the laboratory, and as for the latter, one must not be content with isolated, unconfirmed abnormal blood-sugar reports if they are not consistent with the clinical findings. Two cases are worthy of comment in this connection. Case 4534 came to us in 1925 with 3 per cent sugar in the urine and we found a blood sugar of 0.14 per cent fasting. The child even went to a diabetic camp and took insulin nine years under the supervision of a whole group of doctors. As years went by, however, it was noted that repeatedly blood-sugar tests were normal and we finally proved that she had renal glycosuria. Incidentally, the insulin did no harm. She is alive and well in 1946.

The second patient, a man aged forty-two years, came because abnormally high blood-sugar values had been reported during a sugar tolerance test performed for a life insurance company. The test had been carried out because of the large amount of insurance applied for and because of the fact that 2 great aunts had had diabetes. Since no sugar had been found in the urine and there had been no symptoms of diabetes or other disease, we repeated the test, giving him 100 grams of glucose, with the results indicated below. Needless to state, the insurance was granted!

Time.	Urinary sugar (per cent).	Blood sugar (per cent).	
		Capillary.	Venous.
Fasting	0	0.10	0.09
100 grams glucose by mouth.			
½ hour after glucose	0	0.15	0.12
1 hour after glucose	0	0.17	0.13
2 hours after glucose	0	0.15	0.10
3 hours after glucose	0	0.13	0.10

C. CLASSIFICATION OF GLYCOSURIAS.

It is helpful to group under definite headings the various conditions in which sugar is found in the urine. Our classification includes four types: (1) Diabetes mellitus, (2) potential diabetes, (3) renal glycosuria and (4) unclassified glycosuria. In Table 110 is listed by successive thousands of cases the number of patients falling into the different groups.

1. **Diabetes Mellitus.**—The percentages of true diabetics have varied between 80.4 and 93.3, or an average of 86.3 per cent.

TABLE 110.—CLASSIFICATION OF 28,000 SUPPOSED DIABETICS.

Case No.	D. M.	P. D.	R. G.	Unc.	Pento-suria.	Levulo-suria.	Deferred.
0 to 5000 .	. 4341	124	23	509[1]	2		
5001 to 10000 .	. 4247	80	20	637	3	1	11[1]
10001 to 15000 .	. 4346	8	9	538	1	1	97
15001 to 20000 .	. 4437	5	12	336	3	1	206
20001 to 25000 .	. 4278	..	7	324	..	1	390
25001 to 28000 .	. 2499	..	5	196	..	..	300
	24148	217	76[2]	2540	9	4	1004

[1] One patient in this 5000 cases numbered twice.
[2] Includes 9 cases of renal glycosuria of pregnancy.

2. **Potential Diabetes.**—Potential diabetes is in a way an unsatisfactory diagnosis, but at times a most convenient one. We formerly used it for those individuals with glycosuria closely related to diet, who easily become sugar-free with slight restrictions, and whose blood sugar is below 0.13 per cent fasting and never reaches 0.17 per cent after a meal. The number of patients listed in this group was formerly fairly large, but later has dwindled to zero not because similar cases are not now seen, but because the diagnosis in doubtful cases has been deferred longer. In other words, many of the cases listed under the heading of "Deferred" in Table 110 might well be classed as potential diabetics.

Those patients originally classified as potential diabetics, included in the first 14,000 cases (first seen between 1900 and 1935), were traced to May 1, 1937. The fact that by this time 16.7 per cent had developed diabetes emphasizes that one must be cautious and remember that time alone can prove a potential diabetes benign.

Patients classified as potential diabetics should be asked to eliminate actual sugar and pastry from the diet and to have the blood and urine examined every three months, for the first year, and at six- or twelve-month intervals thereafter. It is important that potential diabetics keep their body weight at, or slightly below, the average normal figure for age and height.

3. **Renal Glycosuria.**—Renal glycosuria, incorrectly termed "renal diabetes" or "diabetes innocens," is a benign condition characterized by the excretion of glucose in the urine in the presence of a normal

blood sugar. The renal threshold for sugar varies considerably from individual to individual, and under certain circumstances may vary from time to time in the same individual. *We restrict the diagnosis of renal glycosuria to conditions in which the renal threshold is extremely low, as indicated by the fact that all specimens of urine examined, including those after an overnight fast, contain sugar.* In so doing numerous cases are discarded (placed in the "unclassified glycosuria" group) which would be termed renal glycosuria by many workers. However, to include all cases in which the renal threshold is only slightly or moderately lower than the average normal results in an unwieldy hodge-podge of cases difficult to study and follow over a period of years. As may be seen from Table 110, among 28,000 cases of melituria there have been 76 cases of renal glycosuria, using the diagnosis in the limited sense described. This group included 9 cases of renal glycosuria of pregnancy.

This low incidence among our own cases is borne out by the experience of others using the same diagnostic standards. Thus, among 4000 cases of glycosuria studied in the Metabolic Clinic at the Montreal General Hospital, Fowler[1] found only 7 cases with constant glycosuria. Using less strict diagnostic standards, Blotner and Hyde[2] made the diagnosis of renal glycosuria in 33 cases occurring in 367 examinees with melituria found in 45,650 men aged eighteen to forty-five years who appeared for final examination at the Boston Induction Station during World War II.

Renal glycosuria is obviously a condition set apart from diabetes mellitus.[3,4] Glycosuria is always present, the blood sugar is normal, insulin has little or no effect on the output of urinary sugar, the rate of utilization of carbohydrate (as determined by the respiratory metabolism) is normal, ketosis develops during starvation rather than following dietary excesses, diabetic symptoms, including polyuria, are absent and the condition, without treatment, is not progressive. Renal glycosuria is asymptomatic except that some patients complain of easy fatigability and lassitude. Whether these symptoms are to be attributed to the disorder *per se* is difficult to decide.

As far as we have been able to discover, there is no published report of an autopsy in a case of renal glycosuria (with a threshold low enough to permit constant glycosuria even in the fasting state) uncomplicated by serious metabolic disease. The case of Grote and Heilman[5] was one of true diabetes mellitus associated with a very low renal threshold; the patient died of pneumonia following resection of the stomach for carcinoma.

[1] Fowler: Ann. Int. Med., **7**, 518, 1933.
[2] Blotner and Hyde: Jour. Am. Med. Assn., **122**, 432, 1943.
[3] Marble: Am. Jour. Med. Sci., **183**, 811, 1932.
[4] Smith and Smith: Arch. Int. Med., **60**, 119, 1937.
[5] Grote and Heilman: Centralbl. f. allg. Path. u. path. Anat., **64**, 65, 1935.

Certain workers[1,2] believe that renal glycosuria may progress to true diabetes. No such case has been seen in this clinic. In the study of approximately 2000 patients included in the first 14,000 cases of glycosuria already referred to, not a single instance of progression to true diabetes was found among the 45 patients with renal glycosuria despite the fact that most of these patients had exhibited glycosuria for ten years or more. It is true that Case 1612 has had at times blood-sugar values above normal but there has been no progression over a period of twenty-nine years. In 1944 following a sugar tolerance test which, except for glycosuria, was unequivocably normal, she was accepted into the WAVES. The patient with renal glycosuria of longest duration is Case 2165, now sixty-two years old, in whom urinary sugar was first discovered at the age of 10.2 years. During the last fifty-two years sugar has been found in sizable amounts at every examination of the urine and at times in quantities as great as 5 per cent or more. Throughout the years he has restricted his diet little, if any. He has remained in good health and has 5 healthy children.

It seems reasonable that if one could follow for a period of years a sufficiently large group of individuals with a very low renal threshold for sugar, some of them possessing certain favoring influences, such as obesity and the presence of diabetes in relatives, would develop diabetes mellitus just as do persons in the general population with an average normal threshold. Such development of diabetes would not necessarily, however, signify any connection between the two conditions. Soisalo[3] and Lawrence[4] likewise regard renal glycosuria and diabetes as two distinct conditions which have nothing to do with each other; they consider the prognosis of renal glycosuria as good. Schnell,[5] basing his argument on the assumption that renal glycosuria (in the limited sense) is inherited as a dominant, and diabetes mellitus as a recessive trait, points to the relative rarity of the former and the relative frequency of the latter condition, as proof of the lack of connection between the two.

It has been stated that renal glycosuria may be a temporary condition and that a normal renal threshold for sugar may be regained. This happens in the disappearance of the renal glycosuria of pregnancy seen following delivery and in the recovery from phloridzin intoxication. However, in our experience, in true idiopathic renal glycosuria, the condition is permanent if allowance be made for the influence of bodily changes, such as those brought about by arteriosclerosis, hypertension and nephritis which may cause an elevation of the renal threshold both in diabetic and non-diabetic individuals. It is quite possible that by a careful follow-up

1 Vegter: Jahrb. f. Kinderh., **150**, 282, 1937–1938.
2 Bertram: P. 25, loc. cit., p. 87.
3 Soisalo: Acta Soc. Med. Fenn. Duodecim, **14**, 1, 1933.
4 Lawrence: Brit. Med. Jour., **1**, 766, 1940.
5 Schnell: Acta med. Scandin., **92**, 153, 1937.

of patients with renal glycosuria over a period of years a tendency toward elevation of the renal threshold may become apparent. In recent years such a shift has seemed to take place in Case 8885, a physician fifty-four years of age in 1946, whose glycosuria is of more than twenty-six years' duration. His renal threshold for sugar seemed definitely higher in 1938 than in 1930. One can only speculate as to the possible influence of the development of tuberculosis in one kidney, removed in 1938.

Brown and Poleshuck[1] point out the familial nature of renal glycosuria and report 4 cases occurring in three generations of one family. Falta[2] mentions a family in which 6 of 7 children have renal glycosuria. He cites also the family reported by Brugsch and Dresel in which 13 of 55 descendants had renal glycosuria. There was an extraordinarily high incidence of glycosuria in the family described by Hjärne;[3] he regarded the instances of true diabetes occurring along with those of renal glycosuria as only coincidences. Among 22 of our own cases of renal glycosuria reported in 1932,[4] there were 15 in which a family history of diabetes was obtained.

It should be kept in mind that, as Lawrence[5] has pointed out, in certain cases of true diabetes mellitus a low renal threshold may exist. Such an individual is Case 8471, who must be content to show small quantities of urinary sugar in order to avoid insulin reactions; other patients include Cases 7317, 13433 and 18061.

It is well worthwhile to attempt to determine as accurately as possible the renal threshold for sugar in those patients suspected of having renal glycosuria. Using strict criteria, this should, of course, be below 100 milligrams per 100 cc. of blood. In 4 patients studied by Steinitz[6] the value ranged from 52 to 80 milligrams per 100 cc. The daily excretion of urinary sugar in these patients was as great as 30 to 50 grams. Thomas and Southworth[7] carried out detailed studies on a woman, aged twenty-nine years, with whom specimens of urine obtained every fifteen minutes continued to show sugar even after the blood sugar had fallen to 56 mg. per cent. In this patient the diuresis resulting from the forcing of fluids seemed to increase the excretion of sugar.

The explanation for the low threshold in renal glycosuria is not altogether clear. It seems certain that the presence of sugar in the urine depends upon the incomplete reabsorption of sugar by the renal tubules. This in turn may be due to some deviation from the average normal in connection with the phosphorylation mechanism, such as a deficiency in tissue phosphatase. Thomas and Southworth[7]

[1] Brown and Poleshuck: Jour. Lab. and Clin. Med., **20**, 605, 1935.
[2] Falta: P. 37, loc. cit., p. 85.
[3] Hjärne: Acta med. Scandin., **67**, 422, 1927.
[4] Marble: Loc. cit., p. 789.
[5] Lawrence: Brit. Med. Jour., **1**, 196, 1929.
[6] Steinitz: Loc. cit., p. 157.
[7] Thomas and Southworth: Ann. Int. Med., **12**, 1560, 1939.

suggest that the renal threshold may be under hormonal control similar to that exerted by posterior pituitary extract on the renal tubules. It has been suggested that the renal glycosuria of pregnancy may be associated with the hormonal imbalance which is present.

Friedman, Seizer and Sokolow[1] found the effective renal blood flow and glomerular filtration to be normal in the individual with renal glycosuria. The lessened tubular reabsorption of glucose did not seem to be due to an organic kidney defect because at levels of plasma glucose above 200 mg. per cent, the efficiency of tubular reabsorption of glucose equalled or exceeded that found in persons without glycosuria.

Treatment of renal glycosuria is unnecessary, although it seems reasonable to urge the patient to eat sparingly of candy, actual sugar, pastry, and to avoid dietary excesses in general. Otherwise a liberal and varied diet should be encouraged. It is important that during the first year of observation the patient report to his physician every three months and thereafter at six- and twelve-month intervals for life. On these occasions, in addition to a general physical examination, the blood and urine should be examined at one hour after an ordinary meal.

Glycosuria of Pregnancy.—Sugar is often found in the urine of pregnant and parturient women. Among 500 cases of pregnancy studied by Williams,[2] sugar was found in the urine at some time during pregnancy in 68 instances, or 13.6 per cent. Urinary sugar was found 4 times as commonly in the second half as in the first half of pregnancy. Williams and Wills[3] found 5.4 per cent of 640 pregnant women to have sugar in the urine. Richardson and Bitter[4] reported that 20 per cent of 247 pregnant women had gross sugar in the urine following an intake of 1.75 grams of glucose per kilogram of body weight without abnormality of the blood-sugar curve. Ninety per cent of the pregnant women showed minimal amounts of glucose in the urine. Frank and Nothmann[5] found that, following the ingestion of 100 grams of glucose by pregnant women, glycosuria without hyperglycemia occurred regularly.

Sugar in the urine during pregnancy is practically always glucose except during the last stages.[6] During lactation, lactosuria is a physiological event. In deciding whether the pregnant woman has a benign or a diabetic type of melituria, the same guiding principles hold as with any patient whose urine contains sugar. Blood-sugar determinations should be made at one hour after a meal liberal in carbohydrate. If these values are all well within a normal range,

1 Friedman, Seizer and Sokolow: Am. Jour. Med. Sci., **204**, 22, 1942.
2 Williams: Boston Med. and Surg. Jour., **192**, 163, 1925.
3 Williams and Wills: Quart. Jour. Med., **22**, 493, 1929.
4 Richardson and Bitter: Am. Jour. Obst. and Gynec., **24**, 362, 1932.
5 Frank and Nothmann: München. med. Wchnschr., **67**, 1433, 1920.
6 Watkins: Jour. Biol. Chem., **80**, 33, 1928.

it is unlikely that true diabetes is present. In doubtful cases, resort may be had to a sugar tolerance test. (See page 158.) Diabetes mellitus may have its onset during pregnancy or a known diabetic may become pregnant. The care of the pregnant diabetic is discussed in Chapter XXIX. It may suffice here to state that every pregnant woman who has sugar in the urine should be carefully studied by means of blood-sugar determinations and kept under close observation during the pregnancy, even though the glycosuria is apparently benign. If the glycosuria persists or if blood-sugar values are not unequivocally normal, she should be asked to report every three months during the first year following delivery and thereafter yearly or at such intervals as the findings to date may dictate. At such visits tests of the blood and urine should be made at one hour after a meal.

4. Unclassified Glycosuria.—Unclassified glycosuria in our classification is the residual group into which all other cases of glycosuria are placed. In Table 111 are listed in detail the various types of unclassified glycosuria (or, more strictly, melituria):

TABLE 111.—TYPES OF "UNCLASSIFIED" MELITURIA.

(a) Glycosuria accompanying activity of glands of internal secretion other than the pancreas. (1) In hyperthyroidism. (2) In hyperpituitarism. (3) In conditions in which the suprarenal glands are stimulated.

(b) Glycosuria due to stimulation of intracranial nerve centers. (1) *Piqûre diabetique* of Claude Bernard. (2) Brain tumors. (3) Cerebral hemorrhage. (4) Injuries of the skull.

(c) Alimentary glycosuria. (1) "Glycuresis" (Benedict). (2) Alimentary glycosuria. (3) Hunger glycosuria.

(d) Glycosuria accompanying infections and toxemias.

(e) Glycosuria in chronic or degenerative conditions. (1) Vascular hypertension. (2) Chronic nephritis and nephrosis. (3) Chronic hepatic disease as cirrhosis of the liver. (4) Malignant disease.

(f) Glycosuria due to chemical agents. (1) Phloridzin. (2) Poisoning as by uranium, curare, carbon monoxide, caffeine, diuretin, morphine, strychnine, chromic salts, bichloride of mercury and chloroform. (3) Anesthesia; asphyxia.

(g) Melituria other than glycosuria. (1) Pentosuria. (2) Lactosuria. (3) Galactosuria. (4) Levulosuria. (5) Sucrosuria. (See page 245.) (6) Mannoheptulosuria. (See page 245.)

(a) **Glycosuria Accompanying Disturbances of Ductless Glands Other Than the Pancreas.**—In diabetes mellitus itself, the influence of hyperfunctioning of the pituitary, adrenal and thyroid glands is a matter of common knowledge. In the field of non-diabetic glycosuria, too, disorders of these glands may often be held responsible for the appearance of sugar in the urine. In the discussion which follows certain of these conditions will be considered in detail. The normoglycemic glycosuria of pregnancy has not been included under this heading, although it has been suggested that the underlying cause may be transient (anatomical or functional) hypertrophy of the pituitary[1] or overactivity of the thyroid gland.[2]

(1) *Hyperthyroidism.*—Glycosuria is a frequent and well-recognized accompaniment of thyrotoxicosis. The literature on the subject has been summarized by Fitz,[3] and by Andersen.[4] The latter found that following the administration of 70 grams of glucose to 30 patients with exophthalmic goiter, there was obtained in general an increase in the height and length of the blood-sugar curve. In 14 instances the maximum value (Hagedorn-Jensen method) was over 200 mg. per cent and in 24 instances it was over 180 mg. per cent. Following operation there was a tendency toward diminution of the alimentary blood-sugar curve, particularly in those instances in which the curve was markedly abnormal before operation. In 7 of 26 patients with marked exophthalmic goiter he found sugar in the twenty-four-hour quantity of urine. When single specimens were tested, however, urinary sugar was found in all cases at one time or another. Andersen regards it as likely that the renal threshold for sugar is lowered in hyperthyroidism.

In a study of 500 cases of thyroid disease, Joslin and Lahey[5] found the incidence of urinary sugar to the extent of 0.1 per cent or more before operation and 0.5 per cent or more following operation to be as follows:

	Per cent.
In 228 cases of primary hyperthyroidism	38.6
In 83 cases of adenomatous goiter with secondary hyperthyroidism	27.7
In 189 cases of non-toxic goiter	14.8
In 500 successive non-thyroid, non-diabetic surgical cases	13.6

Thus, glycosuria was present in secondary hyperthyroidism almost twice as often, and in primary hyperthyroidism almost three times as often, as in the control group. By no means all of these patients had diabetes as is evidenced by the fact that among 2406 cases of hyperthyroidism (primary and secondary) from the Lahey series, in only 75 instances or in 3.15 per cent of cases was it possible to make the diagnosis of true diabetes mellitus. (See page 726.)

In 1926, Wilder[6] reported the results of a study of thyroid disease and diabetes among patients seen at the Mayo Clinic between January 1, 1923, and January 1, 1926. Of 3471 patients with hyperthyroidism, 38, or 1.1 per cent, had diabetes. Of 1249 diabetics, 38, or 3 per cent, had hyperthyroidism. Wilder stresses the action of hyperthyroidism in decreasing carbohydrate tolerance in the diabetic, but expresses doubt as to whether hyperthyroidism

---

[1] Cushing: The Pituitary Body and Its Disorders, Philadelphia, J. B. Lippincott Company, p. 234, 1912.

[2] John: Surg., Gynec. and Obst., **42**, 543, 1926.

[3] Fitz: Loc. cit., p. 726.

[4] Andersen: Studies on Blood Sugar and Glycosuria in Exophthalmic Goiter, Copenhagen, Levin & Munksgaard, 1933.

[5] Joslin and Lahey: Loc. cit., p. 709.

[6] Wilder: Loc. cit., p. 726.

ever precipitates true diabetes except in an individual who already has this condition in a latent form. He, therefore, makes a sharp distinction as to the cause and significance of diabetic and non-diabetic glycosuria during thyrotoxicosis.

It is apparent that care must be taken in making the diagnosis of diabetes in the presence of hyperthyroidism. If the usual diagnostic standards as regards blood sugar are used, it will be found that following operation many cases will be apparently "cured." In the present state of our knowledge of diabetes, it is safer to assume that it is not curable and to regard these instances of "temporary diabetes" in thyrotoxicosis as due to the great burden imposed on the organism by the extra thyroid secretion. Wilder regards it as probable that such "cured" cases represent merely the arrest of a latent diabetic condition. For this reason we make the diagnosis of true diabetes in a patient with hyperthyroidism only when the fasting blood sugar (venous) is 150 mg. per cent or higher or the postprandial blood sugar is 200 mg. per cent or higher.

(2) *Hyperpituitarism.*—Davidoff and Cushing[1] reported that about 25 per cent of 100 patients with acromegaly had sugar in the urine. Later Coggeshall and Root[2] reviewed these original 100 cases plus 53 other cases of acromegaly subsequently studied at the Peter Bent Brigham Hospital. Among the total of 153 cases Coggeshall and Root found in all 55 patients, or 36 per cent with glycosuria (26, or 17 per cent of the 153 acromegalics had diabetes). This frequent association of glycosuria with hyperpituitarism has been the experience of others. Thus, in his review of the literature, Colwell[3] found that about 40 per cent of reported cases of acromegaly had glycosuria and about one-half of these had symptoms suggestive of diabetes.

In the field of carbohydrate metabolism the anterior pituitary now receives much attention. Houssay and his associates[4] were the first to show that severe diabetes does not develop in animals in which both hypophysis and pancreas are removed. Young[5] has produced permanent diabetes in dogs by the intraperitoneal injection of extracts of large amounts of beef pituitaries. In later work by Young, and by others who have confirmed his observations, it has been shown that the pituitary diabetic dogs have suffered marked degeneration of the islet tissue of the pancreas.

(3) *Glycosuria Produced Through Intermediary of Adrenalin Secretion.*—It has long been known that stimulation of the nerves passing to the suprarenal medulla may cause, among other effects, a transient hyperglycemia and glycosuria. The same effect follows the parenteral administration of adrenalin if the dose be large enough. The

[1] Davidoff and Cushing: Loc. cit., p. 713.
[2] Coggeshall and Root: Loc. cit., p. 86.
[3] Colwell: Loc. cit., p. 714.
[4] Houssay: Loc. cit., p. 121.
[5] Young: Loc. cit., p. 121.

rise in blood sugar and the consequent excretion of urinary sugar take place by breakdown of glycogen in the liver.

The classical experiments of Cannon and his associates[1] showed that during emotional excitement or pain, adrenalin is secreted into the blood stream in unusual amounts and, as one of the results of this, glycosuria may occur. Folin, Denis and Smillie[2] found that 18 per cent of 33 presumably normal medical students showed sugar in the urine which was passed immediately after an important examination. Similar results were obtained with a second group of 36 students at a women's college. Cannon and Fiske[3] found that in the urine of 25 members of a football team, immediately after a game sugar was present in 12 instances. Five of the 12 positive tests were among substitutes who had not played. That hyperglycemia and glycosuria under such circumstances are due largely to the emotional stress and not to the exercise *per se* is shown by the studies of Edwards, Richards and Dill.[4] They found that, although in a player on the football field there might be an increase in the blood sugar together with glycosuria, in the same individual when exercising strenuously in the laboratory there was apt to be a decrease rather than an increase in the blood sugar. Thus Levine and his colleagues[5] and Best and Partridge[6] reported the finding of hypoglycemia in runners at the end of a marathon race.

Green and Emery[7] found the effect of emotion upon glycosuria considerably less than reported above. Following a final written examination, the urine of medical and dental students was tested and of 244 samples only 4, or 1.6 per cent, were definitely positive, while 19, or 7.8 per cent, showed a trace of sugar. Divergent results reported by different observers may well reflect variations in emotional stress in the groups studied.

(*b*) **Glycosuria of Intracranial Origin.**—Glycosuria in acromegaly has already been discussed. Some workers believe that the urinary sugar found in conditions of pituitary overgrowth or following operations on or about the hypophysis is due not to disorders of pituitary secretion, but to stimulation of nerve centers or pathways in the hypothalamic region (floor of the third ventricle).[8] Thus in hypophysectomies in dogs, Sachs and MacDonald[9] obtained glycosuria only in those animals in which the region of the floor of the third ventricle was more or less injured and little or no urinary sugar

[1] Cannon: Bodily Changes in Pain, Hunger, Fear and Rage, 2d ed., New York, D. Appleton & Co., 1929.
[2] Folin, Denis and Smillie: Jour. Biol. Chem., **17**, 519, 1914.
[3] Cannon and Fiske: Loc. cit., reference 1 above.
[4] Edwards, Richards and Dill: Am. Jour. Physiol., **98**, 352, 1931.
[5] Levine, Gordon and Derick: Loc. cit., p. 416.
[6] Best and Partridge: Proc. Roy. Soc., London, **105** (Series B), 323, 1929.
[7] Green and Emery: Endocrinology, **30**, 353, 1942.
[8] Colwell: Loc. cit., p. 714.
[9] Sachs and MacDonald: Arch. Neurol. and Psychiat., **13**, 335, 1925.

in those animals in which the base of the brain was carefully avoided at operation.

Early among the experiments in this field was the historic *piqûre diabetique* of Claude Bernard, by which he showed that needle puncture in the floor of the fourth ventricle in dogs caused transient glycosuria. The mechanism is commonly held to be that of stimulation of nerve centers with release of sugar from the liver following glycogenolysis.

The glycosuria accompanying various conditions in which there is increased intracranial pressure, or in which there exists the possibility of local irritation of nerve centers, may possibly be due to stimulation in the hypothalamic region. The mechanism which in this connection is less definite and less well understood, applies in conditions such as brain tumor, cerebral hemorrhage and fractured skull. A case illustrating the glycosuria which may follow subarachnoid hemorrhage has been reported by Courts.[1] Mader[2] found that injection of air for encephalograms by endolumbal puncture gave rise to the same symptoms as the classical sugar and thermal punctures. The hyperglycemia can be controlled and suppressed by insulin.

Davidson and Allen[3] found that in 12 patients with concussion of the brain and in 18 patients with fracture of the skull, blood-sugar curves following the administration of 25 grams of glucose intravenously (within twenty-four to thirty-six hours after the injury) gave in general a value at fifteen minutes after the injection of sugar which was much higher than corresponding values in normal individuals. Furthermore, the curve fell to the fasting level more slowly than in the normal cases. The abnormalities were more striking in the cases with fractured skull than in those with concussion. They regard the mechanism as that of central stimulation of the splanchnic nerves to the suprarenal glands and the liver, with resulting glycogenolysis in the liver. Later studies carried out during the convalescence of their patients showed that the abnormality in carbohydrate metabolism was only a temporary affair. No support was given to the theory of traumatic origin of diabetes mellitus. Still less basis for the traumatic production of glycosuria and diabetes is furnished by the statements of the neuro-surgeons, Cushing and Horrax, who found such complications to be decidedly rare following operations upon the brain. For a more complete discussion see page 84 and the article by Joslin.[4]

(c) **Alimentary Glycosuria.**—Under this heading mention must first be made of the much debated point as to whether normal urine contains traces of sugar. The truth seems to be that normal urine

[1] Courts: Brit. Med. Jour., 1, 190, 1932.
[2] Mader: Klin. Wchnschr., 11, 676, 1932.
[3] Davidson and Allen: Loc. cit., p. 93.
[4] Joslin: New England Jour. Med., 223, 22, 1940.

usually contains very small amounts (less than 0.1 per cent) of substances which reduce alkaline copper solutions. Whether these reducing substances are actually traces of glucose or are unassimilable end-products of carbohydrate metabolism,[1] though a matter of great theoretical interest, is of very little practical importance. The usual Benedict test is not sensitive enough to detect these traces. For a more complete discussion see page 238.

A consideration of straightforward "alimentary" glycosuria is of more practical value. By extreme carbohydrate overloading, the point may be reached at which even the normal organism cannot cope with the situation and small amounts of sugar may appear in the urine. Normal individuals, however, possess a very high tolerance in this respect.

Alimentary glycosuria requires no treatment except: (1) Care to insure that the diagnosis is correct; (2) medical supervision; (3) tests of the blood and urine at least yearly.

The glycosuria which follows the giving of food to a starving man or animal is of interest in this connection. The urinary sugar is presumably due to temporary overloading with carbohydrate of an organism which has not been accustomed to food. Goldblatt and Ellis,[2] from studies on animals and men who were fasted about forty hours, state that the intolerance for carbohydrate is not primarily due to acidosis. However, when such "hunger glycosuria" *is* accompanied by acidosis, a blood-sugar determination may be necessary to rule out diabetes mellitus, although with the giving of food the acidosis of starvation quickly disappears.

Sakauchi[3] states that he has frequently found glycosuria without hyperglycemia in chronically undernourished children. Experimentally he kept young rabbits in a state of undernutrition for weeks. During the first three to five weeks fasting blood sugar values were normal and tolerance curves after the oral administration of sugar were essentially normal. The slight alimentary glycosuria which he observed at times during this period, Sakauchi attributed in part to a lowering of the kidney threshold for sugar. From the third to the fifth week of undernutrition on, sugar tolerance tests gave increasing hyperglycemia and glycosuria. Terminally, however, this effect disappeared and the animals died in hypoglycemia.

Benedict[4] found that his subject who fasted thirty-one days, in 1912, excreted from 296 to 498 milligrams of reducing substances (calculated as glucose) in the twenty-four-hour quantity of urine during the period of starvation. When on the first day after a month

[1] Folin and Berglund: Jour. Biol. Chem., **51**, 213, 1922. See also Benedict and Osterberg: Jour. Biol. Chem., **55**, 769, 1923.

[2] Goldblatt and Ellis: Biochem. Jour., **26**, 991, 1932.

[3] Sakauchi: Japanese Jour. Biochem., **16**, 259, 1932.

[4] Benedict: A Study of Prolonged Fasting, Washington, The Carnegie Institute, p. 292, 1915.

of fasting, about 500 grams of carbohydrate were allowed in a relatively short time, the amount of reducing substances in the urine rose for that day to 4441 milligrams.   On the two subsequent days the values were 267 and 246 milligrams, respectively.

(d) **Glycosuria Accompanying Infections and Toxemias.**—Patients with acute infections often excrete small quantities of sugar in the urine.   This finding of sugar if in a child may be most distressing to apprehensive parents who know about and fear diabetes.   Practically, the situation can be handled best by not making a definite diagnosis until blood-sugar tests have been carried out.   Careful tests of blood and urine should be made after the subsidence of the infection and at three-month intervals during the first year thereafter.

Federer's[1] patient with acute meningitis exhibited transient hyperglycemia, acetonuria and glycosuria.   Ferguson and Barr[2] found transient glycosuria in 30 per cent of 72 cases of meningitis admitted to the New York Hospital over a four year period.   Of the 13 glycosuric cases in which tests for acetone and diacetic acid were made, positive tests were found in 11.

Williams and Dick[3] found glycosuria in 41 per cent of 108 patients with acute infectious diseases following the giving of 100 grams of glucose to adults and approximately 1 gram per pound of body weight to children.   Experimental infections in rabbits were found to lower carbohydrate tolerance as evidenced by abnormal blood-sugar curves following the giving of dextrose.   Strauss[4] has shown that the toxemia produced in rabbits by the intravenous injection of streptococcus filtrates definitely lowered the glucose tolerance. This effect was not obtained when the toxic filtrate was mixed with an excess of erysipelas antiserum before injection.

It is not surprising that glycosuria should be present during infections since they definitely make true diabetes temporarily more severe.   In the laboratory it has been abundantly shown that insulin efficiency is lowered by infections and toxemias.   For further discussion see Chapter XVI.

(e) **Glycosuria in Chronic or Degenerative Conditions.**—There are various "extrainsular" types of glycosuria met with in everyday practice other than those already mentioned. In patients with hypertension, nephritis, or nephrosis, slight glycosuria is not infrequently encountered. Thus, Hiller[5] has identified the presence of dextrose in the urine of patients with kidney disease, thereby confirming the earlier observation that fermentable reducing substances in the urine are frequently increased in all types of nephritis and that in some of

[1] Federer: New England Jour. Med., **233**, 342, 1945.
[2] Ferguson and Barr: Ann. Int. Med , **21**, 173, 1944.
[3] Williams and Dick: Arch. Int. Med., **50**, 801, 1932.
[4] Strauss: Loc. cit., p. 165.
[5] Hiller: Jour. Biol. Chem., **91**, 735, 1931.

the degenerative cases the excretion amounts to gross melituria. In these conditions the urinary sugar is presumably due to kidney damage, although in cases of essential hypertension the influence of overactivity of the sympathetic nervous system must be considered. Brush[1] calls attention to non-diabetic glycosuria in older individuals especially in those who have had some type of obstructive uropathy.

The glycosuria which occasionally accompanies chronic disease of the liver probably arises through impairment of the normal processes of glycogenesis and glycogenolysis in that organ.

The question as to why patients with cancer not infrequently show small amounts of sugar in the urine has received considerable attention. On studying these patients it is often found that, although blood sugar values are normal one hour after a meal, sugar tolerance curves may show definite deviations from the normal. These abnormalities usually are not marked enough to warrant the diagnosis of diabetes, particularly since the symptomatology characteristic of diabetes, is commonly lacking. The most that one can say is that these individuals have an impaired carbohydrate tolerance. Certain clinicians, among them Rohdenburg,[2] Friedenwald[3] and Jackson[4] in this country, have studied the problem with the idea in mind of finding a sugar-tolerance curve characteristic of malignancy which might be used for diagnosis in doubtful cases, but so far results have not been consistent enough to be of much help. In a paper on "Diabetes and Cancer,"[5] this subject is discussed at further length.

(f) **Glycosuria Due to Chemical Agents.**—The glycosuria due to phloridzin poisoning has no practical importance in man. However, as a tool with which to study carbohydrate metabolism has yielded results of such fundamental importance that the glycosuria produced by this agent requires some comment.[6,7,8] Following the parenteral injection of phloridzin into animals or man there occurs a lowering of the renal threshold for sugar so that temporarily (a matter of hours to days, depending on the dose given) there results without hyperglycemia a continuous excretion of sugar in the urine. The condition thus mimics quite closely the spontaneously arising renal glycosuria in man. Evidence is lacking that phloridzin poisoning produces noteworthy metabolic changes other than the effect on the kidney.

[1] Brush: Jour. Urol., 53, 362, 1945.
[2] Rohdenburg, Bernhard and Krehbiel: Am. Jour. Med. Sci., 159, 577, 1920.
[3] Friedenwald and Grove: Am. Jour. Med. Sci., 163, 33, 1922.
[4] Jackson: Texas State Jour. Med., 24, 622, 1929.
[5] Marble: Loc. cit., p. 655.
[6] Lusk: The Science of Nutrition, 4th ed., Philadelphia, W. B. Saunders Company, p. 624, 1928.
[7] Nash: Physiol. Rev., 7, 385, 1927.
[8] McKee and Hawkins: Physiol. Rev., 25, 255, 1945.

In the course of poisoning of animals or man with various chemical agents, glycosuria has been noted. Among these substances are curare, carbon monoxide, caffeine, diuretin, morphine, strychnine, chromic salts, bichloride of mercury, chloroform, uranium salts and potassium dichromate.[1,2]

Lichtwitz[1] states that caffeine, diuretin, morphine, strychnine and chloroform cause glycosuria by stimulation of the central nervous system, whereas curare, carbon monoxide and heavy metals (particularly uranium) act peripherally, probably on the liver cells. Hepler and Simonds[2] found some degree of correlation between the glycosuria due to chemical poisoning and: (*a*) the necrosis of tubular epithelium, (*b*) albuminuria and (*c*) the chemical agent and its dose.

Sugar frequently appears in the urine following anesthesia with ether and chloroform. The action is due, at least in part, to the acidosis produced by the anesthesia. McKittrick and Root[3] have shown that in the diabetic, during anesthesia produced by ether or nitrous oxide and oxygen, the carbon dioxide combining power of the blood falls and the sugar in the blood increases. This is true to a less extent when ethylene is used as an anesthetic and still less when spinal anesthesia is used. Best *et al.*[4] found that the blood of a dog under ether anesthesia contained only one-tenth the amount of insulin per unit of volume as that of a normal dog.

D. MELITURIA OTHER THAN GLYCOSURIA.

In the study of a patient who shows sugar in the urine despite normal blood-sugar values, it is important to ascertain the type of sugar which is excreted. In the overwhelming majority of cases the sugar will be found to be glucose, but in a number large enough to make it definitely worthwhile one can succeed in demonstrating that the sugar is not glucose but instead pentose, fructose, or some other sugar less commonly encountered. In such cases a systematic study is necessary and in carrying this out the following procedures are valuable:

1. *The Benedict Test.*—This is positive for all sugars which may be found in the urine. Lasker and Enklewitz[5] have called attention to the fact that with urine containing pentose, reduction of the copper solution takes place after a few hours at room temperature (*i. e.*, without heating) and within ten minutes at 50° to 60° C. Fructose (levulose), also a ketose, reduces Benedict's solution quickly at 50° to 60° C. but much more slowly than pentose at temperatures

[1] Lichtwitz: Klinische Chemie, 2nd ed., Berlin, Julius Springer, p. 245, 1930.
[2] Hepler and Simonds: Arch. Path., **41**, 42, 1946.
[3] McKittrick and Root: Diabetic Surgery, Philadelphia, Lea & Febiger, Chapter IV, 1928.
[4] Best, Smith and Scott: Am. Jour. Physiol., **68**, 161, 1924.
[5] Lasker and Enklewitz: Loc. cit., p. 244.

below 40° C.   Like pentose and fructose, mannoheptulose reduces Benedict's solution in the cold.[1]

2. Fermentation with bakers' yeast.   Glucose and fructose are always, galactose usually, lactose occasionally, pentose and mannoheptulose never fermented.

3. Bial (Orcinol-HCl) reaction (positive for pentose).

4. Seliwanoff (resorcinol-HCl) reaction (positive for levulose).

5. Characteristic osazone crystals with phenylhydrazine or methylphenylhydrazine (the latter in the case of levulose) can be obtained. This test should be carried further by determining the melting-point of these crystals, since in distinguishing between glucose and pentose the difference between the melting-point of glucosazone (205° C.) and that of pentosazone (157° to 160° C.) is very helpful.

In addition to these tests there are the fermentation reactions with specific bacteria and fungi, as suggested by Castellani,[2] the Tollen (phloroglucinol-HCl) reaction for galactose, the mucic acid test for lactose and galactose and polariscopic and spectroscopic examinations.   These are described in Chapter VII and by Trumper and Cantarow.[3]   Exton[4] recommended a di-sodium-di-nitro-salicylate reagent for the differentiation of the various sugars and stated that the method is simple and rapid.   The reagent is reduced at different rates by different sugars.   By keeping the temperature of a bath constant and noting the presence or absence of reduction after certain stated intervals of time, differentiation of the reducing sugar is possible.

1. **Chronic Essential Pentosuria.**—Chronic essential pentosuria is a rare, benign condition belonging in the group of "inborn errors of metabolism," characterized by the constant presence in the urine of small quantities of pentose, usually xylulose.   All reported cases have been in Jews and predominantly in males.   The condition is harmless, asymptomatic and has no relation to diabetes mellitus. Salzman[5] reports the case of a Jewish girl, aged seventeen years, in whom melituria of thirteen years' standing was shown to be due to the excretion of pentose.   One of Neuman's[6] 4 cases had been observed for twenty-seven years.   The 3 cases reported by us in 1932[7] are alive and well in 1946 following no treatment directed toward the melituria.   The report of Enklewitz and Lasker[8] was followed by a second paper[9] reporting the occurrence in twins of pentosuria of known duration of seventeen years.   The cases had

---

[1] Blatherwick: Loc. cit., p. 245.
[2] Castellani: Jour. State Med., **39**, 621, 1931.
[4] Trumper and Cantarow: Internat. Clin., 41st series, **1**, 38, 1931.
[4] Exton: Loc. cit., p. 244.
[5] Salzman: Jour. Am. Med. Assn., **103**, 483, 1934.
[6] Neuman: Med. Ann. Dist. Columbia, Washington, **1**, 79, 1932; Abstract, Jour. Am. Med. Assn., **99**, 1546, 1932.
[7] Marble: Am. Jour. Med. Sci., **183**, 827, 1932.
[8] Enklewitz and Lasker: Am. Jour. Med. Sci., **186**, 539, 1933.
[9] Enklewitz and Lasker: Jour. Am. Med. Assn., **105**, 958, 1935.

previously been regarded by others as instances of juvenile diabetes, and later of renal diabetes, in twins. Derivaux[1] in 1943 found a total of 163 cases of pentosuria reported in the literature. Blatherwick[2] quoted Margolis[3] as finding 11 cases of pentosuria in 22,000 urine examinations, and stated his own experience in which the incidence was about 1 to 50,000 examinations carried out in connection with applications for life insurance.

Our own series includes 9 patients with chronic essential pentosuria, Cases 1473, 1484, 6629, 6760, 7995, 13676, 16923, 18070 and 18217. All of these patients are Jewish, ranging in age from 2.8 to 31.6 years at the time of the first discovery of sugar, and all but Cases 1484 and 6629 are males. All 9 of these patients have been heard from in 1946; all have continued in good health and have shown no tendency toward progression to diabetes, despite the fact that melituria has been known to exist for at least eight years and in 5 cases (1473, 1484, 6629, 6760, 7995) for nineteen years or more.

It is stated that transient pentosuria occurs after large quantities of certain fruits, as plums, cherries, grapes and prunes, have been eaten. Pentose is also said to occur in the urine along with glucose in certain cases of diabetes mellitus.

Enklewitz and Lasker,[4] in reporting 12 cases of true chronic essential pentosuria, quote W. Voit as obtaining an ozazone with the melting-point of a pentosazone from the urine of 12 of 14 severe diabetics, but they themselves in the examination of the urine of a large number of diabetics failed to obtain a single positive reaction with Bial's reagent. We have encountered one case (Case 6629) of pentosuria in a patient who, on the basis of blood-sugar values, has been classified as having diabetes also. This young Jewish woman was eighteen years of age when sugar was first found in her urine. She has had only occasional blood-sugar values slightly above normal, eats an unrestricted diet, takes no insulin and yet on April 28, 1945 had only 0.3 per cent sugar in the urine and a blood sugar of 80 mg. per cent. Her case is difficult to classify and deserves continued observation and further study.

By the systematic examination of urine specimens of large groups of high school students and by contacts with physicians, Lasker[5] has collected data regarding over 100 cases of pentosuria. There is no doubt but that pentosuria is inherited, apparently as a Mendelian recessive trait. It seems likely that most of the families of pentosurics, at least those in the New York area as studied by Lasker,

[1] Derivaux: Southern Med. Jour., **36**, 587, 1943.
[2] Blatherwick: Xylulosuria (Essential Pentosuria), Practitioner's Library, New York, D. Appleton-Century Company, p. 268, 1937.
[3] Margolis: Am. Jour. Med. Sci., **177**, 348, 1929
[4] Enklewitz and Lasker: Loc. cit., p. 802, ref. 9.
[5] Lasker: Personal communication. See also Lasker, Enklewitz and Lasker, Human Biology, **8**, 243, 1936.

came from foci of relatively limited extent, largely in what was formerly Poland and to a less degree in Germany. In the family studied by Schultsz[1] there were 4 cases of pentosuria; 2 of the patients were brothers and one of these had 2 sons with pentosuria. In a related branch of the family there were 7 instances of renal glycosuria plus 1 case of glycosuria of pregnancy. The pentose was identified as l-xylulose. Schultsz shares the belief of Enklewitz and Lasker[2] that glucuronic acid is the mother-substance of the pentose. He suggests that glucuronic acid is transformed into xylulose in the kidneys. Schultsz believes that pentosuria is transmitted as a dominant trait.

2. **Lactosuria.**—Lactosuria has already been mentioned in the discussion regarding melituria of pregnancy and lactation. As stated there, the sugar appearing in the urine during pregnancy itself (except during the last days) is practically always glucose and not lactose. Therefore, the finding of urinary sugar during pregnancy should be given careful consideration. During lactation, lactosuria occurs physiologically.

Tolstoi[3] found that in diabetic, lactating women, the concentration of lactose in the breast milk remained remarkably constant in spite of very marked elevations or depressions of the blood glucose concentration. Lactose in urine gives a positive Benedict test and may even be fermented by bakers' yeast. Hence its identification may be largely a matter of exclusion of other sugars. Rules for establishing its presence will be found in standard texts and in an article by Trumper and Cantarow.[4]

Watkins[5] carried out an extensive study of lactose metabolism in women. She found that during the last stages of pregnancy there is a more or less constant excretion of lactose and that during the last few days before delivery there is a marked rise in the value obtained with the height reached on the day of delivery. Following delivery the lactose excretion immediately drops to a low level where it remains for from two to five days with then a sudden and often tremendous excretion of lactose. During the first few weeks of lactation fluctuations are very marked. By the end of the first month after delivery a constant and lower level of lactose excretion is assumed and this level slowly approaches normal values. Menstruation causes an increase in the tolerance of women for lactose as does also pregnancy. Watkins gives in detail the method for determination of lactose in urine.

3. **Galactosuria.**—Spontaneous galactosuria is of little importance in clinical medicine. One test of liver function is based on the ability of that organ to metabolize a certain amount of galactose

1 Schultsz: Onderzoekingen over Pentosurie, Amsterdam, N. V. Uitgevers-Maatschappij "Kosmos," 1938.
2 Enklewitz and Lasker: Loc. cit., p. 802, ref. 8.
3 Tolstoi: Jour. Clin. Invest., **14**, 863, 1935.
4 Trumper and Cantarow: Loc. cit., p. 802.
5 Watkins: Loc. cit., p. 792.

(40 grams given orally). Normally 3 grams or less are excreted in the urine within five hours. Excretions of amounts larger than this suggest impairment of liver function.

Bansi[1] reported a case of paroxysmal galactosuria in a woman, aged thirty-two years, with bronchial asthma. The excretion of sugar was noted particularly just before and during menstruation. The patient of Mason and Turner[2] was a maldeveloped and malnourished negro boy observed from the age of six months to three years. He had an enlarged liver and spleen, albuminuria and galactosuria. When milk in the diet was replaced by a soy bean preparation, there occurred a decrease in the size of the liver and spleen and a disappearance of albuminuria and galactosuria. Later trial feedings of milk or lactose provoked albuminuria and galactosuria. Blood studies showed that with a high concentration of blood galactose, hypoglycemic symptoms were absent even though the blood glucose was as low as 13 mg. per 100 cc. A third and similar case was reported by Norman and Fashena.[3] In their patient, chronic hypergalactosemia was associated with galactosuria, albuminuria, nutritional disturbance, enlargement of the liver and spleen, anemia, mild azotemia and osteoporosis. Removal of milk from the diet resulted in the disappearance of all symptoms except the azotemia. Norman and Fashena regard the condition as an inborn error of metabolism in which the essential defect probably lies in the specific enzyme system concerned with the conversion of galactose to glycogen.

For the identification of galactose in the urine the reader is referred to special texts.

4. **Fructosuria (Levulosuria).**—Essential fructosuria is a rare condition. We have discovered only 4 cases, all in young Jewish persons, the only ones so far recognized among over 28,000 cases of melituria: Case 7157, male, 3.7 years in September, 1925; Case 13228, male, 17.8 years in April, 1932; Case 15117, female 1.3 years in July, 1932; and Case 21113, female, 18.3 years in November, 1941. Cases 13228 and 21113 are brother and sister. All are living and well in 1946. Studies of Case 13228 have been reported in detail.[4] We are indebted to Mrs. Margaret Lasker of New York for demonstrating the existence of fructosuria in Case 7157.

Writing in 1937, Blatherwick[5] stated that only 34 cases of essential fructosuria had been recorded in the literature up until that time. Nine of these case reports were by American authors, the first by Strouse and Friedman[8] in 1912, a Dutch case described by Heeres and

[1] Bansi: Klin. Wchnschr., 11, 21, 1932.
[2] Mason and Turner: Am. Jour. Dis. Child., 50, 359, 1935.
[3] Norman and Fashena: Am. Jour. Dis. Child., 66, 531, 1943; see also the article by Bruck and Rapoport: Ibid., 70, 267, 1945.
[4] Marble and Smith: Jour. Am. Med. Assn., 106, 24, 1936.
[5] Blatherwick: p. 264, Loc. cit., p. 803.
[6] Strouse and Friedman: Arch. Int. Med., 9, 99, 1912.

Vos[1] in 1929, 6 others by Silver and Reiner[2] in 1934, and 1 by Marble and Smith[3] in 1936. Blatherwick[4] mentioned that he had studied the metabolism in 2 cases of fructosuria occurring in a sister and a brother. Jacobsen's[5] patients were brothers.

In individuals with essential fructosuria, the rate at which fructose is removed from the blood stream is retarded. As a consequence, a blood fructose level well above the kidney threshold is temporarily maintained and fructosuria results. Presumably the removal of fructose from the blood is normally cared for in large part by the liver and this function is impaired in the patient with fructosuria. The condition is harmless and requires no treatment.

In connection with a detailed study of 3 patients with essential fructosuria, Soisalo[6] carried out fructose tolerance tests on 3 healthy persons, giving 1 gram of fructose per kilogram body weight. He states that the highest percentage of fructose in the blood was 5 to 6 mg. per cent and that in 2 of these subjects the renal threshold for fructose seemed to lie below the level just mentioned. In one normal subject studied by us the renal threshold for fructose seemed to be about 11 mg. per cent.

Levulose as well as dextrose is said to occur in the urine in severe cases of diabetes mellitus. Our experience affords very little data on this point, although in Case 12377, a young Jewish woman with mild diabetes, aged 13.4 years at the time of discovery of melituria in April 1931, levulose was associated with glucose in the urine. Studies in this case have been reported.[3] The patient died July 13, 1938 of cirrhosis of the liver.

E. PROGNOSIS IN NON-DIABETIC GLYCOSURIAS.

What is the likelihood that an individual with apparently benign glycosuria may subsequently develop diabetes? As has been mentioned previously, in 1937 a study was made of 2065 patients who in thirty-eight years between 1897 and 1935 came because of glycosuria which at the time of the original observation was thought not to be diabetic. These patients comprised 14.8 per cent of a total of 14,000 patients who came during this same period for treatment of supposed diabetes. The patients were traced to May 1, 1937 or later; all but 32, or 1.5 per cent of the 2065 patients were traced. Careful preliminary examination of the records led to the discarding of certain cases so that actually 1946 cases were used as the basis of the study. Of these, 1142 were males and 804 females. One thousand six hundred thirty-six patients were living and 310 were

1 Heeres and Vos: Arch. Int. Med., 44, 47, 1929.
2 Silver and Reiner: Arch. Int. Med., 54, 412, 1934.
3 Marble and Smith: Loc. cit., p. 805.
4 Blatherwick: p. 264, Loc. cit., p. 803.
5 Jacobsen: Am. Jour Med. Sci., 200, 304, 1940.
6 Soisalo: Loc. cit., p. 790.

dead. In 193 cases, or 9.9 per cent of the total, true diabetes had developed, which in most instances was mild.

The features favoring the development of diabetes were, in approximately the order named: advancing age, overweight, blood-sugar values above the average normal at first observation (though below a definitely diabetic level) and in the younger patients a family history of diabetes. The percentage becoming diabetic rose with increasing duration since initial observation. It was higher in Jewish than in non-Jewish patients. Adequate study at initial observation, particularly with postprandial blood-sugar tests and glucose tolerance tests, increased greatly the chances of distinguishing diabetic from non-diabetic glycosuria. Thus the diagnosis was subsequently changed in only 6.3 per 1000 per annum among those studied with glucose tolerance tests as compared with 12.6 per 1000 per annum in patients inadequately studied.

A survey of the types of melituria as has just been made may seem at first thought to indicate that a complicated and difficult diagnostic problem presents itself whenever sugar is found in the urine. Such is not the case. Unusual cases there will be, and at times it may be very difficult to state whether a given patient has, or has not, diabetes. Usually, however, a few simple guiding principles will suffice to establish a satisfactory diagnosis. In general, the proper sequence of action in any case should be as follows:

1. A proper evaluation of the patient's history, physical examination and his hereditary background.

2. Examination of the urine for sugar before and after a meal.

3. Determination of the percentage of sugar in the blood at one hour after a meal liberal in carbohydrate.

4. In doubtful cases, the carrying out of a sugar tolerance test.

5. In cases of persistent melituria despite normal blood-sugar values, the identification of the type of sugar excreted.

Such tests should be carried out promptly, once the problem of diagnosis has presented itself. An opinion should be given based on the data available. Delay provokes uncertainty and worry on the part of the patient and leaves the physician in doubt as to the proper treatment. If the melituria seems to be non-diabetic and benign, instructions as to diet and living habits may be given along lines suggested earlier in this chapter. In any case, however, the patient should be kept under observation and requested to report every three months for the first year and at yearly or twice yearly intervals thereafter until such visits no longer seem necessary. On these occasions examinations of the urine and blood for sugar should be made one hour after a meal liberal in carbohydrate.

CHAPTER XXXI.

FOODS AND THEIR COMPOSITION.

THE improvement in the treatment of diabetes owes much to the dissemination of knowledge regarding the composition of foods. To the United States Government we are indebted for an excellent monograph by Atwater and Bryant, entitled "The Chemical Composition of American Food Materials," Bulletin 28, revised edition, which was first issued in 1906. Later government publications have revised and enlarged upon sections of this work, notably Department of Agriculture Circular 50, Proximate Composition of Fresh Fruits, by Chatfield and McLaughlin, Circular 146, Proximate Composition of Fresh Vegetables, by Chatfield and Adams and United States Department of Agriculture Miscellaneous Publication No. 572, 1945. These tables contain average values for food energy, protein, fat, carbohydrate, three minerals and the better known vitamins for a selected list of foods. See pages 294 to 305 for discussion of vitamins and minerals.

The state of Connecticut, from its Agricultural Experiment Station in New Haven, has also published excellent reports on special foods offered for use in the diet of diabetic patients, and from year to year adds analyses of new preparations of this sort as well as analyses of common foods. Professor Street formerly and Professor Bailey recently, who have been intimately concerned in these investigations, have been kindness itself not alone to me, but to my inquisitive patients.

McCance and Lawrence[1] have published an exhaustive study of the carbohydrate content of plant foods, including a discussion of the food value of vegetable carbohydrates.

A suitable diet for a diabetic patient depends upon so many variable factors, particularly the tolerance of the individual, that no general definition of a "diabetic" food can be satisfactorily fixed. The discovery of insulin, for example, materially modified both the theory and practice of diabetic dietetics.

The narrow confines of the diabetic diet in years past greatly stimulated the manufacture of so-called diabetic foods. These were often serviceable, but to be employed with discretion. The patient should never become dependent upon special diabetic foods, for they are often unobtainable, always make him conspicuous, and when he acquires a disgust for foods of this class it is all the harder to abide by the original diet. When the patient buys one of these foods, unfortunately he is often given a list of other diabetic foods and a new diabetic diet list, and confusion in the diet frequently results. The patients under my care who have done best either never use special diabetic foods or use only a few varieties.

[1] The Carbohydrate Content of Foods, Medical Research Council, Special Report Series, No. 134, London, 1929.

(808)

Such foods to be of service to the physician or to the dietitian should bear correct statements of the percentages of protein, fat and carbohydrate which they contain; and under no circumstances should the label bear any statements which convey the impression that such foods may be eaten without restriction.

The high content of protein is one of the most serious drawbacks to diabetic foods. Formerly, when it was not realized that from 100 grams protein 58 grams of carbohydrate might be formed, these special foods with low actual carbohydrate content were considered a great boon. Today we look at the matter differently.

The following food tables were prepared for me under the supervision of Prof. E. M. Bailey of the Connecticut Agricultural Experimental Station, New Haven, Conn. Prof. Bailey makes the following comments upon Table 112:

In the table, "Composition of Common Foods," many of the analyses are based on the authority of Atwater and Bryant's compilation. Professor Sherman's "Food Products,"[1] Leach, "Food Inspection and Analysis,"[2] Winton, "Structure and Composition of Foods," the government bulletins already cited, and various reports of this Station have also been freely consulted. A few analyses have been taken from reports of other Experiment Stations and from other sources. For some of the data for malt beverages the text of Wahl and Henius[3] has been consulted.

In choosing analyses many discrepancies are found between the reports of various authors that are perplexing to the physician and to the dietitian. This is in part due to analytical differences that are bound to occur between various analysts, and in part, and more especially, to actual variations in the composition of the foods examined because of such factors as variety and degree of ripeness or maturity. In this compilation the analysis which represents the average of the greatest number of samples, or the one which for one reason or another seems preferable, has been used.

The significance of the term *protein* as here used is nitrogen multiplied by the conventional factor, 6.25, except in the case of milk and milk products, where the more correct factor, 6.38, has been applied. In the case of gluten products (flour and bread), protein is estimated on the basis of the factor, 5.7. Fat means substances soluble in ether; such ether extract may contain material other than true fat, particularly in the case of fruits and vegetables. The term *carbohydrate* is used in the sense of nitrogen-free extract which is the percentage obtained by deducting the sum of the percentages of water, ash, protein, fat and fiber from 100 per cent. Whenever the significance of "carbohydrate" is known to be other than this the explanation is given in a footnote.

[1] The Macmillan Company, New York, 1918.
[2] Wiley & Sons, New York.
[3] Wahl and Henius: American Handy Book, Brewing and Malting.

The dietitian frequently wishes to know how much of the carbohydrate is "available" in digestion. This question cannot be answered without reservations. That portion which is composed of starch, sucrose and other sugars and dextrin is assimilable; the remainder, consisting of hemicellulose complexes, is of doubtful or undetermined availability.

The carbohydrate values given in Table 112 do not pretend to represent the carbohydrate that is assimilable. They have the significance already explained. Dietary allowances calculated on the bases of such figures will generally be too low, but the error is on the side of safety. As the patient's tolerance is demonstrated, his allowance can be made more liberal. Chatfield and her coworkers have reported sugars and starch for a number of fruits and vegetables in the publications here cited, and this affords an approximate estimate of the carbohydrate that is assimilable.

The dietitian will be impressed, however, by the fact that the total carbohydrate content of fruits and vegetables is of an order of magnitude of 10 or 12 per cent, and often much less, and also by the fact that the natural variations in composition due to variety, degree of maturity and, in cooked foods, method of preparation, are very considerable; so that within this range, distinctions between gross carbohydrate and that which is available are often academic rather than practical. It would appear also that in calculating diets based upon *available* carbohydrate values it would be safer to use maximum figures rather than those representing the average or mean in order that the patient's tolerance may not be overestimated. There is not the same objection to average values representing gross carbohydrate, because these no doubt already provide an ample margin of safety.

In the following tables, where caloric values have been given in the absence of determined values for all constituents, the items not determined are assumed to be negligible. In the case of alcoholic and other beverages the carbohydrate values are in many instances grams per 100 cc., but they have been entered as true percentages because, for practical purposes, the difference is not significant.

TABLE 112.—COMPOSITION OF COMMON FOODS.

MEAT PRODUCTS.

Name and description of food.	Protein, per cent.	Fat, per cent.	Carbohydrate, per cent.	Calories, per 100 gms.
Beef, fresh:				
Brisket, medium fat, edible portion .	15.8	28.5	..	319
Chuck rib, edible portion, all analyses .	19.0	13.4	..	197
Flank, edible portion, all analyses . .	19.6	21.1	..	268
Loin, edible portion, all analyses . .	19.0	19.1	..	247
Neck	20.7	12.7	..	197
Plate	16.8	26.9	..	309
Ribs, edible portion, all analyses . .	17.8	24.6	..	293
Round	20.9	10.6	..	179
Rump, lean	20.9	13.7	..	207

TABLE 112.—COMPOSITION OF COMMON FOODS.—(*Continued.*)

MEAT PRODUCTS—*Continued.*

Name and description of food.	Protein, per cent.	Fat, per cent.	Carbo-hydrate, per cent.	Calories, per 100 gms.
Beef, fresh:—Continued:				
Shank, fore	21.4	8.1	..	158
hind	21.7	8.7	..	165
Shoulder and clod, edible portion, all analyses	20.0	10.3	..	173
Soup stock	5.8	1.5	..	36
Miscellaneous cuts, free from visible fat	22.4	2.9	..	116
Brain, edible portion	8.8	9.3	..	119
Heart, edible portion	16.0	20.4	..	248
Kidney, as purchased	13.7	1.9	Trace	72
Liver, as purchased	20.2	3.1	2.5[1]	119
Lungs, as purchased	16.4	3.2	..	94
Marrow, as purchased	2.2	92.8	..	844
Sweetbreads, as purchased	16.8	12.1	..	176
Suet, as purchased	4.7	81.8	..	755
Tongue, edible portion	18.9	9.2	..	158
Beef, cooked:				
Roast	22.3	28.6	..	347
Steak, round	27.6	7.7	..	180
sirloin	23.9	10.2	..	187
tenderloin	23.5	20.4	..	278
Beef, canned:				
Corned[2]	26.6	11.4	..	209
Dried and smoked[3]	32.6	7.5	..	198
Kidneys, stewed	18.4	5.1	2.1	128
Luncheon beef	27.6	15.9	..	254
Roast	25.9	14.8	..	237
Sweetbreads	20.2	9.5	..	166
Tongue, ground	21.4	25.1	..	312
whole	19.5	23.2	..	287
Tripe	16.8	8.5	..	144
Beef, corned and pickled:				
Corned beef, all analyses, edible portion	15.6	26.2	..	298
Spiced beef, rolled	12.0	51.4	..	511
Tongue, edible portion	12.8	20.5	..	236
Tripe	11.7	1.2	Trace	58
Beef, dried, salted, smoked, edible portion	30.0	6.5	..	179
Veal, fresh:				
Breast, edible portion, all analyses	20.3	11.0	..	180
Chuck, edible portion, all analyses	19.7	5.8	..	131
Flank, edible portion, all analyses	20.1	12.7	..	195
Leg, edible portion, all analyses	20.7	6.7	..	143
cutlets, edible portion	20.3	7.7	..	151
Loin, edible portion, all analyses	19.9	10.0	..	170
Rib	20.2	9.4	..	165
Rump	19.8	16.2	..	225
Shoulder	20.7	4.6	..	124
Heart, as purchased	16.8	9.6	..	154
Kidney, as purchased	16.9	6.4	..	125
Liver, as purchased	19.0	5.3	..	124
Lungs, as purchased	17.1	5.0	..	113
Lamb, fresh:				
Breast, edible portion	19.1	23.6	..	289
Leg, hind, medium fat, edible portion	19.2	16.5	..	225
Loin, without kidney and tallow, edible portion	18.7	28.3	..	330
Shoulder, edible portion	18.1	29.7	..	340

[1] Largely, or in part, glycogen.
[2] Average, 3.4 per cent salt (sodium chloride).
[3] Average, 9.7 per cent salt (sodium chloride).

TABLE 112.—COMPOSITION OF COMMON FOODS.—(*Continued.*)

MEAT PRODUCTS—*Continued.*

Name and description of food.	Protein, per cent.	Fat, per cent.	Carbo-hydrate, per cent.	Calories, per 100 gms.
Lamb, cooked:				
Chops, broiled, edible portion . . .	21.7	29.9	..	356
Leg, roast	19.7	12.7	..	193
Lamb, canned:				
Tongue, spiced, cooked, edible portion	13.9	17.8	..	216
Mutton, fresh:				
Chuck, edible portion, all analyses . .	14.6	36.8	..	390
Leg, hind, medium fat, edible portion .	18.5	18.0	..	236
Loin, without kidney and tallow, edible portion	16.0	33.1	..	362
Shoulder, medium fat, edible portion .	17.7	19.9	..	250
Heart, as purchased	16.9	12.6	..	181
Kidney, as purchased	16.5	3.2	..	95
Liver, as purchased	23.1	9.0	5.0[1]	193
Lungs, as purchased	20.2	2.8	..	106
Mutton, cooked:				
Leg roast, edible portion	25.0	22.6	..	303
Mutton, canned:				
Corned	28.8	22.8	..	320
Tongue	24.4	24.0	..	314
Pork, fresh:				
Ham, lean	25.0	14.4	..	230
Ham, medium fat, edible portion . .	15.3	28.9	..	321
Head cheese, edible portion	19.5	33.8	..	382
Loin (chops), lean, edible portion . .	20.3	19.0	..	252
Loin (chops), medium fat, edible portion	16.6	30.1	..	337
Shoulder, edible portion	13.3	34.2	..	361
Side, lard and other fat included, edible portion	9.4	61.7	..	593
Side, lard and kidneys not included, edible portion	9.1	55.3	..	534
Brains, as purchased	11.7	10.3	..	140
Heart, as purchased	17.1	6.3	..	125
Kidney, as purchased	15.5	4.8	0.7	108
Liver, as purchased	21.3	4.5	1.4[1]	131
Lungs, as purchased	11.9	4.0	..	84
Pork, pickled, salted or smoked:[2]				
Ham, lean, smoked, edible portion . .	19.8	20.8	..	266
Ham, medium fat, smoked, edible portion	16.3	38.8	..	414
Ham, luncheon, cooked	22.5	21.0	..	279
Shoulder, medium fat, smoked, edible portion	15.9	32.5	..	356
Pig's tongue, pickled, edible portion .	17.7	19.8	..	249
Pig's feet, pickled, edible portion . .	16.3	14.8	..	198
Salt pork, clear fat	1.9	86.2	..	783
Bacon, smoked, all analyses, edible portion	10.5	64.8	..	625
Ham, deviled	19.0	34.1	..	383
Sausage:				
Arles, edible portion	26.8	50.6	..	563
Bologna, edible portion	18.7	17.6	0.3[3]	234
Frankfort	19.6	18.6	1.1[4]	250
Pork, as purchased	13.0	44.2	1.1[5]	454

[1] Largely, or in part, glycogen.
[2] The range of salt content for cured pork products may be taken as 3 to 5 per cent.
[3] Carbohydrate range, 0.2 to 3.1 per cent.
[4] Carbohydrate range, 0.0 to 6.6 per cent.
[5] Carbohydrate range, 0.0 to 8.6 per cent.

TABLE 112.—COMPOSITION OF COMMON FOODS.—(*Continued.*)

MEAT PRODUCTS—*Concluded.*

Name and description of food.	Protein, per cent.	Fat, per cent.	Carbo-hydrate, per cent.	Calories, per 100 gms.
Sausage:—Continued:				
Deerfoot Farm, cooked (analysis furnished by manufacturer)	19.9	54.2	0.3	569
Pork and beef, as purchased . . .	19.4	24.1	..	295
POULTRY.				
Poultry, fresh:				
Chicken, broilers, edible portion . .	21.5	2.5	..	109
heart, as purchased . . .	20.7	5.5	..	132
gizzard, as purchased . . .	24.7	1.4	..	111
liver, as purchased . . .	22.4	4.2	2.4[1]	137
Fowls, edible portion	19.3	16.3	..	224
Goose, edible portion	16.3	36.2	..	391
Goose liver, edible portion	16.6	15.9	3.7[1]	224
Turkey, edible portion	21.1	22.9	..	291
FISH PRODUCTS.				
Fish, fresh:				
Alewife, whole, edible portion . . .	19.4	4.9	..	122
Bass, black, edible portion	20.6	1.7	..	98
red, edible portion	16.9	0.5	..	72
sea, edible portion	19.8	0.5	..	84
striped, edible portion . . .	18.6	2.8	..	100
Blackfish, edible portion	18.7	1.3	..	87
Bluefish, edible portion	19.4	1.2	..	88
Butterfish, edible portion	18.0	11.0	..	171
Cod, edible portion	16.7	0.3	..	70
steak, edible portion	18.7	0.5	..	79
Eels, salt water, edible portion . . .	18.6	9.1	..	156
Flounder, edible portion	14.2	0.6	..	62
Haddock, edible portion	17.2	0.3	..	72
Halibut, edible portion	18.6	5.2	..	121
Herring, edible portion	19.5	7.1	..	142
Mackerel, edible portion	18.7	7.1	..	139
Perch, edible portion	19.0	2.4	..	98
Pickerel, edible portion	18.7	0.5	..	79
Porgy, edible portion	18.6	5.1	..	120
Salmon, edible portion	22.0	12.8	..	203
Shad, edible portion	18.8	9.5	..	161
Shad roe, as purchased	20.9	3.8	2.6	128
Smelt, edible portion	17.6	1.8	..	87
Trout, brook, edible portion . . .	19.2	2.1	..	96
Trout, lake, edible portion	17.8	10.3	..	164
Whitefish, edible portion	22.9	6.5	..	150
Fish, preserved or canned:				
Cod, salt, "boneless," as purchased[2] .	27.7	0.3	..	114
Haddock, smoked, edible portion . .	23.3	0.2	..	95
Halibut, smoked, edible portion[3] . .	20.7	15.0	..	218
Herring, smoked, edible portion[4] . .	36.9	15.8	..	290
Mackerel, salt, edible portion[5] . . .	17.3	26.4	..	307
salt, canned, as purchased .	19.6	8.7	..	157
salt, canned in oil, edible portion	25.4	14.1	..	229
Salmon, canned, edible portion . . .	21.8	12.1	..	196
Sardines, canned, edible portion . .	23.0	19.7	..	269

[1] Largely, or in part, glycogen.
[2] Contains 11.0 per cent ash, largely salt.
[3] Contains 15.0 per cent ash, largely (12.1 per cent) salt.
[4] Contains 13.2 per cent ash, largely (11.7 per cent) salt.
[5] Contains 12.9 per cent ash, largely (10.4 per cent) salt.

TABLE 112.—COMPOSITION OF COMMON FOODS.—(*Continued.*)

FISH PRODUCTS—*Concluded.*

Name and description of food.	Protein, per cent.	Fat, per cent.	Carbo-hydrate, per cent.	Calories, per 100 gms.
Fish, preserved or canned:—Continued:				
Sardines, canned in mineral oil, edible portion	22.8	2.7[1]	..	116
Sturgeon, caviare, preserved, Russian, as purchased	30.0	19.7	7.6	328
Tunny (tuna), as purchased . . .	21.7	4.1	..	124
canned in oil, edible portion	23.8	20.0	0.6	278
Turtle meat, canned	23.4	0.7	..	100
Shellfish, etc., fresh:				
Clams, long, in shell, edible portion .	8.6	1.0	2.0[2]	51
round, in shell, edible portion .	6.5	0.4	4.2[2]	46
Crabs, hard shell, whole, edible portion	16.6	2.0	1.2[2]	89
Crayfish, edible portion	16.0	0.5	1.0[2]	73
Lobster, edible portion	16.4	1.8	0.4[2]	83
Mussels, in shell, edible portion . .	8.7	1.1	4.1[2]	61
Oysters, in shell, edible portion . . .	6.2	1.2	3.7[2]	50
Scallops, as purchased	14.8	0.1	3.4[2]	74
Terrapin, edible portion	21.2	3.5	..	116
Turtle, green, edible portion . . .	19.8	0.5	..	84
Shellfish, etc., canned:				
Clams, long, as purchased	8.3	0.4	2.7[2]	48
round, as purchased	8.9	0.8	0.9[2]	46
Crabs, as purchased	15.8	1.5	0.7[2]	80
Lobster, as purchased	18.1	1.1	0.5[2]	84
Oysters, as purchased	8.8	2.4	3.9[2]	72
Shrimp, as purchased	25.4	1.0	0.2	111
Turtle meat	23.4	0.7	..	100
AMPHIBIA.				
Frog's legs, edible portion	15.5	0.2	..	64
GELATIN.				
Gelatin	84.2[3]	0.1	None	338
EGGS.				
Eggs, fresh:[4]				
Hen, whole egg, edible portion . . .	13.4	10.5	..	148
white	12.3	0.2	..	51
yolk	15.7	33.3	..	363
Duck, whole egg, edible portion . .	13.3	14.5	..	184
white	11.1	Trace	..	44
yolk	16.8	36.2	..	393
Goose, whole egg, edible portion . .	13.8	14.4	..	185
white	11.6	Trace	..	46
yolk	17.3	36.2	..	395
Turkey, whole egg, edible portion . .	13.4	11.2	..	154
white	11.5	Trace	..	46
yolk	17.4	32.9	..	366

[1] Total oil present, 13.3 per cent; approximately 20 per cent (= 2.7 per cent), digestible.

[2] Largely, or in part, glycogen.

[3] Nitrogen $\times$ 5.55.

[4] In shell eggs the shell comprises from 10 to 17 per cent of the weight of the whole egg; water content ranges from 60 to 67 per cent. Sea-turtle eggs contain about 76 per cent water.

TABLE 112.—COMPOSITION OF COMMON FOODS.—(*Continued.*)

EGGS—*Concluded.*

Name and description of food.	Protein, per cent.	Fat, per cent.	Carbo-hydrate, per cent.	Calories, per 100 gms.
Eggs, fresh:[1]—*Continued:*				
Guinea fowl, whole egg, edible portion	13.5	12.0	..	162
white	11.6	Trace	..	46
yolk	16.7	31.8	..	353
Plover, whole egg, edible portion	10.7	11.7	..	148
Turtle, fresh water	18.1	11.1	..	172
sea	18.8	9.8	..	163
Eggs, edible portion, cooked:				
Hen, boiled	13.2	12.0	..	161
whites	12.3	0.2	..	51
yolks	15.7	33.3	..	363
Eggs, dehydrated, average	40.0	43.7	..	556

DAIRY PRODUCTS, ETC.

	Protein, per cent.	Fat, per cent.	Carbo-hydrate, per cent.	Calories, per 100 gms.
Milk:				
Milk, whole	3.3	4.0	4.8	68
condensed (evaporated, concentrated)	6.9	8.2	9.9	141
sweetened, condensed (sweetened evaporated, sweetened concentrated)	7.9	9.0	54.6[2]	331
skimmed	3.4	0.3	5.1	37
sweetened, condensed	9.1	1.0	59.1[3]	282
Buttermilk	3.6	0.5	4.1	35
Kephir	3.1	2.0	1.6	37
Kumiss[4]	2.8	2.1	5.4	51
Cream, "heavy" (approximately 40 per cent)	2.1	41.0	1.5	383
"light" (approximately 20 per cent)	2.8	22.0	2.7	220
heavy, sour, Jewish	4.1	41.6	1.5	397
Whey	1.0	0.3	5.0	27
Milk powder (dried milk):				
From whole milk	25.3	25.3	37.5	479
From partly skimmed milk	25.8	14.5	49.9	433
From skimmed milk, average	34.6	1.9	50.9	359
Malted milk (milk powder with malted cereal) average	13.8	6.8	71.9	404
Cheese:				
Brick (soft)	23.8	28.9	..	355
Brie (soft)	18.3	27.5	..	321
Camembert (soft)	19.0	21.5	3.5	284
Cheddar, American	23.7	33.8	..	399
Canadian	23.9	33.8	..	400
English	30.0	30.3	..	393
Cottage (soft)	20.9	1.0	4.3	110
Cream (soft)	25.4	30.3	2.0	382
Edam (American)	24.1	30.3	4.6	388
(Dutch)	29.6	28.0	2.6	381

[1] In shell eggs the shell comprises from 10 to 17 per cent of the weight of the whole egg; water content ranges from 60 to 67 per cent. Sea-turtle eggs contain about 76 per cent water.

[2] Cane sugar, 40.6 per cent; milk sugar, 14 per cent.

[3] Cane sugar, 40.9 per cent; milk sugar, 18.2 per cent.

[4] According to Van Slyke (Leach: Food Inspection and Analysis, p. 174), Kumiss, from cows' milk, contains lactose, 5 per cent; protein, 4.1 per cent; fat (calculated), 1.2 per cent.

TABLE 112.—COMPOSITION OF COMMON FOODS.—*(Continued.)*

DAIRY PRODUCTS, ETC.—*Concluded.*

Name and description of food.	Protein, per cent.	Fat, per cent.	Carbo-hydrate, per cent.	Calories, per 100 gms.
Cheese:—Continued:				
Gorgonozola	25.2	34.7	1.6	420
Gouda	24.4	31.2	..	378
Guyere	30.8	29.3	..	387
Limburger (American)	23.0	29.4	0.4	358
Neufchatel (soft), American	15.0	22.3	2.9	272
Parmesan	35.0	23.0	..	347
Pineapple	29.4	38.1	2.5	471
Roquefort	22.6	29.5	1.8	363
Stilton	23.2	39.0	..	444
Swiss (Emmenthaler)	30.3	30.5	..	396
Ice cream, typical	3.8	12.6[1]	19.6	207

FATS AND OILS.

Fats and Oils:				
Butter,[2] average	1.5	84.6	None	767
Oleomargarine,[3] average	0.8	92.4	None	835
Nut margarine,[4] average	1.4	84.8	None	769
Salad oils and cooking fat, typical	Trace	99.7	None	897

SOUPS AND BROTHS.

Soups, home-made:				
Bean	3.2	1.4	9.4	63
Beef	4.4	0.4	1.1	26
Chicken	10.5	0.8	2.4	59
Clam chowder	1.8	0.8	6.7	41
Meat stew	4.6	4.3	5.5	79
Soups, broths, etc., canned:				
Asparagus, cream of	2.5	3.2	5.5	61
Bouillon, beef	2.2	0.1	0.2	11
clam, typical	1.0	0.1	0.6	7
Celery, cream of	2.1	2.8	5.0	54
Chicken gumbo	3.8	0.9	4.7	42
soup	3.6	0.1	1.5	21
Consommé	1.4	0.1	0.4	8
Corn, cream of	2.5	1.9	7.8	58
Julienne	2.7	..	0.5	13
Mock turtle	3.0	1.0	5.7	44
Mulligatawny	3.7	0.1	5.7	39
Oxtail, edible portion	3.7	1.3	7.1	55
Pea soup	3.6	0.7	7.6	51
Pea, cream of green	2.6	2.7	5.7	58
Tomato	1.8	1.1	5.6	40
Turtle, green	6.1	1.9	3.9	57
Vegetable	2.9	..	0.5	14
Bouillon cubes:				
As purchased, average analysis[5]	11.4	1.8	5.8	85
Prepared as directed, average analysis[6]	0.2	Trace	0.1	1
Clam extract:				
As purchased	23.2	0.2	11.8	142
Prepared as directed[7]	0.5	Trac e	0.3	3
Yeast extract, as purchased	31.3	0.2	12.5	177

[1] Standards for fat in different States vary from 8 to 14 per cent.
[2] Average salt content, 1.6 per cent; range, 0.2 to 4.1 per cent.
[3] Average ash content (largely salt), 0.9 per cent; range, 0.4 to 3.1 per cent.
[4] Average ash content (largely salt), 2.9 per cent; range, 1.1 to 6.1 per cent.
[5] Average salt content, 70.2 per cent.
[6] Average cube weighs 3.8 gms.; 1 cup of broth is assumed to weigh 240 gms.; salt content of prepared broth, 1.1 per cent.
[7] Salt content, 0.4 per cent.

TABLE 112.—COMPOSITION OF COMMON FOODS.—(*Continued.*)
CEREAL PRODUCTS, ETC.

Name and description of food.	Protein, per cent.	Fat, per cent.	Carbo-hydrate, per cent.	Calories per 100 gms.
Alimentary pastes:				
Macaroni	13.4	0.9	74.1[1]	358
" cooked	3.0	1.5	15.8[1]	89
Noodles	11.7	1.0	75.2	357
Spaghetti	12.1	0.4	75.9	356
Vermicelli	10.9	2.0	72.0[1]	350
Bread, soft:				
Bread, alfalfa	10.6	1.3	64.0	310
brown	5.4	1.8	47.1[1]	226
corn (Johnnycake)	7.9	4.7	46.3[1]	259
Graham	8.9	1.8	51.0	256
peanut	33.6	12.8	19.7	328
rye	9.0	0.6	52.7	252
rye, Jewish	9.1	1.1	52.0	254
whole rye	11.9	0.6	34.7	192
rye and wheat	11.9	0.3	51.5[1]	256
wheat, average of many analyses	9.2	1.3	52.6	259
wheat, whole	9.7	0.9	48.5	241
wheat gluten, average	25.0	3.6	28.9	248
Buns, hotcross	7.9	4.8	49.7[1]	274
Biscuit, homemade	8.7	2.6	54.6	277
Maryland	8.4	5.6	58.8	309
soda	9.3	13.7	52.6[1]	371
Rolls, all analyses	8.9	4.1	56.1	297
Bread, hard, and crackers:				
Bread, white, toasted	11.5	1.6	61.2[1]	305
Zwieback	9.8	9.9	73.5[1]	422
Crackers, Boston (split)	11.0	8.5	70.3	402
butter	9.6	10.1	71.2	414
cream	9.7	12.1	69.1	424
egg	12.6	14.0	66.2	441
flatbread	14.9	0.5	73.6[1]	359
Graham	10.0	9.4	72.3	414
oatmeal	11.8	11.1	67.1	416
oyster	11.3	10.5	70.3	421
pilot	11.1	5.0	73.9	385
pretzels	9.7	3.9	72.3	363
saltines	10.6	12.7	68.0	429
soda	9.8	9.1	72.8	412
water	11.7	5.0	75.3	393
Pastry, etc.:				
Cake, coffee	7.1	7.5	62.8	347
cup	5.9	9.0	68.2	377
frosted	5.9	9.0	64.8[1]	364
fruit	5.9	10.9	64.1	378
gingerbread	5.8	9.0	62.6	354
sponge	6.3	10.7	65.9[1]	385
Cookies	7.0	9.7	73.2	408
Doughnuts	6.7	21.0	52.4	425
Fig bars	4.6	6.6	68.1	350
Ginger snaps	6.5	8.6	75.3	405
Lady fingers	8.8	5.0	70.4	362
Macaroons	6.5	15.2	64.1	419
Pie, apple	3.1	9.8	42.8[1]	272
cream	4.4	11.4	51.2[1]	325
custard	4.2	6.3	26.1[1]	178

[1] Includes fiber.

52

TABLE 112.—COMPOSITION OF COMMON FOODS.—(*Continued.*)

CEREAL PRODUCTS, ETC.—*Continued.*

Name and description of food.	Protein, per cent.	Fat, per cent.	Carbo- hydrate, per cent.	Calories, per 100 gms.
Pastry, etc.—Continued:				
Pie,				
lemon	3.6	10.1	37.4[1]	255
mince	5.8	12.3	38.1[1]	286
raisin	3.0	11.3	47.2[1]	303
squash	4.4	8.4	21.7[1]	180
Pudding, Indian meal	5.5	4.8	27.5[1]	175
rice custard	4.0	4.6	31.4[1]	183
tapioca	3.3	3.2	28.2[1]	155
Wafers, miscellaneous	8.7	8.6	74.1	409
vanilla	6.6	14.0	71.3	438
Breakfast foods:				
Corn Preparations:				
Collin's Hulled Corn	7.9	2.0	76.2	354
Corn Kix, General Mills	8.0	1.9	78.9	365
H-O New Process Hominy	8.0	0.3	79.8	354
Jackson's Roman Meal	13.3	3.4	66.1	348
Kellogg's Corn Flakes	8.0	0.3	83.9	370
Nichol's Snow White Samp	7.8	0.3	77.7	345
Post Toasties	8.0	0.2	82.1	362
Quaker Best Yellow Corn Meal	7.5	0.8	78.7	352
Quaker Corn Puffs	8.7	0.3	78.5	352
Quaker Hominy Grits	7.7	0.8	77.6	348
Quaker Toasted Corn Flakes	6.8	0.4	79.9	350
Ralston Hominy Grits	9.0	2.9	75.4	364
Sun Seal Sunnycorn	8.4	0.5	78.3	351
Oat Preparations:				
Coarse American Oatmeal	15.8	5.6	65.3	375
H-O Hornsby's Oats	16.0	6.0	64.4	376
Hornsby's Steam Cooked Oat Meal	16.1	6.7	64.1	381
Irish Oat Meal	15.3	7.2	67.9	398
Irish Oat Meal	15.3	7.0	65.7	387
Quaker Oats	15.9	6.0	64.5	376
Quaker Rolled White Oats	16.6	6.0	63.3	374
Rolled Oats	17.4	6.3	62.8	378
Scotch Oatmeal	11.6	6.4	67.6	374
Scotch Porage Oats	13.3	9.6	64 9	399
Tremont Brand Regular Rolled Oats	15.1	6.5	64.9	379
Rice Preparations:				
B.C. Rice Flakes	6.3	0.3	80.2	349
Comet Cereal	7.2	0.3	80.7	354
Cream of Rice	7.4	0.4	79.6	352
Heinz Rice Flakes	7.5	0.4	78.2	346
Kellogg's Toasted Rice Flakes	10.0	0.4	81.3	369
Quaker Brand Puffed Rice	6.0	0.3	84.0	363
Quaker Puffed Rice	7.6	0.2	79.5	350
Rice Krispies	6.8	0.3	83.9	366
Rye Preparations:				
Cream of Rye	11.1	2.1	72.4	353
Cream of Rye	12.0	1.6	71.8	350
Ry-Krisp	14.0	1.7	74.4	369
Wheat Preparations:				
B-C Vita Wheat	10.9	1.9	76.7	368
Cooked Wheat	10.5	2.4	76.8	371
Cracked Wheat	9.6	2.0	72.1	345
Cream of Wheat	12.6	0.7	74.5	355

[1] Includes fiber.

TABLE 112.—COMPOSITION OF COMMON FOODS.—(*Continued.*)

CEREAL PRODUCTS, ETC.—*Continued.*

Name and description of food.	Protein, per cent.	Fat, per cent.	Carbo-hydrate, per cent.	Calories per 100 gms.
Breakfast foods:—Continued:				
Wheat Preparations:				
Cream of Wheat	11.5	0.9	73.7	349
Enwright's All O'The Wheat Old Fash-				
ioned Cereal	15.0	2.4	66.8	349
Force	10.6	1.1	73.7	347
Force—Toasted Whole Wheat Flakes	9.3	2.2	78.6	371
Grape Nuts	11.5	0.6	74.2	348
Hecker's Cream Farina	12.3	0.9	75.0	357
Hecker's Farina	10.0	0.7	75.9	350
Holland Rusk	12.1	5.1	70.4	376
Huskies Whole Wheat Flakes . .	9.6	1.1	75.2	349
Kellogg's Krumbles	12.0	1.2	72.3	348
Kellogg's Toasted Wheat Biscuit .	14.2	1.4	74.7	368
Kellogg's—Whole Wheat Biscuit .	10.3	1.7	73.6	351
Kellogg's Wheat Krispies	8.8	1.2	77.4	356
Kellogg's Whole Wheat Krumbles .	9.4	2.1	78.0	369
Kellogg's Zwieback	14.3	1.6	76.1	376
Muffets—Whole Wheat Biscuit . .	10.3	1.3	74.8	352
National Biscuit Shredded Biscuit .	9.8	1.3	75.2	352
Overland Wheat Cereal	12.0	0.7	74.8	354
Pettijohn's Rolled Wheat	9.9	1.9	72.0	345
Pillsbury's Farina	11.8	0.7	75.2	354
Post-O The New Wheat Cereal . .	11.6	1.2	70.5	339
Quaker Brand Puffed Wheat . . .	15.5	1.7	71.4	363
Quaker Cracked Wheat	9.3	2.3	73.3	351
Quaker Farina	11.4	0.8	76.1	357
Quaker Puffed Wheat	13.1	1.8	70.2	349
Quaker Wheat Crackels	11.8	1.2	75.0	358
Ralston Wheat Cereal	16.6	2.2	67.7	357
Ralston Wheat Food	11.3	1.8	73.1	354
Shredded Ralston Toasted Whole				
Wheat	9.9	2.3	75.8	364
Shredded Wheat Biscuit	11.0	1.4	75.0	357
Sunshine Rippled Wheat Cereal Biscuit	9.5	1.7	71.8	341
Triscuit	11.0	1.4	73.9	352
Wheatena	11.3	2.8	74.2	367
Wheatena	11.8	2.4	73.8	364
Wheaties	13.2	1.1	72.6	353
Wheatsworth Whole Wheat Cereal .	14.0	2.0	70.8	357
Miscellaneous Preparations:				
B-C Battle Creek "ZO"	15.6	0.8	71.7	356
B-C Cooked Bran	16.4	4.7	54.9	328
B-C Fig and Bran	11.5	2.5	65.2	329
B-C Fig and Bran Flakes	9.5	1.8	73.7	349
B-C Krusty Bran	11.4	2.5	66.4	334
B-C Lima Bean—Rice Flakes . .	13.0	1.5	68.9	341
B-C Toasted Gluten Bran Flakes .	48.8	6.2	25.4	353
B-C Washed Bran	16.9	3.0	52.0	303
Bran-Zos	13.2	2.5	65.6	338
Cellu Breakfast Krisp	4.5	22.4[1]	40.2	179[2]
Ceremel—A Laxative Food . . .	18.3	6.5	54.9	351
Cerevim	19.3	2.2	63.5	351
Educator Bran Cookies	8.9	14.5	64.7	425
Educator Bran Meal	12.3	2.8	66.4	340

[1] Largely mineral oil.
[2] "Fat" not included.

TABLE 112.—COMPOSITION OF COMMON FOODS.—*Continued.*

CEREAL PRODUCTS, ETC.—*Continued:*

Name and description of food.	Protein, per cent.	Fat, per cent	Carbo-hydrate, per cent.	Calories, per 100 gms.
Breakfast foods:—Continued.				
Miscellaneous Preparations:				
Grape Nuts Bran Flakes	10.5	2.7	75.3	368
Grape Nuts	11.3	2.2	77.2	374
Jackson Meal	15.3	2.5	65.8	347
Kellogg's All-Bran	13.0	2.5	62.8	326
Kellogg's 40% Bran Flakes . . .	10.4	1.8	73.5	352
Laxative Biscuit (Kellogg) . . .	16.7	10.8	57.7	395
Lister's Starchless Breakfast Food .	5.9	1.4	72.9	328
Maltex Cereal	15.3	1.5	70.9	358
Maypl Cereal	15.6	4.4	67.9	374
Pep	10.6	1.8	76.5	365
Post's 40% Bran Flakes	12.3	1.8	70.7	348
Roman Meal	15.1	2.7	61.8	332
Sea Moss Farina	9.1	0.3	59.9	279
Trix	14.5	0.2	77.3	369
Uncle Sam Health Food	21.3	24.4	40.9	468
Uncle Sam Laxative Breakfast Food .	18.5	11.4	56.7	403
Weetabix	9.4	2.4	75.0	359
Wheat-Ota—Wheat and Oat Porridge	15.6	4.5	65.8	366
Zed Biscuits	10.3	15.5	64.2	438
Flours, meals, etc.:				
Barley flour	12.3	2.4	71.3	**356**
Buckwheat flour	6.4	1.2	77.5	**346**
Corn flour	8.4	1.8	76.2	**355**
Corn meal	9.2	1.9	74.4	**352**
Oat flour	15.1	6.4	65.7	**381**
Potato flour	0.5	0.1	83.0	335
Rice flour	7.3	0.6	79.3	352
Rye flour	6.8	0.9	78.3	349
Rye meal	13.6	2.0	69.7	351
Soy bean flour	42.5	19.9	24.3	446
Soy bean meal	38.3	14.9	26.6	394
Wheat flour, entire	13.8	1.9	71.0	356
Wheat flour, Graham	13.3	2.2	69.5	351
Wheat flour, patent, average . . .	11.4	1.0	74.8	354
Wheat gluten flour, average . . .	42.1	1.9	46.4	371

VEGETABLES.

	Protein, per cent.	Fat, per cent	Carbo-hydrate, per cent.	Calories, per 100 gms.
Vegetables, fresh (unless otherwise stated):				
Amaranth, leaves and stems . . .	3.0	0.6	4.6	36
Aralia Cordata (Udo)	1.0	0.2	2.6	16
Artichokes, Globe or French . . .	2.9	0.4	11.9[1]	63
Jerusalem	2.9	0.1	16.4[1]	78
cooked . . .	2.4	0.1	16.5[1]	77
Asparagus	2.1	0.2	2.7	21
Bambo shoots	2.5	0.3	4.3	30
Basella, leaves and stems . . .	2.0	0.3	2.4	20
Beans, butter	9.4	0.6	29.1[2]	159
cranberry, young pods . . .	0.4	None	0.6	4
medium	1.3	0.6	1.7	17
fancy	1.0	0.1	2.1	13
Lima	7.1	0.7	20.3	116
Beans, refugee, young pods . . .	0.5	None	0.8	5
medium	1.3	0.1	3.0	18
fancy	1.1	0.1	1.4	11
soy, green, shelled	13.6	6.3	11.0	155
string (carbohydrate range, 3.9 to 10 per cent)	2.3	0.3	5.5	34
string, cooked	0.8	1.1	1.9[2]	21

[1] Chiefly inulin.   [2] Includes fiber.

TABLE 112.—COMPOSITION OF COMMON FOODS.—(*Continued.*)

VEGETABLES—*Continued.*

Name and description of food.	Protein, per cent.	Fat, per cent.	Carbo- hydrate, per cent.	Calories, per 100 gms.
Vegetables, fresh (unless otherwise stated):— Continued:				
Beets (carbohydrate range, 6 to 10 per cent)	1.6	0.1	8.8	43
Broccoli	3.3	0.2	4.2	32
Borage (salad plant)	3.0	0.4	0.4	17
Brussels sprouts	4.4	0.5	7.6	53
Burdock, leaves	4.5	0.1	7.4	49
roots	3.0	0.1	21.1	97
Cabbage (carbohydrate range, 3–6.5 per cent)	1.6	0.3	4.5	27
Chinese	1.2	0.1	2.4	15
Carrots (carbohydrate range, 5.9–11.5 per cent)	1.1	0.4	8.2	41
Cassava, root	1.6	0.2	27.1	117
Cauliflower	1.8	0.5	3.7	27
Celeriac	1.8	0.2	6.0	33
Celery	1.3	0.2	3.0	19
root	2.0	0.4	6.3	37
Chard (Swiss), leaves	2.6	0.4	4.0	30
Chayote (tayote) fruit	0.9	0.1	5.9	28
leaves	3.2	0.7	2.5	29
roots	1.8	0.1	18.8	91
Chenopodium	8.5	1.1	2.7	55
Chicory, root	..	..	15.0	
leaves	1.6	0.3	2.1	27
Chinese vegetables:				
Kai Tsoi	1.7	0.2	1.8	16
Bak Toy	1.2	0.1	1.1	10
Chives, bulbs and tops	3.8	0.6	5.8	44
Collards	4.5	0.6	6.3[1]	49
Corn	3.1	1.1	19.2	99
Cucumbers	0.8	0.2	2.3	14
Dasheen, corms and tubers	2.9	0.2	28.2	126
leaves and stems	2.7	0.7	5.8	40
Dock, leaves and stems	2.1	0.3	2.6	22
Egg plant	1.2	0.3	4.3	25
Endive, leaves	1.6	0.2	3.2	21
Finocchio	1.5	0.1	1.6	13
Garlic, bulbs	4.4	0.2	19 0	95
Greens, beet, cooked	2.2	3.4	3.2[1]	52
dandelion	2.7	0.7	7.0	45
turnip salad	4.2	0.6	6.3[1]	47
Kale	3.9	0.6	6.0	45
sea	1.5	0.2	3.5	22
Kohl-rabi	2.0	0.1	4.2	26
Lambs' quarters	3.8	0.7	5.7	44
Leeks	2.9	0.1	4.0[2]	29
Lettuce	1.2	0.3	2.2	16
Mushrooms[3]	3.5	0.4	6.0	42
Mustard, greens	2.3	0.3	3.2	26
Okra	1.8	0.2	6.4	35
Onions	1.6	0.3	9.1	46
cooked	1.2	1.8	4.9[1]	41
Orach	4.5	0.4	3.7	36
Oyster plant	1.2	0.1	7.0	34

[1] Includes fiber.   [2] Starch and sugar.
[3] Protein and carbohydrates largely unassimilable (E. P. J.).

TABLE 112.—COMPOSITION OF COMMON FOODS.—(*Continued.*)

VEGETABLES—*Continued.*

Name and description of food.	Protein, per cent.	Fat, per cent.	Carbo-hydrate, per cent.	Calories, per 100 gms.
Vegetables, fresh (unless otherwise stated):—Continued:				
Palmetto cabbage	3.3	0.6	6.1	43
cooked	2.9	0.5	5.6	39
Parsley, leaves	3.7	1.0	7.2	53
Parsnips (carbohydrate range, 6–14 per cent)	1.6	0.5	11.0	55
Patience (Rumex Patientia)	2.1	0.2	0.1[2]	11
Peas, green, cooked	6.7	3.4	14.6[1]	116
young	5.4	0.3	10.3	65
medium	6.5	0.4	14.2	86
Peppers, Neapolitan	1.1	0.3	5.7	30
sweet, green	0.8	0.1	4.1	21
Potatoes	2.2	0.1	18.0	82
air (tropical Asia)	1.9	0.4	16.3	76
boiled	2.5	0.1	20.3	92
cooked, chips	6.8	39.8	46.7[1]	572
mashed and creamed	2.6	3.0	17.8[1]	109
sweet	1.8	0.7	26.1	118
cooked	3.0	2.1	42.1[1]	199
Pumpkins	1.2	0.2	6.0	31
Purslane	1.6	0.4	2.5	20
Radishes (carbohydrate range, 2.7–7.5 per cent)	1.3	0.1	5.1	27
Rhubarb	0.6	0.7	2.5	19
Roquette (Rocket salad)	1.1	0.2	2.6	22
Rutabagas (carbohydrate range, 3–12 per cent)	1.3	0.2	7.3	36
Sauerkraut	1.7	0.5	3.8[1]	27
Sorrel (dock)	2.1	0.3	2.6	22
Spinach	2.1	0.3	2.3	20
cooked	2.1	4.1	2.6[1]	56
Squash, summer	0.6	0.1	3.4	17
winter	1.5	0.3	7.4	38
Tomatoes, green	1.2	0.2	2.8	18
ripe	0.9	0.4	3.3	20
juice	0.8	..	3.5	..
Truffles	9.1[3]	0.5	7.0[4]	..
Turnips	1.3	0.2	6.8	34
Vegetable marrow	0.5	0.1	4.0	19
cooked	0.4	0.1	4.1	19
Watercress	1.7	0.3	2.8	21
Yams	2.1	0.2	23.3	103
Vegetables, dried:				
Beans	22.5	1.8	55.2	327
carob	6.3	0.6	80.7	353
frijoles	21.9	1.3	65.1[1]	360
Lima	18.1	1.5	65.9[1]	350
mesquite	12.2	2.5	77.1[1]	380
soy	38.3	14.9	26.6[5]	394
Carrots, evaporated	7.7	3.6	80.3[1]	384
Lentils	25.7	1.0	59.2[1]	349
Peas	24.6	1.0	57.5	337
cow	21.4	1.4	56.7	325
Peppers, green	15.5	8.5	63.0[1]	391
red	9.4	7.7	70.0[1]	387
Potatoes, evaporated	8.5	0.4	80.9[1]	361
Tomatoes	12.9	8.1	62.3[1]	374

[1] Includes fiber.
[3] Largely non-protein.
[5] About one-fourth available.

[2] Starch and sugar.
[4] Largely unavailable.

TABLE 112.—COMPOSITION OF COMMON FOODS.—(Continued.)

VEGETABLES—Continued.

Name and description of food.	Protein, per cent.	Fat, per cent.	Carbo-hydrate, per cent.	Calories, per 100 gms.
Vegetables, canned:				
Artichokes (carbohydrate range, 3.2–6.1 per cent)	0.8	..	4.4	21
Asparagus (carbohydrate range, 1.6–3.3 per cent)	1.5	0.1	2.3	16
Beans, baked	6.9	2.5	17.1	119
haricots verts	1.1	0.1	2.0	13
flageolets (carbohydrate range, 9.8–12.4 per cent)	4.6	0.1	11.5	65
Lima (carbohydrate range, 9.6–16.5 per cent)	4.0	3.0	13.4	97
little green	1.2	0.1	2.8	17
red kidney	7.0	0.2	17.3	99
string (carbohydrate range, 1.5–4.5 per cent)	1.1	0.1	3.3	19
wax	1.0	0.1	2.5	15
Brussels sprouts	1.5	0.1	2.9	19
Corn[1] (carbohydrate range, 11.7–25.1 per cent)	2.8	1.2	18.2	95
and tomatoes	1.6	0.4	9.1	46
Macedoine (mixed vegetables)	1.4	..	3.9	21
Okra[2]	0.7	0.1	2.9	15
Peas[3] (carbohydrate range, 4.3–17.2 per cent)	3.6	0.2	8.6	51
Potatoes, sweet	1.9	0.4	40.6	174
Pumpkins (carbohydrate range, 3.6–7.3 per cent)	0.8	0.2	5.6	27
Squash (carbohydrate range, 3.6–12.8 per cent)	0.9	0.5	9.8	47
Succotash (carbohydrate range, 13.9–21.3 per cent)	3.6	1.0	17.7	94
Tomatoes (carbohydrate range, 1–4.5 per cent)	1.2	0.2	3.5	21
Pickles, condiments, etc.:				
Capers	3.2	0.5	5.0	37
Catsup, tomato (carbohydrate range, 3–26 per cent)	1.8	0.2	10.0	49
Chili sauce (carbohydrate range, 14–28 per cent)	..	..	20.0	..
Horseradish	1.4	0.2	10.5[4]	49
Mayonnaise dressing (average of 10 commercial brands)	1.7	77.8	2.9	719
Mineral oil dressing (average of 3 commercial brands)	1.3	76.0[5]	4.5	..
Mustard, prepared	4.7	4.1	5.0	76
cereal added (carbohydrate range, 4–15 per cent)	3.5	1.9	7.0	59
Olives, green, edible portion (10 samples)[6]	1.3	12.1	2.5	124
ripe, edible portion (8 samples)[7]	1.4	18.0	2.0	176
Pickles, cucumber	0.5	0.3	2.7[4]	16
mixed	1.1	0.4	4.0[4]	24
spiced	0.4	0.1	21.0	87

[1] Average, 0.4 per cent salt (NaCl).
[2] Average, 1.1 per cent salt (NaCl).
[3] Average, 0.7 per cent salt (NaCl).
[4] Includes fiber.
[5] Practically all unavailable.
[6] Salt, 5.9 per cent.
[7] Salt, 2.1 per cent.

TABLE 112.—COMPOSITION OF COMMON FOODS.—(*Continued.*)

VEGETABLES—*Continued.*

Name and description of food.	Protein, per cent.	Fat, per cent.	Carbo-hydrate, per cent.	Calories, per 100 gms.
Pickles, condiments, etc.—Concluded.				
Vinegar, cider (carbohydrate range, 0.3–				
1.5 per cent)	None	None	0.3	1
distilled	None	None	None	..
malt	..	..	0.5[1]	..
spiced salad	..	..	10.0	..
Tarragon	..	..	0.2[1]	..
wine	..	..	0.4	..

FRUITS, BERRIES, ETC.
(*Analyses are of edible portion.*)

	Protein, per cent.	Fat, per cent.	Carbo-hydrate, per cent.	Calories, per 100 gms.
Fruits, berries, etc., fresh:				
Apples (carbohydrate range, 7–16 per cent)	0.3	0.4	13.9	60
Apple juice	0.1	..	12.5	50
Apricots	1.0	0.1	12.3	54
Avocados (alligator pears)	2.1	20.1	7.4	219
Bananas	1.3	0.6	21.0	95
Blackberries	1.3	1.0	8.4	48
Blueberries	0.6	0.6	13.9	63
Cherries	1.0	0.8	16.5	77
Citrang juice	1.3	..	6.9	33
Crabapples	0.4	0.3	17.1	73
Cranberries	0.4	0.6	8.4	41
Currants	1.6	0.4	9.5	48
Egg fruit	3.4	1.9	41.0	195
Figs	1.4	0.4	17.9	81
Gooseberries	0.8	0.4	7.6	37
Grapes	1.3	1.6	14.9	79
Grapejuice (carbohydrate range, 11–20 per cent)	0.4	..	18.5	76
Grapefruit[2]	0.8	..	7.2	32
Grapefruit juice	0.4	0.1	9.8	42
Guavas	1.0	0.6	11.6	56
Huckleberries	0.6	0.6	16.6[6]	74
Lemons	1.0	0.7	7.4	40
juice	..	..	9.8	..
Limes	0.8	0.1	12.3	53
juice	0.5	..	7.8	33
Loganberries[3]	4.6	0.6	7.2[4]	53
juice[5]	0.6	..	6.8	..
Loquat	0.3	..	23.0	..
Mangoes	0.7	0.2	16.2	69
Mulberries	1.2	0.6	12.6	61
Muskmelons	0.6	0.3	7.2	34
Nectarines	0.5	0.1	15.6	65
Oranges	0.9	0.2	10.6	48
Orange juice	0.6	..	13.1	55
Papaw	5.2	0.9	16.8	96
Papaya	0.6	0.1	9.1	40
Peaches.	0.5	0.1	11.4	49
Pears	0.6	0.5	11.4	53
Persimmons	0.8	0.7	29.7	128
Pineapple	0.4	0.2	13.3	57

[1] Manufacturer's analysis.
[2] Florida, California and Puerto Rico, carbohydrate range, 6.6–8.2 per cent (E. M. Frankel).
[3] Jour. Ind. and Eng. Chem., **10**, 30, 1918.   [4] Invert sugar.
[5] Jour. Ind. and Eng. Chem., **9**, 1043, 1917.
[6] Includes fiber.

TABLE 112.—COMPOSITION OF COMMON FOODS.—(*Continued.*)

FRUITS, BERRIES, ETC.—*Concluded.*

Name and description of food.	Protein, per cent.	Fat, per cent.	Carbo-hydrate, per cent.	Calories, per 100 gms.
Fruits, berries, etc., fresh:—Continued:				
Plums	0.7	0.2	12.4	54
Pomegranates	1.5	1.6	16.8	88
Prunes	0.9	0.2	21.3	91
Quince	0.3	0.1	13.2	55
Raspberries, black	1.5	1.6	12.1	69
red	1.1	..	11.6	..
Sapodilla	0.6	1.4	19.4	93
Sour sop	0.8.	0.1	17.2	73
Strawberries	1.0	0.6	6.0	33
Tangelo juice	0.7	..	9.0	..
Watermelons	0.4	0.2	6.7[1]	30
Whortleberries	0.7	0.3	10.0	46
Fruits, berries, etc., dried:				
Apples	1.6	2.2	66.1[1]	291
Apricots	4.7	1.0	62.5[1]	278
Citron	1.5	1.5	78.1[1]	332
Currants	2.4	1.7	74.2[1]	322
Dates	2.1	2.8	78.4[1]	347
Figs	4.3	0.3	74.2[1]	317
Prunes	2.1	..	73.3[1]	..
Raisins	2.6	3.3	76.1[1]	345
Raspberries	7.3	1.8	80.2[1]	366
Fruits, berries, etc., canned; jellies and preserves:[2]				
Apples, crab	0.3	2.4	54.4[1]	240
Apple sauce	0.2	0.8	37.2[1]	157
Apricots	0.9	..	17.3[1]	..
Apricot sauce	1.9	1.3	48.8[1]	215
Bakapple (cloudberry)	1.9	0.3	9.7	49
Blackberries	0.8	2.1	56.4[1]	248
Blueberries	0.6	0.6	12.8[1]	59
Cherries	1.1	0.1	21.1[1]	90
Cherry jelly	1.1	..	77.2[1]	..
Figs, stewed	1.2	0.3	40.9[1]	171
Grape butter	1.2	0.1	58.5[1]	240
Grapefruit	0.5	0.1	8.3	36
Marmalade, orange	0.6	0.1	84.5[1]	341
Peaches	0.7	0.1	10.8[1]	47
Pears	0.3	0.3	18.0[1]	76
Pineapple	0.4	0.7	36.4[1]	154
Prune sauce	0.5	0.1	22.3[1]	92
Strawberries, stewed	0.7	..	24.0[1]	..
Tomato preserves	0.7	0.1	57.6[1]	234

NUTS.

(*Analyses are of edible portion.*)

Almond	21.0	54.9	15.3	639
Almond butter	22.1	61.5	7.9	674
Beechnuts	21.9	57.4	13.2[1]	657
Brazil nuts	16.8	69.4	5.0	712
Butternuts	27.9	61.2	3.5	676
Cashew nuts	19.1	47.1	26.2	605

[1] Includes fiber.

[2] Jams, jellies, preserves and marmalade contain 47 per cent or more carbohydrate. There is a wide variation in the sugar content of canned fruits. Pie peaches are packed in water while other grades may be found in 30, 40 or even 50 per cent syrup.

TABLE 112.—COMPOSITION OF COMMON FOODS.—(Continued.)

NUTS—Concluded.

(Analyses are of edible portion.)

Name ond description of food.	Protein, per cent.	Fat, per cent.	Carbo-hydrate, per cent.	Calories, per 100 gms.
Chestnuts	6.2	5.4	40.3	235
Cocoanuts	5.7	50.6	27.9[1]	590
Cocoanut milk	0.4	1.5	4.6	34
prepared	6.3	57.4	31.5[1]	668
Filberts	15.6	65.3	13.0[1]	702
Hickory nuts	15.4	67.4	11.4[1]	714
Lichi nuts	2.9	0.2	77.5[1]	323
Peanuts	25.8	38.6	21.9	538
Peanut butter	29.3	46.5	17.1[1]	604
Pecans	9.6	70.5	15.3[1]	734
Pine nuts, Pignolias	36.5	47.9	4.8	596
Piniones	6.5	60.7	26.2[1]	677
Pinon	14.6	61.9	17.3[1]	685
Sabine	28.1	53.7	8.4[1]	629
Pistachios	24.3	51.1	14.3	614
Walnuts, California	18.4	64.4	11.6	700
black	27.6	56.3	10.0	657
soft shell	16.6	63.4	13.5	691

ALCOHOLIC BEVERAGES.[2]

	Protein, per cent.	Fat, per cent.	Carbo-hydrate, per cent.	Calories, per 100 gms.
Beer (alcohol usually 3–5 per cent by weight)	0.5	Trace	5.0	50
Ale (alcohol usually 4–6 per cent by weight)	0.5	Trace	5.2	58
Porter (alcohol usually 4–5 per cent by weight)	0.6	..	6.3	60
Stout (alcohol usually 5–7 per cent by weight)	0.5	..	7.0	72
Malt extract (alcohol 2–7.3 per cent by weight; carbohydrate range, 4.8–14 per cent)	0.7	..	7.1	65
Wines,[3] dry (alcohol range, 6–15.5 per cent by weight; carbohydrate range, 0.1–3.6 per cent)	0.2	..	0.3	..
sweet (alcohol range, 10–24 per cent by weight):				
California: Port (carbohydrate range, 0.2–13.6 per cent)	..	..	4.8	..
Madera and Sherry (carbohydrate range, 0.1–17.2 per cent)	..	..	5.4	..
French (carbohydrate range, 0.7–12.4 per cent)	..	..	5.4	..
German (carbohydrate range, 0.6–12.1 per cent)	..	..	4.6	..
Madeira (carbohydrate range, 2.5–3.9 per cent)	..	..	3.0	..
Port (carbohydrate range, 3.8–8.2 per cent)	..	..	6.0	..
Rhine (carbohydrate range, 1.8–10.7 per cent)	..	..	6.4	..

[1] Includes fiber.
[2] Caloric values for alcoholic beverages may be approximated by reckoning protein and carbohydrate as yielding 4 calories per gram, and alcohol, 7.1 calories per gram.
[3] Natural wines contain less than 18 per cent alcohol by weight; wines containing over 18 per cent are usually fortified.

TABLE 112.—COMPOSITION OF COMMON FOODS.—(*Concluded.*)

ALCOHOLIC BEVERAGES.—*Concluded.*

Name and description of food.	Protein, per cent.	Fat, per cent.	Carbo-hydrate, per cent.	Calories, per 100 gms.
Wines, sweet, concluded:				
Champagne (carbohydrate range, 6.5–18.5)	..	..	9.6	..
Tokay: True (carbohydrate range, 1.9–20.5 per cent)	..	..	12.6	..
Commercial (carbohydrate range, 2.7–40.7 per cent)	..	..	19.8	..
Vermouth (carbohydrate range, 3.5–14.4 per cent)	..	..	4.5	..
Distilled liquors: Whiskey (alcohol, 30–45 per cent by weight); brandy (alcohol, 21–51 per cent); rum (alcohol, 25–43 per cent); gin (alcohol, 30–43 per cent) .	None	None	None[1]	..
Cordials (alcohol range, 30–50 per cent by weight):				
Absinthe	..	..	Trace	..
Angostura	..	..	4.2	..
Creme de Menthe	..	..	27.7	..
Kümmel	..	..	31.2	..
Benedictine	..	..	32.6	..
Anisette	..	..	34.4	..
Chartreuse	..	..	34.4	..
Maraschino	..	..	52.3	..

OTHER BEVERAGES.

Name and description of food.	Protein, per cent.	Fat, per cent.	Carbo-hydrate, per cent.	Calories, per 100 gms.
Tea (0.5 ounce to 1 pint water)	..	..	0.6	..
Coffee (1 ounce to 1 pint water)	..	..	0.7	..
Cocoa (0.5 ounce to 1 pint water) . . .	..	..	1.1	..
(0.5 ounce to 1 pint milk) . . .	..	..	6.0	..
Chocolate[2]	12.4	52.2	24.8[3]	..
Cocoa[2]	18.3	26.7	37.5[4]	..
Carbonated drinks (bottled soda, sarsaparilla, birch beer, root beer)	..	..	11.5	..
Ginger ale (sugar range, 5.8–12.3 per cent)	..	..	9.0	..
Cider,[5] sweet	1.0	..	12.5	..

[1] Sugar is sometimes added to brandy.

[2] Analysis of the food itself; not as prepared for drinking. Sweetened chocolate contains from 50 to 60 per cent of sugar; sweetened cocoa contains from 25 to 50 per cent of sugar.

[3] Starch and sugars about 10 per cent; availability of remainder undetermined.

[4] Starch and sugars about 14 per cent; availability of remainder undetermined.

[5] Sugar decreases as fermentation proceeds. Well-fermented cider will contain less than 1 per cent of sugar and about 5 per cent of alcohol.

APPENDIX.

TABLE 113.—HEIGHTS AND WEIGHTS OF CHILDREN BETWEEN ONE AND
FOUR YEARS OF AGE (WITHOUT CLOTHES).[1]

5602 boys			4821 girls	
Height, inches.	Weight, pounds.	Age, months.	Height, inches.	Weight, pounds.
26.5	18.0	6	25.9	16.8
27.3	19.1	7	26.5	17.4
27.6	19.8	8	27.0	18.3
28.1	20.4	9	27.6	19.1
28.5	20.9	10	27.9	19.5
29.0	21.4	11	28.4	20.1
29.4	21.9	12	28.9	20.8
29.9	22.9	13	29.4	21.0
30.3	23.0	14	29.5	21.6
30.8	23.6	15	30.1	21.9
31.1	24.1	16	30.5	22.6
31.4	24.5	17	30.8	22.9
31.8	24.6	18	31.1	23.4
32.3	25.5	19	31.5	23.8
32.6	25.8	20	32.0	24.1
32.9	25.8	21	32.3	24.8
33.3	26.9	22	32.6	25.3
33.6	27.0	23	32.9	25.6
33.8	27.1	24	33.4	26.4
34.0	27.9	25	33.8	26.9
34.1	28.3	26	33.9	27.3
34.8	29.0	27	33.9	27.3
35.1	29.1	28	34.6	27.8
35.4	29.3	29	34.8	27.8
35.4	29.5	30	34.9	28.3
35.5	30.5	31	35.1	28.8
36.0	30.6	32	35.4	29.0
36.1	30.6	33	35.6	29.1
36.5	31.1	34	36.5	30.1
36.8	31.9	35	36.5	30.3
37.1	32.3	36	36.8	30.5
37.4	32.3	37	36.8	30.8
37.5	32.4	38	37.0	31.0
37.9	33.1	39	37.3	31.6
38.5	33.5	40	37.5	32.0
38.6	33.6	41	37.8	32.3
38.6	33.8	42	38.0	32.5
38.8	33.8	43	38.3	32.8
38.9	34.3	44	38.5	33.0
39.0	34.5	45	38.5	33.5
39.0	34.8	46	38.8	33.5
39.3	35.8	47	38.9	33.5
39.5	35.9	48	39.0	33.8

[1] Crum, F. S.: Quarterly Publication of the American Statistical Association, Boston, September, 1916, N. S., No. 115, 15, 332.

TABLE 114.—HEIGHTS AND WEIGHTS OF BOYS BETWEEN FIVE AND FOURTEEN YEARS (WITHOUT CLOTHES).[1]

BOYS — Weight in Pounds — Height in Feet and Inches — Without Clothes — Without Shoes

AGE	3-3	3-4	3-5	3-6	3-7	3-8	3-9	3-10	3-11	4	4-1	4-2	4-3	4-4	4-5	4-6	4-7	4-8	4-9	4-10	4-11	5	5-1	5-2	5-3	5-4	5-5	5-6	5-7	5-8	5-9	5-10	6	6-1
5	35	38	39	41	42	46																												
6		36	39	41	42	44	46	48																										
7				42	43	46	48	49	54																									
8						45	48	50	53	54	57	59																						
9								50	53	55	58	60	62	62	65																			
10									53	55	58	60	62	65	68	69	71																	
11												61	61	65	68	71	77	77	78															
12													63	67	70	75	76	79	84	84	85													
13														67	71	75	78	80	85	86	91	98	99	100										
14															67	71	76	79	82	86	90	94	97	103	107	114	122							
15																		79	82	87	91	95	99	106	112	118	119	121	126	133				
16																						90	96	104	112	120	122	125	129	133	134	136		
17																								104	110	117	122	125	128	130	136	140	140	
18																										118	120	126	131	136	139	143	146	
19																										120	126	129	134	136	139	144	146	149
20																										125	130	132	135	139	145	146	154	165

TABLES 115.—HEIGHTS AND WEIGHTS OF GIRLS BETWEEN FIVE AND FOURTEEN YEARS (WITHOUT CLOTHES).[1]

GIRLS — Weight in Pounds — Height in Feet and Inches — Without Clothes — Without Shoes

AGE	3-3	3-4	3-5	3-6	3-7	3-8	3-9	3-10	3-11	4	4-1	4-2	4-3	4-4	4-5	4-6	4-7	4-8	4-9	4-10	4-11	5-0	5-1	5-2	5-3	5-4	5-5
5		34	37	38	41	43	45																				
6			35	37	39	41	43	45	48																		
7					39	42	44	45	47	50																	
8							42	45	47	49	51	53	56														
9									49	51	53	56	59	63													
10											54	57	58	62	61	69											
11													60	62	63	68	70	75									
12															63	66	69	71	75	78	83	88	94				
13																65	69	73	76	80	86	89	94	99	104		
14																		78	83	88	93	96	100	104	107	112	114
15																				89	97	100	102	106	109	118	118
16																					100	104	109	111	116	116	121
17																						109	109	110	110	117	125
18																						103	106	107	112	114	120
19																						99	105	111	113	119	123
20																						99	111	114	114	115	125

[1] Wood, T. D.: The ninth yearbook of the National Society of the Study of Education, Part I, Health and Education, Chicago, 1910, p. 34.

TABLE 116.—HEIGHTS AND WEIGHTS OF 221,819 MEN OF FIFTEEN OR MORE YEARS OF AGE (WITH CLOTHES).[1]

Age.	Graded average weight in pounds with clothes. Feet and inches with shoes.																	
	5-0	5-1	5-2	5-3	5-4	5-5	5-6	5-7	5-8	5-9	5-10	5-11	6-0	6-1	6-2	6-3	6-4	6-5
15	107	109	112	115	118	122	126	130	134	138	142	147	152	157	162	167	172	177
16	109	111	114	117	120	124	128	132	136	140	144	149	154	159	164	169	174	179
17	111	113	116	119	122	126	130	134	138	142	146	151	156	161	166	171	176	181
18	113	115	118	121	124	128	132	136	140	144	148	153	158	163	168	173	178	183
19	115	117	120	123	126	130	134	138	142	146	150	155	160	165	170	175	180	185
20	117	119	122	125	128	132	136	140	144	148	152	156	161	166	171	176	181	186
21	118	120	123	126	130	134	138	141	145	149	153	157	162	167	172	177	182	187
22	119	121	124	127	131	135	139	142	146	150	154	158	163	168	173	178	183	188
23	120	122	125	128	132	136	140	143	147	151	155	159	164	169	175	180	185	190
24	121	123	126	129	133	137	141	144	148	152	156	160	165	171	177	182	187	192
25	122	124	126	129	133	137	141	145	149	153	157	162	167	173	179	184	189	194
26	123	125	127	130	134	138	142	146	150	154	158	163	168	174	180	186	191	196
27	124	126	128	131	134	138	142	146	150	154	158	163	169	175	181	187	192	197
28	125	127	129	132	135	139	143	147	151	155	159	164	170	176	182	188	193	198
29	126	128	130	133	136	140	144	148	152	156	160	165	171	177	183	189	194	199
30	126	128	130	133	136	140	144	148	152	156	161	166	172	178	184	190	196	201
31	127	129	131	134	137	141	145	149	153	157	162	167	173	179	185	191	197	202
32	127	129	131	134	137	141	145	149	154	158	163	168	174	180	186	192	198	203
33	127	129	131	134	137	141	145	149	154	159	164	169	175	181	187	193	199	204
34	128	130	132	135	138	142	146	150	155	160	165	170	176	182	188	194	200	206
35	128	130	132	135	138	142	146	150	155	160	165	170	176	182	189	195	201	207
36	129	131	133	136	139	143	147	151	156	161	166	171	177	183	190	196	202	208
37	129	131	133	136	140	144	148	152	157	162	167	172	178	184	191	197	203	209
38	130	132	134	137	140	144	148	152	157	162	167	173	179	185	192	198	204	210
39	130	132	134	137	140	144	148	152	157	162	167	173	179	185	192	199	205	211
40	131	133	135	138	141	145	149	153	158	163	168	174	180	186	193	200	206	212
41	131	133	135	138	141	145	149	153	158	163	168	174	180	186	193	200	207	213
42	132	134	136	139	142	146	150	154	159	164	169	175	181	187	194	201	208	214
43	132	134	136	139	142	146	150	154	159	164	169	175	181	187	194	201	208	214
44	133	135	137	140	143	147	151	155	160	165	170	176	182	188	195	202	209	215
45	133	135	137	140	143	147	151	155	160	165	170	176	182	188	195	202	209	215
46	134	136	138	141	144	148	152	156	161	166	171	177	183	189	196	203	210	216
47	134	136	138	141	144	148	152	156	161	166	171	177	183	190	197	204	211	217
48	134	136	138	141	144	148	152	156	161	166	171	177	183	190	197	204	211	217
49	134	136	138	141	144	148	152	156	161	166	171	177	183	190	197	204	211	217
50	134	136	138	141	144	148	152	156	161	166	171	177	183	190	197	204	211	217
51	135	137	139	142	145	149	153	157	162	167	172	178	184	191	198	205	212	218
52	135	137	139	142	145	149	153	157	162	167	172	178	184	191	198	205	212	218
53	135	137	139	142	145	149	153	157	162	167	172	178	184	191	198	205	212	218
54	135	137	139	142	145	149	153	158	163	168	173	178	184	191	198	205	212	219
55	135	137	139	142	145	149	153	158	163	168	173	178	184	191	198	205	212	219

[1] Association of Life Insurance Directors and Actuarial Society of America, New York, 1912, p. 38. Published by a committee. Allow 1 inch for shoes and 10 pounds for clothes.

Table 117.—Heights and Weights of 136,504 Women of Fifteen or More Years of Age (With Clothes).[1]

Age	Graded average weight in pounds with clothes. Feet and inches with shoes.																
	4–8	4–9	4–10	4–11	5–0	5–1	5–2	5–3	5–4	5–5	5–6	5–7	5–8	5–9	5–10	5–11	6–0
15	101	103	105	106	107	109	112	115	118	122	126	130	134	138	142	147	152
16	102	104	106	108	109	111	114	117	120	124	128	132	136	139	143	148	153
17	103	105	107	109	111	113	116	119	122	125	129	133	137	140	144	149	154
18	104	106	108	110	112	114	117	120	123	126	130	134	138	141	145	150	155
19	105	107	109	111	113	115	118	121	124	127	131	135	139	142	146	151	155
20	106	108	110	112	114	116	119	122	125	128	132	136	140	143	147	151	156
21	107	109	111	113	115	117	120	123	126	129	133	137	141	144	148	152	156
22	107	109	111	113	115	117	120	123	126	129	133	137	141	145	149	153	157
23	108	110	112	114	116	118	121	124	127	130	134	138	142	146	150	153	157
24	109	111	113	115	117	119	121	124	127	130	134	138	142	146	150	154	158
25	109	111	113	115	117	119	121	124	128	131	135	139	143	147	151	154	158
26	110	112	114	116	118	120	122	125	128	131	135	139	143	147	151	155	159
27	110	112	114	116	118	120	122	125	129	132	136	140	144	148	152	155	159
28	111	113	115	117	119	121	123	126	130	133	137	141	145	149	153	156	160
29	111	113	115	117	119	121	123	126	130	133	137	141	145	149	153	156	160
30	112	114	116	118	120	122	124	127	131	134	138	142	146	150	154	157	161
31	113	115	117	119	121	123	125	128	132	135	139	143	147	151	154	157	161
32	113	115	117	119	121	123	125	128	132	136	140	144	148	152	155	158	162
33	114	116	118	120	122	124	126	129	133	137	141	145	149	153	156	159	162
34	115	117	119	121	123	125	127	130	134	138	142	146	150	154	157	160	163
35	115	117	119	121	123	125	127	130	134	138	142	146	150	154	157	160	163
36	116	118	120	122	124	126	128	131	135	139	143	147	151	155	158	161	164
37	116	118	120	122	124	126	129	132	136	140	144	148	152	156	159	162	165
38	117	119	121	123	125	127	130	133	137	141	145	149	153	157	160	163	166
39	118	120	122	124	126	128	131	134	138	142	146	150	154	158	161	164	167
40	119	121	123	125	127	129	132	135	138	142	146	150	154	158	161	164	167
41	120	122	124	126	128	130	133	136	139	143	147	151	155	159	162	165	168
42	120	122	124	126	128	130	133	136	139	143	147	151	155	159	162	166	169
43	121	123	125	127	129	131	134	137	140	144	148	152	156	160	163	167	170
44	122	124	126	128	130	132	135	138	141	145	149	153	157	161	164	168	171
45	122	124	126	128	130	132	135	138	141	145	149	153	157	161	164	168	171
46	123	125	127	129	131	133	136	139	142	146	150	154	158	162	165	169	172
47	123	125	127	129	131	133	136	139	142	146	151	155	159	163	166	170	173
48	124	126	128	130	132	134	137	140	143	147	152	156	160	164	167	171	174
49	124	126	128	130	132	134	137	140	143	147	152	156	161	165	168	172	175
50	125	127	129	131	133	135	138	141	144	148	152	156	161	165	169	173	176
51	125	127	129	131	133	135	138	141	144	148	152	157	162	166	170	174	177
52	125	127	129	131	133	135	138	141	144	148	152	157	162	166	170	174	177
53	125	127	129	131	133	135	138	141	144	148	152	157	162	166	170	174	177
54	125	127	129	131	133	135	138	141	144	148	153	158	163	167	171	174	177
55	125	127	129	131	133	135	138	141	144	148	153	158	163	167	171	174	177

[1] Association Life Insurance Directors and Actuarial Society of America, New York, 1912, p. 67. Published by a committee. Allow 1½ inches for shoes and 6 pounds for clothes.

INDEX.

A

53

(833)

CAUSES OF DEATH, arranged according to periods, 229
arteriosclerosis, 230, 481
cancer, 17, 231, 235, 654
cardio-vascular-renal, 230
children, in, 767
coma, 230, 234, 421, 445
  autopsy findings, 447
  during coma and after discharge from hospital, 446
  without, 230
death, certificates, errors and omissions on, 23, 230
gangrene, 230, 495, 496
inanition, 231
infections, 231
insulin reactions, during, 228
miscellaneous, 231
needless diabetic deaths, 232, 339, 447
Registration area, in, 27
suicide, 231
summary of diagnoses, George F. Baker Clinic, 233–235
surgical diabetics, of, 668
tuberculosis, 17, 231, 636
OF DIABETES. See ETIOLOGY.
CENTRAL NERVOUS SYSTEM. See NERVOUS SYSTEM.
CEREAL PRODUCTS, composition of, 817
CEREBRAL HEMORRHAGE, 229, 231, 495, 573
CESAREAN SECTION, 779
CHARCOT JOINTS, 567
CHEESE, composition of, 815
CHEMOTHERAPY, 530, 531, 612, 701, 705, 707
CHILD OF DIABETIC MOTHER, effect of diabetes upon, 773
  size of, 205, 773, 775
CHILDREN, DIABETES IN, 741–768
adrenals and, 765
age at onset, 742
allergy to insulin, 477, 752
arteriosclerosis in, 217, 492, 747, 763
asthma in, 478
behavior problems, 754
blood lipids in, 172–174
caloric requirements, 748
camps for, 5, 753
carbohydrate, impairment of tolerance for, 745
cataracts in, 623, 761
coma in, 420, 454, 755
  cause of death, 230, 450, 767
  signs and symptoms, 755
  treatment, 756
complications in, 14, 755–766
  of insulin treatment, 751
congenital anomalies in, 744, 755
control, standards of, 753
course of disease, 766
deficiency diseases, 759
diagnosis of, 745

CHILDREN, DIABETES IN, diagnosis of, faulty, 745
diet, 748–750
duration of life in, 317, 321
dwarfism, 545, 759
economic status, 764
endocrine imbalance, 743
enlargement of the liver, 545, 757
epilepsy, 568, 759
etiology of, 742–745, 763
eyes in, 761–763
fatty atrophy in, 752
follicle stimulating hormone (FSH), 743, 765
gonads and, 765
growth and development, retardation of, 759
height-weight relationship, 743
hepatomegaly in, 757
heredity, 59, 742
hyperpituitarism, evidence of, 743, 744
hypoglycemia in, 751
incidence of, 741
infancy, diabetes in, 766
infections, 742, 756
  preceding onset, 742
inheritance in ancestry, 59, 742
insulin, use of, with, 750
intelligence of, 754
intercapillary glomerulosclerosis, 747, 762
keto-steroids, 744, 765
lipodystrophy, 752
long duration—20-year cases, 763
menstruation, abnormalities and, 765
mortality, 767
nephritis, 747, 762
neuropathies, 759
obesity, 56, 71, 743
occupations for, 14, 764
onset of, 313
  type of, 745
pathology of diabetes in, 746
physical examination of diabetic child, 754
potential diabetes, 746
prognosis, 321, 768
protamine insulin in treatment of, 750
psychological problem, 754
retinal hemorrhages, 761
retinitis proliferans, 762
secondary sex characteristics, 743, 755, 759
sepsis in, 747, 756
skin lesions, 758
symptoms and signs of, 745
syphilis and, 664
thyroid and, 765
trauma, 743
treatment of, 748–754
  attempts at alleviation, 767
  diet, 748

54